Textbook of Interventional Neurology

Textbook of Interventional Neurology

Edited by

Adnan I. Qureshi
Zeenat Qureshi Stroke Research Center Minneapolis, MN

Associate Editor

Alexandros L. Georgiadis
Zeenat Qureshi Stroke Research Center Minneapolis, MN

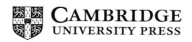

CAMBRIDGE
UNIVERSITY PRESS

CAMBRIDGE UNIVERSITY PRESS
Cambridge, New York, Melbourne, Madrid, Cape Town, Singapore,
São Paulo, Delhi, Dubai, Tokyo, Mexico City

Cambridge University Press
The Edinburgh Building, Cambridge CB2 8RU, UK

Published in the United States of America by
Cambridge University Press, New York

www.cambridge.org
Information on this title: www.cambridge.org/9780521876391

First published 2011

Printed in the United Kingdom at the University Press, Cambridge

A catalog record for this publication is available from the British Library

Library of Congress Cataloging-in-Publication Data

Textbook of interventional neurology / edited by Adnan I. Qureshi ; associate
editor, Alexandros L. Georgiadis.
      p.   cm.
Includes bibliographical references and index.
ISBN 978-0-521-87639-1 (Pbk.)
1. Brain–Endoscopic surgery.   2. Brain–Blood-vessels–Endoscopic surgery.
3. Brain–Tumors–Endoscopic surgery.   4. Cerebrovascular disease–
Endoscopic surgery.   I. Qureshi, Adnan I.   II. Georgiadis, Alexandros L.
III. Title.
[DNLM: 1. Cerebrovascular Disorders–surgery.   2. Brain Neoplasms–
surgery.   3. Catheterization–methods.   4. Endoscopy–methods.
5. Surgical Procedures, Minimally Invasive–methods.   6. Vascular Surgical
Procedures–methods.   WL 355 T3546 2011]
RD594.2.T49 2011
617.4′810597–dc22   2010023938

ISBN 978-0-521-87639-1 Hardback

Contents

Contributors

Alex Abou-Chebl MD
Director of Neurointerventional Services and
Assistant Professor of Neurology and Neurosurgery
University of Louisville
Louisville, KY
USA

Andrei V. Alexandrov MD
Director, Division of Cerebrovascular Disease
Director, Comprehensive Stroke Research Center and
Professor of Neurology,
University of Alabama Hospital
Birmingham, AL
USA

Carlos E. Baccin MD
Clinical Fellow
Department of Interventional Radiology
Hospital Beneficência Portuguesa
Sao Paulo
Brazil

Deepak L. Bhatt MD
Chief of Cardiology, VA Boston Healthcare System
Associate Professor of Medicine,
Harvard Medical School and
Director, Integrated Interventional Cardiovascular Program
Brigham and Women's Hospital and
VA Boston Healthcare System
Boston, MA
USA

Kirk Conrad MD
Austin Radiological Association,
Austin, TX
USA

Steve M. Cordina MD
Endovascular Surgical Neuroradiology Fellow
Department of Neurology
University of Minnesota
Minneapolis, MN
USA

Randall C. Edgell MD
Assistant Professor of Neurology and Neurosurgery
Department of Neurology
St. Louis University
St. Louis, MO
USA

Mustapha A. Ezzeddine MD
Associate Professor of Neurology and Neurosurgery
Department of Neurology
Zeenat Qureshi Stroke Research Center
University of Minnesota
Minneapolis, MN
USA

Matthew D. Ford PhD
Postdoctoral Fellow
Biomedical Stimulation Laboratory
University of Toronto
Toronto, ON
Canada

Alexandros L. Georgiadis MD
Adjunct Assistant Professor of Neurology
Department of Neurology
Zeenat Qureshi Stroke Research Center
University of Minnesota
Minneapolis, MN
USA

Camilo R. Gomez MD, MBA
Director, Alabama Neurological Institute
Birmingham, AL
USA

Nancy Gruell RN
St. David's Medical Center
Austin, TX
USA

Stephen J. Haines MD
Lyle A. French Chair, Professor and Head
Department of Neurosurgery

University of Minnesota
Minneapolis, MN
USA

Ameer E. Hassan DO
Endovascular Surgical Neuroradiology Fellow
Zeenat Qureshi Stroke Research Center
University of Minnesota
Minneapolis, MN
USA

L. Nelson Hopkins MD
Department of Neurosurgery
Kaleida Health
Buffalo, NY
USA

Haitham H. Hussein MD
Zeenat Qureshi Stroke Research Center
Resident of Neurology
University of Minnesota
Minneapolis, MN
USA

Tudor G. Jovin MD
Co-Director, UPMC Stroke Unit
Co-Director, UPMC Center for
Neuroendovascular Therapy
UPMC Stroke Institute
Pittsburgh, PA
USA

Stanley H. Kim MD
Director of Neurovascular Surgery
Neurosurgery, Endovascular and Spine Center
Austin, TX
USA

Osman Kozak MD
Associate Director Neurointerventional and
Neurocritical Care
Abington Memorial Hospital
Willow Grove, PA
USA

Giuseppe Lanzino MD
Professor of Neurosurgery
Mayo clinic
Rochester, MN
USA

Alberto Maud MD
Endovascular Surgical Neuroradiology
Assistant Professor
Department of Neurology

Paul L. Foster School of Medicine
Texas Tech University Health Science Center
El Paso, TX
USA

Muhammad Z. Memon MD
Pre-residency Fellow
Department of Neurosurgery
Zeenat Qureshi Stroke Research Center
University of Minnesota
Minneapolis, MN
USA

Jefferson T. Miley MD
Vascular and Interventional Neurology
Neurosurgery, Endovascular & Spine Center
Austin, TX
USA

Herbert B. Newton MD
Professor of Neurology, Neurosurgery and Oncology
James Cancer Hospital
Columbus, OH
USA

Thanh N. Nguyen MD
Assistant Professor Neurology
Boston University Medical Center
Boston, MA
USA

YihLin Nien MD
Stroke Fellow
Boston University Medical Center
Natick, MA
USA

Raul G. Nogueira MD
Assistant Professor in Neurology and Radiology
Department of Interventional Neuroradiology
Massachusetts General Hospital
Boston, MA
USA

Alexander M. Norbash MD
Professor and Chair of Radiology
Boston University Medical Center
Boston, MA
USA

Anant I. Patel MD
Neurosurgeon
Endovascular and Spine Center
Austin, TX
USA

Edgard Pereira MD
Director, Interventional Neuroradiology Service
Department of Radiology
JFK Medical Center
Atlantis, FL
USA

Johnny C. Pryor MD
Instructor in Neurosurgery
Harvard Medical School
Director of Interventional Neuroradiology and Endovascular
Neurosurgery
Massachusetts General Hospital
Boston, MA
USA

Rabia Qaiser MD
Resident, Department of Neurosurgery
University of Minnesota
St. Louis Park, MN
USA

Adnan I. Qureshi MD
Associate Head and Professor
Zeenat Qureshi Stroke Research Center
Department of Neurology
University of Minnesota
Minneapolis, MN
USA

Mushtaq H. Qureshi MD
Research Fellow
Zeenat Qureshi Stroke Research Center
University of Minnesota
Minneapolis, MN
USA

Jean Raymond MD
Interventional Neuroradiology Research Laboratory
Centre hospitalier de l'Université de Montréal-Hôpital
Notre-Dame
Montreal, Quebec
Canada

José Rafael Romero MD
Assistant Professor, Neurology
Boston University Medical Center
Boston, MA
USA

Daniel Roy MD
Professor of Radiology
Centre hospitalier de l'Université de Montréal-Hôpital
Notre-Dame
Montreal, Quebec
Canada

Qaisar A. Shah MD
Director, Neurointerventional and Neurocritical Care
Neurovascular Association of Abington
Willow Grove, PA
USA

Farhan Siddiq MD
Neurosurgery Resident
Zeenat Qureshi Stroke Research Center
Department of Neurology
University of Minnesota
Minneapolis, MN
USA

Amit Singla MD
Neurosurgery Resident
Department of Neurosurgery
SUNY Upstate University Hospital
Syracuse, NY
USA

David A. Steinman PhD
Professor of Mechanical and
Biomedical Engineering
University of Toronto
Toronto, ON
USA

Dorothea Strozyk MD
Interventional Neuroradiology Fellow
New York Presbyterian Hospital
Columbia University College of Physicians
and Surgeons
New York, NY
USA

Jose I. Suarez MD
Professor of Neurology
Baylor College of Medicine
Houston, TX
USA

M. Fareed K. Suri MD
Assistant Professor of Neurology
University of Minnesota
Minneapolis, MN
USA

Nauman Tariq MD
Clinical Research Fellow
Zeenat Qureshi Stroke Research Center

University of Minnesota
Minneapolis, MN
USA

Robert A. Taylor MD
Assistant Professor
Zeenat Qureshi Stroke Research Center
Departments of Neurology,
Neurosurgery and Radiology
University of Minnesota
Minneapolis, MN
USA

Georgios Tsivgoulis MD
Lecturer of Neurology
Democritus University of Thrace

Alexandroupolis
Greece

Young J. Yu MD
Neurosurgeon
Mount Saint Mary's Hospital
Niagara Falls
New York, NY USA

Haralabos Zacharatos MD
Neurology Resident
Zeenat Qureshi Stroke Research Center
Department of Neurology
University of Minnesota
Minneapolis, MN
USA

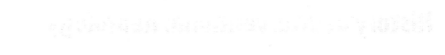

History of interventional neurology

Adnan I. Qureshi MD

Interventional neurology is a subspecialty of neurology that uses catheter technology, radiological imaging, and clinical expertise to diagnose and treat diseases of the central nervous system.[1] Interventional Neurology was a term that was used by Dr. Kori[2] in his article on issues of neurological practice section in Neurology entitled "Interventional neurology: a subspecialty whose time has come." He recommended performance of computed tomographic and magnetic resonance imaging guided procedures including nerve blocks, biopsies, aspirations, and destructive procedures; intra-arterial procedures including carotid angioplasty, carotid thrombolysis, embolizations, chemotherapy, and blood–brain barrier modification; interventional neurosonology; eletromyographic guided procedure including Botulinum toxin injections, trigger point injections; and nerve finder guided procedures to be included in this subspecialty. Over the last two decades, the definition has evolved to a more focused definition, which only includes procedures that are recognized as part of the training requirements of the "Endovascular Surgical Neuroradiology" fellowship according to Accreditation Council for Graduate Medical Education (ACGME). The advent of interventional neurology as a subspecialty has created an opportunity for vascular neurologists to play an active role in the procedural aspects of diagnosis and management of cerebrovascular diseases. However, the above-mentioned description appears to oversimplify the history of interventional neurology, which includes a complex chain of events since 1927. Dr. Qureshi at the Interventional Section of American Academy of Neurology (AAN) in 2006 remarked that "the history of interventional neurology has been a saga of unwavering determination and unparalleled comradeship. What continues to bind us together as a community is the sense of pride. Pride in our heritage of neurology, pride in the sacrifices we made, pride in standing side by side, and finally pride in our vision of the future." This chapter summarizes the events in a chronological order and captures the political and academic aspects of change and evolution over the last 80 years.

The journey starts: Egas Moniz and cerebral angiography

In 1928, Egas Moniz became a Professor of Medicine and subsequently Chair of Neurology at University of Lisbon in Portugal.[3] Since 1927, Dr. Moniz had attempted percutaneous injection of internal carotid artery in four patients, but was limited by irritation of tissue by contrast, intravascular contrast dilution, and radiological equipment. Subsequently, direct injection was attempted after surgical exposure of the internal carotid artery. In his paper in Revue Neurologique[4] in 1927, Dr. Moniz states the objective of his initial work to identify an opaque, non-oily substance which can easily pass through the capillaries for visualization of arteries. Iodides (compared with bromides) performed better as contrast media because of higher radio-opacity when injected in carotid arteries of cadavers in 30%, 20%, 10%, and 7.5% solutions. All solutions were found to opacify intracranial arteries despite the presence of cranium. Dr. Moniz then injected strontium bromide, lithium bromide, and sodium iodide into the common carotid arteries of dogs to obtain radiographs and determine toxicity and effect of dilution from ongoing blood flow. Further cadaveric work was done in collaboration with Almeida Dias and Almeida Lima to understand the radioanatomical appearances of cerebral arteries as described in his paper in Journal de Radiologie in 1927. Subsequently, Dr. Moniz tried to puncture the internal carotid artery in humans using 0.5–0.6 mm needles at the point of entry into the carotid orifice without success. He starting using the landmarks formed by the sternomastoid, digastric, and omohyoid muscles to access the artery under direct exposure. The first six patients were injected with sodium bromide, but the last patient died 8 hours after the procedure due to a stroke. Dr. Moniz changed the injections to sodium iodide injection (22%–25%) in the next four patients, one of whom was not injected because of puncturing a bad artery. The final case of a 20-year-old boy produced a satisfactory result with adequate visualization of intracranial arteries. In 1931, Dr. Moniz

Textbook of Interventional Neurology, ed. Adnan I. Qureshi. Published by Cambridge University Press. © Cambridge University Press 2011.

presented his results at the First International Neurological Congress in Bern. He subsequently published his book *Diagnostic des tomeurs cerebrales et epreuve de l'encephalographie arterielle* in 1931 that described his experience with the first 180 cerebral angiograms. The role of neurologists in diagnostic imaging was further enhanced by Karl Theodore Dussik, who was a neurologist at Allgemeine Poliklinik (General Polyclinic) and University of Vienna Medical School. He was the first to propose the use of ultrasound as a diagnostic device in a paper he wrote in 1941. He also developed the quartz ultrasound generator with help from engineers F Seidl and C Reisinger at the Physics Institute of the University of Vienna.

Transition to transfemoral approach and exclusion of neurology

The next two decades witnessed more emphasis on accessing the arteries through percutaneous puncture using needle-assisted small diameter cannulas followed by advancement of catheters to sites distant to the point of entry. The changing patterns also resulted in a movement which would eventually exclude neurologists from performance of these procedures. In 1941, Dr. Farinas[5] passed a urethral catheter through a trocar inserted in the exposed femoral artery and advanced it into the aorta. In 1947, Dr. Radner[6] performed angiography of the vertebral artery after catheterizing exposed and ligated radial artery. In 1949, Jonsson[7] from Roentgen Diagnostic Department in Karolinska Sjukuset, Stockholm, Sweden performed a percutaneous puncture of the common carotid artery using a blunt cannula with an inner sharp needle. The cannula was directed downwards using a silver thread to inject and visualize thoracic aorta. In 1953, Dr. Sven Seldinger[8] from Roentgen Diagnostic Department in Karolinska Sjukuset, Stockholm, Sweden described a new technique for acquiring percutaneous vascular access by placing a catheter subsequent to the needle puncture and therefore establishing a platform for diagnostic and therapeutic procedures. In the original 40 arterial catheterizations, 37 were performed through a femoral artery puncture. Three were performed after puncture of the brachial artery via the antecubital fossa with subsequent angiography of the subclavian arteries. However, neurological and neurosurgical services continued to carry out angiography using percutaneous puncture of the common carotid artery, and serial films were made by identical roentgenological techniques up to the early 1970s.[9] Selective angiography of the carotid and vertebral arteries by the femoral route was introduced into practice in the early 1960s. These procedures were performed only by radiologists and competed with angiography using percutaneous puncture of the common carotid artery. Hans Newton,[10] a radiologist, at the Karolinska Hospital, Sweden, started occasionally using the femoral route with subsequent catheterization of the carotid arteries in 1963. Cerebral angiography through the femoral route with subsequent catheterization of all supra-aortic arteries was described by Norwegian neuroradiologist, Per Amundsen[11,12] at the Ullevål Hospital in

Norway in 1964. Subsequently, Amundsen' arrived at University of California at San Francisco, CA in 1965, to start teaching trainees in neuroradiology his technique in the United States.[13] A National Institute of Neurological Diseases and Blindness (NINDB) traineeship in neuroradiology in July 1965 involving 11 departments nationally[14] officially consolidated the neuroradiology based practice of cerebral angiography. The training grants were continued by the National Institute of Neurological Disorders and Stroke (NINDS) until about 1976, at which time they were discontinued along with other fellowship programs emphasizing clinical training.[15]

In 1970, Drs. Takahashi and Kawanami[16] reported the results of 422 cerebral angiographic examinations using femoral artery based catheterization. In 1973, Dr. Vitek reported the results for 2000 consecutive examinations[17] and in 1976, Drs. Bradac and Simon reported upon 965 examinations. All three reports suggested that selective angiography of the carotid and vertebral arteries by the femoral route was superior to direct puncture of the vessels in the neck and to retrograde brachial angiography.[18] Several reports were subsequently published with selective angiography of the carotid and vertebral arteries by the femoral route confirming similar findings.[19] By the early 1970s, cerebral angiography through direct carotid puncture by neurologists was an obsolete practice.

Therapeutic procedures: aneurysm embolization and intra-arterial thrombolysis

In 1941, Werner, who was faculty in the Department of Medicine, along with Blakemore, and King[20] from Columbia University College of Physicians and Surgeons, the Presbyterian Hospital and the Neurological Institute of New York, inserted silver wires into an intracranial aneurysm by use of a transorbital approach to prevent rupture by protecting the susceptible wall of the aneurysm from the stress of pulsatile blood flow. They reported a 15-year-old girl who presented to Vanderbilt clinic with diplopia, nausea, and vomiting for 5 months on September 25, 1936. On April 17, 1937, the patient was admitted to the Neurological Institute, New York with severe headaches. An aneurysm of the right internal carotid artery was suspected, based on atrophy of the anterior and posterior clinoid processes and destruction of the lateral and inferior wall of the right optic foramen on skull X-rays. A pneumoencephalogram demonstrated displacement of chiasmatic cistern. The patient was treated using a metal clip placed in the cervical internal carotid artery, with progressive occlusion over the next 5 days. However, the treatment did not improve the patient's symptoms. The patient's symptoms continued to progress with new bruit that could be auscultated over the right eye, visual loss in the right eye, and pituitary dysfunction resulting in multiple admissions. Additional ligations of the right external and superior thyroid arteries and common carotid artery were unsuccessful. On January 21, 1939, 2 years and 9 months after the first symptom, the procedure was carried out as follows:[20] "Under procaine hydrochloride anesthesia an incision was made through the lateral canthus of the right eye. Anesthetic solution was introduced into the orbital tissues. The eye was displaced medially. This gave access to the aneurysm, which had eroded the posterior orbit. Thirty feet of No. 34 gauge coin silver enameled wire was introduced into the aneurysm through a special needle. The velocity of blood flow through the aneurysm was measured and found to be low. The wire was heated to an average temperature of 80 °C. for a total of forty seconds. The aneurysm no longer bled when the needle was cleared at the conclusion of the operation." However, there was progressive diminution of the vision of the left eye after the procedure.

In 1958, Sussmann and Fitch[21] from the Division of Neurosurgery at Muhlenberg Hospital in Plainfield, New Jersey reported the results of slow intravenous infusion of fibrinolysin in three patients with hemiplegia. The site of occlusion of the cerebral vessels was located in each patient by angiography. The first patient was admitted to the hospital on September 6, 1957, because of the abrupt appearance of hemiplegia of the right side and inability to speak. Cerebral angiography on the sixth day of admission demonstrated no filling of the internal carotid artery beyond the bifurcation of the common carotid artery. On the same day, 50 000 units of fibrinolysin were given intravenously over a 3-hour period. Simultaneously, 25 000 units in 100 ml³ were given after 1 hour, over a 15-minute period, into the left carotid artery. This was repeated on 3 of the next 4 days. A second left carotid angiogram taken 10 days after admission showed an incomplete 2 cm column of dye in the proximal internal carotid artery. An Additional 75 000 units of fibrinolysin were given daily, intravenously, over a 2-hour period for the following 6 days. Another angiogram after 18 days of admission demonstrated some improvement in filling of the left internal carotid artery. In another case, the angiogram demonstrated no filling of the middle cerebral arteries before treatment, while on the eighth day after beginning treatment good filling of the middle cerebral arteries was obtained. This patient showed the most favorable results, which could be attributed to starting treatment within 6 hours after the onset of symptoms. No complications were observed related to the diagnostic angiography or to the administration of fibrinolysin in any of these patients.

Entering the intracranial circulation

In 1963, Drs. Luessenhop and Velasquez[22] from the Division of Neurosurgery at Georgetown University Hospital, Washington, DC reported the results of manipulation of catheters and emboli within the intracranial arteries. The initial experiments comprised testing various existing improvised plastic and rubber catheters within glass models of internal carotid artery. The catheters with optimal performance (particularly those with flexible tips) were successfully manipulated to the terminal segment of the internal carotid artery in cadavers. The investigators found that a flow-directed Silastic tube directed by a 2.5 mm embolus at its end could be introduced through a 22 gauge needle in the common carotid arteries of the dogs and subsequently used to catheterize the thoracic aorta. They subsequently demonstrated that a catheter led by an embolus could be maneuvered through the internal carotid and middle cerebral arteries in a 33-year-old woman with cerebral arteriovenous malformation. A subsequent patient was a 51-year-old woman with an arteriovenous malformation and a right internal carotid artery intracranial aneurysm. The investigators were able to introduce flexible Silastic tubing with an enlarged inflatable tip and maneuver the catheter to the neck of the aneurysm using Polaroid films. The balloon was deflated and the catheter was withdrawn with brief occlusion in the common carotid artery to induce flow reversal. The technique was tested in the third patient with a ruptured intracranial aneurysm.

In 1959, Fedor Andreevitch Serbinenko who was a neurosurgeon in N.N. Burdenko Neurosurgery Institute in Moscow, Russia, organized a small laboratory to design a balloon catheter using materials including polyvinyl chloride, polyethylene, nylon materials, silicone, and latex. He had been performing cerebral angiography through direct carotid punctures since 1954 at the institute. On February 8, 1964, the first selective external carotid angiogram in a patient was performed with the assistance of temporary internal carotid balloon occlusion.[23,24] Serbinenko extended his work to permanent therapeutic occlusion of cervical and intracranial arteries. The first such reported vessel occlusion was performed on April 24, 1970 by Serbinenko,[24] to sacrifice an internal carotid artery and treat a carotid cavernous fistula.

Simultaneous work by Dr. G. Debrun from Serv Neuroradiol, Hop-Henri-Mondor, Creteil, Paris, France documented the use of inflatable detachable balloons to obliterate experimental carotid jugular fistulas and aneurysms in dogs.[25] The technique was then applied in a patient with vertebral artery fistula. He subsequently reported the results of intravascular detachable balloons in 17 post-traumatic carotid-cavernous sinus fistulas and 14 intracranial aneurysms.[26] By 1987, Jungreis and colleagues showed that catheters can be advanced and maneuvered in the intracranial circulation using steereable microguidewire to the extent that catheterization of intracranial arteries was no longer dependent upon the use of flow-directed catheters.[27] In 1991, Dr. Guido Guglielmi from the Department of Neurological Sciences, University of Rome Medical School, Rome, Italy and his colleagues from the Department of Radiological Sciences, Endovascular Therapy, University of California Medical Center, Los Angeles, California reported the use of a soft detachable platinum coil delivered through a microcatheter to treat experimental saccular aneurysms created on the common carotid artery of swine. The detachable platinum coil was soldered to a stainless steel delivery guidewire and manufactured by Target Therapeutics, San Jose, California. Thrombosis occurred because of the attraction of negatively charged white blood cells, red blood cells, platelets, and fibrinogen to the positively charged platinum coil positioned within the aneurysm.[28] The investigators reported the results of using electrically detachable coils introduced via an endovascular approach in 15 patients with intracranial saccular aneurysms. Thrombosis of the aneurysm (70% to 100%) was achieved in all 15 patients, with preservation of the parent artery in 14 patients.[29]

Advancements in image acquisition

Concomitant advancement in image acquisition promoted the possibility of real time imaging of catheters and device manipulations. Initially, images were obtained on a manual-pull or a power-driven (Sanchez Perez) film changer when cerebral angiography was performed using common carotid artery injections. Three or four film hard copies were obtained, and separate injections were required for each plane. In the 1960s, a serial roll film changer was used at the Neurological Institute at Columbia Presbyterian in New York, which allowed multiple images to be acquired rapidly, usually two per second for 3 seconds and then one per second for 6 seconds.[30] In 1979, Charles Mistretta invented the "digital vascular imaging" (DVI) technique that is now generally known as digital subtraction angiography (DSA). The subtraction of an image recorded without the use of contrast medium, and one with contrast medium, created a subtracted image that only demonstrated the contrast medium opacification.[31,32]

Sherry and colleagues in 1983 designed a system incorporating continuous recursive digital video filtration, allowing the operator to view a subtracted fluoroscopic image of each control angiographic sequence in real time.[33,34]

Modern era of interventional neurology

The era of modern interventional neurology started with Dr. Gomez and his colleagues. In 1991, Dr. Camilo R. Gomez was an Associate Professor at St. Louis University, St. Louis, Missouri (Fig. 1.1). He along with Dr. Mark Malkoff had set up an interventional protocol for treatment of acute ischemic stroke. Dr. Gomez had just returned from a conference in Argentina where he had met with Dr. Vinuela and had a productive and motivating discussion about the role of neurologists in interventional neuroradiology. Subsequently, Dr. Gomez, with the support of Chairman of Neurology, John B. Selhorst, MD at the Department of Neurology and Souers Stroke Institute, St. Louis University School of Medicine, St. Louis, Missouri, started performing neurointerventional procedures in collaboration with the Head of interventional cardiology, Morton J. Kern MD. The first procedure was performed by Dr. Gomez in the cardiac catheterization laboratory in December 1993. Drs. Gomez and Malkoff successfully incorporated acute response team or "Code Stroke"[35] and neurocritical care as essential components of management of patients undergoing neurointerventional procedures. They successfully connected all pagers of stroke team members to a common access number and instructed the emergency department staff to activate that number immediately upon arrival of a stroke patient (Code Stroke). This step allowed the

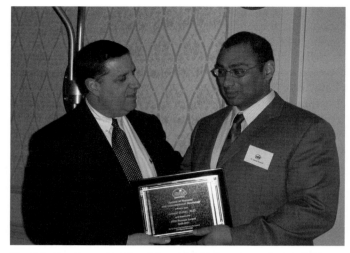

Fig. 1.1. Drs. Gomez (right) and Qureshi (left) share the podium in 2007.

integration of stroke neurologists in all aspects of care including evaluation, endovascular treatment, and post-procedural care. Subsequently, several diagnostic and interventional procedures were performed by Dr. Gomez in the cardiac catheterization laboratory at St. Louis University until July 1994. Later, a change in leadership in the medical school led to circumstances that resulted in Dr. Gomez moving to University of Alabama.

The Department of Neurology under the leadership of Dr. John N. Whitaker, who was Chairman of Neurology and President of the Health Services Foundation, provided Dr. Gomez with the opportunity to start another neurointerventional program in collaboration with interventional cardiologists at University of Alabama. The program was initiated on March 1, 1995 and Dr. Gomez started performing procedures in the cardiac catheterization laboratory. He was also able to build strong relationships with Dr. Jay S. Yadav, who was an interventional cardiology fellow and Dr. Gary S Roubin, who was a leading interventional cardiologist. Dr. Yadav had already completed a residency in neurology and fellowship in neuroimaging. Dr. Gomez was visiting Argentina for a meeting when he met with Dr. Marco Zenteno from Mexico. Dr. Gomez started visiting the Comprehensive Stroke Center, Hospital Angeles del Pedregal, Department of Neurological Endovascular Therapy, Instituto Nacional de Neurología y Neurocirugía, Mexico City, Mexico (National Institute of Neurology and Neurosurgery and Hospital LA at Mexico City) several times a year and performed interventional procedures with Dr. Zenteno.[36] Dr. Morgan Cambell joined Dr. Gomez at the University of Alabama as his first fellow for a 3-year fellowship in 1996, which included a combination of vascular neurology, neurocritical care, and neurointerventional procedures.

Dr. Adnan I. Qureshi (Fig. 1.1) was a neurology resident at Emory University in Atlanta, GA in 1994. Dr. Qureshi in 1996 joined a 2-year fellowship in neurocritical care at Johns

Hopkins Medical Institutions with the incorporation of some aspects of neuroradiology training within the fellowship. Dr. Qureshi subsequently joined the endovascular neurosurgical fellowship at University at Buffalo, State University of New York in July 1998. He was one of the first neurologists along with Edgard Pereira MD to join a formal fellowship program in neurointerventional procedures. The program at University of Buffalo was led by the Chairman of Neurosurgery, Dr. L. Nelson Hopkins, who was one of the most imminent neurosurgeons and considered to be the founder of the modern discipline of endovascular neurosurgery. Drs. Lee R. Guterman (neurosurgeon) and Ajay Wakhloo (neuroradiologist) were both well-reputed neurointerventionalists and formed the other faculty in the program. Dr. Qureshi had an opportunity to train with other neurosurgical fellows such as Drs. Lanzino, Fessler, Ringer, and Lopez, who all subsequently gained prominence in the field. His training included a wide spectrum of endovascular procedures for acute ischemic stroke, extra- and intracranial stent placement, and embolization of arteriovenous malformations and aneurysms. Dr. Qureshi worked diligently to incorporate academic research within the program at the University of Buffalo.

When Dr. Qureshi completed his fellowship in June 2000, he was invited to stay as faculty in the Department of Neurosurgery and trained several neurosurgery fellows during his two and half years at the University of Buffalo. He also developed an angiographic classification scheme for assessing initial severity of arterial occlusion in patients with acute ischemic stroke.[37] The classification scheme has been validated at multiple institutions since its first description and is currently referred to as the "Qureshi grading scheme."[38,39] In December 2002, Dr. Qureshi joined the University of Medicine and Dentistry of New Jersey, Newark, as a Professor of Neurology and Director of the Cerebrovascular Program on the invitation of Patrick Pullicino MD, who was Chairman of Neurology and Neurosciences at that time. An interventional neurology training program was simultaneously initiated, with Drs. Kirmani and Xavier starting as the first fellows in the program. In 2004, Nazli Janjua MD joined the program, becoming one of the first women to enter interventional neurology. Dr. Qureshi also received an RO-1 grant as principal investigator from the National Institutes of Health in 2004, starting a track of extramural funded research by interventional neurologists. The Zeenat Qureshi Stroke Research Center was initiated in 2004. Since its inauguration, the center has led the way in cutting-edge research in epidemiology, clinical trials, and basic research pertaining to cerebrovascular diseases. Zeenat Qureshi Stroke Research Center was transferred to the University of Minnesota in 2006. In 2007, the research center was ranked in the top 20 academic facilities for conducting biomedical research selected from hundreds of institutions representing several disciplines of biological sciences in the United States by *The Scientist*. Teaching, mentoring, and policies were ranked as the strengths of the center.

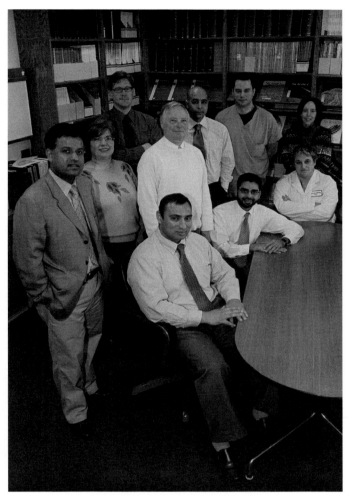

Fig. 1.2. The Minnesota Stroke Initiative team in 2007.

In November 2006, Dr. Qureshi joined the University of Minnesota in Minneapolis, Minnesota as a Professor of Neurology, Neurosurgery, and Radiology and Executive Director of the Minnesota Stroke Initiative.[40] An endovascular surgical neuroradiology fellowship was initiated (Fig. 1.2). Drs. Georgiadis, Shah, and Suri formed the first group of fellows in the newly started program. The ACGME in June 2000 had officially approved the Guidelines for Training in endovascular surgical neuroradiology. Subsequently, the program requirements for neurology were approved by the ACGME in May 2003. On January 1, 2008[41], the criterion for program directorship was modified to include physicians with current certification in the specialty by the American Board of Psychiatry and Neurology. In anticipation of this change, an application was submitted to the Neurosurgery Residency Review Committee at ACGME to request formal accreditation of the endovascular surgical neuroradiology fellowship at the University of Minnesota. The application was subsequently forwarded to a special committee of the Neurology Residency Review Committee with members from the

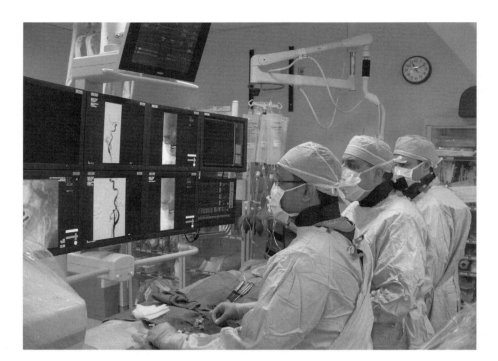

Fig. 1.3. Dr. Shah performing an endovascular procedure with Dr. Gomez (visiting professor) in 2008.

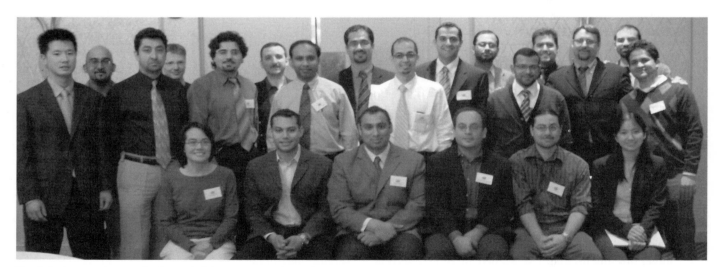

Fig. 1.4. A group photograph of several of the interventional neurology trainees in 2007.

Neurosurgery and Radiology Residency Review Committees. In May 2008, University of Minnesota became the first program to be accredited by the Neurology Residency Review Committee and Dr. Qureshi became the first neurologist to be a program director of an accredited endovascular surgical neuroradiology fellowship program. A total of three fellowship positions per year were approved. Over the years, the fellowship program has graduated outstanding fellows, who have received national awards and federal grants. The program has hosted world renowned visiting professors such as Dr. Gomez (Fig. 1.3), who was the President of the American Society of Neuroimaging (seen in the picture teaching fellows new techniques during his visit to University of Minnesota). In April 2008, Dr. M. Fareed K. Suri (Fig. 1.2) became the first interventional neurologist to receive the extramural K grant from National Institutes of Health for career development.

Interventional neurology: the national and international front

Interventional neurology was simultaneously gaining acceptance into the organized societies of Neurology (Fig. 1.4). In 1996, an "interventional section" was started within the American Academy of Neurology. The section was chaired

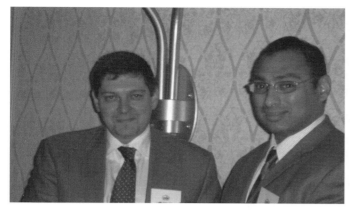

Fig. 1.5. Drs. Jovin (left) and Qureshi (right), Associate Editors of the *Journal of Neuroimaging*, share the podium in 2007.

by prominent interventional neurologists over the years including Kori (1996–1998), Gomez (1998–2000), Yadav (2000–2002), Hauser (2002–2004), Qureshi (2004–2006), and Pereira (2006–2008) leading to unprecedented growth. The interventional neurology field gained prominence in the programs of the annual meeting of the American Academy of Neurology and American Society of Neuroimaging. Dr. Gomez initiated the "Endovascular Therapy and Critical Care Course" and Dr. Suarez initiated the "Interventional Treatment of Acute Ischemic Stroke" course at the 55th Annual Meeting of the American Academy of Neurology, Honolulu, Hawaii, in March 2003. In January 2004, Dr. Qureshi initiated a course on angiography and interventional neurology at the 27th Annual Meeting of the American Society of Neuroimaging, in Phoenix, AZ. In April 2006, Dr. Qureshi initiated the half-day course on "Update on Endovascular Treatment of Cerebrovascular Disease" at the 58th Annual Meeting of the American Academy of Neurology, San Diego, CA. The interventional section of the American Academy of Neurology (AAN) had 267 active members by 2006. A plenary session dedicated to interventional neurology was the highlight of the American Society of Neuroimaging Annual Meeting in Miami in January 2007. The *Journal of Neuroimaging*, the official journal of the Society of Neuroimaging started an interventional section in 2007 with Drs. Qureshi and Jovin (Fig. 1.5) as Associate Editors dedicated to the section. Drs. Qureshi and Georgiadis edited the *Atlas of Interventional Neurology* that was published by Demos Medical Publishing, New York, NY, 2008 becoming the first textbook of interventional neurology. In January 2008, the *Journal of Vascular and Interventional Neurology* was published starting the first periodical for interventional neurology. Interventional neurology was also gaining recognition in other countries and was one of the highlights of the 45th Turkish Neurology Congress, Ulusal Noroloji Kongresi, Antalya, Turkey, 10–15 Kasim, 2009. In November 2009, the International Society of Interventional Neurology was started, with Drs. Qureshi (President), Pereira

(Vice-President), Taylor (Secretary), and Shah (Treasurer) as the first office holders. The society started coordinating the efforts of interventional neurology groups within and outside the United States.

Collaboration also started between professional organizations of various specialties. The Neurovascular Coalition was formed in November 2004, led by John J. Connors, III, MD as the first Immediate Past President of the American Society of Interventional and Therapeutic Neuroradiology to ensure excellence in medical education, training, and research related to vascular conditions affecting the brain and thus promote high-quality patient care. The coalition members included the American Academy of Neurology, American Association of Neurological Surgeons, American Society of Interventional and Therapeutic Neuroradiology, American Society of Neuroradiology, Congress of Neurological Surgeons. AANS/CNS Cerebrovascular Section, and Society of Interventional Radiology. The coalition prepared a multi-society landmark consensus document[42] entitled "Training, competency, and credentialing standards for diagnostic cervicocerebral angiography, carotid stent placement, and cerebrovascular intervention" that defines minimum standards for the training, knowledge, and experience necessary to perform carotid stent placement and other diagnostic and therapeutic cerebrovascular procedures. This was followed by another document "Qualification requirements for performing neuro-interventional procedures: A report of the Practice Guidelines Committee of the American Society of Neuroimaging and the Society of Vascular and Interventional Neurology" that was authored by Qureshi, Abou-Chebl, and Jovin.[43] The document summarized the existing data derived from regulatory bodies, professional organizations, and clinical trials with direct pertinence to indications and qualifications required for performing neurointerventional procedures and provided recommendations regarding qualifications required for performing individual neurointerventional procedures. Such efforts have led to an increased recognition of interventional neurology as a subspecialty of neurology over the last decade.

The future

With sights set on excellence, interventional neurology will continue to grow and prosper. The enduring legacy of any effort or journey is not what we have achieved, but what we have become as a consequence. In the address to the interventional section at the American Academy of Neurology 59th Annual Meeting, Boston, MA, on May 2007, Dr. Qureshi summarized the evolution of Interventional Neurologist as follows: "Any organization that commits to self-sacrifice for the greater good has already taken the first step to greatness. The ramifications of this commitment will shake any organization to the core but their desire to seek greatness will bond them together into an eternal legacy that will last longer than their mortal existence."

References

1. Qureshi AI. Endovascular treatment of cerebrovascular diseases and intracranial neoplasms. *Lancet* 2004;363:804–13.

2. Kori SH. Interventional neurology: a subspecialty whose time has come. *Neurology* 1993;43:2395–9.

3. Wilkins Rh ME. Wilkins Rh. Moniz E. Neurosurgical classic. Xvi. Arterial encephalography. Its importance in the localization of cerebral tumors. *J Neurosurg* 1964;21:144–56.

4. Moniz E. L'encephalographie arterielle, son importance dans la localisation des tumeurs cerebrales. *Revue Neurologique* 1927;2:72–89.

5. Farinas PL. A new technique for the arteriographic examination of the abdominal aorta and its branches. *Am J Roentgenol* 1941;46.

6. Radner S. Intracranial angiography via the vertebral artery; preliminary report of a new technique. *Acta Radiol* 1947;28:838–42.

7. Jonsson G. Thoracic aortography by means of a cannula inserted percutaneously into the common carotid artery. *Acta Radiol* 1949;31: 376–86.

8. Seldinger SI. Catheter replacement of the needle in percutaneous arteriography; a new technique. *Acta Radiol* 1953;39:368–76.

9. Fletcher TM, Taveras JM, Pool JL. Cerebral vasospasm in angiography for intracranial aneurysms. Incidence and significance in one hundred consecutive angiograms. *Arch Neurol* 1959;1:38–47.

10. Newton TH, Kramer RA. Clinical used of selective external carotid arteriography. *Am J Roentgenol Radium Ther Nucl Med* 1966;97:458–72.

11. Amundsen P, Dietrichson P, Enge I, Williamson R. Cerebral angiography by catheterization–complications and side effects. *Acta Radiol Ther Phys Biol* 1963;1:164–72.

12. Amundsen P, Dugstad G, Noyes W. Cerebral angiography via the femoral artery with particular reference to cerebrovascular disease. *Acta Neurol Scand* 1967;43:Suppl 31:115.

13. Rosenbaum AE, Eldevik OP, Mani JR, Pollock AJ, Mani RL, Gabrielsen TO. In re: Amundsen P. Cerebral angiography via the femoral artery with particular reference to cerebrovascular disease. *Acta Neurol Scand* 1967; Suppl. 31:115. *Am J Neuroradiol* 2001;22:584–9.

14. Kieffer SA. Harold O. Peterson, MD: a life in neuroradiology. *AJNR Am J Neuroradiol* 1993;14:1427–35.

15. Taveras JM. Development of the first fellowship training program in neuroradiology in North America. *Am J Neuroradiol* 1991;12:587–90.

16. Takahashi M, Kawanami H. Femoral catheter techniques in cerebral angiography – an analysis of 422 examinations. *Br J Radiol* 1970;43: 771–5.

17. Vitek JJ. Femoro-cerebral angiography: analysis of 2,000 consecutive examinations, special emphasis on carotid arteries catheterization in older patients. *Am J Roentgenol Radium Ther Nucl Med* 1973;118:633–47.

18. Bradac GB, Simon RS. [Routine use of a catheter technique for cerebral angiography (965 examinations) (author's transl)]. *Rofo* 1976;125:66–9.

19. Caresano A, Del Favero C, Crivelli G, Tenti L, Bianchi M. [Selective arteriography of the carotid and vertebral arteries by the femoral route: review of 225 patients (author's transl)]. *Radiol Med* 1977;63:225–32.

20. Werner SCBA, King BG. Aneurysm of the internal carotid artery within the skull: wiring and electrothermic coagulation. *JAMA* 1941;116:578–82.

21. Sussman BJFT. Thrombolysis with fibrinolysis in cerebral arterial occlusion. *JAMA* 1958;167:1705–9.

22. Luessenhop AJ, Velasquez AC. Observations on the tolerance of the intracranial arteries to catheterization. *J Neurosurg* 1964;21:85–91.

23. Serbinenko FA. [Catheterization and occlusion of major cerebral vessels and prospects for the development of vascular neurosurgery]. *Vopr Neirokhir* 1971;35:17–27.

24. Serbinenko FA. Balloon catheterization and occlusion of major cerebral vessels. *J Neurosurg* 1974;41:125–45.

25. Debrun G, Lacour P, Caron JP, Hurth M, Comoy J, Keravel Y. Inflatable and released balloon technique experimentation in dog – application in man. *Neuroradiology* 1975;9:267–71.

26. Debrun G, Lacour P, Caron JP, Hurth M, Comoy J, Keravel Y. Detachable balloon and calibrated-leak balloon techniques in the treatment of cerebral vascular lesions. *J Neurosurg* 1978;49:635–49.

27. Jungreis CA, Berenstein A, Choi IS. Use of an open-ended guidewire: steerable microguidewire assembly system in surgical neuroangiographic procedures. *Am J Neuroradiol* 1987;8:237–41.

28. Guglielmi G, Vinuela F, Sepetka I, Macellari V. Electrothrombosis of saccular aneurysms via endovascular approach. Part 1: Electrochemical basis, technique, and experimental results. *J Neurosurg* 1991;75:1–7.

29. Guglielmi G, Vinuela F, Dion J, Duckwiler G. Electrothrombosis of saccular aneurysms via endovascular approach. Part 2: Preliminary clinical experience. *J Neurosurg* 1991;75:8–14.

30. Leeds NE, Kieffer SA. Evolution of diagnostic neuroradiology from 1904 to 1999. *Radiology* 2000;217:309–18.

31. Ergun DL, Mistretta CA, Kruger RA, Riederer SJ, Shaw CG, Carbone DP. A hybrid computerized fluoroscopy technique for noninvasive cardiovascular imaging. *Radiology* 1979;132:739–42.

32. Brant-Zawadzki M, Gould R, Norman D, Newton TH, Lane B. Digital subtraction cerebral angiography by intraarterial injection: comparison with conventional angiography. *AJR Am J Roentgenol* 1983;140:347–53.

33. Sherry RG, Anderson RE, Kruger RA, Nelson JA. Real-time digital subtraction angiography for therapeutic neuroradiologic procedures. *Am J Neuroradiol* 1983;4:1171–3.

34. Strother CM. Interventional neuroradiology. *Am J Neuroradiol* 2000;21:19–24.

35. Gomez CR, Malkoff MD, Sauer CM, Tulyapronchote R, Burch CM, Banet GA. Code stroke. An attempt to shorten inhospital therapeutic delays. *Stroke* 1994;25:1920–3.

36. Zenteno MA, Murillo-Bonilla LM, Guinto G, *et al.* Sole stenting bypass for the treatment of vertebral artery aneurysms: technical case report. *Neurosurgery* 2005;57:E208; discussion E.

37. Qureshi AI. New grading system for angiographic evaluation of arterial occlusions and recanalization response to intra-arterial thrombolysis in acute ischemic stroke. *Neurosurgery* 2002;50:1405–14; discussion 14–5.

38. Mohammad YM, Christoforidis GA, Bourekas EC, Slivka AP. Qureshi grading scheme predicts subsequent volume of brain infarction following intra-arterial thrombolysis in patients with acute anterior circulation ischemic stroke. *J Neuroimaging* 2008;**18**:262–7.

39. Mohammad Y, Xavier AR, Christoforidis G, Bourekas E, Slivka A. Qureshi grading scheme for angiographic occlusions strongly correlates with the initial severity and in-hospital outcome of acute ischemic stroke. *J Neuroimaging* 2004;**14**:235–41.

40. Qureshi AI, Janardhan V, Memon MZ, *et al.* Initial experience in establishing an academic neuroendovascular service:

program building, procedural types, and outcomes. *J Neuroimaging* 2009;**19**:72–9.

41. Program requirements for residency education in endovascular surgical neuroradiology (Accessed last accessed on September 12, 2007, at, www.acgme.org/acWebsite/RRC_160/160_prIndex.asp.)

42. Connors JJ, 3rd, Sacks D, Furlan AJ, *et al.* Training, competency, and credentialing standards for diagnostic cervicocerebral angiography, carotid stenting, and cerebrovascular intervention: a joint statement from the American Academy of Neurology, the American Association of Neurological

Surgeons, the American Society of Interventional and Therapeutic Neuroradiology, the American Society of Neuroradiology, the Congress of Neurological Surgeons, the AANS/CNS Cerebrovascular Section, and the Society of Interventional Radiology. *Neurology* 2005;**64**:190–8.

43. Qureshi AI, Abou-Chebl A, Jovin TG. Qualification requirements for performing neurointerventional procedures: a Report of the Practice Guidelines Committee of the American Society of Neuroimaging and the Society of Vascular and Interventional Neurology. *J Neuroimaging* 2008;**18**:433–47.

Chapter 2

Diagnostic cerebral angiography

Adnan I. Qureshi and Ameer E. Hassan

Cerebral angiography is a procedure by which the intracranial and extracranial head and neck circulation is evaluated.[1] It entails the placement of a catheter selectively into extracranial cerebral vessels using fluoroscopic guidance, followed by contrast material injection and image acquisition to delineate anatomy and abnormalities.

Utilization of cerebral angiography

The use of non-invasive cerebrovascular imaging was increased while the use of cerebral angiography has declined since 1985.[2] A prominent decrease was seen in pre-procedure cerebral angiograms among patients undergoing carotid endarterectomy.[3,4] According to the most recent Medicare data show that, in 2002, at least 92 000 cervicocerebral arteriograms (Current Procedural Terminology codes 75680 and 75676, respectively, for bilateral or unilateral cervical carotid arteriography) were performed, compared with 109 000 performed 5 years previously. However, in a recent study we found evidence that the overall use of cerebral angiography increased between 1990 and 1991 and 2000 and 2001. We used data from the Nationwide Inpatient Sample, the largest all-payer inpatient care database in the United States.[5] International Classification of Disease, 9th Revision, Clinical Modification primary diagnosis codes were used to identify the patients admitted with stroke and stroke subtypes and secondary codes to identify those with stroke-associated complications and related procedures. In a 2-year period, 1990 to 1991, there were 1 736 352 admissions for cerebrovascular diseases, and in another 2-year period, 2000 to 2001, there were 1 958 018 admissions. Cerebral angiography during hospitalization was performed in 126 572 (7.3%) patients in 1990–1991 and in 161 256 (8.3%) patients in 2000–2001. The rate of cerebral angiography increased most prominently for patients with subarachnoid hemorrhage, from 32% in 1990–1991 to 54% in 2000–2001. The recent increase in utilization during hospitalization is attributed to the increase in neurointerventional procedures among patients with cerebrovascular diseases.[6] Interventional angiography is cerebral angiography that is performed either prior to or during neurointerventional procedures to guide patient selection, planning technical aspects of the procedure, and monitoring the results of these procedures. Another reason for increased rates of angiography may be found in recent data suggesting that, in practice, the reliability of non-invasive studies may be inferior to angiography for appropriate guidance in patient selection.[7,8]

Recommended indications from professional organizations

The practice guidelines from the Stroke Council of the American Heart Association recommend cerebral angiography for imaging in transient ischemic attacks and acute stroke under selected conditions. Patients with retinal ischemic events or transient ischemic attacks are deemed to be candidates for cerebral angiography when there is reasonable evidence of carotid atherosclerotic disease that warrants consideration of endarterectomy. Evidence of luminal reduction greater than or equal to 70% on ultrasound, magnetic resonance angiography, or computed tomographic arteriography, is usually a strong indication for cerebral angiography in symptomatic patients who are candidates for endarterectomy. Some stenotic lesions measured at 50% to 69% by non-invasive techniques may show luminal reduction greater than or equal to 70% on cerebral angiography, making them eligible for endarterectomy. Conversely, occlusion on non-invasive testing may correlate with a residual hairline lumen on cerebral angiography in as many as 9% of patients (Class II, see Table 2.1). Cerebral angiography also is required to evaluate intracranial stenosis or occlusion. Selective subclavian and/or vertebral cerebral angiography remains the reference procedure for imaging of vessels in vertebrobasilar occlusive disease. The outline of arteries that are diseased, whether from stenotic or occlusive atherosclerosis, dissection, or arterial dysplasias, can be characterized more accurately than by current magnetic resonance angiography techniques. Selective cerebral angiography is the recommended procedure for diagnosis of cerebral aneurysm in patients with subarachnoid hemorrhage (type A). Cerebral angiography is recommended to detect beading, stenosis, or aneurysm, particularly in medium sized and small cerebral

Textbook of Interventional Neurology, ed. Adnan I. Qureshi. Published by Cambridge University Press. © Cambridge University Press 2011.

Table 2.1. Criteria for grading the quality of evidence ratings for diagnostic tests by the Stroke Council, American Heart Association**

Class I	Evidence provided by one or more well-designed clinical studies of a diverse population using a gold standard reference test in a blinded evaluation appropriate for the proposed diagnostic application.
Class II	Evidence provided by one or more clinical studies of a restricted population using a reference test in a blinded evaluation of diagnostic accuracy.
Class III	Evidence provided by expert opinion, non-randomized historical controls, or observation(s) from case series.
Strength of recommendations rating	
Type A	Strong positive recommendation, based on Class I evidence or overwhelming Class II evidence when circumstances preclude randomized clinical trials.
Type B	Positive recommendation, based on Class II evidence.
Type C	Positive recommendation, based on strong consensus of Class III evidence.
Type D	Negative recommendation, based on inconclusive or conflicting Class II evidence.
Type E	Strong negative recommendation, based on evidence of ineffectiveness or lack of efficacy, based on Class I or Class II evidence.
Classification of recommendations	
Class I	Conditions for which there is evidence for and/or general agreement that the procedure or treatment is useful and effective.
Class II	Conditions for which there is conflicting evidence and/or a divergence of opinion about the usefulness/efficacy of a procedure or treatment.
IIa	The weight of evidence or opinion is in favor of the procedure or treatment.
IIb	Usefulness/efficacy is less well established by evidence or opinion.
Class III	Conditions for which there is evidence and/or general agreement that the procedure or treatment is not useful/effective and in some cases may be harmful.
Level of evidence	
Level of evidence A	Data derived from multiple randomized clinical trials.
Level of evidence B	Data derived from a single randomized trial or non-randomized studies.
Level of evidence C	Consensus opinion of experts.

**Guidelines from the American Heart Association/American Stroke Association Stroke Council

vessels affected by vasculitis (type C). Where magnetic resonance imaging and magnetic resonance angiography are not available, cerebral angiography is a diagnostic option to be used independently or in combination with other tests for diagnosis of deep vein, cortical vein, or dural sinus thrombosis (type C). Cerebral angiography may be done if the diagnosis from magnetic resonance imaging/magnetic resonance angiography is unclear and there is strong suspicion of arterial dissection (type C). Cerebral angiography also continues to be the "gold standard" in the diagnostic evaluation of unruptured intracranial aneurysms[10] and provides the most information about small perforating vessels by producing higher-resolution images than other imaging modalities.

The Brain Attack Coalition recommends the following regarding cerebral angiography (grade 1A).[11] Cerebral angiography is the gold standard for the detection and characterization of cerebral aneurysms, arteriovenous malformations, and arteriovenous fistulas, and for measuring the exact degree of stenosis in extracranial and intracranial arteries (grade IA). It is the procedure of choice for evaluating the third- and fourth-order intracranial branches to make a diagnosis of central nervous system vasculitis. Because of the emergent nature of some of the stroke types discussed above, cerebral angiography must be available at a comprehensive stroke center on a 24/7 basis, with support personnel available to come in from home for a procedure within 60 minutes of being called. A comprehensive stroke center must demonstrate a peri-procedure stroke and death rate of less than 1% and an overall serious complication rate of less than or equal to 2% for cerebral angiography.

The Quality Improvement Guidelines[12] for Adult Diagnostic Neuroangiography from the Society of Cardiovascular and Interventional Radiology, the American Society of Interventional and Therapeutic Neuroradiology, and the American Society of Neuroradiology defined appropriate indications for performance of cerebral angiography (see Table 2.2). The threshold for these indications is 99%. When fewer than 99% of procedures are performed for these indications, the institution should review the process of patient selection.

Technical aspects of the procedure

The cerebral angiography is comprised of six steps as outlined below:

Percutaneous access

Percutaneous access is secured through two main routes for a cerebral angiogram. The femoral artery is the most common route followed by radial artery access. Brachial and carotid artery access are rarely used. Femoral artery access requires insertion of an 18 or 19 gage needle in the common femoral artery below the inguinal ligament. The inguinal ligament runs from the anterior superior iliac spine to the pubic tubercle.

The site for percutaneous insertion is determined by one of three methods. The first requires manual identification of the pubic symphysis and the anterior superior iliac spine to

Table 2.2. Indications for cerebral angiography: Guidelines of the Society of Cardiovascular and Interventional Radiology, the American Society of Interventional and Therapeutic Neuroradiology, and the American Society of Neuroradiology[12]

Indications
1. Define presence/extent of vascular occlusive disease and thromboembolic phenomena.
2. Define etiology of hemorrhage (subarachnoid, intraventricular, parenchymal, craniofacial).
3. Define presence, location, and anatomy of intracranial aneurysms and vascular malformations.
4. Evaluate vasospasm related to subarachnoid hemorrhage.
5. Define presence/extent of trauma to cervicocerebral vessels (e.g., dissection, pseudoaneurysm).
6. Define vascular supply to tumors.
7. Define presence/extent of vasculitis (infectious, inflammatory, drug-induced).
8. Diagnose and/or define congenital or anatomic anomalies (e.g., vein of Galen fistula).
9. Define presence of venous occlusive disease (e.g., dural sinus cortical, deep).
10. Outline vascular anatomy for planning and determining the effect of therapeutic measures.
11. Perform physiologic testing of brain function (e.g., WADA).

Table 2.3. Various catheters used for cerebral angiography in 150 consecutive studies in adult patients

Diagnostic catheters	Frequency
Single catheter used in study	74 procedures
Multiple catheters used in study	76 procedures
4 F vertebral catheter	10
5 F Davis catheter	95
5 F Simmons II catheter	40
5 F Simmons I catheter	10
5 F Headhunter catheter	20

determine the position of the inguinal ligament. An imaginary line is drawn between the two anatomic points and femoral artery pulsation is sought four inches below the line. The second method uses fluoroscopy to identify the center of the femoral bone head and uses the identified site for palpation. The third method requires an ultrasound probe to visualize the common femoral artery and the needle is manipulated under direct ultrasound guidance. The modified Seldinger's technique is used which requires needle insertion in the artery, passage of an introducer wire, and introduction of an introducer sheath over the wire in to the artery.[13] Fluoroscopic visualization of the direction and location of the introducer wire provides confirmation of adequate positioning of the wire.

Introducer sheaths are available from 4 to 8 French in diameter and are selected based on the requirements of the catheters intended for use. The sheaths are available in 20 cm, 40 cm, and 80 cm length, and usually the 40 cm or 80 cm sheaths are reserved for patients with tortuous femoral and iliac vessels. A randomized trial compared introduction of diagnostic catheters through introducer sheaths to direct introduction without sheaths, for cerebral angiography.[14] The ease of catheter manipulation was greater with an introducer sheath and a lower incidence of bleeding at the femoral puncture site during the procedure was observed (2%, versus 36%). Because of bleeding, conversion to sheath insertion was necessary in 39% of 421 patients in the control group. Therefore, use of arterial sheaths is recommended for cerebral angiography.

Radial artery access is used in patients with difficult femoral artery access usually due to occlusive disease of the femoral and/or iliac arteries. The radial artery may also be preferred for visualization of the right subclavian artery which may be difficult to catheterize in patients with tortuous vessels through the femoral route. The radial and ulnar arteries supply blood to the musculoskeletal tissue and skin of the hand. In most patients, the ulnar artery can supply both territories in case of radial artery compromise, through the palmar arch. Before considering radial artery access, patients are examined to confirm patency of the palmar arch.[15] A visual Allen test is performed, for which blanching of the palm subsides within 7 seconds after release of the ulnar artery, while still compressing the radial artery.[16] In addition, a Doppler probe is placed over the expected region of the palmar arch to determine whether arterial signal intensity remains present during compression of the radial artery.[15] Our preferred method requires a pulse oximeter placed on the patient's thumb while the radial artery is compressed, and patency of the palmar arch is considered present if a strong waveform remains and the percentage of oxygen saturation remains unchanged. Puncture of the radial artery (on the right in most procedures) is performed approximately 2 cm cephalad to the radial styloid using a 21 gauge needle. Immediately after sheath insertion, a mixture of heparin (5000 IU/ml), verapamil (2.5 mg), lidocaine (2%, 1.0 ml), and nitroglycerin (0.1 mg) is infused through the introducer sheath to relieve and/or prevent vasospasm.[17]

Aortic placement and selective catheterization of supra-aortic arteries

Most diagnostic cerebral angiograms are performed using either a 4 or 5 French diagnostic catheter with tapered tip and wire braiding for enhanced torque control. For practical purposes, five diagnostic catheters with different configuration are used for cerebral angiography (see Table 2.3 and Fig. 2.1). 1) The Pigtail catheter which has ring-shaped multiple side-holes at its distal end for large volume injections with minimal catheter movement and is used for aortic arch injections or aortograms. 2) The vertebral curve (Davis) catheter (see Fig. 2.2) with a simple hockey-stick design, normally used for selective

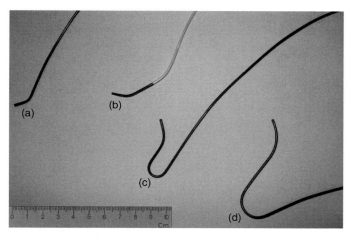

Fig. 2.1. Various types of diagnostic catheters used in cerebral angiography: (a) Davis catheter; (b) Simmons II catheter; (c) Simmons I catheter; (d) Headhunter catheter.

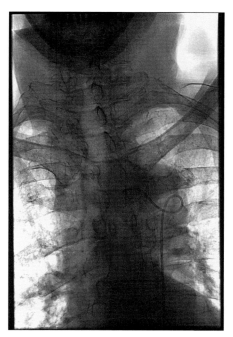

Fig. 2.2. A Davis catheter in the arch of the aorta with tip turned cephalad to engage supra-aortic vessel origin.

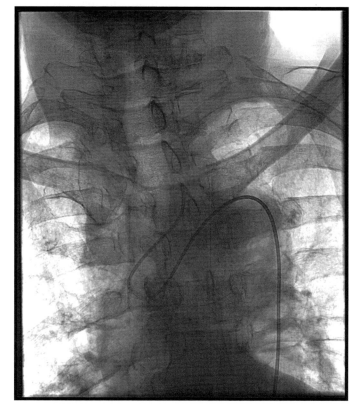

Fig. 2.3. A constituted Simmons II catheter in the arch of the aorta with tip turned cephalad to engage supra-aortic vessel origin.

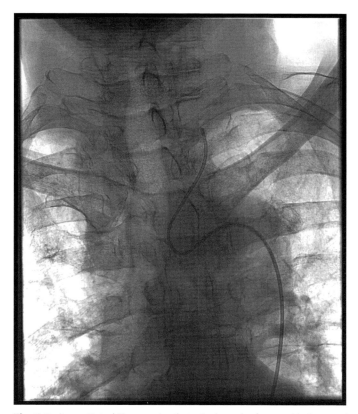

Fig. 2.4. A constituted Simmons I catheter in the arch of aorta with tip turned cephalad to engage supra-aortic vessel origin.

studies of the carotid or vertebral arteries, but also for innominate and subclavian artery injections. Simmons II catheter (see Fig. 2.3), with a tip that curves back upon the body of the catheter for selection of vessels, is used for older patients with tortuous aortas and/or great vessel origins particularly for selection of the left common carotid, innominate, or left subclavian arteries. The Simmons I catheter (see Fig. 2.4), with a

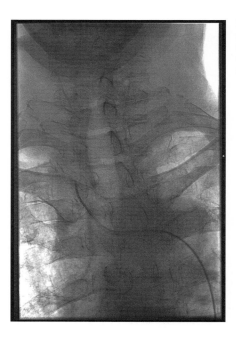

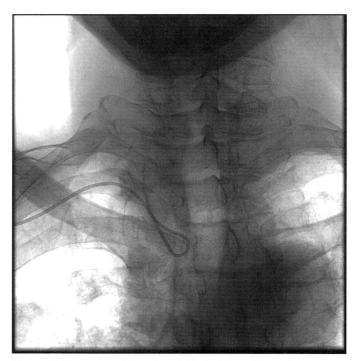

Fig. 2.5. A Headhunter catheter in the arch of aorta with tip turned cephalad to engage supra-aortic vessel origin.

Fig. 2.6. The sequence of steps required to constitute the Simmons II catheter in the aorta.

tip that curves back upon the body of the catheter once reconstituted, allows for placement in tortuous origins off the arch. Because of the shorter curve (as compared to the Simmons II), the Simmons I catheter is preferred for angiography performed through the radial artery. 5) The Headhunter catheter, which is cobra-shaped (see Fig. 2.5), has greater stiffness than the above mentioned catheters and is used for catheterizing difficult right subclavian arteries.

The diagnostic catheter is advanced over a 0.035 inch wire with a gentle curve at the distal end that can be manipulated from the proximal end of the guidewire. The guidewire is advanced into the abdominal aorta, thoracic aorta, and the arch of aorta. The diagnostic catheter is then advanced over the guidewire into the arch of the aorta. The guidewire is withdrawn into the diagnostic catheter and the catheter pulled back with the angulated tip pointed cephalad in a direction that allows engagement of the origin of the supra-aortic vessels. Once the origin is engaged, the guidewire is advanced towards the distal common carotid artery or subclavian artery. The diagnostic catheter is advanced over the guidewire into the desired position and the guidewire is withdrawn.

In patients with a tortuous aorta, as is commonly found in elderly patients, a Simmons II catheter is routinely employed. The Simmons II catheter is reconstituted by pulling and rotating the catheter in the arch of the aorta until a loop is formed (see Fig. 2.6). A guidewire is passed through the catheter and the catheter assumes the shape of a hook due to retropulsion created by the passage of the wire. Reconstitution can also be achieved by advancing the Simmons II catheter into a supra-aortic vessel over a wire. Subsequently, the wire is withdrawn and the catheter is pushed forward until it enters into the arch of the aorta assuming its desired configuration. The Simmons II catheter is then manipulated until it engages the origin of the

supra-aortic vessels. Once the origin is engaged, the catheter is pulled back resulting in the advancement of the catheter towards the distal common carotid artery or subclavian artery. The catheter may be removed from a selected vessel by pushing and reforming a curve in the arch or by pulling and straightening a curve in the arch.

A Headhunter catheter is used for catheterizing a challenging right subclavian artery. The Headhunter configuration allows stable placement and manipulation of the catheter in the right innominate artery to allow access to the right subclavian artery.

A Simmons I catheter may be helpful in circumstances where tortuous proximal segments of the supra-aortic vessels may not permit advancing the angulated or Simmons II catheter. The Simmons I is required for a radial artery approach. In that case, the Simmons I catheter is advanced over a 0.035 inch guidewire through the brachial, axillary, subclavian, and innominate arteries into the arch of the aorta. The Simmons I catheter is reconstituted into the desired configuration by pulling and rotating the catheter in the arch of the aorta until a loop is formed. A guidewire is passed through the catheter and the catheter assumes the shape of a hook due to retropulsion created by the passage of the wire. The Simmons I catheter can also be reconstituted by pushing the catheter towards the heart and deflecting it off the aortic valve.

The diagnostic catheters are advanced into the internal or external carotid artery or vertebral arteries over a guidewire after the origin of these vessels is visualized and their patency

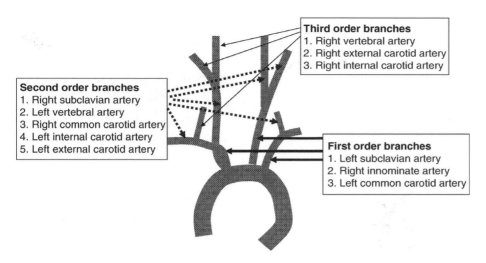

Third order branches
1. Right vertebral artery
2. Right external carotid artery
3. Right internal carotid artery

Second order branches
1. Right subclavian artery
2. Left vertebral artery
3. Right common carotid artery
4. Left internal carotid artery
5. Left external carotid artery

First order branches
1. Left subclavian artery
2. Right innominate artery
3. Left common carotid artery

Fig. 2.7. An illustration of first-, second-, and third-order vessels that are catheterized during cerebral angiography.

confirmed. Roadmapping techniques allow adequate positioning of guidewires and diagnostic catheters under direct visualization, with knowledge of the underlying vessel location and configuration.

From a practical standpoint, two anatomic variants are frequently encountered and need to be considered during catheterization. The left common carotid artery may originate from the right innominate artery and selective catheterization may require passage of the diagnostic catheter (usually Simmons II) into the right innominate artery and then into the left common carotid artery. The left vertebral artery may originate from the arch of the aorta and the origin is then usually between the origin of the left common carotid artery and left subclavian artery.

Vessels catheterized for contrast injections

Depending upon the diagnostic question, the diagnostic catheter is placed in the common carotid artery, internal carotid artery, or external carotid artery for the anterior circulation. For the posterior circulation, the catheter may be placed in the subclavian or vertebral artery. The catheter is usually placed in the most distal vessel possible to avoid runoff of contrast into vessels that do not need to be visualized. Advancing the catheter into the internal carotid or vertebral artery requires caution to avoid traversing diseased segments and causing vessel spasm or dissection. Where to place the catheter in the internal carotid or vertebral artery is chosen with consideration of catheter stability and direction of contrast flow. Special caution is required in introducing diagnostic catheters through tortuous origins of vertebral arteries and small vessels such as the external carotid artery and vertebral artery, which are prone to vasospasm. Contrast injections into the external carotid artery may cause facial flushing and discomfort and therefore diluted contrast is preferred.

The identification of all catheter introduction sites and all the vessels catheterized is important for reimbursement (see Fig. 2.7). The highest-order vascular family catheterized is used to determine the requested charges. This means identifying the final destination of a catheter, whether it is first-, second-, or third-order in a vascular family. Also, any additional second- or third-order vessels catheterized in a vascular family are reported. The vessels are classified as follows: The first-order vessels are the right innominate, left common carotid, and left subclavian arteries. Second-order vessels are the right subclavian, right common carotid, left internal carotid, left external carotid, and left vertebral arteries. Third-order vessels are the right internal carotid, right external carotid, and right vertebral arteries.

Contrast injection

The injection of contrast agent must be at a rate and volume that safely and adequately opacifies the vascular territory of interest. Contrast may be injected through the diagnostic catheter either by hand injection of 5–10 ml or by a programmed injector. The recommended injection volume and rate in our practice are 8 ml at 6 ml/s for the internal carotid or vertebral artery, 6 ml at 4 ml/s for the external carotid artery, and 10–12 ml at 8 ml/s for the common carotid or subclavian artery. For an aortogram, 40 ml of contrast are injected at a rate of 15 ml/s into the aortic arch. A programmed injector is definitely required for acquisition of multiple images for rotational reconstruction. In a survey of 63 program directors of neuroradiology programs[18] the following mean injection rates and total volumes (± standard deviations) were reported for specific vessels:

- Common carotid arteries: 7.2 (± 1.8) ml/s and 9.9 (± 2.0) ml total
- Internal carotid arteries: 5.8 (± 1.4) ml/s and 7.9 (± 1.5) ml total
- Vertebral arteries: 5.4 (± 1.2) ml/s and 7.8 (± 1.7) ml total.

The modes (rate/total) for the common carotid, internal carotid, and vertebral arteries were 7/12, 6/8, and 5/8, respectively.

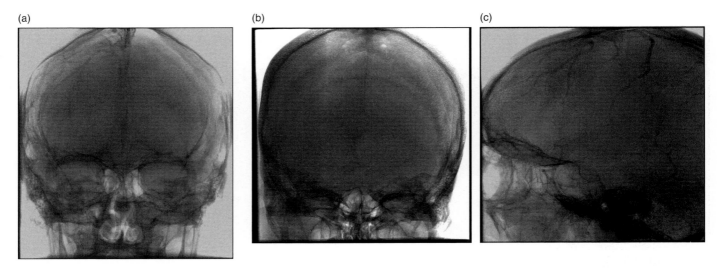

Fig. 2.8. Unsubtracted images demonstrating: (a) anterio-posterior projection; (b) Townes and (c) lateral projection.

Projections for image acquisition

Optimal positioning, magnification, and filming rates are necessary to provide sufficient information regarding the disease and vascular territory being studied. A suggested frame rate is 2 per second during the arterial phase and 1 per second during the capillary and venous phases.

Several projections may be necessary to best detect and characterize the targeted lesion, but a minimum of two perpendicular projections is essential. An aortic arch study is performed in the 20–25 degree left anterior oblique projection to include the arch, proximal great vessels, vertebral origins, and carotid bifurcations. A right anterior oblique projection may be obtained simultaneously if the examination is performed on a biplane digital unit but this is rarely necessary. Cervical images of the carotid bifurcation and vertebral arteries are usually acquired in the antero-posterior and lateral projections. In the antero-posterior projection, the central X-ray passes from the front to the back of the body or part, with the film at the back. In the lateral projection, the central ray enters the body or part from the side and is perpendicular to the medial or axial plane. Additional modified views (obliques) may be obtained, if required.

A standard set of projections is used for image acquisition of the intracranial vessels during contrast injection (see Fig. 2.8). The antero-posterior projection for the anterior cerebral circulation is obtained in half-axial projection, with the central ray at an angle to the frontal and medial planes. The symmetrical structures should be projected evenly on either side of the midline. The posterior circulation is visualized in a Townes projection which is a radiographic projection of the head in which the central ray enters obliquely through the frontal bone, yielding a view of facial structures and the occipital bone. The skull is projected without geometric distortion, which normally elongates the occiput. The posterior clinoid processes should be visible in the round foramen magnum. Caldwell's projection is a postero-anterior projection with the head turned 20–45° away from the side of the injection or the image intensifiers turned toward the side of the injection to provide an alternate view of the anterior communicating artery and middle cerebral artery bifurcation. Carotid or Townes-angle biplane obliques are acquired with the head turned 20–45° away from the side of the injection or the image intensifiers turned 20–45° toward the side of the injection to optimally visualize the posterior inferior cerebellar artery origins, the vertebrobasilar junction, the anterior communicating artery, and the middle cerebral artery bifurcation. The submentovertex projection is a radiographic projection of the head with the central ray entering under the chin and directed toward the vertex, and is used for visualizing the anterior communicating artery. A tilt lateral view can be used to project the middle cerebral artery vessels above the supraclinoid carotid. The lateral tube or image intensifier is caudal on the side of the injection and cephalad on the side opposite to the injection.

Note that, if the anterior communicating artery does not fill or fills poorly, the cross-compression technique may be employed. During injection of one carotid artery, the operator or assistant compresses the opposite carotid, promoting collateral flow across the anterior communicating artery. A similar compression of the carotid artery during injection of the vertebral artery promotes flow through the posterior communicating artery to facilitate its visualization.

Three-dimensional rotational angiography has recently emerged as a substitute for the multiple image acquisition projections described above[19]. Rotational cerebral angiography provides continuously changing projections, with excellent visualization of lesions such as aneurysms or other vascular malformations requiring special or oblique views[20] (see Fig. 2.9). Rotational angiography as part of routine angiography gives a three-dimensional impression with one injection and

(a)

(b)

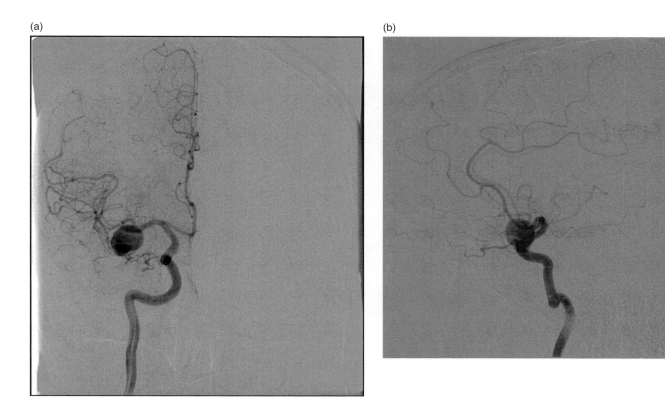

(c)

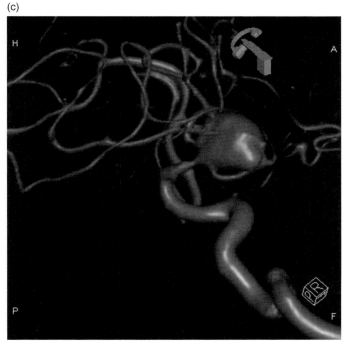

Fig. 2.9. A comparison of images provided by antero-posterior and lateral images of an intracranial aneurysm with images acquired and reconstructed using 3D cerebral angiography.

one series of films. However, the number of frames required to produce a 3-D rotational angiography volume reconstruction (100–300 frames) is much higher than a typical biplanar series (20–40 frames).[21] Images for 3-D rotational angiography are acquired by rotating the frontal C-arm in two arcs, one for mask acquisition and another with injection of contrast material. Image acquisition goes from 100° left anterior oblique to 100° right anterior oblique with the X-ray tube traveling

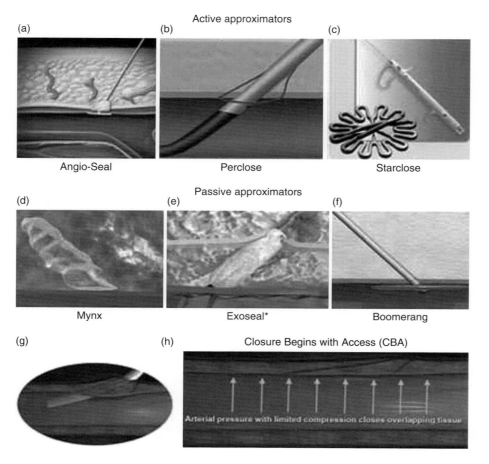

Active approximators

(a)   (b)   (c)

Angio-Seal   Perclose   Starclose

Passive approximators

(d)   (e)   (f)

Mynx   Exoseal*   Boomerang

(g)   (h)   Closure Begins with Access (CBA)

Arterial pressure with limited compression closes overlapping tissue

Fig. 2.10. Vascular closure devices by mechanism of action (a)–(f). In the bottom row, cartoons (g), (h) depict the effects of Arstasis* access and closure. On the left (g), the sheath has been placed across a shallow diagonal entry path. A small "pilot" track was used for access for the Arstasis device. On the right (h), the sheath has been pulled from the diagonal track, which has sealed. Devices including SuperStitch (Sutura, Fountain Valley,CA), X-Site (St. Jude), and FemoSeal* (St. Jude). Other passive approximation devices include VasoSeal/On-Site (St. Jude) and Duett (Vascular Solutions). Other CBA: FISH (Femoral Introducer Sheath and Hemostasis, Morris Innovative Research, Bloomington, IN). (*Investigational device). See plate section.

under the patient. Three-dimensional rotational angiography has been demonstrated to provide superior visualization of cerebral aneurysms[22–24] and other neurovascular lesions.[25,26]

Hemostasis at the site of percutaneous access

After the procedure, the catheters and sheath are removed, and manual pressure is applied at the site of femoral puncture. A 6-hour bed rest is recommended after removal of the introducer sheath, although a shorter period of 4 hours may be adequate.[27,28] For radial artery access, a superficial pressure dressing is applied to the radial artery puncture site. Patients are observed for 2 hours before discharge. During this observation period, bed rest is not required.[17] In the endovascular procedure setting, vascular closure devices have emerged as an alternative to mechanical compression in order to achieve vascular hemostasis after puncture of the femoral artery.[29] Vascular closure devices (see Figs. 2.10 and 2.11, Table 2.4) are categorized based on the mechanism of hemostatic action, which includes biodegradable plug, suture, staples, or ultrasound. Vascular closure devices offer advantages over mechanical compression including shorter time to hemostasis and patient ambulation, high rate of patient satisfaction, and greater cost-effectiveness. Complications related to the site of femoral access are still a concern despite use of closure devices.

A meta-analysis of randomized, case-controlled, and cohort studies compared access-related complications with vascular closure devices versus mechanical compression in 37 066 patients.[30] No difference was revealed in complication rates between Angio-Seal and mechanical compression for diagnostic procedures or percutaneous coronary interventions. Meta-analysis limited to randomized trials only showed a trend toward fewer complications using Angio-Seal in a setting of percutaneous coronary intervention. No differences were observed regarding Perclose in either diagnostic procedures or percutaneous coronary interventions. An increased risk in complication rates using VasoSeal was found in the percutaneous coronary interventions setting. The overall analysis favored mechanical compression over vascular closure devices, supporting use of vascular closure devices in selected patients.

Technically successful cerebral angiography

A successful examination is defined as study that provides sufficient selective neuroangiographic technical evaluation and image interpretation to establish or exclude pathology of the extracranial and intracranial circulation[12] preferably in one session. Rarely, more than one session may be necessary due to limitation of vascular access, contrast agent dose limit, patient intolerance, inadequate anesthesia, or comorbid

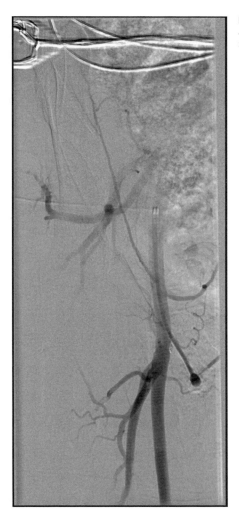

Fig. 2.11. Femoral angiogram demonstrating star close patch.

conditions such as congestive heart failure that obviates prolonged supine positioning.[12]

Intravascular contrast agents
Basic properties of intravascular contrast agents

The original radiological contrast media were salt solutions of very high osmolality, several fold greater than that of tissue cells, plasma, or tissue fluid (all of which have an osmolality of 300 mOsmols per kg water). The high osmolality causes a sensation of heat and discomfort or even pain during contrast injection. Erythrocytes and vascular endothelium are adversely affected by the high osmolality of intravascular contrast agents, resulting in tissue anoxia and increased capillary permeability, and disruption of the blood–brain barrier. Vasodilatation, systemic hypotension, and osmotic hypervolemia can occur due to the high osmolality of contrast media. Numerous chemical modifications have allowed a shift from high to low osmolality and from ionic to non-ionic contrast agents[31,32] (see Table 2.5). Low osmolality contrast agents are synthesized with a non-ionizing radical (such as amide or amine) instead

of the carboxyl group of a tri-iodinated substituted benzoic acid. Use of low osmolality contrast agents is associated with reduced chemotoxic effects on red blood cells, histamine release, electrocardiographic changes, and hemodynamic changes, compared with use of conventional agents. Low osmolality contrast agents are recommended especially in patients with alteration of the blood–brain barrier (major trauma, tumor, or stroke), prior contrast media reactions, or marked anxiety.[33,34] Other benefits include decreased osmotic load, which can be important in infants or severely dehydrated patients. We recommend routine use of low osmolality contrast agents for cerebral angiography.

Hypersensitivity reactions to contrast agents

Contrast agents can cause allergic reactions with vasomotor, vagal-type, or anaphylactoid symptoms.[35] Hypersensitivity allergic reactions (predominantly minor) occur in 1% to 6% of patients who receive contrast agents.[36] The rate of severe reactions range from 0.01% to 0.02%.[35] The rate is higher with ionic agents. Vasomotor effects include self-limited warmth, nausea, and emesis. Vagal-type reactions include hypotension associated with bradycardia. Anaphylactoid reactions are classified as minor, moderate, or severe. Minor reactions involve limited nausea, vomiting, limited urticaria, pruritus, and diaphoresis. Moderate anaphylactoid reactions include faintness, severe vomiting, profound urticaria, facial edema, laryngeal edema, and mild bronchospasm. Mild or moderate anaphylactoid reactions usually occur within 30 minutes. Severe or fatal reactions usually develop rapidly (94% within 20 minutes and 60% in the first 5 minutes) following contrast exposure. Significant risk factors for hypersensitivity reactions include a history of asthma/bronchospasm, a previous hypersensitivity reaction, and a history of allergy or atopy.

Patients with risk factors should receive prednisone, 50 mg orally, at 13, 7, and 1 hours before the procedure; diphenhydramine, 50 mg orally or intramuscularly, 1 hour before the procedure; or ephedrine sulfate, 25 mg orally, 1 hour before the procedure to reduce the risk of hypersensitivity reaction.[37] H_2 blockers are adjunctive agents with marginal benefit. Premedication does not eliminate the possibility of a fatal reaction on re-administration of radiocontrast media, because reactions can occur despite pretreatment.[38–41] Therefore, at-risk patients should be observed for 20 to 30 minutes following the procedure. Emergent treatment for anaphylactoid reactions requires maintenance of an adequate airway, breathing, and circulation, plus appropriate pharmacologic use of intravenous fluids and epinephrine if necessary.

Delayed (late) adverse reactions, consisting of nausea, emesis, headache, itching, skin rash, musculoskeletal pain, and fever, may occur within 1 hour to 1 week in 2.8% of patients following the administration of iodinated contrast media.[42] Oral steroids maybe helpful for delayed contrast reactions, although there are no controlled trials to confirm benefit.[35]

Table 2.4. Closure devices taken with permission from Endovascular Today 2009

Company name	Product name	Type	Puncture size (F)	Maximum wire compatibility (inch)	FDA approved	Comments
Abbott Vascular	Perclose A-T	Suture	5–8	0.038	Yes	Automated knot for secure, mechanical vascular closure of 5- to 8-F access sites; braided polyester suture closure can be challenged and confirmed at the table
	Perclose ProGlide					Automated knot for secure, mechanical vascular closure of 5- to 8-F access sites; monofilament polypropylene suture closure can be challenged and confirmed at the table
	Prostar XL		8.5–10			Designed to close up to 10-F access sites; braided polyester suture for secure, mechanical closure; closure can be challenged and confirmed at the table
	StarClose	Nitinol clip	5, 6			An extravascular nitinol clip that mechanically closes the arteriotomy to ensure rapid hemostasis; closure can be challenged and confirmed at the table
	StarClose SE					Next-generation StarClose with enhanced ease-of-use design; extravascular nitinol clip that mechanically closes the arteriotomy to ensure rapid hemostasis; closure can be challenged and confirmed at the table
AccessClosure, Inc.	Mynx	Extravascular polyethylene glycol (PEG) sealant	5, 6, 7	Utilizes existing procedural sheath	Yes	Designed to minimize pain; uses extravascular, conformable PEG sealant that provides durable hemostasis; dissolves within 30 days, leaving no residue
Cardiva Medical, Inc.	Cardiva Catalyst II	Arteriotomy tamponade	5, 6, 7	Works through existing sheath	Yes	Deployable nitinol disc that provides temporary hemostasis at the arteriotomy, allowing it to recoil to the size of an 18-gauge needle; hemostatic coating on the wire accelerates the clotting cascade facilitating vessel closure, preserving the artery, and leaving no residue
Morris Innovative	FISH (Femoral Introducer Sheath and Hemostasis Device)	Biomaterial (SIS) seal allows for remodeling of host tissue at the arteriotomy	5, 6, 8	Works through existing sheath	Yes	Closure begins with access as the biomaterial sealant is introduced through the procedural sheath; the biomaterial actively approximates the arteriotomy for sealing where it is most effective, completely healing the vessel without scar tissue formation
St. Jude Medical, Inc.	Angio-Seal VIP, Angio-Seal STS Plus	Mechanical seal	6, 8	6 F = 0.035; 8 F = 0.038	Yes	Suture, collagen, and anchor sandwich of the arteriotomy; all components reabsorb within 90 days; FDA labeling for immediate restick
	Angio-Seal Evolution		4–8			Next-generation Angio-Seal with automated collagen compaction and

Table 2.4. (cont.)

Company name	Product name	Type	Puncture size (F)	Maximum wire compatibility (inch)	FDA approved	Comments
						enhanced ease-of-use design; suture, collagen, and anchor sandwich of the arteriotomy; all components reabsorb within 90 days; FDA labeling for immediate restick
	VasoSeal VHD, ES, Elite	Extravascular collagen sponge	5, 6, 7, 8	0.038		Extravascular: no permanent intra-arterial component; bioabsorbable, collagen supports the natural healing process
	VasoSeal Low Profile		4, 5			Smaller design than VHD to accommodate 4- and 5-F puncture tracts
Sutura	SuperStitch	Polypropylene suture and knot	6–12	Works through existing sheath	Yes	True 6- and 8-F suture delivery through the sheath; does not enlarge arteriotomy; available in 6-, 8-, and 12-F, as well as 12-F extended length
Vascular Solutions, Inc.	Duett Pro, Diagnostic Duett Pro	Thrombin and collagen procoagulant	5–9	Works through existing sheath	Yes	Utilizes the existing sheath, a balloon catheter, and a procoagulant to achieve hemostasis; Duett Pro is approved for use with GP IIb/IIIa inhibitors and ACT of <400

Table 2.5. Intravascular contrast agents, their chemical and physical properties, and associated complications

Type	Example	w/v%*	Iodine (mg/ml)	Osmolality (mOsm/kg)	Rates of contrast induced nephropathy
High osmolar Ionic	Meglumine diatrizoate	65%	306	1530	7%[93]
Low osmolar Non-ionic	Iopamidol	61.2%	300	616	3.5%[94]
	Iohexol	64.6%	300	640	
	Ioversol	63.6%	300	645	
Iso-osmolar Non-ionic	Iodixanol	65.2%	320	290	1.4%[94]

*weight/volume %

Contrast-induced nephropathy

Contrast-induced nephropathy is commonly defined as an acute decline in renal function following the administration of parenteral contrast in the absence of other causes.[43,44] For research purposes, a definition such as a rise in serum creatinine 25% or 50% above the baseline value is often used.[43] The most common presentation consists of an acute rise in serum creatinine in the absence of oliguria at 24 to 48 hours after contrast administration. Serum creatinine elevation peaks at 3 to 5 days and returns to baseline values by 7 to 10 days. In the USA and Europe, contrast induced nephropathy is the third leading cause of acute renal failure in hospitalized patients, accounting for 10% of such cases.[45] The estimates of

the incidence of contrast-induced nephropathy vary due to differences in the definition of renal failure, patient comorbidities, and the presence of other potential causes of acute renal failure. A recent epidemiologic study reported a rate of 14.5% among approximately 1800 consecutive patients undergoing invasive cardiac procedures.[46]

Contrast induced nephropathy is a consequence of both direct renal tubular epithelial cell toxicity and renal medullary ischemia.[43] The nature of the contrast, associated ions, concentration, and concomitant hypoxia contribute to the cellular damage with unclear contribution of the osmolality of the solution. Contrast exposure induces a biphasic hemodynamic change in the kidney, with an initial, transient increase and then a more prolonged decrease in renal blood flow.[43] The elimination half-life following intravascular administration in patients with normal renal function is about 2 h, so 75% of the administered dose is excreted in urine within 4 h. After 24 h, 98% of the injected contrast medium is out of the body.[44] Mild, transient decreases in glomerular filtration rate occur after contrast administration in almost all patients.[43] Whether a patient develops clinically significant acute renal failure, however, depends very much on the presence or absence of certain risk factors.[47]

The risk of renal failure rises with the number of risk factors present. In one study, the frequency of renal failure rose progressively from 1.2% to 100% as the number of risk factors went from zero to four.[48] Another study estimated that patients without any risk factors have a much lower risk, of approximately 3%.[49] The most important risk factor is pre-existing renal failure. A multivariate analysis of prospective trials demonstrated that baseline renal impairment, diabetes mellitus, congestive heart failure, and higher doses of contrast media increase the risk of contrast induced nephropathy.[43] Patients with diabetes mellitus and renal impairment, however, have a substantially higher risk of contrast nephropathy than patients with renal impairment alone.[50] Other risk factors include hydration status and concurrent use of potentially nephrotoxic drugs such as non-steroidal anti-inflammatory agents and angiotensin-converting enzyme inhibitors. Although higher contrast volume is associated with a higher risk of contrast-induced nephropathy, the maximum tolerated volume is not known but is estimated between 300 and 400 ml per procedure.[43] The ratio of the volume of administered contrast media to creatinine clearance (V/CrCl)>3.7[51] has been demonstrated to be an independent predictor of an early increase in serum creatinine following contrast exposure.

Many strategies have been evaluated to prevent contrast induced nephropathy including volume expansion; hydration with intravenous administration of sodium chloride (0.9% or 0.45%); infusion of mannitol; administration of atrial natriuretic peptide, loop diuretics, calcium antagonists, theophylline, dopamine, acetylcysteine, or the dopamine-1 receptor antagonist fenoldopam; use of low-osmolar non-ionic contrast media instead of high-osmolar ionic contrast media; rapid hemodialysis after contrast administration; injection of small volume of contrast medium; gadolinium-based contrast media instead of iodine-based contrast media for radiography; and, avoiding short intervals (less than 48 h) before repeat administration of contrast media. Based on the existing evidence, there have been thirteen guidelines proposed for prevention of contrast induced nephropathy.[52] A review of most recent guidelines is presented in Table 2.5.[53–56] Hydration, cessation of intake of nephrotoxic drugs, and administration of the lowest possible dose of contrast medium is consistently emphasized,[52] but recommendations on the prophylactic use of drugs, and the iso-osmolar dimer vary.

The administration of intravenous fluids before, during, and after the contrast procedure is the main strategy for prevention contrast-induced nephropathy[52,56] based on the results of eight randomized controlled trials. The first trial[57] on the effect of hydration reported that forced diuresis with furosemide or mannitol was inferior to hydration with 0.45% saline alone in patients with preexisting renal disease. A second trial[58] showed that, in patients with normal renal function, a hydration protocol with 0.9% saline was superior to one with 0.45% saline. To date, three randomized trials[59] have demonstrated that use of isotonic sodium bicarbonate was superior to standard hydration with saline. The underlying hypothesis is that the alkalinization of tubular fluid diminishes the production of free oxygen radicals, which are mediators of contrast induced nephropathy. This regimen may therefore become more widely acceptable in the next few years.

Meta-analyses of randomized trials have suggested a potential benefit of low osmolar contrast medium[62] (22 randomized trials); iso-osmolar contrast medium[63] (16 randomized trials); theophylline, an adenosine antagonist, with a trend toward reduction[64] (9 randomized trials); and N-acetyl cysteine, having antioxidant and vasodilatory effects, with a significant reduction[65] (13 studies). However, these findings were heterogeneous across studies suggesting benefit in selected patients.

In most cases the injury resulting from contrast induced nephropathy is mild and renal impairment resolves spontaneously.[43] Avoidance of further nephrotoxic insults and careful control of fluid and electrolyte balance is usually adequate. Dialysis may be required in more severe cases. No specific therapy has been found to be of benefit in the treatment of contrast induced nephropathy. A randomized trial of atrial natriuretic peptide as a treatment for acute renal failure did not demonstrate an overall reduction in the need for dialysis in a subgroup of 65 patients with contrast induced nephropathy.[66] Another trial[67] randomized 72 patients who developed contrast induced nephropathy to receive 0.45% saline with or without dopamine 1 ml/kg per hour until serum creatinine returned to its baseline value. Patients in the dopamine treatment group had higher peak serum creatinine and required dialysis more frequently suggesting a detrimental effect.

Complications related to cerebral angiography

The clinical practice guidelines of the Society of Cardiovascular and Interventional Radiology, the American Society of Interventional and Therapeutic Neuroradiology, and the American Society of Neuroradiology recommend that all major complications resulting from adult diagnostic neuroangiography should be less than 2%.[12] This threshold refers to any complication which requires or causes major therapy, unplanned increase in level of care, prolonged hospitalization, permanent adverse sequelae or death. The following are the predominant complications associated with cerebral angiography.

Vascular complications related to percutaneous access

Vascular complications arising after percutaneous access can be local hematomas, femoral pseudoaneurysms, and retroperitoneal hemorrhages. The rates differ depending upon the definition used in studies pertaining to cerebral angiography and can vary from 1%–4% (see Table 2.7). More thorough data is available through a review of 30 studies[30] that included a total of 37 066 patients undergoing coronary angiography and percutaneous coronary intervention. The rate of femoral access complications excluding local hematomas was 2.7% an among 12 596 treated with closure devices and 3.0% among 24 470 patients who underwent compression. In another analysis, the rate of femoral access complications requiring transfusion or surgery among 1377 patients recruited in various clinical trials evaluating neurointerventional procedures was 2.1%.

Femoral punctures can lead to pseudoaneurysms,[68,69] a dilatation in the wall of the femoral artery at the site of entry. The presentation consists of local swelling and varying degrees of local infection or bleeding. The majority of femoral pseudoaneurysms less than 3 cm in diameter will spontaneously thrombose and may be simply observed with serial Doppler ultrasound exams in asymptomatic patients. Symptomatic pseudoaneurysms, pseudoaneurysms with a diameter greater than 3 cm, and those found in patients who are anticoagulated may require treatment. Ultrasound-guided thrombin injection has become the preferred method for treating femoral pseudoaneurysms because of its low risk, high success rate, and efficacy in the setting of anticoagulation.[70–72] Ultrasound-guided compression is an alternative less effective method[73] that may be considered when thrombin products are contraindicated. Surgical repair maybe preferred in the presence of infection, rapid expansion, or if less invasive methods are not technically feasible. In a study of 75 patients with post-catheterization pseudoaneurysms,[71] the results of surgical repair, local compression and thrombin injection methods were compared. Thrombin injection into pseudoaneurysms caused closure of the cavity and neck in all patients. However, five patients required additional thrombin injection during the same session, and two patients in a follow-up procedure. No peri-procedural complications were observed. The mean hospital stay was 27 days in surgically treated patients, 8 days in those treated with compression, and 5 days in those treated with thrombin.

Neurological complications

Patients undergoing cerebral angiography can develop ischemic stroke or transient ischemic attack during or after the procedure.[8,74–88] Table 2.6 demonstrates the rates of neurological complications reported in recent large clinical studies. The rates of transient and permanent complications following cerebral angiography are less than 3% and 1%, respectively. The most common reasons are thrombosis within the catheter with subsequent embolization, mechanical disruption of aortic or supra-aortic vessel plaque, or dissection of the catheterized vessel with subsequent thrombosis and embolization secondary to wire or catheter manipulation. Most clinical events consist of a recurrence or worsening of a pre-existing neurological deficit.

Most clinical events occur within the first 72 hours following cerebral angiography. In a prospective review of 1002 procedures[75] the ischemic event rate between 0 and 24 hours was 1.3% (0.1% permanent) and another 1.8% of the patients suffered an ischemic event (0.3% permanent) between 24 and 72 hours after angiography. Another study prospectively reviewed the rates of transient, reversible, and permanent neurological complications in 2899 consecutive angiograms.[85] There was a 1.3% rate of any neurological complications; 0.7% were transient, 0.2% were reversible (resolved within 7 days), and 0.5% were permanent. In a single center review of 19 826 consecutive patients[78] undergoing diagnostic cerebral angiography from 1981 through 2003, neurological complications occurred in 2.6% of examinations; 0.1% of these resulted in permanent disability. In another prospective study of 2,924 diagnostic cerebral angiography procedures[88] there were no permanent neurological complications, although asymptomatic technical complications (10 dissections) were reported.

Risk factors for neurologic complications have been reported in many studies (see Table 2.7) including patient's age, presence of atherosclerotic cerebrovacular disease (particularly located in the arch of the aorta or in the internal carotid arteries), fluoroscopic time, number and size of catheters, type and number of vessels injected, and operator experience. Neurological complications have decreased in recent years,[78] because of improvements in technology and lower proportion of patients undergoing evaluation for atherosclerotic diseases such as carotid stenosis because of increasing use of non-invasive imaging modalities. In another analysis of three prospective studies[89] the combined risk of permanent and transient neurological complications was significantly lower in patients with subarachnoid hemorrhage compared with patients with transient ischemic attack or stroke (1.8% versus 3.7%). The combined risk of permanent and transient neurological complications was also significantly lower in patients with aneurysm/arteriovenous malformation without subarachnoid hemorrhage compared with patients with transient ischemic attack or stroke (0.3% versus 3.7%).

Recently, asymptomatic ischemic events (detected on magnetic resonance imaging) during cerebral angiography have gained more attention[90] (see Table 2.6). One study prospectively evaluated a total of 107 consecutive patients undergoing cerebral angiography using diffusion weighted magnetic resonance imaging.[91] Fifty-one angiographies were performed by experienced neuroradiologists and 56 by neuroradiologists in training. In 12 patients (11%), a total of 17 new lesions without any clinical symptoms were identified. Of these 12 patients, 11 (92%) with 16 lesions had procedures performed by neuroradiologists in training. In 11 of 12 patients (92%) with

Table 2.6. Summary of recent recommendations for preventing contrast induced nephropathy from various professional organizations[53]

Organization	Summary of recommendations
Canadian Association of Radiologists	1. Consider alternative imaging that does not require contrast. 2. Fluid volume loading is the single most important protective measure. 3. Nephrotoxic medications should be discontinued 48 h prior to the study. 4. Contrast agent volume and frequency of administration should be minimized. 5. High-osmolar contrast should be avoided in patients with renal impairment. 6. There is some evidence to suggest that iso-osmolar contrast reduces the risk of nephropathy among patients with renal impairment. 7. Acetylcysteine has been advocated to reduce the incidence of CIN; however, not all studies have shown a benefit, and it is difficult to formulate evidence-based recommendations at this time. Its use may be considered in high-risk patients but is not considered mandatory.
Alberta Kidney Disease Network	1. Consider alternative imaging procedures that do not require contrast. 2. If the patient has ≥ 2 risk factors for CIN then consider acetylcysteine 600–1200 mg orally twice daily for 2 doses before the procedure and 2 doses after the procedure; or Ascorbic acid 3 g orally 2 h before the procedure and 2 g orally twice daily after procedure. 3. IV normal saline 1 ml/kg per hour for 6–12 h before the procedure or IV 5% dextrose and water plus sodium bicarbonate 154 mEq/L, 3 ml/kg for 1 h before the procedure with monitoring for metabolic alkalosis. 4. Use minimum possible volume of iso-osmolar or low-osmolar contrast during the procedure. 5. IV normal saline 1 ml/kg per hour for 6–12 h or IV 5% dextrose and water plus sodium bicarbonate 154 mEq/L, 1 ml/kg for 6 h with careful monitoring for fluid overload.
Consensus panel for contrast induced nephropathy	1. All patients receiving contrast agents should be evaluated for their risk of contrast induced nephropathy. 2. All patients receiving contrast agents should be in optimal volume status at the time of exposure to contrast agents. 3. High-risk patients should only be considered for pharmacologic prophylaxis with therapies supported by clinical evidence. 4. Low osmolality contrast agents should be used in all patients. 5. Drugs that adversely affect renal function should be withheld prior to and immediately following contrast agent exposure. 6. In all high-risk patients, a follow-up serum creatinine should be obtained at not less than 24 h or more than 72 h following contrast agent exposure.
European Society of Urogenital Radiology	1. NSAIDs and diuretics should be stopped 24 h before the procedure and can be reintroduced 24 h thereafter. 2. Metformin should be discontinued on the morning of the procedure and restarted if contrast induced nephropathy has not developed. 3. If serum creatinine has risen after a procedure, the next procedure should be delayed until serum creatinine has peaked and stabilized or, ideally, has returned to baseline. 4. After the contrast study, serum creatinine levels should be followed for 24–48 h in medium-risk or high-risk patients. 5. All patients undergoing a contrast procedure should be administered water or IV normal saline at least 500 ml before the procedure and 2500 ml for 24 h after the procedure. 6. In patients with higher risk (i.e. dehydration, circulatory collapse or congestive heart failure) the procedure should be delayed pending correction of the hemodynamic status. 7. The amount of contrast should be kept as low as possible and low-osmolar or iso-osmolar contrast medium should be used. 8. Although controversial, the use of 1200 mg acetylcysteine twice daily on the day of contrast procedure and the day before can be defended. For emergency procedures, an intravenous bolus of 1200 mg can replace the first oral dose. 9. High-risk patients should have nephrological advice before the contrast agent exposure, requiring an individualized protocol. 10. In patients unable to receive appropriate hydration and/or admitted to the intensive care unit, the administration of 200 mg theophylline 30 min before the procedure can be defended.

Abbreviations used: IV, intravenous; NSAID, non-steroidal anti-inflammatory drug; CIN, contrast-induced nephropathy.

Table 2.7. Table providing rates of neurological and percutaneous access complications in various studies

Study	Number of patients	Permanent neurological deficits	Transient neurological deficits	Percutaneous access complications	Time frame of complication ascertainment	Risk factors for neurological complications
Kaufmann TJ, et al.[78]	19 826	39 (0.2%)	522 (2.6%)	832 (4.2%)	Within 24 hours	1. Atherosclerotic cerebrovascular disease; 2. Indication of subarachnoid hemorrhage; 3. The comorbidity of frequent transient ischemic attacks; 4. Operator experience
Willinsky RA, et al.[85]	2899	14 (0.5%)	20 (0.7%)	14 (0.4%)	Transient, lasting <24 h, Permanent, lasting >7 days	1. Age of 55 years or older; 2. Patients with cardiovascular disease; 3. Fluoroscopic times exceeds 10 min or longer
Dawkins AA, et al.[88]	2924	0	10 (0.3%)	12 (0.4%)	Until discharge	1. Emergency procedures; 2. Angiography procedures performed for intracerebral hemorrhage and subarachnoid hemorrhage.
Cloft HJ, et al.[89] (meta-analysis)	3517	32 (0.9%)	11 (0.3%)	11 (0.3%)	Within 24 h	1. Patient's age; 2. Total volume of contrast used; 3. Length of procedure; 4. Use of more than one catheter; 5. Presence of systolic hypertension; 6. History of TIA/stroke.
Heiserman JE, et al.[90]	91	0	0 [but 23 (25%) had asymptomatic DW-MRI lesions]	Not reported	Within 7 days	1. Contrast volume used; 2. Fluoroscopy time; 3. Frequent additional catheters; 4. Number of vessels catheterized; 5. History of vasculopathy
Krings T, et al.[91]	107	0	0 [but 12 (11%) had asymptomatic DW-MRI lesions]	0	Within 24 h	1. Underlying vessel disease; 2. Practitioner level of experience
Bendszus M, et al.[92]	150	0	0 [but 17 (11.3%) had DW-MRI lesions without neurological deficits]	0	Within 3 days	1. Not using heparin or air filters during angiography; 2. History of vasculopathy; 3. Fluoroscopy time; 4. Difficulty catheterizing appropriate vessels

Abbreviations used: DW-MRI, diffusion-weighted magnetic resonance imaging; TIA, transient ischemic attack.

abnormalities seen on diffusion-weighted imaging, risk factors could be identified (atherosclerotic vessel wall disease, vasculitis, and hypercoagulable states). The rate of diffusion abnormalities in patients with risk factors was 11/48 (23%) which was higher than in patients without any risk factors (1/59; 2%).

To prevent the risk of neurological events, non-invasive modalities should be preferentially used in patients with highest risk of neurological complications (i.e., patients aged 55 years or greater or those being investigated for ischemic cerebrovascular diseases). If diagnostic angiography is necessary in these patients, practitioners with higher level of experience should perform these studies. Pre-treatment with aspirin has been recommended for patients at risk for neurological complications prior to undergoing cerebral angiography. Air filters and heparin have been advocated during cerebral angiography. In a prospective study, diffusion-weighted magnetic resonance imaging before and after cerebral angiography and transcranial Doppler ultrasound during angiography were used to evaluate the frequency of cerebral embolism. One hundred and fifty patients undergoing diagnostic cerebral angiography[92] were randomized into three groups: conventional angiographic technique, systemic heparin treatment throughout the procedure, or air filters between the catheter and both the contrast medium syringe and the catheter flushing. There were no neurological complications reported during or after angiography. Overall, 26 new ischemic lesions were detected in 17 patients (11%) on magnetic resonance imaging. In the control group, 11 patients showed a total of 18 lesions. In the heparin group, 3 patients showed a total of four lesions. In the air filter group, 3 patients exhibited a total of four lesions. The reduced incidence of ischemic events in the heparin and air filter groups compared with the control group was significant. Transcranial Doppler ultrasound demonstrated a large number of microembolic signals that was significantly lower in the air filter group compared with the heparin and control groups.

We recommend that diagnostic catheters have continuous saline infused through the central lumen for the duration of the procedure. For high risk patients, we administer aspirin prior to the procedure if they are not already using aspirin and we use high dose heparin (5000 U/L) in the saline infused through the catheter. Air filters are routinely employed in the diagnostic catheters.

Summary

Cerebral angiography has been the gold standard for diagnosis of cerebrovascular diseases. In recent years, non-invasive imaging has started to replace cerebral angiography. However, the use of interventional engiography is expected to continue to increase along with the use of neuro-interventional procedures.

References

1. Quality improvement guidelines for adult diagnostic neuroangiography. Cooperative study between the asnr, asitn, and the scvir. American Society of Neuroradiology. American Society of Interventional and Therapeutic Neuroradiology. Society of Cardiovascular and Interventional Radiology.[see comment][reprint in *J Vasc Interv Radiol.* 2003 Sep;14(9 pt 2):S257–62; pmid: 14514829]. *Am J Neuroradiol* 2000;**21**:146–50.

2. Gehlbach SH, Adamache KW, Cromwell J. Changes in the use of diagnostic technologies among medicare patients, 1985 and 1990. *Inquiry* 1996;**33**:363–72.

3. Holloway RG, Jr., Witter DM, Jr., Mushlin AI, Lawton KB, McDermott MP, Samsa GP. Carotid endarterectomy trends in the patterns and outcomes of care at academic medical centers, 1990 through 1995. *Archiv Neurol* 1998;**55**: 25–32.

4. Collier PE. Changing trends in the use of preoperative carotid arteriography: the community experience. *Cardiovasc Surg* 1998;**6**:485–9.

5. Qureshi AI, Suri MFK, Nasar A, *et al.* Changes in cost and outcome among US patients with stroke hospitalized in 1990 to 1991 and those hospitalized in 2000 to 2001. *Stroke* 2007;**38**:2180–4.

6. Qureshi AI. Ten years of advances in neuroendovascular procedures. *J Endovasc Ther* 2004;**11** Suppl 2:II1–4.

7. Johnston DC, Goldstein LB. Clinical carotid endarterectomy decision making: Noninvasive vascular imaging versus angiography.[see comment]. *Neurology* 2001;**56**:1009–15.

8. Qureshi AI, Suri M, Ali Z, *et al.* Role of conventional angiography in evaluation of patients with carotid artery stenosis demonstrated by doppler ultrasound in general practice.[see comment]. *Stroke* 2001;**32**:2287–91.

9. Culebras A, Kase CS, Masdeu JC, *et al.* Practice guidelines for the use of imaging in transient ischemic attacks and acute stroke. A report of the stroke council, american heart association. *Stroke* 1997;**28**:1480–97.

10. Bederson JB, Awad IA, Wiebers DO, *et al.* Recommendations for the management of patients with unrupted intracranial aneurysms: A statement for healthcare professionals from the stroke council of the american heart association. *Circulation* 2000;**102**:2300–08.

11. Alberts MJ, Latchaw RE, Selman WR, *et al.* Recommendations for comprehensive stroke centers: a consensus statement from the brain attack coalition. *Stroke* 2005;**36**: 1597–616.

12. Quality improvement guidelines for adult diagnostic neuroangiography. Cooperative study between the asnr, asitn, and the scvir. American Society of Neuroradiology. American Society of Interventional and Therapeutic Neuroradiology. Society of Cardiovascular and Interventional Radiology. *Am J Neuroradiol.* 2000;**21**:146–50.

13. Seldinger SI. Catheter replacement of the needle in percutaneous arteriography; a new technique. *Acta Radiol* 1953;**39**:368–76.

14. Moran CJ, Milburn JM, Cross DT, 3rd, Derdeyn CP, Dobbie TK, Littenberg B. Randomized controlled trial of sheaths in diagnostic neuroangiography. *Radiology* 2001;**218**:183–7.

15. Nohara AM, Kallmes DF. Transradial cerebral angiography: Technique and outcomes. *Am J Neuroradiol* 2003;**24**:1247–50.

16. Benit E, Vranckx P, Jaspers L, Jackmaert R, Poelmans C, Coninx R. Frequency of a positive modified allen's test in 1,000 consecutive patients undergoing cardiac catheterization. *Cathet Cardiovasc Diagn* 1996;**38**: 352–4.

17. Levy EI, Boulos AS, Fessler RD, *et al.* Transradial cerebral angiography: an alternative route. *Neurosurgery* 2002;**51**:335–40; discussion 340–2.

18. Yousem DM, Trinh BC. Injection rates for neuroangiography: Results of a survey.[see comment]. *Am J Neuroradiol* 2001;**22**:1838–40.

19. Gailloud P, Oishi S, Carpenter J, Murphy KJ. Three-dimensional digital angiography: new tool for simultaneous three-dimensional rendering of vascular and osseous information during rotational angiography. *Am J Neuroradiol* 2004;**25**:571–3.

20. Thron A, Voigt K. Rotational cerebral angiography: procedure and value. *Am J Neuroradiol* 1983;**4**:289–91.

21. Schueler BA, Kallmes DF, Cloft HJ. 3d cerebral angiography: Radiation dose comparison with digital subtraction angiography. *Am J Neuroradiol* 2005;**26**:1898–901.

22. Beck J, Rohde S, Berkefeld J, Seifert V, Raabe A. Size and location of ruptured and unruptured intracranial aneurysms measured by 3-dimensional rotational angiography. *Surg Neurol* 2006;**65**: 18–25; discussion 25–17.

23. Raabe A, Beck J, Rohde S, Berkefeld J, Seifert V. Three-dimensional rotational angiography guidance for aneurysm surgery. *J Neurosurg* 2006;**105**:406–11.

24. Lauriola W, Nardella M, Strizzi V, Cali A, D'Angelo V, Florio F. 3D angiography in the evaluation of intracranial aneurysms before and after treatment. Initial experience. *Radiol Med* 2005;**109**:98–107.

25. Racadio JM, Fricke BL, Jones BV, Donnelly LF. Three-dimensional rotational angiography of neurovascular lesions in pediatric patients. *Am J Roentgenol* 2006;**186**:75–84.

26. Hoit DA, Malek AM. Three-dimensional rotational angiographic detection of in-stent stenosis in wide-necked aneurysms treated with a self-expanding intracranial stent. *Neurosurgery* 2005;**57**:1228–36; discussion 1228–36.

27. Searle MM, Hoff L. Bedrest after elective cardiac catheterisation. *Professional Nurse* 2000;**15**:588–91.

28. Lim R, Anderson H, Walters MI, Kaye GC, Norell MS, Caplin JL. Femoral complications and bed rest duration after coronary arteriography. *Am J Cardiol* 1997;**80**:222–3.

29. Lasic Z, Nikolsky E, Kesanakurthy S, Dangas G. Vascular closure devices: A review of their use after invasive procedures. *Am J Cardiovasc Drugs* 2005;**5**:185–200.

30. Nikolsky E, Mehran R, Halkin A, *et al.* Vascular complications associated with arteriotomy closure devices in patients undergoing percutaneous coronary procedures: a meta-analysis.[see comment]. *J Am Coll Cardiol* 2004;**44**:1200–9.

31. Solomon R, Biguori C, Bettmann M. Selection of contrast media. *Kidney Int – Suppl* 2006:S39–S45.

32. Matthai WH, Jr., Kussmaul WG, 3rd, Krol J, Goin JE, Schwartz JS, Hirshfeld JW, Jr. A comparison of low- with high-osmolality contrast agents in cardiac angiography. Identification of criteria for selective use. *Circulation* 1994;**89**:291–301.

33. Bettmann MA. Guidelines for use of low-osmolality contrast agents. *Radiology* 1989;**172**:901–3.

34. Matthai WH, Jr., Hirshfeld JW, Jr. Choice of contrast agents for cardiac angiography: Review and recommendations based on clinically important distinctions. *Cathet Cardiovasc Diagn* 1991;**22**:278–89.

35. Hagan JB. Anaphylactoid and adverse reactions to radiocontrast agents. *Immunol Allergy Clini N Am* **24**:507–19.

36. Juergens CP, Khaing AM, McIntyre GJ, *et al.* Adverse reactions of low osmolar non-ionic and ionic contrast media when used together or separately during percutaneous coronary intervention. *Heart, Lung Circ* 2005;**14**:172–7.

37. Wittbrodt ET, Spinler SA. Prevention of anaphylactoid reactions in high-risk patients receiving radiographic contrast media. *Annals of Pharmacotherapy.* 1994;**28**:236–41.

38. Marshall GD, Jr., Lieberman PL. Comparison of three pretreatment protocols to prevent anaphylactoid reactions to radiocontrast media. *Ann Allergy* 1991;**67**:70–4.

39. Morcos SK, Thomsen HS, Webb JA, Contrast Media Safety Committee of the European Society of Urogenital R. Prevention of generalized reactions to contrast media: a consensus report and guidelines. *Eur Radiol* 2001;**11**:1720–8

40. Freed KS, Leder RA, Alexander C, DeLong DM, Kliewer MA. Breakthrough adverse reactions to low-osmolar contrast media after steroid premedication.[see comment]. *Am J Roentgenol* 2001;**176**:1389–92.

41. Thomsen HS, Morcos SK, Contrast Media Safety Committee of European Society of Urogenital R. Management of acute adverse reactions to contrast media. *Eur Radiol* 2004;**14**:476–81.

42. Munechika H, Hiramatsu Y, Kudo S, *et al.* Delayed adverse reactions to nonionic contrast medium (iohexol) in iv use: Multicentric study. *Acad Radiol* 2002;**9** Suppl 1:S69–71.

43. Murphy SW, Barrett BJ, Parfrey PS. Contrast nephropathy. *J Am Soc Nephrol* 2000;**11**:177–82.

44. Thomsen HS, Morcos SK. Contrast media and the kidney: European society of urogenital radiology (esur) guidelines. *Br J Radiol* 2003;**76**:513–18.

45. Nash K, Hafeez A, Hou S. Hospital-acquired renal insufficiency. *Am J Kidney Dis* 2002;**39**:930–6.

46. McCullough PA, Wolyn R, Rocher LL, Levin RN, O'Neill WW. Acute renal failure after coronary intervention: Incidence, risk factors, and relationship to mortality. *Am J Med* 1997;**103**: 368–75.

47. Thomsen HS, Morcos SK, Members of Contrast Media Safety Committee of European Society of Urogenital R. In which patients should serum creatinine be measured before iodinated contrast medium administration? *Eur Radiol* 2005;**15**:749–54.

48. Rich MW, Crecelius CA. Incidence, risk factors, and clinical course of acute renal insufficiency after cardiac catheterization in patients 70 years of age or older. A prospective study. *Arch Intern Med* 1990;**150**:1237–42.

49. Rudnick MR, Berns JS, Cohen RM, Goldfarb S. Contrast media-associated nephrotoxicity. *Semin Nephrol* 1997;**17**:15–26.

50. Parfrey PS, Griffiths SM, Barrett BJ, *et al.* Contrast material-induced renal failure in patients with diabetes mellitus, renal insufficiency, or both. A prospective controlled study. [see comment]. *N Engl J Med* 1989;**320**:143–9.

51. Laskey WK, Jenkins C, Selzer F, *et al.* Volume-to-creatinine clearance ratio: a pharmacokinetically based risk factor for prediction of early creatinine increase after percutaneous coronary

intervention. *J Am Coll Cardiol* 2007;**50**:584–90.

52. Thomsen HS, Morcos SK. Contrast-medium-induced nephropathy: is there a new consensus? A review of published guidelines. *Eur Radiol* 2006;**16**:1835–40.

53. Benko A, Fraser-Hill M, Magner P, *et al.* Canadian Association of R. Canadian association of radiologists: Consensus guidelines for the prevention of contrast-induced nephropathy. *Can Assoc Radiol J* 2007;**58**:79–87.

54. Pannu N, Wiebe N, Tonelli M; for the Alberta Kidney Disease Network. Prophylaxis strategies for contrast-induced nephropathy. *J Am Med Assoc* 2006;**295**:2765–79.

55. Solomon R, Deray G, Consensus Panel for CIN. How to prevent contrast-induced nephropathy and manage risk patients: practical recommendations. *Kidney Int – Suppl* 2006:S51–3.

56. Morcos SK, Thomsen HS, Webb JA. Contrast-media-induced nephrotoxicity: a consensus report. Contrast media safety committee, European Society of Urogenital Radiology (esur).[see comment]. *Eur Radiol* 1999;**9**:1602–13.

57. Solomon R, Werner C, Mann D, D'Elia J, Silva P. Effects of saline, mannitol, and furosemide to prevent acute decreases in renal function induced by radiocontrast agents.[see comment]. *N Engl J Med* 1994;**331**:1416–20.

58. Mueller C, Buerkle G, Buettner HJ, *et al.* Prevention of contrast media-associated nephropathy: Randomized comparison of 2 hydration regimens in 1620 patients undergoing coronary angioplasty.[see comment]. *Archi Intern Med* 2002;**162**:329–36.

59. Merten GJ, Burgess WP, Gray LV, *et al.* Prevention of contrast-induced nephropathy with sodium bicarbonate: a randomized controlled trial.[see comment]. *JAMA* 2004;**291**:2328–34.

60. Ozcan EE, Guneri S, Akdeniz B, *et al.* Sodium bicarbonate, n-acetylcysteine, and saline for prevention of radiocontrast-induced nephropathy. A comparison of 3 regimens for protecting contrast-induced nephropathy in patients undergoing coronary procedures. A single-center prospective controlled trial. *Am Heart J* 2007;**154**:539–44.

61. Masuda M, Yamada T, Mine T, *et al.* Comparison of usefulness of sodium bicarbonate versus sodium chloride to prevent contrast-induced nephropathy in patients undergoing an emergent coronary procedure. *Am J Cardiol* 2007;**100**:781–6.

62. Solomon R, Dumouchel W. Contrast media and nephropathy: Findings from systematic analysis and food and drug administration reports of adverse effects. *Investi Radiol* 2006;**41**:651–60.

63. McCullough PA, Bertrand ME, Brinker JA, Stacul F. A meta-analysis of the renal safety of isosmolar iodixanol compared with low-osmolar contrast media.[see comment]. *J Am Coll Cardiol* 2006;**48**:692–9.

64. Bagshaw SM, Ghali WA. Theophylline for prevention of contrast-induced nephropathy: a systematic review and meta-analysis. *Arch Intern Med* 2005;**165**:1087–93.

65. Zagler A, Azadpour M, Mercado C, Hennekens CH. N-acetylcysteine and contrast-induced nephropathy: a meta-analysis of 13 randomized trials. *Am Heart J* 2006;**151**:140–5.

66. Lewis J, Salem MM, Chertow GM, *et al.* Atrial natriuretic factor in oliguric acute renal failure. Anaritide acute renal failure study group.[see comment]. *Am J Kidney Dis* 2000;**36**:767–74.

67. Abizaid AS, Clark CE, Mintz GS, *et al.* Effects of dopamine and aminophylline on contrast-induced acute renal failure after coronary angioplasty in patients with preexisting renal insufficiency. *Am J Cardiol* **83**:260–3.

68. Corriere MA, Guzman RJ. True and false aneurysms of the femoral artery. *Semin Vasc Surg* 2005;**18**:216–23.

69. Demirbas O, Batyraliev T, Eksi Z, Pershukov I. Femoral pseudoaneurysm due to diagnostic or interventional angiographic procedures. *Angiology* 2005;**56**:553–6.

70. Imsand D, Hayoz D. Current treatment options of femoral pseudoaneurysms. *Vasa* 2007;**36**:91–5.

71. Kablak-Ziembicka A, Przewlocki T, Plazak W, *et al.* Treatment options for post-catheterisation femoral pseudoaneurysm closure. *Kardiologia Polska* 2005;**62**:229–39.

72. Luedde M, Krumsdorf U, Zehelein J, *et al.* Treatment of iatrogenic femoral pseudoaneurysm by ultrasound-guided compression therapy and thrombin injection. *Angiology* 2007;**58**:435–9.

73. Tisi PV, Callam MJ. Surgery versus non-surgical treatment for femoral pseudoaneurysms. *Cochrane Database Syst Rev* 2006:CD004981

74. Earnest FT, Forbes G, Sandok BA, *et al.* Complications of cerebral angiography: prospective assessment of risk. *Am J Roentgenol* 1984;**142**:247–53.

75. Dion JE, Gates PC, Fox AJ, Barnett HJ, Blom RJ. Clinical events following neuroangiography: a prospective study. *Stroke* 1987;**18**:997–1004.

76. Grzyska U, Freitag J, Zeumer H. Selective cerebral intraarterial dsa. Complication rate and control of risk factors. *Neuroradiology* 1990;**32**:296–9.

77. Johnston DC, Chapman KM, Goldstein LB. Low rate of complications of cerebral angiography in routine clinical practice. *Neurology* 2001;**57**:2012–14.

78. Kaufmann TJ, Huston J, 3rd, Mandrekar JN, Schleck CD, Thielen KR, Kallmes DF. Complications of diagnostic cerebral angiography: evaluation of 19,826 consecutive patients. *Radiology* 2007;**243**:812–19.

79. Komiyama M, Yamanaka K, Nishikawa M, Izumi T. Prospective analysis of complications of catheter cerebral angiography in the digital subtraction angiography and magnetic resonance era. *Neurol Med-Chir* 1998;**38**:534–9; discussion 539–40.

80. Leow K, Murie JA. Cerebral angiography for cerebrovascular disease: The risks. *Br J Surg* 1988;**75**:428–30.

81. Mani RL, Eisenberg RL, McDonald EJ, Jr., Pollock JA, Mani JR. Complications of catheter cerebral arteriography: analysis of 5,000 procedures. I. Criteria and incidence. *Am J Roentgenol* 1978;**131**:861–5.

82. Mani RL, Eisenberg RL. Complications of catheter cerebral arteriography: Analysis of 5,000 procedures. II. Relation of complication rates to clinical and arteriographic diagnoses. *Am J Roentgenol* 1978;**131**:867–9.

83. Mani RL, Eisenberg RL. Complications of catheter cerebral arteriography: analysis of 5,000 procedures. III. Assessment of arteries injected, contrast medium used, duration of procedure, and age of patient. *Am J Roentgenol* 1978;**131**:871–4.

84. McIvor J, Steiner TJ, Perkin GD, Greenhalgh RM, Rose FC. Neurological morbidity of arch and carotid

arteriography in cerebrovascular disease. The influence of contrast medium and radiologist. *Br J Radiol* 1987;**60**:117–22.

85. Willinsky RA, Taylor SM, TerBrugge K, Farb RI, Tomlinson G, Montanera W. Neurologic complications of cerebral angiography: Prospective analysis of 2,899 procedures and review of the literature. *Radiology* 2003; **227**:522–8.

86. Heiserman JE, Dean BL, Hodak JA, *et al*. Neurologic complications of cerebral angiography.[see comment]. *Am J Neuroradiol* 1994;**15**:1401–7; discussion 1408–11.

87. Leffers AM, Wagner A. Neurologic complications of cerebral angiography. A retrospective study of complication rate and patient risk factors. *Acta Radiol* 2000;**41**:204–10.

88. Dawkins AA, Evans AL, Wattam J, *et al*. Complications of cerebral angiography: a prospective analysis of 2,924 consecutive procedures. *Neuroradiology* 2007;**49**:753–9.

89. Cloft HJ, Joseph GJ, Dion JE. Risk of cerebral angiography in patients with subarachnoid hemorrhage, cerebral aneurysm, and arteriovenous malformation: a meta-analysis. *Stroke* 1999;**30**:317–20.

90. Heiserman JE. Silent embolism after cerebral angiography – what harm? [comment]. *Lancet.* 1999;**354**:1577–8.

91. Krings T, Willmes K, Becker R, *et al*. Silent microemboli related to diagnostic cerebral angiography: a matter of operator's experience and patient's disease. *Neuroradiology* 2006;**48**:387–93.

92. Bendszus M, Koltzenburg M, Bartsch AJ, *et al*. Heparin and air filters reduce embolic events caused by intra-arterial cerebral angiography: a prospective, randomized trial. *Circulation* 2004;**110**:2210–15.

93. Rudnick MR, Goldfarb S, Wexler L, *et al*. Nephrotoxicity of ionic and nonionic contrast media in 1196 patients: A randomized trial. The iohexol cooperative study. *Kidney Int.* 1995;**47**:254–61.

94. McCullough PA, Bertrand ME, Brinker JA, Stacul F. A meta-analysis of the renal safety of isosmolar iodixanol compared with low-osmolar contrast media. *J Am Coll Cardiol* 2006;**48**:692–9.

Pathophysiological and pharmacological treatment of thromboembolic and ischemic complications associated with endovascular procedures

Ameer E. Hassan DO, Steve M. Cordina MD, Haitham H. Hussein MD, Deepak L. Bhatt MD, MPH and Adnan I. Qureshi MD

Introduction

Thromboembolic and ischemic complications are not uncommon sequelae of endovascular procedures. In this chapter, we review the pathophysiology and treatment of those complications. The following aspects are discussed: (1) arterial injury and thrombosis; (2) pharmacological agents used for the prevention and treatment of thromboembolism; (3) thrombogenicity of catheters, contrast agents and implanted devices.

It should be noted that the preventive and therapeutic regimens described are empirically derived.

Pathophysiological features of thrombosis after arterial injury

The intact arterial endothelium provides a protective barrier that separates blood cells and plasma factors from highly thrombogenic elements in the deeper layers of the vessel wall. These subendothelial elements include collagen, von Willebrand factor, and tissue factor (coagulation Factor III or tissue thromboplastin), which is a membrane protein located in fibroblasts and macrophages. After arterial injury exposes blood to subendothelial structures, platelet adhesion and activation occur, accompanied by activation of coagulation factors. The magnitude of the thrombotic response depends on the severity of the injury and the degree of subendothelial exposure.[1]

Platelet adhesion, activation, and aggregation

Damage to the vessel wall and local exposure of the subendothelium trigger platelet adhesion, the first step in the process of hemostasis (Fig. 3.1). Platelets have specific membrane glycoproteins (GPs) that bind to exposed proteins in the subendothelial layers.[2,3] Platelet adhesion is followed by platelet activation, which is mediated by several mechanical and chemical processes. Platelet activation causes morphological changes in the shape of platelets and activation of membrane GP IIb/IIIa receptors.[4] Activated GP IIb/IIIa receptors bind to fibrinogen molecules, which subsequently form bridges between adjacent platelets and facilitate platelet aggregation (Fig. 3.2). Platelet activation also releases adenosine diphosphate (ADP), serotonin, and thromboxane A_2, which trigger the recruitment and activation of surrounding platelets (Fig. 3.3).[5]

Tissue factor-induced activation of thrombin and fibrinogen

Tissue factor, a component of arterial subendothelium and atherosclerotic plaque, is exposed through vascular injury.[6] When exposed to blood, tissue factor binds to coagulation Factors VII and VIIa, resulting in the assembly of a functional tissue factor – Factor VIIa complex and the activation of Factors IX and X. Factor X can be stimulated via this complex or through a cascade of serial activation of Factors VIII, XII, XI, and IX. These steps occur concomitantly with platelet activation. Activated Factor X then converts prothrombin to thrombin. Thrombin hydrolyzes fibrinogen into fibrin monomers, which undergo spontaneous polymerization to form the fibrin clot.

Fibrinolysis of thrombus

A series of proteases in plasma inhibit coagulation and promote fibrinolysis. One of them, antithrombin III (AT III), neutralizes thrombin and Factors IX and X by forming a complex with them.[7] Fibrinolysis represents the major pathway for limitation of clot formation.[8] The endothelium has a major role in the regulation of fibrinolytic activity. The fibrinolytic system contains an inactive precursor proenzyme, plasminogen, which is present in plasma. Plasminogen activators convert plasminogen to the active protease plasmin, which degrades the fibrin in the clot to soluble degradation

Textbook of Interventional Neurology, ed. Adnan I. Qureshi. Published by Cambridge University Press. © Cambridge University Press 2011.

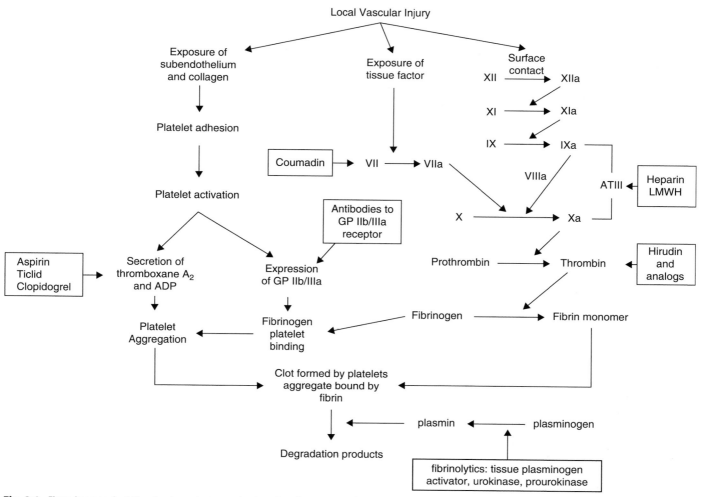

Fig. 3.1. Flow diagram depicting the important steps in thrombus formation and the sites in the cascade that are amenable to therapeutic intervention. Platelet adhesion, activation, and aggregation occurring at the site of arterial injury are mediated by local factors, including thromboxane A_2 (inhibited by aspirin) and ADP (inhibited by ticlopidine and clopidogrel). Concomitantly, thrombin is formed by serial activation of clotting factors via contact with subendothelial tissue factor. Thrombin cleaves fibrinogen into fibrin. Thrombin activation is indirectly blocked by heparin and its analogs. However, after thrombin is clot bound (with fibrin), it is relatively protected from heparin and is effectively blocked only by direct thrombin inhibitors (hirudin and its analogs). The final common pathway in clot formation is the binding of fibrinogen to platelets via platelet GP IIb/IIIa receptors, which is inhibited by antibodies to platelet GP IIb/IIIa receptors.

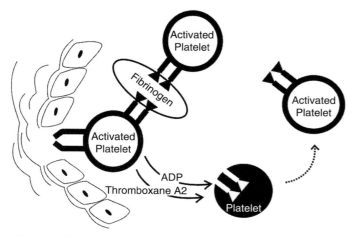

Fig. 3.2. Adhesion of platelets to the injured vessel wall. Activation of platelets leads to the expression of platelet GP IIb/IIIa receptors, which bind to fibrinogen to form bridges between platelets.

products.[9] Two immunologically distinct physiological plasminogen activators, i.e., tissue-type plasminogen activator (t-PA) and urokinase-type plasminogen activator, have been identified. Plasminogen activators are regulated by plasma plasminogen activator inhibitors (PAIs) (mainly PAI-1) and active plasmin is regulated in plasma by [alpha]$_2$-antiplasmin.[8,10] A delicate balance between activation and inhibition of fibrinolysis exists in the circulation.

Duration of procoagulant activity after arterial injury

An important determinant of the duration of prophylactic and treatment regimens is the persistence of the procoagulant activity of the injured vessel wall. The initial response to arterial injury involves platelet adhesion, aggregation, and activation, as well as activation of the coagulation system.

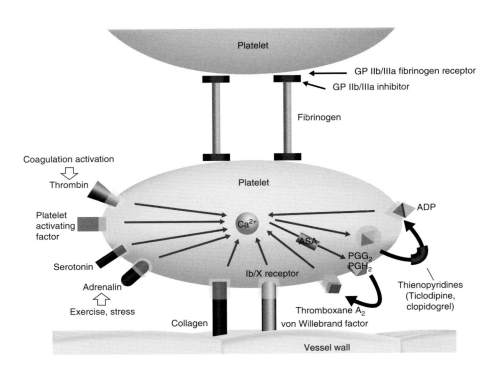

Fig. 3.3. Sites of action of the available antiplatelet agents – aspirin (ASA), thienopyridines, glycoprotein IIb/IIIa inhibitors.

Subsequent development of thrombus is dependent on platelet and fibrin recruitment which is primarily dependent on local thrombin and tissue factor expression. Local expression of tissue factor and thrombin continues for up to 24 hours after injury.[11,12] The prolonged expression of tissue factor seems to be related to delayed induction of tissue factor messenger ribonucleic acid and protein in the vessel wall in response to injury.[12] The origin of delayed induction of tissue factor is unknown, but it may be mediated by smooth muscle cells in the media or monocytes that are recruited to the exposed subendothelium and readily express tissue factor. Although there is a marked decrease in the thrombin and procoagulant activity of injured blood vessels after the first 24 hours, elevated levels of thrombin are detected for up to 72 hours.[11] The persistent activation of thrombin may contribute to the thrombotic complications observed early after endovascular procedures.[11] Treatment with aspirin reduces this late expression of thrombin, presumably by attenuation of platelet-bound Factor Xa/Va activity.[13]

Re-endothelialization of injured blood vessels

Regrowth of the endothelial cell monolayer abolishes the thrombogenic activity of the injured vascular segment, because of the intrinsic fibrinolytic activity of the endothelium and the covering of thrombogenic subendothelial surfaces.[10] Endothelial cells synthesize and secrete plasminogen activators (the main source of t-PA) and PAIs.[14] Re-endothelialization of the injured arterial wall occurs from areas of intact endothelium[15,16] and is almost complete 2 weeks after arterial injury.[16] However, the regenerated cells have irregular sizes and polygonal shapes and lack the typical alignment in the direction of blood flow. The functional capacity of the endothelium is impaired for almost 4 weeks after injury. The process of endothelial regrowth ceases 6 weeks after injury.[15] Some areas of extensive denudation are not covered with endothelium but instead form a non-thrombogenic "pseudoendothelium" composed of phenotypically altered smooth muscle cells.[15] Endothelialization may require at least 4 weeks to cover foreign surfaces, such as metallic stents.[17] Stents become completely covered with endothelium because their open lattice configuration allows surviving patches of endothelium to spread in a multicentric approach.[18] In contrast, aneurysm coil surfaces are mainly covered with a thin cell layer with fibrous tissue within the coil meshwork. Endothelialization over coil surfaces is often incomplete.[19]

Pharmacological features of agents used for thrombosis prophylaxis

Thrombosis can be prevented by inhibiting two major steps, i.e., platelet adhesion and aggregation and tissue factor-induced activation of thrombin and fibrinogen. The information provided in this section is derived mainly from studies of either ischemic stroke or coronary intervention. Because the use of most of these agents in neurointerventional procedures is new, data for that patient population are limited. The information from ischemic stroke trials can be used primarily to define the side-effect profiles of various pharmacological agents without allowing definitive statements regarding efficacy. Interventional cardiology literature, however, allows conclusions on drug efficacy as well. We think that the similarities between some coronary and neurointerventional procedures support the extrapolation of efficacy results.

Inhibition of platelet adhesion and aggregation

Antiplatelet therapy is used extensively for prophylaxis of thromboembolic events in the acute and chronic periods after endovascular procedures (Table 3.1). Antiplatelet activity occurs primarily via inhibition of thromboxane A_2 or ADP release or via blockade of GP IIb/IIIa receptors.

Aspirin

Aspirin is the most extensively used platelet inhibitor for both coronary and cerebrovascular diseases. Aspirin exerts its antiplatelet activity via irreversible inhibition of platelet cyclooxygenase-1 and production of thromboxane A_2.[20,21] Single oral doses of 5 to 100 mg of aspirin result in dose-dependent inhibition of platelet cyclooxygenase activity, with 100 mg almost completely suppressing thromboxane A_2 biosynthesis.[22] This inhibitory effect is rapid and, because the platelets cannot synthesize new protein, the aspirin-induced defect is permanent (lasting the 8–10 day lifespan of the platelets). With respect to the most effective dose of aspirin for stroke prevention, direct comparisons revealed no differences in efficacy between doses of 300 and 1200 mg daily,[23] or between doses of 30 and 283 mg daily,[24] although small differences might not have been detected because of the limited sample sizes. Some authors have argued that higher doses are more effective[25] because those doses might influence interactions between platelets and endothelia that might help prevent or limit thrombus formation.[26] The systematic overview of the Antiplatelet Trialists' Collaboration provides unequivocal evidence that aspirin therapy reduces by one-half the odds of arterial or graft occlusion among patients who have undergone a range of vascular operations, including coronary artery or peripheral vessel surgery and angioplasty.[27] Individuals who regularly take aspirin have increased risk of serious gastrointestinal complications resulting in hospitalization or death, such as bleeding, perforation, or other adverse events.[28] Variables that influence the overall incidence of gastrointestinal side effects during prolonged aspirin therapy include the dose and dosing interval, the duration of treatment, and the type of formulation used (plain versus enteric coated). In the antiplatelet trials, there was a statistically non-significant 20% increase in the risk of hemorrhagic stroke associated with the use of aspirin.[27]

Aspirin is a weak platelet inhibitor and does not inhibit platelet aggregation by thromboxane A_2-independent pathways or affect platelet adhesion or secretion.[21] Therefore, aspirin has no effect on thrombin, which is thought to play a major role in acute ischemic syndromes. Aspirin, unlike the newer antiplatelet agents, does not affect platelet secretion and thus has no effect on local accumulation of platelet-derived mitogenic factors.[21] These mitogenic factors promote cellular proliferation and lead to restenosis and accelerated atherosclerosis after angioplasty. Another limitation of aspirin therapy is that individual responses to aspirin vary considerably. "Aspirin resistance" is a controversial term that refers to the occurrence of stroke in a patient who is being treated with aspirin. One study classified the reason for admission in 5.7% of patients consecutively admitted for ischemic stroke as failure to respond to aspirin therapy, since the patients were on aspirin at the time of the new ischemic stroke. The group studied the characteristics and risk factors and suggested that individuals with greater risk factors for occlusive disease might benefit less from aspirin.[29] Another group tested whether "aspirin resistance" might develop over time and looked for aspirin's effects on platelet aggregation.[30] Maximal effect of aspirin was tested and increased doses were given to obtain maximal inhibition. Even at 1300 mg per day, about 8% of patients showed aspirin resistance. One study tested 129 consecutive patients with stroke, transient ischemic attack (TIA) or vascular cognitive impairment and assessed relationships between aspirin resistance and thromboembolic events using platelet function assay. They found that aspirin resistance determined by PFA-100 did not predict new thrombotic events in patients with stable ischemic cerebrovascular disease.[31]

Clopidogrel

Clopidogrel is a thienopyridine derivative that inhibits platelet aggregation. The agent is administered orally and converted into a metabolite in the liver. The active metabolites are excreted by the kidneys. Clopidogrel inhibits the binding of ADP to its platelet receptor. This ADP receptor blockade leads to direct inhibition of fibrinogen binding to the GP IIb/IIIa complex. The inhibition of platelet aggregation is concentration dependent. Adequate inhibition with clopidogrel (75 mg, daily) requires 2 to 3 days after the initiation of therapy.[32] Maximal inhibition occurs after 4 to 7 days. The antiplatelet action is irreversible and lasts for 7 to 10 days. Concomitant aspirin use results in synergistic inhibition of platelet aggregation, presumably because of potentiation of the effect of aspirin on collagen-induced platelet aggregation.[33] Comparative studies of ticlopidine (first generation thienopyridine) and clopidogrel show similar efficacy, but better safety and tolerability with clopidogrel.[34]

A major side effect of ticlopidine and clopidogrel is bleeding. Among patients with ischemic stroke enrolled in the Ticlopidine Aspirin Stroke Study and the Canadian American Ticlopidine Study, the rates of major hemorrhage and minor bleeding with ticlopidine were 0.2 to 0.5% and 6.5 to 9%, respectively.[35–37] In the Clopidogrel versus Aspirin in Patients at Risk for Ischemic Events study, the frequency of major bleeding associated with clopidogrel was 1.4%.[38] In comparison, the rate of major bleeding associated with aspirin in the Ticlopidine Aspirin Stroke Study and the Clopidogrel versus Aspirin in Patients at Risk for Ischemic Events study was 1.4 to 1.6%.[35,37,38] Other adverse effects that can occur with ticlopidine are neutropenia, gastrointestinal symptoms, and skin rashes. However, in coronary stent studies, the rates of neutropenia among patients receiving ticlopidine did not differ

Table 3.1. Antiplatelet agents used in endovascular procedures[a]

Agent	Commercial name (Company)	Mechanism of action	Indications in EVP	Dose	Complications	Monitoring	Half-life	Reversal
Abciximab	ReoPro (Eli Lilly & Co., Indianapolis,IN)	Inhibits platelet aggregation by binding to GP IIb/IIIA receptor sites (non-competitive)	Adjunct to PTA and stent placement	0.25 mg/kg IV bolus followed by 10 μm/min infusion for 12 h	Bleeding complications, thrombocytopenia	Not performed as standard CBC 4 h after bolus	10 min, platelet dysfunction for 48 h	Platelet transfusion
Eptifibatide	Integrilin (Cor Therapeutics, South San Francisco, CA)	Inhibits platelet aggregation by preventing binding to GP IIb/IIIa receptor sites (competitive)	Adjunct to PTA and stent placement	135 μg/kg IV bolus followed by 0.5 μg/kg/min infusion for 20–24 h	Bleeding complications	Not performed as standard CBC 4 h after bolus	90–120 min	Platelet transfusion
Aspirin	Ecotrin (SmithKline Beecham Consumer, Pittsburgh, PA), Acuprin (Richwood Pharmaceuticals, Florence, KY)	Inhibits platelet aggregation by blocking thromboxane A_2 production	Used for long-term prevention of post-procedure thromboembolism	325–1300 mg, orally, daily	GI bleeding, gastritis	Bleeding time	Platelet inhibition for 11 d	Platelet transfusion
Ticlopidine hydrochloride	Ticlid (Roche, Nutley, NJ)	Inhibits platelet aggregation by inhibiting ADP-induced platelet-fibrinogen interaction	Used for long-term prevention of post-procedure thromboembolism	250 mg, orally, twice daily	Neutropenia, bleeding complications, maculopapular rash, diarrhea, GI bleeding, liver enzyme elevations	Not performed as CBC standard every 2 weeks for the first 3 months	12.6 h, platelet inhibition for 11 d	Platelet transfusion, IV methyl prednisolone, 20 mg
Clopidogrel	Plavix (Roche, Nutley, NJ)	Inhibits platelet aggregation by inhibiting ADP-induced platelet-fibrinogen interaction	Used for long-term prevention of post-procedure thromboembolism	75 mg, orally, daily	Bleeding	Not performed as standard	Platelet inhibition for 11 d	Platelet transfusion IV methyl prednisolone 20 mg
Dipyridamole USP	Persantine (Boehringer Ingelheim, Gaithersburg, MD)	Inhibits platelet adhesion	Not defined	75–100 mg, four times per day	Dizziness, abdominal distress, rash	Not required	α, 40 min; β, 10 h	Platelet transfusion

[a]ADP, adenosine diphosphate; EVP, endovascular procedures; GI, gastrointestinal; GP, glycoprotein; IV, intravenous; PTA, percutaneous transluminal angioplasty; USP, United States Pharmacopeia; min, minutes; h, hours; d, days; CBC, complete blood count.

from those of the control group.[39] This was attributed to the short duration of treatment (1 mo) in these studies. In the Clopidogrel versus Aspirin in Patients at Risk for Ischemic Events study, the rate of neutropenia associated with clopidogrel (0.1%) was similar to that for aspirin.[38] Diarrhea or nausea may be observed in the first 2 or 3 weeks after treatment and is often relieved when the medication is taken with meals. Rashes may rarely develop with ticlopidine administration, requiring cessation of treatment and possibly initiation of clopidogrel therapy. Two important interactions of thienopyridines, with cimetidine (which reduces the clearance) and with carbamazepine or phenytoin (the antiepileptic drug dose may require reduction), have been observed.

Prasugrel

Prasugrel is a novel thienopyridine that was shown in a recent trial to be superior to clopidogrel in acute coronary syndrome patients undergoing percutaneous coronary intervention. It was, however, associated with more fatal bleeding. It also caused more intracranial bleeding in the small subgroup of patients with prior stroke or TIA.[40–42]

Ticagrelor

Ticagrelor is an oral, reversible, direct-acting inhibitor of the adenosine diphosphate receptor P2Y12 that has a more rapid onset and more pronounced platelet inhibition than clopidogrel.[43,44] Wallentin et al.[45] compared outcomes in ticagrelor versus clopidogrel use in patients with acute coronary syndromes. At 12 months, the primary end point of the study – a composite of death from vascular causes, myocardial infarction, or stroke – had occurred in 9.8% of patients receiving ticagrelor as compared with 11.7% of those receiving clopidogrel. There was no significant difference in the rates of major bleeding between the ticagrelor and clopidogrel groups, but ticagrelor was associated with a higher rate of major bleeding not related to coronary-artery bypass grafting (4.5% vs. 3.8%, $P = 0.03$), including more instances of fatal intracranial bleeding and fewer instances of fatal bleeding of other types.

Platelet GP IIb/IIIa receptor-specific antibodies

Unlike aspirin, the class of drugs that inhibit GP IIb/IIIa receptors prevent the binding of fibrinogen to these receptors, thereby inhibiting platelet aggregation irrespective of the metabolic pathway responsible for the initiation of platelet aggregation. A murine monoclonal antibody directed against the GP IIb/IIIa receptor inhibits the binding of fibrinogen to platelets and thus inhibits platelet aggregation.[46] A fragment of the antibody was subsequently attached to human immunoglobulin to form a nonimmunogenic compound, abciximab (ReoPro; Eli Lilly and Company, Indianapolis, IN). This compound has undergone extensive clinical evaluation[47] and was approved by the United States Food and Drug Administration for clinical use. Intravenously administered abciximab is a short-acting agent with a half-life of 10 minutes, but its effects on platelets last for almost 48 hours. Eptifibatide (Integrilin; Cor Therapeutics, South San Francisco, CA), a cyclic peptide that may be a more specific inhibitor of GP IIb/IIIa receptors, has also undergone extensive clinical evaluation. Non-peptide inhibitors of GP IIb/IIIa receptors, i.e., tirofiban (Merck, West Point, PA), have been used in interventional neurology and are more selective. Tirofiban, like eptifibatide, the other RGD-based synthetic glycoprotein IIb/IIIa receptor antagonist, is highly selective for the glycoprotein IIb/IIIa integrin resulting in the competitive inhibition of fibrinogen and von Willebrand mediated platelet aggregation by reversibly occupying the glycoprotein IIb/IIIa receptor binding site. This represents an important difference in the mechanism of action of tirofiban when compared to abciximab.[48] Tirofiban has a plasma half-life of approximately 2 hours, compared to the half-life of abciximab that is only 10–30 minutes.[49] Tirofiban and eptifibatide require dose correction for renal insufficiency and are contraindicated in renal failure patients.[50] Orally active inhibitors of GP IIb/IIIa receptors have also been developed, but were found to be associated with excess mortality.[51]

In trials with human subjects, abciximab, eptifibatide, and tirofiban, all of which are administered parenterally, have been demonstrated to be potent inhibitors of platelet aggregation, with acceptable safety profiles. Six randomized, placebo-controlled trials of platelet GP IIb/IIIa inhibitors among patients who underwent coronary balloon angioplasty and atherectomy have been reported. In these trials, patients received aspirin, and reductions in the rates of myocardial infarctions (MIs) were observed. Four trials tested abciximab and demonstrated a significant decrease (approximately 50%) in all cardiac events at 30 days.[52–55] The other two trials tested the GP IIb/IIIa inhibitors eptifibatide and tirofiban and demonstrated strong positive but non-significant trends.[56,57] The TARGET (Tirofiban and ReoPro Give Similar Efficacy Outcomes Trial) study was intended to demonstrate the non-inferiority of tirofiban compared to abciximab, although the study findings demonstrated that tirofiban offered less protection from major ischemic events.[58] The optimal duration of treatment with drugs that inhibit GP IIb/IIIa receptors has not been determined. The benefit of abciximab was most pronounced in the Evaluation of 7E3 for Prevention of Ischemic Complications trial[53] in which abciximab administration was initiated 1 hour before the procedure and continued for 12 hours; this is currently the most accepted administration regimen.

The principal and most serious adverse effect of drugs that inhibit GP IIb/IIIa receptors is bleeding. In the Evaluation of 7E3 for Prevention of Ischemic Complications trial, the rate of major bleeding was two times higher for the abciximab-treated group than for the placebo-treated group.[53] Patients who were older and those with lower body weight seemed to be at increased risk.[59] Bleeding may be minimized with lower doses of the drug and shorter courses of concomitant heparin therapy, together with early removal of the sheath after the procedure.[60] Thrombocytopenia occurs infrequently with abciximab, and even less often with eptifibatide or tirofiban.[55]

von Willebrand factor (vWF)

The two mediators of primary hemostasis are vWF and platelets. Platelet activation and aggregation is mediated by vWF when platelets adhere to exposed vascular subendothelial collagen. The simultaneous exposure of tissue factor leads to initiation of the process of secondary hemostasis; i.e., activation of the procoagulant cascade and eventual formation of a hemostatic fibrin clot.[61] This interaction between vWF and platelets is mediated via the A1 or C3 domain of the vWF. Under the high shear force conditions that are encountered in the arterial circulation, vWF is activated via a physical deformation which exposes its A1 domain and enables its binding to the platelet glycoprotein Ib receptor. It also binds to exposed collagen directly via its A3 domain. During ischemic stress, platelets are exposed to subendothelial matrix proteins. These increase platelet adhesion to vessel walls by stimulating binding of collagens to the GP VI receptor on platelets.[62,63]

Selective GP Ib receptor inhibition

There is experimental evidence that selective inhibition of the GP Ib receptor has a different impact on outcome and risk of ICH as compared with GP IIb/IIIa inhibition.[64] This is on the basis of the molecular properties of vWF. Its A1 domain gets exposed solely under high shear conditions and then binds to the GP Ib platelet receptor, causing platelet aggregation to proceed. There is thus a more precise target of action as compared with irreversible platelet inhibition, as seen under the effect of GP IIb/IIIa inhibitors. GP Ib receptor inhibition leads to an effective vWF-mediated activation pathway inhibition.

Kleinschnitz et al.[64] found that selective GP Ib and VI monoclonal inhibition in a mouse model which then subsequently underwent a temporary total middle cerebral artery occlusion led to decreased infarct volume and absence of any hemorrhagic transformation of the stroke. This was in contrast to the hemorrhagic transformations which one can see with final common pathway inhibition. The selective inhibition of both GP Ib and VI was tested both pre- and post-occlusion and benefit was shown both times. This holds promise for possible antiplatelet therapy applications in stroke prevention and treatment.

vWF antagonists

High vWF levels have been also implicated in increased risk of a first ischemic stroke.[65] This further reinforces the need to develop a drug that targets the vWF component of the clotting process. A number of anti-vWF compounds are already available, as monoclonal antibodies or as aptamers, for example the aptamer ARC 1779.

Aptamers are nucleic acid species that have been engineered through repeated rounds of in vitro selection until they bind to pre-determined molecular targets. The usefulness of these compounds lies in their molecular specificity, much like antibodies. The advantage of aptamers over antibodies is that they are easily produced and elicit little to no immunogenic response in live organisms.

ARC 1779 binds competitively to the A1 domain of activated vWF, with a resultant inhibition of interaction with the GP Ib receptor and thus of all vWF-platelet activation pathways. This inhibition is selective in that it is clinically evident only during periods of platelet activation due to pathological thrombosis. A recent evaluation of this compound in humans showed effective vWF and platelet inhibition which was time-limited, dose-dependent and well tolerated.[66]

Inhibition of tissue factor-induced activation of thrombin and fibrinogen

Activation of thrombin can be inhibited by any of the following approaches: with direct thrombin inhibitors such as hirudin and its analogs hirulog and hirugen, with AT III-dependent inhibitors such as standard heparin and low-molecular weight heparin (LMWH) preparations, or with indirect inhibitors such as warfarin (Table 3.2).

Heparin

Heparin is a glycosaminoglycan, which is administered intravenously and is composed of a mixture of polysaccharides, each weighing between 3000 and 40 000 daltons. The most commonly accepted actions of heparin are activation and modulation of AT III activity, which result in thrombin neutralization and inactivation of Factors IXa, Xa, XIa, and XIIa.[67] Indirect actions that contribute to the anticoagulant effects of heparin include the specific inhibition of thrombin by heparin Cofactor II and the restoration of endothelial surface electronegativity. Heparin also has antiplatelet effects in vivo, by preventing thrombin-induced platelet aggregation and inhibiting von Willebrand factor.[68] The anticoagulant effects of heparin are immediate after injection. Its half-life is approximately 1.5 hours.

The two major complications associated with heparin treatment, are, hemorrhage and idiosyncratic, immunologically induced thrombocytopenia,[69] which is associated with elevated platelet immunoglobulin G levels or a heparin-dependent platelet aggregating factor.[70] Thrombocytopenia is observed 3 to 15 days after treatment initiation and usually resolves within 4 days after treatment cessation. In 1979, Gruntzig et al.[71] empirically used heparin with an antiplatelet agent during coronary balloon angioplasty. Because various degrees of resistance to heparin can be encountered and clinical effectiveness is correlated with the magnitude of anticoagulation, regular monitoring is required to adjust the infusion rate. Measurement of the activated coagulation time (ACT) is the preferred

Table 3.2. Anticoagulant agents used in endovascular procedures[a]

Agent	Commercial Name (Company)	Mechanism of action	Indications in EVP	Dose	Complications	Monitoring	Half-life	Reversal
Heparin sodium	Heparin (Wyeth-Ayerst, Philadelphia, PA)	Inhibits thrombosis by preventing Factor X activation	Adjunct to most interventional procedures	70–100 U/kg IV bolus during procedures, post-procedure 18 U/kg/h and titrated	Bleeding, thrombocytopenia	ACT of 250–350 s, monitored every hour during procedure; APTT 1.5–2.5 × control, monitored every 6 h	90 min	Protamine sulfate, 1 mg for 100 units (not to exceed 50 mg total)
Ardeparin sodium	Normiflo (Wyeth-Ayerst, Philadelphia, PA)	Inhibits thrombosis by inactivating Factor Xa	Not defined	50 U/kg twice daily SC for venous thromboembolism	Bleeding, thrombocytopenia	No monitoring required	3.3 h	Protamine sulfate, 1 mg for 100 U ardeparin not to exceed 50 mg total)
Enoxaparin sodium	Lovenox (Rhone-Poulenc Rorer, Collegeville, PA)	Inhibits thrombosis by inactivating Factor Xa	Not defined	1 mg/kg twice daily SC	Bleeding, liver enzyme elevations	No monitoring required	4.5 h	Protamine sulfate, 1 mg for 1 mg (not to exceed 50 mg total)
Warfarin sodium	Coumadin (DuPont Pharmaceuticals, Wilmington, DE)	Inhibits formation of vitamin K-dependent clotting factors (Factors II, VII, IX, and X)	Used for long-term prevention of post-procedure thromboembolism	Usual range, 5–15 mg, orally, daily	Bleeding complications, hypersensitivity, adverse drug interactions (phenytoin, prednisone, phenobarbital)	PT (or INR) 2–3 times control values	35 h	IM vitamin K, fresh frozen plasma

[a]ACT, activated clotting time; APTT, activated partial thromboplastin time; EVP, endovascular procedures; IM, intramuscular; INR, international normalized ratio; IV, intravenous; PT, prothrombin time; SC, subcutaneously; U, units; s, seconds; h, hours.

method for evaluation of responses to heparin, because the ACT demonstrates a linear heparin dose–response curve, even at the higher doses used during interventional procedures.[72] In contrast, the activated partial thromboplastin time demonstrates a logarithmic response and is inaccurate at higher doses. Two commercial systems are currently available for automated measurement of ACT values, i.e., the Medtronic HemoTec ACT (Medtronic HemoTec, Englewood, CO) and Hemochron (International Technidyne, Edison, NJ) systems. Ferguson et al.[73] and Narins et al.[74] recently demonstrated the importance of titrating intravenous heparin administration on the basis of ACT values, to ensure adequate antithrombin activity.

Two studies have demonstrated that acute thrombosis immediately after coronary stent placement is correlated with low ACTs.[74,75] Both studies recommended administration of a 10 000-unit bolus dose and repeated bolus doses to achieve an ACT of more than 300 seconds (HemoTec) or 350 seconds (Hemochron) during the procedure. The use of intravenously administered heparin during the post-procedural period is more controversial. Small randomized trials have failed to demonstrate a benefit of continuing intravenous heparin therapy for a 24-hour period after coronary angioplasty.[76,77] In reducing thrombotic complications, furthermore, continuing heparin therapy after the procedure can increase the risk of bleeding from the site of the sheath.[78]

LMWH

LMWH is formed by fractionation of the heterogeneous heparin mixture (M_r 3000–40 000 daltons) to heparin molecules (M_r 4000–5500 daltons). The high-molecular weight heparin chains bind to endothelial cells and a variety of plasma proteins (and possibly to macrophages), where they are rapidly cleaved by a saturable, dose-dependent mechanism[79]. This non-specific binding limits the amount of heparin available to interact with AT III and decreases the anticoagulant effect of heparin. In contrast, LMWH preparations have lower affinity for both endothelial cells and the heparin-binding proteins observed in plasma.[79] The decreased non-specific binding of LMWH explains why LMWH has greater bioavailability at low doses and produces more predictable anticoagulant responses than does standard heparin. In fact, the anticoagulant effects of weight-adjusted doses are so predictable that little or no laboratory monitoring is required. LMWH, unlike standard unfractionated heparin, has little or no effect in global tests of coagulation. It retains the ability to inhibit thrombosis but is associated with fewer bleeding complications.[80] An additional advantage of LMWH is a lower risk of heparin-induced thrombocytopenia.[81] Two preparations, i.e., enoxaparin and dalteparin, have been approved for use in the United States.

Direct inhibitors of thrombin

LMWH overcomes many of the pharmacokinetic limitations of standard heparin. However, both LMWH and standard heparin are relatively ineffective inhibitors of thrombin after its binding to fibrin.[79,83] These indirect thrombin inhibitors are used for standard anticoagulation during cardiac catheterization and neuro-endovascular procedures to prevent procedural thrombotic complications. More recently, direct thrombin inhibitors have been extensively evaluated as anticoagulants during percutaneous coronary interventions (PCI) to reduce the negative peri-procedural clinical events including ischemia, bleeding, and mortality associated with indirect thrombin inhibitors. Bivalirudin (Angiomax®, The Medicines Company, NJ) (previously known as Hirulog®), is a reversible direct thrombin inhibitor that has been shown to have (1) shorter half-life (25 vs. 90 minutes) and a better safety profile,[84] (2) ability to inhibit free- and clot-bound thrombin,[85] (3) avoidance of platelet activation,[86] (4) avoidance of heparin-induced thrombocytopenia (HIT),[87] and (5) a significant reduction of bleeding without a reduction in thrombotic or ischemic endpoints when compared to heparin.[88,89] Due to the above advantages it is replacing heparin and other indirect thrombin inhibitors as the anticoagulant of choice in patients presenting with ACS. In coronary interventions, however, target ACT values are usually higher, and tight ACT control is not as critical as in neuro-endovascular procedures. Bivalirudin's ACT values are more predictable, and therefore rates of cerebral hemorrhagic complications might prove to be lower in future neuroendovascular trials. The optimal ACT value for neuro-endovascular procedures is still a subject of debate. In high-risk procedures such as angioplasty and stenting we use the 300–350 second range.[90] It is clear that avoiding ACT values in excess of 350 is important if hemorrhagic complications are to be avoided.[91]

Warfarin

Among the derivatives of naturally occurring lactones (coumarins), warfarin is the most widely used agent because of its pharmacodynamic profile. Coumarins modulate anticoagulant activity by retarding thrombin generation through inhibition of the vitamin K/epoxide reductase activity-dependent coagulation Factors II, VII, IX, and X. Warfarin is rapidly absorbed from the gastrointestinal tract, with peak plasma values being reached within 90 minutes; its half-life is approximately 40 hours. Because the dose–response relationship for warfarin differs among individuals and many other drugs can interfere with its pharmacokinetics, close monitoring is required. The anticoagulant effects of warfarin appear when the normal clotting factors are cleared from the circulation (within 8 h for Factor VII but only after 72–96 h for Factors II, IX, and X). Although loading doses more rapidly prolong the prothrombin time, the risk of bleeding is enhanced. Therefore, loading doses are not recommended. The thrombogenic potential may be higher at the initiation of therapy, because of the rapid depletion of vitamin K-dependent anticoagulant protein C (half-life, 6 h). The major risk associated with warfarin use is bleeding. Low rates of intracranial hemorrhage (0.3% annually) or other major hemorrhage (1%–2% annually) were documented in seven studies of stroke prevention using warfarin in cases of atrial fibrillation.[92]

Is antiplatelet therapy superior to anticoagulant therapy in endovascular procedures?

This question has been raised with respect to patients undergoing stent placement and angioplasty for treatment of coronary or cerebral vascular diseases. Patients were treated with a variety of anticoagulant agents in initial attempts to reduce the high risk of thrombosis associated with coronary artery angioplasty and stent placement. Between 1989 and 1993, the standard regimens consisted of aspirin, dipyridamole, dextran, heparin, and warfarin. These aggressive regimens produced considerable bleeding complications, especially hematomas at the insertion sites for femoral sheaths, at rates of 3% to 16%.[93] Furthermore, these anticoagulant regimens did not effectively prevent subacute thrombosis; the rate remained approximately 7% and was as high as 28% when stenting was used to salvage angioplasty procedures. Coupled with these disadvantages were prolonged hospital stays.[82,94] The high complication rates and the failure to prevent subacute thrombosis prompted a search for alternative antithrombotic regimens, with the emphasis on antiplatelet agents (aspirin and ticlopidine) rather than anticoagulants. This was supported by evidence suggesting that local platelet deposition and activation are the major factors in thrombosis after angioplasty and stent placement.[95] Several groups in France cooperated to assess regimens that could replace anticoagulants with antiplatelet agents.[96] In 1993 and 1994, when the aspirin dose was lowered, heparin was administered only as a bolus dose and was followed by LMWH, ticlopidine was introduced, and dipyridamole, dextran, and warfarin were discontinued, the rate of bleeding complications was reduced by two-thirds and the frequency of subacute thrombosis was decreased to approximately one-eighth of the previous level (from 10.4% to 1.3%–1.8%). In a study comparing aspirin/warfarin and aspirin/ticlopidine regimens[39] patients were randomized to receive ticlopidine (250 mg, twice daily, for 28 days) plus aspirin (200 mg, daily) or phenprocoumon (for 28 days; target international normalized ratio, 3.5–4.5) plus aspirin (200 mg, daily). Clinical cardiac events (MIs, events requiring emergency coronary intervention, and deaths) were significantly less common for the aspirin/ticlopidine group (1.6% versus 6.2%), as were stent occlusions (0.8% versus 5.4%). Preliminary (but unpublished) data from the larger Stent Antithrombotic Regimen Study were presented at the American Heart Association meeting in 1997.[82] A total of 1652 patients were randomized to receive aspirin plus warfarin, aspirin plus ticlopidine, or aspirin alone. The composite clinical event (death, Q-wave MI, emergency surgery, subacute closure, and repeat angioplasty) rate was significantly lower for the aspirin/ticlopidine group (0.6%) than for the other two groups (both 2.4%). In conclusion, during coronary artery stent deployment, the introduction of antiplatelet therapy (aspirin and ticlopidine), as opposed to anticoagulant therapy, has resulted in fewer bleeding complications, shorter hospital stays, and reduced stent thrombotic closure rates.

Is combination antiplatelet therapy superior to monotherapy?

Because of potential synergistic action, a combination of aspirin and clopidogrel has been evaluated for use for carotid artery stent placement. In one study, a randomized, controlled trial in 47 patients with high-grade carotid artery stenosis (> 70% NASCET [North American Symptomatic Carotid Endarterectomy Trial] criteria), it was shown that dual antiplatelet therapy with clopidogrel and aspirin significantly reduced the 30-day incidence of adverse neurologic outcomes after carotid artery stent placement compared with aspirin and heparin (0 versus 25%; $P = 0.02$). These results were found without an additional increase in bleeding complications.[97] The 30-day 50%–100% restenosis rates were lower in the dual antiplatelet group compared with the aspirin plus heparin group (5% versus 26%; $P = 0.01$). The study was terminated prematurely due to an overall unacceptable level of complications in the aspirin plus heparin group,

favoring clopidogrel and aspirin. The present preprocedural management of patients for percutaneous transluminal angioplasty or stent placement is the administration of aspirin 325 mg/day and clopidogrel 75 mg/day p.o. starting 3 days before the procedure.[90,98] If clopidogrel was not initiated 3 days before the procedure, then a loading-dose of 300 mg is administered. Post-procedural management consists of aspirin 325 mg/day and clopidogrel 75 mg/day, which are prescribed on discharge. Clopidogrel is discontinued 1–3 months for bare metal stents or 3–6 months after discharge for drug-eluting stents, but aspirin is continued indefinitely.[98] Harker et al.[99] observed marked reduction in the deposition of platelets and fibrinogen on the stent surface in a baboon model of arterial thrombosis when clopidogrel was used in combination with aspirin (compared with clopidogrel alone).

Mechanical protection against thromboembolic phenomena

Small case series have reported the efficacy of temporary occlusion of the internal carotid artery distal to the manipulation of ulcerated plaques, to prevent inadvertent embolization in the cerebral circulation. Initial attempts to use this technique during carotid angioplasty required bilateral femoral artery catheterization.[100] Théron et al.[101] simplified this method by designing a triple coaxial catheter that enables temporary carotid artery occlusion, aspiration of debris, and flushing of the working site via the same catheter. In their preliminary study, angioplasty with balloon protection was performed for 136 patients. No embolic complications were observed during angioplasty. Two embolic complications occurred during stent placements performed without balloon protection. A similar approach has been described for aneurysm coiling, in which a balloon is inflated in front of the aneurysm neck during electrothrombosis of coils placed within the aneurysmal sac.[102] Preliminary results suggest that balloon protection prevents the protrusion of coils into the lumen of the main vessels. Theoretically, this approach should prevent embolization from the aneurysmal sac, particularly in aneurysms with wide necks.

Factors affecting thrombogenesis during endovascular procedures
Thrombogenicity of contrast materials

Two major forms of angiographic contrast materials are used during endovascular procedures, low-osmolar contrast agents (LOCAs) and high-osmolar contrast agents. The LOCAs can be divided into ionic and non-ionic agents.[103] The majority of evidence regarding the risk of thrombosis with contrast materials is derived from experiments measuring the rate of clot formation in syringes containing a mixture of contrast agent and blood.[104,105] In vitro studies suggest that all contrast materials reduce platelet aggregation. This platelet inhibitory effect is more pronounced with ionic contrast agents (both high-osmolar contrast agents and LOCAs).[106] Some in vitro evidence suggests that non-ionic contrast agents may be weaker anticoagulants than ionic contrast agents.[104] Ionic contrast agents (both high-osmolar contrast agents and LOCAs) cause greater prolongation of activated partial thromboplastin times than do non-ionic LOCAs.[107] Furthermore, non-ionic contrast agents may promote clotting in catheters and angiography syringes, placing patients at risk of thromboembolism.[104,107–109] Despite in vitro evidence suggesting that contrast agents may influence the thromboembolic risk during endovascular procedures, no definite evidence from clinical studies has been documented to support these observations. Stormorken[107] measured platelet aggregation at the beginning and end of routine cerebral angiographic procedures. The aggregation of platelets was unchanged at the conclusion of the procedures. The inhibitory effect of contrast materials that was previously demonstrated in vitro did not yield clinical effects in that study, presumably because of rapid dilution of contrast agents by blood. In another study, which evaluated 42 patients undergoing intra-arterial administration of contrast agents, platelet function in both arterial and venous blood was not altered, regardless of the agent used.[106] In contrast, Gasperetti et al.[110] observed that the use of non-ionic contrast material during coronary angioplasty was associated with a higher risk of intravascular thrombosis. This difference may become significant if there is prolonged exposure[103] or a large amount of intravascular thrombus.[110,111] During cerebral angiography, there is probably no benefit of ionic contrast material, compared with non-ionic contrast material, because of the limited exposure. For more extensive procedures, such as angioplasty, ionic contrast materials are probably preferable.

Thrombogenicity of angiographic catheters and guidewires

The basic equipment used during endovascular procedures includes angiographic catheters, guidewires, and microcatheters. Several investigators have suggested that vascular catheters used for diagnostic and therapeutic purposes are not biologically inert but may serve as nidi for thrombosis.[112,113] The physiochemical properties of the catheter surface, including physical irregularities[114,115] and the chemical composition[116,117] determine the thrombogenic potential of the catheter. Wilner et al.[118] investigated the thrombogenic properties of various catheters in a dog model, by studying the fibrinopeptide A response (index of thrombin action) and local deposition of fibrin and platelets on the surface of the catheters. Polyurethane and woven Dacron catheters elicited profound elevations in fibrinopeptide A levels and marked deposition of platelets and fibrin on the catheter surface. The least thrombogenic response was observed with thin-walled polyethylene catheters.[119] To measure the effect of catheter coating layers, the thrombogenic properties of polyethylene with and without

lead oxide and Teflon were compared. Thrombogenesis, as measured by the deposition of radiolabeled platelets, was most pronounced for polyethylene with lead oxide after intra-arterial exposure in dogs. Using electron microscopy, Bourassa et al.[114] studied thrombus deposition in various catheters after coronary angiography among human subjects. Polyurethane catheters exhibited more regular external surfaces and a lower tendency for thrombogenesis. The internal surfaces of both polyurethane and polyethylene catheters were smoother than the external surfaces and exhibited fewer thrombi adhering to the surfaces. Heparin is a mucopolysaccharide with a negative electrical charge and decreases the interaction of non-biological surfaces with blood. Preliminary results suggest that the application of heparin[120,121] or a benzalkonium-heparin complex[122] to external catheter surfaces reduces thrombus deposition on the catheter surfaces. Kido et al.[121] suggested that heparin-coated catheters be used when extended angiographic procedures are performed.

Anderson et al.[123] observed that guidewires (both stainless steel and Teflon-coated) also exhibited surface irregularities that retained blood constituents despite aggressive cleaning. Although mechanical irregularities on guidewires may promote platelet aggregation and fibrin deposition, the clinical significance of this observation is not clear. However, repeated use of the same guidewire is discouraged.[124]

Presently, microcatheters and guidewires have hydrophilic coatings. Hydrophilic coatings have reduced the thrombogenicity of polyurethane catheters. Anderson et al.[123] suggested, on the basis of in vitro evidence, that hydrophilic surfaces bind less fibrinogen and fewer platelets than do either non-hydrophilic or heparin-coated catheters, but this has not been supported in other studies.[125] Kallmes et al.[126] compared the thrombogenicity of various microcatheters after short-, medium-, and long-term implantation. The following catheters were evaluated: hydrophilic, FasTracker 18 (Target Therapeutics, Fremont, CA) and Transit (Cordis Endovascular Systems, Miami Lakes, FL); non-hydrophilic, Tracker 18 (Target Therapeutics) and Magic 1.8 (Balt, Montmorency, France). Those authors observed that some hydrophilic coatings diminished thrombogenicity; for example, the hydrophilic FasTracker microcatheter accumulated fewer depositions than did its non-hydrophilic counterpart, the Tracker microcatheter. However, the Transit microcatheter (also hydrophilic) seemed more thrombogenic than the hydrophilic FasTracker microcatheter. The authors concluded that differences in catheter materials may account for differences in thrombogenicity. In addition, they observed that polyvinylchloride was the most thrombogenic of the microcatheter materials evaluated.

Thrombogenicity of vascular coils and stents

When blood first contacts a foreign surface, the sequence of events initiated often ends in blood coagulation and thrombus formation.[127] Initially, a thin layer of platelets and fibrinogen covers the surface of the foreign material. The magnitude of the initial reaction depends on the surface charge, chemical properties, and topographic features of the vascular device and the pattern of blood flow in the vicinity. Both coils and stents are intravascularly implanted devices that invoke thrombogenic responses when placed in vessels.

The coils most commonly used in endovascular procedures are platinum Guglielmi detachable coils.[128] The purpose of the coils is to induce thrombosis at the site of deployment, via electrothrombosis. Electrothrombosis occurs because white and red blood cells, platelets, and fibrinogen are negatively charged. If a positively charged electrode is placed in the bloodstream, it attracts negatively charged blood components, promoting clot formation. The size and weight of the thrombus formed are directly proportional to the coulombs (milliamperes × minutes) of electricity delivered. Platinum is used for electrothrombosis because the positive end does not dissolve, unlike metals with a high dissociation constant. Furthermore, platinum is three to four times more thrombogenic than stainless steel. The platinum coil is delivered by a stainless steel delivery system, which is detached by electrolysis. Numerous experimental and human studies have indicated that the thrombotic reaction induced by electrothrombosis is not complete.[129,130] Therefore, modifications of the coil surface to enhance the thrombogenic potential are being developed.[129] Although the initial thrombotic reaction after coil placement is important for aneurysm obliteration, fresh thrombus in the aneurysmal sac can embolize to distal distributions. Such complications are not uncommon and are discussed later.

Intravascular stents are used to prevent restenosis after percutaneous angioplasty. Three classes of stents are currently available,[131] i.e., self-expanding or spring-loaded stents, which can be constrained to small diameters and then expanded to a predetermined dimension; balloon-expandable stents (e.g., Palmaz stents; Johnson & Johnson, Warren NJ), in which plastic deformation of the metal beyond its elastic limits is used for permanent expansion; and thermal expansion-deployed stents composed of materials that expand from small to large diameters with exposure to heat, such as nitinol (nickel-titanium alloy). In vivo studies have demonstrated that platelets rapidly accumulate on the stent surface after placement.[132] Platelet accumulation is most pronounced when stents are placed within a mechanically injured arterial surface. The thrombogenicity is partly attributable to the 316L stainless steel used in stents. Both platelets and fibrinogen adhere to stainless steel after contact with blood. The surface material and geometric configuration of the stent are other important determinants of thrombosis. In an animal model, thrombosis was related to the number of strut–strut intersections within the stent.[20] Coating the stent surface with polymer material reduced the observed thrombogenicity. Other factors that contribute to stent thrombogenicity are plaque around the stent and the surface area of the stent. A smaller stent surface area is associated with a higher risk of thrombosis.[133] Thermal expansion is associated with a lower risk of platelet adhesion in vitro but not in vivo.[134]

Thrombogenic potential of artificial embolic materials

Many types of embolic materials, including microfibrillar collagen, Gelfoam (Upjohn Co., Kalamazoo, MI) powder, and polyvinyl alcohol, are used in therapeutic embolization of the head and neck. Microfibrillar collagen is a topical hemostatic agent prepared from purified bovine collagen. Gelfoam is available as a powder, with particles ranging from 40 to 60 μm. Vessel occlusion is caused by the emboli and the thrombus that form within and around the particles. The emboli migrate distally, and distal obstruction may be observed for up to 4 months.[135] Polyvinyl alcohol is a sponge-like material that is hardened with formaldehyde[136] and is thrombogenic because of a high friction coefficient.

Pharmacological features of agents used for thrombosis treatment

Pharmacological dissolution of blood clots may be accomplished with intravenous or intra-arterial infusion of plasminogen activators that activate the fibrinolytic system. Multiple thrombolytic agents have been approved for clinical use or are under clinical investigation. The first generation agents were streptokinase and two-chain urokinase(two-chain urokinase-type plasminogen activator or urokinase). Second generation agents included recombinant t-PA (prepared as alteplase), and prourokinase (recombinant single-chain urokinase-type plasminogen activator) which the FDA did not approve for use in stroke therapy. Third generation agents include reteplase and tenecteplase (both are modified forms of alteplase) with longer half-life and greater fibrin specificity. All thrombolytic agents act by converting the proenzyme plasminogen into the active enzyme plasmin (Table 3.3). Plasmin lyses fibrin clots into soluble degradation products. Streptokinase, two-chain urokinase, and anisoylated plasminogen streptokinase activator complex result in extensive systemic activation of plasminogen (not clot-specific). In contrast, t-PA and single-chain urokinase activate plasminogen preferentially at the fibrin surface (clot-specific). Plasmin associated with the fibrin surface is protected from rapid inhibition by [alpha]$_2$-antiplasmin and thus produces more effective clot dissolution.[137]

A major limitaton of currently available drugs agents is thrombolytic resistance, which can be observed in almost one-fourth of patients.[137] This phenomenon is attributed to release of plasminogen activator inhibitor 1 (PAI 1) by platelets and platelet activation.[138] Although these agents can lyse the fibrin component of the clot, the dispersion of other components, including platelets, may not be adequate.

Table 3.3. Some of the thrombolytic agents used in endovascular procedures[a]

Agent	Commercial name (Company)	Mechanism of action	Indications in EVP	IA dose	Complications	Monitoring	Half-life	Reversal
Urokinase	Abbokinase (Abbott, Chicago, IL)	Converts plasminogen to plasmin, fibrin non-specific	IA for acute arterial occlusion	150 000–1 300 000 U	Intracranial hemorrhage	Total fibrinogen and fibrin degradation products	14–20 min	Fresh frozen plasma
Recombinant t-PA (alteplase)	Activase (Cenenlech, South San Francisco, CA)	Converts plasminogen to plasmin, fibrin specific	IA for acute arterial occlusion	5–40 mg	Intracranial hemorrhage	Total fibrinogen and fibrin degradation products	<5 min	Fresh frozen plasma
Recombinant t-PA (reteplase)	Retavase (Boehringer Mannheim, Gaithersburg, MD)	Converts plasminogen to plasmin, fibrin specific	Not defined			Total fibrinogen and fibrin degradation products	13–16 min	Fresh frozen plasma
Recombinant prourokinase	Prolyse (Abott, Chicago, IL)	Converts plasminogen to plasmin, fibrin specific	IA for acute arterial occlusion	6–9 mg	Intracranial hemorrhage	Total fibrinogen and fibrin degradation products	α, 6–8 min; β, 90–200 min	Fresh frozen plasma

[a]EVP, endovascular procedures; IA, intra-arterial(ly); t-PA, tissue plasminogen activator; U, units; min, minutes.

The most important side effect of thrombolysis is bleeding. The risk is increased with the concomitant use of aspirin and heparin. The rate of intracranial bleeding with intra-arterial administration of thrombolytic agents has not been documented in large studies. In a meta-analysis of 12 trials involving patients with ischemic stroke who received intravenously administered thrombolytic agents (recombinant t-PA, urokinase, or streptokinase), a high incidence of early symptomatic (10%) or fatal (6%) intracranial hemorrhaging was reported.[139] Treatment of life-threatening bleeding associated with thrombolytic therapy should include discontinuation of heparin therapy and administration of protamine (if required), cryoprecipitate (particularly if fibrinogen is depleted), and fresh frozen plasma.

No clear advantage of using antithrombotic combination therapy with aspirin and heparin as a routine adjunct to thrombolysis has been demonstrated. Both aspirin and heparin have limited effects on the rate of coronary thrombolysis and do not consistently prevent reocclusion. These results are attributed to aspirin's non-selective inhibition of the synthesis of both proaggregatory and antiaggregatory prostaglandins and the ineffectiveness of heparin in the inhibition of clot-associated thrombin. Because of a lack of confirmatory evidence supporting the use of heparin to maintain vessel patency after thrombolysis, no widely accepted guidelines for combination therapy exist. In a meta-analysis, the early use of aspirin with intravenous thrombolytic therapy for ischemic stroke treatment was associated with higher odds of death than observed in trials that tended to avoid early aspirin use (odds ratio, 2.06 versus 1.01).[139] The specific properties of applicable thrombolytic agents are discussed below.

t-PA

Two recombinant forms of t-PA are commercially available, Activase (Genentech, South San Francisco, CA) and Retavase (Boehringer Ingelheim, Gaithersburg, MD). Recombinant t-PA is a poor enzyme in the absence of fibrin, but it strikingly enhances the plasminogen activation rate in the presence of fibrin. This increased activity seems to result from a conformational change in recombinant t-PA after its attachment to fibrin. However, the clot specificity is incomplete, and some degree of systemic fibrinolysis does occur. Circulating recombinant t-PA is taken up and degraded by hepatocytes. The half-lives of Activase and Retavase are less than 5 minutes and 13 to 16 minutes, respectively. Studies have demonstrated that higher doses and faster administration are associated with more potent thrombolytic effects.[140] Because of the higher risk of bleeding complications associated with fixed-dose recombinant t-PA administration among patients with low body weights, weight adjustment of the dose has been recommended.[141]

Urokinase

Urokinase (Abbokinase, Abbott, Chicago, IL) is a two-chain serine protease, which, like streptokinase, lacks fibrin specificity. It directly activates plasminogen, without forming an activator complex. It is metabolized by the liver and its half-life is between 14 and 20 minutes. Although current interest in systemic administration of urokinase is limited because of the systemic lytic state it induces, local delivery of urokinase is still widely used for endovascular procedures.

Prourokinase

Prourokinase (non-glycosylated human single-chain urokinase) is a relatively fibrin-specific thrombolytic agent. A variable amount (6%–22%) of prourokinase is converted to two-chain urokinase in vivo.[142] The exact mechanism by which prourokinase exerts its action is not fully understood. It is not clear whether conversion to urokinase is required for thrombolysis induced by prourokinase. Prourokinase is rapidly cleared from plasma, and the half-life of the first exponential phase is 6 to 8 minutes; the terminal half life ranges from 90 to 200 minutes. Prourokinase is cleared primarily by the liver.[143] In recent clinical trials that evaluated the use of intra-arterially administered prourokinase in the treatment of acute middle cerebral artery occlusion, both a higher rate of recanalization and improved outcomes were observed.[144] However, a higher rate of symptomatic intracranial hemorrhage was observed for patients who received prourokinase (10.2%, compared with 1.8% for patients treated with intravenously administered heparin).

Combined use of thrombolytic agents and platelet GP IIa/IIIb-specific antibodies

Thrombolytic agents target the fibrin mesh component of thrombus, which paradoxically leads to an increase in thrombin activity and platelet activation.[145] Thrombin activates platelets, which release a series of agonists, including PAI-1.[145] Therefore, a platelet-rich thrombus, which is more resistant to thrombolytic agents, is formed after successful initial thrombolysis. Strong antiplatelet agents, such as GP IIb/IIIa-specific antibodies, increase the potential for initial thrombolysis and reduce the risk of reocclusion. Ohman et al.[146] reported a twofold higher recanalization rate with the concurrent use of alteplase and Integrilin (bolus of 180 μg/kg and infusion of 0.75 μg/kg per min for 24 h) for patients with acute MIs. Similarly, the Thrombolysis in Myocardial Infarction 14 investigators [145] reported that the most complete recanalization was achieved with a combination of low-dose alteplase (50 mg) and abciximab (bolus of 0.25 mg/kg and infusion of 10 μg/kg per min for 12 h) for patients with acute MIs. Qureshi et al.[147] reported a combination of intra-arterial recombinant t-PA and intravenous abciximab within 3 to 6 hours of stroke onset that resulted in partial or complete recanalization in 13 of the 20 patients. Thirteen patients demonstrated early neurological improvement, and favorable outcome at 1 month was observed in six patients. This approach provides new capacities to enhance the success of thrombolysis in the intracranial circulation by increasing the rate of recanalization and preventing reocclusion.

Complications of antiplatelet and anticoagulant agents

A set of complications can be seen with antiplatelet and anticoagulant agents. These are briefly described below:

Bone marrow suppression and agranulocytosis

Thienopyridines of which ticlopidine and clopidogrel are the most known are well known to cause myelotoxicity. Ticlopidine causes more myelotoxicity than clopidogrel and needs frequent monitoring of hematologic laboratory values. This, along with a narrower range of indications and less convenient dosing schedule, has led to its supplantation by clopidogrel, and it is not in common clinical use any longer. While the mechanism for clopidogrel-associated myelotoxicity is unknown,[148] it is infrequent, and typically happens weeks to months after start of therapy, with a rate of incidence of agranulocytosis, granulocytopenia and aplastic anemia that is <1% for all patients on clopidogrel.[38] This possibility should be entertained if a patient on clopidogrel presents with fever and/or infection. Post-marketing cases of fatal hemorrhage, thrombocytopenic purpura with some fatalities, and ophthalmic hemorrhage have been reported.

Thrombocytopenia

The use of anticoagulants or antiplatelet drugs leads to an increased risk of bleeding and thrombocytopenia. This is true of heparin, glycoprotein IIb/IIIa receptor inhibitors, and thienopyridines.[149]

The CRUSADE (Can Rapid Risk Stratification of Unstable Angina Patients Suppress Adverse Outcomes With Early Implementation of the American College of Cardiology/American Heart Association Guidelines) trial evaluated over 36 000 patients with non-ST segment elevation acute coronary syndrome. Of these, a total of 4697 (13%) of patients developed a new thrombocytopenia that was defined as a platelet count of $<150 \times 10^9$/L during their hospitalization.[150] This was associated with increased risk of hemorrhage and mortality. The CAPRIE (Clopidogrel versus Aspirin in Patients at Risk of Ischemic Events) trial [151] showed that thrombocytopenia was identical in the clopidogrel and aspirin groups with a non-significant difference in incidence of severe thrombocytopenia (0.19% vs 0.10% for clopidogrel and aspirin, respectively).

Glycoprotein IIb/IIIa associated thrombocytopenia

Thrombocytopenia (defined as a platelet count less than 100 000 cells per ml[3]) and severe thrombocytopenia (less than 50 000 cells per ml[3]) have been reported as complications of abciximab use. [54,152-154] The overall incidence of thrombocytopenia related to abciximab is 5%. The incidence of severe thrombocytopenia ranges from 0.4% to 1%. [154] Acute thrombocytopenia (platelets less than 20 000 per ml^3 within 24 hours of abciximab initiation) has also been reported. The risk increases with concomitant administration of heparin. Platelet transfusion was necessary in 2.1% to 5.5% of the patients. [153] Thrombocytopenia after abciximab re-administration is presumed to be immune mediated. [155,156] Approximately 7% of patients develop antibodies (IGg) to abciximab after first exposure. [156] Available data suggest abciximab (c7E3 Fab) has considerably less immunogenic potential than murine 7E3 Fab (m7E3 Fab). [157,158] Over 50% of patients demonstrated human antimurine antibody responses to m7E3 Fab in one study. [158]

Thrombocytopenia has also been reported following eptifibatide and tirofiban infusion. A pooled analysis of eight major prospective, placebo-controlled, randomized, multicenter trials of intravenous GP IIb/IIIa receptor inhibitors demonstrated a greater risk of thrombocytopenia ($n = 42$) with abciximab than with eptifibatide and tirofiban. [159]

Heparin-induced thrombocytopenia

Heparin-induced thrombocytopenia (HIT), is an immune mediated thrombocytopenia following heparin administration. HIT is essentially a prothrombotic disorder mediated by an IgG antiplatelet factor 4/heparin antibody, which induces platelet, endothelial cell, monocyte, and other cellular activation, leading to thrombin generation and thrombotic complications. [160] HIT can complicate unfractionated as well as low molecular weight heparin administration; however, the incidence is less in low molecular weight heparin patients. HIT can be a life- and limb-threatening condition with severe and extensive thromboembolism (both venous and arterial) rather than with bleeding. Venous thrombosis is more common than arterial thrombosis. Diagnosis is based on a drop in platelet count; therefore, a baseline platelet count should be obtained prior to initiation of treatment. A drop in platelet count by 50%, a drop of 30% with concomitant thrombosis, or more should prompt investigation. Heparin-dependent IgG antibodies are positive in the serum. [81] Management of patients with HIT should start by discontinuing any heparin products, which should be replaced with a non-heparin anticoagulant such as a direct thrombin inhibitor or danaparoid followed by a vitamin K antagonist for long-term treatment. The new anti-factor Xa drugs (fondaparinux, rivaroxaban, apixaban) and other non-heparin antithrombotic agents can potentially be used for the treatment of HIT if clinically validated.

Because early detection of heparin-induced thrombocytopenia seems to improve outcome, all patients on heparin should have a platelet count measured before the start of heparin treatment, on the first day thereafter, and then regularly on every second day from day 5 to day 20 of treatment. [161]

Thrombotic thrombocytopenic purpura

This condition is a complication of thienopyridine therapy, which consists of thrombocytopenia, microangiopathic hemolytic anemia, renal dysfunction, neurologic abnormalities, and fever. The treatment is therapeutic plasma exchange (TPE), which should be promptly instituted, especially when this is related to thienopyridine therapy. This ensures that the likelihood of survival is increased. [162] In the RADAR project (Research on Adverse Drug and Events and Reports), two separate mechanisms for thienopyridine-induced TTP were identified. The first is an immunologic pathway, associated with more than two weeks of thienopyridine use and the other is a non-immunologic pathway which is associated with less than 2 weeks of thienopyridine use. When compared with ticlopidine, TTP associated with clopidogrel was more likely to fall in the less than two weeks category. Also, clopidogrel-related TTP usually presents with less severe thrombocytopenia, and is associated with renal insufficiency in more cases. There is a 70% survival rate in patients who are treated with TPE versus a 66.7% survival rate for those not treated in the less than two weeks cohort. Survival rate for patients who developed TTP after 2 weeks, and received TPE is 77.8%. In other words, overall mortality for thienopyridine associated TTP is 25.8%, with an increased rate seen in patients with abnormal neurologic status (P-value < 0.02), serum creatinine > 2.5 mg/dL ($P < 0.04$) and not being treated with TPE ($P < 0.0006$). Patients with von Willebrand factor cleaving protease ADAMTS13 activity of $>15\%$ at the time of diagnosis with TTP had a four times higher likelihood of dying (41.9% vs 9.1%, $P < 0.036$).

Hemolytic uremic syndrome (HUS)

HUS is a syndrome characterized by the triad of microangiopathic hemolytic anemia, thrombocytopenia, and acute renal failure. Two cases of clopidogrel-associated hemolytic uremic syndrome have been reported. The onset was in the first 2 weeks of therapy in both cases. The clinical picture of HUS includes fatigue, petechial rash, hematuria, and non-cardiogenic pulmonary edema. Laboratory findings suggestive of HUS include drop of hematocrit and platelet count, rise of serum creatinine and lactate dehydrogenase, decrease in haptoglobin, and peripheral blood smear showing erythrocyte fragmentation and polychromasia. Treatment is with plasmapheresis and steroid therapy. [163,164]

Pseudothrombocytopenia

Pseudothrombocytopenia is a laboratory artifact due to in vitro anticoagulation interaction seen with abciximab. To exclude pseudothrombocytopenia, the manufacturer recommends blood samples be taken in three separate tubes containing ethylenediaminetetraacetic acid (EDTA), citrate, and heparin. A low platelet count in EDTA but not in heparin and/or citrate is supportive of a diagnosis of pseudothrombocytopenia. [165] The frequency of pseudothrombocytopenia was 2.1%

(117 out of 5476 patients) and 0.6% (17 out of 3079 patients) (P < 0.001) for abciximab-treated patients and placebo-treated patients, respectively, in an evaluation of four major clinical trials. Of all of the abciximab-treated patients with low platelet counts, 36.3% were determined to be pseudothrombocytopenia. Pseudothrombocytopenia does not increase bleeding, stroke, transfusion requirements or the need for repeat revascularization and does not require specific treatment or early discontinuation of abciximab.[166]

Allergic reactions

Allergic reaction to aspirin

Two variants of aspirin sensitivity have been described. Both reactions typically have a rapid onset within 15 minutes after aspirin ingestion, but can be delayed for up to 3 hours.[167]

The urticaria-angioedema type occurs more frequently in patients with chronic urticaria (incidence about 23%) and is present overall in about 3.8% of adults and 0.3% in children.

The other variation is a bronchospastic type, characterized by acute bronchospasm, severe rhinitis, and nasal polyps, which are present in about 50%.[168] This type is predominantly found in adults with asthma. Up to 19% of asthmatics develop positive challenges if spirometry is performed. The incidence increases to 40% in asthmatics with pansinusitis and nasal polyps.[169] Women are more susceptible than men.

Other dermatologic manifestations are far less common; for example, eczema (2.4%), purpura (1.5%), and erythema multiforme (1.0%).[170]

The incidence of cross-reactivity between aspirin and other analgesics appears to be related to the extent of cyclo-oxygenase inhibition. Aspirin cross-reacts with virtually all potent non-salicylate inhibitors, including diflunisal, indomethacin, sulindac, tolmetin, naproxen, diclofenac, fenoprofen, ibuprofen, ketoprofen, piroxicam, and mefenamic acid. Non-aspirin salicylates with weak anticyclo-oxygenase activity are generally well tolerated by aspirin-intolerant individuals.[171]

Allergic reaction to clopidogrel

Allergic reactions to clopidogrel have been reported rarely (less than 1%). From worldwide postmarketing experience, very rare cases of hypersensitivity reactions, including anaphylactoid reactions, have been reported.[172] Severe hypersensitivity reaction included neutropenia, rash, fever, tachycardia, nausea, and vomiting.[173] In the CAPRIE study, there were significantly more patients with rash in the clopidogrel group (6.0%) compared with the aspirin group (4.6%) However, these events were generally mild and transient in nature.[151]

A recent study treated clopidogrel-induced skin reactions using a short course of prednisolone and chlorpheniramine (5 days oral prednisolone and chlorpheniramine (4 mg three times daily) for 7 days), without stopping or substituting clopidogrel. There was complete resolution seen in the majority (89%) of patients within an average of 3.2 days following treatment. One patient had partial resolution, and one had no response to treatment, but both were able to continue clopidogrel.[174] Desensitization can be considered in patients who have exhibited allergic reactions to the drug.

Allergic reaction to abciximab

Hypersensitivity and allergic reactions to abciximab were evaluated in the phase 3 clinical trials[175–177] in 8556 treated patients undergoing coronary angioplasty. No excess hypersensitivity or anaphylactic reactions were observed in patients treated with abciximab compared with placebo. However, a few isolated cases of anaphylactic shock attributed to abciximab have been reported. The clinical picture included generalized exanthema, cervicofacial swelling, thrombocytopenia, hypotension, bradycardia, and shock. The immunohistologic study indicated a T-cell mediated allergy.[178] Overall, abciximab appears to possess a low immunogenic potential.[157] Abciximab-induced thrombocytopenia is thought to be immune mediated, as mentioned above.

Special considerations in pregnancy and breast feeding (Table 3.4)

One characteristic of the FDA definitions of the pregnancy categories is that the FDA requires a relatively large amount of high-quality data on a pharmaceutical for it to be defined as Pregnancy Category A. As a result of this, many drugs that would be considered Pregnancy Category A in other countries are allocated to Category C by the FDA

Anticoagulants

The use of anticoagulant therapy during pregnancy is challenging because the potential for fetal, as well as maternal, complications must be considered. LMWH, UFH heparinoid, and danaparoid, are safe for the fetus. Limited data are available about the safety of new anticoagulants (e.g., direct thrombin inhibitors, fondaparinux) during pregnancy.[179] Vitamin K antagonists are fetopathic especially when administered between the sixth week and twelfth week of gestation. Warfarin passes through the placental barrier and may cause fatal hemorrhage to the fetus in utero. Furthermore, there have been reports of birth malformations in children born to mothers who have been treated with warfarin during pregnancy. In a systematic review of the literature examining fetal and maternal outcomes of pregnant women with prosthetic valves, Chan and colleagues found that the use of vitamin K antagonists throughout pregnancy was associated with congenital anomalies in 35 of 549 live births (6.4%; 95% confidence interval [CI], 4.6%–8.9%). The most common fetal anomaly seen was characteristic coumarin embryopathy, consisting of nasal hypoplasia and/or stippled epiphyses, and limb hypoplasia. Vitamin K antagonists have also been associated with CNS abnormalities after exposure during any trimester

Table 3.4. US FDA pharmaceutical pregnancy categories

Pregnancy Category A	Adequate and well-controlled studies have failed to demonstrate a risk to the fetus in the first trimester of pregnancy (and there is no evidence of risk in later trimesters).
Pregnancy Category B	Animal reproduction studies have failed to demonstrate a risk to the fetus and there are no adequate and well-controlled studies in pregnant women OR Animal studies have shown an adverse effect, but adequate and well-controlled studies in pregnant women have failed to demonstrate a risk to the fetus in any trimester.
Pregnancy Category C	Animal reproduction studies have shown an adverse effect on the fetus and there are no adequate and well-controlled studies in humans, but potential benefits may warrant use of the drug in pregnant women despite potential risks.
Pregnancy Category D	There is positive evidence of human fetal risk based on adverse reaction data from investigational or marketing experience or studies in humans, but potential benefits may warrant use of the drug in pregnant women despite potential risks.
Pregnancy Category X	Studies in animals or humans have demonstrated fetal abnormalities and/or there is positive evidence of human fetal risk based on adverse reaction data from investigational or marketing experience, and the risks involved in use of the drug in pregnant women clearly outweigh potential benefits.

and fetal wastage. UFH and LMWH do not cross the placenta and, therefore, do not have the potential to cause fetal bleeding or teratogenicity, although bleeding at the uteroplacental junction is possible.[180]

Aspirin

Although animal studies have shown that aspirin may increase the risk of congenital anomalies, data from human studies are conflicting. Aspirin has been assigned to pregnancy category C by the FDA. However, aspirin is considered to be in pregnancy category D by the FDA if full dose aspirin is taken in the third trimester due to effects on the fetal cardiovascular system (closure of the ductus arteriosus). Aspirin use during pregnancy has been associated with certain risks such as alterations of maternal and newborn hemostasis, increased perinatal mortality, intrauterine growth retardation, premature closure of ductus arteriosus, pulmonary hypertension, and teratogenic effects.[167]

On the other hand, there are data suggesting that aspirin is safe in pregnancy. The most compelling data come from a meta-analysis of 14 randomized studies including a total of 12 416 women that reported that low-dose (50 to 150 mg/d) aspirin therapy administered during the second and third trimesters of pregnancy to women at risk for pre-eclampsia was safe for the mother and fetus. The authors of this meta-analysis also reviewed observational studies including >96 000 pregnancies and found no evidence of teratogenicity or long-term adverse effects of aspirin during pregnancy.[181] Another meta-analysis of eight studies (seven observational and one randomized) that evaluated the risk of congenital anomalies with aspirin exposure during the first trimester found no evidence of an increase in the overall risk of congenital malformations associated with aspirin use, suggesting that aspirin is safe even when used early in pregnancy.[182]

Current American Heart Association recommendations state "Pregnant women (with non-cardioembolic stroke) may be considered for treatment with unfractionated heparin (UFH) or low molecular weight heparin (LMWH) in the first trimester, followed by low-dose aspirin for the remainder of the pregnancy."[183]

Clopidogrel

Clopidogrel's ability to cross the placenta is unknown. There are no controlled studies in pregnant women. Studies conducted in animals at doses much higher than those used in humans revealed no evidence of impaired fertility or fetal toxicity as a result of clopidogrel.[172] Clopidogrel is classified as category B.

Direct thrombin inhibitors

The use of direct thrombin inhibitors in pregnant women should be limited to those with severe allergic reactions (including HIT) to heparin who cannot receive danaparoid. Investigations have documented placental transfer of r-hirudin in rabbits and rats. Although small numbers of case reports of successful outcomes with r-hirudin use in pregnancy have been published, there are insufficient data to evaluate its safety in this setting.

Abciximab studies in animals have revealed adverse effects on the fetus (teratogenic or embryocidal or other) and there are no controlled studies in women. The drug is classified as category C and should be given only if the potential benefit outweighs the potential risk to the fetus. Eptifibatide does not cross the placenta and animal-reproduction studies have not demonstrated a fetal risk. It is classified as category B.

Lactation

Aspirin

Some available data have suggested that low intermittent doses of aspirin can be used safely in the breast feeding mother.[184] However, others have suggested that breastfeeding is contra-indicated during aspirin administration due to the increasing connection between salicylates and Reye's syndrome.[185] Neonates should be observed for possible abnormal platelet function especially following use of high doses of aspirin in nursing mothers. Sensitivity rashes have also been observed in breast feeding infants.[184]

Clopidogrel

Because human data are lacking regarding the use of clopidogrel during breast feeding, caution is advised. Due to its molecular weight, it is theoretically possible that clopidogrel-would be excreted in breast milk. Studies in rats have shown that clopidogrel and/or its metabolites are excreted in the milk.[172]

Warfarin

Despite a lack of data suggesting any harmful effect to breast feeding infants, many obstetricians remain reluctant to pre-scribe warfarin to lactating women. There have been two convincing reports demonstrating that warfarin is not detected in breast milk and does not induce an anticoagulant effect in the breast-fed infant when nursing mothers consume the drug. Therefore, the use of warfarin in women who require post-partum anticoagulant therapy is safe.

Unfractionated heparin (UFH)

Because of its high molecular weight and strong negative charge, UFH does not pass into breast milk and can be safely given to nursing mothers.[186]

Low molecular weight heparin (LMWH)

In a case series of 15 women receiving 2500 IU of LMWH after cesarean section, there was evidence of excretion of small amounts of LMWH into the breast milk in 11 patients.[186] However, given the very low bioavailability of orally ingested heparin, there is unlikely to be any clinically relevant effect on the nursing infant.

Direct thrombin inhibitors

Very little is known about the passage of danaparoid into breast milk. A small number of case reports have reported none or very low anti-Xa activity in the breast milk of dana-paroid-treated women.[187] As Danaparoid is not absorbed after oral intake, it is unlikely that any anticoagulant effect would appear in breast-fed infants. In a single case report, no hirudin was detected in the breast milk of a nursing mother with a therapeutic plasma hirudin level. Enteral absorption of r-hirudin appears to be low.[188] Therefore, it is unlikely that exposed infants would experience a significant anticoagulant effect, even if small amounts of hirudin appear in breast milk.

Glycoprotein IIb/IIIa inhibitors

Available evidence and expert consensus are inconclusive or are inadequate for determining infant risk during breast feeding. It is unknown whether abciximab, upon ingestion, is absorbed systemically or excreted into human milk. Until further data are available, caution is advised if abciximab is administered to a nursing woman.[165] No reports describing the use of eptifibatide during human lactation are available and the effects on the nursing infant from exposure to the drug in milk are unknown.

Measurement of platelet response to antiplatelet therapy

Antiplatelet therapy reduces, but does not eliminate, the risk of ischemic events, and the biological effects of aspirin and clopidogrel vary among individuals, giving rise to the concept of "aspirin/clopidogrel resistance." Clinically, resistance is defined as the failure of therapy to prevent acute vascular thrombotic events despite fully compliant intake of appropriate doses. In the laboratory, resistance theoretically encompasses the drug's failure to attain a particular level of platelet inhibition in ex vivo studies. Although platelet testing was originally developed to identify patients at risk for platelet dysfunction,[189] there has been considerable focus on using ex vivo platelet testing to identify patients whose platelets may be poorly responsive to antiplatelet therapy.[190] Several platelet function tests are available, including bleeding time, optical aggregometry, PFA-100, and VerifyNow (Table 3.5). However, agreement among tests is poor, definitions of non-response vary, and there is currently no reference standard. For example, work performed by Lordkipanidzé et al.[191,192] showed the prevalence of aspirin and clopidogrel resistance to be highly assay – specific and the tests themselves to have poor sensitivity to detect resistant subjects. However, there are no published data that address the clinical utility of changing antiplatelet therapy regimens based on ex vivo laboratory findings of non-responsiveness to aspirin or clopidogrel.[189]

Potential causes of variability of platelet responsiveness

The apparent variability of platelet response to antiplatelet therapy may be explained by patient- or agent-specific factors.

Table 3.5. Platelet function assays[190]

Platelet function assay tests	Advantages	Disadvantages
Optical aggregometry	Historical gold standard	Time consuming; requires sample preparation and operator expertise; expensive
Whole blood aggregometry	Whole blood assay; small sample volume; sample can be hemolyzed, icteric, or lipemic	Time consuming; expensive
Bleeding time	Inexpensive; in vivo	Paining; time consuming; operator dependent; may leave scar
Urinary 11-dehydro-TXB2	Non-invasive; used to estimate TXA2 inhibition; stable metabolite of TXA2	Reproducibility and biologic variability uncertain; dependent on renal function; indirect measurement
Serum TXB2	Used to estimate TXA2 inhibition; stable metabolite of TXA2	Indirect measurement
PFA-100 assay	Point of care; whole-blood assay; simple; small sample volume; high-shear condition	Comparability with other methods uncertain; dependent on platelet count and hematocrit
VerifyNow device	Point of care; whole-blood assay; small sample volume; rapid; simple	Comparability with other methods uncertain
Cone-and-plate analyzer	High-shear condition; whole-blood assay; rapid; simple; higher sensitivity than aggregometry	Not well studied; comparability with other methods uncertain

Non-platelet factors include bioavailability, genetic polymorphisms, and multiple ADP receptors (Table 3.6). Suboptimal dosing and drug–drug interactions may also contribute to variable platelet response to aspirin and clopidogrel.[193] Variability in intestinal absorption and hepatic conversion of clopidogrel to its active metabolite may explain differences observed between clopidogrel and prasugrel in platelet function tests.[194] In some patients, drug–drug interactions may be operative. Although some interactions are known to be clinically significant, e.g., certain non-steroidal anti-inflammatory drugs [NSAIDs] and aspirin,[195] the clinical significance of others, e.g., clopidogrel[196,197] is uncertain. Non-steroidal anti-inflammatory drugs, particularly ibuprofen, block the access of aspirin to its binding site on the platelet cyclooxygenase-1 enzyme, an interaction that has been shown to lead to treatment failure.[198,199] This drug–drug interaction can be reduced by administering the NSAID 30 minutes after taking aspirin (immediate release, not enteric-coated) or >8 hours before aspirin.[198] Consideration of concomitant drug use is therefore an important factor in assessing true aspirin resistance. Similarly, because clopidogrel is metabolized by cytochrome P450 (CYP), other drugs metabolized, induced, or inhibited by CYP may be clinically relevant.[200] Clopidogrel is a prodrug that is converted to its active metabolite by the highly polymorphic CYP. In a study of healthy volunteers, polymorphisms CYP2C19 and CYP2C9 were associated with blunted antiplatelet response to clopidogrel.[201] In a study of patients undergoing PCI, CYP22C19 polymorphism was associated with more platelet reactivity, which was associated with poor clinical outcomes after stent placement.[202] CYP3A is another

Table 3.6. Factors associated with low platelet responsiveness on ex vivo platelet function testing[190,209]

Mechanism/factor
• Bioavailability (metabolism or absorption)
• Genetic (receptor polymorphism)
• Drug–drug interactions
• Suboptimal dosing
• Multiple ADP receptors (P2Y12, P2Y1, P2X1)
• Platelet–erythrocyte interaction
• Exercise/mental stress
• Diabetes
• Smoking
• Hyperlipidemia
• Age
• Gender
• Hypertension

important isozyme that is relevant to potential drug–drug interactions with clopidogrel. A multivariable analysis showed that the CYP3A5 polymorphism was a predictor of cardiovascular events among clopidogrel users receiving CYP3A substrates.[203]

Compliance is another important consideration. Among 500 patients enrolled in the Prospective Registry Evaluating

Myocardial Infarction: Events and Recovery, who received a DES, patients who discontinued clopidogrel therapy within 1 month of PCI (13.6%) were nine times as likely to die within the year compared to those who maintained clopidogrel past 1 month (hazard ratio 9.02, 95% CI 1.3–60.6; $P = 0.02$).[204] Results of two studies of 19 167 ACS patients showed 8%–9% of patients stop taking aspirin within 3–6 months of hospital discharge.[205,206] In two separate studies, patients who were previously assessed as resistant to antiplatelet therapy were found to be "sensitive" after reinforcing adherence or directly observing administration.[207,208] Because adherence clearly influences measurement of antiplatelet resistance, it is important to put in place a reliable method of determining patient adherence.

Clinical implications of variable platelet response

Several studies report a link between lack of response to aspirin or clopidogrel upon ex vivo platelet testing and occurrence of ischemic events. A meta-analysis ($n = 3000$) comparing patients who are responsive and resistant to aspirin suggests that the latter group faces a nearly four-fold greater risk of adverse cardiovascular events.[210] The risk remained elevated in non-responders whether or not they were taking another antiplatelet agent in addition to aspirin.[210] Although such studies link aspirin non-responsiveness to clinical events, there remains large measurement variability, depending on the platelet assay being used. More importantly, there is no proven course of action once non-responsive patients are identified.

Problems with study design and the non-standardization of testing methods limit interpretation of the data. For example, studies that suggest a relationship between lack of platelet responsiveness to clopidogrel and adverse clinical outcomes generally include small cohort sizes and use retrospective approaches, surrogate end points and outcome measures, and non-conforming techniques and definitions to determine lack of responsiveness on ex vivo platelet testing.[211] Thus, there is no accumulated body of evidence definitively linking results of ex vivo platelet testing to subsequent ischemic events. Large, randomized studies with appropriately designed end points are needed. It is uncertain whether measuring inhibition of platelet aggregation (IPA) to achieve greater platelet inhibition via corresponding dose adjustment or medication change in patients whose platelets are hyporesponsive will result in better outcomes. Preliminary evidence from a randomized clinical trial suggests that providing additional clopidogrel loading doses to percutaneous coronary intervention patients who have a vasodilator-stimulated phosphoprotein phosphorylation (VASP) index >50% may lower the risk of adverse events.[212] However, confirmation in a larger patient population is necessary before VASP-guided dosing is recommended as part of routine care.

The effect of modulating aspirin dose also remains controversial. One study found the highest levels of aspirin resistance at doses <100 mg/d compared with doses >300 mg/d, suggesting that resistance may be overcome with higher aspirin dosing.[213] A better understanding of aspirin resistance patterns may lead to more aggressive dosing strategies, but currently, there is insufficient evidence to recommend dosing escalation.

The failure of oral glycoprotein (GP) IIb/IIIa inhibitors,[51] which profoundly alter platelet aggregation, highlights the importance of prospective clinical data and the limitations of platelet function testing. Furthermore, recent results of studies comparing the IPA and clinical efficacy of prasugrel and clopidogrel show that although higher IPA may result in greater clinical efficacy, this is achieved at the cost of increased fatal bleeding.[194,214] Overall, given the absence of clear guidelines on the optimal approach to measuring platelet function and interpreting the findings in relation to clinical risk, routine laboratory testing for platelet function is not recommended for patients receiving antiplatelet therapy.[215,216]

Measurement of intensity of anticoagulation
The activated partial thromboplastin time (APTT) and the activated clotting time (ACT)

There are two ways to monitor anticoagulation: one is the activated partial thromboplastin time (APTT) and the other is activated clotting time (ACT). APTT is the most commonly used method to monitor therapy with heparin. This is despite its log linear relationship to heparin dose and also individual patient variations.[217–219] ACT is employed in the monitoring of anticoagulation in situations where a high level of anticoagulation is necessary. Examples of this include cardiopulmonary bypass, cardiac, and cerebral catheterization procedures. It is preferable because it has a linear relationship to heparin dose.[220] ACT has a poor correlation with actual heparin concentrations, but is a reliable indicator of fibrin monomer formation.[221–223] Kubalek et al.[224] compared the effectiveness of ACT as compared with APTT in monitoring anticoagulation in patients undergoing neuroradiological procedures after a 2500U–5000U heparin bolus. In the case of APTT, it was found that the measurements were out of range in 67% of patients using bedside monitoring equipment and 76.5% using laboratory testing. On the other hand, there was reliable ACT measurement in all patients. These results indicated that ACT is the method of choice for monitoring anticoagulation in neuroangiographic procedures. Kurec et al.[225] found that manual-activated clotting time correlated best with the whole blood clotting time, was sensitive to low concentrations of heparin, formed a discernible clot within a convenient time period in blood containing high concentrations of heparin, was reproducible and was easily performed.

Methods of measuring ACT

ACT is measured with either kaolin or Celite as activators.[226] This leads to the two machines commonly used for this purpose, Hemotec and Hemochron, having highly significant differences, in both in vitro tests (modified APTT with whole blood in a neutral coagulometer), and ACT where aprotinin and heparin were used, as well as with parallel measurements with the two machines with blood from patients undergoing cardiopulmonary bypass with high dose aprotinin therapy ($P < 0.001$).[227] Of note, the Hemotec machine with kaolin as activator is not affected by aprotinin throughout surgery, while the Hemochron clotting times almost double as soon as aprotinin and heparin are combined. Doherty et al.[228] shows that in ACT measurements, in cases where aprotinin is being used, only kaolin activation yields accurate results. Svenmaker et al.[229] concluded that ACT is not a standardized measure and that test results are strongly associated with the specific compounds used to initiate the coagulation process. This does translate into a more accurate way to avoid clot formation during cardiopulmonary bypass, given the variability in dose-related heparin effects. Its use led to less overall utilization of heparin and protamine, and ultimately decreased the incidence of transfusions by up to 30%.

Site and timing of measuring ACT

The site of administration and timing of venous sampling markedly affects the measured ACT during interventions. Operators should be aware of these effects when assessing the accuracy of the ACT during coronary and intracranial interventions.[230,231]

Effect of platelet glycoprotein IIB/IIIa on ACT

Based on previous evidence suggesting that abciximab may have a more potent anticoagulant effect than small-molecule glycoprotein (GP) IIb/IIIa inhibitors, Casserly et al.[232] prospectively reviewed collected heparin dose, activated clotting time (ACT), and corresponding clinical outcome data from the Do Tirofiban and ReoPro Give Similar Efficacy Outcome Trial (TARGET), which was a direct comparison of tirofiban versus abciximab in 4809 patients who underwent percutaneous intervention. When stratified by ACT quartile, no statistically significant difference in bleeding or ischemic end points between the tirofiban and abciximab cohorts was observed. There was no observed difference in the anticoagulant effect of tirofiban and abciximab, as measured by the ACT, or in the incidence of bleeding or ischemic complications in each ACT quartile.

Conclusions

In endovascular procedures, arterial injury and the use of catheters, contrast agents, and implanted devices with thrombogenic potential place patients at risk for thrombosis and embolization. Extensive research has been performed to elucidate the pathophysiological features underlying thrombosis associated with endovascular procedures. Recognition of the important role of platelet aggregation in arterial thrombosis has led to the development of antiplatelet agents such as ticlopidine, prasugrel clopidogrel, and inhibitors of the GP IIb/IIIa receptor. Administration of these agents should be initiated before the procedure for optimal antiplatelet effects. A combination of aspirin with clopidogrel provides the best oral antiplatelet therapy. Treatment should be continued until endothelialization has occurred (4–6 wk after the procedure). For patients at high risk, the use of antibodies to GP IIb/IIIa receptors during the period of maximal local prothrombotic activity (initial 24 h) may be a reasonable alternative. The intraoperative use of heparin is well established; however, post-procedural use is restricted because of hemorrhagic complications and limited benefits. A better understanding of the limitations of standard treatments (such as aspirin and heparin) and the benefits of newer available agents will further the development of improved strategies for prophylaxis and treatment of thromboembolic complications associated with endovascular procedures.

References

1. Parsons TJ, Haycraft DL, Hoak JC, Sage H. Interaction of platelets and purified collagens in a laminar flow model. *Thromb Res* 1986;**43**:435–43.

2. Hynes RO. Integrins: a family of cell surface receptors. *Cell.* 1987;**48**(4):549–54.

3. Smyth SS, Joneckis CC, Parise LV. Regulation of vascular integrins. *Blood* 1993;**81**:2827–43.

4. Lefkovits J, Plow EF, Topol EJ. Platelet glycoprotein IIb/IIIa receptors in cardiovascular medicine. *N Engl J Med* 1995;**332**:1553–9.

5. Fuster V, Jang IK. Role of platelet-inhibitor agents in coronary artery disease. In Topol EJ, ed. *Textbook of Interventional Cardiology.* 2nd edn. Philadelphia: W.B. Saunders Co.; 1994. 3–22.

6. Barry WL, Sarembock IJ. Antiplatelet and anticoagulant therapy in patients undergoing percutaneous transluminal coronary angioplasty. *Cardiol Clin* 1994;**12**:517–35.

7. Weitz JI, Hudoba M, Massel D, Maraganore J, Hirsh J. Clot-bound thrombin is protected from inhibition by heparin-antithrombin III but is susceptible to inactivation by antithrombin III-independent inhibitors. *J Clin Invest* 1990;**86**:385–91.

8. Booth NA. The natural inhibitors of fibrinolysis. In Bloom AL, Forbes CD, Thomas DP, Tuddenham EGD, eds. *Haemostasis and Thrombosis.* 3rd edn. Edinburgh: Churchill Livingstone, 1994.

9. Granger CB, Califf RM, Topol EJ. Thrombolytic therapy for acute myocardial infarction. A review. *Drugs* 1992;**44**(3):293–325.

10. Lijnen HR, Collen D. Endothelium in hemostasis and thrombosis. *Prog Cardiovasc Dis* 1997;**39**:343–50.

11. Ghigliotti G, Waissbluth AR, Speidel C, Abendschein DR, Eisenberg PR. Prolonged activation of prothrombin on the vascular wall after arterial injury. *Arterioscler Thromb Vasc Biol* 1998;**18**:250–7.

12. Speidel CM, Eisenberg PR, Ruf W, Edgington TS, Abendschein DR. Tissue factor mediates prolonged procoagulant activity on the luminal surface of balloon-injured aortas in rabbits. *Circulation* 1995;**92**:3323–30.

13. Theroux P, Waters D, Lam J, Juneau M, McCans J. Reactivation of unstable angina after the discontinuation of heparin. *N Engl J Med* 1992;**327**:141–5.

14. Lijnen HR, Collen D. Fibrinolytic agents: mechanisms of activity and pharmacology. *Thromb Haemost* 1995;**74**:387–90.

15. Ferns GA, Stewart-Lee AL, Anggard EE. Arterial response to mechanical injury: balloon catheter de-endothelialization. *Atherosclerosis* 1992;**92**:89–104.

16. More RS, Rutty G, Underwood MJ, Brack MJ, Gershlick AH. A time sequence of vessel wall changes in an experimental model of angioplasty. *J Pathol* 1994;**172**:287–92.

17. Van Belle E, Tio FO, Chen D, Maillard L, Kearney M, Isner JM. Passivation of metallic stents after arterial gene transfer of phVEGF165 inhibits thrombus formation and intimal thickening. *J Am Coll Cardiol* 1997;**29**:1371–9.

18. Palmaz JC. Intravascular stenting: from basic research to clinical application. *Cardiovasc Intervent Radiol* 1992;**15**:279–84.

19. Reul J, Weis J, Spetzger U, Konert T, Fricke C, Thron A. Long-term angiographic and histopathologic findings in experimental aneurysms of the carotid bifurcation embolized with platinum and tungsten coils. *Am J Neuroradiol* 1997;**18**:35–42.

20. Roth GJ, Stanford N, Majerus PW. Acetylation of prostaglandin synthase by aspirin. *Proc Natl Acad Sci USA* 1975;**72**:3073–6.

21. Theroux P. Antiplatelet therapy: do the new platelet inhibitors add significantly to the clinical benefits of aspirin? *Am Heart J* 1997;**134**:S62–70.

22. Patrignani P, Filabozzi P, Patrono C. Selective cumulative inhibition of platelet thromboxane production by low-dose aspirin in healthy subjects. *J Clin Invest* 1982;**69**:1366–72.

23. Farrell B, Godwin J, Richards S, Warlow C. The United Kingdom transient ischaemic attack (UK-TIA) aspirin trial: final results. *J Neurol Neurosurg Psychiatry* 1991;**54**:1044–54.

24. A comparison of two doses of aspirin (30 mg vs. 283 mg a day) in patients after a transient ischemic attack or minor ischemic stroke. The Dutch TIA Trial Study Group. *N Engl J Med* 1991;**325**:1261–6.

25. Dyken ML, Barnett HJ, Easton JD, *et al.* Low-dose aspirin and stroke. "It ain't necessarily so". *Stroke* 1992;**23**:1395–9.

26. Ratnatunga CP, Edmondson SF, Rees GM, Kovacs IB. High-dose aspirin inhibits shear-induced platelet reaction involving thrombin generation. *Circulation* 1992;**85**:1077–82.

27. Collaborative overview of randomised trials of antiplatelet therapy–II: Maintenance of vascular graft or arterial patency by antiplatelet therapy. Antiplatelet Trialists' *Collaboration. BMJ* 1994;**308**:159–68.

28. Patrono C. Aspirin as an antiplatelet drug. *N Engl J Med* 1994;**330**:1287–94.

29. Bornstein NM, Karepov VG, Aronovich BD, Gorbulev AY, Treves TA, Korczyn AD. Failure of aspirin treatment after stroke. *Stroke* 1994;**25**:275–7.

30. Helgason CM, Bolin KM, Hoff JA, *et al.* Development of aspirin resistance in persons with previous ischemic stroke. *Stroke* 1994;**25**:2331–6.

31. Boncoraglio GB, Bodini A, Brambilla C, Corsini E, Carriero MR, Parati EA. Aspirin resistance determined with PFA-100 does not predict new thrombotic events in patients with stable ischemic cerebrovascular disease. *Clin Neurol Neurosurg* 2009;**111**:270–3.

32. Coukell AJ, Markham A. Clopidogrel. *Drugs* 1997;**54**:745–50; discussion 51.

33. Harker LA, Bruno JJ. Ticlopidine's mechanism of action on platelets. In Hass WK, Easton JD, eds. *Platelets and Vascular Diseases.* New York: Springer-Verlag, 1993:41–59.

34. Bhatt DL, Bertrand ME, Berger PB, *et al.* Meta-analysis of randomized and registry comparisons of ticlopidine with clopidogrel after stenting. *J Am Coll Cardiol* 2002;**39**:9–14.

35. Bellavance A. Efficacy of ticlopidine and aspirin for prevention of reversible cerebrovascular ischemic events. The Ticlopidine Aspirin Stroke Study. *Stroke* 1993;**24**:1452–7.

36. Gent M, Blakely JA, Easton JD, *et al.* The Canadian American Ticlopidine Study (CATS) in thromboembolic stroke. *Lancet* 1989;**1**:1215–20.

37. Hass WK, Easton JD, Adams HP, Jr., *et al.* A randomized trial comparing ticlopidine hydrochloride with aspirin for the prevention of stroke in high-risk patients. Ticlopidine Aspirin Stroke Study Group. *N Engl J Med* 1989;**321**:501–7.

38. A randomised, blinded, trial of clopidogrel versus aspirin in patients at risk of ischaemic events (CAPRIE). CAPRIE Steering Committee. *Lancet* 1996;**348**:1329–39.

39. Schomig A, Neumann FJ, Kastrati A, *et al.* A randomized comparison of antiplatelet and anticoagulant therapy after the placement of coronary-artery stents. *N Engl J Med* 1996;**334**:1084–9.

40. Wiviott SD, Braunwald E, McCabe CH, *et al.* Prasugrel versus clopidogrel in patients with acute coronary syndromes. *N Engl J Med.* 2007;**357**:2001–15.

41. Bhatt DL. Intensifying platelet inhibition–navigating between Scylla and Charybdis. *N Engl J Med* 2007;**357**:2078–81.

42. Bhatt DL. Prasugrel in clinical practice. *N Engl J Med* 2009;**361**:940–2.

43. Storey RF, Husted S, Harrington RA, *et al.* Inhibition of platelet aggregation by AZD6140, a reversible oral P2Y12 receptor antagonist, compared with clopidogrel in patients with acute coronary syndromes. *J Am Coll Cardiol* 2007;**50**:1852–6.

44. Husted S, Emanuelsson H, Heptinstall S, Sandset PM, Wickens M, Peters G. Pharmacodynamics, pharmacokinetics, and safety of the oral reversible P2Y12 antagonist AZD6140 with aspirin in patients with atherosclerosis: a double-blind comparison to clopidogrel with aspirin. *Eur Heart J* 2006;**27**:1038–47.

45. Wallentin L, Becker RC, Budaj A, *et al.* Ticagrelor versus clopidogrel in patients with acute coronary syndromes. *N Engl J Med* 2009;**361**:1045–57.

46. Coller BS, Peerschke EI, Scudder LE, Sullivan CA. A murine monoclonal antibody that completely blocks the binding of fibrinogen to platelets

produces a thrombasthenic-like state in normal platelets and binds to glycoproteins IIb and/or IIIa. *J Clin Invest* 1983;**72**:325–38.

47. Scarborough RM, Rose JW, Hsu MA, *et al.* Barbourin. A GPIIb-IIIa-specific integrin antagonist from the venom of Sistrurus m. barbouri. *J Biol Chem* 1991;**266**:9359–62.

48. Tam SH, Sassoli PM, Jordan RE, Nakada MT. Abciximab (ReoPro, chimeric 7E3 Fab) demonstrates equivalent affinity and functional blockade of glycoprotein IIb/IIIa and alpha(v)beta3 integrins. *Circulation* 1998;**98**:1085–91.

49. Gowda RM, Khan IA, Vasavada BC, Sacchi TJ. Therapeutics of platelet glycoprotein IIb/IIIa receptor antagonism. *Am J Ther* 2004;**11**:302–7.

50. Bhatt DL, Topol EJ. Current role of platelet glycoprotein IIb/IIIa inhibitors in acute coronary syndromes. *JAMA* 2000;**284**:1549–58.

51. Chew DP, Bhatt DL, Sapp S, Topol EJ. Increased mortality with oral platelet glycoprotein IIb/IIIa antagonists: a meta-analysis of phase III multicenter randomized trials. *Circulation* 2001;**103**:201–6.

52. Randomised placebo-controlled trial of abciximab before and during coronary intervention in refractory unstable angina: the CAPTURE Study. *Lancet* 1997;**349**:1429–35.

53. Use of a monoclonal antibody directed against the platelet glycoprotein IIb/IIIa receptor in high-risk coronary angioplasty. The EPIC Investigation. *N Engl J Med* 1994;**330**:956–61.

54. Platelet glycoprotein IIb/IIIa receptor blockade and low-dose heparin during percutaneous coronary revascularization. The EPILOG Investigators. *N Engl J Med* 1997;**336**:1689–96.

55. Vorchheimer DA, Badimon JJ, Fuster V. Platelet glycoprotein IIb/IIIa receptor antagonists in cardiovascular disease. *JAMA* 1999;**281**:1407–14.

56. Randomised placebo-controlled trial of effect of eptifibatide on complications of percutaneous coronary intervention: IMPACT-II. Integrilin to Minimise Platelet Aggregation and Coronary Thrombosis-II. *Lancet* 1997;**349**:1422–8.

57. Effects of platelet glycoprotein IIb/IIIa blockade with tirofiban on adverse cardiac events in patients with unstable angina or acute myocardial infarction undergoing coronary angioplasty. The RESTORE Investigators. Randomized Efficacy Study of Tirofiban for Outcomes and REstenosis. *Circulation* 1997;**96**:1445–53.

58. Topol EJ, Moliterno DJ, Herrmann HC, *et al.* Comparison of two platelet glycoprotein IIb/IIIa inhibitors, tirofiban and abciximab, for the prevention of ischemic events with percutaneous coronary revascularization. *N Engl J Med* 2001;**344**:1888–94.

59. Aguirre FV, Ferguson JJ, Califf RM for the EPIC Investigators. Clinical predictors of bleeding complications in high risk angioplasty patients: results from the EPIC Study Group (abstract). *Circulation* 1993;**88**, 1–252.

60. Lincoff AM, Tcheng JE, Bass T. A multicenter, randomized, double-blind pilot trial of standard versus low dose weight-adjusted heparin inpatients treated with the platelet GP IIb/IIIa receptor antibody c7E3 during percutaneous coronary revascularization. (abstract). *J Am Coll Cardiol* 1995;**25**:80A–1A.

61. Andrews RK, Berndt MC. Platelet physiology and thrombosis. *Thromb Res* 2004;**114**:447–53.

62. Savage B, Saldivar E, Ruggeri ZM. Initiation of platelet adhesion by arrest onto fibrinogen or translocation on von Willebrand factor. *Cell* 1996;**84**:289–97.

63. Kehrel B. Platelet-collagen interactions. *Semin Thromb Hemost* 1995;**21**:123–9.

64. Kleinschnitz C, Pozgajova M, Pham M, Bendszus M, Nieswandt B, Stoll G. Targeting platelets in acute experimental stroke: impact of glycoprotein Ib, VI, and IIb/IIIa blockade on infarct size, functional outcome, and intracranial bleeding. *Circulation* 2007;**115**:2323–30.

65. Bongers TN, de Maat MP, van Goor ML, *et al.* High von Willebrand factor levels increase the risk of first ischemic stroke: influence of ADAMTS13, inflammation, and genetic variability. *Stroke* 2006;**37**:2672–7.

66. Gilbert JC, DeFeo-Fraulini T, Hutabarat RM, *et al.* First-in-human evaluation of anti von Willebrand factor therapeutic aptamer ARC1779 in healthy volunteers. *Circulation* 2007;**116**:2678–86.

67. Hirsh J. Heparin. *N Engl J Med* 1991;**324**(22):1565–74.

68. Sobel M, McNeill PM, Carlson PL, *et al.* Heparin inhibition of von Willebrand factor-dependent platelet function in vitro and in vivo. *J Clin Invest* 1991;**87**:1787–93.

69. Bell WR, Tomasulo PA, Alving BM, Duffy TP. Thrombocytopenia occurring during the administration of heparin. A prospective study in 52 patients. *Ann Intern Med* 1976;**85**:155–60.

70. Kelton JG, Sheridan D, Brain H, Powers PJ, Turpie AG, Carter CJ. Clinical usefulness of testing for a heparin-dependent platelet-aggregating factor in patients with suspected heparin-associated thrombocytopenia. *J Lab Clin Med* 1984;**103**:606–12.

71. Gruntzig AR, Senning A, Siegenthaler WE. Nonoperative dilatation of coronary-artery stenosis: percutaneous transluminal coronary angioplasty. *N Engl J Med* 1979;**301**:61–8.

72. Bowers J, Ferguson JJ, 3rd. The use of activated clotting times to monitor heparin therapy during and after interventional procedures. *Clin Cardiol* 1994;**17**:357–61.

73. Ferguson JJ, Dougherty KG, Gaos CM, Bush HS, Marsh KC, Leachman DR. Relation between procedural activated coagulation time and outcome after percutaneous transluminal coronary angioplasty. *J Am Coll Cardiol* 1994;**23**:1061–5.

74. Narins CR, Hillegass WB, Jr., Nelson CL, *et al.* Relation between activated clotting time during angioplasty and abrupt closure. *Circulation* 1996;**93**:667–71.

75. Bittl JA, Ahmed WH. Relation between abrupt vessel closure and the anticoagulant response to heparin or bivalirudin during coronary angioplasty. *Am J Cardiol* 1998;**82**:50PV–6P.

76. Ellis SG, Roubin GS, Wilentz J, Douglas JS, Jr., King SB, 3rd. Effect of 18- to 24-hour heparin administration for prevention of restenosis after uncomplicated coronary angioplasty. *Am Heart J* 1989;**117**:777–82.

77. Friedman HZ, Cragg DR, Glazier SM, *et al.* Randomized prospective evaluation of prolonged versus abbreviated intravenous heparin therapy after coronary angioplasty. *J Am Coll Cardiol* 1994;**24**:1214–19.

78. Lincoff AM, Tcheng JE, Califf RM, *et al.* Standard versus low-dose weight-adjusted heparin in patients treated with the platelet glycoprotein IIb/IIIa receptor antibody fragment abciximab (c7E3 Fab) during percutaneous coronary revascularization. PROLOG Investigators. *Am J Cardiol* 1997;**79**:286–91.

79. Weitz JI. Low-molecular-weight heparins. *N Engl J Med* 1997; **337**:688–98.

80. Cade JF, Buchanan MR, Boneu B, *et al.* A comparison of the antithrombotic and haemorrhagic effects of low molecular weight heparin fractions: the influence of the method of preparation. *Thromb Res* 1984;**35**:613–25.

81. Warkentin TE, Levine MN, Hirsh J, *et al.* Heparin-induced thrombocytopenia in patients treated with low-molecular-weight heparin or unfractionated heparin. *N Engl J Med* 1995;**332**:1330–5.

82. Zidar JP. Rationale for low-molecular weight heparin in coronary stenting. *Am Heart J* 1997;**134**:S81–7.

83. Hogg PJ, Jackson CM. Fibrin monomer protects thrombin from inactivation by heparin-antithrombin III: implications for heparin efficacy. *Proc Natl Acad Sci USA* 1989;**86**:3619–23.

84. Arora UK, Dhir M. Direct thrombin inhibitors (part 1 of 2). *J Invasive Cardiol* 2005;**17**:34–8.

85. Bittl JA. Comparative safety profiles of hirulog and heparin in patients undergoing coronary angioplasty. The Hirulog Angioplasty Study Investigators. *Am Heart J* 1995;**130**: 658–65.

86. Ramana RK, Lewis BE. Percutaneous coronary intervention in patients with acute coronary syndrome: focus on bivalirudin. *Vasc Health Risk Manag.* 2008;**4**:493–505.

87. Chamberlin JR, Lewis B, Leya F, *et al.* Successful treatment of heparin-associated thrombocytopenia and thrombosis using Hirulog. *Can J Cardiol* 1995;**11**:511–14.

88. Lincoff AM, Bittl JA, Kleiman NS, *et al.* Comparison of bivalirudin versus heparin during percutaneous coronary intervention (the Randomized Evaluation of PCI Linking Angiomax to Reduced Clinical Events [REPLACE]-1 trial). *Am J Cardiol* 2004;**93**: 1092–6.

89. Bittl JA, Strony J, Brinker JA, *et al.* Treatment with bivalirudin (Hirulog) as compared with heparin during coronary angioplasty for unstable or postinfarction angina. Hirulog Angioplasty Study Investigators. *N Engl J Med* 1995;**333**:764–9.

90. Qureshi AI, Luft AR, Sharma M, Guterman LR, Hopkins LN. Prevention and treatment of thromboembolic and ischemic complications associated with endovascular procedures: Part II–Clinical aspects and recommendations. *Neurosurgery* 2000;**46**:1360–75; discussion 75–6.

91. Georgiadis AL, Shah QS, Suri MFK, Qureshi AI. Adjunct bivalirudin dosing protocol for neuro-endovascular procedures. *J Vasc Intervent Neurol* 2008;**1**:50–3.

92. Cleland JG, Cowburn PJ, Falk RH. Should all patients with atrial fibrillation receive warfarin? Evidence from randomized clinical trials. *Eur Heart J* 1996;**17**:674–81.

93. Schatz RA, Baim DS, Leon M, *et al.* Clinical experience with the Palmaz-Schatz coronary stent. Initial results of a multicenter study. *Circulation* 1991;**83**:148–61.

94. Karrillon GJ, Morice MC, Benveniste E, *et al.* Intracoronary stent implantation without ultrasound guidance and with replacement of conventional anticoagulation by antiplatelet therapy. 30-day clinical outcome of the French Multicenter Registry. *Circulation* 1996;**94**:1519–27.

95. Inoue T, Sakai Y, Fujito T. Expression of activation dependent platelet membrane protein after coronary stenting: A comparison with balloon angioplasty (abstract). *Circulation* 1996;**94**:I–1523.

96. Jordan C, Carvalho H, Fajadet J, *et al.* Reduction of subacute thrombosis rate after coronary stenting using a new anticoagulant protocol (abstract). *Circulation* 1994;**90**:I–125.

97. McKevitt FM, Randall MS, Cleveland TJ, Gaines PA, Tan KT, Venables GS. The benefits of combined anti-platelet treatment in carotid artery stenting. *Eur J Vasc Endovasc Surg* 2005;**29**:522–7.

98. Qureshi AI, Kirmani JF, Harris-Lane P, *et al.* Vertebral artery origin stent placement with distal protection: technical and clinical results. *Am J Neuroradiol* 2006;**27**:1140–5.

99. Harker LA, Marzec UM, Kelly AB, *et al.* Clopidogrel inhibition of stent, graft, and vascular thrombogenesis with antithrombotic enhancement by aspirin in nonhuman primates. *Circulation* 1998;**98**:2461–9.

100. Theron J, Courtheoux P, Alachkar F, Bouvard G, Maiza D. New triple coaxial catheter system for carotid angioplasty with cerebral protection. *Am J Neuroradiol* 1990;**11**:869–74; discussion 75–7.

101. Theron JG, Payelle GG, Coskun O, Huet HF, Guimaraens L. Carotid artery stenosis: treatment with protected balloon angioplasty and stent placement. *Radiology* 1996;**201**:627–36.

102. Mericle RA, Wakhloo AK, Rodriguez R, Guterman LR, Hopkins LN. Temporary balloon protection as an adjunct to endosaccular coiling of wide-necked cerebral aneurysms: technical note. *Neurosurgery* 1997;**41**:975–8.

103. Matthai WH, Jr., Hirshfeld JW, Jr. Choice of contrast agents for cardiac angiography: review and recommendations based on clinically important distinctions. *Cathet Cardiovasc Diagn* 1991;**22**:278–89.

104. Engelhart JA, Smith DC, Maloney MD, Westengard JC, Bull BS. A technique for estimating the probability of clots in blood/contrast agent mixtures. *Invest Radiol* 1988;**23**:923–7.

105. Kimball JP, Sansone VJ, Diters LA, Wissel PS. Red blood cell aggregation versus blood clot formation in ionic and nonionic contrast media. *Invest Radiol* 1988;**23** Suppl 2:S334–9.

106. Grabowski EF. A hematologist's view of contrast media, clotting in angiography syringes and thrombosis during coronary angiography. *Am J Cardiol* 1990;**66**:23F–5F.

107. Stormorken H. Effects of contrast media on the hemostatic and thrombotic mechanisms. *Invest Radiol* 1988;**23**:S318–25.

108. Grollman JH, Jr., Liu CK, Astone RA, Lurie MD. Thromboembolic complications in coronary angiography associated with the use of nonionic contrast medium. *Cathet Cardiovasc Diagn* 1988;**14**:159–64.

109. Hwang MH, Piao ZE, Murdock DK, Messmore HL, Giardina JJ, Scanlon PJ. Risk of thromboembolism during diagnostic and interventional cardiac procedures with nonionic contrast media. *Radiology* 1990;**174**:453–7.

110. Gasperetti CM, Feldman MD, Burwell LR, et al. Influence of contrast media on thrombus formation during coronary angioplasty. *J Am Coll Cardiol* 1991;**18**:443–50.

111. Mabin TA, Holmes DR, Jr., Smith HC, et al. Intracoronary thrombus: role in coronary occlusion complicating percutaneous transluminal coronary angioplasty. *J Am Coll Cardiol* 1985;**5**:198–202.

112. Jacobsson B, Schlossman D. Angiographic investigation of formation of thrombi on vascular catheters. *Radiology* 1969;**93**:355–9.

113. Jacobsson B, Bergentz SE, Ljungqvist U. Platelet adhesion and throms formation on vascular catheters in dogs. *Acta Radiol Diagn* (Stockh) 1969;**8**:221–7.

114. Bourassa MG, Cantin M, Sandborn EB, Pederson E. Scanning electron microscopy of surface irregularities and thrombogenesis of polyurethane and polyethylene coronary catheters. *Circulation* 1976;**53**:992–6.

115. Nachnani GH, Lessin LS, Motomiya T, Jensen WN. Scanning electron microscopy of thrombogenesis on vascular catheter surfaces. *N Engl J Med* 1972;**286**:139–40.

116. Lyman DJ, Brash JL, Klein KG. The effects of chemical structure and surface properties of synthetic polymers on the coagulation of blood. *Proceedings of the Artificial Heart Program Conference*. Washington, DC: National Institutes of Health; 1998. pp. 113–22.

117. Wasiewski W, Fasco MJ, Martin BM, Detwiler TC, Fenton JW. Thrombin adsorption to surfaces and prevention with polyethylene glycol 6,000. *Thromb Res* 1976;**8**:881–6.

118. Wilner GD, Casarella WJ, Baier R, Fenoglio CM. Thrombogenicity of angiographic catheters. *Circ Res* 1978;**43**:424–8.

119. Schlossman D. Thrombogenic properties of vascular catheter materials in vivo. The differences between materials. *Acta Radiol Diagn* (Stockh) 1973;**14**:186–92.

120. Eldh P, Jacobsson B. Heparinized vascular cathers: a clinical trial. *Radiology* 1974;**111**:289–92.

121. Kido DK, Paulin S, Alenghat JA, Waternaux C, Riley WD. Thrombogenicity of heparin- and non-heparin-coated catheters: clinical trial. *Am J Roentgenol* 1982;**139**:957–61.

122. Cramer R, Moore R, Amplatz K. Reduction of the surgical complication rate by the use of a hypothrombogenic catheter coating. *Radiology* 1973;**109**:585–8.

123. Anderson JH, Gianturco C, Wallace S, Dodd GD. A scanning electron microscopic study of angiographic catheters and guide wires. *Radiology* 1974;**111**:567–71.

124. Rashid A, Hildner FJ, Fester A, Javier R, Samet P. Thromboembolism associated with pigtail catheters. *cathet Cardiovasc Diagn* 1975;**1**:183–94.

125. Leach KR, Kurisu Y, Carlson JE, Repa I, Epstein DH, Urness M, et al. Thrombogenicity of hydrophilically coated guide wires and catheters. *Radiology* 1990;**175**:675–7.

126. Kallmes DF, McGraw JK, Evans AJ, et al. Thrombogenicity of hydrophilic and nonhydrophilic microcatheters and guiding catheters. *Am J Neuroradiol* 1997;**18**:1243–51.

127. Baier RE, Dutton RC. Initial events in interactions of blood with a foreign surface. *J Biomed Mater Res* 1969;**3**:191–206.

128. Guglielmi G, Vinuela F, Sepetka I, Macellari V. Electrothrombosis of saccular aneurysms via endovascular approach. Part 1: Electrochemical basis, technique, and experimental results. *J Neurosurg* 1991;**75**:1–7.

129. Byrne JV, Hope JK, Hubbard N, Morris JH. The nature of thrombosis induced by platinum and tungsten coils in saccular aneurysms. *Am J Neuroradiol* 1997;**18**:29–33.

130. Horowitz MB, Purdy PD, Burns D, Bellotto D. Scanning electron microscopic findings in a basilar tip aneurysm embolized with Guglielmi detachable coils. *Am J Neuroradiol* 1997;**18**:688–90.

131. Salam TA, Taylor B, Suggs WD, Hanson SR, Lumsden AB. Reaction to injury following balloon angioplasty and intravascular stent placement in the canine femoral artery. *Am Surg* 1994;**60**:353–7.

132. Krpski WC, Bass A, Kelly AB, Marzec UM, Hanson SR, Harker LA. Heparin-resistant thrombus formation by endovascular stents in baboons. Interruption by a synthetic antithrombin. *Circulation* 1990;**82**:570–7.

133. Werner GS, Gastmann O, Ferrari M, et al. Risk factors for acute and subacute stent thrombosis after high-pressure stent implantation: a study by intracoronary ultrasound. *Am Heart J* 1998;**135**:300–9.

134. Post MJ, de Graaf-Bos AN, van Zanten HG, de Groot PG, Sixma JJ, Borst C. Thrombogenicity of the human arterial wall after interventional thermal injury. *J Vasc Res* 1996;**33**:156–63.

135. Kunstlinger F, Brunelle F, Chaumont P, Doyon D. Vascular occlusive agents. *Am J Roentgenol* 1981;**136**:151–6.

136. Nakabayashi K, Negoro M, Handa T, Keino H, Takahashi M, Sugita K. Evaluation of particulate embolic materials with MR imaging, scanning electron microscopy, and phase-contrast microscopy. *Am J Neuroradiol* 1997;**18**:485–91.

137. Collen D, Lijnen HR. Basic and clinical aspects of fibrinolysis and thrombolysis. *Blood* 1991;**78**:3114–24.

138. DeWood MA, Spores J, Notske R, et al. Prevalence of total coronary occlusion during the early hours of transmural myocardial infarction. *N Engl J Med* 1980;**303**:897–902.

139. Wardlaw JM, Warlow CP, Counsell C. Systematic review of evidence on thrombolytic therapy for acute ischaemic stroke. *Lancet* 1997;**350**:607–14.

140. Topol EJ. Ultrathrombolysis. *J Am Coll Cardiol* 1990;**15**:922–4.

141. Califf RM, Topol EJ, George BS, et al. Hemorrhagic complications associated with the use of intravenous tissue plasminogen activator in treatment of acute myocardial infarction. *Am J Med* 1988;**85**:353–9.

142. de Boer A, Kluft C, Gerloff J, et al. Pharmacokinetics of saruplase, a recombinant unglycosylated human single-chain urokinase-type plasminogen activator and its effects on fibrinolytic and haemostatic parameters in healthy male subjects. *Thromb Haemost* 1993;**70**:320–5.

143. Kounnas MZ, Henkin J, Argraves WS, Strickland DK. Low density lipoprotein receptor-related protein/alpha 2-macroglobulin receptor mediates cellular uptake of pro-urokinase. *J Biol Chem* 1993;**268**:21862–7.

144. del Zoppo GJ, Higashida RT, Furlan AJ, Pessin MS, Rowley HA, Gent M. PROACT: a phase II randomized trial of recombinant pro-urokinase by direct arterial delivery in acute middle cerebral artery stroke. PROACT Investigators. Prolyse in Acute Cerebral Thromboembolism. *Stroke* 1998;**29**:4–11.

145. Antman EM, Giugliano RP, Gibson CM, *et al.* Abciximab facilitates the rate and extent of thrombolysis: results of the thrombolysis in myocardial infarction (TIMI) 14 trial. The TIMI 14 Investigators. *Circulation* 1999;**99**: 2720–32.

146. Ohman EM, Kleiman NS, Gacioch G, *et al.* Combined accelerated tissue-plasminogen activator and platelet glycoprotein IIb/IIIa integrin receptor blockade with Integrilin in acute myocardial infarction. Results of a randomized, placebo-controlled, dose-ranging trial. IMPACT-AMI Investigators. *Circulation* 1997;**95**:846–54.

147. Qureshi AI, Harris-Lane P, Kirmani JF, *et al.* Intra-arterial reteplase and intravenous abciximab in patients with acute ischemic stroke: an open-label, dose-ranging, phase I study. *Neurosurgery* 2006;**59**:789–96; discussion 96–7.

148. McCarthy MW, Kockler DR. Clopidogrel-associated leukopenia. *Ann Pharmacother* 2003;**37**:216–19.

149. Kilickiran Avci B, Oto A, Ozcebe O. Thrombocytopenia associated with antithrombotic therapy in patients with cardiovascular diseases: diagnosis and treatment. *Am J Cardiovasc Drugs* 2008;**8**:327–39.

150. Wang TY, Ou FS, Roe MT, *et al.* Incidence and prognostic significance of thrombocytopenia developed during acute coronary syndrome in contemporary clinical practice. *Circulation* 2009;**119**:2454–62.

151. Harker LA, Boissel JP, Pilgrim AJ, Gent M. Comparative safety and tolerability of clopidogrel and aspirin: results from CAPRIE. CAPRIE Steering Committee and Investigators. Clopidogrel versus aspirin in patients at risk of ischaemic events. *Drug Saf* 1999;**21**:325–35.

152. Adgey AA. An overview of the results of clinical trials with glycoprotein IIb/IIIa inhibitors. *Eur Heart J* 1998;**19**:D10–21.

153. Gammie JS, Zenati M, Kormos RL, *et al.* Abciximab and excessive bleeding in patients undergoing emergency cardiac operations. *Ann Thorac Surg* 1998;**65**:465–9.

154. Berkowitz SD, Harrington RA, Rund MM, Tcheng JE. Acute profound thrombocytopenia after C7E3 Fab (abciximab) therapy. *Circulation* 1997;**95**:809–13.

155. O'Shea JC, Madan M, Cantor WJ, *et al.* Design and methodology of the ESPRIT trial: evaluating a novel dosing regimen of eptifibatide in percutaneous coronary intervention. *Am Heart J* 2000;**140**:834–9.

156. Tcheng JE. A symposium: safety issues concerning the use of glycoprotein IIb-IIIa inhibitors in the management of acute coronary syndromes. *Am Heart J* 1999;**138**:261–2.

157. Simoons ML, de Boer MJ, van den Brand MJ, *et al.* Randomized trial of a GPIIb/IIIa platelet receptor blocker in refractory unstable angina. European Cooperative Study Group. *Circulation* 1994;**89**:596–603.

158. Kleiman NS, Ohman EM, Califf RM, *et al.* Profound inhibition of platelet aggregation with monoclonal antibody 7E3 Fab after thrombolytic therapy. Results of the Thrombolysis and Angioplasty in Myocardial Infarction (TAMI) 8 Pilot Study. *J Am Coll Cardiol* 1993;**22**:381–9.

159. Dasgupta H, Blankenship JC, Wood GC, Frey CM, Demko SL, Menapace FJ. Thrombocytopenia complicating treatment with intravenous glycoprotein IIb/IIIa receptor inhibitors: a pooled analysis. *Am Heart J* 2000;**140**:206–11.

160. Shantsila E, Lip GY, Chong BH. Heparin-induced thrombocytopenia. A contemporary clinical approach to diagnosis and management. *Chest* 2009;**135**:1651–64.

161. Kahl K, Heidrich H. The incidence of heparin-induced thrombocytopenias. *Int J Angiol* 1998;**7**:255–7.

162. Bennett CL, Kim B, Zakarija A, *et al.* Two mechanistic pathways for thienopyridine-associated thrombotic thrombocytopenic purpura: a report from the SERF-TTP Research Group and the RADAR Project. *J Am Coll Cardiol* 2007;**50**:1138–43.

163. Moy B, Wang JC, Raffel GD, Marcoux JP, 2nd. Hemolytic uremic syndrome associated with clopidogrel: a case report. *Arch Intern Med* 2000;**160**:1370–2.

164. Oomen PH, Tulleken JE, Zijlstra JG. Hemolytic uremic syndrome in a patient treated with clopidogrel. *Ann Intern Med* 2000;**132**:1006.

165. ReoPro (R) product information. *Eli Lilly Co.*; 2003.

166. Sane DC, Damaraju LV, Topol EJ, *et al.* Occurrence and clinical significance of pseudothrombocytopenia during abciximab therapy. *J Am Coll Cardiol* 2000;**36**:75–83.

167. Dukes M. *Meyler's Side Effects of Drugs.* 11th edn. Amsterdam: Elsevier, 1988.

168. Samter M, Beers RF, Jr. Intolerance to aspirin. Clinical studies and consideration of its pathogenesis. *Ann Intern Med* 1968;**68**:975–83.

169. McDonald JR, Mathison DA, Stevenson DD. Aspirin intolerance in asthma. Detection by oral challenge. *J Allergy Clin Immunol* 1972;**50**:198–207.

170. Speer F, Denison TR, Baptist JE. Aspirin allergy. *Ann Allergy.* 1981;**46**:123–6.

171. Mathison DA, Stevenson DD, Simon RA. Precipitating factors in asthma. Aspirin, sulfites, and other drugs and chemicals. *Chest* 1985;**87**:50S–4S.

172. Plavix(R) product information Bristol-Myers Squibb/Sanofi Pharmaceuticals Partnership; 2005.

173. Doogue MP, Begg EJ, Bridgman P. Clopidogrel hypersensitivity syndrome with rash, fever, and neutropenia. *Mayo Clin Proc* 2005;**80**:1368–70.

174. McKenzie DB, Rao U, Hobson A, Levy T, Talwar S, Swallow R. A novel strategy for managing clopidogrel-induced adverse skin reactions. *EuroIntervention* 2009;**5**:470–4.

175. Topol EJ, Lincoff AM, Kereiakes DJ, *et al.* Multi-year follow-up of abciximab therapy in three randomized, placebo-controlled trials of percutaneous coronary revascularization. *Am J Med* 2002;**113**:1–6.

176. Lincoff AM, LeNarz LA, Despotis GJ, *et al.* Abciximab and bleeding during coronary surgery: results from the EPILOG and EPISTENT trials. Improve Long-term Outcome with abciximab GP IIb/IIIa blockade. Evaluation of Platelet IIb/IIIa Inhibition in STENTing. *Ann Thorac Surg* 2000;**70**:516–26.

177. Hamm CW, Heeschen C, Goldmann B, *et al.* Benefit of abciximab in patients with refractory unstable angina in

55

relation to serum troponin T levels. c7E3 Fab Antiplatelet Therapy in Unstable Refractory Angina (CAPTURE) Study Investigators. *N Engl J Med* 1999;**340**:1623–9.

178. Moneret-Vautrin DA, Morisset M, Vignaud JM, Kanny G. T cell mediated allergy to abciximab. *Allergy* 2002;**57**:269–70.

179. Bates SM, Greer IA, Pabinger I, Sofaer S, Hirsh J. Venous thromboembolism, thrombophilia, antithrombotic therapy, and pregnancy: American College of Chest Physicians Evidence-Based Clinical Practice Guidelines (8th Edition). *Chest* 2008;**133**:844S–86S.

180. Chan WS, Anand S, Ginsberg JS. Anticoagulation of pregnant women with mechanical heart valves: a systematic review of the literature. *Arch Intern Med* 2000;**160**:191–6.

181. Coomarasamy A, Honest H, Papaioannou S, Gee H, Khan KS. Aspirin for prevention of preeclampsia in women with historical risk factors: a systematic review. *Obstet Gynecol* 2003;**101**:1319–32.

182. Kozer E, Nikfar S, Costei A, Boskovic R, Nulman I, Koren G. Aspirin consumption during the first trimester of pregnancy and congenital anomalies: a meta-analysis. *Am J Obstet Gynecol* 2002;**187**:1623–30.

183. Sacco RL, Adams R, Albers G, *et al.* Guidelines for prevention of stroke in patients with ischemic stroke or transient ischemic attack: a statement for healthcare professionals from the American Heart Association/American Stroke Association Council on Stroke: co-sponsored by the Council on Cardiovascular Radiology and Intervention: the American Academy of Neurology affirms the value of this guideline. *Stroke* 2006;**37**:577–617.

184. Chaplin S, Sanders G, Smith J. Drug excretion in human breast milk. *Adv Drug React Ac Pois Rev* 1982;**1**:255–87.

185. Unsworth J, d'Assis-Fonseca A, Beswick DT, Blake DR. Serum salicylate levels in a breast fed infant. *Ann Rheum Dis* 1987;**46**:638–9.

186. Richter C, Sitzmann J, Lang P, Weitzel H, Huch A, Huch R. Excretion of low molecular weight heparin in human milk. *Br J Clin Pharmacol* 2001;**52**:708–10.

187. Schindewolf M, Magnani HN, Lindhoff-Last E [Danaparoid in pregnancy in cases of heparin intolerance – use in 59 cases]. *Hamostaseologie* 2007;**27**:89–97.

188. Lindhoff-Last E, Willeke A, Thalhammer C, Nowak G, Bauersachs R. Hirudin treatment in a breastfeeding woman. *Lancet* 2000;**355**:467–8.

189. Harrington RA, Kleiman NS, Granger CB, Ohman EM, Berkowitz SD. Relation between inhibition of platelet aggregation and clinical outcomes. *Am Heart J* 1998;**136**:S43–50.

190. Faxon DP, Freedman JE. Facts and controversies of aspirin and clopidogrel therapy. *Am Heart J* 2009;**157**:412–22.

191. Lordkipanidze M, Pharand C, Nguyen TA, Schampaert E, Palisaitis DA, Diodati JG. Comparison of four tests to assess inhibition of platelet function by clopidogrel in stable coronary artery disease patients. *Eur Heart J* 2008;**29**:2877–85.

192. Lordkipanidze M, Pharand C, Schampaert E, Turgeon J, Palisaitis DA, Diodati JG. A comparison of six major platelet function tests to determine the prevalence of aspirin resistance in patients with stable coronary artery disease. *Eur Heart J* 2007;**28**:1702–8.

193. Guthikonda S, Lev EI, Kleiman NS. Resistance to antiplatelet therapy. *Curr Cardiol Rep* 2005;**7**:242–8.

194. Brandt JT, Payne CD, Wiviott SD, *et al.* A comparison of prasugrel and clopidogrel loading doses on platelet function: magnitude of platelet inhibition is related to active metabolite formation. *Am Heart J* 2007;**153**: 66 e9–16.

195. Catella-Lawson F, Reilly MP, Kapoor SC, *et al.* Cyclooxygenase inhibitors and the antiplatelet effects of aspirin. *N Engl J Med* 2001;**345**:1809–17.

196. Saw J, Steinhubl SR, Berger PB, *et al.* Lack of adverse clopidogrel-atorvastatin clinical interaction from secondary analysis of a randomized, placebo-controlled clopidogrel trial. *Circulation* 2003;**108**:921–4.

197. Wienbergen H, Gitt AK, Schiele R, *et al.* Comparison of clinical benefits of clopidogrel therapy in patients with acute coronary syndromes taking atorvastatin versus other statin therapies. *Am J Cardiol* 2003;**92**:285–8.

198. Administration USFaD. Concomitant use of ibuprofen and aspirin: potential for attenuation of the anti-platelet effect of aspirin. 2006 [cited April 2008]; Available from: www.fda.gov/CDER/Drug/InfoSheets/HCP/ibuprofen_aspirinHCP.htm

199. Kurth T, Glynn RJ, Walker AM, *et al.* Inhibition of clinical benefits of aspirin on first myocardial infarction by nonsteroidal antiinflammatory drugs. *Circulation* 2003;**108**:1191–5.

200. Lau WC, Gurbel PA. Antiplatelet drug resistance and drug-drug interactions: Role of cytochrome P450 3A4. *Pharm Res* 2006;**23**:2691–708.

201. Brandt JT, Close SL, Iturria SJ, *et al.* Common polymorphisms of CYP2C19 and CYP2C9 affect the pharmacokinetic and pharmacodynamic response to clopidogrel but not prasugrel. *J Thromb Haemost* 2007;**5**:2429–36.

202. Trenk D, Hochholzer W, Fromm MF, *et al.* Cytochrome P450 2C19 681G>A polymorphism and high on-clopidogrel platelet reactivity associated with adverse 1-year clinical outcome of elective percutaneous coronary intervention with drug-eluting or bare-metal stents. *J Am Coll Cardiol* 2008;**51**:1925–34.

203. Suh JW, Koo BK, Zhang SY, *et al.* Increased risk of atherothrombotic events associated with cytochrome P450 3A5 polymorphism in patients taking clopidogrel. *CMAJ* 2006;**174**:1715–22.

204. Spertus JA, Kettelkamp R, Vance C, *et al.* Prevalence, predictors, and outcomes of premature discontinuation of thienopyridine therapy after drug-eluting stent placement: results from the PREMIER registry. *Circulation* 2006;**113**:2803–9.

205. Eagle KA, Kline-Rogers E, Goodman SG, *et al.* Adherence to evidence-based therapies after discharge for acute coronary syndromes: an ongoing prospective, observational study. *Am J Med* 2004;**117**:73–81.

206. Newby LK, Bhapkar MV, White HD, *et al.* Aspirin use post-acute coronary syndromes: intolerance, bleeding and discontinuation. *J Thromb Thrombolysis* 2003;**16**:119–28.

207. Schwartz KA, Schwartz DE, Ghosheh K, Reeves MJ, Barber K, DeFranco A. Compliance as a critical consideration in patients who appear to be resistant to aspirin after healing of myocardial infarction. *Am J Cardiol* 2005;**95**:973–5.

208. von Pape KW, Strupp G, Bonzel T, Bohner J. Effect of compliance and

dosage adaptation of long term aspirin on platelet function with PFA-100 in patients after myocardial infarction. *Thromb Haemost* 2005;**94**:889–91.

209. Barsky AA, Arora RR. Clopidogrel resistance: myth or reality? *J Cardiovasc Pharmacol Ther* 2006;**11**(1):47–53.

210. Krasopoulos G, David TE, Armstrong S. Custom-tailored valved conduit for complex aortic root disease. *J Thorac Cardiovasc Surg* 2008;**135**:3–7.

211. Wiviott SD. Clopidogrel response variability, resistance, or both? *Am J Cardiol* 2006;**98**:18N–24N.

212. Bonello L, Camoin-Jau L, Arques S, et al. Adjusted clopidogrel loading doses according to vasodilator-stimulated phosphoprotein phosphorylation index decrease rate of major adverse cardiovascular events in patients with clopidogrel resistance: a multicenter randomized prospective study. *J Am Coll Cardiol* 2008;**51**:1404–11.

213. Hovens MM, Snoep JD, Eikenboom JC, van der Bom JG, Mertens BJ, Huisman MV. Prevalence of persistent platelet reactivity despite use of aspirin: a systematic review. *Am Heart J* 2007;**153**:175–81.

214. Wiviott SD, Trenk D, Frelinger AL, et al. Prasugrel compared with high loading- and maintenance-dose clopidogrel in patients with planned percutaneous coronary intervention: the Prasugrel in Comparison to Clopidogrel for Inhibition of Platelet Activation and Aggregation-Thrombolysis in Myocardial Infarction 44 trial. *Circulation* 2007;**116**:2923–32.

215. Burns TL, Mooss AN, Hilleman DE. Antiplatelet drug resistance: not ready for prime time. *Pharmacotherapy* 2005;**25**:1621–8.

216. Michos ED, Ardehali R, Blumenthal RS, Lange RA, Ardehali H. Aspirin and clopidogrel resistance. *Mayo Clin Proc* 2006;**81**:518–26.

217. Fujii Y, Takeuchi S, Koike T, Nishimaki K, Ito Y, Tanaka R, et al. Heparin administration and monitoring for neuroangiography. *Am J Neuroradiol* 1994;**15**:51–4.

218. Scott JA, Berenstein A, Blumenthal D. Use of the activated coagulation time as a measure of anticoagulation during interventional procedures. *Radiology* 1986;**158**:849–50.

219. Reiner JS, Coyne KS, Lundergan CF, Ross AM. Bedside monitoring of heparin therapy: comparison of activated clotting time to activated partial thromboplastin time. *Cathet Cardiovasc Diagn* 1994;**32**:49–52.

220. Aylsworth CL, Stefan F, Woitas K, Rieger RH, LeBoutillier M, 3rd, DiSesa VJ. New technology, old standards: disparate activated clotting time measurements by the Hemochron Jr compared with the standard Hemochron. *Ann Thorac Surg* 2004;**77**:973–6.

221. Verska JJ. Control of heparinization by activated clotting time during bypass with improved postoperative hemostasis. *Ann Thorac Surg* 1977;**24**:170–3.

222. Young JA, Kisker CT, Doty DB. Adequate anticoagulation during cardiopulmonary bypass determined by activated clotting time and the appearance of fibrin monomer. *Ann Thorac Surg* 1978;**26**:231–40.

223. Niles SD, Sutton RG, Ploessl J, Pennell B. Correlation of ACT as measured with three commercially available devices with circulating heparin level during cardiac surgery. *J Extra Corpor Technol* 1995;**27**:197–200.

224. Kubalek R, Berlis A, Schwab M, Klisch J, Schumacher M. Activated clotting time or activated partial thromboplastin time as the method of choice for patients undergoing neuroradiological intervention. *Neuroradiology* 2003;**45**:325–7.

225. Kurec AS, Morris MW, Davey FR. Clotting, activated partial thromboplastin and coagulation times in monitoring heparin therapy. *Ann Clin Lab Sci* 1979;**9**:494–500.

226. Bechtel JF, Prosch J, Sievers HH, Bartels C. Is the kaolin or celite activated clotting time affected by tranexamic acid? *Ann Thorac Surg* 2002;**74**:390–3; discussion 3.

227. Wendel HP, Heller W, Gallimore MJ, Bantel H, Muller-Beissenhirtz H, Hoffmeister HE. The prolonged activated clotting time (ACT) with aprotinin depends on the type of activator used for measurement. *Blood Coagul Fibrinolysis* 1993;**4**:41–5.

228. Doherty TM, Shavelle RM, French WJ. Reproducibility and variability of activated clotting time measurements in the cardiac catheterization laboratory. *Catheter Cardiovasc Interv* 2005;**65**:330–7.

229. Svenmarker S, Appelblad M, Jansson E, Haggmark S. Measurement of the activated clotting time during cardiopulmonary bypass: differences between Hemotec ACT and Hemochron Jr apparatus. *Perfusion* 2004;**19**:289–94.

230. Zisman E, Rozenberg B, Katz Y, Ziser A. A comparison between arterial- and venous-sampled activated clotting time measurements. *Isr J Med Sci* 1997;**33**:786–8.

231. Kerensky RA, Azar GJ, Jr., Bertolet B, Hill JA, Kutcher MA. Venous activated clotting time after intra-arterial heparin: effect of site of administration and timing of sampling. *Cathet Cardiovasc Diagn* 1996;**37**:151–3.

232. Casserly IP, Topol EJ, Jia G, et al. Effect of abciximab versus tirofiban on activated clotting time during percutaneous intervention and its relation to clinical outcomes–observations from the TARGET trial. *Am J Cardiol* 2003;**92**:125–9.

Alexandros L. Georgiadis MD, Mustapha A. Ezzeddine MD and Adnan I. Qureshi MD

Introduction

The post-procedure care of patients undergoing endovascular procedures is essential in order to achieve good outcomes and prevent potentially catastrophic complications.

The intensivist taking over the care of the patient must have knowledge of:

- Basic principles of neuroendovascular procedures, especially with regard to peri-procedural medications that are commonly used
- The specific procedure performed and medications administered
- The result of the procedure and other relevant findings
- Potential complications
- The results of post-procedural neuroimaging studies if any were performed
- Essential medications for the post-procedural period (such as anti-platelets, renal prophylaxis, etc.)
- The patient's neurological and medical history.

We will first review some general principles and then discuss the post-procedure management of specific interventions.

Important aspects of endovascular interventions

Use of medications

Anticoagulation

Intravenous heparin is used in all neuro-interventional procedures. All sheaths and catheters are continuously flushed with heparinized saline in order to prevent clot formation. Prior to microcatheter insertion, a heparin bolus is administered to achieve a target activated clotting time (ACT) of 250–300 or 300–350 seconds, depending on the procedure and institutional practice. ACT is maintained at that level for the duration of catheter manipulation. The total dose of heparin administered is usually in the 3000 to 10 000 Unit range. Inadvertent excessive anticoagulation is not an infrequent occurrence. In the absence of serious hemorrhagic complications, anticoagulation is not

reversed at the end of the procedure to avoid potential thromboembolic complications.

Anti-platelet medications

Aspirin and clopidogrel are used routinely in patients undergoing angioplasty and/or stent placement. Those agents are initiated 3 to 5 days prior to scheduled procedures so that optimal anti-platelet effect has been achieved by the time of the intervention. To avoid thrombotic complications, it is essential that both medications continue to be administered in the post-procedure period. Intravenous antiplatelets glycoprotein ((GP) IIB/IIIA inhibitors) are used in patients who are deemed to be at high risk for thrombosis or re-thrombosis. A bolus is administered during or at the end of the procedure and is followed by continuous infusion typically for 12–24 hours.

Sedatives, analgesics and anesthetics

Neuro-interventional procedures that do not involve catheterization of the intra-cerebral vasculature are performed, when possible, in awake, sedated patients. This approach offers the advantage of continuous neurological monitoring and avoids the risks of general anesthesia. Extracranial artery angioplasty and stent placement and embolization for epistaxis and extracranial tumors fall into this category. Intra-arterial thrombolysis can also be performed without general anesthesia in patients who are cooperative. More elaborate intracerebral procedures, such as aneurysm and AVM embolization and intracranial angioplasty and stent placement are usually performed under general anesthesia.

In awake patients, intravenous benzodiazepines and opiates are commonly used for two reasons: (1) to achieve anxiolysis and sedation so as to minimize agitation and movement, and (2) to relieve the back pain that is frequent in longer procedures, especially among the elderly patients.

When assessing the patients' neurological status following the procedure, knowledge of the dosing and timing of such medications is essential. Table 4.1 lists some important characteristics of the most commonly used drugs.

Textbook of Interventional Neurology, ed. Adnan I. Qureshi. Published by Cambridge University Press. © Cambridge University Press 2011.

Table 4.1. Pharmacological properties of commonly used analgesic and hypnotic agents

	Pharmacological effect (minutes)		Half life	Approximate duration of action	Prolonged effect with repeated or prolonged dosing	Cardio-vascular effects	Usual mode of administration	Usual dose	Dose adjustment necessary	
	Onset	Peak							Hepatic failure	Renal failure
Morphine	2–5	15	2 h	1 h	Yes	++	IV bolus	2–4 mg	Yes	Yes
Fentanyl	<1	5	3–4 h	30–60 mins	Yes	+	IV bolus	25–50 µg	Yes	Yes
Remifentanil	<1	2–3	8–20 mins	15 mins	No	+	Infusion	0.05–01 µg/kg/min	No	No
Propofol	<1	<1	3–12 h	3–10 mins	Yes	++	Infusion and IV bolus	0.5–1 mg/kg 5–50 µg/kg/min	No	No
Midazolam	1.5–5	20–60	3 h	2–6 h	Yes	+	IV bolus	1–2 mg	Yes	Yes

Please note that elderly patients may require lower doses. In general, cautious incremental dosing is the preferred practice. In case of continuous infusions the time period listed reflects the duration of action after discontinuation of the infusion. Abbreviations used: min = minute; h = hour; IV = intravenous.

Intravenous fluids

As mentioned above, the sheaths and catheters are continuously flushed with heparinized saline. Depending on the length of the procedure and the number and gauge of the catheters used, a patient can receive between 1000 mL and 5000 mL of infusions. Unlike in surgical procedures, blood products are not commonly used. It is important to note urinary output, so as to assess the fluid balance during the procedure, especially for patients with cardiac compromise.

Renal prophylaxis

In order to minimize the risk of contrast-induced nephropathy in susceptible patients, *N*-acetylcysteine is administered twice before and twice after the procedure at a dose of 600–1200 mg.[1] Maintaining adequate hydration before and after the procedure is also of great importance.[1] More details are provided in Chapter 2.

Potential sources of complications

Even in successful procedures, difficulties are sometimes encountered that can lead to immediate or delayed complications. Moreover, some techniques that may be applied can also be inherently associated with specific risks. Table 4.2 gives an overview of techniques and inadvertent events and the complications that can be associated with them.

Post-procedure imaging

Post-procedure imaging is performed routinely following intra-arterial thrombolysis. Non-contrasted computed tomographic (CT) is the imaging of choice. The main purpose of post-thrombolysis CT scan is to exclude intracerebral hemorrhage, but in some occasions, other important information, such as the presence of early edema and mass effect can be ascertained. It must be noted that the interpretation of

potential hemorrhagic findings is often confounded by the presence of extravasated contrast.

Following all other procedures, CT scan is performed only when there is suspicion of a complication, or if the patient cannot be clinically assessed. The scan is then examined for the presence of intraparenchymal or subarachnoid hemorrhage and accompanying hydrocephalus. Early ischemic changes are generally not discernible on CT scans. Scans are best performed prior to the patient's transfer to the intensive care unit (ICU).

General principles of post-procedure monitoring

State-of-the-art care is provided in a dedicated neuro-ICU led by a trained neurointensivist and specialized nurses. In the absence of complications, monitoring extends over 24 hours.

Monitoring of neurological status

Immediately after the procedure, or following recovery from anesthesia, a full neurological assessment has to be performed and documented by the endovascular team. A brief neurological examination is then performed hourly by the nursing staff as is standard practice for all neuro-ICU patients. Any change in examination should prompt immediate assessment by the neuro-intensivist team.

Cardiovascular and respiratory monitoring

Tight blood pressure control is crucial in the care of endovascular patients, especially following AVM embolization, thrombolysis, and carotid artery angioplasty and/or stent placement (see p. 00).

Table 4.2. Intra-procedure techniques and events and the associated complications

Event	Possible complication
Supra-inguinal puncture	Retroperitoneal hematoma
Multiple punctures	Access site hematoma
Intra-vascular entrapment of a wire or device	Thromboembolic complications
Excessive instrumentation (e.g. use of "buddy wires", use of dual microwire or microcatheter techniques)	Dissection or vasospasm
Distal positioning of guidecatheters necessitated by system instability	
Difficulty encountered when crossing a stenotic lesion	
Difficulty in stent delivery requiring multiple attempts or multiple angioplasties	
Visible intravascular thrombus formation	
Significant atherosclerosis of navigated vessels	
Coil protrusion/prolapse	
Stent-assisted coil-embolization	
Balloon-assisted coil-embolization	
Reflux of therapeutic embolic material into normal arteries	
Aneurysm puncture/rupture	Subarachnoid hemorrhage
Incomplete filling of the aneurysm	
Reflux of therapeutic embolic material into the venous system	Intraparenchymal hemorrhage
Intra-procedure hemodynamic instability	Post-procedure hemodynamic instability

While blood pressure monitoring using automated cuff measurements every 10 to 15 minutes might suffice in some cases, continuous intra-arterial blood pressure assessment is recommended for patients with unstable blood pressure, or patients requiring frequent administration of medication in order to stay in the desired blood pressure range. For such patients, radial artery catheterization is the first choice, followed by brachial artery catheterization. Femoral artery catheters are generally used only in unstable patients. If the femoral sheath has been left in place, then blood pressure readings can be transduced from the existing catheter.

Heart rate and rhythm are recorded on a continuous basis using standard ICU monitoring systems. Hemodynamic instability should be anticipated in patients who have undergone carotid angioplasty and/or stent placement. On the other hand, significant changes in hemodynamic parameters may indicate a neurologic event and warrant prompt neurologic assessment.

Most endovascular patients do not require ventilatory support during their ICU stay. As mentioned above, some procedures are performed under conscious sedation and when general anesthesia has been used, patients are generally extubated following recovery, provided that there are no major neurologic complications. In most cases where respiratory compromise is encountered, it is either secondary to large doses of opiates or benzodiazepines administered during the procedure, or secondary to neurologic deterioration. Continuous assessment of respiratory rate and oxygen saturation is performed as a standard practice for almost all ICU patients.

Percutaneous access site monitoring
Following removal of the arterial sheath

The arterial sheath is removed at the end of the procedure provided that ACT is less than 200 seconds. If it is slightly above 200 seconds, the patient can remain in the angio suite until a repeat measurement shows the desired value. If the ACT is excessively high, or if intravenous anti-platelet agents have been initiated, removal of the sheath is deferred. The same is true if a repeat procedure is anticipated.

After the sheath is removed, manual pressure is applied for a minimum of 15 minutes, focally, just proximal to the insertion site. Use of a closure device can reduce this time to 2 to 5 minutes. In a minority of patients, the pain related with the intense pressure can lead to a vagal response of bradycardia and hypotension, which may require administration of intravenous atropine.

Before the patient is transported, it is essential that the site has been inspected for swelling and/or bleeding for an additional 5 to 10 minutes. Thereafter, the relevant extremity needs to be immobilized for 6 hours (or 2 to 3 hours if a closure device has been used). The insertion site is inspected every 15 minutes for the first hour and at least once hourly for the following 5 hours. Pedal pulses, temperature, and coloration of the limb are assessed. Bleeding and swelling around the insertion site should be recognized immediately. If mild bleeding or oozing is noted, manual pressure must be applied as needed, and can be followed by application of a pressure dressing. If mechanical pressure devices are used, adequate perfusion of the distal limb has to be ensured.

In cases of severe or refractory bleeding, red blood cells should be held available and anticoagulation may need to be reversed. Surgical exploration is to be considered if hemostasis cannot be achieved within 2 hours or if the patient becomes hemodynamically unstable.

Retroperitoneal hemorrhage can ensue if the anterior or posterior wall of the common femoral artery is punctured proximal or adjacent to the inguinal ligament. The most common manifestation is hypotension which may be refractory to fluid boluses and require administration of vasopressors. The patients may complain of abdominal or flank pain. In the initial phase, hemoglobin levels may still be normal. Definitive diagnosis is made by CT scan of the abdomen. Surgical exploration should be considered in cases of significant hemodynamic instability.

With indwelling arterial sheath

In patients with an indwelling arterial sheath, typically in the common femoral artery, the goal is to prevent sheath thrombosis, which could result in distal limb ischemia. The sheath is flushed continuously with a solution containing 1000 to 5000 Units of heparin in 1000 mL of normal saline. The rate of infusion is adjusted to maintain minimal antegrade flow and thus prevent backflow of blood into the sheath. The limb must be inspected every hour as described above.

If oozing or bleeding is present, the first measure should be application of local pressure. With the sheath in place, the perfusion or pressure applied should be moderate to avoid thrombotic complications. The same principle is true for pressure dressings; and mechanical pressure devices should be used cautiously. If the bleeding cannot be stopped, then there are three options available. One is to reverse anticoagulation if feasible, leave the sheath in place and observe further. The second is to exchange the sheath over the wire for a larger gauge sheath (e.g., a 5-F for a 6-F sheath). The final option is to remove the sheath with or without previous reversal of anticoagulation. The decision how to proceed is made on a case-by-case basis.

Post-procedure management for specific neuro-endovascular interventions

Each neuro-endovascular intervention has unique post-procedure management requirements because of the differences in baseline characteristics of the selected patients, in the pathophysiology of the underlying disease, and in devices and medications used.

Intra-arterial thrombolysis for acute ischemic stroke
Management of intracranial hemorrhage

Intra-arterial thrombolysis is always followed by a CT scan of the head. If intracranial hemorrhage is present, protamine is administered in order to reverse heparin-mediated anticoagulation. Thrombolytics have very short half-lives and no specific agent is available to reverse their effect. If GP IIB/IIIA inhibitors have been used, it is necessary to transfuse platelets.

Blood pressure management

The available data on the effect of blood pressure control is derived from studies of intravenous thrombolysis. It is, however, reasonable to presume that these principles apply to intra-arterial thrombolysis as well. It must be noted that available data are limited by the fact that patients with refractory hypertension were excluded from thrombolysis and that some of the newer anti-hypertensive agents were not used.

Hypertension and ICH

Based on the criteria of the NINDS recombinant tissue plasminogen activator (rt-PA) efficacy trial[2] blood pressure elevations are tolerated up to 180/105 mmHg. Lack of strict blood pressure control following intravenous thrombolysis has been shown to be associated with an increased risk of ICH. Some of the studies that have shown the association between hypertension and ICH are quoted below.

In a large audit of practices and outcomes of 29 hospitals in the Cleveland area,[3] NINDS blood pressure parameters were not followed in 52% of 70 patients treated with intravenous thrombolysis. The rate of symptomatic ICH among those patients was 16%. After a quality improvement program was implemented in nine of those hospitals, non-compliance to blood pressure parameters dropped to 6%.[4] Symptomatic ICH was observed in only 6% of the 47 patients that were treated.

In the Australian Streptokinase Trial,[5] baseline systolic blood pressure in excess of 165 mmHg was associated with a 25% increased risk of major ICH among the treated patients.

In a multi-center retrospective and prospective analysis[6] of data from 1205 patients treated in routine clinical practice with intravenous rt-PA within 3 hours from symptom onset, elevated pre-treatment mean arterial pressure led to an increased rate of ICH.

Hypertension as an independent outcome predictor

In the NINDS rt-PA trial,[7] the frequency, course, and treatment of hypertension were recorded during the first 24 hours after randomization. It was shown that patients with post-randomization hypertension (24% of all rt-PA treated patients) did not have higher ICH rates if they were treated appropriately. However, their rates of favorable outcomes at 3 months were lower. Sudden or prolonged blood pressure drops that could in part account for this finding were not noted. The correlation between persistent hypertension and poor prognosis has also been established in a systematic review by Willmot and colleagues,[8] while Mattle *et al.* have produced data that suggest that systolic blood pressure is inversely associated with recanalization.[9] It is therefore reasonable to assume that hypertension in the setting of acute stroke is a marker of poor outcome because it reflects lack of recanalization.

How long should blood pressure be monitored closely?

In a recent retrospective chart review, Aiyagari and colleagues[10] found that hypertension is unlikely to develop if it is not seen before treatment or in the first 6 hours post-treatment. This data suggests that a subset of patients could potentially be closely monitored for 6 hours only and then be transferred out of the ICU. Pending accumulation of further data, it is at this time reasonable to continue monitoring all patients for 24 hours.

How should blood pressure be managed?

Based on all of the above, blood pressure should be kept below 180/105 mmHg in order to avoid ICH, but overzealous treatment should be avoided so as not to compromise collateral circulations.

In a subset of patients, recanalization is not achieved and tissue perfusion is dependent on collateral circulations. Avoiding hypotension and volume depletion in those patients is important to prevent neurologic deterioration. In fact, induced hypertension[11] can be considered if the patient is already hypotensive, provided that the 180/105 mmHg cut-off is not reached.

Use of GP IIb/IIIa inhibitors

The American Stroke Association recommends not using antiplatelet or anticoagulant medications for 24 hours following thrombolysis. Routine use of such agents in this time period should therefore be avoided. However, the safety of GP IIb/IIIa inhibitors associated with intra-arterial thrombolysis has been documented in several studies.[14,15]

In our practice, we consider using intravenous antiplatelet agents if:

1. The patient has not received intravenous thrombolysis
2. There is partial recanalization after intra-arterial thrombolysis

3. Intra-vascular, non-occlusive thrombus is visualized
4. Re-occlusion is observed during or after administration of thrombolytics

We prefer to obtain a CT scan of the head to rule out ICH prior to initiating intravenous anti-platelet agents.

Regulation of temperature and glucose level

Hyperglycemic patients who are treated with thrombolysis have a worse outcome in terms of neurological deficits, size of stroke and incidence of ICH.[16–18] Fever also independently predicts a poor prognosis after stroke.[19] It is therefore essential that temperature and glucose are monitored closely (every 4 hours) and maintained at normal levels. Hyperglycemia is usually treated with an infusion or frequent subcutaneous injection of insulin titrated to serum glucose levels. Fever is treated with acetaminophen or non-steroidal anti-inflammatory medications. In refractory cases, cooling blankets or intravascular cooling devices can be useful.

Carotid angioplasty and stent placement

The post-procedure care of those patients should be geared towards avoiding and early recognition of three major complications: thromboembolic events, hypotension, and cerebral hyperperfusion syndrome.

Thromboembolic events

Angioplasty induces intimal damage with exposure of thrombogenic subintimal tissue. Stents provoke a foreign body reaction. Platelets bind to the subintima and stent surface followed by activation and aggregation. The highest levels of thrombogenicity are seen in the first 72 hours after the procedure. Dual anti-platelet treatment (aspirin and clopidogrel) is paramount in this period in order to avoid complications which can range from minor embolic events to complete stent thrombosis. A randomized controlled trial,[20] which included 47 patients with >70% internal carotid artery (ICA) stenosis by NASCET criteria found that dual antiplatelet treatment was superior to aspirin plus heparin. Thirty-day incidence of adverse neurologic outcomes was 0% vs. 25%, $P = 0.02$ and 30-day incidence of >50% in-stent restenosis was 5% vs. 26%, $P = 0.01$. There was no significant difference in hemorrhagic complications. The study was terminated prematurely. The superiority of dual antiplatelet prophylaxis was confirmed in a single-center carotid stent registry study performed by interventional cardiologists.[21] The patients ($n = 162$) were ineligible for endarterectomy and had severe symptomatic (>70%) or asymptomatic (>80%) ICA stenosis. The patients on dual antiplatelets had fewer ischemic events and lower rates of stent thrombosis (0% vs. 20%). ICH rates were not significantly different between the groups.

Current practice is to start aspirin (325 mg daily) and clopidogrel (75 mg daily) 3–5 days prior to a scheduled procedure.[22,23] In emergent cases, a clopidogrel bolus of 300–600 mg can be administered, along with 325 mg of aspirin. Following the procedure, clopidogrel is continued for 1–3 months (bare metal stents) or 3–12 months (drug-eluting stents). The patients stay on aspirin indefinitely.[22]

Patients who develop new neurologic deficits while in the hospital can be treated with intra-arterial infusion of lytics or GP IIb/IIIa inhibitors after ICH has been ruled out by a CT scan. Intravenous thrombolysis is not advised because of the recent femoral puncture. Moreover, in this scenario, intra-arterial thrombolysis can be performed promptly and the dose of thrombolytics can be titrated to achieve recanalization.

Hemodynamic depression (hypotension and bradycardia)

During carotid angioplasty there is acute distension of parts of the ICA wall where baroreceptors are located. Acute hypotension and bradycardia to the point of cardiac asystole can ensue. Intravenous atropine is the treatment of choice. In patients who are particularly prone to such a response, glycopyrrolate or atropine may be used prophylactically.[24]

Risk factors that have been identified include severely calcified or ulcerated lesions, lesions located at the bulb, de novo lesions, and history of myocardial infarction.[25,26]

The occurrence of hemodynamic depression (HD) during the procedure predicts hemodynamic instability in the post-procedure period due to persisting changes in compliance of the artery wall which result in excessive vagal tone. Gupta and colleagues[25] studied 500 patients who had undergone ICA stent placement. HD was found in 42% of cases, and persistent HD in 17%. Patients with persistent HD were at a significantly higher risk of developing adverse clinical events, including stroke.

Knowledge of the status of other cerebral arteries is important in determining treatment. In the absence of other hemodynamically significant stenotic lesions, the threshold to intervene is higher. Medications such as phenylephrine that can exacerbate bradycardia should be avoided. Our agent of choice is dopamine. For most patients, it is appropriate to maintain systolic blood pressure in the range of 120–140 mmHg.

Cerebral hyperperfusion syndrome (CHS)

Cerebral hyperperfusion syndrome is a rare, albeit very important complication of carotid revascularization procedures. The term was coined by Sundt and colleagues in 1981.[27] Most of the data on CHS stem from studies of patients who underwent carotid endarterectory (CEA). However, since the underlying etiology of CHS is the same for both procedures, it is reasonable to assume that these data are valid for CAS as well.

Pathophysiology

Cerebral autoregulation refers to the propensity of cerebral arterioles to maintain distal perfusion at constant levels by dilating when regional cerebral blood flow (rCBF) decreases and constricting when the opposite occurs. Their capacity to dilate in order to augment perfusion establishes what is called "cerebrovascular reserve." Distal to a severe ICA stenosis, arterioles may be maximally dilated, in which case the cerebrovascular reserve (CVR) is diminished or lost. In addition to

this, exposure to chronic hypoperfusion can lead to loss of autoregulation, so that increases in rCBF cannot be met with an appropriate vasoconstrictive response. When, following revascularization, such vessels are exposed to increased perfusion pressure, the result is relative hyperperfusion which is believed to be the pathophysiologic basis of CHS. Post-revascularization increases in cerebral perfusion in the range of 20%–40% are to be expected[28]. Frank hyperperfusion is defined as an increase of CBF of >100% compared to baseline.[27,29] By transcranial doppler (TCD) criteria, hyperperfusion is present when there is a >100% increase of peak systolic velocities in the MCA or a >100% increase of the pulsatility index.[30] Patients who exhibit hyperperfusion post-procedure, are at least ten times more likely to develop CHS.[29]

Pathology

The pathologic changes that are associated with CHS range from cerebral edema due to transudation of fluid[31] to frank ICH. In some cases, intraventricular[32] and subarachnoid hemorrhages[33,34] have been reported.

Incidence and timing

The commonly reported incidence of hyperperfusion as defined by the criteria mentioned above in CEA studies ranges between 8% and 14.5%.[29,30,35–40] The respective CHS rates usually range between 0.5% and 3.6%.[27,30,35–39]

In a large retrospective study of 450 patients who were treated with ICA stent placement, Abou-Chebl and colleagues[42] reported a 1.1% incidence of CHS and a 0.67% incidence of ICH.

Osagawara and colleagues[34] recently reported on their experience with 4494 patients who had undergone ICA revascularization procedures (1596 CEA, 2898 stent placement). CHS was seen in 1.9% of post-CEA patients and in 1.1% of post-stenting patients, ICH rates were 0.4% and 0.7%, respectively.

Following CEA, there is typically a latency period of a few days before CHS develops. The peak incidence appears to be between the fifth and eighth post-operative day.[30,31,34] Cases have been reported as late as a month after the procedure. In contrast to this, the peak incidence of CHS following stent placement is in the first post-procedure day.[34,42] In the series by Abou-Chebl and colleagues, the range was 6 hours to 4 days.[42] In the Osagawara series[34] 15/31 patients developed CHS in the first day. There was one case on day 7 and one case on day 10.

When autoregulation will be re-established cannot be accurately predicted. However, in one study[29] CBF had returned to normal in all CHS patients a month after the procedure and a TCD study has suggested that autoregulation normalizes within 6 weeks.[43]

Clinical manifestations

Common clinical manifestations are changes in level of consciousness, new focal deficits, headache, and seizures.[27,31,41]

Identifying patients at risk

- Assessment of CVR prior to the procedure

CVR is assessed by comparing baseline rCBF to rCBF after acetazolamide challenge. If the resulting increase in rCBF is below a defined level, then CVR is said to be diminished. In some cases, rCBF actually drops. This is interpreted as intra-cerebral steal, i.e., the dilation of normal arterioles with preserved autoregulation channels redirecting blood away from the affected territory. Intracerebral steal is a stronger predictor of CHS than diminished CVR.[29]

- Assessment of perfusion after the procedure

TCD and single photon emission computed tomographic (SPECT) scan can be used after the procedure to identify hyperperfusion. As mentioned above, patients with hyperperfusion are at much higher risk of developing CSH.

- Angiographic features

Pre-treatment ICA stenosis of >90% and contralateral stenosis of >80% are important predictors of CSH.[42]

Treatment

Post-procedure hypertension is a common occurrence. Qureshi and colleagues[26] reported an incidence of 38.8% among 51 patients who underwent carotid stent placement. Intra-procedural hypertension predicts hypertension in the post-procedure period.[26]

Strict control of blood pressure has been shown to prevent clinical deterioration and ICH in multiple series.[29,30,42] In patients who have documented hyperperfusion with no clinical signs, systolic blood pressure (SBP) should be kept below 120 mmHg if possible. In patients who have developed clinical signs of CHS, we would recommend lowering the SBP as tolerated until clinical signs regress and/or there is normalization of rCBF or middle cerebral artery (MCA) peak velocities. Agents that can augment rCBF, such as hydralazine, should be avoided. There is no data to support that withholding anti-platelet treatment may reduce the risk of ICH. On the other hand, if ICH is present, antiplatelet medications should be withheld and their action reversed by means of platelet transfusion and administration of intravenous methylprednisolone (25 mg). If repeat CT 24 hours later shows no extension of ICH, aspirin can be restarted. Clopidogrel can be re-initiated 5–7 days later (opinion-based recommendation).

General measures for the treatment of cerebral edema, such as hyperventilation and hyperosmotic agents, can be considered, although there are no reports on their use for CHS.[28]

Since delayed CHS does occur, albeit infrequently, following carotid stent placement, it is paramount to instruct patients to comply strictly with their medication regimen, to measure their blood pressure daily for at least a week and to call and report any symptoms that could be suggestive of CHS.

Figure 4.1 offers an algorithm for the management of neurological complications following stent placement.

Coil-embolization of aneurysms

The two main complications of aneurysm coil embolization are thromboembolism and aneurysm rupture. The International Study of Unruptured Intracranial Aneurysms Invesigators reported a hemorrhage rate of 2% and a cerebral infarction rate of 5% among endovascularly treated patients.[44]

Table 4.2 lists factors that can increase the risk of those complications.

Thromboembolism

The thrombogenicity of coils, stents, and intravascular balloons is the main cause of thromboembolic events. Preventing such events is challenging particularly in patients who present with ruptured aneurysms. On one hand, subarachnoid hemorrhage (SAH) is *per se* associated with increased clotting tendency. On the other hand, aggressive use of anti-platelet agents may in theory induce re-bleeding, especially before the aneurysm is secured. While we do not have adequate data to support any practice paradigm, it is probably safe to initiate anti-platelet agents in anticipation of stent-assisted coiling a few hours before the procedure, provided that the patient is beyond the first 24 hours post SAH when re-rupture is most likely. After the aneurysm has been obliterated, the risk of re-bleeding is probably very low, even with use of dual anti-platelet treatment. This is supported by low rates of re-bleeding in case series describing the use of self-expanding stents in patients with recently ruptured aneurysms[45,46] and small case reports and case series describing the use of intravenous anti-platelet agents in patients with recent SAH and peri-procedural thromboembolic events.[47]

Based on the above data, and until more data becomes available, we would recommend starting anti-platelet agents shortly before coil placement if the patient is 24 hours out of SAH and stent placement seems unavoidable, or immediately after stent-assisted coil placement if need for stent is determined during the procedure.

If thromboembolism is recognized during the procedure, treatment options include intra-arterial thrombolysis,[48] intravenous antiplatelets,[49] and intra-arterial antiplatelets.[50,51] Our current practice is to administer small intra-arterial boluses (2.5–5 mg) of GP IIb/IIIa inhibitors up to a total dose of 15 mg or until recanalization is achieved. We follow this with a 12–24 hour intravenous infusion in selected patients.

Aneurysm rupture

Aneurysm rupture can occur during endovascular treatment and can generally be diagnosed without help of CT scan. It appears to be more common when previously ruptured aneurysms are treated (3.6% vs. 2% incidence in two separate large series of ruptured[52] and unruptured aneurysms).[44] In the majority of cases, rupture occurs during insertion of the first coil.[52]

The most common finding in an awake patient is deteriorating level of consciousness. During the procedure, when

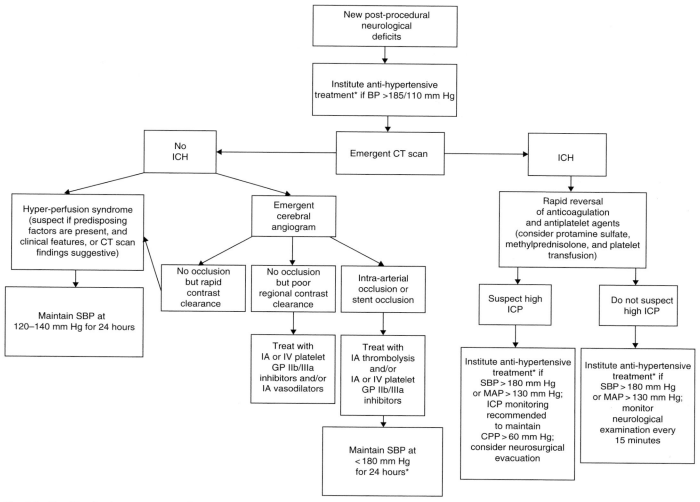

Fig. 4.1. Algorithm for the management of neurological deficits after stent placement. Abbreviations used: SBP, systolic blood pressure; CT, computed tomographic; ICP, intracranial pressure; MAP, mean arterial pressure; ICH, intracrenial hemorrhage.

patients are under anesthesia, the most common manifestation is a sudden increase in blood pressure with a concurrent intracranial pressure (ICP) increase. There is usually visible extravasation of contrast upon selective injection. Fresh blood can be sometimes in cerebrospinal fluid seen if an intraventricular drain is in place. Signs of herniation can evolve rapidly, depending on the severity of the acute aneurysmal bleeding.

Appropriate measures must be undertaken immediately. In a best case scenario, a physician is there to evaluate the patient, while the endovascular surgeon continues with embolization of the aneurysm. The goal is to stop extravasation, and this can sometimes be achieved with placement of even one additional coil. At the same time, if the patient shows signs of herniation, the following steps are undertaken:

- Intravenous push of 1 g/kg mannitol
- Hyperventilation
- Hemodynamic stabilization, without overzealous blood pressure control in order to maintain cerebral perfusion pressure

- Reversal of anticoagulation with protamine sulfate
- Emergent ventriculostomy if an intraventricular drain is not already in place
- Transfusion of platelets if antiplatelet agents have been used
- Administration of 25 mg intravenous methylprednisolone if clopidogrel has been used.[53]

The next step is to perform CT scan of the head. If there is intraparenchymal hematoma that can be evacuated, then neurosurgical intervention should be considered. Surgery in this scenario also offers the advantage of surgical obliteration of the aneurysm, if the embolization procedure was prematurely terminated. Alternatively, the patients can return for further embolization after they have been stabilized.

Vasospasm

A further question in management is how safe it is to treat vasospasm in the face of a recently embolized ruptured aneurysm. Current data do not demonstrate an increased risk of rebleeding following any of the commonly used treatments of vasospasm: induced hypervolemia, induced hypertension, intra-arterial vasodilators, or balloon angioplasty.

Increase in mass effect

Rarely, following coil-embolization of large aneurysms, new or increased mass effect signs can develop. Those include cranial neuropathies and obstructive hydrocephalus. Treatment is symptomatic. As fibrosis develops within the aneurysmal sac, mass effect reduces without need for intervention.

Embolization of arterio-venous malformations (AVM)s

Complications arise when there is inadvertent embolization of normal arteries or of the venous draining system. The former can result in ischemic stroke. The later is more common and can result in increased outflow resistance, which can manifest angiographically as delayed contrast clearance. Since outflow obstruction can lead to ICH, prompt reversal of anticoagulation following the procedure is recommended.

The vessels that lie in the vicinity of the nidus are exposed to chronic hypoperfusion due to the vascular steal effect of the AVM. This holds true especially for larger, high-flow AVMs.[54] The chronic hypoperfusion leads to impaired autoregulation.[54] Embolization decreases flow through the nidus and exposes the neighboring vessels to increased flow and hemodynamic stress. In the absence of strict blood pressure control, cerebral edema and ICH can ensue. This phenomenon is referred to as normal perfusion pressure breakthrough.[55] It is recommended that SBP be maintained at or below 120 mmHg for the first 24 hours after the procedure.

Early detection of ICH by CT can allow for prompt surgical evacuation (as indicated) and prompt clinical measures to reduce the sequelae of mass effect and herniation.

Intracranial angioplasty and stent placement

Ischemic infarction is the main adverse event to be anticipated following intracranial angioplasty and stent placement. Stroke usually occurs during or shortly after the procedure. Apart from the reasons outlined in the carotid angioplasty and stent section, stroke in intracranial procedures can also be due to compromise of perforators arising from the treated vessel segment. Table 4.2 lists other procedure-related factors that increase stroke risk.

If a patient develops a new neurologic deficit, emergent CT scan is performed to rule out ICH. If there is no ICH, emergent angiography is performed and treatment with intra-arterial thrombolytics and/or intravenous antiplatelets can be administered.

CHS can occur following intracranial angioplasty stenting. The etiology and treatment are the same as described above in the ICA angioplasty and stenting section.

Conclusions

A successful endovascular procedure is only the first step towards a good patient outcome. Knowledge of the specific problems that can arise after a given procedure and close monitoring by a trained neuro-ICU team is paramount. Good communication between the endovascular and intensive care teams can ensure that potential complications can be anticipated and thus prevented or treated early.

References

1. Pannu N, Wiebe N, Tonelli M. Prophylaxis strategies for contrast-induced nephropathy. *JAMA* 2006; **295**: 2765–79.

2. Tissue plasminogen activator for acute ischemic stroke. The National Institute of Neurological Disorders and Stroke rt-PA Stroke Study Group. *N Engl J Med* 1995; **333**: 1581–7.

3. Katzan IL, Furlan AJ, Lloyd LE, *et al.* Use of tissue-type plasminogen activator for acute ischemic stroke: the Cleveland area experience. *JAMA* 2000; **283**: 1151–8.

4. Katzan IL, Hammer MD, Furlan AJ, *et al.* Quality improvement and tissue-type plasminogen activator for acute ischemic stroke: A Cleveland update. *Stroke* 2003; **34**: 799–800.

5. Gilligan AK, Markus R, Read S, *et al.* Baseline blood pressure but not early computed tomography changes predicts major hemorrhage after streptokinase in acute ischemic stroke. *Stroke* 2002; **33**: 2236–42.

6. Tanne D, Kasner SE, Demchuk AM, *et al.* Markers of increased risk of intracerebral hemorrhage after intravenous recombinant tissue plasminogen activator therapy for acute ischemic stroke in clinical practice: The Multicenter rt-PA Stroke Survey. *Circulation* 2002; **105**: 1679–85.

7. Brott T, Mei L, Rashmi K, *et al.* Hypertension and its treatment in the NINDS trial. *Stroke* 1998; **29**: 1504–9.

8. Willmot M, Leonardi-Bee J, Bath PMW. High blood pressure in acute stroke and subsequent outcome. A systematic review. *Hypertension* 2004; **43**: 18–24.

9. Mattle HP, Kappeler L, Arnold M, *et al.* Blood pressure and vessel recanalization in the first hours after ischemic stroke. *Stroke* 2005; **36**: 264–9.

10. Aiyagari V, Gujjar A, Zazulia AR, Diringer MN. Hourly blood pressure monitoring after intravenous tissue plasminogen activator for ischemic stroke. Does everyone need it? *Stroke* 2004; **35**: 2326–30.

11. Rordorf G, Koroshetz WJ, Ezzeddine MA, Segal AZ, Buonanno FS. A pilot study of drug-induced hypertension for treatment of acute stroke. *Neurology* 2001; **56**: 1210–13.

12. Marzan AS, Hungerbuehler H-J, Studer A, Baumgartner RW, Georgiadis D. Feasibility and safety of norepinephrine-induced arterial hypertension in acute ischemic stroke. *Neurology* 2004; **62**: 1193–5.

13. Georgiadis AL, Al-Kawi A, Janjua N, Kirmani JF, Ezzeddine MA, Qureshi AI. Cerebral angiography can demonstrate

changes in collateral flow during induced hypertension. *Radiology Case Reports [Online]* 2007; **2**:37.

14. Gupta R, Vora NA, Horowitz MB, *et al.* Multimodal reperfusion therapy for acute ischemic stroke: factors predicting vessel recanalization. *Stroke* 2006; **37**:986–90.

15. Eckert B, Koch C, Thomalla G, *et al.* Aggressive therapy with intravenous abciximab and intra-arterial rt-PA and additional PTA/stenting improves clinical outcome in acute vertebrobasilar occlusion: combined local fibrinolysis and intravenous abciximab in acute vertebrobasilar stroke treatment (FAST): results of a multicenter study. *Stroke* 2005; **36**:1160–5.

16. Demchuk AM, Morgenstern LB, Krieger DW, *et al.* Serum glucose level and diabetes predict tissue plasminogen activator-related intracerebral hemorrhage in acute ischemic stroke. *Stroke* 1999; **30**: 34–9.

17. Els T, Klisch J, Orszagh M, *et al.* Hyperglycemia in patients with focal cerebral ischemia after intravenous thrombolysis: Influence on clinical outcome and infarct size. *Cerebrovasc Dis* 2002; **13**: 89–94.

18. Parsons MW, Barber PA, Desmond PM, *et al.* Acute hyperglycemia adversely affects stroke outcome: a magnetic resonance imaging and spectroscopy study. *Ann Neurol* 2002; **52**: 20–8.

19. Azzimondi G, Bassein L, Nonino F, *et al.* Fever in acute stroke worsens prognosis. A prospective study. *Stroke* 1995; **26**: 2040–3.

20. McKevitt FM, Randall MS, *et al.* The benefits of combined antiplatelet treatment in carotid artery stenting. *Eur J Endovasc Surg* 2005; **29**: 522–7.

21. Bhatt DL, Kapadia SR, *et al.* Dual antiplatelet therapy with clopidogrel and aspirin after carotid artery stenting. *J Invasive Cardiol* 2001; **13**: 772–3.

22. Qureshi AI, Kirmani JF, *et al.* Vertebral artery origin stent placement with distal protection: technical and clinical results. *Am J Neuroradiol* 2006; **27**: 1140–5.

23. Qureshi AI, Luft AR, *et al.* Prevention and treatment of thromboembolic and ischemic complications associated with endovascular procedures: Part II – Clinical aspects and recommendations. *Neurosurgery* 2000; **46**: 1360–75.

24. Chakravarti S. Carotid artery angioplasty and stenting: anesthetic implications. *Can J Anesth* 2007; **54**: 44024.

25. Gupta R, Abou-Chebl A, Bajzer CT, Schumacher HC, Yadav JS. Rate, predictors and consequences of hemodynamic depression after carotid artery stenting. *J Am Coll Cardiol* 2006; **47**: 1538–43.

26. Qureshi AI, Luft AR, Mudit S, *et al.* Frequency and determinants of postprocedural hemodynamic instability after carotid angioplasty and stenting. *Stroke* 1999; **30**: 2086–93.

27. Sundt TM, Sharbrough FW, Piepgras DG, *et al.* Correlation of cerebral blood flow and electroencephalographic changes during carotid endarterectomy. *Mayo Clin Proc* 1981; **56**: 533–43.

28. Van Mook WNKA, Rennenberg RJMW, Schurink GW, *et al.* Cerebral hyperperfusion syndrome. *Lancet Neurol* 2005; **4**: 877–88.

29. Hosoda K, Kawaguchi T, Shibata Y, et al. Cerebral vasoreactivity and internal carotid artery flow help to identify patients at risk for hyperperfusion after carotid endarterectomy. *Stroke* 2001; **32**: 1567–73.

30. Dalman JE, Beenakkers ICM, Moli FL, Leusink JA, Ackerstaff RGA. Transcranial Doppler monitoring during carotid endarterectomy helps to identify patients at risk of portoperative hyperperfusion. *Eur J Vasc Endovasc Surg* 1999; **18**: 222–7.

31. Breen JC, Caplan LR, DeWitt LD, Belkin M, Mackey WC, O'Donnell TP. Brain edema after carotid surgery. *Neurology* 1996; **46**: 175–81.

32. Mori T, Fukuoka M, Kazita K, Mima T, Mori K. Intraventricular hemorrhage after carotid stenting. *J Endovasc Surg* 1999; **6**: 337–41.

33. Hartmann M, Weber R, Zoubaa S, Schranz C, Knauth M. Fatal subarachnoid hemorrhage after carotid stenting. *J Neuroradiol* 2004; **31**: 63–6.

34. Osagawara K, Sakai N, Kuroiwa T, *et al.* Intracranial hemorrhage associated with cerebral hyperperfusion syndrome following carotid endarterectomy and carotid artery stenting: retrospective review of 4494 patients. *J Neurosurg* 2007; **107**: 1130–6.

35. Piepgras DG, Morgan MK, Sundt TM, Yanagihara T, Mussman LM. Intracerebral hemorrhage after carotid endarterectomy. *J Neurosurg* 1988; **68**: 532–6.

36. Keunen R, Nijmeijer HW, Tavy D, *et al.* An observational study of pre-operative transcranial Doppler examinations to predict cerebral hyperperfusion following carotid endarterctomies. *Neurol Res* 2001; **23**: 593–8.

37. Osagawara K, Konno H, Yukawa H, Endo H, Inoue T, Ogawa A. Transcranial regional cerebral oxygen saturation monitoring during carotid endarterectomy as a predictor of postoperative hyperperfusion. *Neurosurgery* 2003; **53**: 309–14.

38. Osagawara K, Yukawa H, Kobayashi M, *et al.* Prediction and monitoring of cerebral hyperperfusion after carotid endarterectomy by using single-photon emission computerized tomography scanning. *J Neurosurg* 2003; **99**: 504–10.

39. Ogasawara K, Inoue T, Kobayashi M, *et al.* Cerebral hyperperfusion following carotid endarterectomy: diagnostic utility of intraoperative transcranial Doppler ultrasonography compared with single-photon emission computed tomography study. *Am J Neuroradiol* 2005; **26**: 252–7.

40. Hosoda K, Kawaguchi T, Ishii K, *et al.* Prediction of hyperperfusion after carotid endarterectomy by brain SPECT analysis with semiquantitative statistical mapping method. *Stroke* 2003; **34**: 1187–93.

41. Ho DS, Wang Y, Chui M, Ho SL, Cheung RT. Epileptic seizures attributed to cerebral hyperperfusion after percutaneous transluminal angioplasty and stenting of the internal carotid artery. *Cerebrovasc Dis* 2000; **10**: 374–9.

42. Abou-Chebl A, Yadav JS, Reginelli JP, Bajzer C, Bhatt D, Krieger DW. Intracranial hemorrhage and hyperperfusion syndrome following carotid artery stenting. Risk factors, prevention and treatment. *J Am Coll Cardiol* 2004; **43**: 1596–601.

43. Magee TR, Davies AH, Baird RN, Horrocks M. Transcranial Doppler measurement before and after carotid endarterectomy. *J R Coll Surg Edinb* 1992; **37**: 311–12.

44. International Study of Unruptured Intracranial Aneurysms Investigators.

Unruptured Intracranial aneurysms: natural history, clinical outcome, and risks of surgical and endovascular treatment. *Lancet* 2003; **362**: 103–10.

45. Fiorella D, Albuquerque FC, Deshmukh VR, McDougall CG. Usefulness of the neuroform stent for the treatment of cerebral aneurysms: results at initial (3–6-mo) follow-up. *Neurosurgery* 2005; **56**: 1191–202.

46. Fitzpatrick D, Chen M, Meyers PM. Horizontal neuroform stent deployment for a ruptured basilar terminus aneurysm via the posterior communicating artery. *J Vasc Interv Radiol* 2006; **17**: 1687–91.

47. Aviv RI, O'Neill RO, Patel MC, Colquhoun IR. Abciximab in patients with ruptured aneurysms. *Am J Neuroradiol* 2005; **26**: 1744–50.

48. Cronqvist M, Pierot L, Boulin A, *et al.* Local intraarterial fibrinolysis of thromboembolic occurring during endovascular treatment of intracerebral aneurysms: a comparison of anatomic results and clinical outcome. *Am J Neuroradiol* 1998; **19**: 157–65.

49. Aviv RI, O'Neill R, Patel MC, Colquhoun IR. Abciximab in patients with ruptured intracranial aneurysms. *Am J Neuroradiol* 2005; **26**: 1744–50.

50. Mounayer C, Piotin M, Baldi S, Spelle L, Moret J. Intraarterial administration of abciximab for thromboembolic events occurring during aneurysm coil placement. *Am J Neuroradiol* 2003; **24**: 2039–43.

51. Park JH, Kim JE, Sheen SH, *et al.* Intrarterial abciximab for treatment of thromboembolism during coil embolization of intracranial aneurysms: outcome and fatal hemorrhagic complications. *J Neurosurg* 2008; **108**: 450–7.

52. Gallas S, Pasco A, Cottier J-P, *et al.* A multicenter study of 705 ruptured intracranial aneurysms treated with Guglielmi Detachable Coils. *Am J Neuroradiol* 2005; **26**: 1723–31.

53. Tiffany BR, Barrali R. Advances in the pharmacology of acute coronary syndrome. Platelet inhibition. *Emerg Med Clin North Am* 2000; **18**: 723–43.

54. Nagasawa S, Kawanishi M, Kondoh S, Kajimoto S, Yamaguchi K, Ohta T. Hemodynamic simulation study of cerebral arteriovenous malformations. Part 2. Effects of impaired autoregulation and induced hypotension. *J Cereb Blood Flow Metab* 1996; **16**(1): 162–9.

55. Spetzler RF, Wilson CB. Perfusion pressure breakthrough theory. *Clin Neurosurg* 1978; **25**: 651–72.

Chapter 5

Acute ischemic stroke

Alexandros L. Georgiadis, Georgios Tsivgoulis, Andrei V. Alexandrov, Adnan I. Qureshi and José I. Suarez

Introduction

The endovascular treatment of acute ischemic stroke encompasses a heterogeneous group of treatment modalities directed towards achieving recanalization of intravascular occlusions through an intra-arterial approach. The applied treatments can be pharmacological, mechanical, or a combination of both. Intra-arterial (IA) interventions have been promoted because a high concentration of thrombolytic agents can be delivered into the thrombus complemented by mechanical disruption to facilitate thrombolysis.[1] However, despite the uncontrolled observation that recanalization rates may be higher with IA thrombolysis compared with intravenous (IV) thrombolysis,[2] clinical benefit may be counter-balanced by the delay to initiate treatment.

IV administration of alteplase (recombinant tissue plasminogen activator, rt-PA) has become standard of care for patients with ischemic stroke who present within 3 hours (more recently 4.5 hrs) of symptom onset. The National Institute of Neurological Disorders and Stroke (NINDS) rt-PA trial[3] evaluated the efficacy of IV rt-PA in a two-part study. The first part demonstrated that a higher rate of the primary end point of early improvement can be observed among patients treated with rt-PA (47%) than in the placebo-treated group (39%). The second part was conducted with the 3-month outcome as the primary end point and was designed as the pivotal efficacy trial. The pre-specified end point, a global outcome statistic, was highly in favor of rt-PA treatment. As compared with patients given placebo, patients treated with rt-PA were at least 30% more likely to have minimal or no disability at three months on the assessment scales. The United States Food and Drug Administration (FDA) approval for IV rt-PA came in June 1996 and since then, both the Stroke Council of the American Heart Association and the Quality Standards Subcommittee of the American Academy of Neurology have issued guidelines to improve the utilization of thrombolysis in patients with ischemic stroke.[4,5] However, the rate of death and disability associated with acute ischemic stroke despite treatment with IV rt-PA remains at >50%.[3,6,7] This high burden of death and disability mandates that new treatments for acute ischemic stroke be explored further with particular emphasis on endovascular treatment.

Medications and devices used in the endovascular treatment of acute ischemic stroke

Thrombolytics

All currently available thrombolytic agents are plasminogen activators. The clinical properties of those agents have evolved over four generations of drugs.[8] Plasminogen is an inactive enzyme that circulates in the body. Plasminogen activators cleave the Arg560-Val561 bond of plasminogen, thus converting it in its active form, plasmin. The major physiological plasminogen activators are tissue-type plasminogen activator (t-PA) and urokinase-type plasminogen activator (u-PA).[9] Plasmin breaks fibrin down into fibrin degradation products and split products (fibrinolysis), thus dissolving clots which are mainly composed of fibrin-bound platelets. However, plasmin is capable of degrading fibrin that is not bound to thrombi and also circulating fibrinogen with the potential of inducing a lytic state with uncontrolled bleeding. Therefore, ideally, a plasminogen activator used for thrombolysis should only generate plasmin at the interface with clot-bound fibrin, i.e., have high fibrin (or clot) specificity.[10] First-generation thrombolytics (urokinase and streptokinase) had no clot specificity. Second-generation thrombolytics (rt-PA, pro-urokinase) were genetically engineered to be fibrin-specific. Recombinant t-PA still causes systemic plasminogen consumption and fibrinogenolysis, but its activity is enhanced 72-fold by fibrin.[11] Trials comparing the safety and efficacy of first and second generation thrombolytics in patients with acute myocardial infarction (MI) have demonstrated higher recanalization rates and lower incidence of intra-cranial hemorrhage (ICH) associated with the second generation drugs.[12]

Third-generation thrombolytics (e.g., reteplase, tenecteplase) have even higher affinity to fibrin, and longer half-lives.

Textbook of Interventional Neurology, ed. Adnan I. Qureshi. Published by Cambridge University Press. © Cambridge University Press 2011.

Reteplase has not been shown to have any clear benefit over rt-PA regarding safety or efficacy in the treatment of MI.[13] Tenecteplase has been studied in acute MI in three phase II trials and in one large Phase III trial.[14] It was found to be equivalent to rt-PA as regards recanalization, mortality and rates of ICH.[14] However, it was associated with significantly lower overall bleeding complications. A Phase I, dose-escalating study of intravenous tenecteplase in acute ischemic stroke,[15] has shown that doses between 0.1 and 0.4 mg/kg are safe when administered within 3 hours from symptom onset. A phase IIB study comparing three different tenecteplase doses to rt-PA has been recently completed, but the results have not yet been published.

Desmoteplase, considered a fourth-generation agent, comes closest to the ideal profile of a thrombolytic drug. Its efficiency is enhanced 13 000-fold by fibrin. Also, unlike rt-PA, it has not been shown to have neurotoxic effects, it has a half-life long enough to allow bolus administration, and has no interaction with β-amyloid (a possible cause of ICH).[11,16] However, the initial promising results in patients treated with IV desmoteplase within 3 to 9 hours from stroke onset[16,17] were not replicated in the Phase III trial DIAS 2.[18]

Heparin and direct thrombin inhibitors

There are two ways to achieve thrombin inhibition: with direct thrombin inhibitors such as hirudin, its analogs hirulog and hirugen and bivalirudin, and with antithrombin III-dependent drugs such as standard (unfractionated) and low molecular weight heparin preparations.[19]

Unfractionated heparin is still the drug that is most commonly used in endovascular procedures, including intra-arterial thrombolysis. The dosing of heparin is controversial, the current trend being towards using lower doses.

Multiple studies have shown that higher heparin doses are associated with increased risk of hemorrhage. In the Prolyse in Acute Cerebral Thromboembolism (PROACT) I trial[20] the heparin dosing was reduced based on a recommendation from the External Safety Committee. This led to a significant reduction in hemorrhage rates and the same dosing regimen was carried over to PROACT II.[21]

In a single-center experience, the rate of ICH in patients undergoing intra-arterial thrombolysis was reduced when the dose of intra-procedural heparin was changed from 50 U/kg[22] to 30 U/kg,[23] albeit with a concurrent reduction in the dose of reteplase.

A prospective randomized trial with acute MI patients undergoing primary angioplasty (HEAP 2)[24] also showed more bleeding complications in the high-dose heparin group. Whereas higher heparin dosing was associated with higher likelihood of recanalization of cerebral vessels in PROACT, this finding was not confirmed in HEAP 2 for the coronary vasculature.

Drawbacks of heparin include that it does not sufficiently suppress thrombin generation or inhibit clot-bound thrombin and that its effect cannot be predicted with accuracy.[25] Direct thrombin inhibitors are more effective experimentally in inhibiting platelet deposition and thrombus formation. Studies of prevention of re-occlusion in experimental thrombotic and embolic stroke are showing promising results.[26] However, the risk of hemorrhage in patients with cerebrovascular disease is not known for these agents. In the Hirudin for the Improvement of Thrombolysis (HIT 4) study,[27] 1028 MI patients treated with streptokinase were randomized to concurrent therapy with heparin or hirudin. Patients treated with hirudin showed an accelerated restoration of blood flow and a reduction of re-infarction over the first 5 days. However, there was no difference in 30-day mortality or in the incidence of bleeding complications.

Platelet glycoprotein IIb/IIIa (GP IIb/IIIa) inhibitors

Platelet activation causes morphological changes in the shape of platelets and activation of membrane GP IIB/IIIA receptors.[19] Activated GP IIB/IIIA receptors bind to fibrinogen molecules, which subsequently form bridges between adjacent platelets and facilitate platelet aggregation. The final common pathway in clot formation is the binding of fibrinogen to platelets via platelet GP IIB/IIIA receptors. GP IIB/IIIA inhibitors prevent the binding of fibrinogen to these receptors, thereby inhibiting platelet aggregation irrespective of the activation pathway responsible for its initiation. Thrombolytic agents target the fibrin mesh component of the thrombus, which paradoxically leads to an increase in thrombin activity and platelet activation. Strong antiplatelet agents, such as GP IIB/IIIA-specific antibodies, increase the potential for initial thrombolysis and reduce the risk of reocclusion.[28,29] GP IIB/IIIA inhibitors alone have led to recanalization in patients with acute MI presumably by augmenting the effect of intrinsic thrombolytic factors.[30,31] In patients with acute MI, combination treatment of low dose thrombolytics and GP IIB/IIIA inhibitors increases recanalization rates but also increases the rates of systemic bleeding complications. In phase III trials involving patients with MI,[32,33] significant improvement in clinical outcomes with combination treatment compared with thrombolytics alone has not been demonstrated. In acute ischemic stroke, combination treatment has been evaluated in phase I and phase II studies with adequate demonstration of safety of this paradigm as discussed later.

Mechanical devices

The mechanical devices used for the treatment of acute ischemic stroke are divided into two groups: (1) thrombectomy devices, which are intended for disruption and fragmentation of thrombi and usually used as adjunctive therapy along with pharmacological thrombolysis; and (2) thrombus retrieval devices, which are intended to engage the thrombus and remove it from the intravascular compartment. A closer description of individual devices is provided below.

Microvena snare

The snare is a collapsible loop of wire (2 mm or 4 mm in diameter) attached to a straight wire that can be introduced through a micro-catheter (inner diameter of 0.021″ or greater).[34] The micro-catheter is placed across the occlusion over a micro-wire and subsequently the snare is introduced through the micro-catheter. The ideal method involves advancing the snare until it reaches the distal end of the micro-catheter and subsequently withdrawing the micro-catheter to expose the snare and allow it to achieve its spheroidal shape. The snare is opened and closed by withdrawing and advancing the micro-catheter over the snare within the thrombus.

Angioplasty balloon catheters

The angioplasty balloon catheters are used to perform angioplasty within the segment of intravascular occlusion. Primary angioplasty as an adjunct to pharmacological thrombolysis is particularly beneficial in occlusions with an underlying atherosclerotic lesion. The angioplasty catheters are advanced over a micro-wire that has been placed across the occlusion using a micro-catheter. Traversing the occlusion with a micro-catheter first, gives the opportunity to perform a super-selective contrast injection distal to the occlusion in order to qualitatively and quantitatively assess the tortuosity and diameter of vessel. This assessment helps in selecting the length and diameter of the balloon. A submaximal angioplasty is performed by undersizing the angioplasty balloon in reference to the vessel diameter. If needed, several angioplasties may be performed in order to cover the entire length of the occluded arterial segment.

Intravascular stents

Intravascular stents have been used to achieve recanalization in arterial occlusions that are resistant to other treatment modalities.[35] In acute MI, primary stent placement has provided the best treatment outcomes.[36] Both balloon-expandable and self-expanding stents have been used in patients with acute ischemic stroke. Balloon-expandable stents are more effective in achieving recanalization but their use is limited at times due to the length of the occluded segment and excessive tortuosity of the proximal vessels. Stent placement as an adjunct to pharmacological thrombolysis is particularly beneficial in occlusions with an underlying atherosclerotic lesion. The stent has to adequately extend beyond the length of the occluded segment to achieve successful recanalization which limits the intracranial use to short segments of occluded arteries. Traversing the occlusion using a micro-catheter to perform a super-selective contrast injection distal to the occlusion to qualitatively and quantitatively assess the tortuosity and diameter of the vessel is strongly recommended. Balloon-expandable stents are slightly undersized compared to the reference vessel, while self-expanding stents are slightly oversized. In the setting

of acute stroke, the risk of re-occlusion following stent placement is particularly high due to the pre-existing high thrombus burden and inability to use aggressive antiplatelet treatment. The most conclusive evidence of benefit with stent placement is seen in the treatment of acute cervical internal carotid artery (ICA) occlusions.

EKOS ultrasound catheter

The EKOS ultrasound catheter will be discussed later.

Angiojet rheolytic catheter

The device works by emitting a powerful saline jet that creates a low pressure zone around the catheter tip inducing a vacuum effect.[37,38] Thrombus is drawn into the catheter, where it is fragmented by the jet, and subsequently removed from the body. The Angiojet has three components: (1) drive unit, to monitor system performance to ensure patient safety; (2) pump set, to achieve isovolumetric balance between fluid delivery and removal; (3) disposable catheters that are compatible with 4- to 6-French guide catheters indicated for use in coronary arteries and bypass grafts, arteriovenous access conduits, and/or peripheral arteries. The device is intended for the control and selective infusion of physician-specified fluids, including thrombolytic agents, into the peripheral vascular system.

Rheolytic thrombectomy has been used for recanalization in cases where the clot burden is high, such as in acute ICA occlusion and in sinus thrombosis. However, existing data are limited to case reports and case series.[39–42]

The NeuroJet was a smaller device, designed for the intracranial circulation. However, development of the device never went forward owing to complications that arose in the initial feasibility and safety study.[43]

Merci retrieval system

The Merci retrieval system consists of a balloon guide catheter (8F or 9F), the Merci retriever (L5, X5, X6), and a Merci micro-catheter (MC 14X or MC 18L). The guide catheter has a large 2.1 mm lumen and a balloon located at its distal tip. The Merci retriever is a tapered wire made of nitinol with five helical loops of decreasing diameter (from 2.8 mm to 1.1 mm) at its distal end. The Merci retriever is advanced through the micro-catheter in its straight configuration and resumes its pre-imposed helical shape once it is delivered into the occluded intracranial artery in order to ensnare the thrombus. X5 and X6 are first-generation devices, whereas the L5 is second generation system. The X5 and X6 have five helical loops with a 0.012 and 0.014 inch outer diameter, respectively. The L5 differs from the X5 and X6 devices in the inclusion of a system of arcading filaments attached to a non-tapering helical nitinol coil in a sidewinder configuration. The device is advanced so the distal loops of the helix are deployed distal to the clot. The micro-catheter and the device are pulled back so as to fully engage the clot, then the proximal loops of the device are deployed by further retraction of the micro-catheter. Subsequently, the balloon of the balloon guide catheter is inflated to arrest flow within the proximal arterial segment and the micro-catheter and embolectomy device are gently withdrawn into the body of the guide catheter while aspirating with a syringe. Finally, the balloon is deflated and the clot is retrieved.

Penumbra system

The Penumbra System® (Penumbra, Alameda, CA) has been designed to revascularize large vessel occlusions in the intracranial circulation. It consists of three main components which can be delivered via a standard 6-French guide catheter: a reperfusion catheter, a separator, and a thrombus removal ring. The components are available in different sizes to be used according to the target vessel. The device can remove clot through two mechanisms: aspiration and extraction. The reperfusion catheter, which is connected to an aspiration pump, is passed through the guide catheter and brought in position just proximal to the clot over a guide-wire. The guide-wire is then exchanged for the separator and the aspiration pump is turned on, generating a vacuum of -20 mmHg. During aspiration, the separator is used to debulk the thrombus by repeated manipulation of its proximal surface. If adequate revascularization is not achieved, the thrombus removal ring is used to extract additional clot under flow arrest induced by inflation of a proximal balloon guide catheter. The system was approved by the FDA for use in ischemic stroke in January 2008.

Overview of existing data for the various treatment modalities

Intra-arterial pharmacological thrombolysis vs. placebo

PROACT

The phase II PROACT trial[20] randomized 40 patients with middle cerebral artery (MCA) stroke to recombinant pro-urokinase ($n = 26$) or placebo ($n = 14$). All patients were treated within 6 hours of symptom onset. The initial protocol included administration of 100 U/kg intravenous heparin, followed by a continuous infusion at a rate of 1000 U/hour over 4 hours. Among the first 16 patients treated, the rate of symptomatic ICH was 27.3% in the pro-urokinase group and 20% in the placebo group. The heparin regimen was then altered to a 2000 U bolus, followed by a 500 U/hour infusion over 4 hours. The 24 patients subsequently treated exhibited lower ICH rates (6.7% for the pro-urokinase group, 0% for the placebo group). However, high-dose heparin was also associated with greater recanalization rates (81.8% vs. 40% in the low-dose group).

The overall recanalization rate was significantly higher in the treated group (58% vs. 14% in non-treated patients). There was a trend to better clinical outcomes and lower 90-day mortality, but the differences did not reach clinical significance.

Conclusions

- The use of IV heparin is associated with increased risk of ICH and with higher rates of recanalization. Both are dose related.
- Intra-arterial thrombolysis with low-dose heparin is safe and increases recanalization rates in patients with MCA stroke treated within 6 hours of symptom onset. However, clinical benefit could not be demonstrated.

PROACT II

PROACT II[21] was a phase III, randomized, multi-center trial. It included 180 patients within 6 hours of onset of an acute ischemic stroke and angiographically confirmed MCA occlusion. All patients had a microcatheter placed in the matrix of the thrombus. The patients were randomized to receive 9 mg of IA pro-urokinase plus low-dose heparin (as defined in PROACT) or IA placebo plus low-dose heparin alone. Although treated patients suffered more symptomatic ICH (10% vs. 2% in the heparin-only group), their likelihood of recanalization and good clinical outcome was significantly higher (66% vs. 18% recanalization, 40% vs. 25% modified Rankin scale (mRS) of 2 or less).

Conclusions

- IA thrombolysis is safe and improves clinical outcomes in patients with MCA ischemic stroke treated within 6 hours of symptom onset.

Other studies

Recently, a case-control analysis was reported using data from 16 922 acute ischemic stroke patients that were enrolled into Japan's Multicenter Stroke Investigator's Collaboration (J-MUSIC).[44] Ninety-one patients had presented within 4.5 hours after symptom onset and received IA urokinase. All patients had cardioembolic stroke in the carotid artery distribution with an National Institutes of Health Stroke Scale (NIHSS) score ranging from 5 to 22. They were compared to a control group of 182 patients without IA treatment matched for NIHSS score, gender, and age. The mRS score at discharge was lower in the IA urokinase treated group than in the control group and the rate of favorable outcome (mRS of 0–2) was higher in the urokinase treated group (51%) than in the control group (34%).

Macleod et al.[45] randomized patients with angiographic evidence of posterior circulation vascular occlusion that presented within 24 hours of symptom onset to either IA treated urokinase or conservative management. Sixteen patients were randomized, and there was some imbalance between groups, with greater severity of deficits at baseline observed in the treatment arm. A good outcome was observed in four of eight patients who received intra-arterial urokinase compared with one of eight patients in the control group.

Combined intravenous and intra-arterial thrombolysis (bridging approach), single-arm studies

A reduced dose of thrombolytic is administered intravenously, so as to reserve a smaller dose for IA administration.

The theoretical advantage of this approach is that it combines the rapid administration of IV thrombolytic medication with the selective IA thrombolysis that offers enhanced local lytic activity. The comparison between different studies is limited by differences in methods of administration, thrombolytic agents, and doses.

Suarez and colleagues[46] treated a series of 45 patients with 0.6 mg/kg of IV rt-PA followed by IA urokinase or rt-PA after they were triaged based on magnetic resonance imaging (MRI) findings. The incidence of symptomatic ICH was low at 4.4%, and favorable clinical outcomes were observed in 77% of patients.

Interventional Management of Stroke (IMS)

The IMS study[47] was an open-label, single-arm, NINDS-funded pilot study. Patients included ($n = 80$) had a NIHSS score of 10 or greater and were treated within 3 hours from onset of stroke symptoms. They received 0.6 mg/kg of IV rt-PA, followed by up to 22 mg of rt-PA given IA at the site of the thrombus. The patients were compared to the NINDS rt-PA and placebo-treated patients. No significant difference was found between NINDS rt-PA treated patients and IMS patients as regards 3-month mortality, 3-month clinical outcome and rate of symptomatic ICH. Asymptomatic ICH was more common ($P<0.0001$) among the IMS patients. The high rates of asymptomatic ICH that are commonly observed in studies that involve intra-arterial thrombolysis are generally attributed to high resolution advanced computed tomography (CT) scanners and the presence of contrast that can be mistaken for blood.

IMS II

IMS II[48] used similar patient selection criteria and administered IV rt-PA using a protocol similar to IMS. If an arterial occlusion was detected at angiography, additional rt-PA was administered via the EKOS micro-infusion catheter or a standard micro-catheter at the site of the thrombus up to a total dose of 22 mg. The 3-month mortality among the 81 IMS II patients was 16% as compared with the mortality of placebo (24%) and rt-PA-treated subjects (21%) in the NINDS rt-PA Stroke trial. IMS II patients had significantly better outcomes at 3 months than NINDS placebo-treated subjects for all end points and better outcomes than NINDS rt-PA-treated subjects in selected endpoints.

Combined intravenous and intra-arterial thrombolysis vs. intravenous thrombolysis

EMS

The Emergency Management of Stroke (EMS) trial[49] included 35 patients within 3 hours from stroke onset. The patients were randomized to combined IV and IA rt-PA (0.6 mg/kg IV followed by up to 20 mg IA, $n = 17$) or placebo and IA rt-PA ($n = 18$). In the IV/IA group there were higher recanalization rates, but clinical outcomes were not significantly better, and there were also more hemorrhagic complications.

IMS III

The IMS III trial which is currently underway compares combined IV/IA treatment with IV thrombolysis alone. Aside from standard micro-catheters and the EKOS micro-catheter, the Mechanical Embolus Removal in Cerebral Ischemia (MERCI) retriever is also being studied.

IA vs. IV thrombolysis

BASICS

BASICS[50] was a multi-center study that enrolled 619 consecutive patients with basilar artery occlusion. Of the 592 patients who were ultimately analyzed, 183 were treated conservatively, 121 with IV thrombolysis (including 41 patients who received additional IA treatment), and 288 were treated with multimodal, IA thrombolysis. In patients with mild to moderate deficits, IA treatment was inferior to IV, and in patients with severe deficits there was no significant difference.

Other studies

A randomized multicenter trial[51] compared IV urokinase with IA urokinase within the first 6 hours of acute ischemic stroke. Patients fulfilling the selection criteria were randomly assigned to receive urokinase 900 000 units via the IV ($n = 14$) or IA ($n = 13$) approach. The study was terminated when 27 patients had been included because of the overall high mortality rate. Seven patients (26%) died, four in the IV group, three in the IA group. Although IA-treated patients showed greater and earlier improvement there was no significant difference in primary and secondary outcomes.

IA thrombolysis following full-dose treatment with IV rt-PA

Use of IA thrombolysis in patients who have not responded to full dose IV rt-PA was recently reported in a series of 69 patients.[52] The rate of ICH (5.8%) was comparable to that reported in the NINDS rt-PA trial. Recanalization was achieved in 72% of patients and outcome was favorable (discharge home or to an inpatient rehabilitation facility) in 55%.

In a recent meta-analysis,[53] patients who had received full-dose IV rt-PA followed by IA intervention were compared to patients who had received 0.6 mg/kg IV rt-PA followed by IA intervention. Patients who had been treated with 0.9 mg/kg of IV rt-PA had higher rates of favorable outcome [odds ratio; OR = 1.60, 95% confidence interval; 95% CI = 1.07–2.40, $P = 0.022$] and similar rates of symptomatic ICH (OR = 0.86, 95% CI 0.41–1.83, $P = 0.70$).

Mechanical thrombolysis

MERCI I

The MERCI I trial[54] investigated the safety and efficacy of an embolectomy device (Merci retriever) used within 8 hours of symptom onset in patients who were ineligible for IV rt-PA in a prospective, non-randomized, multicenter trial. Angiographic recanalization was achieved in 48% of patients, while clinically significant procedural complications occurred in 7% of the patients. Good neurological outcome (mRS of 0–2) was associated with successful recanalization.

Multi-MERCI

The Multi MERCI[55,56] was an international, multicenter, prospective, single-arm trial of patients with large vessel stroke treated within 8 hours of symptom onset. Baseline stroke severity was high (median NIHSS score 19, range 15–23). Patients were recruited if they had received IV rt-PA with no improvement or were ineligible for IV rt-PA. Treatment with the Retriever alone resulted in successful recanalization in 54% of treated vessels and in 69% after adjunctive therapy (IA thrombolysis). Clinically significant procedural complications occurred in 5% of the patients. The symptomatic ICH rate was not significantly different between patients who had and patients who had not received IV rt-PA (7% vs 10%).

Pooled MERCI and multi-MERCI data analyses

Systolic blood pressure of < 150 mmHg and M2 occlusion were independent predictors of recanalization.[57] The strongest predictors of mortality and good outcome were recanalization status, baseline NIHSS score, and age. ICA occlusion was an additional predictor of mortality, but did not appear to influence the chance of good outcome.

Flint and colleagues[58] identified 80 patients with intracranial internal carotid artery (ICA) occlusion among the MERCI and Multi-MERCI subjects. The achieved recanalization rates were not significantly different from the overall rates (54% without and 63% with adjunct endovascular treatment). Patients with angiographic recanalization had at 90 days a 30% mortality rate and a 39% chance of good outcome as opposed to a 73% mortality rate ($P < 0.001$) and a 3% chance of good outcome ($P < 0.001$) among patients who failed to recanalize.

In a different subgroup analysis, Lutsep et al.[59] looked at patients with vertebrobasilar occlusions. Among 27 patients, recanalization was achieved in 78% and among those subjects there was a trend towards better outcome. At 90 days, good outcome was seen in 41% and mortality was 44%.

Nogueira and colleagues[60] reported on the outcomes among patients with abnormal hemostasis as defined by an international normalized ratio (INR) of >1.7, an aPTT of >45 seconds, or a platelet count of <100 000. There was no significant difference in their rates of symptomatic ICH, recanalization, and mortality, but their rate of good outcome was only 9% (vs. 35% in patients with normal hemostasis; $P = 0.002$).

Penumbra system

The first report published on the Penumbra system was by Bose and colleagues.[61] Twenty-one target vessels were treated in 20 consecutive patients presenting within 8 hours from symptom onset. Stroke severity was high, with 11 patients having an NIHSS score of greater than 20. Six of the patients had received IV thrombolysis without response. The primary endpoint of a Thrombolysis in Myocardial Infarction (TIMI) score of ≥ 2 (partial or complete recanalization) in the affected vessel was met by all patients. At 30-day follow-up, 45% had an mRS score of ≤ 2. The all-cause mortality rate was also 45%.

The Penumbra Pivotal Stroke Trial, published in the following year, included 125 patients presenting within 8 hours of symptom onset with an NIHSS score of ≥ 8 and an angiographically verified occlusion of a large intracranial vessel.[62] The revascularization rate to TIMI 2 or 3 was 81.6%. At 90 days, 25% of the patients had an mRS score of ≤ 2, and the mortality rate was 32.8%. Recanalization was strongly associated with good clinical outcome at 30 days, but the association declined to borderline significance by 90 days.

The remaining available published data also demonstrate high recanalization rates (80%–93%) and acceptable rates of symptomatic ICH (0%–7%).[63-65] Further studies will be needed to assess the significance of this intervention for patient outcome.

Intravenous GPIIB/IIIA inhibitors and intra-arterial thrombolytics

Use of platelet GPIIB/IIIA inhibitors has been suggested to prevent platelet activation and reocclusion and is being evaluated in several studies as adjunctive therapy to IA thrombolysis.

Qureshi et al.[66] enrolled 20 patients presenting at 3–6 hours in a dose-ranging Phase I study with 4 escalating tiers of IA reteplase (0.5, 1, 1.5, and 2 units). The patients received IV abciximab as a 0.25 mg/kg bolus followed by 0.125 µg/kg per min continuous infusion. There was only 1 ICH (in the 1 unit tier). Recanalization was achieved in 13/20 patients and favorable outcome at one month (mRS ≤ 2) was observed in six patients.

A multicenter study[67] reported the results of treating patients with acute vertebrobasilar occlusion using a combination of IV bolus of abciximab (0.25 mg/kg) followed by a 12-hour infusion therapy (0.125 µg/kg per minute) and low-dose IA rt-PA (median dosage: 20 mg) in 47 patients. The results were compared with a retrospective cohort of 41 patients, treated by IA rt-PA monotherapy (median dosage: 40 mg). The rate of symptomatic ICHs was 13% and 12% for combination treatment and thrombolytic treatment alone, respectively. The combination treatment had higher rates of complete recanalization (45% vs. 22%), favorable outcomes (34% vs. 17%), and survival (62% vs. 32%) compared with thrombolysis alone.

Nagel and colleagues[68] studied 75 patients with basilar artery occlusion who had been treated at a single center over a period of 8 years. Thirty-two patients who had received IA rt-PA only were compared to 45 patients who had received IV abciximab and IA rt-PA. Patients in the combined treatment group had significantly higher recanalization rates (83.7% vs. 62.5%, $P = 0.03$), survival rates (58.1 vs. 25%, $P = 0.01$) and favorable outcome (mRS $\leq$ 3; 34.9% vs. 12.5%, $P = 0.02$). Symptomatic ICH rates were similar in both groups.

IA GPIIB/IIIA inhibitors

GPIIB/IIIA inhibitors have been administered intra-arterially in the setting of multi-modal thrombolysis, but there are no data derived from prospective studies yet.

Hypothermia

New efforts are directed towards delaying irreversible ischemic injury in the period prior to recanalization using IA thrombolysis[69] and to avoid the "futile recanalization phenomenon". Hypothermia is a promising adjunct to endovascular treatment due to its neuroprotective effect. Results of a pilot study suggested that moderate hypothermia (32–34 °C) induced by surface cooling was technically feasible and safe for patients with acute ischemic strokes who were undergoing IV or IA thrombolytic therapy.[69] In a subsequent multicenter study,[70] endovascular cooling using a heat exchange catheter to a core body temperature of 33 °C was feasible in patients with moderate to severe anterior circulation territory ischemic stroke. Among the 18 patients who underwent hypothermia, IV and IA thrombolysis was used in ten and three patients, respectively. The rate of ICH was not different compared with the group that was treated with normothermia.

Cerebral perfusion augmentation devices

Specific devices have also been developed to augment cerebral perfusion such as dual inflatable balloons that are positioned in supra-renal and infra-renal locations[71] and sequentially inflated to improve rCBF. Studies are underway to assess the feasibility and efficacy of this approach to maintain residual flow prior to IA thrombolysis.

Selection of patients for endovascular treatment

There is no evidence yet to support that IA treatment following IV thrombolysis is beneficial for all stroke patients and IV thrombolysis remains the standard of care for patients who present within the treatment window. Criteria that have been proposed or used for selection of patients to undergo endovascular intervention have included presentation between 3 h and 8 h after symptom onset, severe neurological deficits (NIHSS score ≥ 10), recent history of major surgical procedures (within 14 days), and occlusion of major cervical or intracranial vessels. A list of available evidence and indications is presented in Table 5.1.[21–23,44–46,51,54,55,58,67,72–102]

Time from stroke onset

Patients presenting 3 hours or more after onset of symptoms have not been eligible for IV rt-PA. In the Alteplase Thrombolysis for Acute Noninterventional Therapy in Ischemic Stroke (ATLANTIS) study,[103] patients with ischemic stroke who received IV alteplase (0.9 mg/kg) 3 to 5 hours after onset of symptoms had similar outcomes as those observed in patients who received placebo. However, the ECASS III trial showed significant benefit for patients treated at 3–4.5 hours from symptom onset[104] and the American Stroke Association has therefore recently recommended expanding the IV treatment window to 4.5 hours.[105]

IA therapy demonstrated a benefit up to 6 hours after onset of symptoms in the PROACT II trial.[21] Therefore, IA therapy is currently the only proven treatment available to patients presenting 4.5 hours or more after onset of symptoms.

Severity of neurological deficits on presentation

The predicted clinical response to intravenously administered rt-PA was analyzed in the Standard Treatment with Alteplase to Reverse Stroke (STARS) study.[6] A total of 389 patients with a mean age of 69 years (range 28–100 years) were treated with intravenously administered rt-PA within 3 hours of onset of symptoms. The analysis demonstrated a 22% decrease in the odds of recovery for every five-point increase in baseline NIHSS score; patients with baseline NIHSS scores of more than 10 experienced a 75% decrease in the odds of recovery. Similarly, Tomsick et al.[106] reported on 55 patients with acute ischemic stroke who were treated with intravenously administered rt-PA within 90 minutes of onset of symptoms. Patients with major neurological deficits (NIHSS score ≥ 10) experienced a significantly lower frequency of favorable outcomes.

Patients with contra-indications for intravenous thrombolysis

Super-selective IA administration of thrombolytics reduces overall systemic exposure to thrombolytics. Therefore, patients who have undergone major surgery within the past 14 days and are ineligible for IV rt-PA may be treated with IA thrombolysis.[107] No major hemorrhagic complications related to surgical sites have been observed in previous series.[76,108]

Patients who are therapeutically anticoagulated are also ineligible for IV rt-PA. In a recent case series of three patients, anticoagulation was reversed with fresh frozen plasma transfusion and small-dose IA reteplase was administered without complications.[109]

Radiological criteria
Diffusion-weighted imaging (DWI)

Acute DWI changes are widely used to assess irreversible tissue damage in the setting of acute stroke.[110] In order to make an estimate of the penumbra, i.e., the salvageable ischemic tissue,

Table 5.1. Summary of evidence of efficacy of IA thrombolysis for ischemic stroke patients depending on clinical and radiological features, site of vascular occlusion and IA treatment used

Indications	Recanalization	Safety	Better than conservative management	Comparison to IV rt-PA
Clinical features				
All ischemic strokes within 3 hours of SO	Level III[86,87]	Level III[87]	Level III[87]	Equivalent, Level III[87]
All ischemic strokes within 6 hours of SO	Level V[51,81–85,88]	Level II[51,81–85,88]	Level V[51,81–85,88]	Equivalent, Level II[85]
All anterior circulation ischemic strokes within 6 hours of SO	Level III[44]	Level III[44]	Level III[44]	Level V[80]
All posterior circulation ischemic strokes within 6 hours (or 24 hours) of SO	Level II[45]	Level II[45]	Level II[45,79]	Equivalent within 3 hours of SO, Level V[78]
Ineligible for iv rt-PA within 6 hours of SO	Level V[22,23,77]	Level V[22,23,77]	Level V[22,23,77]	Iv rt-PA contraindicated
Perioperative stroke within 6 hours of SO	Level V[75,76]	Level V[75,76]	Level V[75,76]	Iv rt-PA contraindicated
Radiological features				
Hyperdense artery sign on CT scan	Level III[74]	Level III[74]	Level V[74]	Superior to iv rt-PA (Level III)[74]
Early ischemic changes on CT scan	Level II[72]	Level II[72]	Level II[72,73]	Superior to iv rt-PA (level III)[73]
Perfusion deficits on CT perfusion	Level V[89]	Level V[89]	Level V[89]	N/A
PWI–DWI mismatch in MRI	Level V[46,87,90]	Level V[46,87,90]	Level V[46,87,90]	N/A
Deficits on SPECT scan	Level V[91]	Level V[91]	Level V[91]	N/A
Site of occlusion				
ICA occlusion within 8 hours of SO	Level V[23,58,75,92]	Level V[23,58,75,92]	Level V[23,58,75,92]	N/A
MCA occlusions within 6 hours of SO	Level I[20,21,93]	Level I[20,21,93]	Level I[21]	N/A
Vertebral/basilar occlusions within 24 hours of SO	Level II[45,93–95]	Level II[45,93–95]	Level II[4593–95]	Equivalent within 3 hours of SO, Level V[78]
Technique				
IA pro-urokinase	Level I[20,21]	Level I[20,21]	Level I[20,21]	N/A
IA urokinase	Level III[44,45,85,88]	Level III[44,45,85,88]	Level III[44,45,85,88]	N/A
IA alteplase (rt-PA)	Level IV[86,87,96]	Level IV[86,87,96]	Level IV[86,87,96]	Level IV[86,87,96]
IA reteplase	Level V[51,88,97]	Level V[51,88,97]	Level V[51,88,97]	N/A
IA thrombolysis with IV abciximab	Level IV[67,98,99]	Level IV[67,98,99]	Level IV[67,98,99]	N/A
IA thrombolysis with mechanical disruption of thrombus	Level V[22,51,88,100]	Level V[22,51,88,100]	Level V[22,51,88,100]	N/A
IV rt-PA followed by IA thrombolysis	Level IV[86,87,101]	Level IV[86,87,101]	Level IV[86,87,101]	Level IV[86,87,101]
Mechanical clot retrieval	Level IV[54,55,58,102]	Level IV[54,55,58,102]	Level IV[54,55,58,102]	IV contraindicated
IV followed by mechanical clot retrieval	Level IV[55]	Level IV[55]	Level IV[55]	N/A
Definitions of levels of evidence				
Level I. Data from randomized trials with low false-positive and low false-negative errors				
Level II. Data from randomized trials with high false-positive and high false-negative errors				
Level III. Data from non randomized concurrent cohort studies				
Level IV. Data from non randomized cohort studies using historical controls				
Level V. Data from anecdotal case series (Adapted from Adams HP[1])				

Abbreviations used: N/A, No comparison available; SO, symptom onset; rt-PA, recombinant tissue plasminogen activator; MRI, magnetic resonance imaging; CT, computed tomography; IA, intra-arterial; IV, intravenous.

Symbols used: *Evidence not strong for preferential use over intravenous rt-PA in appropriate candidates.

abnormalities on DWI images are compared to those detected by perfusion weighted images (PWI). The area of PWI–DWI mismatch (PWI abnormalities exceed DWI abnormalities) provides an estimate of the hypoperfused but viable tissue. This estimate is not entirely accurate because DWI lesions can regress[111] and PWI abnormalities include areas of benign oligemia which are likely to survive in any scenario.[111] Patients with significant mismatch are ideal candidates for endovascular intervention.

If PWI cannot be obtained, the clinical-diffusion mismatch (CDM) is an acceptable surrogate. CDM, defined as an NIHSS score of ≥ 8 combined with an ischemic (DWI) volume of $\leq 25\,\mathrm{mL}$ has been shown to predict PWI–DWI mismatch[112] (specificity 93%, sensitivity 53%), infarct growth, and early neurological deterioration.[113]

CT perfusion

With the onset of ischemia, regional cerebral blood flow (rCBF) decreases. Penumbral tissue can still auto-regulate, and thus maintain regional cerebral blood volume (rCBV). Infarcted tissue loses the ability to autoregulate (vasodilate) and exhibits a reduction in rCBF and rCBV. Therefore, the mismatch between rCBF and rCBV changes can be used to assess the penumbra similarly to DWI–PWI mismatch.[43,114]

Non-contrast CT scan

A study compared outcomes of patients treated with IV–IA rt-PA, IV rt-PA, and placebo within 3 hours of symptom onset stratified by the baseline CT scan appearance.[73] The CT scans were scored using the Alberta Stroke Program Early CT (ASPECT) score and dichotomized into ASPECT score > 7 (favorable scan) and ASPECT score ≤ 7 (unfavorable scan). A multiplicative interaction effect was shown indicating that patients with an ASPECT score > 7 in the IV–IA cohort were more likely to have a good outcome compared with IV rt-PA and with placebo.

Another study compared outcomes of 83 patients with and without hyperdense artery sign on initial CT scan treated with IV or IA rt-PA.[74] A favorable outcome, indicated by a significant improvement in the discharge NIHSS score, was noted in patients treated with IA rt-PA, irrespective of the presence or absence of hyperdense artery sign. A less favorable outcome in discharge NIHSS score was noted with IV rt-PA in patients with hyperdense artery sign than those without the hyperdense artery sign. The observation suggests that the differential response to IV rt-PA in patients with hyperdense artery sign on initial CT scan is not seen with IA thrombolysis. Other radiological criteria proposed as seen in Table 5.1 lack any direct or indirect evidence for preferential use of IV or IA thrombolysis.

Endovascular treatment protocols
Initial angiography

The initial diagnostic angiography is very important. Emphasis must be placed on identifying the site of occlusion and collateral supply to the affected region. An infusion catheter is placed in the aortic arch and contrast is injected using a programmed infusion system.[115] Concomitant cranial images are acquired in Townes projection (antero-posterior axis) using rapid frame acquisition. This technique allows visualization of all intracranial vessels and thus rapid identification of the site of occlusion and an initial estimate of collateral supply. In patients who already have undergone a CT angiogram, such global assessment of cerebral arteries may not be necessary. In order to further localize and quantify the occlusive lesion and collaterals, selective angiography follows.

Angiographic findings can be incorporated into a scheme that stratifies patients according to expected rate of recanalization and short-term outcome following IA thrombolysis (Table 5.2).[2,116,117] Two prognostic variables were incorporated into this grading scheme: anatomic site of occlusion and collateral supply.[2,116] The grades have been assigned according to recanalization response and clinical outcome associated with IA thrombolysis in previous studies. Patients with similar outcomes have been graded in the same categories. An attempt has been made to recognize the importance of collateral supply for occlusion sites where collaterals are found commonly and affect overall outcome. Previous studies have suggested that the clinical outcome after thrombolysis varies with the anatomic location of the occlusion. An ICA occlusion could result in an infarction that involves the distributions of both the anterior and middle cerebral arteries and is associated with poor outcome. Similarly, a complete occlusion of the basilar artery could result in an infarction involving the midbrain, pons, and cerebellum and is associated with poor outcome. The rate of recanalization also varies depending on the anatomic site of occlusion.

On the basis of the existing data, the grading scheme was designed to identify occlusions at sites with documented differences in rates of recanalization and clinical outcome. The five sites of occlusion that were identified were the internal carotid artery, main trunk of the MCA (M1 segment), superior or inferior division of the MCA (M2 segments), and MCA branches (M3 segments). Further sub-categorization of the MCA (M1) segment occlusion is based on the observation that occlusion of the MCA with involvement of lenticulostriate arteries (compared with lenticulostriate-sparing M1 occlusion) has a worse prognosis when treated with IA thrombolysis as regards outcome and risk of ICH. This observation is attributed to the fact that the lenticulostriate arteries are terminal vessels lacking collaterals; irreversible ischemic changes develop rapidly in the distribution of lenticulostriate arteries and delayed revascularization is associated with a high rate of ICH. On the basis of existing evidence, basilar artery occlusion was divided into either proximal (complete) occlusion or distal (partial) occlusion in the proposed classification scheme. To provide an objective criterion, basilar artery occlusion was considered partial if the basilar trunk was visualized along with filling of three or more major branches.

Table 5.2. Grading scheme for stratification of patients with acute ischemic stroke based on initial site of occlusion and collateral supply[2,116,117]

Grade 0	No occlusion		
Grade 1	MCA occlusion (M3 region)	ACA occlusion (A2 or distal segments)	1 BA/VA branch occlusion
Grade 2	MCA occlusion (M2 region)	ACA occlusion (A1 or A2 segments)	2 or more BA/VA branch occlusion
Grade 3	MCA occlusion (M1 Region)		
A	Lenticulostriate arteries spared and/or leptomeningeal collaterals visualized		
B	No sparing of lenticulostriate arteries nor leptomeningeal collaterals visualized		
Grade 4	ICA occlusion (collaterals present)	BA occlusion (partial filling direct or via collaterals)	
A	Collaterals fill MCA	Anterograde filling*	
B	Collaterals fill ACA	Retrograde filling*	
Grade 5	ICA occlusion (no collaterals)	BA occlusion (complete)	

Abbreviations used: *ACA*, anterior cerebral artery; *BA*, basilar artery; *VA*, vertebral artery.
*Predominant pattern of filling.

The inter-observer variability and correlation with recanalization, and short-term favorable outcome and mortality have been described in patients with acute ischemic stroke undergoing IA thrombolysis previously.[116,117]

Multiple studies have shown that residual perfusion in the affected distribution is an important determinant of clinical recovery and ICH after thrombolysis (see later section). The magnitude of the collateral circulation determines the reduction in rCBF that occurs within the affected distribution. Because of anastomotic connections between anterior and posterior portions of the craniocervical circulation and between hemispheres through the circle of Willis, collateral sources of supply may develop in patients with ICA and/or basilar artery occlusion. In patients with ICA occlusion, collateral supply through the anterior communicating artery may preserve the anterior cerebral artery distribution or the posterior circulation may provide supply to the anterior circulation through the posterior communicating artery. The grading scheme incorporates information regarding collateral supply to the anterior circulation in the presence of an ICA occlusion. A further subcategory (4A) is included to define the magnitude of collateral supply depending on the presence or absence of collateral filling of the ipsilateral MCA. A subcategory has been added to occlusion of the M1 segment of the MCA (Grade 3A) to include the favorable prognostic significance of leptomeningeal collaterals from cortical branches of the anterior cerebral artery to the MCA distribution. In the grading scheme, adequate collateralization of the posterior circulation was defined as visualization of the basilar trunk and three or more basilar artery branches through collateral filling from the anterior circulation. A definition for partial basilar occlusion was provided. The risk of infarction is dependent on the number of branches that are occluded and the number of branches that are patent. The basilar artery usually has a total of six major branches. Angiographic filling of three or more branches is an indication that at least half of the major branches are filling directly or via collateral pathways.

The Qureshi grading scale has been shown to correlate with the initial stroke severity, the volume of infarction in patients with anterior circulation stroke following IA thrombolysis, and in-hospital outcomes.[117,118]

Multimodal treatment: pharmacological thrombolysis and mechanical thrombectomy

A 6-French guide catheter is placed in the ICA or vertebral artery proximal to the occlusion site.[23] Each patient receives intravenously administered heparin (30 U/kg body weight) to achieve an activated clotting time (ACT) of more than 200 seconds. The ACT is checked periodically throughout the procedure and heparin boluses are administered as needed to keep it above 200 seconds. A 2.3-French microcatheter is advanced to the occluded vessel just proximal to the thrombus through the guide catheter over a micro-wire. A micro-catheter injection is used to confirm correct placement. The micro-wire is introduced again and passed through the clot. The micro-catheter is advanced past the clot and the micro-wire is removed. By means of a simultaneous injection through the guide-catheter and micro-catheter, the proximal and distal margins of the thrombus are visualized, allowing an assessment of the extent of the thrombus.[119] The micro-catheter injection past the clot is also useful for assessing distal vessel size. Thrombolytic (alteplase, reteplase, tenecteplase, or urokinase) is then infused at a rate of approximately one bolus over 5 minutes. Angiography is performed after each dose of thrombolytic is delivered to evaluate the status of recanalization. The dose of thrombolytic is titrated to angiographic recanalization with boluses also delivered into the clot and proximal to the clot. Mechanical disruption of the clot is undertaken after the first doses of thrombolytic have been administered and there is persistent partial or complete occlusion. In large vessels, including the ICA, proximal MCA (M1 segment), and basilar artery, angioplasty is performed using an angioplasty balloon catheter. The diameter of the balloon is selected on the basis of measurements of the vessel immediately proximal and distal to the occlusion. The size of the balloon should be roughly 80% of the smaller vessel diameter. One or, infrequently, two inflations of the angioplasty balloon are performed. In smaller vessels including the distal MCA (M2 and M3 segments), anterior cerebral artery, and posterior cerebral artery, a 2- or 4- mm snare is introduced through the 2.3-French micro-catheter and advanced into the clot matrix. Multiple passes are made through the clot using the fully extended loop of the snare to fragment, but not to capture, the clot. Snare maneuvers are permissible for proximal vessels if the distal end of the thrombus extends into distal vessels not amenable to angioplasty such as the M2 segment of the MCA. Additional thrombolytics are administered if required for further recanalization until a pre-determined maximal dose is reached. No heparin is given after the procedure is completed.

Multimodal treatment: pharmacological thrombolysis and mechanical thrombectomy using the MERCI retrieval device

The balloon guide catheter is inserted via the femoral route and placed either in the proximal ICA or the subclavian or vertebral arteries.[55] With the balloon of the guide catheter deflated, a 0.014-inch guide-wire is advanced through the clot within the occluded intracranial vessel. The micro-catheter is then advanced over this wire through the clot as described above. A selective angiogram is performed after traversing the thrombus to evaluate the size and tortuosity of the distal arteries. Once the micro-catheter is in correct position, the guide-wire is exchanged for the embolectomy device. The X5 or X6 Merci Retriever is advanced through the micro-catheter until 2 to 3 helical loops are deployed beyond the thrombus.[102] The retriever is then retracted and the proximal loops are deployed within the thrombus. Five clockwise rotations are applied to the retriever to ensnare the thrombus. The balloon at the outside of the guide-catheter is inflated to institute regional flow arrest in the path of thrombus withdrawal (to prevent distal embolization). The Merci retriever with the ensnared thrombus, and the micro-catheter are retrieved together into the guide catheter lumen. The L5 retriever device is used in a manner similar to the first generation of retriever devices.[55] The L5 retriever is advanced so that up to four of the distal loops of the helix are deployed distal to the thrombus. The micro-catheter and the device are then pulled back to fully engage the thrombus and the proximal loops of the device are deployed by further retraction of the micro-catheter. The balloon of the guide catheter is inflated to initiate flow arrest within the proximal arterial segment, and the micro-catheter and embolectomy device are gently withdrawn into the lumen of the guide catheter while aspirating with a syringe. The balloon is then deflated and the clot is retrieved. Up to six Retriever passes within the vessel were allowed in previous clinical trials to achieve recanalization.[55] An illustrative case is presented in Fig 1 (A-J).

Multimodal treatment: internal carotid artery occlusion with or without tandem occlusion

Acute extracranial ICA occlusion resulting in ischemic stroke is different from other forms of acute occlusion of the cerebral blood vessels.[120] The occluded segment of the ICA consists of predominantly atherosclerotic plaque with a superimposed thrombus. In acute occlusions of intracranial vessels an embolus usually blocks a vessel that was previously normal. Because of the presence of pre-existing atherosclerotic disease, ICA occlusion should be approached with the intention to place a self-expanding stent. Visualization of the ICA distal to the occlusion must be performed prior to treatment for two reasons: to confirm patency of the distal vessel which could be occluded from embolization or clot propagation (especially in the supraclinoid region) and to obtain vessel measurements so as to select stent size accurately.

A 6-F guide sheath is advanced over a stiff 0.035 inch guide-wire into the arch of the aorta. The ICA is catheterized using a 120–125 cm 5- or 6-F Simmons I or II catheter placed through the guide sheath. The sheath is subsequently advanced over the catheter until it reaches the distal common carotid artery. The patient is given IV heparin before the occlusion is traversed. A steerable guide wire is gently advanced from the ipsilateral common carotid artery through the occlusion into the distal cervical ICA. Attempts should be made to cross the lesion with a 0.014-inch or 0.018-inch micro-wire. However, in some cases, a 0.035-inch wire might be neccesary.[121] A micro-catheter or diagnostic catheter is advanced over the wire into the distal cervical ICA. Repeat angiography of the ICA distal to the occlusion is performed to assess for tandem occlusion and obtain vessel measurements. Subsequently, through the catheter, an exchange length wire is placed in the high-cervical segment of the ICA. Over this wire, a balloon catheter is placed across the lesion and a pre-stent sub-maximal angioplasty is performed so as to facilitate passage of the stent. The balloon catheter is then exchanged for the stent catheter and the stent is brought in position and deployed. Details on stent sizing and positioning are presented in Chapter 4. Post-stent angioplasty maybe required, depending on the residual stenosis. After the cervical ICA is recanalized, treatment of the tandem lesion is undertaken in the manner described above.

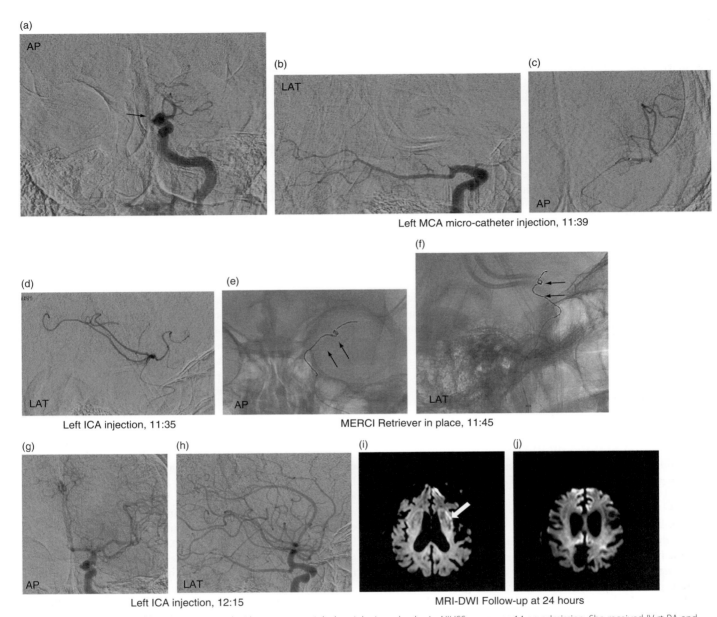

Left MCA micro-catheter injection, 11:39

Left ICA injection, 11:35

MERCI Retriever in place, 11:45

Left ICA injection, 12:15

MRI-DWI Follow-up at 24 hours

Fig. 5.1. (a)–(j). A 94-year old woman presented with acute-onset right hemiplegia and aphasia. NIHSS score was 14 on admission. She received IV rt-PA and was taken to angio suite for possible intervention. Diagnostic angiography revealed occlusion of the left ICA intracranially (arrow) (a), (B). An 8-French concentric balloon guide-catheter was positioned in the cervical ICA. A MERCI 18 L micro-catheter was introduced over a Synchro 2 standard micro-wire and positioned in the superior division of the left MCA (c), (d). The MERCI retriever was then deployed (see arrows) (e), (f) and the system was pulled back. Once the system was in the supraclinoid portion of the ICA, the guide-catheter balloon was inflated and suction was applied. The micro-catheter and retriever were removed. Subsequent guide-catheter injections showed complete recanalization of the ICA (g), (h). Follow-up MRI at 24 hours (i), (j) showed a small region of diffusion restriction (arrow, i). The patient had only a mild residual deficit. Abbreviations used: ICA, internal carotid artery; MCA, middle cerebral artery; DWI, diffusion-weighted imaging; NIHSS, National Institutes of Health Stroke Scale; IV, intravenous; rt-PA, recombinant tissue plasminogen activator.

Ultrasound-enhanced thrombolysis

Enhancement of thrombolysis through ultrasound: experimental evidence

The ability of ultrasonic mechanical pressure waves to enhance thrombolysis was first documented in the 1970s,[122,123] and has been confirmed by several investigators in experimental in vitro and in vivo models.[124–128] Various ultrasound energies ranging from 0.2–2.0 W/cm^2 and frequencies ranging from 20 kHz to 2 MHz were used in these studies. Moreover, ultrasound can promote the motion of fluid around a thrombus, an effect called microstreaming.[129] It is possible that the application of ultrasound energy agitates the blood close to the occluding thrombus and promotes the mixing of rt-PA, effectively increasing the concentration of the agent that is in contact with the thrombus. Consequently, it has been hypothesized that in stroke patients, ultrasound can promote rt-PA delivery to the areas with stagnant flow near the occlusion.

Although low kiloHertz frequencies better potentiate rt-PA effects,[130] these systems are not available for clinical practice due to safety concerns and inability to image vasculature with this frequency/wavelength range. Meanwhile, 1–2.2 MHz frequencies can also enhance rt-PA-induced thrombus dissolution utilizing various mechanisms such as fluid streaming around clot surface, disaggregation of fibrin fibers, and creating more binding sites for rt-PA without heating or cavitation.[131,132]

Diagnostic applications of ultrasound in acute cerebral ischemia

Portable diagnostic 2 MHz TCD equipment can be used in the emergency department for continuous monitoring during the infusion of rt-PA in acute ischemic stroke patients.[133] With prior training and experience in the interpretation of TCD, this test, particularly in combination with urgent carotid/vertebral artery duplex scanning, can yield a high degree of accuracy for bedside detection and localization of arterial occlusion and recanalization.[134,135] In addition, TCD can provide complementary information to other imaging modalities such as CT angiography by showing real-time flow findings (embolization, collateralization of flow, alternating flow signals indicative of steal phenomenon).[136]

Once abnormal residual flow signals are identified, an ultrasound beam can be steadily focused at the presumed intra-cranial thrombus location, and arterial recanalization can be monitored in real time.[135] When IV rt-PA infusion was continuously monitored with 2 MHz TCD, there was higher rates of early recanalization and dramatic recovery.[135] Two other studies conducted by separate groups in Germany[137,138] and France[139] also reported higher rates of recanalization than expected in patients with acute MCA occlusion who were not eligible for rt-PA and received

2 MHz color-coded TCD continuous monitoring. This intriguing finding suggested a potential therapeutic effect of diagnostic TCD ultrasound in the setting of acute cerebral ischemia and led to the design of prospective randomized clinical trials.

Therapeutic applications of ultrasound in acute cerebral ischemia
Transcranial Doppler

The CLOTBUST (Combined Lysis of Thrombus in Brain ischemia using transcranial Ultrasound and Systemic rt-PA) was a phase II clinical randomized multi-center international trial.[140] It had pre-specified safety and efficacy end-points and a pre-determined sample size of 63 patients per group. All enrolled patients had acute ischemic stroke due to MCA occlusion and were treated with the standard 0.9 mg/kg dose of IV rt-PA therapy within 3 hours of symptom onset. They were randomized (1:1) to a target group receiving continuous TCD-monitoring or to a control group with monitoring at pre-specified intervals. The safety end-point was symptomatic ICH resulting in worsening of the neurologic deficit by 4 or more points on the NIHSS score. The primary combined activity end-point was complete recanalization on TCD or dramatic clinical recovery, defined as NIHSS score $\leq$ 3, or improvement by $\geq$ 10 points on the NIHSS within 2 hours following the rt-PA bolus.

All projected 126 patients received rt-PA and were randomized 1:1 to target (median pre-treatment NIHSS score 16) or control (median NIHSS score 17).[140] Age, occlusion location by TCD and time to rt-PA bolus were similar between groups. Symptomatic ICH occurred in 4.8% in both groups. The primary end-point was achieved by 31 (49%) target vs. 19 (30%) control patients, $P = 0.03$. The rate of sustained complete recanalization at the end of TCD-monitoring was 38% in the active and 13% in the control group. At 3 months, 42% of the target and 29% of the control patients achieved favorable outcomes (mRS 0–1, $P = 0.20$). CLOTBUST was not powered to evaluate the efficacy of ultrasound-enhanced thrombolysis in improving functional outcome, but was designed to establish the safety of this treatment and to provide preliminary data for the design of a larger clinical efficacy trial. Indeed, the detected trend towards better functional outcomes in patients treated with continuous TCD-monitoring, indicates the feasibility of a pivotal phase III clinical trial that, at 274 patients per group, would be properly powered to detect this difference in 3-month outcomes. The main limitation of the CLOTBUST trial was related to the extreme dependency on the skill of the operator who performed TCD, which makes these results difficult to generalize. It is unrealistic to expect that the average clinician can quickly develop the skills for the rapid localization of occlusions with this hand-held diagnostic method. Therefore, very few stroke centers are

Table 5.3. Reported controlled clinical trials of microsphere-potentiated ultrasound-enhanced systemic thrombolysis for acute ischemic stroke using Trancranial Doppler (TCD) and Transcranial Color-Coded (TCCD) Ultrasonography

Trial	F	Microspheres	Design	R	REC**	AsxICH**	sICH**	Outcome at 3 months
TCD								
Molina et al.[151]	2 MHz	galactose-based	US/MS/rt-PA (n = 38) vs. US/rt-PA (n = 37) vs. TPA (n=36)	N	55%	23%	3%	56% (mRS 0–2)
Alexandrov et al.[150]	2 MHz	perfultren-lipid	US/MS/rt-PA (n = 12) vs. US/rt-PA (n = 3)	Y	42%	25%	0%	40% (mRS 0–1)
TCCD								
Larrue et al.[149]	2 MHz*	galactose-based	US/MS/rt-PA (n = 9) vs. rt-PA (n = 11)	Y	48%	78%	0%	NA
Perren et al.[148]	2 MHz*	phospholipid-encapsulated sulphur hexafluoride	US/MS/rt-PA (n = 11) vs. rt-PA (n = 15)	N	64%	NA	9%	NA

Abbreviations used: US, Continuous Ultrasound Monitoring; MS, gaseous microspheres; rt-PA recombinant tissue plasminogen activator; R, Randomization; REC, recanalization at the end of TCD monitoring; sICH, symptomatic intracranial hemorrhage; AsxICH, asymptomatic intracranial hemorrhage; mRS, modified Rankin Scale; NA, not available; Y, yes; N, no; F, Frequency; ECA,
*patients received monitoring with a pulsed wave 2 MHz phased array Doppler and intermittent exposure to dual frequency duplex
**complete recanalization in the active treatment group (microsphere-potentiated ultrasound-enhanced systemic) thrombolysis.

qualified to participate in CLOTBUST and other future trials evaluating the efficacy of ultrasound-enhanced thrombolysis. The great majority of CLOTBUST patients (121 of 126) were enrolled by 2 of the 4 participating centers.

Transcranial color-coded duplex

Transcranial duplex technology was recently tested in a smaller randomized clinical trial. Duplex transducers are different from the ones used in CLOTBUST since they generate multiple small beams at dual emitting frequencies, one for Doppler and one for gray scale imaging (Table 5.3). One of the major limitations of this technology is that there are no reliable head frames for transducer fixation, and most studies are carried out using hand-held probes. In addition, the mechanical index of these scanners is higher than TCD and no dose escalation study was performed to determine what dose of ultrasound is needed to enhance thrombolysis without safety concerns that will be outlined below.

Eggers et al.[138] evaluated 25 patients (11 treated with rt-PA and duplex monitoring vs. 14 control patients treated with rt-PA alone) and reported a trend in the target group towards higher recanalization rates, more hemorrhagic transformations (18% symptomatic ICH rate), and better neurologic outcomes at 3 months compared to patients who received rt-PA alone. This study did not have a pre-determined sample size, and the results may be affected by the small number of patients enrolled. More studies are needed to evaluate the potential of transcranial duplex technology to enhance thrombolysis.[138]

The same group and others[137–139,141] reported the provocative finding that patients who are not eligible for systemic rt-PA therapy may potentially benefit from continuous monitoring with ultrasound alone since, hypothetically, ultrasound may help facilitate the endogenous thrombolytic process that leads to spontaneous recanalization in patients with acute stroke. It is unclear if only partial recanalization can be induced by ultrasound alone, and if this exposure would result in a significant difference at 3 months justifying a large clinical trial. In any case, there are no clear data regarding the benefit of ultrasound monitoring without rt-PA. Therefore, rt-PA treatment should not be substituted by ultrasound alone in patients who are eligible for IV thrombolysis. Furthermore, different experimental strategies are being tested in an extended time window for acute stroke treatment, and continuous exposure to ultrasound may find its application in combination with other strategies such as GPIIB/IIIA antagonists, direct thrombin inhibitors or as an adjunct to IA thrombolysis.

Intra-arterial ultrasound devices

Ultrasound transducers have been incorporated into catheters for intra-arterial delivery of thrombolytic drugs (EKOS® NeuroWave™ Catheter, EKOS Corporation, Bothell, WA). The EKOS MicroLysUS infusion catheter is a 2.5F standard micro-infusion catheter with a 2 mm, 2.1 MHz pulsed-wave ring sonography transducer (average power 0.21–0.45 W, average SPTA intensity 400 mW/cm^2) at its distal tip. This transducer generates a 360° circumferential pulse wave around the distal tip and is designed to be used in conjunction with IA thrombolytic infusion.

A pilot study found that the use of the EKOS microcatheter is feasible in the treatment of acute ischemic stroke.[100] In 14 subjects, the average time to recanalization was 46 minutes with eight patients achieving TIMI flow grades of 2 (partial recanalization) or 3 (complete recanalization) within the first hour. Overall clinical outcomes as measured by mRS grades of ≤ 2 were similar to historical controls. Mortality (36%) and symptomatic ICH (14%) rates compared reasonably to those reported in previous trials of IA thrombolysis.

The EKOS catheter has been tested in the IMS II trial. The rate of symptomatic ICH in IMS II subjects (9.9%)[48] was not significantly different from that of rt-PA treated subjects in the NINDS rt-PA Stroke Trial (6.6%). Interestingly, IMS II subjects had significantly better outcomes at 3 months than NINDS placebo-treated subjects for all end points (OR ≥ 2.7) and better outcomes than NINDS rt-PA–treated subjects as measured by the Barthel Index and Global Test Statistic. Finally, the rate of any recanalization (TIMI grades 2 or 3) at the specific site of arterial occlusion at the end of the procedure in EKOS-treated subjects was 73% (24 of 33) as compared with subjects treated with standard micro-catheter in IMS I[47] (56%; 33 of 59; $P = 0.11$). These promising findings have led to the design of a randomized trial (IMS III) comparing standard intravenous rt-PA with a combined IV and IA (assisted by EKOS ultrasound device) approach.

Therapeutic low-frequency ultrasound

In experimental models, using lower frequencies (20 kHz to 1 MHz), rt-PA-mediated clot degradation was as much as 50% more efficient when ultrasound was added.[124–130] Consequently, it has been postulated that the use of therapeutic, i.e., non-imaging ultrasound, in combination with IV thrombolytic therapy might be a feasible, safe, and potentially an effective acute stroke treatment option.[142] This hypothesis was tested in the TRanscranial low-frequency Ultrasound-Mediated thrombolysis in Brain Ischemia (TRUMBI) trial.[143] First, the investigators used a very low kHz system (< 40 kHz) that produced intolerable tinnitus and was withdrawn from clinical testing (M. Daffertshofer, personal communication). It was replaced by a mid kHz system operating at 300 kHz. Low-frequency ultrasound (300 kHz $\pm$ 1.5 kHz to avoid standing-waves) with an intensity of 700 mW/cm^2 (temporal average spatial peak intensity) was applied simultaneously with IV administration of rt-PA and for 30 minutes after rt-PA infusion (total insonation time of 90 minutes). The trial was terminated after 26 patients were enrolled with a 36% rate of symptomatic hemorrhage in the target group and no signal of efficacy on early recanalization or clinical outcomes at 3 months. The investigators found a high rate of atypical hemorrhages in the rt-PA plus ultrasound group either in the subarachnoid or in the ventricular space or at remote parenchymal locations distant to the infarct core. The underlying mechanism causing the high rate of hemorrhage was not clear. The high rates of subarachnoid hemorrhage particularly lead to speculation of some mechanical action from the ultrasound disrupting small vessels in the subarachnoid space. In conclusion, the TRUMBI trial demonstrated adverse bio-effects of mid-KHz ultrasound promoting ICH both in areas affected and unaffected by ischemia.

Microsphere-potentiated ultrasound-enhanced thrombolysis

Experimental data have suggested that ultrasound-enhanced thrombolysis can be further amplified by the addition of gaseous microspheres. Gaseous microspheres, used as ultrasound contrast agents, are micron-sized lipid or albumin shells that when exposed to ultrasound, expand and produce stable cavitation with strong reflected echoes.[144–146] They are used to generate ultrasound images with better contrast. At the same time, microspheres agitate fluid where they are activated by ultrasound and this is useful in drug delivery and mechanical "grinding" of a thrombus. Microspheres with ultrasound can lyse thrombi without a lytic drug. In addition, entrapment of rt-PA in echogenic liposomes has been recently demonstrated to be feasible and effective in lysing porcine clots using ultrasound.[147]

Several studies have been reported with different types of commercially available microspheres (Table 5.3).[148–151] Molina et al. pioneered this approach in stroke patients and reported the largest study to date that compared the CLOTBUST Target arm to the CLOTBUST Target insonation protocol (2 MHz continuous TCD-monitoring) combined with Levovist air microspheres.[151] The Barcelona group demonstrated that, at 2 hours after rt-PA bolus, the rt-PA+TCD+Levovist group achieved a 55% sustained recanalization rate compared with 38% in the rt-PA+TCD group of the CLOTBUST trial. The safety and feasibility of infusion of new and more stable C_3F_8 perfultren-lipid microspheres in patients treated with ultrasound-enhanced thrombolysis has recently been reported in a small phase IIA randomized clinical trial.[150] Interestingly, in 75% of patients, microspheres permeated to areas with no pre-treatment residual flow, and in 83%, residual flow velocity improved at a median of 30 min from start of microsphere infusion (range 30 s–120 min) by a median of 17 cm/s, or 118% above pre-treatment values. There was no symptomatic ICH both in the target (rt-PA+2MHz continuous TCD-monitoring+microspheres) and control group (rt-PA+2MHz continuous TCD-monitoring). A total of three asymptomatic ICH occurred in the target group. Moreover, after evaluation of TCD tracings as part of a secondary analysis, microspheres were moving at velocities higher than surrounding residual red blood cell flow in patients with MCA occlusions (39.8 $\pm$ 11.3 vs. 28.8 $\pm$ 13.8 cm/s, $P < 0.001$).[152]

Larrue et al. recently randomized patients with acute (<3 hours) MCA main stem occlusion as demonstrated by CT or MR angiography to either transcranial duplex ultrasound continuous monitoring combined with intravenous galactose-based gaseous microspheres and rt-PA (combined treatment group), or rt-PA alone (control group).[149] Their trial was prematurely discontinued on the basis of safety reasons, since a high rate of asymptomatic ICHs was demonstrated on gradient-echo MRI in the combined treatment group (78%).

Perren *et al.* studied the safety and feasibility of TCD ultrasound monitoring combined with a second generation, phospholipid-encapsulated sulphur hexafluoride microsphere (SonoVue®, Bracco Diagnostics, Inc., Princeton, NJ) and IV systemic thrombolysis in patients with acute MCA occlusion.[148] All patients were monitored with continuous hand-held 2 MHz TCD (Pulsed wave mode power output: 189 mW/cm^2; sample volume 10 mm; Acuson Sequoia, Siemens Inc., Malvern, PA) over 60 minutes. Patients who received microspheres-potentiated ultrasound-enhanced thrombolysis had higher rate of improvement in NIHSS score and of experienced higher rates of recanalization (complete recanalization rate of 64%) in comparison to patients treated with rt-PA only (complete recanalization rate of 53%). Unfortunately, functional outcomes at three months following stroke onset were unavailable and this methodological shortcoming prohibited the investigators from comparing the rates of functional independence between the two groups.

Currently, a phase I–II randomized placebo-controlled, open-label international multi-center study (TUCSON trial) of new and more stable perfultren-lipid microspheres (MRX 801, Imarx Therapeutics, Inc., Tuscon, AZ) is underway.[153] A total of 72 patients with acute intracranial arterial occlusion will be randomized to microspheres-potentiated ultrasound-enhanced thrombolysis (four groups with increasing doses of perfultren-lipid microspheres) versus IV rt-PA alone.

Complications of endovascular treatment
Treatment-related intracranial hemorrhage

The reported rates of symptomatic ICH seen in patients undergoing endovascular interventions within 24 hours following treatment range between 6% and 14%.[154,155] Asymptomatic ICH is seen in 26%–58% of the patients treated endovascularly.[155] The high rates of asymptomatic ICH are often attributed in part to misinterpretation of extravasated contrast dye for blood.

Stroke-related ICH is linked to activation of matrix metalloproteases (MMP) secondary to ischemia.[156] Thrombolytics are also potent activators of MMP.[157] The activation of MMP leads to degradation of subendothelial connective tissue in the capillary wall matrix. The degradation of matrix leads to breakdown of the blood–brain barrier which is formed by capillary endothelium, subendothelial tissue, and astrocyte foot processes. ICH results from the combination of blood–brain barrier breakdown and thrombolytic induced temporary coagulopathy. Stroke severity, older age, higher thrombolytic doses, adjunctive use of heparin or platelet GP IIB/IIIA inhibitors, hyperglycemia, large perfusion deficits, and delayed recanalization[158] have been linked to increased likelihood of ICH.

Pharmacological strategies to reduce ICH related to thrombolytics under pre-clinical investigation include hypothermia, free radical-spin trap compounds,[159] and MMP inhibitors.[160] Possible reduction in ICH rates in patients treated with intravenous rt-PA by the free radical-trapping agent NX-059 was suggested by the Stroke-Acute Ischemic NXY Treatment (SAINT I) trial.[161] Among the 480 rt-PA-treated cases, those who received NXY-059 had significantly lower rates of symptomatic ICH than those receiving placebo (6.4% vs. 2.5%). However, this effect was not confirmed in the larger SAINT II trial.[162]

Once ICH has occurred, there is no clear treatment strategy. The half-life of thrombolytics is very short and no direct antagonists are available. However, intra-procedural heparin should be reversed using IV protamine sulphate. Platelet transfusion is recommended if GP IIB/IIIA inhibitors were concurrently used. Routine use of blood products in these patients has not been demonstrated to be of any benefit. In the NINDS rt-PA trial, 13 of the 22 patients with symptomatic ICH received blood products (fresh frozen plasma, cryoprecipitate, or platelets);[163] however, 12 of the 13 patients were dead at 90 days. Surgical treatment of these ICHs is controversial. Only one patient with symptomatic ICH in the NINDS rt-PA trial had operative removal of the ICH, and he subsequently died. In the GUSTO-I trial, a total of 268 patients with acute MI had an ICH following thrombolytic treatment.[164] Mortality rate at 30 days for all patients with ICH was 60%. Surgical evacuation was associated with significantly higher 30-day survival and a trend toward improved functional status. However, a selection bias cannot be excluded and the results simply raise the possibility of surgical evacuation in selected patients. In patients with ischemic stroke, the operative site is complicated by the presence of pre-existing ischemic tissue intermingled with the ICH. The value of other hemostatic agents such as aprotinin remains unknown. Aprotinin reduces bleeding through its effects on fibrinolytic pathways, coagulation pathways, the inflammatory response, and platelet function.[165] By preserving the adhesive glycoproteins on the platelet membrane, it also promotes platelet adhesion. Aprotinin is approved for prophylactic use to reduce perioperative blood loss in patients undergoing coronary artery bypass grafting[165] and recommended in hip and spine surgery.[166]

Complete or partial failure of recanalization

In a review of 53 studies[167] encompassing 2066 patients, recanalization rates for IA thrombolysis (63.2%), combined intravenous and intra-arterial thrombolysis (67.5%), and mechanical thrombolysis (83.6%) were reported. Recanalization was strongly associated with improved functional outcome and reduced mortality.

Recanalization rates depend on the site of occlusion, the substrate of thrombus, thrombus burden, time between symptom onset and treatment, and treatment modalities used. Theoretically, occlusions with underlying atherosclerotic substrate are less likely to respond to thrombolytics because of high thrombogenicity and platelet activation. A similar resistance to thrombolytics may be observed with organized thrombi that have a high fibrous content. Over time, the thrombus evolves by formation of adhesions with the surrounding artery through binding of platelets and endothelium and subendothelium. Secondary thrombus forms around the primary thrombus due to stasis of flow and locally generated thrombogenecity. Therefore, the chances of achieving recanalization decrease over time.

The chances of achieving recanalization improve with higher doses of thrombolytics, concurrent use of high dose heparin, GP IIB/IIIA inhibitors, mechanical thrombus disruption, and use of stent placement.[168] However, this has to be counterbalanced with the higher risk of ICH and other complications possibly associated with these additional maneuvers.

Recanalization is sometimes associated with a "no-reflow phenomenon."[169–171] In the presence of ischemia, there is activation of integrin receptors on the endothelial cells of the capillaries leading to platelet and monocyte aggregation within those vessels. This plugging of the capillaries prevents adequate perfusion at the tissue level even when the medium size arteries have been recanalized. In patients with acute MI, delay in contrast transit is used as an index for establishing the presence of no-reflow phenomenon.[88] This phenomenon can also be observed following IA thrombolysis in patients with acute ischemic stroke. In one study, partial or complete normalization of diffusion imaging abnormalities on MRI occurred in 8 of 18 (44%) ischemic stroke patients following angiographic recanalization.[172] Among the eight patients with early diffusion imaging reversal, late secondary injury was observed in five patients on repeat imaging on day 7. Use of GP IIB/IIIA platelet inhibitors and local vasodilators[173] has been proposed to reverse the no-reflow phenomenon.

Re-occlusion and distal fragmentation

Arterial re-occlusion and distal embolization are known complications of ischemic stroke intervention,[97,174,175] impacting on treatment strategies and device design. Thrombolytic agents lyse the fibrin meshwork of the thrombus, but result in both increased thrombin activity and platelet activation.[19,66] As part of the activation response to thrombin, platelets express GP IIb/IIIa receptors on their surface, which can bind to ligands, such as fibrinogen, thereby promoting thrombus formation and additional thrombin generation. Therefore, platelet activation leads to resistance to thrombolysis and promotes re-occlusion. We have observed re-occlusion in experimental models of ischemic stroke treated with intra-arterial thrombolysis (reteplase), even without mechanical disruption of clot.[176] These experimental findings in conjunction with our clinical observations suggest that clot formation and lysis is a very dynamic process. The use of mechanical disruption (such as balloon angioplasty, snare manipulation, or stent placement) may lead to disruption of atherosclerotic plaques or endothelial erosion that triggers platelet activation, adherence and aggregation, and also the exposure of tissue factor, which, in turn, activates the clotting cascade. Because of the

prominent involvement of platelet activation in this process, platelet GP IIB/IIIA inhibitors have been recommended for preventing reocclusion.[176]

In a study of 46 consecutive patients[97] who underwent IA thrombolysis, re-occlusion was observed in eight (17%) patients. The re-occlusions were treated by using additional doses of reteplase alone ($n = 1$), reteplase with snare maneuver and/or angioplasty ($n = 5$), reteplase with angioplasty or snare and then stent placement ($n = 1$), and angioplasty with stent placement ($n = 1$). The re-occlusions resolved in six of eight patients after further treatment. Independent functional outcome scores were significantly lower among patients with angiographically shown re-occlusion than in those without.

In a retrospective analysis of data from four prospective acute stroke protocols,[175] "distal embolization" defined qualitatively as appearance of an occlusion on a downstream vessel and "arterial re-occlusion" defined as subsequent re-occlusion of the target vessel after initial recanalization had been achieved were reported. Arterial re-occlusion occurred in 18% of these patients, whereas distal embolization occurred in 16% of the 91 patients treated in these protocols. Arterial re-occlusion, but not distal embolization, was associated with a lower likelihood of favorable outcome at 1–3 months.

Futile recanalization phenomenon

Recanalization has been recognized as the main measure of re-establishing flow and salvaging ischemic tissue.[167] However, a proportion of patients do not improve or improve to a such a small extent that the outcome remains poor despite adequate recanalization.[177,173] This phenomenon is referred to as the "futile recanalization phenomenon." The major reason behind the syndrome of failed recanalization is presence of irreversibly damaged tissue in the ischemic distribution.[130] Therefore, re-establishing rCBF does not help the tissue recover. The initial severity of deficits, time to recanalization, and age of the patient have been associated with poor clinical outcome despite angiographic recanalization.[178,179] The time that a tissue is salvagable depends upon the residual blood flow in the affected distribution mantained by collateral blood vessels. Severe reduction of rCBF subsequent to an intravascular occlusion is usually associated with rapid irreversible injury and not asociated with meaningful tissue salvage despite restoration of regional blood flow. Many measures have been proposed to identify the presence of salvagable tissue prior to attempting recanalization particularly in patients in whom treatment is considered after 6 hours of symptom onset. These include angiographic visualization of collaterals,[173] perfusion–diffusion mismatch on MRI,[116,173] preserved rCBV on CT perfusion scans,[131] or partial flow documented by TCD ultrasound.[132] Other factors that have been implicated in the syndrome of failed recanalization are reocclusion, no-reflow phenomenon, and ICH.

New efforts are being directed towards delaying the onset of irreversible ischemia until recanalization can be achieved.[130]

Table 5.4. Regulatory approvals from the FDA for neurovascular devices

Device	Type of approval	Date of approval	Approved indication
Merci® Retriever (Concentric Medical, Inc) X5, X6	510(k)	August 2004	Restoration of blood flow in the neurovasculature by removing thrombus in patients experiencing ischemic stroke. Can be used in patients who are ineligible for or have failed intravenous rt-PA treatment. Can also be used for the retrieval of foreign bodies misplaced during intravascular procedures.
EKOS Peripheral Infusion System	510(k)	March 2005	Controlled and selective infusion of physician-specified fluids, including thrombolytics, into the peripheral vasculature
Penumbra System™ (Penumbra Inc, San Leandro, CA)	510(k)	August 2007	Revascularization of patients with acute ischemic stroke secondary to intracranial large vessel occlusive disease within 8 hours of symptom onset
Modified Merci® Retriever	510(k)	August 2007	Same as for the X5 and X6 Retriever
Merci® L6 Retriever	510(k)	August 2007	Same as for the X5 and X6 Retriever

Hypothermia is a promising adjunct to endovascular interventions due to its neuroprotective effect.

Incorporation of existing data into a practical protocol

We use a protocol for selecting acute ischemic stroke patients for endovascular treatment stratified by time. For patients who present within 3 hours of symptom onset, we administer IV thrombolysis (rt-PA 0.9 mg) consistent with the recommendations of the ASA, Stroke Council.[5] For patients with initial NIHSS score of 10 or greater, we perform an emergent cerebral angiogram to identify any arterial occlusion.[30] We subsequently proceed with endovascular treatment relying on mechanical disruption and low dose IA thrombolytics to achieve further recanalization. In patients who present between 3 and 6 hours and have a NIHSS score of 4 or greater,[17] we perform endovascular treatment by performing an emergent cerebral angiogram followed by appropriately selected endovascular treatment. In patients who present after 6 hours, we perform either a CT perfusion to identify presence of relatively preserved rCBV[87] or diffusion-weighted MRI to identify a clinical diffusion mismatch.[93] If there is evidence of either, we perform endovascular treatment. In patients with posterior circulation ischemic stroke who present between 6 and 24 hours or those with progressive ischemic deficits, we perform an emergent diffusion weighted MRI to identify presence of salvagable tissue in the brain stem prior to using endovascular treatment. In patients in whom IV thrombolysis is contraindicated, such as patients with recent surgery (within 2 weeks)[94] or those with elevated international normalized ratio, we consider endovascular treatment up to 6 hours following symptom onset.

Recommendations from professional societies

The 2003 guidelines by the Stroke Council of the ASA[1] concluded that IA administration of at least one specific thrombolytic agent appears to be of some benefit in the treatment of carefully selected patients with acute ischemic stroke secondary to occlusion of the MCA (Class I, see Table 2.1 definitions). This conclusion was based on the results of a prospective, randomized, placebo-controlled phase III study demonstrating the efficacy of IA thrombolysis with pro-urokinase among patients with stroke of < 6 hours duration secondary to occlusion of the middle cerebral artery (Class I). The FDA has not approved the drug, and pro-urokinase is not currently available for clinical use. The guidelines recommended that IA thrombolysis is an option for treatment of selected patients with major stroke of < 6 hours duration due to large vessel occlusions of the middle cerebral artery (grade B). Therefore, extrapolation to the available thrombolytic drug (rt-PA) is based on consensus as supported by case series data. The guidelines acknowledged that case series data suggest this approach may also be of benefit in patients with basilar artery occlusion treated at longer intervals. The availability of IA thrombolysis should generally not preclude the administration of IV rt-PA in otherwise eligible patients.

The Brain Attack Coalition[184] recognizes that there has been extensive experience with this technique, which is commonly used at many medical centers, and is recommended in the current AHA *Advanced Cardiac Life Support* handbook. Based on all of these factors and the consensus of the Brain Attack Coalition, IA lytics are considered a recommended component of a comprehensive stroke center (grade IIB). Complication rates should be monitored closely. Mechanical thrombectomy techniques for the cerebral circulation are also being developed that use a variety of devices such as

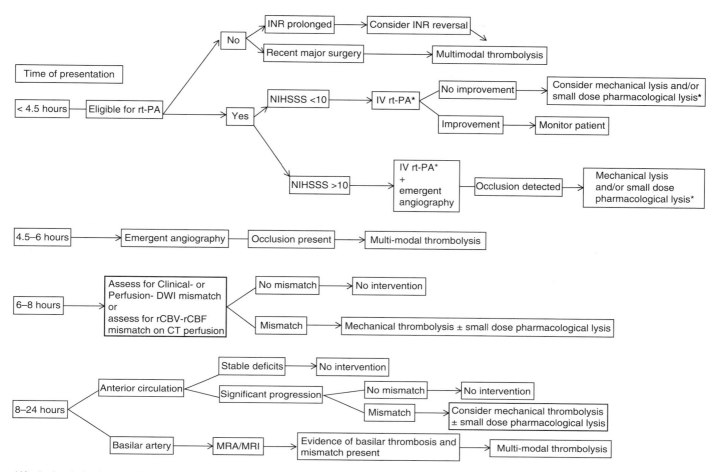

*After having obtained approval from our Institutional Review Board, we can administer small dose intra-arterial thrombolytics even after full dose IV rt-PA. An alternate approach is bridging treatment, where only 2/3 of the rt-PA dose are administered IV if intra-arterial intervention is anticipated. The remaining rt-PA dose can be given intra-arterially.

Fig. 5.2. Algorithm for triaging patients for endovascular intervention.

microcatheters, snares, clot retrievers, and angioplasty catheters (grade VC). Administration of lytic agents into the sinuses may also be efficacious in treating selected cases of cerebral venous thrombosis, although this therapy has not been studied in a rigorous manner (grade VC).

The 2007 guideline from the American Heart Association/American Stroke Association Stroke Council[5] recommended that treatment should require the patient to be at an experienced stroke center with immediate access to cerebral angiography and qualified interventionalists. Facilities are encouraged to define criteria to credential individuals who can perform IA thrombolysis procedures (Class I, Level of Evidence C). IA thrombolysis is reasonable in patients who have contraindications to the use of IV thrombolysis, such as recent surgery (Class IIa, Level of Evidence C). Although the MERCI device is a reasonable intervention for extraction of IA thrombi in carefully selected patients, the panel also recognizes that the utility of the device in improving outcomes after stroke is unclear (Class IIb, Level of Evidence B). The panel also

recommends that the device be studied in additional clinical trials that will define its role in the emergency management of stroke.

There is currently no fibrinolytic agent with an FDA label indication for IA administration for the treatment of acute ischemic stroke. In August 2004, the FDA approved the Merci® retriever (Concentric Medical, Inc) (see Table 5.4). Since then, newer generations of the MERCI retriever have been approved (Table 5.4).

Utilization of endovascular treatments

Our group obtained national estimates of thrombolysis, associated in-hospital outcomes, and mortality from National Hospital Discharge Survey data from 1999 to 2001.[185] There were 1 796 513 admissions for ischemic stroke between 1999 and 2001. Of these admitted patients, 1 314 (0.07%) underwent IA thrombolysis and 11 283 (0.6%) underwent IV thrombolysis. We observed a trend toward a higher frequency of use of IV and IA thrombolysis and hospitals with greater number of beds (P < 0.01). Another estimate was obtained from a total of 282 276 patients with ischemic stroke in the Nationwide Inpatient Sample between 1999 and 2002.[186] Of those, 3358 patients (1.19%) underwent IV thrombolysis and 477 patients (0.17% of the total cohort or 14% of all thrombolysis cases) received an angiogram and presumably underwent endovascular treatment. Among the patients who underwent endovascular treatment, 15% died, and approximately 50% were discharged home or to rehabilitation facilities. ICH occurred in 6% of these patients. However, despite its limited use, endovascular treatment for acute ischemic stroke has the largest potential to increase due to the large number of untreated but potentially eligible patients.[187]

Another estimate was derived from patients between the ages of 1 and 17 years, entered in the Nationwide Inpatient Sample between 2000 and 2003.[188] An estimated 2904 children were admitted with ischemic stroke, of which 46 (1.6%) received thrombolytic therapy. Of those who received thrombolysis, IA thrombolysis was used in 41%. The children who received thrombolysis were less likely to be discharged home with higher rates of death and dependency, although the differences in clinical severity from those who had not received thrombolysis were not known.

Conclusions

The FDA approval of IV rt-PA for acute cerebral ischemia marked the onset of a new era in our approach to stroke. IA treatments have since been developed that serve two purposes: They can be used in patients ineligible for IV rt-PA or as adjunctive treatment in patients with poor response to rt-PA. The current standard of practice in most academic stroke centers is applying different treatment modalities sequentially, as indicated, until satisfactory recanalization is achieved. Currently, recanalization is considered the best surrogate marker for positive clinical outcome. This approach has been termed "multi-modal thrombolysis." Figure 5.2 offers a simplified algorithm that can be used in triaging the patients for IA treatments. It is important to keep in mind the risk to benefit ratio for each procedure which is undertaken in each specific patient, always taking into consideration the wishes of the family regarding to ensure "aggressive" treatment efforts are appropriately used.

All acute stroke interventions are currently underutilized. Efforts should be directed towards offering treatment to more eligible patients in the future. More randomized data are needed to help define future treatment guidelines.

References

1. Adams HPJ, Adams RJ, Brott T, *et al.* Guidelines for the early management of patients with ischemic stroke: A scientific statement from the Stroke Council of the American Stroke Association. *Stroke* 2003;**34**:1056–83.

2. Qureshi AI. Endovascular treatment of cerebrovascular diseases and intracranial neoplasms. *Lancet* 2004;**363**:804–13.

3. Tissue plasminogen activator for acute ischemic stroke. The National Institute of Neurological Disorders and Stroke rt-PA Stroke Study Group. *N Engl J Med* 1995;**333**:1581–7.

4. Practice advisory: thrombolytic therapy for acute ischemic stroke-summary statement. Report of the Quality Standards Subcommittee of the American Academy of Neurology. *Neurology*. 1996;**47**:835–9.

5. Adams HPJ, del Zoppo G, Alberts MJ, *et al.* Guidelines for the early management of adults with ischemic stroke: a guideline from the American Heart Association/American Stroke Association Stroke Council, Clinical Cardiology Council, Cardiovascular Radiology and Intervention Council, and the Atherosclerotic Peripheral Vascular Disease and Quality of Care Outcomes in Research Interdisciplinary Working Groups: the American Academy of Neurology affirms the value of this guideline as an educational tool for neurologists. *Stroke* 2007;**38**:1655–711.

6. Albers GW, Bates VE, Clark WM, *et al.* Intravenous tissue-type plasminogen activator for treatment of acute stroke: the Standard Treatment with Alteplase to Reverse Stroke (STARS) study. *JAMA* 2000;**283**:1145–50.

7. Hacke W, Kaste M, Fieschi C, *et al.* Randomised double-blind placebo-controlled trial of thrombolytic therapy with intravenous alteplase in acute ischaemic stroke (ECASS II). Second European-Australasian Acute Stroke Study Investigators. *Lancet* 1998;**352**:1245–51.

8. Qureshi AI, Pande RU, Kim SH, *et al.* Third generation thrombolytics for the treatment of ischemic stroke. *Curr Opin Investig Drugs* 2002;**3**:1729–32.

9. Baker WFJ. Thrombolytic therapy: current clinical practice. *Hematol Oncol Clin North Am* 2005;**19**:147–81, vii.

10. Liberatore GT, Samson A, Bladin C, Schleuning W-D, Medcalf RL. Vampire bat salivary plasminogen activator (desmoteplase): a unique fibrinolytic enzyme that does not promote neurodegeneration. *Stroke* 2003;**34**:537–43.

11. An international randomized trial comparing four thrombolytic strategies for acute myocardial infarction. The GUSTO investigators. *N Engl J Med* 1993;**329**:673–82.

12. A comparison of reteplase with alteplase for acute myocardial infarction. The Global Use of Strategies to Open Occluded Coronary Arteries (GUSTO III) Investigators. *N Engl J Med* 1997;**337**:1118–23.

13. Van De Werf F, Adgey J, Ardissino D, *et al.* Single-bolus tenecteplase compared with front-loaded alteplase in acute myocardial infarction: the ASSENT-2 double-blind randomised trial. *Lancet* 1999;**354**:716–22.

14. Haley ECJ, Lyden PD, Johnston KC, Hemmen TM. A pilot dose-escalation safety study of tenecteplase in acute ischemic stroke. *Stroke* 2005;**36**:607–12.

15. Hacke W, Albers G, Al-Rawi Y, *et al.* The Desmoteplase in Acute Ischemic Stroke Trial (DIAS): a phase II MRI-based 9-hour window acute stroke thrombolysis trial with intravenous desmoteplase. *Stroke*. 2005;**36**:66–73.

16. Furlan AJ, Eyding D, Albers GW, *et al.* Dose Escalation of Desmoteplase for Acute Ischemic Stroke (DEDAS):

evidence of safety and efficacy 3 to 9 hours after stroke onset. *Stroke* 2006;37:1227–31.

17. Hacke W, Furlan AJ, Al-Rawi Y, *et al.* Intravenous desmoteplase in patients with acute ischaemic stroke selected by MRI perfusion-diffusion weighted imaging or perfusion CT (DIAS-2): a prospective, randomised, double-blind, placebo-controlled study. *Lancet Neurol* 2009;8:141–50.

18. Qureshi AI, Luft AR, Sharma M, Guterman LR, Hopkins LN. Prevention and treatment of thromboembolic and ischemic complications associated with endovascular procedures: Part I– Pathophysiological and pharmacological features. *Neurosurgery* 2000;46:1344–59.

19. del Zoppo GJ, Higashida RT, Furlan AJ, *et al.* PROACT: a phase II randomized trial of recombinant pro-urokinase by direct arterial delivery in acute middle cerebral artery stroke. PROACT Investigators. Prolyse in Acute Cerebral Thromboembolism. *Stroke* 1998;29:4–11.

20. Furlan A, Higashida R, Wechsler L, *et al.* Intra-arterial prourokinase for acute ischemic stroke. The PROACT II study: a randomized controlled trial. Prolyse in Acute Cerebral Thromboembolism. *JAMA* 1999;282:2003–11.

21. Qureshi AI, Ali Z, Suri MF, *et al.* Intra-arterial third-generation recombinant tissue plasminogen activator (reteplase) for acute ischemic stroke. *Neurosurgery* 2001;49:41–8; discussion 48–8; discussion 48–50.

22. Qureshi AI, Siddiqui AM, Suri MFK, *et al.* Aggressive mechanical clot disruption and low-dose intra-arterial third-generation thrombolytic agent for ischemic stroke: a prospective study. *Neurosurgery.* 2002;51:1319–27; discussion 1327–1327; discussion 1327–9.

23. Liem A, Zijlstra F, Ottervanger JP, *et al.* High dose heparin as pretreatment for primary angioplasty in acute myocardial infarction: the Heparin in Early Patency (HEAP) randomized trial. *J Am Coll Cardiol.* 2000;35:600–4.

24. Zeymer U, Neuhaus KL. Clinical trials in acute myocardial infarction. *Curr Opin Cardiol.* 1999;14:392–402.

25. Albers GW. Antithrombotic agents in cerebral ischemia. *Am J Cardiol* 1995;75:34B–8B.

26. Neuhaus KL, Molhoek GP, Zeymer U, *et al.* Recombinant hirudin (lepirudin) for the improvement of thrombolysis with streptokinase in patients with acute myocardial infarction: results of the HIT-4 trial. *J Am Coll Cardiol* 1999;34:966–73.

27. Szabo S, Walter T, Etzel D, *et al.* Benefical effects of reteplase in combination with abciximab: platelet/ leukocyte interactions and coagulation system. *Int J Clin Pharmacol Res* 2003;23:37–40.

28. Manoharan G, Adgey AAJ. Considerations in combination therapy: fibrinolytics plus glycoprotein IIb/IIIa receptor inhibitors in acute myocardial infarction. *Clin Cardiol* 2004;27:381–6.

29. Antman EM, Gibson CM, de Lemos JA, *et al.* Combination reperfusion therapy with abciximab and reduced dose reteplase: results from TIMI 14. The Thrombolysis in Myocardial Infarction (TIMI) 14 Investigators. *Eur Heart J* 2000;21:1944–53.

30. Ibbotson T, McGavin JK, Goa KL. Abciximab: an updated review of its therapeutic use in patients with ischaemic heart disease unde?going percutaneous coronary revascularisation. *Drugs* 2003;63:1121–63.

31. Chan AW, Moliterno DJ. Defining the role of abciximab for acute coronary syndromes: lessons from CADILLAC, ADMIRAL, GUSTO IV, GUSTO V, and TARGET. *Curr Opin Cardiol* 2001;16:375–383.

32. Topol EJ. Reperfusion therapy for acute myocardial infarction with fibrinolytic therapy or combination reduced fibrinolytic therapy and platelet glycoprotein IIb/IIIa inhibition: the GUSTO V randomised trial. *Lancet* 2001;357:1905–14.

33. Qureshi AI, Janjua N, Kirmani JF, *et al.* Mechanical disruption of thrombus following intravenous tissue plasminogen activator for ischemic stroke. *J Neuroimaging* 2007;17:124–30.

34. Levy EI, Mehta R, Gupta R, *et al.* Self-expanding stents for recanalization of acute cerebrovascular occlusions. *Am J Neuroradiol* 2007;28:816–22.

35. Bouzamondo A, Damy T, Montalescot G, Lechat P. Revascularization strategies in acute myocardial infarction: a meta-analysis. *Int J Clin Pharmacol Ther* 2004;42:663–671.

36. Antoniucci D. Rheolytic thrombectomy in acute myocardial infarction: the Florence experience and objectives of the multicenter randomized JETSTENT trial. *J Invasive Cardiol* 2006;18: 32C–4C.

37. Simonton CA3rd, Brodie BR, Wilson H, *et al.* AngioJet experience from the multi-center STENT Registry. *J Invasive Cardiol.* 2006;18 Suppl C:C22–3.

38. Chow K, Gobin YP, Saver J, *et al.* Endovascular treatment of dural sinus thrombosis with rheolytic thrombectomy and intra-arterial thrombolysis. *Stroke.* 2000;31:1420–5.

39. Kirsch J, Rasmussen PA, Masaryk TJ, Perl J 2nd, Fiorella D. Adjunctive rheolytic thrombectomy for central venous sinus thrombosis: technical case report. *Neurosurgery* 2007;60:E577–8; discussion E578.

40. Opatowsky MJ, Morris PP, Regan JD, Mewborne JD, Wilson JA. Rapid thrombectomy of superior sagittal sinus and transverse sinus thrombosis with a rheolytic catheter device. *Am J Neuroradiol* 1999;20:414–17.

41. Bellon RJ, Putman CM, Budzik RF, *et al.* Rheolytic thrombectomy of the occluded internal carotid artery in the setting of acute ischemic stroke. *AJNR Am J Neuroradiol* 2001;22:526–30.

42. Molina CA, Saver JL. Extending reperfusion therapy for acute ischemic stroke: emerging pharmacological, mechanical, and imaging strategies. *Stroke* 2005;36:2311–20.

43. Inoue T, Kimura K, Minematsu K, Yamaguchi T. A case-control analysis of intra-arterial urokinase thrombolysis in acute cardioembolic stroke. *Cerebrovasc Dis* 2005;19:225–8.

44. Macleod MR, Davis SM, Mitchell PJ, *et al.* Results of a multicentre, randomised controlled trial of intra-arterial urokinase in the treatment of acute posterior circulation ischaemic stroke. *Cerebrovasc Dis* 2005;20:12–17.

45. Suarez JI, Zaidat OO, Sunshine JL, *et al.* Endovascular administration after intravenous infusion of thrombolytic agents for the treatment of patients with acute ischemic strokes. *Neurosurgery.* 2002;50:251–9; discussion 259–60.

46. Combined intravenous and intra-arterial recanalization for acute ischemic stroke: the Interventional

Management of Stroke Study. *Stroke* 2004;**35**:904–11.

47. The Interventional Management of Stroke (IMS) II Study. *Stroke* 2007;**38**:2127–35.

48. Lewandowski CA, Frankel M, Tomsick TA, *et al.* Combined intravenous and intra-arterial r-TPA versus intra-arterial therapy of acute ischemic stroke: Emergency Management of Stroke (EMS) Bridging Trial. *Stroke* 1999;**30**:2598–605.

49. Schonewille WJ, Wijman CAC, Michel P, *et al.* Treatment and outcomes of acute basilar artery occlusion in the Basilar Artery International Cooperation Study (BASICS): a prospective registry study. *Lancet Neurol* 2009;**8**:724–30.

50. Ducrocq X, Bracard S, Taillandier L, *et al.* Comparison of intravenous and intra-arterial urokinase thrombolysis for acute ischaemic stroke. *J Neuroradiol* 2005;**32**:26–32.

51. Shaltoni HM, Albright KC, Gonzales NR, *et al.* Is intra-arterial thrombolysis safe after full-dose intravenous recombinant tissue plasminogen activator for acute ischemic stroke?. *Stroke* 2007;**38**:80–4.

52. Georgiadis AL, Memon MZ, Shah QA, *et al.* Comparison of partial (0.6 mg/kg) versus full-dose (0.9 mg/kg) intravenous recombinant tissue plasminogen activator followed by endovascular treatment for acute ischemic stroke: a meta-analysis. *J Neuroimaging* 2009;in press:online.

53. Smith WS, Sung G, Starkman S, *et al.* Safety and efficacy of mechanical embolectomy in acute ischemic stroke: results of the MERCI trial. *Stroke* 2005;**36**:1432–8.

54. Smith WS. Safety of mechanical thrombectomy and intravenous tissue plasminogen activator in acute ischemic stroke. Results of the multi Mechanical Embolus Removal in Cerebral Ischemia (MERCI) trial, part I. *Am J Neuroradiol* 2006;**27**:1177–82.

55. Smith WS, Sung G, Saver J, *et al.* Mechanical thrombectomy for acute ischemic stroke: final results of the Multi MERCI trial. *Stroke* 2008;**39**:1205–12.

56. Nogueira RG, Liebeskind DS, Sung G, Duckwiler G, Smith WS. Predictors of good clinical outcomes, mortality, and successful revascularization in patients with acute ischemic stroke undergoing thrombectomy: pooled analysis of the Mechanical Embolus Removal in Cerebral Ischemia (MERCI) and Multi MERCI Trials. *Stroke* 2009;**40**:3777–83.

57. Flint AC, Duckwiler GR, Budzik RF, Liebeskind DS, Smith WS. Mechanical thrombectomy of intracranial internal carotid occlusion: pooled results of the MERCI and Multi MERCI Part I trials. *Stroke* 2007;**38**:1274–80.

58. Lutsep HL, Rymer MM, Nesbit GM. Vertebrobasilar revascularization rates and outcomes in the MERCI and multi-MERCI trials. *J Stroke Cerebrovasc Dis* 2008;**17**:55–7.

59. Nogueira RG, Smith WS. Safety and efficacy of endovascular thrombectomy in patients with abnormal hemostasis: pooled analysis of the MERCI and multi MERCI trials. *Stroke* 2009;**40**:516–22.

60. Bose A, Henkes H, Alfke K, *et al.* The Penumbra System: a mechanical device for the treatment of acute stroke due to thromboembolism. *AJNR Am J Neuroradiol* 2008;**29**:1409–13.

61. The penumbra pivotal stroke trial: safety and effectiveness of a new generation of mechanical devices for clot removal in intracranial large vessel occlusive disease. *Stroke* 2009;**40**: 2761–8.

62. Grunwald IQ, Walter S, Papanagiotou P, *et al.* Revascularization in acute ischaemic stroke using the penumbra system: the first single center experience. *Eur J Neurol* 2009;**16**: 1210–16.

63. Struffert T, Kohrmann M, Engelhorn T, *et al.* Penumbra Stroke System as an "add-on" for the treatment of large vessel occlusive disease following thrombolysis: first results. *Eur Radiol* 2009;**19**:2286–93.

64. Penumbra system: a novel mechanical thrombectomy device for large-vessel occlusions in acute stroke. *Am J Neuroradiol.* 2009;in press:online.

65. Qureshi AI, Harris-Lane P, Kirmani JF, *et al.* Intra-arterial reteplase and intravenous abciximab in patients with acute ischemic stroke: an open-label, dose-ranging, phase I study. *Neurosurgery.* 2006;**59**:789–96; discussion 796–7.

66. Eckert B, Koch C, Thomalla G, *et al.* Aggressive therapy with intravenous abciximab and intra-arterial rtPA and additional PTA/stenting improves clinical outcome in acute vertebrobasilar occlusion: combined local fibrinolysis and intravenous abciximab in acute vertebrobasilar stroke treatment (FAST): results of a multicenter study. *Stroke* 2005;**36**:1160–5.

67. Nagel S, Schellinger PD, Hartmann M, *et al.* Therapy of acute basilar artery occlusion: intraarterial thrombolysis alone vs bridging therapy. *Stroke* 2009;**40**:140–6.

68. Krieger DW, De Georgia MA, Abou-Chebl A, *et al.* Cooling for acute ischemic brain damage (cool aid): an open pilot study of induced hypothermia in acute ischemic stroke. *Stroke* 2001;**32**:1847–54.

69. De Georgia MA, Krieger DW, Abou-Chebl A, *et al.* Cooling for Acute Ischemic Brain Damage (COOL AID): a feasibility trial of endovascular cooling. *Neurology* 2004;**63**:312–17.

70. Hill MD, Rowley HA, Adler F, *et al.* Selection of acute ischemic stroke patients for intra-arterial thrombolysis with pro-urokinase by using ASPECTS. *Stroke* 2003;**34**:1925–31.

71. Hill MD, Demchuk AM, Tomsick TA, Palesch YY, Broderick JP. Using the baseline CT scan to select acute stroke patients for IV-IA therapy. *Am J Neuroradiol* 2006;**27**:1612–16.

72. Agarwal P, Kumar S, Hariharan S, *et al.* Hyperdense middle cerebral artery sign: can it be used to select intra-arterial versus intravenous thrombolysis in acute ischemic stroke?. *Cerebrovasc Dis* 2004;**17**:182–190.

73. Qureshi AI, Ziai WC, Yahia AM, *et al.* Stroke-free survival and its determinants in patients with symptomatic vertebrobasilar stenosis: a multicenter study. *Neurosurgery* 2003;**52**:1033–9; discussion 1039–40.

74. Chalela JA, Katzan I, Liebeskind DS, *et al.* Safety of intra-arterial thrombolysis in the postoperative period. *Stroke* 2001;**32**:1365–9.

75. Schreiber TLCS, Massop D, Kumar V, *et al.* Report of the CASES-PMS study: patient demographics and 30-day major adverse events for the Cordis PRECISE nitinol stent and Angioguard TM Emboli capture guidewire condition of approval surveillance study. 2006; American College of Cardiology 55th Annual Scientific Session; Atlanta, Georgia.

76. Lindsberg PJ, Soinne L, Tatlisumak T, *et al.* Long-term outcome after intravenous thrombolysis of basilar artery occlusion. *JAMA* 2004;**292**: 1862–6.

77. Schonewille WJ, Algra A, Serena J, Molina CA, Kappelle LJ. Outcome in patients with basilar artery occlusion treated conventionally. *J Neurol Neurosurg Psychiatry* 2005;**76**:1238–41.

78. del Zoppo GJ, Poeck K, Pessin MS, *et al.* Recombinant tissue plasminogen activator in acute thrombotic and embolic stroke. *Ann Neurol* 1992;**32**:78–86.

79. Casto L, Caverni L, Camerlingo M, *et al.* Intra-arterial thrombolysis in acute ischaemic stroke: experience with a superselective catheter embedded in the clot. *J Neurol Neurosurg Psychiatry* 1996;**60**:667–70.

80. Gonner F, Remonda L, Mattle H, *et al.* Local intra-arterial thrombolysis in acute ischemic stroke. *Stroke* 1998;**29**:1894–900.

81. Jahan R, Duckwiler GR, Kidwell CS, *et al.* Intraarterial thrombolysis for treatment of acute stroke: experience in 26 patients with long-term follow-up. *Am J Neuroradiol* 1999;**20**:1291–9.

82. Brekenfeld C, Remonda L, Nedeltchev K, *et al.* Endovascular neuroradiological treatment of acute ischemic stroke: techniques and results in 350 patients. *Neurol Res* 2005;**27** Suppl 1:S29–35.

83. Suarez JI, Sunshine JL, Tarr R, *et al.* Predictors of clinical improvement, angiographic recanalization, and intracranial hemorrhage after intra-arterial thrombolysis for acute ischemic stroke. *Stroke* 1999;**30**:2094–100.

84. Hacke W, Donnan G, Fieschi C, *et al.* Association of outcome with early stroke treatment: pooled analysis of ATLANTIS, ECASS, and NINDS rt-PA stroke trials. *Lancet* 2004;**363**:768–74.

85. Ostrem JL, Saver JL, Alger JR, *et al.* Acute basilar artery occlusion: diffusion-perfusion MRI characterization of tissue salvage in patients receiving intra-arterial stroke therapies. *Stroke* 2004;**35**:e30–4.

86. Akasaka T, Yoshida K, Kawamoto T, *et al.* Relation of phasic coronary flow velocity characteristics with TIMI perfusion grade and myocardial recovery after primary percutaneous transluminal coronary angioplasty and

rescue stenting. *Circulation* 2000;**101**:2361–7.

87. Lev MH, Segal AZ, Farkas J, *et al.* Utility of perfusion-weighted CT imaging in acute middle cerebral artery stroke treated with intra-arterial thrombolysis: prediction of final infarct volume and clinical outcome. *Stroke* 2001;**32**:2021–8.

88. Uno M, Harada M, Yoneda K, *et al.* Can diffusion- and perfusion-weighted magnetic resonance imaging evaluate the efficacy of acute thrombolysis in patients with internal carotid artery or middle cerebral artery occlusion?. *Neurosurgery* 2002;**50**:28–34; discussion 34–5.

89. Ogasawara K, Ogawa A, Doi M, *et al.* Prediction of acute embolic stroke outcome after local intraarterial thrombolysis: value of pretreatment and posttreatment 99mTc-ethyl cysteinate dimer single photon emission computed tomography. *J Cereb Blood Flow Metab* 2000;**20**:1579–86.

90. Endo S, Kuwayama N, Hirashima Y, *et al.* Results of urgent thrombolysis in patients with major stroke and atherothrombotic occlusion of the cervical internal carotid artery. *Am J Neuroradiol* 1998;**19**:1169–75.

91. Molyneux AJ, Kerr RSC, Yu L-M, *et al.* International subarachnoid aneurysm trial (ISAT) of neurosurgical clipping versus endovascular coiling in 2143 patients with ruptured intracranial aneurysms: a randomised comparison of effects on survival, dependency, seizures, rebleeding, subgroups, and aneurysm occlusion. *Lancet* 2005;**366**:809–17.

92. Brandt T, von Kummer R, Muller-Kuppers M, Hacke W. Thrombolytic therapy of acute basilar artery occlusion. Variables affecting recanalization and outcome. *Stroke* 1996;**27**:875–81.

93. Sliwka U, Mull M, Stelzer A, Diehl R, Noth J. Long-term follow-up of patients after intraarterial thrombolytic therapy of acute vertebrobasilar artery occlusion. *Cerebrovasc Dis* 2001;**12**:214–19.

94. Qureshi AI, Suri MF, Shatla AA, *et al.* Intraarterial recombinant tissue plasminogen activator for ischemic stroke: an accelerating dosing regimen. *Neurosurgery* 2000;**47**:473–6; discussion 477–9.

95. Qureshi AI, Siddiqui AM, Kim SH, *et al.* Reocclusion of recanalized arteries during intra-arterial thrombolysis for acute ischemic stroke. *Am J Neuroradiol* 2004;**25**:322–8.

96. Lee P-Y, Chen W-H, Ng W, *et al.* Low-dose aspirin increases aspirin resistance in patients with coronary artery disease. *Am J Med* 2005;**118**:723–7.

97. Qureshi AI. Interventional Section 2006–2007, American Academy of Neurology. 2006:

98. Mahon BR, Nesbit GM, Barnwell SL, *et al.* North American clinical experience with the EKOS MicroLysUS infusion catheter for the treatment of embolic stroke. *Am J Neuroradiol* 2003;**24**:534–8.

99. Ernst R, Pancioli A, Tomsick T, *et al.* Combined intravenous and intra-arterial recombinant tissue plasminogen activator in acute ischemic stroke. *Stroke* 2000;**31**:2552–7.

100. Gobin YP, Starkman S, Duckwiler GR, *et al.* MERCI 1: a phase 1 study of Mechanical Embolus Removal in Cerebral Ischemia. *Stroke* 2004;**35**:2848–54.

101. Clark WM, Wissman S, Albers GW, *et al.* Recombinant tissue-type plasminogen activator (Alteplase) for ischemic stroke 3 to 5 hours after symptom onset. The ATLANTIS Study: a randomized controlled trial. Alteplase Thrombolysis for Acute Noninterventional Therapy in Ischemic Stroke. *JAMA* 1999;**282**:2019–26.

102. Hacke W, Kaste M, Bluhmki E, *et al.* Thrombolysis with alteplase 3 to 4.5 hours after acute ischemic stroke. *N Engl J Med* 2008;**359**:1317–29.

103. Del Zoppo GJ, Saver JL, Jauch EC, Adams HPJ. Expansion of the time window for treatment of acute ischemic stroke with intravenous tissue plasminogen activator: a science advisory from the American Heart Association/American Stroke Association. *Stroke* 2009;**40**:2945–8.

104. Tomsick T, Brott T, Barsan W, *et al.* Prognostic value of the hyperdense middle cerebral artery sign and stroke scale score before ultraearly thrombolytic therapy. *Am J Neuroradiol.* 1996;**17**:79–85.

105. Katzan IL, Masaryk TJ, Furlan AJ, *et al.* Intra-arterial thrombolysis for perioperative stroke after open heart surgery. *Neurology.* 1999;**52**:1081–4.

106. Zaidat OO, Slivka AP, Mohammad Y, *et al.* Intra-arterial thrombolytic therapy in peri-coronary angiography ischemic stroke. *Stroke.* 2005;**36**: 1089–1090.

107. Janjua N, Alkawi A, Georgiadis A, *et al.* Feasibility of IA thrombolysis for acute ischemic stroke among anticoagulated patients. *Neurocrit Care* 2007;**7**:152–5.

108. Baird AE, Warach S. Magnetic resonance imaging of acute stroke. *J Cereb Blood Flow Metab* 1998;**18**: 583–609.

109. Kidwell CS, Alger JR, Saver JL. Beyond mismatch: evolving paradigms in imaging the ischemic penumbra with multimodal magnetic resonance imaging. *Stroke* 2003;**34**:2729–35.

110. Prosser J, Butcher K, Allport L, *et al.* Clinical-diffusion mismatch predicts the putative penumbra with high specificity. *Stroke* 2005;**36**:1700–4.

111. Davalos A, Blanco M, Pedraza S, *et al.* The clinical-DWI mismatch: a new diagnostic approach to the brain tissue at risk of infarction. *Neurology* 2004;**62**:2187–92.

112. Wintermark M, Reichhart M, Thiran J-P, *et al.* Prognostic accuracy of cerebral blood flow measurement by perfusion computed tomography, at the time of emergency room admission, in acute stroke patients. *Ann Neurol* 2002;**51**:417–32.

113. Divani AA, Qureshi AI, Hoffman KR, Suri MFK, Kirmani JF. Comparison of asymmetry in cerebral blood flow between brain hemispheres using digital subtraction angiography. *J Neuroimaging* 2006;**16**:139–45.

114. Qureshi AI. New grading system for angiographic evaluation of arterial occlusions and recanalization response to intra-arterial thrombolysis in acute ischemic stroke. *Neurosurgery* 2002;**50**:1405–14; discussion 1414–15.

115. Mohammad Y, Xavier AR, Christoforidis G, Bourekas E, Slivka A. Qureshi grading scheme for angiographic occlusions strongly correlates with the initial severity and in-hospital outcome of acute ischemic stroke. *J Neuroimaging* 2004;**14**:235–41.

116. Mohammad YM, Christoforidis GA, Bourekas EC, Slivka AP. Qureshi grading scheme predicts subsequent volume of brain infarction following intra-arterial thrombolysis in patients with acute anterior circulation ischemic stroke. *J Neuroimaging* 2008;**18**:262–7.

117. Qureshi AI, Alkawi A, Hussein HM, Divani AA. Angiographic analysis of intravascular thrombus volume in patients with acute ischemic stroke. *J Endovasc Ther* 2007;**14**:475–82.

118. Qureshi AI. Endovascular revascularization of symptomatic acute extracranial internal carotid artery occlusion. *Stroke* 2005;**36**:2335–6.

119. Jovin TG, Gupta R, Uchino K, *et al.* Emergent stenting of extracranial internal carotid artery occlusion in acute stroke has a high revascularization rate. *Stroke* 2005;**36**:2426–30.

120. Trubestein G, Engel C, Etzel F, *et al.* Thrombolysis by ultrasound. *Clin Sci Mol Med Suppl* 1976;**3**:697s–8s.

121. Tachibana KTS. Ultrasonic vibration for boosting fibrinolytic effects of urokinase in vivo. *Thromb Haemost* 1981:**46**;211.

122. Behrens S, Daffertshofer M, Spiegel D, Hennerici M. Low-frequency, low-intensity ultrasound accelerates thrombolysis through the skull. *Ultrasound Med Biol* 1999;**25**:269–73.

123. Suchkova V, Siddiqi FN, Carstensen EL, *et al.* Enhancement of fibrinolysis with 40-kHz ultrasound. *Circulation* 1998;**98**:1030–5.

124. Akiyama M, Ishibashi T, Yamada T, Furuhata H. Low-frequency ultrasound penetrates the cranium and enhances thrombolysis in vitro. *Neurosurgery* 1998;**43**:828–32; discussion 832–3.

125. Kimura M, Iijima S, Kobayashi K, Furuhata H. Evaluation of the thrombolytic effect of tissue-type plasminogen activator with ultrasonic irradiation: in vitro experiment involving assay of the fibrin degradation products from the clot. *Biol Pharm Bull* 1994;**17**:126–30.

126. Lauer CG, Burge R, Tang DB, *et al.* Effect of ultrasound on tissue-type plasminogen activator-induced thrombolysis. *Circulation* 1992;**86**:1257–64.

127. Polak JF. Ultrasound energy and the dissolution of thrombus. *N Engl J Med* 2004;**351**:2154–5.

128. Sakharov DV, Barrertt-Bergshoeff M, Hekkenberg RT, Rijken DC. Fibrin-specificity of a plasminogen activator affects the efficiency of fibrinolysis and responsiveness to ultrasound: comparison of nine plasminogen activators in vitro. *Thromb Haemost* 1999;**81**:605–12.

129. Blinc A, Francis CW, Trudnowski JL, Carstensen EL. Characterization of ultrasound-potentiated fibrinolysis in vitro. *Blood* 1993;**81**:2636–43.

130. Ishibashi T, Akiyama M, Onoue H, Abe T, Furuhata H. Can transcranial ultrasonication increase recanalization flow with tissue plasminogen activator?. *Stroke* 2002;**33**:1399–404.

131. Francis CW, Blinc A, Lee S, Cox C. Ultrasound accelerates transport of recombinant tissue plasminogen activator into clots. *Ultrasound Med Biol* 1995;**21**:419–24.

132. Chernyshev OY, Garami Z, Calleja S, *et al.* Yield and accuracy of urgent combined carotid/transcranial ultrasound testing in acute cerebral ischemia. *Stroke* 2005;**36**:32–7.

133. Alexandrov AV, Demchuk AM, Felberg RA, *et al.* High rate of complete recanalization and dramatic clinical recovery during tPA infusion when continuously monitored with 2-MHz transcranial doppler monitoring. *Stroke* 2000;**31**:610–14.

134. Tsivgoulis G, Sharma VK, Lao AY, Malkoff MD, Alexandrov AV. Validation of transcranial Doppler with computed tomography angiography in acute cerebral ischemia. *Stroke.* 2007;**38**:1245–9.

135. Eggers J, Seidel G, Koch B, Konig IR. Sonothrombolysis in acute ischemic stroke for patients ineligible for rt-PA. *Neurology* 2005;**64**:1052–4.

136. Eggers J, Koch B, Meyer K, Konig I, Seidel G. Effect of ultrasound on thrombolysis of middle cerebral artery occlusion. *Ann Neurol* 2003;**53**: 797–800.

137. Cintas P, Le Traon AP, Larrue V. High rate of recanalization of middle cerebral artery occlusion during 2-MHz transcranial color-coded Doppler continuous monitoring without thrombolytic drug. *Stroke* 2002;**33**: 626–8.

138. Alexandrov AV, Molina CA, Grotta JC, *et al.* Ultrasound-enhanced systemic thrombolysis for acute ischemic stroke. *N Engl J Med* 2004;**351**:2170–8.

139. Skoloudik DBMHPVDSO. Safety and efficacy of thrombotripsy- Acceleration of thrombolysis by TCCS, 2003;

Proceedings of the NSRG Meeting, Germany:CD-Rom.

140. Daffertshofer M, Hennerici M. Ultrasound in the treatment of ischaemic stroke. *Lancet Neurol* 2003;**2**:283–90.

141. Daffertshofer M, Gass A, Ringleb P, *et al.* Transcranial low-frequency ultrasound-mediated thrombolysis in brain ischemia: increased risk of hemorrhage with combined ultrasound and tissue plasminogen activator: results of a phase II clinical trial. *Stroke* 2005;**36**:1441–6.

142. Wu Y, Unger EC, McCreery TP, *et al.* Binding and lysing of blood clots using MRX-408. *Invest Radiol* 1998;**33**:880–5.

143. Tsutsui JM, Xie F, Johanning J, *et al.* Treatment of deeply located acute intravascular thrombi with therapeutic ultrasound guided by diagnostic ultrasound and intravenous microbubbles. *J Ultrasound Med* 2006;**25**:1161–8.

144. Unger EC, Porter T, Culp W, *et al.* Therapeutic applications of lipid-coated microbubbles. *Adv Drug Deliv Rev* 2004;**56**:1291–314.

145. Tiukinhoy-Laing SD, Huang S, Klegerman M, Holland CK, McPherson DD. Ultrasound-facilitated thrombolysis using tissue-plasminogen activator-loaded echogenic liposomes. *Thromb Res* 2007;**119**:777–84.

146. Perren F, Loulidi J, Poglia D, Landis T, Sztajzel R. Microbubble potentiated transcranial duplex ultrasound enhances IV thrombolysis in acute stroke. *J Thromb Thrombolysis* 2008;**25**:219–223.

147. Larrue V, Viguier A, Arnaud C, *et al.* Transcranial ultrasound combined with intravenous microbubbles and tissue plasminogen activator for acute ischemic stroke: a randomized controlled study. *Stroke* 2007;**38**:472.

148. Alexandrov AV, Mikulik R, Ribo M, *et al.* A pilot randomized clinical safety study of sonothrombolysis augmentation with ultrasound-activated perflutren-lipid microspheres for acute ischemic stroke. *Stroke* 2008;**39**:1464–9.

149. Molina CA, Ribo M, Rubiera M, *et al.* Microbubble administration accelerates clot lysis during continuous 2-MHz ultrasound monitoring in stroke patients treated with intravenous tissue plasminogen activator. *Stroke* 2006;**37**:425–9.

150. Sharma VK, Tsivgoulis G, Lao AY, *et al.* Quantification of microspheres appearance in brain vessels: implications for residual flow velocity measurements, dose calculations, and potential drug delivery. *Stroke* 2008;**39**:1476–81.

151. Kase CS, Furlan AJ, Wechsler LR, *et al.* Cerebral hemorrhage after intra-arterial thrombolysis for ischemic stroke: the PROACT II trial. *Neurology* 2001;**57**:1603–10.

152. Khatri P, Wechsler LR, Broderick JP. Intracranial hemorrhage associated with revascularization therapies. *Stroke* 2007;**38**:431–40.

153. Kahles T, Foerch C, Sitzer M, *et al.* Tissue plasminogen activator mediated blood-brain barrier damage in transient focal cerebral ischemia in rats: relevance of interactions between thrombotic material and thrombolytic agent. *Vascul Pharmacol* 2005;**43**:254–9.

154. Burggraf D, Martens HK, Dichgans M, Hamann GF. rt-PA causes a dose-dependent increase in the extravasation of cellular and non-cellular blood elements after focal cerebral ischemia. *Brain Res* 2007;**1164**:55–62.

155. Lansberg MG, Albers GW, Wijman CAC. Symptomatic intracerebral hemorrhage following thrombolytic therapy for acute ischemic stroke: a review of the risk factors. *Cerebrovasc Dis* 2007;**24**:1–10.

156. Maier CM, Hsieh L, Crandall T, Narasimhan P, Chan PH. Evaluating therapeutic targets for reperfusion-related brain hemorrhage. *Ann Neurol* 2006;**59**:929–38.

157. Pfefferkorn T, Rosenberg GA. Closure of the blood–brain barrier by matrix metalloproteinase inhibition reduces rtPA-mediated mortality in cerebral ischemia with delayed reperfusion. *Stroke* 2003;**34**:2025–30.

158. Lees KR, Zivin JA, Ashwood T, *et al.* NXY-059 for acute ischemic stroke. *N Engl J Med* 2006;**354**:588–600.

159. Shuaib A, Lees KR, Lyden P, *et al.* NXY-059 for the treatment of acute ischemic stroke. *N Engl J Med* 2007;**357**:562–71.

160. The NINDS t-PA Stroke Study Group. Intracerebral hemorrhage after intravenous t-PA therapy for ischemic stroke. *Stroke.* 1997;**28**:2109–18.

161. Mahaffey KW, Granger CB, Sloan MA, *et al.* Neurosurgical evacuation of intracranial hemorrhage after thrombolytic therapy for acute myocardial infarction: experience from the GUSTO-I trial. Global Utilization of Streptokinase and tissue-plasminogen activator (tPA) for Occluded Coronary Arteries. *Am Heart J* 1999;**138**:493–9.

162. Sedrakyan A, Treasure T, Elefteriades JA. Effect of aprotinin on clinical outcomes in coronary artery bypass graft surgery: a systematic review and meta-analysis of randomized clinical trials. *J Thorac Cardiovasc Surg* 2004;**128**:442–8.

163. Kokoszka A, Kuflik P, Bitan F, Casden A, Neuwirth M. Evidence-based review of the role of aprotinin in blood conservation during orthopaedic surgery. *J Bone Joint Surg Am* 2005;**87**:1129–36.

164. Rha J-H, Saver JL. The impact of recanalization on ischemic stroke outcome: a meta-analysis. *Stroke* 2007;**38**:967–73.

165. Gupta R, Vora NA, Horowitz MB, et al. Multimodal reperfusion therapy for acute ischemic stroke: factors predicting vessel recanalization. *Stroke* 2006;**37**:986–90.

166. Wang CX, Yang T, Shuaib A. Clot fragments formed from original thrombus obstruct downstream arteries in the ischemic injured brain. *Microcirculation* 2006;**13**:229–36.

167. Reffelmann T, Kloner RA. The no-reflow phenomenon: a basic mechanism of myocardial ischemia and reperfusion. *Basic Res Cardiol* 2006;**101**:359–72.

168. van Gaal WJ, Banning AP. Percutaneous coronary intervention and the no-reflow phenomenon. *Expert Rev Cardiovasc Ther.* 2007;**5**:715–31.

169. Kidwell CS, Saver JL, Starkman S, *et al.* Late secondary ischemic injury in patients receiving intraarterial thrombolysis. *Ann Neurol* 2002;**52**:698–703.

170. Quintana M, Kahan T, Hjemdahl P. Pharmacological prevention of reperfusion injury in acute myocardial infarction. A potential role for adenosine as a therapeutic agent. *Am J Cardiovasc Drugs* 2004;**4**:159–67.

171. Saqqur M, Molina CA, Salam A, *et al.* Clinical deterioration after intravenous recombinant tissue plasminogen activator treatment: a multicenter transcranial Doppler study. *Stroke* 2007;**38**:69–74.

172. Janjua N, Alkawi A, Suri MFK, Qureshi AI. Impact of arterial reocclusion and distal fragmentation during thrombolysis among patients with acute ischemic stroke. *Am J Neuroradiol.* 2008;**29**:253–8.

173. Qureshi AI, Suri MFK, Ali Z, *et al.* Intraarterial reteplase and intravenous abciximab for treatment of acute ischemic stroke. A preliminary feasibility and safety study in a non-human primate model. *Neuroradiology* 2005;**47**:845–54.

174. Zaidat OO, Suarez JI, Sunshine JL, *et al.* Thrombolytic therapy of acute ischemic stroke: correlation of angiographic recanalization with clinical outcome. *Am J Neuroradiol* 2005;**26**:880–4.

175. Higashida RT, Furlan AJ, Roberts H, *et al.* Trial design and reporting standards for intra-arterial cerebral thrombolysis for acute ischemic stroke. *Stroke* 2003;**34**:e109–37.

176. Hussein HM, Georgiadis AL, Vazquez G, *et al.* Occurrence and predictors of futile recanalization following endovascular treatment among patients with acute ischemic stroke: a multicenter study. *Am J Neuroradiol* 2010;in press:online.

177. Lee T-Y, Murphy BD, Aviv RI, *et al.* Cerebral blood flow threshold of ischemic penumbra and infarct core in acute ischemic stroke: a systematic review. *Stroke* 2006;**37**:2201; author reply 2203.

178. Lev MH, Nichols SJ. Computed tomographic angiography and computed tomographic perfusion imaging of hyperacute stroke. *Top Magn Reson Imaging* 2000;**11**:273–87.

179. Sekoranja L, Loulidi J, Yilmaz H, *et al.* Intravenous versus combined (intravenous and intra-arterial) thrombolysis in acute ischemic stroke: a transcranial color-coded duplex sonography–guided pilot study. *Stroke* 2006;**37**:1805–9.

180. Sacco RL, Chong JY, Prabhakaran S, Elkind MSV. Experimental treatments for acute ischaemic stroke. *Lancet* 2007;**369**:331–41.

181. Alberts MJ, Latchaw RE, Selman WR, *et al.* Recommendations for comprehensive stroke centers: a consensus statement from the Brain Attack Coalition. *Stroke* 2005;**36**:1597–616.

182. Qureshi AI, Suri MFK, Nasar A, *et al.* Thrombolysis for ischemic stroke in the United States: data from National Hospital Discharge Survey 1999–2001. *Neurosurgery* 2005;**57**:647–54; discussion 647–54.

183. Choi JH, Bateman BT, Mangla S, *et al.* Endovascular recanalization therapy in acute ischemic stroke. *Stroke* 2006;**37**:419–24.

184. Qureshi AI. Ten years of advances in neuroendovascular procedures. *J Endovasc Ther* 2004;**11** Suppl 2:II1–4.

185. Janjua N, Nasar A, Lynch JK, Qureshi AI. Thrombolysis for ischemic stroke in children: data from the nationwide inpatient sample. *Stroke* 2007;**38**:1850–4.

Chapter

6

Cervical internal and common carotid artery stenosis

Adnan I. Qureshi MD and L. Nelson Hopkins MD

Incidence, prevalence, and screening

Prevalence of symptomatic and asymptomatic carotid artery stenosis

A review of patients identified in all secondary care services in Oxfordshire and a nested population-based study of incidence of transient ischemic attack (TIA) and stroke (the Oxford vascular study-OXVASC)[1] found that the incidence of 50% or greater symptomatic carotid artery stenosis increased with age, particularly in persons aged 80 years or greater. Of the 65 persons with symptomatic 50%–99% carotid stenosis identified from 575 patients, 42 underwent carotid endarterectomy (CEA). The incidence of carotid artery stenosis 50% or greater ranged from 0.5 per 1000 for persons aged 60–69 years to 1.5 per 1000 for patients aged 80 years or greater. A second analysis from the prospective Northern Manhattan Stroke Study (NOMASS) ($n = 431$) and the Berlin Cerebral Ischemia Databank (BCID) ($n = 483$)[2] estimated the prevalence of high-grade carotid stenosis ($\geq 60\%$ diagnosed by Doppler ultrasound). High-grade carotid stenoses were found in 14% and 21% of the NOMASS and BCID patients, respectively. A multicenter study[3] estimated the prevalence of symptomatic internal carotid artery stenosis $\geq 50\%$ or occlusion in young adults (aged 15–44 years) and reported a prevalence of 16% in patients with a recent TIA or stroke in the carotid territory.

A detailed review of prevalence of asymptomatic stenosis in general population and selected patient population is summarized based on a detailed review (see Table 6.1). Barnett et al.[4] estimated that approximately two million people living in North America and Europe have asymptomatic carotid artery stenosis that are candidates for treatment.[5]

The prevalences vary depending upon the definitions used to define carotid artery disease.

Prevalence of carotid endarterectomy

We estimated that there were 1 126 997 admissions for ischemic stroke in US hospitals in 1990 to 1991 and 1 259 740 in

Table 6.1 Prevalence of extracranial carotid artery disease in general population and selected patient population based on Qureshi et al.

Patient category	Prevalence
General population	2%–18%
Anticipating open heart surgery	8%–21%
Peripheral vascular disease	15%–37%
Post-radiation therapy for head or neck cancer	12%–35%

2000 to 2001.[6] The rates of CEA were 13% and 22% among patients admitted in 1990–1991 and 2000–2001, respectively. An estimated 151 000 CEAs are performed every year,[7] which provides some data regarding the prevalence of carotid artery stenosis in the US. A study[8] calculated the annual rate of CEA in the US states of California and New York and in the Canadian province of Ontario from 1983 through 1995. After the results of the clinical trials in the 1990s became available, a dramatic increase in the rates of the procedure from 1989 to 1995 (from 66 to 99 per 100 000 in California, from 40 to 96 per 100 000 in New York, and from 15 to 38 per 100 000 in Ontario) was observed. The executive committee of the Carotid Revascularization Endovascular versus Stent Trial (CREST) examined Medicare Provider Analysis and Review (MEDPAR) data[9] on the number of CEAs performed at each medical center in the US. In 2002, Medicare billing for CEA was documented in 89 860 patients as compared with billings for carotid stent placement in 3909 patients. MEDPAR data included Medicare billing only and probably underestimated the total number of patients undergoing either procedure.

Pathology of cervical internal carotid artery atherosclerosis

Pathology

Internal carotid artery atherosclerosis consists of the atherosis (intra-and extra-cellular lipid deposition) and sclerosis

---

Textbook of Interventional Neurology, ed. Adnan I. Qureshi. Published by Cambridge University Press. © Cambridge University Press 2011.

(fibrosis, reduced compliance, and endothelial dysfunction) within the vessel wall. Morphological analysis of lumen narrowing revealed that only 28% of plaques had circular lumens; 50% had elliptical lumens, and 22% had either crescentic or multi-lobular lumens.[10] Histological analysis of specimens removed during endarterectomy for ulceration, inflammation, size of necrotic core, thickness of fibrous cap, hemorrhage and luminal thrombosis suggested a relationship between a thin fibrous cap and a large necrotic core, irregular plaque contour, and ulceration. Another relationship was identified between a large necrotic core and ulceration and inflammation. Increasing amounts of necrosis were associated with greater surface thrombosis.

Pathological correlates of ischemic symptoms

The relationship between ulceration, thrombus, and calcification within atherosclerotic plaques and ipsilateral or contralateral ischemic stroke were examined in one study.[11] Plaques were analyzed from 241 subjects: 170 patients enrolled in the Asymptomatic Carotid Atherosclerosis Study (ACAS) and 71 patients enrolled in the North American Symptomatic Carotid Endarterectomy Trial (NASCET); 128 subjects had no history of stroke symptoms, 80 subjects had ipsilateral ischemic symptoms, and 33 had contralateral symptoms. Plaque ulceration was more common in plaques obtained during endarterectomy from symptomatic patients than asymptomatic patients (36% vs. 14%). Thrombus was most commonly observed in plaques obtained from patients with both ipsilateral symptoms and ulceration. The extent of calcification and frequency of ulceration were not associated with ischemic stroke symptoms.

Intraplaque hemorrhages were associated with ischemic symptoms. Among 89 atheromatic plaques removed following endarterectomy,[12] intraplaque hemorrhage was identified in 72% and 38% of symptomatic and asymptomatic patients, respectively. The incidence of ulceration of the intima, with or without the presence of thrombus, was associated with intraplaque hemorrhages but without any significant relationship with ischemic symptoms. A high incidence of intraplaque hemorrhage was found in both the symptomatic (94%) and asymptomatic (71%) patients in another study of CEA specimens from 33 symptomatic and 14 asymptomatic patients with >70% stenosis.[13] The plaques obtained from the symptomatic patients contained more fibrosis than lipids, compared with those obtained from the asymptomatic patients. Overall, intraluminal thrombosis and calcification were rare. Another histological study of plaques obtained following endarterectomy from 526 consecutive symptomatic patients[14] demonstrated that dense plaque inflammation (especially infiltration with macrophages) was most strongly associated with both cap rupture and time since stroke. Plaque inflammation and overall instability persisted with time after a transient ischemic attack but decreased with time after a stroke.

Pathophysiology of ischemic events related to carotid stenosis

Pathological studies

Using the pathologic and clinical data, embolism and hemodynamic failure have been implicated in the mechanism of the ischemic events associated with carotid stenosis. Embolization from the plaque has been proposed as the main mechanism for ischemic lesions.[15] In the pathological study by Fisher and Ojemann,[16] the occurrence of TIAs correlated with severity of carotid stenosis (1 mm or less), but less so with the presence of mural thrombus. Carotid plaques resected from symptomatic patients are more frequently ulcerated and have intraluminal thrombus (compared with asymptomatic plaques) and, therefore, are at greater risk for distal embolization of thrombus and atherosclerotic debris.[17]

Transcranial Doppler ultrasound studies

Several transcranial Doppler ultrasound studies have demonstrated the presence of emboli (transient high intensity signal) during insonation of the middle cerebral artery ipsilateral to carotid arery stenosis. In a study of 105 patients with carotid artery stenosis ranging from 20%–99% or occlusion, 1 hour insonation of the ipsilateral middle cerebral artery was performed.[18] The presence of multiple embolic signals was more frequent in symptomatic patients (33%) than in asymptomatic patients (10%). The detection of emboli was likely in patients with increasing degree of stenosis. No emboli were detected in carotid artery stenosis below 80%. There was a decline in multiple embolic signals with increasing interval between ischemic event and insonation. In another study of 111 patients with >60% carotid artery stenosis (69 symptomatic, 42 asymptomatic), embolic signal was detected in 37% of the patients during 1 hour insonation of the ipsilateral middle cerebral artery.[19] In symptomatic patients there was a significant inverse relationship between the number of embolic signal detected per hour and time elapsed since last ischemic event. The detection of embolic signal predicted TIA and stroke during follow-up in both symptomatic and asymptomatic patients. Asymptomatic embolization predicted new ischemic events after controlling for other cardiovascular risk factors, degree of stenosis, symptomatic status, and aspirin or warfarin use.[19] Another study of 64 asymptomatic patients with unilateral 70% to 90% carotid artery stenosis (mean follow-up, 72 weeks)[20] demonstrated that a microembolic rate of ≥ 2 per hour in the ipsilateral middle cerebral artery was associated with a substantially increased risk of developing cerebral ischemic events.

Regional cerebral hypoperfusion

Ipsilateral regional cerebral hypoperfusion is a contributing mechanism to ischemic events associated with stenosis.[21] There is some evidence that regional hypoperfusion and embolization may act synergistically to cause ischemic events. The flow territory of the ipsilateral carotid artery in patients with carotid artery stenosis are smaller, compared with territories of the contralateral carotid artery and vertebrobasilar arteries.[25] The regional hypoperfusion improves after revascularization of the artery.[22] Both carotid stent placement and endarterectomy results in a normalization of the territorial distribution and regional cerebral blood flow.[25] Impaired vasodilatory capacity related to maximal dilatation of arterioles in presence of hypoperfusion may further increase the susceptibility to ischemia in the distribution of the stenotic artery.[26] Impaired vasodilatory response to CO_2 inhalation has been demonsatrated among patients with unilateral > 70% carotid artery stenosis.[27] The regional hypoperfusion may become more prominent during vasodilatory challenge such as CO_2 inhalation. In another study, cerebral perfusion on the side ipsilateral to the internal carotid artery occlusion was decreased compared with the contralateral side in the basal ganglia, frontal lobe and parietal lobe.[28] During a CO_2 inhalation, the ipsilateral frontal lobe demonstrated a perfusion decrease compared with the contralateral frontal lobe. Furthermore, in patients without collateral flow via the anterior communicating artery, the perfusion of the ipsilateral frontal lobe was significantly decreased during the CO_2 inhalation. Hemodynamic response during neural activation may be impaired in the presence of carotid artery stenosis.[29] The effect of internal carotid artery occlusive disease on the pattern of cerebral blood flow response during visual stimulation using positron emission tomography demonstrated reduced regional cerebral blood flow activation in regions surrounding the visual cortex in 9 of the 13 patients with carotid artery steno-occlusive lesions. The hemispheric values of oxygen extraction fraction in the carotid artery distribution negatively correlated with the cerebral blood flow change in the surrounding region.

Angiographic characteristics of carotid artery stenosis

Quantification, characterization, and vessel size determinations

The basis for angiographic quantitative measurement involves expressing the measurement of minimum vessel lumen as a fraction of a reference lumen diameter. A uniform technique for measuring carotid artery stenosis is as follows: % stenosis = [1 − minimum residual lumen/normal distal cervical internal carotid artery (ICA) diameter] × 100. The definition was used in the North American Symptomatic Carotid Endarterectomy Trial (NASCET) and since has been widely used in practice.[30] The technique requires measurement of: (1) minimum lumen diameter within the stenosis identified on either antero-posterior or lateral projection; and (2) diameter of the internal carotid artery distal to the stenosis when both the vessel walls become parallel (avoid measuring carotid bulb or post-stenotic dilatation) as the reference diameter (see

Fig. 6.1). Another method used in the European Carotid Surgery Trial (ECST) required the reference diameter derivation by measuring the distance between two lines connecting arterial segments proximal and distal to the stenosis. A third method involves using the diameter of the proximal common carotid artery to be used as the reference diameter (common carotid (CC) method). One study compared the three methods[31] in 1001 patients recruited in the ECST. The ECST and CC methods overestimated the stenosis compared with the NASCET method. The ability of the derived measurements in the prediction of ipsilateral carotid distribution ischemic stroke was subsequently assessed in 1001 consecutively selected patients randomly assigned to medical treatment in the ECST.[32] There was little difference in the ability of the three methods to predict ipsilateral carotid distribution ischemic stroke.

A previous study demonstrated a very high interobserver reliability in categorizing carotid artery stenosis using the NASCET method (kappa = 0.73 to 0.79).[33] Another study demonstrated a high interrater agreement for carotid artery stenosis measurements in patients undergoing CEA.[34] The correlation co-efficient was 0.74 and 0.72 for NASCET and ECST criteria, respectively. Another study compared the reliability of measuring stenosis using the three methods.[35] The relationship between the NASCET and CC methods was linear; the mean ratio of distal internal carotid artery to common carotid diameter of 0.62 (SD of 0.11). The relationships between the ECST and NASCET methods or CC methods were parabolic. Despite comparable reproducibility, the authors concluded that converting from the NASCET method to the CC method, in the absence of superiority or simplicity, was not justified.

There are some limitations with the NASCET method. The criteria depends upon adequately visualizing the internal carotid artery distal to the stenosis. The visualization maybe obscured in the presence of near occlusion and poor distal flow. The resulting poststenotic reduction in luminal diameter would underestimate the stenosis. In the NASCET, a calculated degree of stenosis for recognized near-occlusion cases was not performed. Instead, these cases were arbitrarily assigned value of 95%, representing a very severe stenosis. The point of minimum stenosis may not be adequately visualized due to overlying vessels, heavy calcification, or inadequate views of the distal internal carotid artery or carotid bulb. A study comparing angiographic measurements with measurements on histological specimens in intact carotid plaques removed during surgery demonstrated that angiographic images underestimated the stenosis.[36] Another study compared postmortem angiography with computerized planimetric analysis of the cross-sections of fixed tissue[37] and demonstrated moderate accuracy and reproducibility in detecting and measuring carotid artery stenosis independent of the technique of measurement used.

Other measures for quantitative measurement of internal carotid artery stenosis have been proposed. In the 119 angiograms, the minimum residual lumen diameter of the stenosis

(a)

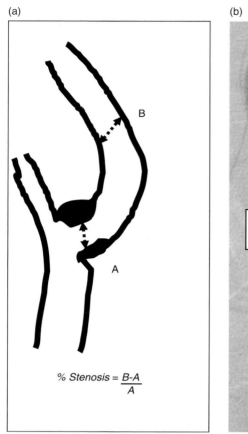

(b)

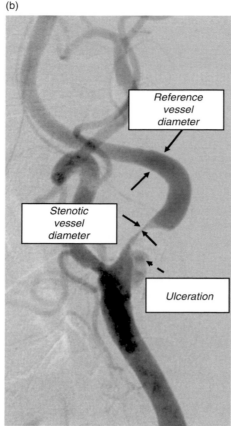

(c)

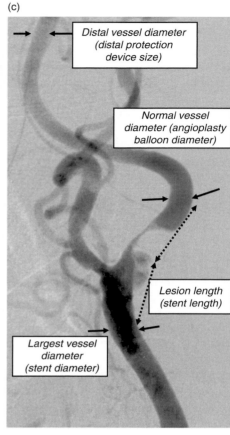

Fig. 6.1. (a) The schematic (left) illustrates the method of measuring the severity of stenosis according to the NASCET method; (b) the middle picture demonstrates the method of measuring the stenosis based on an angiographic image in lateral view: and, (c) the right picture demonstrates the measurements necessary for planning the carotid angioplasty and stent procedure.

was compared with the calculated percentage area of stenosis, the percentage diameter of stenosis, and the qualitative estimates of stenosis. The measurement of the minimum residual lumen diameter performed better in theoretical modeling for quantifying the severity of carotid stenoses.[38] Another index, the Carotid Stenosis Index (CSI), is based on the known anatomic relationship between the CCA and ICA (1.2 x CCA diameter = proximal ICA diameter).[39] In a blinded measurement of angiograms of 57 patients (114 carotid arteries), the NASCET method could only be applied correctly in 89% and the ECST method in 95% of cases because of overlying vessels or inadequate views of the distal ICA or carotid bulb. An additional 9% of NASCET cases had a "negative" stenosis, in which the stenosis is wider than the distal ICA. The CSI method was applicable in 99% of cases. However, other methods have not been widely adopted since the benefits of CEA for patients with 70% to 99% stenosis as determined by the NASCET method have been established.

Ulcerations

Angiographic ulceration can be present in up to 14% of the patients, usually proximal to the point of maximum stenosis.[40]

Data from the medical treatment group of the Aspirin in TIA study were reviewed, and prospective analysis of patients with asymptomatic bruits was performed to determine whether carotid stenosis (0% to 49% or 50% to 99%) or ulceration resulted in an increased risk of ipsilateral TIA or infarct.[41] In symptomatic arteries, greater than 50% stenosis implied a higher risk of subsequent symptoms; ulceration was associated with an increased risk only in non-stenotic vessels. The frequency of embolic signal detected in the middle cerebral artery has also been correlated with ulceration.[42]

In the NASCET[43] the presence of angiographic ulceration among medically treated symptomatic patients was associated with an increased risk of stroke. The risk of stroke was greater than two fold at higher degrees of stenosis. The risk of ipsilateral stroke at 24 months for medically treated patients with ulcerated plaques increased incrementally from 26.3% to 73.2% as the degree of stenosis increased from 75% to 95%. For patients with no ulcer, the risk of stroke remained constant at 21.3% for all degrees of stenosis. Angiographic evidence of ulceration of the target lesion has been associated with a higher rate of new lesions seen on diffusion-weighted imaging (DWI)[44] and with ischemic stroke in the peri-procedural period after carotid stent placement in some[45] but not all studies.[46]

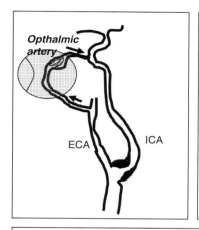

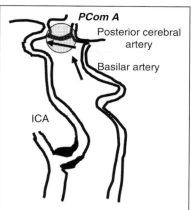

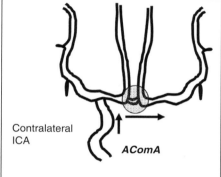

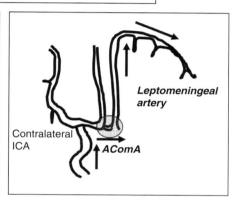

Fig. 6.2. Various collateral pathways that result in relative preservation of blood flow to variable extent in hemisphere ipsilateral to carotid artery stenosis are illustrated. The primary collateral pathway is highlighted in bold and underlined. Abbreviations used: PCom, posterior communicating artery; ACom A, anterior communicating artery; ECA, external carotid artery; and, ICA, internal carotid artery.

It should be noted that the correlation between angiographic ulceration and ulceration identified during pathological evaluation is not good.[15] The assessment of plaque surface ulceration varies depending on the type of angiography and the quality of visualization of the stenosis.[47] The detection of ulceration during Doppler ultrasound may be better than that observed in cerebral angiography.[48,49] The detection of ulceration by angiography was compared with observations during endarterectomy in the first 500 patients recruited into the NASCET.[50] Sensitivity and specificity of detecting ulcerated plaques were 45.9% and 74.1%, respectively. The positive predictive value of identifying an ulcer was 72%. These observations from a multicenter study confirm that little agreement exists between angiography and surgical observation for detecting carotid plaque ulceration.

Lesion irregularity

A correlative study[10] evaluated the relationship between presenting neurologic symptoms of patients with high-resolution magnetic resonance imaging (MRI; 200 microm) studies of ipsilateral plaque surface invaginations and ledges, lumen shape, and the location of the plaque bulk creating the stenosis after surgical removal. Thirty-five plaques were graded as having major surface contour irregularities, and 45 plaques were graded as having minor irregularities. There was a

significant correlation between major surface irregularity and TIA or stroke. Surface irregularities identified by high resolution imaging of the carotid plaques with magnetic resonance imaging (MRI) were common, but only the presence of major irregularities correlated with TIA or stroke. Irregular plaques can be identified but underestimated in extent with angiography. In the ESCT[51] a total of 1897 symptomatic stenoses (63.1%) had surface irregularity on the angiogram. Angiographic plaque irregularity and plaque surface thrombus at endarterectomy increased in frequency as the degree of stenosis increased. However, the degree of stenosis was still predictive of the 2-year risk of stroke on medical treatment after correction for plaque surface irregularity. Angiographic plaque irregularity was an independent predictor of ipsilateral ischemic stroke in medically treated patients with any severity of stenosis. Neither the degree of stenosis nor plaque surface irregularity was predictive of stroke risk after endarterectomy or the risk of non-stroke vascular events.

Calcification

There is an association between the presence of carotid calcification and atheromatous disease.[52] Current emphasis on detection of calcification within the plaque is predominantly using computed tomography (CT) angiography.[53,54] Extracranial carotid artery calcified plaques causing stenosis are significantly less likely to be symptomatic and thus may be more stable than non-calcified plaques.[55] Calcium scores in the cervical carotid arteries may represent an independent marker for luminal stenosis and ischemic symptoms.[54] Angiographic evidence of calcification of the target lesion has not been associated with ischemic stroke in the peri-procedural period after carotid stent placement.[46,56] There is a relationship between post-procedural hypotension and carotid artery calcification detected by Doppler ultrasound,[57] but such relationship is not seen with angiographic calcification.[58] Some investigators advocate the use of calcification within the plaque to stratify risk and treatment modalities.[59] Carotid angioplasty with stent placement is less preferable as an option for patients with concentric calcification due to high recoil and resistance to angioplasty.

Angiographic collaterals

In the NASCET,[60] angiographic collateral filling through anterior communicating (ACoA) and posterior communicating arteries (PCoA) and retrograde filling through ophthalmic arteries were determined in the 2885 patients recruited into NASCET. Of these, 280 (9.7%) patients were identified by angiography to have collateral pathways toward the symptomatic ICA: 195 through the ACoA only, 25 through the PCoA only, 5 retrograde through the ophthalmic arteries only, and 55 with multiple collateral pathways. The presence of collaterals supplying the symptomatic ICA increased with severity of stenosis (3% for stenosis of 50%–69% and 64% for ≥95% stenosis). Two-year risk of ipsilateral ischemic stroke in medically treated patients with severe ICA stenosis was reduced in the presence of collaterals: 28% to 11%. Similar reductions were observed for ipsilateral TIA (36% vs. 19%) and disabling or fatal strokes (13% vs. 6%). For surgically treated patients, the perioperative risk of ipsilateral stroke was 1% in the presence of collaterals vs. 5% when collaterals were absent. The 2-year stroke risks for surgical patients with and without collaterals were 6% vs. 8%, respectively.

Absence of collateral pathways is associated with hypoperfusion and reduced vasodilatory reserve. In patients without collateral flow via the anterior circle of Willis, the perfusion of the ipsilateral frontal lobe was significantly decreased during the CO_2 challenge.[28] No regional cerebral blood flow (rCBF) differences were related to presence or absence of collateral flow via the posterior communicating artery. Patients with decreased vasodilatory reserve had significantly greater dependence on either the retrograde opthalmic or leptomeningeal collaterals (42%) than did patients without decreased reserve (7%).[61] Similarly, the cerebral hemispheres with decreased cerebrovascular resistance showed a higher prevalence of 70% or greater stenosis or occlusion (74%) than did hemispheres without such increase in resistance (16%). Collateral flow in the circle of Willis in subjects with ICA stenosis occurs equally often in symptomatic and asymptomatic patients; however, it is more efficient in patients without

symptoms[62] based on assessment of flow velocities. The rate of development of collateral circulation depends on ICA stenosis severity. The presence of chronic hypertension adversely affects the formation of collaterals.[63]

The collateral pathways are modified after revascularization. CEA reduces the caliber of compensatory collateral channels to normal levels as measured by magnetic resonance (MR) angiography in the presence of severe unilateral stenosis.[64] Luft et al.[65] evaluated the frequency and predictors of changes in inflow of contrast medium before and after carotid stent placement: In 31 patients: (36%) initial angiogram showed contralateral anterior cerebral artery (ACA) filling, and in 39% of these, normal filling was restored after stent placement. Lesser contralateral carotid stenosis was associated with crossed ACA filling and with restoration of normal filling pattern after stent placement.

Near occlusion or pseudo-occlusion

The 106 patients with carotid-near-occlusion in NASCET[66] were subdivided into those with a string-like lumen ($n = 29$) and those without a string-like lumen ($n = 77$). Of the 48 patients with near occlusion treated with CEA, 3 (6.3%) had perioperative strokes, similar to the 70%–94% stenosis group. Only 1 of 58 patients (2%) with near occlusion treated medically had a stroke in the first month, suggesting that CEA is not needed on an emergent basis under these circumstances. For medically treated patients, the 1-year risk of stroke increases with escalating degrees of carotid stenosis, where the risk is 35% for patients with 90%–94% stenosis. For patients with near occlusion, the 1-year stroke risk diminishes to 11%, which approximates the risk for patients with 70%–89% stenosis. A comparison of treatment differences indicates that CEA reduces the risk of stroke at 1 year by approximately one-half, regardless of the degree of stenosis or the subcategory of carotid near occlusion.

Another analysis reviewed 1216 patients with severe (≥ 70%) stenosis on angiography in the NASCET and ECST.[67] One of 5 ($n = 262$) had two or more criteria for near occlusion: (1) delayed filling of contrast in ICA compared with external carotid artery (ECA); (2) intracranial collaterals seen as cross-filling of contralateral vessels or ipsilateral contrast dilution; (3) obvious diameter reduction of ICA compared with opposite ICA; or (4) ICA diameter reduction compared with ipsilateral ECA. The 3-year risk of ipsilateral stroke for medically treated patients with near occlusion was 15% vs. 11% for surgically treated. Patients who continued to receive treatment in the medical arm for the trial's duration had a 3-year risk of 18%. Medically treated patients with severe stenosis but without near occlusion had a 3-year risk of 26% vs. surgically treated of 8%.

In another study, three different types of pseudo- or segmental occlusion were identified.[68] In most cases, a subtotal stenosis (near-occlusion) at the carotid bifurcation is the underlying lesion (type I). In approximately 35% the internal carotid artery is totally occluded at the bifurcation, but collaterals prevent downstream occlusion (type II), or retrograde flow from the circle of Willis and ophthalmic artery preserves a patent petrous part and siphon (type III). Among 79% of 128 patients, the patency of the arteries could be restored using CEA. Three patients (2.3%) died perioperatively, nine (7%) developed ischemic stroke (seven ipsilateral, two contralateral), and one developed intracerebral hemorrhage. The combined stroke-mortality rate was 9%.

Post-stenotic narrowing and string sign

The diameter of the internal carotid artery is 0.5–1.0 times the common carotid artery.[69] As the atherosclerotic plaque circumferentially enlarges, it eventually causes a critical hemodynamically significant stenosis. Perfusion pressures distal to the stenosis are reduced, which leads to subsequent collapse of the distal ICA vessel lumen and production of post-stenotic narrowing and subsequently the string sign.[70] This collapse is often a result of decreased flow and reduced arterial pressure rather than atherosclerotic disease. However, structural changes beyond flow reduction related vessel collapse are frequently observed. However, there is usually opportunity for successful revascularization once the proximal lesion is repaired with CEA. Post-stenotic narrowing or string sign can be mimicked by collateral channels through vasa vasorum or ascending pharyngeal artery or hypoplastic internal carotid artery.[71] The ECST and NASCET have also shown that the "string sign" is not associated with a high risk of stroke, and emergent CEA is not indicated.[74,75]

Contralateral carotid occlusion

The prevalence of contralateral occlusion is relatively low among patients undergoing CEA in systematic review (407/8626; 4.7%).[76] Contralateral internal carotid artery occlusion has been associated with higher risk of stroke and death following CEA,[77] although not all studies have confirmed this observation.[80,81] The risk may be increased for ischemic events on the side of occluded internal carotid artery.[82,83] In a systematic review,[76] occlusion of the contralateral internal carotid artery (14 studies) was significantly associated with an increased risk of operative stroke and death following CEA. In the NASCET,[84] a total of 659 patients were grouped into one of three categories according to the extent of stenosis in the contralateral carotid artery: less than 70% (559 patients), 70% to 99% (57 patients), and occlusion (43 patients). Medically treated patients with an occluded contralateral artery were at two-fold greater risk to suffer an ipsilateral stroke at 2 years compared with patients with either severe or mild-to-moderate contralateral artery stenosis. The perioperative risk of stroke and death was higher in patients with an occluded contralateral artery or mild-to-moderate contralateral stenosis. Despite higher perioperative morbidity in the presence of an occluded contralateral artery, the longer-term outlook for patients who had CEA performed on the recently symptomatic, severely

stenosed ipsilateral carotid artery was considerably better than for medically treated patients.

In the asymptomatic carotid atherosclerosis study (ACAS),[85] 163 participants who had a baseline contralateral occlusion documented by Doppler ultrasound (77 medically and 86 surgically treated) were compared with 1485 participants without contralateral carotid occlusion (748 medically and 737 surgically treated) for the risk of a combined end point of perioperative (30-day) death or stroke or long-term (5-year) ipsilateral stroke. For those without contralateral occlusion, surgery was associated with a 6.7% absolute reduction in the 5-year risk, while for those with a contralateral occlusion, surgery was associated with a 2.0% absolute increase in risk. The findings suggest that CEA in asymptomatic subjects with contralateral occlusion may not provide any long-term benefit. However, in another study over a 10-year period, patients with ≤70% asymptomatic carotid stenosis with contralateral carotid occlusion were entered into a protocol of clinical examination and Duplex surveillance every 6 months.[86] The ipsilateral stroke-free survival rates at l, 2, 3, 4, and 5 years were 94%, 88%, 78%, 70%, and 63%. Due to the higher incidence of ipsilateral strokes and all strokes than that reported by the ACAS study among patients with asymptomatic carotid stenosis and contralateral occlusion with maximal medical therapy, prophylactic CEA may be justified in these patients.

Presence of bilateral carotid disease may also have implications for medical management. In another analysis of the ECST and NASCET,[87] the relationship between blood pressure and stroke risk in patients with unilateral carotid occlusion and patients with bilateral ≥70% carotid stenosis suggested that the blood pressure reduction is associated with higher risk of ischemic stroke in patients with bilateral ≥70% carotid stenosis but not with unilateral carotid occlusion. The observations suggest that aggressive blood pressure lowering may not be advisable in this group prior to revascularization.

Ipsilateral intracranial stenosis and external carotid artery stenosis

A systematic review of all studies[76] published since 1980, which related risk of stroke and death to various pre-operative clinical and angiographic characteristics, including unpublished data on 1729 patients from the ECST identified risk factors for operative stroke and death from CEA. Stenosis of the ipsilateral internal carotid siphon (five studies), and stenosis of the ipsilateral external carotid artery (one study) were associated with higher rate of peri-operative stroke and death. A multicenter review of 1160 patients who underwent CEA found internal carotid artery stenosis near the carotid siphon was a risk factor for peri-operative stroke and death.[88] Other studies have not been able to confirm the increased risk of stroke and death following CEA in the presence of intracranial vascular disease.[89,90]

Randomized trials evaluating the benefit of carotid endartectomy

The North American Symptomatic Carotid Endarterectomy Trial (NASCET)

The NASCET was a randomized trial conducted at 50 clinical centers throughout the US and Canada. Recruitment occured in two predetermined strata based on the severity of carotid stenosis −30% to 69% and 70% to 99%.[60] The study included patients who had had a hemispheric or retinal transient ischemic attack or a non-disabling stroke within the 120 days before entry. Patients were randomized to optimal medical care, including antiplatelet therapy alone or in combination with CEA. All patients were examined by neurologists 1, 3, 6, 9, and 12 months after entry and then every 4 months thereafter. Study end points were assessed by blinded, independent case review. The study arm recruiting patients with stenosis 70%–99% was prematurely terminated after 659 patients were recruited because CEA was found to be highly beneficial in this group of patients.[91] Life-table estimates of the cumulative risk of any ipsilateral stroke at two years were 26% in the 331 medically treated patients and 9% in the 328 patients treated with CEA. For a major or fatal ipsilateral stroke, the corresponding estimates were 13.1% and 2.5%.

A subsequent report[92] assessed the benefit of CEA in patients with symptomatic moderate stenosis, defined as stenosis of less than 70%. Patients who had moderate carotid artery stenosis were stratified according to the degree of stenosis (50%–69% or < 50%) and randomly assigned either to undergo CEA (1108 patients) or to receive medical care alone (1118 patients). Among patients with stenosis of 50% to 69%, the five-year rate of any ipsilateral stroke was 15.7% among patients treated with CEA and 22.2% among those treated with medical treatment alone. Among patients with less than 50% stenosis, the event rate was 18.7% and 14.9% in the medically treated and those treated with CEA, respectively. In an analysis of durability of the benefit of CEA in patients with severe stenosis over 8 years of follow-up, the 30-day rate of death or disabling ipsilateral stroke persisting at 90 days was 2.1% and 6.7% at 8 years. The highest benefit was seen among men, patients with recent stroke as the qualifying event, and patients with hemispheric symptoms.

The European Carotid Surgery Trial (ECST)

The European Carotid Surgery Trial[93] was a multicenter trial that recruited 2518 patients with a stenotic lesion in the relevant (ipsilateral) carotid artery who had experienced at least one transient or mild symptomatic ischamic vascular event in the distribution of one or both carotid arteries within the previous 6 months. The first report provided data on 778 patients with "severe" (70%–99%) stenosis. Although 7.5% of the patients who underwent CEA had a stroke (or died) within 30 days of surgery, during the next 3 years the risks of

ipsilateral ischemic stroke were (by life-table analysis) an additional 2.8% for those randomized to CEA and 16.8% for medically treated patients. At 3 years, the cumulative risk of surgical death, surgical stroke, ipsilateral ischemic stroke, or any other stroke was 12.3% and 21.9% for CEA treated and medically treated patients, respectively. The total 3-year risk of any disabling or fatal stroke (or surgical death) was 6.0% for those randomized to CEA and 11.0% in those randomized to medical treatment. For 374 patients with only "mild" (0%–29%) stenosis the rate of 3-year risk of ipsilateral ischemic stroke was very low in the medically treated patients to gain any benefit from CEA with its perioperative risks.

The second report[94] presented data on 3024 patients; 1811 patients were randomized to CEA and 1213 to medical treatment. The overall rate of major stroke or death was 37% in CEA-treated patients and 37% in medically treated patients after a mean follow-up of 6.1 years. The risk of perioperative major stroke or death (7.0%) did not vary substantially with severity of stenosis. However, the risk of major ipsilateral ischemic stroke in the medically treated group increased with severity of stenosis, particularly above 80% of the original luminal diameter, in the first 2–3 years after randomization. For patients with stenosis of 80% or greater, the rate of a major stroke or death at 3 years was 26.5% for the medically treated patients and 14.9% for the CEA treated patients, an absolute benefit from CEA of 11.6%.

Pooled data from the randomized controlled trials of CEA for symptomatic carotid stenosis

An analysis pooled data[95] from the ECST, NASCET, and Veterans Affairs trial 309 was conducted. The severity of stenosis in patients included in the ECST was re-measured by the method used in the other two trials. Data for 6092 patients, with 35 000 patient-years of follow-up, were analyzed. CEA increased the 5-year risk of ipsilateral ischemic stroke in patients with less than 30% stenosis, had no benefit in patients with 30%–49% stenosis, was of marginal benefit in those with 50%–69% stenosis, and was highly beneficial in those with 70% stenosis or greater without near-occlusion. There was a trend towards benefit from surgery in patients with near-occlusion at 2 years' follow-up.

A second pooled analysis[96] from the ECST and NASCET determined the risk of ipsilateral ischemic stroke for medically treated patients, the perioperative risk of stroke and death, and the overall benefit from CEA in patient subgroups. Among the 5893 patients with 33 000 patient–years of follow-up, benefit from CEA was greatest in men, patients aged 75 years or older, and those randomized within 2 weeks after their last ischemic event. For patients with 50% or greater stenosis, the number of patients needed to undergo CEA (i.e., number needed to treat) to prevent one ipsilateral stroke in 5 years was nine for men vs. 36 for women, five for age 75 years or older vs. 18 for younger than 65 years, and five for those randomized within 2 weeks after their last ischemic event, vs. 125 for patients randomized after more than 12 weeks.

The Asymptomatic Carotid Atherosclerosis Study (ACAS)

The ACAS[97] randomized a total of 1662 patients with asymptomatic carotid artery stenosis of 60% or greater to CEA or best medical management. The severity of stenosis was defined by angiography, Doppler examination using cut point with 95% positive predictive value, or Doppler examination using a local laboratory cut point with 90% positive predictive value confirmed by ocular pneumo-plethysmographic examination (that has been subsequently eliminated from clinical practice), performed within the previous 60 days. After a median follow-up of 2.7 years, with 4657 patient–years of observation, the aggregate risk over 5 years for ipsilateral stroke and any perioperative stroke or death was estimated to be 5.1% for patients randomized to CEA and 11.0% for patients treated medically (aggregate risk reduction of 53%; absolute risk reduction of approximately 1% per year). The benefit was dependent upon CEA being performed with less than 3% perioperative stroke or death.

The Asymptomatic Carotid Surgery Trial (ACST)

The ACST[98] randomized 3120 asymptomatic patients with significant carotid stenosis to immediate CEA and indefinite deferral of any CEA. The degree of ICA stenosis recorded at randomization was based on carotid Duplex ultrasound. The risk of stroke or death within 30 days of CEA was 3.1%. The mean follow-up was 3.4 years. The cumulative 5-year risks were 6% vs. 12% for all strokes, 4% vs. 6% for fatal or disabling strokes, and 2% vs. 4% for only fatal strokes. There was no significant heterogeneity in the perioperative risk or in the long-term postoperative benefits in various patient subgroups. These benefits were separately significant for men and women; for those with 70% or greater carotid artery narrowing on ultrasound; and for those younger than 65 and 65–74 years of age. In asymptomatic patients younger than 75 years of age with ICA stenosis of 70% or more, immediate CEA reduced the 5-year stroke risk from about 12% to about 6% (including the 3% perioperative risk).

Pooled data from the randomized controlled trials of CEA for asymptomatic carotid stenosis

A meta-analysis of three trials[99] with a total of 5223 patients reported that, despite about a 3% perioperative stroke or death rate, CEA for asymptomatic ICA stenosis reduces the risk of ipsilateral stroke, and any stroke, by approximately 30% over 3 years. For the outcome of any stroke or death, there was a non-significant trend towards fewer events in the CEA group. In subgroup analysis, CEA appeared more beneficial in men than in women and more beneficial in younger

patients than in older patients, although the data for effect of age were inconclusive. There was no statistically significant difference between the treatment effect estimates in patients with different grades of stenosis but the data were insufficient.

Randomized trials comparing the benefit of endovascular carotid stenosis treatment with carotid endarterectomy

The Carotid and Vertebral Artery Transluminal Angioplasty Study (CAVATAS)

CAVATAS was a multicenter clinical trial[100] that randomized 504 patients to endovascular treatment ($n = 251$) or CEA ($n = 253$). Endovascular treatment consisted of balloon angioplasty alone or stent placement in 88% and 22% of the patients, respectively. The rates of stroke and/or death within 30 days of treatment did not differ significantly between endovascular treatment and CEA (6% vs. 6%, respectively, for disabling stroke or death; 10% vs. 10% for any stroke lasting more than 7 days, or death). Cranial neuropathy was reported in 9% of patients treated with CEA and in none after endovascular treatment. Major hematomas in the groin or neck occurred less often after endovascular treatment (1% vs. 7%). At 1 year after treatment, severe recurrent (70%–99%) ipsilateral carotid stenosis was more frequent after endovascular treatment. However, no substantial difference in the rate of ipsilateral stroke was detected with survival analysis up to 3 years after randomization. Follow-up standardized Doppler ultrasound criteria at approximately 1 month ($n = 283$) and 1 year ($n = 347$) after treatment were used to determine the rates of asymptomatic and symptomatic restenosis.[101] The rate of ipsilateral restenosis ≥70% at 1 year after endovascular treatment was higher than after CEA (18.5% vs. 5.2%). Residual severe stenosis was present in 7% of patients at 1 month and restenosis ≥70% occurred in 11% of the endovascular group occurred between 1 month and 1 year. After CEA, 2% had residual severe stenosis at 1 month, and 3% developed restenosis ≥70% between 1 month and 1 year. Recurrent ipsilateral symptoms were more common in endovascular patients with severe stenosis but most were TIAs and none were disabling or fatal strokes.

The Stenting and Angioplasty with Protection in Patients at High Risk for Endarterectomy (SAPPHIRE)

The Stenting and Angioplasty with Protection in Patients at High Risk for Endarterectomy (SAPPHIRE)[102] compared carotid artery stent placement with concomitant use of an emboli-protection device with CEA in 334 patients considered high surgical risk for CEA. Patients were eligible if they either had a symptomatic stenosis ≥50% or an asymptomatic stenosis ≥80%. The primary end point was the cumulative incidence of death, stroke, or myocardial infarction within 30 days after the procedure or death or ipsilateral stroke between 31 days and 1 year. The primary end point occurred in 20 patients (12%) randomized to carotid stent placement and in 32 patients (20%) randomized to CEA. For patients with asymptomatic carotid artery stenosis, the cumulative incidence of the primary end point at 1 year was lower among those who were treated with stent placement (10%) than among those who underwent CEA (22%). The peri-procedural incidence of death, myocardial infarction, or stroke among patients with asymptomatic carotid artery stenosis was 5% and 10% among those who underwent stent placement or CEA, respectively.

At 3 years, data were available for 260 patients (78%) that comprised 86% of patients in the stent treated and 70% of endarterectomy treated patients.[92] The prespecified major secondary end point was a composite of death, stroke, or myocardial infarction within 30 days after the procedure or death or ipsilateral stroke between 31 days and 1080 days (3 years). The prespecified major secondary end point occurred in 41 patients in the stent placement group (cumulative incidence, 25%) and 45 patients in the CEA group (cumulative incidence, 27%). There were 15 strokes in each of the two groups; of which 11 and 9 were ipsilateral in the stent placement and CEA groups, respectively.

Endarterectomy vs. Angioplasty in Patients with Symptomatic Severe Carotid Stenosis (EVA-3S) trial

The Endarterectomy vs. Angioplasty in Patients with Symptomatic Severe Carotid Stenosis (EVA-3S) trial[103] was a multicenter, randomized, non-inferiority trial comparing stent placement with CEA in patients with symptomatic carotid stenosis ≥60%. Patients were eligible if they suffered a hemispheric or retinal TIA or a non-disabling stroke (or retinal infarct) within 120 days before enrollment. CEA and stent placement was to be performed within 2 weeks after randomization and the primary end point of any stroke or death was ascertained within 30 days after treatment. The trial started recruiting in November 2000. In January 2003, the safety committee recommended mandatory use of distal protection devices because of a higher risk of stroke in patients treated without distal protection. Although initially recruiting patients with stenosis ≥ 70%, the trial started recruiting patients with stenosis ≥ 60% in October 2003. In September 2005, the safety committee recommended stopping enrollment after 527 patients (intended target recruitment of 872 patients) had been randomized. The interim analysis based on the observed 30-day risk of stroke or death after CEA suggested that > 4000 patients were required to adequately test the non-inferiority of stent placement. Given the observed 30-day event rate among patients randomized to stent placement, the committee considered it to be extremely unlikely that the trial would reach its objectives despite further enrollment.

The 30-day incidence of any stroke or death was 4% and 10% after CEA or stent placement, respectively. The rate of disabling stroke or death was 2% and 3% after CEA and after stent placement, respectively. At 6 months, the incidence of any stroke or death was 6% after CEA and 12% after stent placement. The higher rates of stroke or death undermined the lower rates of cranial nerve injury and shorter duration of hospital stay observed in patients treated with stent placement. Post-hoc analyses demonstrated lower rates of 30-day stroke or death among patients who underwent stent placement with distal protection. However, most patients in the trial underwent the procedure with distal protection (227 of 247 patients) and the relative risk of stroke or death for stent placement did not change significantly after use was mandated. No significant differences in outcome were observed related to the number of stent procedures performed in individual centers or to the experience of the interventional physicians, although these analyses were able to detect only large differences. There were five different carotid stent devices and seven different distal protection devices used in the study that added an undefined bias. A follow-up study[104] found the rates of ipsilateral stroke from 31 days to 4 years were very low in both groups – 11% for CAS and 6% for CEA – a difference that was not statistically significant.

Stent-Protected Angioplasty vs. Carotid Endarterectomy (SPACE) trial

SPACE was a multinational (Germany, Austria, and Switzerland), multicenter (35 centres) randomized trial.[105] A total of 1200 patients with symptomatic ICA stenosis were randomly assigned within 180 days of TIA or moderate stroke to carotid artery stent placement (n = 605) or CEA (n = 595). Severe stenosis required for eligibility was defined as at least 70% stenosed in duplex ultrasound, corresponding to a stenosis level of ≥50% according to the NASCET criteria or ≥70% according to the ECST criteria. The primary endpoint was ipsilateral ischemic stroke or death from time of randomization to 30 days after the procedure. The non-inferiority margin was defined as less than 3% on the basis of an expected event rate of 5%. Patients allocated to carotid artery stent placement received 100 mg aspirin plus 75 mg clopidogrel daily for at least 3 days before and 30 days post-procedure. For patients allocated CEA, surgeons used their usual operative technique. All patients had to be given at least 100 mg aspirin before, during, and after CEA. Certain aspects of the procedure such as use of protection devices, predilation, and balloon size for stent placement and use of shunting and general anesthesia for CEA were left up to the discretion of treating physicians. In the carotid stent group, 151 (27%) patients were treated with an embolic protection device. Median delay from randomization to treatment was 4 days and 5 days in patients assigned to endovascular treatment and those assigned to CEA, respectively.

The rate of death or ipsilateral ischemic stroke from randomization to 30 days after the procedure was 7% with carotid stent placement and 6% with CEA. The rate of ipsilateral ischemic stroke only from randomization to 30 days after the procedure was 7% and 5% with carotid stent placement and with CEA, respectively. The rate of disabling stroke (modified Rankin score ≥ 3) or death between randomization and 30 days after treatment, and the overall stroke incidence did not differ between the two groups. A comparison of rate of primary endpoint events between those who underwent carotid stent placement with or without use of distal protection device suggested a equal rates of approximately 7% in 151 and 416 of those treated with and without such a device, respectively.

The 2-year follow-up[106] results found the rate of any peri-procedural stroke or death, and/or ipsilateral ischemic stroke within two years, was very similar, at 9% each in the CEA and stent treated group. Furthermore, the investigators reported the absolute number of recurrent ischemic events after the peri-procedural period at 2-year follow-up was low – 10 events after CEA (2%) and 12 after carotid stent placement (2%).

Carotid Revascularization Endarterectomy vs. Stent Trial (CREST)

The CREST[107,108] was a prospective, randomized, parallel, two-arm, multi-center trial with blinded endpoint adjudication. Primary endpoints are analyzed using standard time-to-event statistical modeling with adjustment for major baseline covariates. Patients with symptomatic stenosis of 50% or more stenosis by angiography, 70% or more by ultrasonography, or 70% or more by computed tomography or magnetic resonance angiography (later in the trial) were eligible. Asymptomatic patients had 60% or more lesions by angiography, 70% or more by ultrasonography, or 80% or more on computed tomography or magnetic resonance angiography were also eligible. The primary outcome is the occurrence of any stroke, myocardial infarction, or death during a 30-day peri-procedural period, and ipsilateral stroke during follow-up of up to 4 years. Secondary outcomes include restenosis and health-related quality of life. The study randomized 2502 patients from 117 US and Canadian centers and included 1321 symptomatic and 1181 asymptomatic patients (http://www.medscape.com/view-article/717669). The patients were randomized to receive either carotid artery stent and distal protection devices or CEA. The results of the study are summarized in Table 6.2. The composite primary endpoint of any stroke, myocardial infarction, or death during the peri-procedural period or ipsilateral stroke on follow-up, was observed in 7.2% and 6.8% of the patients randomized to carotid artery stent placement and CEA, respectively. At 30 days, the rate of stroke was significantly higher with carotid artery stent placement compared with CEA. The proportion of subjects who suffered from major stroke at 1 month was similar (<1% in both groups). Conversely, myocardial infarction was significantly higher with CEA compared with carotid artery stent placement. However,

Table 6.2 A summary of results from CREST with regards to primary, secondary, and safety endpoints

Endpoint	CAS	CEA	Hazard ratio (95% CI)	P Value
Primary endpoint ≤4 years	7.2	6.8	1.11 (0.81 – 1.51)	.51
Primary endpoint: peri-procedural components	5.2	4.5	1.18 (0.82 – 1.68)	.38
Peri-procedural stroke and MI				
Any peri-procedural stroke	4.1	2.3	1.79 (1.14 – 2.82)	.01
Peri-procedural major stroke	0.9	0.7	1.35 (0.54 – 3.36)	.52
Peri-procedural MI	1.1	2.3	0.50 (0.26 – 0.94)	.03
Cranial nerve palsies	0.3	4.8	0.07 (0.02 – 0.18)	.0001
Ipsilateral stroke after peri-procedural period ≤4 years	2.0	2.4	0.94 (0.50 – 1.76)	.85

Abbreviations used: CREST, Carotid Revascularization Endarterectomy vs. Stent Trial; CAS, carotid stent placement; CEA, carotid endarterectomy; MI, myocardial infarction.

patients who had an myocardial infarction reported a better quality of life after recovery than those who had a stroke. In an interaction test, patients 69 years and younger, carotid artery stent placement results were superior to CEA results; for patients older than 70, CEA results were better than carotid artery stent placement.

International Carotid Stenting Study (ICSS)

The International Carotid Stenting Study (ICSS) was a multi-center, international, randomized controlled trial in which patients with recently symptomatic carotid artery stenosis were randomly assigned to receive carotid artery stent placement or CEA.[222] The primary outcome measure of the trial is the 3-year rate of fatal or disabling stroke in any territory, which has not been reported. Among the 1713 patients (855 to carotid stent and 858 to CEA), the 120-day incidence of stroke, death, or procedural MI was 8.5% in the stent group compared with 5.2% in the CEA group (hazards ratio of 1.7 $p = 0.006$). Risks of any stroke and all-cause death were higher in the stent group than in the CEA group. A subset of patients underwent MRI 1–7 days before treatment, and 1–3 days after treatment (post-treatment scan).[223] Among 231 patients who participated in the substudy, at least one new DWI lesion detected on post-treatment MRI in 62 (50%) of 124 patients in the stent group and 18 (17%) of 107 patients in CEA group. The rate of new DWI lesions was similar in patients treated at centers using and not using routine distal protection devices (73% and 34%). When the data was pooled with EVA-3S and SPACE studies,[224] 3433 patients with symptomatic carotid artery stenosis were analyzed. Age significantly modified the treatment effect with no difference observed in 120-day risk of stroke or death between carotid stent placement and CEA in patients younger than 70 years, but two-fold higher rates observed in patients aged ≥70 years undergoing carotid stent placement.

Potential explanation for differences in results

There are several explanations for these somewhat discrepant results between trials. Inclusion of asymptomatic patients, mandatory use of distal protection devices, use of standardized peri-procedural antiplatelet regimen, and rigorousness of credentialing requirement for physicians performing the procedure were all cited as possible reasons why the results of stent placement differed between trials.

Neuropsychological consequences of CEA and stent placement for treatment of symptomatic carotid stenosis: a prospective randomized study

The investigators compared the neuropsychological consequences of carotid artery stent placement and CEA and additionally measured the serum S100beta protein, a marker of cerebral damage.[109] A total of 48 patients with symptomatic carotid artery stenosis >70% (according to ECST criteria) were enrolled and 45 patients participated in the follow-up. The patients were randomly assigned for CEA (24 patients) or carotid artery stent placement (21 patients). Patients were assessed before treatment, and again 6 and 30 days after treatment using a comprehensive neuropsychological test battery. Following previously used criteria, a cognitive change in patients was assumed to have occurred when there was a decline of more than one standard deviation in two or more tests assessing various cognitive domains. Patients treated with carotid artery stent and those treated with CEA did not significantly differ in terms of age, gender, education, degree of carotid artery stenosis, neurological symptoms, and vascular risk factors. A comparison of measures acquired at 6 days and 30 days after the treatment showed a comparable number of patients with cognitive changes compared to baseline in both groups. There were no significant differences in S100beta protein values either 2 hours prior to or 1 and 2 hours after the procedure.

Meta-analysis and pooled analysis

A meta-analysis[110] was performed using a random effects model because significant heterogeneity was observed. A literature search of MEDLINE, PubMed, and Cochrane databases for randomized clinical trials comparing carotid artery stent placement and CEA for treatment of carotid artery stenosis supplemented by a review of bibliographies of relevant articles and personal files. Five randomized trials totaling 1154 patients (577 randomized to CEA and 577 randomized to carotid artery stent placement) were included. The composite end point of 1-month stroke or death rate was not different between patients treated with carotid artery stent compared with those treated with CEA (relative risk [RR], 1.3; 95% confidence interval [CI], 0.6–2.8; $P = 0.5$). The 1-month stroke rate (831 patients analyzed: RR, 1.3; 95% CI, 0.4–3.6; $P = 0.7$) and disabling stroke rate (831 patients analyzed: RR, 0.9; 95% CI, 0.2–3.5; $P = 0.9$) was similar for carotid artery stent and CEA treated patients. The 1-month rates of myocardial infarction (814 patients analyzed: RR, 0.3; 95% CI, 0.1–0.9) and cranial nerve injury (918 patients analyzed: RR, 0.05; 95% CI, 0.01–0.3) were significantly lower for CAS. No significant differences were observed in 1-year rates of ipsilateral stroke (814 patients analyzed: RR, 0.8; 95% CI, 0.5–1.2; $P = 0.2$).

A second meta-analysis[111] was performed after two further large-scale trials were completed. Two sets of analysis were performed: one with trials and one with large trials including only symptomatic patients. In total, 2985 patients were included in eight trials of which 89% were symptomatic. In contrast to previous analyses, this meta-analysis found a significantly lower odds for rate of any stroke or death within 30 days after treatment with a disadvantage of endovascular treatment when analyzing all trials (odds ratio [OR], 1.4; 95% confidence interval [CI] 1.–1.8; $P = 0.02$). Significant heterogeneity was found for this analysis. The increase of the odds of suffering from disabling stroke or death in the endovascular compared with the surgical group was not significant in the analysis of all trials; no heterogeneity was found for this analysis. Inclusion of only the large trials with symptomatic patients, the odds ratio (OR) for the endpoint any stroke or death was 1.3 (95% CI 0.9–1.8; $P = 0.11$); with some heterogeneity. For the endpoint disabling stroke or death, the OR was 1.3 (95% CI 0.9–1.9; $P = 0.2$) without any heterogeneity.

Another pooled analysis[112] of eight prospective trials including only high surgical risk patients, analyzed 3282 patients (3115 treated with stent placement and 167 treated with CEA). The composite end point of 1-month stroke, myocardial infarction, or death was significantly lower among patients treated with stent placement (5%) compared with those treated with CEA (10%) (odds ratio, 0.5; 95% confidence interval, 0.3–0.9; $P < 0.05$). The 1-month stroke rate and death rate were similar for carotid stent and CEA treated patient. The 1-month rates of myocardial infarction were significantly lower for patients treated with stent placement (1%) compared with those treated with CEA (6%).

A review of 206 articles with 54 713 patients[113] treated with carotid stent placement published between January 1990 and June 2008 reported an overall 30-day risk of stroke or death of 4.7% (95% CI, 4.1 to 5.2) with substantial heterogeneity across studies. The 30-day risk of stroke or death was two folds higher among symptomatic (7.6%; 95% CI 3.6 to 9.1%) than in asymptomatic (3.3%; 95% CI 2.6 to 4.1%) patients. Risks increased with age, hypertension, and history of coronary artery disease, and were unrelated to sex and the presence of contralateral carotid artery occlusion. The risk associated with carotid stent placement was lower in patients who were treated for carotid restenosis after CEA and in those treated with the use of a distal protection device. There was also a trend for a higher risk of complications in patients who had calcified plaque. The absolute 30-day risk of stroke or death was not significantly higher in studies where there was an independent neurologic assessment by an independent neurologist.

Data from registries evaluating the benefit of carotid stent placement in high-risk patients

There are several stent registries evaluating carotid artery stent placement with distal protection. A total of 29 multicenter prospective studies were identified in one review (http://content.onlinejacc.org/cgi/content/full/49/1/126/TBL10).

The high-risk registries are single arm that include patients considered at high surgical risk for CEA due to prespecified anatomical criteria and/or medical comorbidities. The primary endpoint (all stroke, death, or Q-wave myocardial infarction [MI] is assessed through 30 days; non-Q-wave MI through 24 h; and ipsilateral stroke or neurologic death through 1 year) is compared with a proportionally weighted objective performance criterion (OPC) of 12.6% for published CEA results in similar patients, plus a pre-specified non-inferiority margin of 4%. The success of procedure in the registry is determined by the upper 95% confidence limit of event rate for the primary composite endpoint to meet the pre-specified criteria for non-inferiority relative to the calculated OPC plus non-inferiority margin (14.4%–16.6% depending upon the trial) for historical CEA treated patient outcomes with similar characteristics.

Five studies that were overseen by Food and Drug Administration with an independent Data and Safety Monitoring Board were reviewed in this chapter: Boston Scientific EPI: A Carotid Stenting Trial for High-risk Surgical Patients (BEACH);[114] Carotid Artery Revascularization Using the Boston Scientific EPI FilterWire EXTM and the EndoTex TM Nexstent (CABERNET);[115] Acculink for Revascularization of Carotids in High-Risk Surgical Patients (ARCHER);[116] Medtronic AVE Self-expanding Carotid Stent System with Distal Protection in the Treatment of Carotid Stenosis (MAVERIC),[117] and A Registry Study to Evaluate the NeuroShield Bare Wire Cerebral Protection System and X.act Stent in Patients at High Risk for CarotId EndarTerectomY (SECURITY).[118]

Boston Scientific EPI: a carotid stenting trial for high-risk surgical patients (BEACH)

The BEACH trial[114] evaluated the outcomes of carotid artery stent placement with distal emboli protection, using the Carotid Wallstent and the FilterWire EX/EZ(TM), in 747 patients at high surgical risk for CEA. The trial included both patients with symptomatic (> 50%) and asymptomatic (> 80%) carotid artery stenosis. The study was conducted in three phases: (1) roll-in (R) group ($n = 189[25\%]$) consisting

of up to nine initial patients per site for device and protocol experience; (2) pivotal (P) group ($n = 480[65\%]$) intended for device approval presentation to the FDA; and (3) a bilateral (B) registry group ($n = 78 [10\%]$) for patients with bilateral carotid artery disease. The technical success rate for stent deployment and FilterWire EX/EZ deployment and retrieval was 98%. The overall procedure success rate (< 50% residual diameter stenosis) after stent deployment was 98%. The 30-day composite MI, stroke and/or rate for the entire cohort of 747 patients was 6% (all death = 2%, all stroke = 4%, and all MI = 1%). The event rates in the bilateral group was similar to the Roll-in and pivotal groups suggesting that staged sequential treatment of bilateral stenoses may be comparable to unilateral lesions only. A 1-year follow-up[119] of 480 patients in the pivotal arm demonstrated that the composite primary end point occurred in 9% (40 of 447), with a repeat revascularization rate of 5%.

Acculink for Revascularization of Carotids in High-Risk Surgical Patients (ARCHER)

The ARCHeR (ACCULINK for Revascularization of Carotids in High-Risk patients) trial was a series of three sequential, multicenter, non-randomized, prospective studies[116] enrolling 581 high-surgical-risk patients at 48 sites. Patients with symptomatic ≥ 50%, or asymptomatic ≥ 80% were treated with ACCULINK stent. The ACCUNET filter embolic protection system was used in the last two studies (422 patients). The primary efficacy end point was a composite of death, stroke, and MI within 30 days, and ipsilateral stroke between 31 and 365 days. The 30-day rate of death, stroke, and/or MI was 8% and stroke and/or death was 7%; most (23/32) strokes were minor. The 30-day major or fatal stroke rate was 2%. Ipsilateral strokes occurred in 1% of the treated patients after 30 days. The primary composite end point of 30-day death, stroke, and MI and ipsilateral stroke at 1 year was 10%. Target lesion revascularization at 12 months and 2 years was 2% and 3%, respectively.

Medtronic AVE Self-expanding Carotid Stent System with Distal Protection in the Treatment of Carotid Stenosis (MAVERIC)

The MAVERIC[117] evaluated the Medtronic Self-Expanding Carotid Stent (Exponent) in combination with the Medtronic Interceptor Carotid Filter System for the treatment of carotid artery stenosis among patients at high risk for CEA. Carotid duplex scans were performed at baseline and at 30 days and 6 months. Fifty-two carotid procedures were performed in 51 patients (mean age, 69 years; 84% of patients were men). The delivery success rate was 94% for the Interceptor Filter System and 96% for the Exponent Stent. The combined rate of death, stroke, and/or MI at 30 days was 6%, and was 6% and 12% at 6 and 12 months, respectively.

NeuroShield Bare Wire Cerebral Protection System and X.act Stent in Patients at High Risk for Carotid EndarTerectomY (SECURITY)

The SECuRITY trial was a prospective, multi-center registry reporting upon 305 high-risk patients at 30 sites[120] treated with the EmboShield bare wire filter and the Xact carotid stent. Patients with symptomatic ≥50%, or asymptomatic ≥80% were treated. Overall, 28% of the treated patients were ≥80 years. The combined rate of death, stroke, and/or MI at 30 days was 7.2%. The Xact carotid stent was successfully deployed with <50% residual in 96% and the EmboShield device was successfully delivered and removed in 97% of the treated patients. A histological analysis identified embolic debris in 66% of filters, and platelets and fibrin in another 23% of 143 filters used.

Distal protection devices

Concept of distal protection devices

The concept of distal protection involves using devices to prevent emboli released at the site of angioplasty or stent placement from entering the intracranial circulation and reduce cerebral ischemic complications. The distal protection devices are classified into three broad categories (see Fig. 6.2); (1) occlusive, based on temporary occlusion of flow distal to the procedure site followed by aspiration at completion of procedure; (2) filter, relying on non-occlusive porous filter basket placed distal to the procedure site followed by removal of device in a collapsed form; and (3) flow reversal, consisting of temporary occlusion proximal to the procedure site with flow redirected in a retrograde direction from intracranial into the extracranial circulation. The filter devices have become the predominant form of distal protection in clinical use.

Evidence supporting use of distal protection devices

Distal protection devices were incorporated into clinical practice based on indirect comparative evidence. Multiple studies have compared the rates of peri-procedural stroke associated with carotid stent placement with or without distal protection devices. These studies were not randomized and procedures without distal protection device were conducted at a time carotid stent placement was not a widely available procedure. Iyer et al.[121] reported that rate of procedural and 30-day events was 0.9% and 2.3% among 3160 patients treated with and without a distal protection device, respectively (unmatched case-control design). Another study of 651 consecutive patients enrolled in a registry[122] reported a combined 30-day stroke/death rate of 1% and 4% for patients who underwent carotid stent placement with ($n = 471$) or without distal protection ($n = 180$), respectively. Another study[123] reported that rate of all-stroke and/or death rates within 30 days were

4% and 11% in patients treated with ($n = 75$) and without ($n = 75$) distal protection, respectively. In a systematic review[124] of 2537 carotid artery stent procedures treated without distal protection devices, and 896 procedures with distal protection devices, the combined stroke and death rate within 30 days was 2% and 6% in patients treated with or without distal protection devices, respectively. This effect was mainly due to a decrease in the occurrence of minor strokes (4% vs. 1%) and major strokes (1% vs. 0.3%). A random effects meta-analysis of 134 studies with concurrently reported data on carotid artery stent placement (12 263 patients with distal protection patients and 11 198 patients without distal protection) was performed.[125] Using pooled analysis of all 134 reports, the relative risk for stroke was lower estimated at 0.62 (95% CI 0.54 to 0.72) among patients treated with carotid stent placement with distal protection. Subgroup analysis revealed a significant benefit among carotid stent placement with distal protection in both symptomatic and asymptomatic patients.

Experience from EVA-3S and SPACE trials

In the EVA 3S trial,[126] the safety committee recommended mandatory use of distal protection devices after 80 patients were randomized to stent treatment in a randomized trial comparing CEA with stent placement in symptomatic patients. The 30-day stroke rate was four times higher in patients treated without distal protection devices (26% versus 9%). However, most patients in the trial underwent the procedure with distal protection (227 of 247 patients) and the relative risk of stroke or death for stent placement did not change significantly after mandatory use was instituted. However in the contemporary SPACE trial,[105] stroke and/or death occurred in 7% of 151 patients treated with, and in 7% of 416 treated without, such a device of the 567 patients randomized to stent placement.

Post-marketing carotid stent studies

The post-marketing studies examined outcomes of carotid stent placement after introduction into general practice based on pivotal studies conducted in high-surgical-risk patients treated by highly selected physicians and hospitals. The primary endpoint of major stroke, death, and/or MI was ascertained and compared for non-inferiority with an objective performance criterion (OPC) of 6.3% established from the rates observed in the stent treated patients within the pivotal trials.

The CASES-PMS study

The Cases-PMS study evaluated the results of treating patients at high surgical risk who were either symptomatic ≥50% or asymptomatic ≥ 80% stenosis of the common or internal carotid artery using PRECISE Nitinol Stent and the ANGIOGUARD XP Emboli Capture Guidewire. The physicians were qualified based on either prior experience or following participation in a formal training program.[127] The 30-day stroke, death and/or MI rate was 5%. Asymptomatic patients ($n = 1,158$, 78%) had an event rate of 5%. Outcomes were similar across levels of physician experience, carotid stent volume, geographic location, and presence or absence of training program.

Carotid Acculink/Accunet Post-Approval Trial to Uncover Unanticipated or Rare Events (CAPTURE)

The CAPTURE was a prospective, multi-center registry[128] assessing the procedural results among physicians with varying levels of experience as a measure of the adequacy of physician training, and the identification of rare/unexpected device-related complications. A total of 3500 patients were enrolled by 353 physicians at 144 sites. The 30-day primary endpoint of death, any stroke, and/or MI within 30 days post-procedure was 6% and did not differ among the three operator experience levels from most to least experienced, respectively. There were no differences in outcomes among physician specialties when adjusted for case mix. There were no unanticipated device related adverse events.

Patient selection

Stent placement is considered for patients with symptomatic ≥50% or asymptomatic ≥ 60% internal carotid artery stenosis. The high surgical risk characteristics are summarized in the Table 6.3. The conditions or characteristics discussed predispose patients to a higher perioperative risk of stroke and death in various CEA reports.[129] The data is predominantly derived from case series because patients with one or more of these risk factors generally were excluded from enrollment in prospective CEA trials. CAS may provide a practicable alternative for treating carotid artery stenosis in these patients.

Demographic factors and co-morbidities

Age

Elderly patients appear to have a higher rate of post-operative stroke or death with CEA, although carotid stent placement also appears to have a high risk of peri-procedural stroke or death in this age group. An assessment of the perioperative mortality of 113 300 Medicare patients undergoing CEA found that patients aged ≥ 85 years were three times more likely to die than those younger than 70 years.[133] A multicenter review of 1160 CEA procedures found a postoperative stroke or death rate of 8% in asymptomatic patients aged ≥ 75 years compared with 2% in patients aged < 75 years.[129,130] Similarly, the risk of postoperative MI associated with CEA was 7% in symptomatic patients aged ≥ 75 years compared with 2% in patients aged < 75 years. However, a NASCET subgroup analysis found no evidence of a decremented benefit with CEA among patients aged ≥ 75 years than those in younger age groups.[134] The absolute risk reduction was 29% for 71 patients aged ≥ 75 years, 15% for 285 of those aged between 65 and 74 years, and 10% for

303 patients < 65 years. Although CEA definitely seems to benefit older patients, it is possible that CAS may provide similar benefits in symptomatic patients with acceptable rates of perioperative complications.[96,129] The margin of benefit is lower in asymptomatic patients, therefore, carotid stent placement or any carotid procedure requires more careful assessment.

Severe coronary artery disease

The coexistence of severe carotid artery stenosis and symptomatic coronary artery disease is not uncommon.[132,135] Coronary angiography demonstrated one, two, and three vessel disease and left main coronary artery stenoses in 17%, 15%, 22%, and 7%, respectively, among the 444 patients who underwent carotid stent placement at one center.[136] A total of 23% of the patients had symptomatic coronary artery disease. Underlying coronary artery disease adversely affects the perioperative risk among patients undergoing CEA. In an analysis of the NASCET results, a history of treatment of coronary artery disease was associated with a lower CEA complication rate when compared with those with previously undiagnosed coronary artery disease.[79] Presence of underlying coronary artery disease increased the 30 day risk of stroke and death (OR, 1.5) in the New York Carotid Artery Surgery (NYCAS) Study, a population-based cohort of 9308 CEAs performed in Medicare patients.[137] The high-risk registries of CAS have consistently included patients with moderate to severe underlying coronary arteries including BEACH,[114] CABERNET,[115] ARCHER,[116] MAVERIC,[117] and SECURITY[118] and have demonstrated stroke and death rates below the acceptable threshold set in these studies (discussed earlier).

Adjunct to coronary artery bypass surgery

Significant carotid artery diseases among patients who are undergoing coronary artery bypass grafting (CABG) increases the risk for perioperative stroke. A study of 539 patients reported that carotid artery stenosis > 75% detected by non-invasive tests was an independent predictor of stroke risk (OR, 9.9) during CABG.[138] The American Heart Association/ American College of Cardiology (AHA/ACC) guidelines in 2004 recommended that carotid artery screening should be performed in the following subset of patients: age greater than 65 years, left main coronary artery stenosis, peripheral vascular disease, history of smoking, history of TIA or stroke, or carotid bruit on examination.[139]

The timing of the procedures is controversial when both procedures are considered necessary for patients with severe coexistent disease of the carotid and coronary arteries. In the past, options have included the performance of both procedures simultaneously or in a staged approach in which one procedure is performed several days after the other. Reports of combined CEA and CABG procedures suggest a perioperative stroke or death rate ranging from 7% to 9%, approximately 1.5 to 2.0 times the risk of each procedure performed separately.[132] In a multicenter review, the composite risk of stroke and death was 19% among patients who had CEA and CABG performed simultaneously as opposed to the 2% rate among those who had CEA alone.[130] However, patients who undergo CEA before CABG also have a higher risk of perioperative complications.[135,140] A meta-analysis of 56 studies reporting on patients treated by both CEA and CABG reported a composite incidence of stroke, MI, and death of 16% for simultaneous operations, 26% for CEA followed by CABG, and 16% for CABG followed by CEA.[141] Therefore, a less invasive procedure such as carotid artery stent placement may provide another option in this high-risk subgroup, avoiding a major operation or general anesthesia.[142]

The short-term stroke and death rate appear to be relatively lower with carotid artery stent placement followed by CABG than those associated with combined CABG and CEA or with CABG followed by CEA. In a report of carotid artery stent placement was performed before planned CABG in 49 patients with coexistent disease of the coronary and carotid arteries (carotid artery stenosis≥70%).[142] The 30-day mortality and stroke rates for the carotid stent placement followed by CABG was 8% and 2%, respectively. In addition, no clinically significant recurrent carotid artery stenosis was noted during a mean follow-up interval of 27 months. These results support the consideration of carotid artery stent placement as an adjunct to CABG in patients with coexistent severe coronary artery disease. In a review of six studies reporting on 277 patients treated with carotid stent placement followed by staged CABG,[143] the incidence of stroke and death associated with the stent procedure was 5% and subsequently 2% stroke rate during CABG. The mean time interval between carotid stent placement and CABG was 32 days. The overall combined 30-day event rate after CABG, including all events that occurred during carotid stent placement, was 12% which included 3% minor stroke, 3% major stroke, and 8% mortality.

Congestive heart failure

Patients with pre-existing congestive heart failure have a higher rate of perioperative stroke or death with CEA. A multicenter review of patients undergoing CEA found a perioperative stroke or death rate of 9% in patients with congestive heart failure compared with 2% in patients without congestive heart failure.[129,130] The high-risk registries of CAS have consistently included small proportions of patients with severe congestive heart failure including BEACH,[114] CABERNET,[115] ARCHER,[116] MAVERIC,[117] and SECURITY[118] and have demonstrated stroke and death rates below the acceptable threshold set in these studies (discussed earlier).

Anatomical features
High- or low-lying lesions

High-lying lesions that extend higher than cervical vertebrae (C2) level can be difficult to expose surgically with a cervical excision during CEA. These include a high carotid bifurcation

near the cranial base, especially in a patient with a short or thick neck, or a long carotid artery stenosis that extends to the cranial base. Low lesions that extend close to or below the clavicle can also be technically difficult by a cervical approach. Endovascular approach is superior in overcoming these anatomical challenges.

Tandem lesions

The presence of tandem lesions in which the distal lesion was more severe than the proximal lesion was an exclusion in NASCET.[91] In a multicenter review of 1160 procedures among symptomatic patients, the risk of postoperative stroke or death associated with CEA was 14% versus 8% in patients with ipsilateral and without intra cranial carotid siphon stenosis.[129] In a systematic review of 36 studies, an increased risk for perioperative stroke or death was reported with CEA in patients with stenosis of the ipsilateral siphon.[76] In another report, angioplasty was performed with and without stent placement in 11 patients with tandem lesions.[144] The proximal lesion was the only lesion treated in ten of these patients. Both lesions were treated in the remaining patients. No perioperative stroke or cardiac event or deaths occurred in this group of patients.

Ipsilateral intraluminal thrombus

In a multicenter review of 1160 procedures, the risk of postoperative stroke or death with CEA was found to be 18% in symptomatic patients with intraluminal thrombus compared with 8% rate observed in those without thrombus.[129] In a subgroup analysis of 53 patients enrolled in the NASCET who had intraluminal clot superimposed on atherosclerotic plaque identified by angiography, the 30-day risk of stroke was 11% in those randomly assigned to receive medical treatment and 12% in those who underwent CEA.[145] The high morbidity rate with CEA in this subgroup is related to thrombo-embolic phenomena occurring due to presence of fresh thrombus and the substantial risk of emboli dislodgement during surgical dissection of the carotid artery. Aggressive use of high dose of heparin and concomitant glycoprotein IIB/IIIA inhibitors during carotid stent placement may limit embolic events without an excessive risk of bleeding from surgical sites.

Contralateral carotid occlusion

Patients with symptomatic severe carotid artery stenosis and concurrent contralateral carotid artery occlusion have a high risk of ipsilateral ischemic stroke with medical treatment, although the rate of stroke and death following CEA is high. The risk of ipsilateral stroke in medically treated patients with severe stenosis of the symptomatic carotid artery and occlusion of the contralateral carotid artery was 69% at 2 years in a subgroup analysis of NASCET.[84] Although CEA led to a significant reduction in stroke risk in this group, the perioperative risk of stroke or death in the presence of contralateral carotid artery occlusion was 14%. This increased risk may be related to temporary bilateral ischemia despite the high frequency of carotid artery shunting used during CEA.[84] For these patients, carotid stent placement represents a valid alternative to CEA, obviating the need for temporary occlusion in the presence of an already reduced cerebrovascular reserve.

Postendarterectomy restenosis

Repeat CEA for recurrent carotid artery stenosis after CEA[146] is technically more challenging than the initial procedure because of scarring around the arteries, friability of the recurrent plaque, and the necessity for complex anastomosis techniques. Among 82 patients undergoing CEAs for recurrent carotid stenosis at one institution, the composite rate of major morbidity and mortality was 11%, a five-fold higher rate than the risk associated with primary CEA at the same institution.[146] Similar findings at another institution suggested an increased risk of cerebral ischemic events associated with CEA performed for recurrent stenosis.[147] The 30-day rates of perioperative stroke was 5% in the retreatment group, as compared with 0.8% in the primary CEA group. These investigators also found a high rate (17%) of cranial nerve palsy with second CEA. However, in a study reviewing the results of carotid artery stent placement performed among 18 patients with postendarterectomy recurrent carotid stenosis was found with only a single case of TIA and no peri-procedural stroke.[148] A multicenter review of post-CEA restenosis reported that the 30-day stroke and death rate was 3.7% among 338 patients treated with carotid artery stent placement.[149]

Radiation-induced carotid stenosis

Accelerated, radiation-induced carotid artery stenosis presents an increased risk for perioperative complications with CEA. The presence of a long lesion, lack of well-defined dissection planes, and scarring around the vessels adds substantial challenge to CEA,[150,151] resulting in a higher risk of wound infections and cranial nerve palsies. Additionally, restenosis occurs more frequently after CEA in patients with radiation-induced atheromatous disease.[152,153] Carotid stent placement could provide a more effective method for the treatment of carotid stenosis associated with radiation therapy.[154,155]

Timing of procedure

An analysis of pooled data[96] from the ECAS and NASCET trials evaluated the overall benefit from surgery in relation to timing of procedure from index ischemic event. A total of 5893 patients with 33 000 patient-years of follow-up were analyzed. A longer time from the last symptomatic event to randomization reduced the effectiveness of CEA. Benefit from CEA was greatest in patients randomized within 2 weeks after their last ischemic event, and declined rapidly with increasing delay. These results were consistent across the individual trials. In a systematic review of 11 studies,[156] there was no difference between early (<3 to 6 weeks) and late (>3 to 6 weeks) CEA for stroke in stable patients. It is important to note that there is almost a "time window" for carotid intervention, which is based on high aggregation of recurrent ischemic events during the first 2 weeks after index event. While, the procedural risk may be reduced in delayed procedures, the risk of recurrent ischemic stroke while awaiting procedure can lead to poor patient outcome despite better procedural results. Therefore, for patients with TIA or minor ischemic stroke related to carotid artery stenosis, carotid intervention within 2 weeks is recommended in ASA Stroke Council guidelines.[157]

Technique of extracranial internal carotid artery stenosis treatment

The percutaneous approach

A stable access to the extracranial carotid artery is necessary for carotid artery procedures. For almost all procedures, a femoral approach is adequate. Most operators would place a smaller diameter introducer sheath in the femoral artery to confirm adequate position prior to replacing it with a larger 6F system required for the procedure. For right extracranial carotid artery lesions, a consideration may be given to the right radial approach in rare circumstances such as extensive femoral–iliac occlusive disease or aortic disease such as dissection. A direct common carotid artery percutaneous approach is rarely used for bypassing tortuous aortic arch.

Guidesheath placement

Most extracranial internal carotid artery stent procedures are performed using a 6F guidesheath. Special guidesheaths for the carotid procedure are available which include Cook Shuttle (100 cm). The guidesheath can be introduced into the target common carotid artery through several methods (see Fig. 6.3): (1) a Simmons II diagnostic catheter can be used to catheterize the external carotid artery. Subsequently, a super-stiff 0.035 inch or 0.038 inch exchange length guidewire is placed in the external carotid artery through the 5 F Simmons II catheter. The Simmons catheter is removed and the 6F guidesheath with the introducing obturator is advanced over the guidewire into the common carotid artery; (2) the guidecatheter can be introduced into the common carotid artery using a 0.035 inch guidewire and co-axial placement using a 5F 120 cm Simmons I catheter. The 6 F carotid sheath is placed in the arch of aorta and Simmons I catheter is passed through the sheath and used to select the target carotid artery. Subsequently, the guidewire and Simmons I catheter are advanced into the common carotid artery prior to advancing the guide sheath; or (3) the 6 F guide sheath is placed in the arch of aorta and 6F Simmons II 120 cm catheter is passed through the sheath and used to select the carotid artery. Subsequently, the guidewire and Simmons II catheter are advanced into the common carotid artery prior to advancing the guide sheath. Co-axial placement of 0.018 inch stiff microwire may be

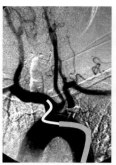
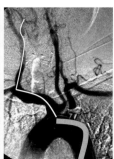
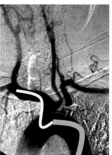
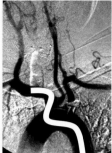

| 6 F guide sheath introduced over 5 F 125 cm SIMMONS I catheter (Vitek) | 6 F guide sheath introduced over 0.035 inch 260 cm superstiff wire placed in external carotid artery by a diagnostic catheter | 6 F guide sheath introduced over 6 F 120 cm SIMMONS II catheter | 8 F guide catheter with SIMMONS II curve over a 0.035 inch guidewire |

Fig. 6.3. Schematic depiction of various methods used for accessing and placing the guide-sheath or guide-catheter in the common carotid artery for carotid angioplasty and stent procedure.

required to create a more stable platform for advancing the 6F guide sheath. An 8 F guidecatheter may be necessary in very tortuous aortic arches to access the common carotid artery and provide an inner lumen large enough to allow passage of stent and balloon catheters.

Intravenous anticoagulation and antiplatelet agents

Patients are administered intravenous heparin during the procedure to reduce the risk of thrombo-embolism associated with the procedure.[158] Activated coagulation time is used to monitor the level of anticoagulation during the procedure. The level of anti-coagulation is controversial. Some investigators recommend a 70 U/kg bolus at the beginning of the procedure to achieve an activated coagulation time between 300 and 350 seconds.[159] In a retrospective analysis of 605 patients who underwent carotid artery stent placement using unfractionated heparin,[160] the optimal peak procedural activated clotting time associated with the lowest combined incidence of death, stroke, or myocardial infarction was 250 to 299 seconds. Preliminary data about the use of intravenous direct thrombin inhibitors instead of heparin is also encouraging.

Intravenous antiplatelet agents (platelet glycoprotein [GP] IIB/IIIA inhibitors) including abciximab,[161] and high,[162] and low[163] dose eptifibatide have been used as adjunctive treatment with intravenous heparin during the procedure. The use of these agents has become relatively uncommon[164] due to risk of intracerebral hemorrhage[165] and unclear benefit in reducing ischemic complications associated with the procedure. In one study,[166] the all stroke/neurological death rate in 216 patients treated with heparin and GP IIB/IIIA inhibitors was 6% compared with 2% in the 334 patients in the heparin-only control group. From 01/2000 to 06/2005 1322 carotid stent placement's were registered registry of the Arbeitsgemeinschaft Leitende Kardiologische Krankenhausarzte (ALKK).[167] In 94 (7%) procedures a GPII B/IIIA was used.

The use of a GPII b/IIIa during stent placement decreased significantly over time: from 18% in 2000 to 3% in 2005. There was no significant difference in the combined death or stroke rate between the two groups (5% vs. 3%), which was confirmed by logistic regression analysis after adjusting for possible confounders. Currently, the use of GP IIB/IIIA inhibitors is restricted to patients with intravascular thrombus or new neurological deficits during the procedure (rescue treatment).[168,169] It should be noted that, if GP IIB/IIIA inhibitors are to be used, heparin dose should be reduced to maintain activated coagulation time below 200 seconds.

Morphological assessment of the carotid artery target segments

The target segments are best visualized in lateral views. The optimal view should avoid the overlap between internal carotid and external carotid artery origins. The views that identify the point of greatest stenosis and provide the best images for the segments of the target arteries may not be the same. Therefore, the operator must carefully assess the value of various projections to determine the projection to use for traversing the origin. A careful assessment of the tortuosity and extent of lesion is required to decide on the segments that require to be covered with stent. Almost invariably, the bifurcation is involved to the extent that to ensure that the margins of the stent extend from normal to normal segments, the proximal end of the stent needs to be placed in the common carotid artery. Identifying the distal most part of the lesion in the internal carotid artery is necessary to avoid stent placement proximal to the end of lesion or avoid unnecessary placement in distal segment increasing the risk of dissection or vasospasm. If distal segment of the internal carotid artery cannot be visualized from common carotid artery injection due to near occlusive stenosis, the lesion may need to be traversed by a microcatheter for contrast injection and visualization of arterial segment distal to the lesion.

Morphological assessment of the lesion

Most lesions in the internal carotid artery origin are athero-sclerotic in nature. However, dissections can also occur at similar locations. Certain aspects of the procedure may differ depending upon the underlying substrate (atherosclerosis versus dissection), such as the use of balloon angioplasty and choice of stents. The operator must review the demographic and clinical characteristics of the patient and supplement it with angiographic data. A lesion that extends beyond 20 mm after the origin of the internal carotid artery or involves multiple segments distal to the origin lesion is unlikely to be atherosclerotic. Involvement of other extracranial vessels and lesion appearances may also provide diagnostic information. Therefore, careful visualization of other extracranial vessels is required (through review of angiographic images or other non-invasive tests performed as part of diagnostic evaluation) prior to performing the procedure. Lesion characteristics such as calcification have direct implications for choosing angioplasty catheters.

Traversing the lesion and placement of distal protection device

The vessel diameter is measured at the intended site of the distal protection device in the distal internal carotid artery. There are several types of distal protection devices available. Currently, almost all procedures are done with filter based distal protection devices that have a radio-opaque inlet with an attached basket that faces the lesion and attached in some manner to a 0.014 inch microwire (see Figs. 6.4 and 6.5). A portion of the microwire precedes the basket for navigation and entry in a graded manner. The filter device is introduced in a collapsed manner contained within a delivery catheter. After reaching the target segment, the device is deployed by withdrawal of the delivery catheter. The size of the distal protection device is selected based on the measured diameter. The selection of device is highly dependent upon availability, participation in a clinical protocol, and infrequently on profile. The preferred site for placement is usually high cervical to avoid excessive intracranial placement of microwire distal to the filter. The deployment site must be in a segment of the internal carotid artery that has a diameter large enough to allow adequate unfolding and in a segment that is relatively straight to allow proper alignment. Distal occlusive devices and proximal occlusion with flow reversal devices are used in rare cases with intravascular thrombus or mobile lesions to create an absolute seal. The use of these devices is complicated by interruption of cerebral blood flow through the ipsilateral carotid artery.

There may be resistance to passage of distal protection device in the presence of severe stenosis. The operator may place a 0.014 inch microwire across the lesion and than advance a distal protection device over the microwire or perform a predilation with a small angioplasty balloon to create an orifice large enough for passage of the device. The distal protection device may not advance if the distal internal carotid artery is very tortuous. The operator must decide preferably based on initial angiographic assessment or following intra-procedural device failure to straighten the internal carotid artery segment to select the next step: (1) abandon the use of distal protection device and perform the procedure using a standard 0.014 inch microwire; (2) place a support 0.014 inch microwire parallel to the existing distal protection device and advance it ahead of the device to straighten the target segment. Advancing the microwire in the distal tortuous extracranial segments may rarely require microcatheter support to facilitate navigation. After treatment of the stenosis, the distal protection device is retrieved using a standard retrieval catheters provided by the manufacturer. In the event of failure of using the retriever catheter provided by the manufacturers, 4-F angiographic catheter (MPA1-TempoTM4, length 125 cm, inner diameter 0.038 inch, Cordis Corporation, Miami, FL) can be used to retrieve the device.

No clear difference in rate of events has been demonstrated between different distal protection devices. An in vitro model[170] tested passage of particles (150–250 micro m [small], 355–500 micro m [medium], 710–1000 micro m [large]; 5 mg each) through Angioguard (AG), Filter Wire EX (EX(A), EX (B)), Trap, Neuroshield (NS), and GuardWire Plus (GW). None of the tested devices or modifications completely prevented embolization. An occlusion balloon leads to increased embolization into the ECA in this in vitro model. The risk of procedural and 30-day events was compared between the different types of distal protection devices among 3160 CAS procedures using nine different devices.[121] Compared with the most frequently used device (FilterWire, Boston Scientific, Natick, MA), there was no significant difference in the risk of peri-procedural adverse events with any of the other distal protection device. There was no significant difference in risk of peri-procedural events between eccentric and concentric filters, although there was a trend towards lower events with eccentric filters. In another study of 304 patients,[171] close cell stent design and eccentric filter devices were found to have lower rates of 30-day stroke, death, or TIA. Another study[172] compared the GuardWire distal occlusion system ($n = 19$) and the distal FilterWire EX ($n = 12$) in 31 consecutive patients monitored with transcranial Doppler for microembolic signals before, during, and after CAS. Compared to the GuardWire, the use of the FilterWire was associated with more microembolic signals during stent deployment, postdilation, and retrieval of the protection device. However, there was no difference in clinical event rates.

Pre-stent angioplasty

The purpose of the pre-stent angioplasty is to create adequate lumen diameter within the lesion to allow passage of stent delivery catheter without resistance. Primary angioplasty alone is avoided due to the high risk of recoil and dissections. The

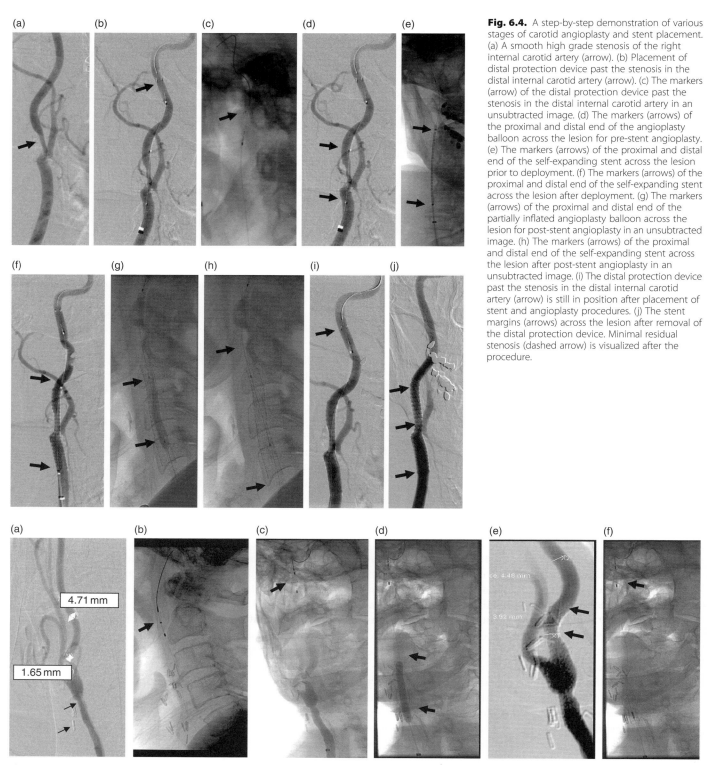

Fig. 6.4. A step-by-step demonstration of various stages of carotid angioplasty and stent placement. (a) A smooth high grade stenosis of the right internal carotid artery (arrow). (b) Placement of distal protection device past the stenosis in the distal internal carotid artery (arrow). (c) The markers (arrow) of the distal protection device past the stenosis in the distal internal carotid artery in an unsubtracted image. (d) The markers (arrows) of the proximal and distal end of the angioplasty balloon across the lesion for pre-stent angioplasty. (e) The markers (arrows) of the proximal and distal end of the self-expanding stent across the lesion prior to deployment. (f) The markers (arrows) of the proximal and distal end of the self-expanding stent across the lesion after deployment. (g) The markers (arrows) of the proximal and distal end of the partially inflated angioplasty balloon across the lesion for post-stent angioplasty in an unsubtracted image. (h) The markers (arrows) of the proximal and distal end of the self-expanding stent across the lesion after post-stent angioplasty in an unsubtracted image. (i) The distal protection device past the stenosis in the distal internal carotid artery (arrow) is still in position after placement of stent and angioplasty procedures. (j) The stent margins (arrows) across the lesion after removal of the distal protection device. Minimal residual stenosis (dashed arrow) is visualized after the procedure.

Fig. 6.5. Selected steps of various stages of carotid angioplasty and stent placement for restenosis following previous carotid endarterectomy. (a) A smooth high grade stenosis of the right internal carotid artery (arrows). The stenosis measures 65% by NASCET criteria. The arrows demonstrate stigmatas of previous endarterectomy such as surgical clips and dilatation at site of patch placement. (b) Placement of distal protection device past the stenosis in the distal internal carotid artery in a compressed manner (arrow). (c) Deployment allowing expansion of the device visualized by the markers (arrow) of the distal protection device past the stenosis in the distal internal carotid artery in an unsubtracted image. (d) The markers (arrows) of the proximal and distal end of the inflated angioplasty balloon across the lesion for pre-stent angioplasty in an unsubtracted image. (e) The markers (arrows) of the proximal and distal end of the self-expanding stent across the lesion after deployment. (f) The distal protection device past the stenosis in the distal internal carotid artery (arrow) is compressed by the advancement of retrieval catheter after completion of stent placement and angioplasty procedures.

A summary of selected stents and distal protection devices used during carotid stent placement			
Stent	Closed cell (all struts are interconnected)	Wallstent-1.08 mm^2 (Boston Scientific Corp.), Xact-2.74 mm^2 (Abbott Vascular), Nexstent-4.7 mm^2 (Endotex)	
	Open cell (all struts are not interconnected)	Precise-5.89 mm^2 (Cordis), Acculink-11.48 mm^2 (Guidant), Protégé-10.71 mm^2 (ev3), Exponent-6.51 mm^2 (Medtronic)	
Distal protection device	Occlusive (balloon)	Distal occlusion	Percusurge (Medtronic)
		Proximal occlusion	Parodi Anti Emboli System (Gore)
	Non-occlusive (filter)	Symmetric	AngioGuard-100 micron (Cordis), Rx Accunet-115 micron (Guidant), EmboShield-140 micron (Abbott)
		Asymmetric	Filterwire EX-110 micron (Boston Scientific), Epi Filterwire EX-80 micron (Boston Scientific)- Spider-110 micron-(ev3)

Fig. 6.6. A summary of selected distal protection devices and stents according to their mechanical properties. The free stent area is provided in front of each stent in mm^2 derived from Bosier M et al.[173] The pore sizes are provided for each distal protection device.

pre-stent angioplasty is performed using a balloon with a nominal diameter of 3.0–4.0 mm. The length of the balloon is usually selected as 30 mm to 40 mm to ensure adequate extension of the balloon on both ends of the lesion. Larger diameter balloons or cutting balloons may be rarely required if the lesion is very resistant to angioplasty. An angiographic assessment after the angioplasty is required to ensure that adequate dilation has occurred. Usually, a lumen diameter of at least 2 mm is necessary for passage of stent device.

It should be noted that pre-stent angioplasty may lead to stimulation of carotid baro-receptors with subsequent brady-cardia and hypotension. The bradycardia is instantaneous and may progress to asystole. Immediate deflation of the balloon is necessary and recovery of heart rate follows concurrently. If bradycardia is anticipated due to low baseline heart rate, intravenous atropine (0.5–1.0 mg) or glycopyrrolate (0.1–0.2 mg) may be administered prior to angioplasty. The inflation is undertaken when an increase in heart rate is documented. Care must be undertaken in patients with underlying coronary artery disease to avoid provoking myocardial ischemia. Rarely, angioplasty may lead to dissection within the lesion. Therefore, the decision on stent must be made prior to the angioplasty and preferably the stent should be readily available for quick use.

Stent deployment

Currently, only self-expanding stents are being used for treating carotid artery stenosis. The largest diameter of the

target segments that requires opposition of the stent is measured. The nominal diameter of the stent must exceed the vessel diameter. In almost all circumstances, the common carotid artery is the reference vessel. The principles of stent deployment are similar between various stents. Once the stent is in position, the outer sheath of the delivery device is withdrawn allowing the stent to expand from distal to proximal end. The stents are compressed within the inner core and outer sheath prior to delivery and expand due to its biomechanical properties. The stents are made of nitinol and have a memory shape that allows the stent to take a pre-defined configuration after exposure to body temperature.

The stent design (see Fig. 6.6) may affect the scaffolding and subsequent post-procedural plaque embolization through the stent struts. Stents with a smaller free cell area and hence a greater percentage of wall coverage may result in lower rates of embolic events. In a review of 3179 patients who underwent carotid stent placement with various stents, post-procedural complication rates are highest for the open cell types and increased with larger free cell area.[173] In a secondary analysis of the SPACE trial, ipsilateral stroke or ipsilateral stroke death within 30 days was significantly lower in 127 patients treated with a closed cell stent (5.6%) compared with 436 of those treated with an open cell stent (11.0%).[174]

The length of the stent must be selected to: (1) adequately cover the lesion; (2) consider the position of the distal end to avoid angulated or unopposed placement due to tortuosity or post-stenotic dilatation; and (3) consider the consequences of deployment into the distal internal carotid artery (size mismatch). The vessel diameter of the distal internal carotid artery may be much smaller than the stent size mandated by the diameter of the common carotid artery. A tapered stent that provides two differing diameters at each end or a sheet stent that allows variable levels of unfolding may be necessary.

The stent delivery device may not traverse the lesion despite pre-stent angioplasty. A second angioplasty may be required to increase the diameter of the stenotic segment to facilitate passage. If tortuousity within the segment is the reason for resistance, strategies such as advancing the carotid sheath, breath holding, or manual neck compression to change the trajectory of entry for the stent delivery catheter maybe helpful. The operator should be aware of the risk of dissection or vasospasm at the site of distal end of the stent due to diameter mismatch or straightening of tortous segment. A second stent may be required to treat the dissection if it is flow limiting or clinically symptomatic. A portion of the lesion may remain outside the stent due to malposition requiring a second stent. An overlap between the two stents is required to avoid restenosis between the stents.

Covered stents are not used for treatment of carotid stenosis. A trial randomized 14 asymptomatic patients comparing the rates of cerebral microembolism during and after carotid stent placement using either a self-expanding covered ($n = 8$) or a bare ($n = 6$) carotid stent.[175] A significant reduction in ipsilateral microembolic signals by transcranial Doppler ultrasound was observed with the covered stent as compared with the bare stent. Comparison of the pre-procedural and 24-hour post-procedural DW-MRI images showed no new ipsilateral lesions but one new lesion was detected in the contralateral hemisphere in the covered stent group, resulting in an overall 7% rate of new ischemic lesions. No neurological complications occurred up to 6 months. Restenosis ($> 70\%$) occurred in three (38%) of eight patients treated with the covered stent and none of the patients treated with bare stents ($P = 0.21$). The trial was stopped when the third restenosis of a covered stent was detected.

Post-stent angioplasty

Post-stent angioplasty is performed to treat any residual stenosis that may be left after stent placement. The ideal residual stenosis that correlates with clinical endpoints is not known, but most studies have considered a residual stenosis of less than 30% as an adequate angiographic result. The diameter of the balloon that is selected is based on the diameter of the distal internal carotid artery (estimated normal diameter of the arterial segment with the stenosis in the absence of disease). The length of the balloon is selected to ensure expansion within the stent but not exceed beyond the ends of the stent. The struts at the end of the stent may damage the balloon during inflation.

Post-stent angioplasty may lead to stimulation of carotid baro-receptors with subsequent bradycardia and hypotension. A similar management as outlined for pre-stent angioplasty is recommended. The likelihood is higher if bradycardia was observed during pre-stent angioplasty and prophylactic administration of atropine or glycopyrrolate is strongly recommended. Post-stent angioplasty also is associated with a high risk of embolization. The balloon shears off plaque material that may be protruding through the struts of the stent. Therefore, the balance between near ideal angiographic results and risk of multiple post-stent angioplasty procedures must be carefully determined.

Choice of stent and stent sizes in stenosis related to dissections

An attempt should be made to determine if the dissection is acute or chronic based on the clinical presentation, MRI findings of thrombus within the wall (observed in acute dissections), or angiographic findings such as pseudoaneurysm (observed in chronic dissections). Any angioplasty should be avoided in acute dissections if possible and self-expanding stents alone can result in adequate expansion. Chronic dissections may require a concomitant angioplasty followed by self expanding stent for adequate results. The procedure is described in more detail in the "Chapter on Dissections."

Post-procedure angiography

Angiographic images are acquired to visualize the treated segment. Intracranial views are obtained to identify any intravascular occlusion or segmental delay in contrast opacification. A brief neurological examination is performed to identify any new deficits. In the absence of any new deficits, the distal protection device is retrieved using a retrieval catheter as described above. Angiographic imaging after retrieval of distal protection device is recommended to identify any spasms or dissection at the site of device placement. The vessel configuration also changes when the relative straightening of the vessel after removal of the 0.014 inch microwire disappears. The alignment and opposition of the stent may change after removal of the microwire.

Post-procedural management

A complete neurological examination is performed immediately as well as 24 hours after the procedure. Thirty-eight major events or death (inclusive of all neurologic events and any complications that required treatment) were recorded in the first 30 days after 201 CAS in one study.[176] These were 7 (3.4%) major access site complications (3%); 18 (8.8%) neurological events (9%) including 10 (4.9%) were TIAs (5%) and strokes (4%), cardiovascular complications (4%), and others (3%). Of the events recorded, 53% of events occurred in the first 6 hours, 5% between 6 and 12 hours, 8% between

12 and 24 hours, and 34% between 24 hours to 30 days post-procedure. Aspirin (325 mg daily) and clopidogrel (75 mg daily) are prescribed at discharge and continued for a period of 1 month. Subsequently, aspirin is continued indefinitely. On the basis of The Stroke Prevention by Aggressive Reduction in Cholesterol Levels (SPARCL) Trial,[177] AHA/ASA stroke council[178] recommended statin therapy with intensive lipid-lowering effects for patients with atherosclerotic ischemic stroke or TIA and without known coronary artery disease to reduce the risk of stroke and cardiovascular events (Class I, Level of Evidence B). For those patients with atherosclerotic ischemic stroke or TIA and a history of coronary artery disease, statin agents are recommended with a target LDL-cholesterol level of <100 mg/dL; and an LDL-cholesterol of < 70 mg/dL is recommended for very high-risk patients with multiple risk factors. A detailed account of the peri-procedural management is presented in the chapter on peri-procedural management.

Follow-up

The usual clinic follow-ups are scheduled at 1 month, 6 months, and 1 year and then subsequently at yearly intervals. An early follow-up may be required with the primary care physician or internist if the patient's antihypertensive medication was withheld during hospitalization due to post-procedural hypotension. The blood pressure progressively increases in the days following the procedure and antihypertensive medication will need to be re-instituted. Routine screening using Doppler ultrasound of all patients who have undergone carotid angioplasty and stent placement cannot be mandated based on the low prevalence of restenosis and lack of correlation between restenosis and late stroke. Angioplasty and rarely stent placement has been considered for patients with symptomatic restenosis or selected high-grade asymptomatic restenosis, although there is lack of evidence demonstrating benefit from intervening in patients with restenosis using these indications. The optimal duration interval between carotid stent placement and ultrasound remains unclear however data derived from CEA studies suggest that the highest yield appears to be in studies performed between 3 and 18 months. Some investigators recommend the practice of performing ultrasound screening at 1 month and 12 months following carotid stent placement. Screening is recommended for all patients who develop ipsilateral ischemic stroke, retinal ischemic events or TIAs. Serial screening should be considered for patients with contralateral carotid artery stenosis ≥50% or even for those with contralateral disease <50%. Because progression of stenosis in the contralateral artery has a higher likelihood of becoming symptomatic, annual screening may be considered. Studies are required to develop Doppler ultrasound criteria with higher specificity to screen patients following carotid stent placement.

Table 6.3 Risk factors for peri-procedural ischemic stroke associated with carotid stent placement

Age[188,191,192]
Symptomatic stenosis[193,194]
Renal insufficiency[193]
Baseline systolic blood pressure >180 mmHg[189]
Baseline C-reactive protein (CRP) values >5 mg/dl[190]
Multiple showers of microemboli (>5) at postdilation after stent deployment, particulate
Macroembolus, and massive air embolism on TCD[187]
Angioplasty-induced asystole[187]
Prolonged hypotension[187,195]
Absence of statin therapy[196]
Length of the lesion[191,194]

Complications associated with carotid stent placement

The complications associated with carotid stent placement are described below.

Peri-procedural cerebral ischemic events

Peri-procedural cerebral ischemic events range from transient ischemic events to minor and major ischemic stroke. The causes range from embolization of plaque material from aortic arch atheromas and carotid plaque during device manipulation; thrombosis and embolization related to subintimal fissures created by angioplasty or reaction to intravascular foreign body such as stents; stasis due to flow interruption by devices in near occlusive lesions or vasospasm, and hypotension in presence of flow limiting vascular lesions.[158] In a study of 471 consecutive patients[179] who underwent elective carotid stent placement (without distal protection) for high-grade symptomatic (n = 147) or asymptomatic (n = 324) ICA stenosis, neurological events were observed in 33 patients (7%). These included 15 TIAs, eight minor strokes, and ten major strokes that led to death in two patients (combined stroke and death rate, 4%). Prior to introduction of distal protection devices, in a review of 14 studies and 834 patients, thromboembolic events were observed in 73 (8.8%) patients; 26 events were TIAs and 47 were strokes.[159] The outcomes of the 47 strokes were categorized as 20 with full recovery, 15 with good recovery, 6 with poor recovery, 2 with no recovery, and 4 deaths. The majority of thromboembolic events occurred postoperatively among patients who underwent carotid stent placement. A study[180] reviewed the 1-month stroke and death rate for symptomatic and asymptomatic treated patients in SAPPHIRE, ARCHER, and BEACH (all studies that used distal protection). The rate of stroke or death was 8% (n = 31) for 375 symptomatic patients and 6%

($n = 67$) for 1105 asymptomatic patients treated with carotid stent placement with distal protection. An analysis of the 30-day event rate for 3500 patients in the CAPTURE registry[181] found 5% of patients experienced a stroke (4% ipsilateral and 1% non-ipsilateral, 2% major). The timing of events was as follows: 22% were intraprocedural, 58% were detected post-procedure and pre-discharge, and 20% occurred after discharge. Overall, 41% (69 of 170) of all strokes were major. Major strokes were more frequent among symptomatic compared with asymptomatic patients, 5% and 2%, respectively. Major strokes constituted almost half (44%) of ipsilateral strokes and overall, 23% of the major strokes were hemorrhagic in nature.

The prevalence of new ischemic lesions on DWI MRI is relatively high although most of these lesions are clinically asymptomatic. A study reported the results of MRI performed 48 hours before and 48 hours after carotid stent placement using distal protection in 50 patients with symptomatic, high grade ($> 70\%$) carotid stenosis.[182] New punctate DWI lesions with a median diameter of 2 mm were detected in 14 cases ipsilateral to stent placement and in 7 cases in other vascular territories. In another study, DWI was performed immediately before and after carotid artery stent placement in 68 patients with and 175 without distal protection.[183] The proportion of patients with new ipsilateral DWI lesion(s) was significantly lower after carotid artery stent placement with (52%) than without (68%) distal protection device. The frequency of DWI lesions was also more frequent in symptomatic patients (74% vs. 56%) or those at or ≥ 75 years of age (67% vs. 46%). In another study of 53 procedures,[184] new DWI lesions were identified in 22 patients (42%) and atheromatous plaque and/or fibrin was found in 21 filter devices (40%). However, no clear relationship between the presence of debris captured by the filter device and new lesions detected by DWI was found.

A study used multifrequency transcranial Doppler (TCD) to detect solid microemboli in the ipsilateral middle cerebral artery during carotid stent placement in 27 consecutive patients with symptomatic high-grade carotid stenoses.[185] A total 484 solid microemboli in 17 patients (63%) were detected. On MR imaging 24 hours after the procedure, six patients (22%) had developed 13 new clinically silent DWI lesions within the ipsilateral middle cerebral artery territory. Patients in whom microemboli were detected during procedure were more likely to develop new DWI lesions (29% versus 10%). Another study compared the incidence of microemboli in 151 patients treated with distal protection devices, and 197 patients treated without distal protection devices.[186] Median number of microemboli in various phases of the procedure in patients with and without distal protection devices was as follows: wiring, 51 vs. 27; predilation, 19 vs. 13; stent deployment, 64 vs. 49; and postdilation, 24 vs. 16. A subsequent analysis of 550 patients determined the association between TCD detected microemboli and occurrence of ischemic stroke within 7 days of stent procedure.[187] Multiple showers of microemboli (> 5) at postdilation after stent deployment,

particulate macroembolus, and massive air embolism were independently associated with ischemic deficits.

Table 6.3 demonstrates the demographic, clinical, and angiographic risk factors for ischemic events associated with carotid stent placement. An analysis of 1196 patients randomized to carotid stent placement or CEA in the SPACE trial.[188] The primary outcome event was death or ipsilateral stroke (ischemic or hemorrhagic) within 30 days after therapy. Six predefined variables were analyzed for relevance as potential risk factors: age, sex, type of qualifying event, side of intervention, degree of stenosis, and presence of high-grade contralateral stenosis or occlusion. Risk of ipsilateral stroke or death increased significantly with age in the carotid stent placement group but not in the CEA group. Classification and regression tree analysis demonstrated that the age cut-off that best distinguished high-risk and low-risk populations who had carotid stent placement was 68 years. The rate of ipsilateral stroke was 3% in patients aged < 68 years and 11% in those aged ≥ 68 years. Other studies have identified severely elevated baseline systolic blood pressure (> 180 mmHg)[189] and baseline C-reactive protein (CRP) elevation (> 5 mg/dl)[190] as risk factors for cerebral ischemic events.

Detailed strategies for management of patients who develop cerebral ischemic events are described in the chapter on peri-procedural management. Briefly, if the event occurs during procedure, a cerebral angiogram is performed to assess the angiographic appearance of intracranial vessels after removal of the distal protection device. In the post-procedure period, an emergent non-contrast computed tomographic (CT) scan is recommended to exclude any intracranial hemorrhage. Subsequently, an emergent cerebral angiogram is recommended. An algorithm for management is presented in the Chapter on "Peri-procedural Management."

Cerebral hyperperfusion

It is hypothesized that reperfusion injury is due to a failure of autoregulation of rCBF. Chronic hypoperfusion results in cerebral arterioles being maximally dilated with subsequent loss of their ability to constrict when normal perfusion pressure is restored. The use of dual antiplatelet therapy (aspirin and clopidogrel) and intraprocedural anticoagulation may further contribute to the hemorrhagic component of the syndrome. Single photon emission CT (SPECT) for rCBF measurements was performed before, and 7 days after procedure in 30 consecutive patients with unilateral severe carotid stenosis who underwent carotid stent placement.[197] Three patients had cerebral hyperperfusion phenomenon immediately after stent placement. One developed status epilepticus 2 weeks after the procedure. Significant predictors of hyperperfusion included patient age, pretreatment cerebrovascular resistance, and pretreatment asymmetry index ([ipsilateral rCBF/contralateral rCBF] $\times$ 100).

In another study[198] blood pressure was maintained $< 140/90$ mmHg in all patients undergoing carotid stent placement, except if there was a contraindication such as known, severe, flow-limiting stenoses in other vascular beds. Blood pressure was maintained less than 120/80 mmHg in patients at high risk for reperfusion syndromes defined by presence of hypertension at baseline, internal carotid artery stenosis of $\geq 90\%$, and poor collateral blood flow. The latter was defined by either contralateral carotid occlusion or contralateral carotid stenosis $\geq 80\%$, or an isolated ipsilateral carotid circulation (i.e., absent anterior and posterior communicating arteries). A total of 836 patients were treated with carotid stent placement, 266 before the initiation of the comprehensive blood pressure management protocol and 570 following initiation of the protocol. The frequency of reperfusion syndrome was greater in patients without comprehensive blood pressure management compared with those treated with comprehensive blood pressure management protocol 2% vs. 1%. There was a significant difference, however, between the two groups in the risk of intracerebral hemorrhage, 1% vs. 0%, respectively.

The EMGREG-International consensus proceedings[199] recommended that systolic blood pressure should be maintained below 140 mmHg in the first 48 hours after carotid stent placement. A more aggressive systolic blood pressure paradigm (below 120 mmHg) may be considered in patients at high risk for reperfusion syndrome but this should be considered with consideration of possible adverse consequences of aggressive blood pressure reduction (e.g., due to presence of other flow-limiting stenosis). Preferred agents include intravenous nicardipine, nitroglycerine, or nitroprusside. Increased propensity for hypotension and bradycardia in the post-procedure period must be recognized when using antihypertensive agents. In patients with new neurological deficits in the post-procedure period, a distinction must be made between reperfusion syndrome (cerebral edema and/or intraparenchymal hemorrhage) and ischemic stroke. The management of blood pressure is completely different for each of the two entities mandated rapid diagnosis using CT scan. Aggressive blood pressure lowering to reduce systolic blood pressure below 120 mmHg is recommended for treating reperfusion syndrome.

Hemodynamic depression

Hemodynamic complications frequently occur during and after carotid stent placement mediated through dysfunction of adventitial baroreceptors in arterial segments by radial expansion induced by angioplasty and stents placement. The baroreceptors are stretch receptors located in the carotid sinus (dilated segment of the ICA at its origin from the common carotid artery). Impulses arising in the carotid sinus travel through the sinus and glossopharyngeal nerves to the nucleus tractus solitarius (NTS) in the caudal medulla. Stimulation of the carotid sinus inhibits sympathetic neurons in the NTS and reduces sympathetic tone to peripheral blood vessels, leading to a reduction in blood pressure. The carotid sinus in one of the main baroreceptors that play a key role in short-term

adjustments of blood pressure when relatively abrupt changes in blood volume, cardiac output, or peripheral resistance occur. Impulses from the carotid sinus also initiate excitatory impulses from the NTS to the nucleus ambiguus and dorsal vagal nucleus. The increase in vagal activity results in a decrease in heart rate.

The most common intra-procedural event is transient bradycardia at the time of angioplasty which resolves after deflation of balloon. The most common post-procedural event is hypotension which resolves after hours. The frequency of these events varies depending upon the definition used and presence of different risk factors. The effect of these events on subsequent neurological events is not consistently demonstrated. In one study, intra-procedural hemodynamic events occurred in 73 of the 256 patients (29%) consisting of hypotension in 9%, bradycardia in 5%, or both in 15% of patients.[200] Persistent post-procedural hemodynamic events occurred in 91 of the 256 patients (36%) consisting of hypotension in 16%, bradycardia in 9%, or both in 11% of patients. Procedural hypotension and bradycardia were not associated with incidence of ischemic stroke, but were associated with an increased duration of hospital stay. Another study[195] reported the rate of hemodynamic depression defined by peri-procedural hypotension (systolic blood pressure < 90 mmHg) or bradycardia (heart rate < 60 beats/s) in 500 consecutive CAS procedures. Hemodynamic depression occurred during 210 procedures (42%), whereas persistent depression developed in 84 procedures (17%). Features that independently predicted hemodynamic depressions included lesions involving the carotid bulb or the presence of a calcified plaque. Prior ipsilateral CEA was associated with reduced risk of hemodynamic depressions. Patients who developed persistent hemodynamic depressions were at increased risk of a peri-procedural major adverse clinical event or stroke.

In a study of 51 patients who underwent carotid angioplasty and stent placement for symptomatic ($n = 29$) or asymptomatic ($n = 22$) carotid artery stenosis,[58] the frequency of postprocedural hemodynamic complications was as follows: hypotension, 22%; hypertension, 39%; and bradycardia, 28%. Intraprocedural hypotension and history of MI independently predicted post-procedural hypotension. Post-procedural hypertension was predicted by intraprocedural hypertension and previous ipsilateral CEA. Post-procedural bradycardia was associated with intraprocedural hypotension and intraprocedural bradycardia. The majority of post-procedural events were temporally separate from the intraprocedural hemodynamic events. Both post-procedural hypotension and bradycardia represented a continuum of intraprocedural events in two patients and one patient, respectively. All events had resolved at the conclusion of the intensive care unit monitoring period. In another study of 31 consecutive patients[57] post-procedural hypotension was observed after treatment 14 patients (42%); medical treatment was necessary in seven (21%). A distance between carotid bifurcation and maximum stenotic lesion (≤ 10 mm) and type of stenosis (eccentric) on angiogram were determined to be independent risk factors of postprocedural hypotension.

Intra-procedural bradycardia is transient but may prevent adequate inflation of balloon and adequate dilation of lesion. Intravenous atropine (0.5–1.0 mg) or glycopyrrolate (0.1–0.2 mg) prior to angioplasty may be necessary. A temporary pacemaker is almost never required. Post-procedural hypotension requires fluid resuscitation and intravenous vasopressors. Intravenous dopamine infusion titrated to systolic blood pressure target (> 100 mmHg) is recommended. Dopamine unlike phenylephrine avoids the bradycardia following carotid angioplasty and stent placement. The infusion can be weaned off within 24 hours except in rare circumstances. Oral sympathomimetics such as midodrine tablets may reduce the duration of prolonged infusion in such events. An important condition to exclude if peri-procedural hypotension is observed is retroperitoneal hemorrhage. The hypotension related to retroperitoneal hemorrhage is usually difficult to treat with vasopressors unlike hypotension related to carotid stent placement.

Peri-procedural myocardial infarction

Post-procedural coronary ischemic events are infrequent. The rate of elevation in serum tropinin concentration was measured in the first 3 post-procedure days in 150 consecutive patients scheduled to undergo CEA ($n = 75$) or carotid stent placement ($n = 75$).[201] The incidence of increase of tropinin (> 0.5 ng/mL) was higher in the CEA group compared with that in the carotid stent placement group (13% vs. 1%). At 5 years, the overall incidence of major cardiac complications (non-fatal myocardial infarction and death related to cardiac origin) was significantly more frequent in the CEA group (20% vs. 5%). In view of concurrent existence, the Councils Stroke Council and the Council on Clinical Cardiology of the AHA/ASA Coronary Risk Evaluation[202] stated that ischemic stroke subtype information provides important information on concomitant cardiac risk, and recommended routine testing for coronary artery disease in patients with carotid or other large vessel disease.

Restenosis

There has been recent data that ultrasound criterion to identify restenosis after carotid stent placement is different from that used for diagnosing de novo stenosis.[203] Reduced compliance in the stent treated artery may result in elevated velocity relative to the native artery regardless of restenosis.[204] Stanziale et al.[205] recommended that to determine ≥70% in-stent stenosis, peak systolic velocity > 350 cm/s and internal carotid artery/common carotid artery ratio ≥ 4.75 are sensitive criteria. The criteria recommended for identifying de novo stenosis > 70% is systolic velocity > 230 cm/s and internal carotid artery/common carotid artery ratio ≥ 4.0, respectively.[206] Groschel et al.[207] documented a systematic analysis of 34 studies that reported on a total of 4185 patients

with a follow-up of 3814 arteries over a median of 13 months (range, 6 to 31 months). The cumulative restenosis rates (> 50%) after 1 and 2 years were approximately 6% and 8% in those studies. The rate was lower (approximately 4%) in the first 2 years in studies defining restenosis by severity > 70% to 80%.

Several large prospective studies[101,102,208–214] have evaluated the rates of restenosis following carotid stent placement. McCabe et al.[101] reported upon patients who were treated by balloon angioplasty alone, stent placement, or CEA, and followed by standardized Doppler ultrasound at approximately 1 month ($n = 283$) and 1 year ($n = 347$) after treatment. More patients had ≥70% stenosis of the ipsilateral carotid artery 1 year after endovascular treatment than after CEA (19% versus 5%). The rates were 22% and 18% in the stent and angioplasty treated groups, respectively. Five of the 32 patients with severe restenosis after endovascular treatment had ipsilateral ischemic symptoms at 1 year.

Recent studies (see Table 6.4) that have used self-expanding stents have not demonstrated high rates of restenosis observed with balloon angioplasty and balloon-expanding stents. Yadav et al.[102] reported the results of follow-up visits with duplex ultrasonography scheduled at 6 and 12 months after the procedure and annually thereafter for 3 years in 334 patients. The secondary endpoint of estimated rate of target-vessel revascularization using of the Kaplan–Meier method at one year were 4% vs. 1% after CEA and carotid stent placement, respectively. In a study of 386 carotid stent placement procedures in 354 patients with median follow-up period of 29 months, the rates of freedom from > 60% restenosis after carotid stent procedures at 12, 24, 36, and 48 months were 97%, 94%, 92%, and 90%, respectively.[215] The rates of freedom from all fatal and non-fatal strokes at 12, 24, 36, and 48 months were 97%, 91%, 89%, and 85%, respectively. In another study, asymptomatic in-stent restenosis developed after 12 procedures (11%)[216] among 101 carotid stent placements. A cumulative freedom from in-stent restenosis at 24 months was estimated at 88%. Risk factors for restenosis include postendarterectomy stenosis,[215] multiple stent placement,[215] radiation exposure,[217] and prior neck cancer.[216]

Repeat endovascular treatment has been considered for patients with symptomatic restenosis or selected high-grade asymptomatic restenosis, although there is lack of evidence demonstrating benefit from intervening in patients with restenosis using these indications. Use of traditional balloon angioplasty with or without stent placement is still considered one of the options. Cutting balloon angioplasty has recently been used as an alternative treatment option for revascularization of in-stent restenosis with higher procedural success rates. A review of 16 patients with restenosis treated with cutting balloon angioplasty[218] suggested that more than 90% of patients showed either complete angiographic resolution or residual stenosis of less than 30%. Additional stent placement or angioplasty was required in only half of the patients, and one patient had recurrent stenosis.

Table 6.4 Rates of restenosis among patients treated with carotid artery stent placement

Study	Number of patients	Definition of carotid artery disease	Prevalence	Retreatment
Roubin et al. (2001)[212]	518 patients treated with CAS	Restenosis requiring treatment (mean follow-up 17±12 months)	16 patients (3%)	15 CA and 1 CEA
Chakhtoura et al. (2001)[214]	50 CAS in 46 patients	In-stent restenoses ≥80% at 3- to 6-month intervals (mean follow-up 18 ± 10 months)	4 (8%)	All required retreatment; 3 CA and 1 CAS
Qureshi et al. (2003)[213]	35 patients enrolled in the Nex stent trial	≥70% residual stenosis on follow-up at 6 and 12 months	1 (3%)	1 restenosis requiring retreatment
Wholey et al. (2003)[209,210]	12 392 CAS patients in the Global Stent Registry	Reported by investigators	3% (first year), 3% (second year), and 2% (third year)	
Wholey et al. (2003)[209]	273 CAS with self expanding stents	≥50%	16% (3 years)	
Setacci et al. (2003)[211]	372 CAS	>80% after 6 months (range 6–40 months)	4%(n = 14)	All required retreatment
McCabe et al. (2005)[101]	173–124 CA and 41 CAS 174 underwent CEA	≥70% (360 days after treatment, range 181 and 540 days after treatment)	18.5% (5.2% in the CEA group), CAS vs. CA (22% versus 18%)	
Yadav et al. (2005)[102]	159 underwent CAS-151 underwent CEA	Restenosis requiring treatment at 12 months	1 (0.7%) in CAS and 6 (4.6%) in CEA treated group	
Levy et al. (2005)[208]	112 CAS in high risk surgical patients	≥80% on follow-up at 1 day, 1 month, 6 months, and yearly (mean follow-up 16 ± 11 months)	5%	Six patients (three symptomatic), 5 CA and 1 CAS

Abbreviations used: CEA, carotid endarterectomy; CA, carotid angioplasty; and CAS, carotid angioplasty and stent placement.
Adapted from Qureshi et al.[5,6] with permission.

Regulatory and professional guidelines

The Brain Attack Coalition[219] acknowledges that stent placement may be an acceptable treatment option in patients at high risk for CEA (i.e., restenosis after CEA, radiation fibrosis, fibromuscular dysplasia, surgically inaccessible stenosis, contralateral carotid disease, and significant cardiac or pulmonary disease). Stent placement in extracranial carotid arteries for atherothrombotic disease is a grade IIB recommendation and is considered an optional element of a comprehensive stroke center. The Brain Attack Coalition recommends that, for patients with average surgical risk, stent placement should be performed as part of a randomized clinical trial or under a local institutional review board approved protocol. The statement also recommended that stent placement be performed by individuals with training and appropriate expertise.

The American Heart Association/American Stroke Association Stroke Council[157] recommended that, among patients with symptomatic severe stenosis (> 70%) in whom other specific circumstances exist such as radiation-induced stenosis or restenosis after endarterectomy, carotid stent placement is not inferior to CEA and may be considered (Class IIb, Level of Evidence B). Carotid stent placement was considered reasonable when performed by operators with established peri-procedural morbidity and mortality rates of 4% to 6%, similar to that observed in trials of CEA and carotid stent placement (Class IIa, Level of Evidence B). The Collaborative Panel of the American Society of Interventional and Therapeutic Neuroradiology, the American Society of Neuroradiology, and the Society of Interventional Radiology[220] recommended stent placement for patients with symptomatic stenosis of 70% or greater by NASCET criteria and asymptomatic stenosis of 90% or greater or "near occlusion" in high-surgical-risk patients or those who refuse to undergo CEA after proper informed consent.

The Centers for Medicare and Medicaid Services[221] concluded that the evidence is adequate to conclude that carotid stent placement with embolic protection is reasonable and necessary for patients who are at high risk for CEA and have symptomatic carotid artery stenosis 70% or greater. Coverage is limited to procedures performed using FDA approved carotid artery stents and embolic protection devices. Patients at high risk for CEA are defined as those having significant comorbidities and/or anatomic risk factors and would be poor candidates for endarterectomy in the opinion of a surgeon.

References

1. Fairhead JF, Rothwell PM. Underinvestigation and undertreatment of carotid disease in elderly patients with transient ischaemic attack and stroke: comparative population based study. *BMJ* 2006;**333**:525–7.

2. Mast H, Thompson JL, Lin IF, *et al.* Cigarette smoking as a determinant of high-grade carotid artery stenosis in Hispanic, black, and white patients with stroke or transient ischemic attack. *Stroke* 1998;**29**:908–12.

3. Carolei A, Marini C, Nencini P, *et al.* Prevalence and outcome of symptomatic carotid lesions in young adults. National Research Council Study Group. *BMJ* 1995;**310**:1363–6.

4. Barnett HJ, Eliasziw M, Meldrum HE, Taylor DW. Do the facts and figures warrant a 10-fold increase in the performance of carotid endarterectomy on asymptomatic patients? *Neurology* 1996;**46**:603–8.

5. Qureshi AI, Alexandrov AV, Tegeler CH, *et al.* Guidelines for screening of extracranial carotid artery disease: a statement for healthcare professionals from the multidisciplinary practice guidelines committee of the American Society of Neuroimaging; cosponsored by the Society of Vascular and Interventional Neurology. *Journal of Neuroimaging* 2007;**17**:19–47.

6. Qureshi AI, Suri MFK, Nasar A, *et al.* Changes in cost and outcome among US patients with stroke hospitalized in 1990 to 1991 and those hospitalized in 2000 to 2001. *Stroke.* 2007;**38**:2180–2184.

7. Qureshi AI. Ten years of advances in neuroendovascular procedures. *J Endovasc Ther.* 2004;**11** Suppl 2:II1–4.

8. Tu JV, Hannan EL, Anderson GM, *et al.* The fall and rise of carotid endarterectomy in the United States and Canada. *N Engl J Med.* 1998;**339**:1441–7.

9. Hobson RW II, Brott TG, Roubin GS, Silver FL, Barnett HJM. Carotid artery stenting: meeting the recruitment challenge of a clinical trial. *Stroke* 2005;**36**:1314–15.

10. Troyer A, Saloner D, Pan XM, *et al.* Major carotid plaque surface irregularities correlate with neurologic symptoms. *Journal of Vascular Surgery* 2002;**35**:741–7.

11. Fisher M, Paganini-Hill A, Martin A, *et al.* Carotid plaque pathology: thrombosis, ulceration, and stroke pathogenesis.[erratum appears in *Stroke* 2005 Oct;36(10):2330 Note: dosage error in text]. *Stroke.* 2005;**36**:253–7.

12. Arapoglou B, Kondi-Pafiti A, Katsenis K, Dimakakos P. The clinical significance of carotid plaque haemorrhage. *Int Angiol.* 1994;**13**:323–6.

13. Montauban van Swijndregt AD, Elbers HR, Moll FL, de Letter J, Ackerstaff RG. Cerebral ischemic disease and morphometric analyses of carotid plaques. *Ann Vasc Surg* **13**:468–74.

14. Redgrave JNE, Lovett JK, Gallagher PJ, Rothwell PM. Histological assessment of 526 symptomatic carotid plaques in relation to the nature and timing of ischemic symptoms: the Oxford plaque study. *Circulation* 2006;**113**:2320–8.

15. Berkovic SF, Bladin PF, Ferguson LR, Royle JP, Thomas DP. Carotid plaques and retinal emboli: a clinical, angiographic and morphological study. *Clin Exp Neurol.* 1983;**19**:177–182.

16. Fisher CM, Ojemann RG. A clinico-pathologic study of carotid endarterectomy plaques. *Rev Neurol (Paris).* 1986;**142**:573–589.

17. Findlay JM. Editorial comment–plaque pathology and patient selection for carotid endarterectomy. *Stroke* 2005;**36**:257–8.

18. Droste DW, Dittrich R, Kemeny V, Schulte-Altedorneburg G, Ringelstein EB. Prevalence and frequency of microembolic signals in 105 patients with extracranial carotid artery occlusive disease. *J Neurol Neurosurg Psychiatry* 1999;**67**:525–8.

19. Molloy J, Markus HS. Asymptomatic embolization predicts stroke and TIA risk in patients with carotid artery stenosis. *Stroke* 1999;**30**:1440–3.

20. Siebler M, Nachtmann A, Sitzer M, *et al.* Cerebral microembolism and the risk of ischemia in asymptomatic high-grade internal carotid artery stenosis. *Stroke* 1995;**26**:2184–6.

21. Turk AS, Grayev A, Rowley HA, *et al.* Variability of clinical CT perfusion measurements in patients with carotid stenosis. *Neuroradiology* 2007;**49**:955–61.

22. Waaijer A, van Leeuwen MS, van Osch MJP, *et al.* Changes in cerebral perfusion after revascularization of symptomatic carotid artery stenosis: CT measurement. *Radiology* 2007;**245**:541–8.

23. Bisdas S, Nemitz O, Berding G, *et al.* Correlative assessment of cerebral blood flow obtained with perfusion CT and positron emission tomography in symptomatic stenotic carotid disease. *Eur Radiol* 2006;**16**:2220–8.

24. Divani AA, Qureshi AI, Hoffman KR, Suri MFK, Kirmani JF. Comparison of asymmetry in cerebral blood flow between brain hemispheres using digital subtraction angiography. *J Neuroimaging* 2006;**16**:139–45.

25. Van Laar PJ, Hendrikse J, Mali WPTM, *et al.* Altered flow territories after carotid stenting and carotid endarterectomy. *J Vas Surg* 2007;**45**:1155–61.

26. Haubrich C, Kruska W, Diehl RR, Moller-Hartmann W, Klotzsch C. Recovery of the blood pressure – cerebral flow relation after carotid stenting in elderly patients. *Acta Neurochir* 2007;**149**:31–6; discussion 137.

27. Russo G, de Falco R, Scarano E, Cigliano A, Profeta G. Non invasive recording of CO_2 cerebrovascular reactivity in normal subjects and patients with unilateral internal carotid artery stenosis. *J Neurosurg Sci* 1994;**38**:147–53.

28. de Boorder MJ, van der Grond J, van Dongen AJ, *et al.* Spect measurements of regional cerebral perfusion and carbondioxide reactivity: correlation with cerebral collaterals in internal carotid artery occlusive disease. *J Neurol* 2006;**253**:1285–91.

29. Yamauchi H, Kudoh T, Sugimoto K, *et al.* Altered patterns of blood flow response during visual stimulation in carotid artery occlusive disease. *Neuroimage* 2005;**25**:554–60.

30. Chaturvedi S, Policherla PN, Femino L. Cerebral angiography practices at US teaching hospitals. Implications for carotid endarterectomy. *Stroke* 1997;**28**:1895–7.

31. Rothwell PM, Gibson RJ, Slattery J, Sellar RJ, Warlow CP. Equivalence of measurements of carotid stenosis. A comparison of three methods on 1001 angiograms. European Carotid Surgery Trialists' Collaborative Group. *Stroke* 1994;**25**:2435–9.

32. Rothwell PM, Gibson RJ, Slattery J, Warlow CP. Prognostic value and

reproducibility of measurements of carotid stenosis. A comparison of three methods on 1001 angiograms. European Carotid Surgery Trialists' Collaborative Group. *Stroke* 1994;**25**:2440–4.

33. Gagne PJ, Matchett J, MacFarland D, *et al.* Can the NASCET technique for measuring carotid stenosis be reliably applied outside the trial? *J Vasc Surg.* 1996;**24**:449–55; discussion 455–6.

34. Stapf C, Hofmeister C, Hartmann A, *et al.* Interrater agreement for high grade carotid artery stenosis measurement and treatment decision. *Eur J Med Res.* 2000;**5**:26–31.

35. Eliasziw M, Smith RF, Singh N, *et al.* Further comments on the measurement of carotid stenosis from angiograms. North American Symptomatic Carotid Endarterectomy Trial (NASCET) Group. *Stroke* 1994;**25**:2445–9.

36. Netuka D, Benes V, Mandys V, *et al.* Accuracy of angiography and Doppler ultrasonography in the detection of carotid stenosis: a histopathological study of 123 cases. *Acta Neurochir.* 2006;**148**:511–20; discussion 520.

37. Schulte-Altedorneburg G, Droste DW, Kollar J, *et al.* Measuring carotid artery stenosis – comparison of postmortem arteriograms with the planimetric gold standard. *J Neurol.* 2005;**252**:575–82.

38. Brown PM, Johnston KW. The difficulty of quantifying the severity of carotid stenosis. *Surgery* 1982;**92**: 468–73.

39. Bladin CF, Alexandrov AV, Murphy J, Maggisano R, Norris JW. Carotid Stenosis Index. A new method of measuring internal carotid artery stenosis. *Stroke* 1995;**26**:230–4.

40. Lovett JK, Rothwell PM. Site of carotid plaque ulceration in relation to direction of blood flow: an angiographic and pathological study. *Cerebrovasc Dis* 2003;**16**:369–75.

41. Grotta JC, Bigelow RH, Hu H, Hankins L, Fields WS. The significance of carotid stenosis or ulceration. *Neurology* 1984;**34**:437–42.

42. Valton L, Larrue V, Arrue P, Geraud G, Bes A. Asymptomatic cerebral embolic signals in patients with carotid stenosis. Correlation with appearance of plaque ulceration on angiography. *Stroke* 1995;**26**:813–15.

43. Eliasziw M, Streifler JY, Fox AJ, *et al.* Significance of plaque ulceration in symptomatic patients with high-grade carotid stenosis. North American Symptomatic Carotid Endarterectomy Trial. *Stroke* 1994;**25**:304–8.

44. Kastrup A, Groschel K, Schnaudigel S, *et al.* Target lesion ulceration and arch calcification are associated with increased incidence of carotid stenting-associated ischemic lesions in octogenarians. *J Vasc Surg* 2008; **47**:88–95.

45. Hofmann R, Niessner A, Kypta A, *et al.* Risk score for peri-interventional complications of carotid artery stenting. *Stroke* 2006;**37**:2557–61.

46. Sayeed S, Stanziale SF, Wholey MH, Makaroun MS. Angiographic lesion characteristics can predict adverse outcomes after carotid artery stenting. *J Vasc Surg* 2008;**47**:81–7.

47. Rothwell PM, Gibson RJ, Villagra R, Sellar R, Warlow CP. The effect of angiographic technique and image quality on the reproducibility of measurement of carotid stenosis and assessment of plaque surface morphology. *Clin Radiol* 1998;**53**: 439–43.

48. Kagawa R, Moritake K, Shima T, Okada Y. Validity of B-mode ultrasonographic findings in patients undergoing carotid endarterectomy in comparison with angiographic and clinicopathologic features. *Stroke* 1996;**27**:700–5.

49. Orlandi G, Parenti G, Landucci Pellegrini L, *et al.* Plaque surface and microembolic signals in moderate carotid stenosis. *Ital J Neurol Sci.* 1999;**20**:179–82.

50. Streifler JY, Eliasziw M, Fox AJ, *et al.* Angiographic detection of carotid plaque ulceration. Comparison with surgical observations in a multicenter study. North American Symptomatic Carotid Endarterectomy Trial. *Stroke* 1994;**25**:1130–2.

51. Rothwell PM, Gibson R, Warlow CP. Interrelation between plaque surface morphology and degree of stenosis on carotid angiograms and the risk of ischemic stroke in patients with symptomatic carotid stenosis. On behalf of the European Carotid Surgery Trialists' Collaborative Group. *Stroke* 2000;**31**:615–21.

52. Doris I, Dobranowski J, Franchetto AA, Jaeschke R. The relevance of detecting carotid artery calcification on plain radiograph. *Stroke* 1993;**24**: 1330–4.

53. Bartlett ES, Walters TD, Symons SP, Fox AJ. Quantification of carotid stenosis on CT angiography. *Am J Neuroradiol* 2006;**27**:13–19.

54. Nandalur KR, Baskurt E, Hagspiel KD, *et al.* Carotid artery calcification on CT may independently predict stroke risk. *Am J Roentgenol* 2006;**186**: 547–52.

55. Nandalur KR, Baskurt E, Hagspiel KD, Phillips CD, Kramer CM. Calcified carotid atherosclerotic plaque is associated less with ischemic symptoms than is noncalcified plaque on MDCT. *Am J Roentgenol* 2005;**184**:295–8.

56. Lam RC, Lin SC, DeRubertis B, *et al.* The impact of increasing age on anatomic factors affecting carotid angioplasty and stenting. *J Vasc Surg* 2007;**45**:875–80.

57. Nonaka T, Oka S, Miyata K, *et al.* Prediction of prolonged postprocedural hypotension after carotid artery stenting. *Neurosurgery* 2005;**57**:472–7; discussion 472–7.

58. Qureshi AI, Luft AR, Sharma M, *et al.* Frequency and determinants of postprocedural hemodynamic instability after carotid angioplasty and stenting. *Stroke* 1999;**30**:2086–93.

59. Schuknecht B. High-concentration contrast media (HCCM) in CT angiography of the carotid system: impact on therapeutic decision making. *Neuroradiology* 2007;**49**:S15–26.

60. Henderson RD, Eliasziw M, Fox AJ, Rothwell PM, Barnett HJ. Angiographically defined collateral circulation and risk of stroke in patients with severe carotid artery stenosis. North American Symptomatic Carotid Endarterectomy Trial (NASCET) Group. *Stroke* 2000;**1**:128–32.

61. Ozgur HT, Kent Walsh T, Masaryk A, *et al.* Correlation of cerebrovascular reserve as measured by acetazolamide-challenged SPECT with angiographic flow patterns and intra- or extracranial arterial stenosis. *Am J Neuroradiol* 2001;**22**:928–36.

62. Kablak-Ziembicka A, Przewlocki T, Pieniazek P, *et al.* Evaluation of cerebral circulation in patients with significant carotid artery stenosis. *Kardiologia Polska* 2005;**63**:381–9; discussion 390.

63. Hedera P, Bujdakova J, Traubner P, Pancak J. Stroke risk factors and

development of collateral flow in carotid occlusive disease. *Acta Neurol Scandi* 1998;**98**:182–6.

64. Hendrikse J, Rutgers DR, Klijn CJM, Eikelboom BC, van der Grond J. Effect of carotid endarterectomy on primary collateral blood flow in patients with severe carotid artery lesions. *Stroke* 2003;**34**:1650–4.

65. Luft AR, Qureshi AI, Suri MF, *et al*. Frequency and predictors for angiographically improved inflow of contrast medium after carotid angioplasty and stenting. *Neuroradiology* 2001;**43**:877–83.

66. Morgenstern LB, Fox AJ, Sharpe BL, *et al*. The risks and benefits of carotid endarterectomy in patients with near occlusion of the carotid artery. North American Symptomatic Carotid Endarterectomy Trial (NASCET) Group. *Neurology* 1997;**48**:911–15.

67. Fox AJ, Eliasziw M, Rothwell PM, et al. Identification, prognosis, and management of patients with carotid artery near occlusion. *Am J Neuroradiol* 2005;**26**:2086–94.

68. Kniemeyer HW, Aulich A, Schlachetzki F, Steinmetz H, Sandmann W. Pseudo- and segmental occlusion of the internal carotid artery: a new classification, surgical treatment and results. *Eur J Vasc & Endovasc Surg* 1996;**12**:310–20.

69. Williams MA, Nicolaides AN. Predicting the normal dimensions of the internal and external carotid arteries from the diameter of the common carotid. *Eur J Vasc Surg* 1987;**1**:91–6.

70. Pappas JN. The angiographic string sign. *Radiology* 2002;**222**:237–8.

71. Martin MA, Marotta TR. Vasa vasorum: another cause of the carotid string sign. *Am J. Neuroradiol.* 1999;**20**:259–62.

72. Brooks AJ, Behm GM, Baxter BT, Lynch TG. Carotid string sign resulting from an aberrant branch of the internal carotid artery. *Journal of Cardiovascular Surgery* 1998;**39**:163–5.

73. Heth JA, Loftus CM, Piper JG, Yuh W. Hypoplastic internal carotid artery mimicking a classic angiographic "string sign". Case report. *Journal of Neurosurgery* 1997;**86**:567–70.

74. Naylor AR, Rothwell PM, Bell PRF. Overview of the principal results and secondary analyses from the European and North American randomised trials of endarterectomy for symptomatic carotid stenosis. *Eur J Vasc & Endovascular surgery* 2003;**26**:115–29.

75. Berman SS, Bernhard VM, Erly WK, *et al*. Critical carotid artery stenosis: diagnosis, timing of surgery, and outcome. *J Vasc Surg.* 1994;**20**:499–508; discussion 508–10.

76. Rothwell PM, Slattery J, Warlow CP. Clinical and angiographic predictors of stroke and death from carotid endarterectomy: systematic review. *BMJ* 1997;**315**:1571–7.

77. Reed AB, Gaccione P, Belkin M, *et al*. Preoperative risk factors for carotid endarterectomy: defining the patient at high risk. *J Vasc Surg* 2003;**37**:1191–9.

78. da Silva AF, McCollum P, Szymanska T, de Cossart L. Prospective study of carotid endarterectomy and contralateral carotid occlusion. *Br J. Surg* 1996;**83**:1370–2.

79. Ferguson GG, Eliasziw M, Barr HW, *et al*. The North American Symptomatic Carotid Endarterectomy Trial: surgical results in 1415 patients. *Stroke* 1999;**30**:1751–8.

80. Pulli R, Dorigo W, Barbanti E, *et al*. Carotid endarterectomy with contralateral carotid artery occlusion: is this a higher risk subgroup?. *Eur J Vasc Endovasc Surg* 2002;**24**:63–8.

81. Karmeli R, Lubezky N, Halak M, *et al*. Carotid endarterectomy in awake patients with contralateral carotid artery occlusion. *Cardiovasc Surg* 2001;**9**:334–8.

82. AbuRahma AF, Robinson P, Holt SM, Herzog TA, Mowery NT. Perioperative and late stroke rates of carotid endarterectomy contralateral to carotid artery occlusion: results from a randomized trial. *Stroke* 2000;**31**:1566–71.

83. Julia P, Chemla E, Mercier F, Renaudin JM, Fabiani JN. Influence of the status of the contralateral carotid artery on the outcome of carotid surgery. *Ann Vasc Surg* 1998;**12**:566–71.

84. Gasecki AP, Eliasziw M, Ferguson GG, Hachinski V, Barnett HJ. Long-term prognosis and effect of endarterectomy in patients with symptomatic severe carotid stenosis and contralateral carotid stenosis or occlusion: results from NASCET. North American Symptomatic Carotid Endarterectomy Trial (NASCET) Group. *J Neurosurg* 1995;**83**:778–82.

85. Baker WH, Howard VJ, Howard G, Toole JF. Effect of contralateral occlusion on long-term efficacy of endarterectomy in the asymptomatic carotid atherosclerosis study (ACAS). ACAS Investigators. *Stroke* 2000;**31**:2330–4.

86. AbuRahma AF, Metz MJ, Robinson PA. Natural history of > or =60% asymptomatic carotid stenosis in patients with contralateral carotid occlusion. *Annals of Surgery.* 2003;**238**:551–61; discussion 561–561; discussion 561–2.

87. Rothwell PM, Howard SC, Spence JD, Carotid Endarterectomy Trialists C. Relationship between blood pressure and stroke risk in patients with symptomatic carotid occlusive disease. *Stroke* 2003;**34**:2583–90.

88. McCrory DC, Goldstein LB, Samsa GP, *et al*. Predicting complications of carotid endarterectomy. *Stroke.* 1993;**24**:1285–91.

89. Schuler JJ, Flanigan DP, Lim LT, *et al*. The effect of carotid siphon stenosis on stroke rate, death, and relief of symptoms following elective carotid endarterectomy. *Surgery* 1982;**92**:1058–1067.

90. Mackey WC, O'Donnell TFJ, Callow AD. Carotid endarterectomy in patients with intracranial vascular disease: short-term risk and long-term outcome. *J Vasc Surg* 1989;**10**:432–8.

91. North American Symptomatic Carotid Endarterectomy Trial Collaborators. Beneficial effect of carotid endarterectomy in symptomatic patients with high-grade carotid stenosis. *N Engl J Med.* 1991; **325**:445–53.

92. Gurm HS, Yadav JS, Fayad P, *et al*. Long-term results of carotid stenting versus endarterectomy in high-risk patients. *N Engl J Med* 2008;**358**: 1572–9.

93. MRC European Carotid Surgery Trial: interim results for symptomatic patients with severe (70–99%) or with mild (0–29%) carotid stenosis. European Carotid Surgery Trialists' Collaborative Group. *Lancet* 1991;**337**:1235–43.

94. Randomised trial of endarterectomy for recently symptomatic carotid stenosis: final results of the MRC European

Carotid Surgery Trial (ECST). *Lancet* 1998;**351**:1379–87.

95. Rothwell PM, Eliasziw M, Gutnikov SA, *et al.* Analysis of pooled data from the randomised controlled trials of endarterectomy for symptomatic carotid stenosis. *Lancet* 2003;**361**:107–16.

96. Rothwell PM, Eliasziw M, Gutnikov SA, Warlow CP, Barnett HJ. Endarterectomy for symptomatic carotid stenosis in relation to clinical subgroups and timing of surgery. *Lancet.* 2004;**363**:915–24.

97. Endarterectomy for asymptomatic carotid artery stenosis. Executive Committee for the Asymptomatic Carotid Atherosclerosis Study. *JAMA* 1995;**273**:1421–8.

98. Halliday A, Mansfield A, Marro J, *et al.* Prevention of disabling and fatal strokes by successful carotid endarterectomy in patients without recent neurological symptoms: randomised controlled trial. *Lancet.* 2004;**363**:1491–502.

99. Chambers BR, Donnan GA. Carotid endarterectomy for asymptomatic carotid stenosis. *Cochrane Database of Syst Revi.* 2005;**4**:CD001923.

100. Endovascular versus surgical treatment in patients with carotid stenosis in the Carotid and Vertebral Artery Transluminal Angioplasty Study (CAVATAS): a randomised trial. *Lancet* 2001;**357**:1729–37.

101. McCabe DJ, Pereira AC, Clifton A, Bland JM, Brown MM. Restenosis after carotid angioplasty, stenting, or endarterectomy in the Carotid and Vertebral Artery Transluminal Angioplasty Study (CAVATAS). *Stroke* 2005;**36**:281–86.

102. Yadav JS, Wholey MH, Kuntz RE, *et al.* Protected carotid-artery stenting versus endarterectomy in high-risk patients. *N Engl J Med* 2004;**351**:1493–501.

103. Mas JL, Chatellier G, Beyssen B, *et al.* Endarterectomy versus stenting in patients with symptomatic severe carotid stenosis. *N Engl J Med* 2006;**355**:1660–71.

104. Endartectomy versus angioplasty in patients with symptomatic severe carotid stenosis (EVA-3S, NCT 00190398): Final results.(Abstract 4). *Eur Stroke Conference*, 2008.

105. Ringleb PA, Allenberg J, Bruckmann H, *et al.* 30 day results from the SPACE trial of stent-protected angioplasty versus carotid endarterectomy in symptomatic patients: a randomised non-inferiority trial. *Lancet* 2006;**368**:1239–47.

106. Two year results of the SPACE study (Stent- protected percutaneous angioplasty of the carotid angioplasty vs endartectomy).(Abstract 5). *Eur Stroke Conference*, May 14, 2008.

107. Hobson RW 2nd. CREST (Carotid Revascularization Endarterectomy versus Stent Trial): background, design, and current status. *Semin Vasc Surg* 2000;**13**:139–43.

108. Clark WM CREST Investigators. Carotid revascularization endarterectomy vs stenting trial. Final results. Presented at the International stroke conference, Feb 23–26, San Antonio, Texas. 2010.

109. Witt K, Borsch K, Daniels C, *et al.* Neuropsychological consequences of endarterectomy and endovascular angioplasty with stent placement for treatment of symptomatic carotid stenosis: a prospective randomised study. *J Neurol* 2007;**254**:1524–32.

110. Qureshi AI, Kirmani JF, Divani AA, Hobson RW 2nd. Carotid angioplasty with or without stent placement versus carotid endarterectomy for treatment of carotid stenosis: a meta-analysis. *Neurosurgery.* 2005;**56**:1171–9; discussion 1179–81.

111. Luebke T, Aleksic M, Brunkwall J. Meta-analysis of randomized trials comparing carotid endarterectomy and endovascular treatment. *Eur J Vasc Endovasc Surg.* 2007; **34**:470–9.

112. Miller AC **RAMSMFKQAI**. Carotid stent placement versus carotid endarterectomy for treatment of high surgical risk patients with carotid stenosis: A pooled analysis of 3282 patients. *The 59th Annual Meeting of American Academy of Neurology.* 2007.

113. Touze E, Trinquart L, Chatellier G, Mas JL. Systematic review of the perioperative risks of stroke or death after carotid angioplasty and stenting. *Stroke* 2009;**40**:e683–93.

114. White CJ, Iyer SS, Hopkins LN, Katzen BT, Russell ME. Carotid stenting with distal protection in high surgical risk patients: the BEACH trial 30 day results. *Catheter Cardiovasc Interv.* 2006;**67**:503–12.

115. Hopkins LN. CABERNET: Carotid artery revascularization using the Boston Scientific filterwire EX/EZ and the EndoTex next stent. *16th Annual Transcatheter Cardiovascular Therapeutics Meeting.*

116. Gray WA, Hopkins LN, Yadav S, *et al.* Protected carotid stenting in high-surgical-risk patients: the ARCHeR results. *J Vasc Surg* 2006;**44**:258–68.

117. Hill MD, Morrish W, Soulez G, *et al.* Multicenter evaluation of a self-expanding carotid stent system with distal protection in the treatment of carotid stenosis. *Am J Neuroradiol* 2006;**27**:759–65.

118. Hobson RWIIBTBRGS. Carotid stenting in the CREST lead-in phase: periprocedural stroke, myocardial infarction, and death rates are lower than reported for preceding stent trials. *Circulation* 2003;**108**:IV-604.

119. Iyer SS, White CJ, Hopkins LN, *et al.* Carotid artery revascularization in high-surgical-risk patients using the Carotid WALLSTENT and FilterWire EX/EZ: 1-year outcomes in the BEACH Pivotal Group. *J Am Coll Cardiol.* 2008;**51**:427–34.

120. Safian RD, Bresnahan JF, Jaff MR, *et al.* Protected carotid Stenting in high-risk patients with severe carotid artery stenosis. *J Am Coll Cardiol* 2006;**47**:2384–9.

121. Iyer V, de Donato G, Deloose K, *et al.* The type of embolic protection does not influence the outcome in carotid artery stenting. *J Vasc Surg* 2007;**46**:251–6.

122. Boltuch J, Sabeti S, Amighi J, *et al.* Procedure-related complications and early neurological adverse events of unprotected and protected carotid stenting: temporal trends in a consecutive patient series. *J Endovasc Ther* 2005;**12**:538–47.

123. Macdonald S, McKevitt F, Venables GS, Cleveland TJ, Gaines PA. Neurological outcomes after carotid stenting protected with the NeuroShield filter compared to unprotected stenting. *J Endovasc Ther* 2002;**9**:777–85.

124. Kastrup A, Groschel K, Krapf H, *et al.* Early outcome of carotid angioplasty and stenting with and without cerebral protection devices: a systematic review of the literature. *Stroke* 2003;**34**:813–19.

125. Garg N, Karagiorgos N, Pisimisis GT, *et al.* Cerebral protection devices reduce periprocedural strokes during carotid

angioplasty and stenting: a systematic review of the current literature. *J Endovasc Ther* 2009;**16**:412–27.

126. Mas JL, Chatellier G, Beyssen B. Carotid angioplasty and stenting with and without cerebral protection: clinical alert from the Endarterectomy Versus Angioplasty in Patients With Symptomatic Severe Carotid Stenosis (EVA-3S) trial. *Stroke* 2004;**35**: e18–20.

127. Katzen BT, Criado FJ, Ramee SR, et al. Carotid artery stenting with emboli protection surveillance study: thirty-day results of the CASES-PMS study. *Catheter Cardiovasc Interv* 2007;**70**:316–23.

128. Gray WA, Yadav JS, Verta P, et al. The CAPTURE registry: results of carotid stenting with embolic protection in the post approval setting. *Catheter Cardiovasc Interv* 2007;**69**:341–8.

129. Goldstein LB, McCrory DC, Landsman PB, et al. Multicenter review of preoperative risk factors for carotid endarterectomy in patients with ipsilateral symptoms. *Stroke* 1994;**25**:1116–21.

130. Goldstein LB, Samsa GP, Matchar DB, Oddone EZ. Multicenter review of preoperative risk factors for endarterectomy for asymptomatic carotid artery stenosis. *Stroke* 1998;**29**:750–3.

131. Ouriel K, Hertzer NR, Beven EG, et al. Preprocedural risk stratification: identifying an appropriate population for carotid stenting. *J Vasc Surg* 2001;**33**:728–32.

132. Paciaroni M, Eliasziw M, Kappelle LJ, et al. Medical complications associated with carotid endarterectomy. North American Symptomatic Carotid Endarterectomy Trial (NASCET). *Stroke* 1999;**30**:1759–63.

133. Wennberg DE, Lucas FL, Birkmeyer JD, Bredenberg CE, Fisher ES. Variation in carotid endarterectomy mortality in the Medicare population: trial hospitals, volume, and patient characteristics. *JAMA* 1998;**279**:1278–81.

134. Alamowitch S, Eliasziw M, Algra A, Meldrum H, Barnett HJ. Risk, causes, and prevention of ischaemic stroke in elderly patients with symptomatic internal-carotid-artery stenosis. *Lancet* 2001;**357**:1154–60.

135. Harbaugh RE, Stieg PE, Moayeri N, Hsu L. Carotid-coronary artery bypass

graft conundrum. *Neurosurgery* 1998;**43**:926–31.

136. Hofmann R, Kypta A, Steinwender C, et al. Coronary angiography in patients undergoing carotid artery stenting shows a high incidence of significant coronary artery disease. *Heart* 2005;**91**:1438–41.

137. Halm EA, Tuhrim S, Wang JJ, et al. Risk factors for perioperative death and stroke after carotid endarterectomy: results of the new york carotid artery surgery study. *Stroke* 2009;**40**:221–9.

138. Faggioli GL, Curl GR, Ricotta JJ. The role of carotid screening before coronary artery bypass. *J Vasc Surg* 1990;**12**:724–9; discussion 729–31.

139. Eagle KA, Guyton RA, Davidoff R, et al. ACC/AHA 2004 guideline update for coronary artery bypass graft surgery: a report of the American College of Cardiology/American Heart Association Task Force on Practice Guidelines (Committee to Update the 1999 Guidelines for Coronary Artery Bypass Graft Surgery). *Circulation* 2004;**110**:e340–437.

140. Del Sette M, Eliasziw M, Streifler JY, et al. Internal borderzone infarction: a marker for severe stenosis in patients with symptomatic internal carotid artery disease. For the North American Symptomatic Carotid Endarterectomy (NASCET) Group. *Stroke* 2000;**31**:631–6.

141. Moore WS, Barnett HJ, Beebe HG, et al. Guidelines for carotid endarterectomy. A multidisciplinary consensus statement from the ad hoc Committee, American Heart Association. *Stroke* 1995;**26**:188–201.

142. Lopes DK, Mericle RA, Lanzino G, et al. Stent placement for the treatment of occlusive atherosclerotic carotid artery disease in patients with concomitant coronary artery disease. *J Neurosurg* 2002;**96**:490–6.

143. Guzman LA, Costa MA, Angiolillo DJ, et al. A systematic review of outcomes in patients with staged carotid artery stenting and coronary artery bypass graft surgery. *Stroke* 2008;**39**:361–5.

144. Kim SHMRALGQAIGLRHLN. Carotid angioplasty and stent placement in patients with tandem stenosis. *Neurosurgery* 1998;**43**.

145. Villarreal JSJEMSBFAHVBHJ. North American Symptomatic Carotid Endarterectomy Trial: prognosis of patients with intraluminal thrombus in

the internal carotid artery. (abstract). *Stroke* 1998;**29**.

146. Meyer FB, Piepgras DG, Fode NC. Surgical treatment of recurrent carotid artery stenosis. *J Neurosurg* 1994;**80**:781–7.

147. AbuRahma AF, Jennings TG, Wulu JT, Tarakji L, Robinson PA. Redo carotid endarterectomy versus primary carotid endarterectomy. *Stroke* 2001;**32**:2787–92.

148. Lanzino G, Mericle RA, Lopes DK, et al. Percutaneous transluminal angioplasty and stent placement for recurrent carotid artery stenosis. *J Neurosurg* 1999;**90**:688–94.

149. New G, Roubin GS, Iyer SS, et al. Safety, efficacy, and durability of carotid artery stenting for restenosis following carotid endarterectomy: a multicenter study. *J Endovasc Ther* 2000;**7**:345–52.

150. Loftus CM, Biller J, Hart MN, Cornell SH, Hiratzka LF. Management of radiation-induced accelerated carotid atherosclerosis. *Arch Neurol* 1987;**44**:711–14.

151. Melliere D, Becquemin JP, Berrahal D, Desgranges P, Cavillon A. Management of radiation-induced occlusive arterial disease: a reassessment. *J Cardiovasc Surg (Torino)* 1997;**38**:261–9.

152. Leseche G, Castier Y, Chataigner O, et al. Carotid artery revascularization through a radiated field. *J Vasc Surg* 2003;**38**:244–50.

153. Cazaban S, Maiza D, Coffin O, et al. Surgical treatment of recurrent carotid artery stenosis and carotid artery stenosis after neck irradiation: evaluation of operative risk. *Ann Vasc Surg* 2003;**17**:393–400.

154. Ting AC, Cheng SW, Yeung KM, et al. Carotid stenting for radiation-induced extracranial carotid artery occlusive disease: efficacy and midterm outcomes. *J Endovasc Ther* 2004; **11**:53–9.

155. Ecker RD, Donovan MT, Hopkins LN. Endovascular management of carotid artery disease after radiation therapy and radical neck dissection. *Neurosurg Focus* 2005;**18**:e8.

156. Bond R, Rerkasem K, Rothwell PM. Systematic review of the risks of carotid endarterectomy in relation to the clinical indication for and timing of surgery. *Stroke* 2003;**34**:2290–301.

157. Sacco RL, Adams R, Albers G, et al. Guidelines for prevention of stroke in patients with ischemic stroke or

transient ischemic attack: a statement for healthcare professionals from the American Heart Association/American Stroke Association Council on Stroke: co-sponsored by the Council on Cardiovascular Radiology and Intervention: the American Academy of Neurology affirms the value of this guideline. *Stroke* 2006;**37**:577–617.

158. Qureshi AI, Luft AR, Sharma M, Guterman LR, Hopkins LN. Prevention and treatment of thromboembolic and ischemic complications associated with endovascular procedures: Part I–Pathophysiological and pharmacological features. *Neurosurgery* 2000;**46**:1344–59.

159. Qureshi AI, Luft AR, Sharma M, Guterman LR, Hopkins LN. Prevention and treatment of thromboembolic and ischemic complications associated with endovascular procedures: Part II–Clinical aspects and recommendations. *Neurosurgery* 2000;**46**:1360–75; discussion 1375–6.

160. Saw J, Bajzer C, Casserly IP, *et al.* Evaluating the optimal activated clotting time during carotid artery stenting. *Am J Cardiol* 2006;**97**:1657–60.

161. Qureshi AI, Suri MFK, Ali Z, *et al.* Carotid angioplasty and stent placement: a prospective analysis of perioperative complications and impact of intravenously administered abciximab. *Neurosurgery* 2002;**50**: 466–73; discussion 473–5.

162. Qureshi AI, Siddiqui AM, Hanel RA, *et al.* Safety of high-dose intravenous eptifibatide as an adjunct to internal carotid artery angioplasty and stent placement: a prospective registry. *Neurosurgery* 2004;**54**:307–16; discussion 316–17.

163. Qureshi AI, Ali Z, Suri MF, *et al.* Open-label phase I clinical study to assess the safety of intravenous eptifibatide in patients undergoing internal carotid artery angioplasty and stent placement. *Neurosurgery* 2001;**48**:998–1004; discussion 1004–5.

164. Qureshi AI. Adjunctive use of platelet glycoprotein IIb/IIIa inhibitors for carotid angioplasty and stent placement: time to say good bye? *J Endovasc Ther: Official J Int Soc Endovasc Specialists.* 2003;**10**:42–4.

165. Qureshi AI, Saad M, Zaidat OO, *et al.* Intracerebral hemorrhages associated with neurointerventional procedures using a combination of antithrombotic agents including abciximab. *Stroke* 2002;**33**:1916–19.

166. Wholey MH, Wholey MH, Eles G, *et al.* Evaluation of glycoprotein IIb/IIIa inhibitors in carotid angioplasty and stenting. *J Endovasc Ther: Official J Int Soc Endovasc Specialists* 2003;**10**:33–41.

167. Zahn R, Ischinger T, Hochadel M, *et al.* Glycoprotein IIb/IIIa antagonists during carotid artery stenting: results from the carotid artery stenting (CAS) registry of the Arbeitsgemeinschaft Leitende Kardiologische Krankenhausarzte (ALKK). *Clin Res Cardiol* 2007;**96**:730–7.

168. Seo KD, Lee KO, Kim DJ, Lee K-Y. Rescue use of tirofiban for acute carotid in-stent thrombosis. *Yonsei Med J.* 2008;**49**:163–6.

169. Tong FC, Cloft HJ, Joseph GJ, Samuels OB, Dion JE. Abciximab rescue in acute carotid stent thrombosis. *Am J Neuroradiol* 2000;**21**:1750–2.

170. Muller-Hulsbeck S, Jahnke T, Liess C, *et al.* Comparison of various cerebral protection devices used for carotid artery stent placement: an in vitro experiment. *J Vasc Int Radiol* 2003;**14**:613–20.

171. Hart JP, Peeters P, Verbist J, Deloose K, Bosiers M. Do device characteristics impact outcome in carotid artery stenting?[erratum appears in *J Vasc Surg* 2007;45(1):226]. *J Vasc Surg* 2006;**44**:725–30; discussion 730–1.

172. Rubartelli P, Brusa G, Arrigo A, *et al.* Transcranial Doppler monitoring during stenting of the carotid bifurcation: evaluation of two different distal protection devices in preventing embolization. *J Endovasc Ther: Official J Int Soc Endovasc Specialists.* 2006;**13**:436–42.

173. Bosiers M, de Donato G, Deloose K, *et al.* Does free cell area influence the outcome in carotid artery stenting?. *Eur J Vasc Endovasc Surg.* 2007;**33**:135–41; discussion 142–3.

174. Jansen O, Fiehler J, Hartmann M, Bruckmann H. Protection or nonprotection in carotid stent angioplasty: the influence of interventional techniques on outcome data from the SPACE Trial. *Stroke* 2009;**40**:841–6.

175. Schillinger M, Dick P, Wiest G, *et al.* Covered versus bare self-expanding stents for endovascular treatment of carotid artery stenosis: a stopped randomized trial. *J Endovasc Ther: Official J Int Soc Endovasc Specialists.* 2006;**13**:312–19.

176. Tan KT, Cleveland TJ, Berczi V, *et al.* Timing and frequency of complications after carotid artery stenting: what is the optimal period of observation?. *J Vasc Surg* 2003;**38**:236–43.

177. Amarenco P, Bogousslavsky J, Callahan A 3rd, *et al.* High-dose atorvastatin after stroke or transient ischemic attack. *N Engl J Med* 2006;**355**:549–59.

178. Adams RJ, Albers G, Alberts MJ, *et al.* Update to the AHA/ASA recommendations for the prevention of stroke in patients with stroke and transient ischemic attack. *Stroke* 2008;**39**:1647–52.

179. Sabeti S, Schillinger M, Mlekusch W, *et al.* Contralateral high-grade carotid artery stenosis or occlusion is not associated with increased risk for poor neurologic outcome after elective carotid stent placement. *Radiology* 2004;**230**:70–6.

180. Qureshi AI, Janardhan V, Bennett SE, *et al.* Who should be screened for asymptomatic carotid artery stenosis? Experience from the Western New York Stroke Screening Program. *J Neuroimaging* 2001;**11**:105–11.

181. Fairman R, Gray WA, Scicli AP, *et al.* The CAPTURE registry: analysis of strokes resulting from carotid artery stenting in the post approval setting: timing, location, severity, and type. *Ann Surg* 2007;**246**:551–6; discussion 556–8.

182. du Mesnil de Rochemont R, Schneider S, Yan B, *et al.* Diffusion-weighted MR imaging lesions after filter-protected stenting of high-grade symptomatic carotid artery stenoses. *Am J Neuroradiol* 2006;**27**:1321–5.

183. Kastrup A, Groschel K, Nagele T, *et al.* Effects of age and symptom status on silent ischemic lesions after carotid stenting with and without the use of distal filter devices. *Am J Neuroradiol* 2008;**29**:608–12.

184. Maleux G, Demaerel P, Verbeken E, *et al.* Cerebral ischemia after filter-protected carotid artery stenting is common and cannot be predicted by the presence of substantial amount of debris captured by the filter device. *Am J Neuroradiol* 2006; **27**:1830–3.

185. Rosenkranz M, Fiehler J, Niesen W, et al. The amount of solid cerebral microemboli during carotid stenting does not relate to the frequency of silent ischemic lesions. *Am J Neuroradiol* 2006;**27**:157–61.

186. Ackerstaff RGA, Suttorp MJ, van den Berg JC, et al. Prediction of early cerebral outcome by transcranial Doppler monitoring in carotid bifurcation angioplasty and stenting. *J Vasc Surg* 2005;**41**:618–24.

187. Vos JA, van den Berg JC, Ernst SMPG, et al. Carotid angioplasty and stent placement: comparison of transcranial Doppler US data and clinical outcome with and without filtering cerebral protection devices in 509 patients. *Radiology* 2005;**234**:493–9.

188. Stingele R, Berger J, Alfke K, et al. Clinical and angiographic risk factors for stroke and death within 30 days after carotid endarterectomy and stent-protected angioplasty: a subanalysis of the SPACE study. *Lancet Neurol* 2008;**7**:216–22.

189. Howell M, Krajcer Z, Dougherty K, et al. Correlation of periprocedural systolic blood pressure changes with neurological events in high-risk carotid stent patients. *J Endovasc Ther: Official J Int Soc Endovasc Specialists.* 2002;**9**:810–16.

190. Groschel K, Ernemann U, Larsen J, et al. Preprocedural C-reactive protein levels predict stroke and death in patients undergoing carotid stenting. *Am J Neuroradiol* 2007;**28**:1743–6.

191. Mathur A, Roubin GS, Iyer SS, et al. Predictors of stroke complicating carotid artery stenting. *Circulation* 1998;**97**:1239–45.

192. Hobson RW, 2nd, Howard VJ, Roubin GS, et al. Carotid artery stenting is associated with increased complications in octogenarians: 30-day stroke and death rates in the CREST lead-in phase. *J Vasc Surg* 2004;**40**:1106–11.

193. Safian RD, Bresnahan JF, Jaff MR, et al. Protected carotid stenting in high-risk patients with severe carotid artery stenosis. *J Am Coll Cardiol* 2006;**47**:2384–9.

194. Qureshi AI, Luft AR, Janardhan V, et al. Identification of patients at risk for periprocedural neurological deficits associated with carotid angioplasty and stenting. *Stroke* 2000;**31**:376–82.

195. Gupta R, Abou-Chebl A, Bajzer CT, Schumacher HC, Yadav JS. Rate, predictors, and consequences of hemodynamic depression after carotid artery stenting. *J Am Coll Cardiol* 2006;**47**:1538–43.

196. Groschel K, Ernemann U, Schulz JB, et al. Statin therapy at carotid angioplasty and stent placement: effect on procedure-related stroke, myocardial infarction, and death. *Radiology* 2006;**240**:145–51.

197. Kaku Y, Yoshimura S-ichi, Kokuzawa J. Factors predictive of cerebral hyperperfusion after carotid angioplasty and stent placement. *Am J Neuroradiol* 2004;**25**:1403–8.

198. Abou-Chebl A, Reginelli J, Bajzer CT, Yadav JS. Intensive treatment of hypertension decreases the risk of hyperperfusion and intracerebral hemorrhage following carotid artery stenting. *Catheterization Cardiovasc Interventions.* 2007; **69**:690–6.

199. Cheung AT, Hobson RW 2nd. Hypertension in vascular surgery: aortic dissection and carotid revascularization. *Ann Emerg Med* 2008;**51**:S28–33.

200. Diehm N, Katzen BT, Dick F, et al. Influence of stent type on hemodynamic depression after carotid artery stent placement. *J Vasc Interventional Radiol* 2008;**19**:23–30.

201. Motamed C, Motamed-Kazerounian G, Merle JC, et al. Cardiac troponin I assessment and late cardiac complications after carotid stenting or endarterectomy. *J Vasc Surg* 2005;**41**:769–74.

202. Adams RJ, Chimowitz MI, Alpert JS, et al. Coronary risk evaluation in patients with transient ischemic attack and ischemic stroke: a scientific statement for healthcare professionals from the Stroke Council and the Council on Clinical Cardiology of the American Heart Association/American Stroke Association. *Circulation* 2003;**108**:1278–90.

203. Robbin ML, Lockhart ME, Weber TM, et al. Carotid artery stents: early and intermediate follow-up with Doppler US. *Radiology* 1997;**205**:749–56.

204. Lal BK, Hobson RW 2nd, Goldstein J, Chakhtoura EY, Duran WN. Carotid artery stenting: is there a need to revise ultrasound velocity criteria?. *J Vasc Surg* 2004;**39**:58–66.

205. Stanziale SF, Wholey MH, Boules TN, Selzer F, Makaroun MS. Determining in-stent stenosis of carotid arteries by duplex ultrasound criteria. *J Endovasc Ther* 2005;**12**:346–53.

206. Grant EG, Benson CB, Moneta GL, et al. Carotid artery stenosis: gray-scale and Doppler US diagnosis–Society of Radiologists in Ultrasound Consensus Conference. *Radiology* 2003;**229**:340–6.

207. Groschel K, Riecker A, Schulz JB, Ernemann U, Kastrup A. Systematic review of early recurrent stenosis after carotid angioplasty and stenting. *Stroke* 2005;**36**:367–73.

208. Levy EI, Hanel RA, Lau T, et al. Frequency and management of recurrent stenosis after carotid artery stent implantation. *J Neurosurg* 2005;**102**:29–37.

209. Wholey MH, Al-Mubarek N, Wholey MH. Updated review of the global carotid artery stent registry. *Catheter Cardiovasc Interv* 2003;**60**:259–66.

210. Wholey MH, Wholey MH, Tan WA, et al. A comparison of balloon-mounted and self-expanding stents in the carotid arteries: immediate and long-term results of more than 500 patients. *J Endovasc Ther* 2003; **10**:171–81.

211. Setacci C, de Donato G, Setacci F, et al. In-stent restenosis after carotid angioplasty and stenting: a challenge for the vascular surgeon. *Eur J Vasc Endovasc Surg* 2005;**29**:601–7.

212. Roubin GS, New G, Iyer SS, et al. Immediate and late clinical outcomes of carotid artery stenting in patients with symptomatic and asymptomatic carotid artery stenosis: a 5-year prospective analysis. *Circulation* 2001;**103**:532–7.

213. Qureshi AI, Knape C, Maroney J, Suri MF, Hopkins LN. Multicenter clinical trial of the NexStent coiled sheet stent in the treatment of extracranial carotid artery stenosis: immediate results and late clinical outcomes. *J Neurosurg* 2003;**99**:264–70.

214. Chakhtoura EY, Hobson RW, 2nd, Goldstein J, et al. In-stent restenosis after carotid angioplasty-stenting: incidence and management. *J Vasc Surg* 2001;**33**:220–5; discussion 225–6.

215. Lin PH, Zhou W, Guerrero MA, et al. Carotid artery stenting with distal

protection using the carotid wallstent and filterwire neuroprotection: single-center experience of 380 cases with midterm outcomes. *Vascularity* 2006;**14**:237–44.

216. Skelly CL, Gallagher K, Fairman RM, *et al*. Risk factors for restenosis after carotid artery angioplasty and stenting. *J Vasc Surg* 2006;**44**:1010–15.

217. Younis GA, Gupta K, Mortazavi A, *et al*. Predictors of carotid stent restenosis. *Catheterization Cardiovasc Interventions* 2007; **69**:673–82.

218. Shah QA, Georgiadis AL, Suri MF, Rodriguez GJ, Qureshi AI. Cutting balloon angioplasty for carotid in-stent restenosis: case reports and review of the literature. *J Neuroimaging* 2008;**18**:428–32.

219. Alberts MJ, Latchaw RE, Selman WR, *et al*. Recommendations for comprehensive stroke centers: a consensus statement from the Brain Attack Coalition. *Stroke* 2005;**36**: 1597–616.

220. Higashida RT, Meyers PM, Connors JJ, *et al*. Intracranial angioplasty & stenting for cerebral atherosclerosis: a position statement of the American Society of Interventional and Therapeutic Neuroradiology, Society of Interventional Radiology, and the American Society of Neuroradiology. *J Vasc Interv Radiol* 2005;**16**:1281–5.

221. Lee RK. A resident's primer of Medicare reimbursement in radiology. *J Am Coll Radiol* 2006;**3**:58–63.

222. International Carotid Stenting Study investigators, Ederle J, Dobson J, Featherstone RL, *et al*. Carotid artery stenting compared with endarterectomy in patients with symptomatic carotid stenosis (International Carotid Stenting Study): an interim analysis of a randomised controlled trial. *Lancet* 2010;**375**:985–97.

223. Bonati LH, Jongen LM, Haller S. *et al*. ICSS-MRI study group. New ischaemic brain lesions on MRI after stenting or endarterectomy for symptomatic carotid stenosis: a substudy of the International Carotid Stenting Study (ICSS). *Lancet Neurol*. 2010;**9**:353–62.

224. Carotid Stenting Trialists' Collaboration, Bonati LH, Dobson J, Algra A, *et al*. Short-term outcome after stenting versus endarterectomy for symptomatic carotid stenosis: a preplanned meta-analysis of individual patient data. *Lancet* 2010;**376**:1062–73.

Extracranial vertebral artery disease

Robert A. Taylor MD, Muhammad Zeeshan Memon MD and Adnan I. Qureshi MD

Introduction

Extracranial vertebral artery disease has been historically thought of as a relatively benign entity due to the capacity to develop collaterals from the contralateral vertebral artery and the capacity to reconstitute the artery from other arteries in the neck, such as the ascending cervical artery or deep cervical artery.[1] Fisher also claimed that vertebral origin atherosclerotic disease likely progresses slowly.[1] However, little rigorous data have been published on the natural history of extracranial vertebral artery disease. Most reports focus on posterior circulation strokes in general or focus on intracranial steno-occlusive disease.

The first reports of endovascular treatment of extracranial vertebral artery disease were published in 1981 with balloon angioplasty as the primary treatment modality.[2,3] Unlike the extracranial carotid artery, surgical accessibility to this site is difficult and has been associated with high peri-operative morbidity and mortality rates of up to 20%.[4] In patients who are refractory to medical therapy, endovascular therapy for steno-occlusive lesions is an increasingly utilized treatment option. The most common types of lesions found in the extracranial vertebral include atherosclerotic lesions and dissections. The endovascular therapy for extracranial vertebral steno-occlusive disease generally includes balloon angioplasty alone, stent placement alone or both.

Anatomical considerations

The extracranial vertebral artery has been classified into 3 segments, V1, V2 and V3 (see Fig. 7.1). The V1 segment is the segment between the origin and where it enters the foramen transversarium bony canal usually at the C6 vertebral body. This segment is located in soft tissue and can be tortuous in some patients. The V2 segment is between the C6 and C2 vertebral bodies where the vessel runs through the bony canals of the vertebral bodies. The V3 segment is between the foramen transversarium of the C2 vertebral body and where it enters the dura. The V4 segment is an intradural segment so is considered intracranial. The V1 and V4 segments are the most

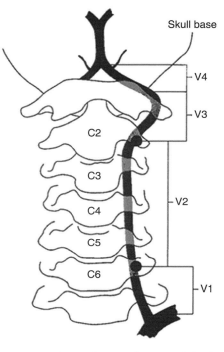

Fig. 7.1. The extracranial vertebral artery segments, V1, V2, and V3 are shown in relation to surrounding vertebral bodies and other anatomical structures.

prone to atherosclerotic disease, while the V2 and V3 segments are more prone to dissections.

One or both vertebral arteries can be hypoplastic (less than 2 mm in diameter), which has been reported to be present in 8% of cases in an early autopsy study.[5] Occasionally, a hypoplastic vertebral artery ends in the posterior inferior cerebellar artery (PICA). The left vertebral artery has been reported to arise from the aortic arch between the left common carotid artery and left subclavian artery in 6% of people.[6]

Potential collaterals

The extracranial vertebral artery may reconstitute in the setting of acute occlusion from a variety of potential collaterals. Typical potential collaterals may include the contralateral vertebral artery, occipital artery to vertebral artery, and ascending cervical artery or deep cervical artery to vertebral artery (see

---

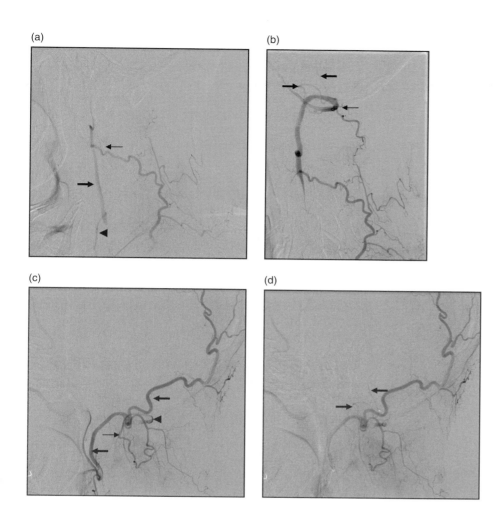

(a) (b) (c) (d)

Fig. 7.2. Potential collaterals to the extracranial vertebral artery. A 52-year-old man who presented with neck pain and a left posterior inferior cerebellar artery (PICA) territory infarction was found to have a left vertebral artery occlusion at the origin (not shown). Digital subtraction angiography from a left subclavian artery injection on the lateral projection (a) demonstrates reconstitution of the left vertebral artery V2 segment (thick arrow) by an ascending cervical artery collateral (thin arrow) and deep cervical artery collateral (arrowhead) vessels. Selective injection of the deep cervical artery demonstrates another small collateral vessels to the V3 vertebral artery segment (thin arrow) with filling of the distal left PICA (thick arrows). Digital subtraction angiography of a left occipital artery injection on the lateral projection (c) demonstrates the left occipital artery (thick arrows) with a small collateral vessel anastomosing with the distal V2 segment of the left vertebral artery (thin arrow). The V3 segment loop is seen to be filling slowly (arrowhead). Delayed images demonstrate slow filling of the left PICA (thick arrows).

Fig. 7.2). These collaterals may sometimes supply sufficient blood to the brain to prevent infarction in the setting of a proximal vertebral artery occlusion.

Clinical signs, symptoms, and underlying mechanisms

The most common clinical signs of posterior circulation ischemia include limb weakness, gait and limb ataxia, oculomotor palsies, and oropharyngeal dysfunction, but may also include vision loss, numbness, dizziness, vertigo, headache, nausea, and vomiting.[7] Patients most frequently present with a constellation of signs and symptoms and rarely just a single sign or symptom, such as isolated vertigo. Less than 1% of the patients in the New England Posterior Circulation Stroke Registry presented with just one sign or symptom.[8] The most common causes of posterior circulation strokes include embolism, large-artery atherosclerotic disease, small vessel disease, and arterial dissection.[8–11] Extracranial vertebral artery steno-occlusive disease may be caused by atherosclerotic lesions, compression by osteophytes, dissections, vessel kinking, and vessel kinking associated with head turning.

Atherosclerotic disease
Prevalence

An estimated 700 000 new or recurrent strokes occur each year in the US.[12] Since about 80% of those strokes are ischemic, about 20% of those ischemic strokes are in the posterior circulation,[7] and about 9% of all posterior circulation strokes are due to extracranial steno-occlusive disease.[13] An estimated 12 000 strokes per year are caused by extracranial vertebral artery steno-occlusive disease. While extracranial vertebral artery steno-occlusive disease of 50% or greater may be the cause of 9% of posterior circulation strokes, it may be found much more commonly, in about 30% of patients with posterior circulation strokes.[8] Extracranial vertebral artery steno-occlusive disease most commonly causes intra-arterial embolism, followed by a hemodynamic compromise resulting in stroke.[8,14,15]

Autopsy studies

Early autopsy studies in the 1960s by Fisher *et al.* evaluated atherosclerosis of the extracranial and intracranial vertebral and carotid arteries in 178 unselected cases.[5] The cause of death included atherosclerotic causes in at least 42 cases, including cerebral infarction in seven cases. Five extracranial vertebral artery occlusions were found, four at the origin and one at the C2–C5 segment, for a prevalence of 2.8%. The vertebral artery that was found to be occluded was generally the smaller one. Severe stenosis ($\geq$50%) of the extracranial vertebral arteries was found in 15 cases, for a prevalence of 8.4%.

Angiographic studies

The Joint Study of Extracranial Arterial Occlusion was a multi-center study that enrolled 4778 patients with signs and symptoms of ischemic cerebrovascular disease to undergo cerebral angiography between 1961 and 1965.[16] Stenosis of the V1 segment of 50% or greater was found in 18.4% of the patients in the right vertebral artery and 22.3% of patients in the left vertebral artery. Stenosis of the extracranial vertebral artery was about half as common as that of the extracranial carotid artery. Occlusions at the V1 segment were found in 4% of patients in the right vertebral artery and 5.7% of patients in the left vertebral artery. Eighty percent of the patients also had inflammation of the intracranial vessels, including V2–V4 vertebral segments. Stenosis of 50% or greater of the V2 or V3 segments was found in 5.4% of patients in the right vertebral artery and 5.6% of patients in the left vertebral artery. Occlusions of these segments were found in 3.2% on the right and 4.4% on the left.

Pathology

Fisher's autopsy study found plaques of the extracranial vertebral artery to be most commonly at the vertebral artery origin, but otherwise relatively evenly distributed throughout the extracranial vertebral artery.[5] Vertebral artery plaques were frequently annular and concentric, fibrous, and smooth with low incidence of ulceration or intramural hemorrhage. This morphological appearance was different from the extracranial carotid circulation where lesions were frequently calcified and ulcerated.

Natural history

The natural history of extracranial vertebral artery stenosis has not been well studied. Overall, the risk of ischemic stroke related to extracranial vertebral artery stenosis is less than that attributed to intracranial vertebral artery disease.

Moufarrij et al. followed 96 patients for an average of 4.6 years who had vertebral artery lesions of 50% or greater found on angiography for various indications.[17] Vertebral artery stenosis was most frequently located at the origin (93%). Eighteen patients were classified as symptomatic from vertebrobasilar transient ischemic attacks (TIAs), while the other 78 patients were found to have lesions on diagnostic workup for unrelated symptoms or signs mostly for asymptomatic carotid bruits, hemispheric TIAs or hemispheric strokes. In follow-up, possible vertebrobasilar TIAs occurred in 19 patients (19.8%) and strokes occurred in 23 patients (24%). Of the ischemic strokes, only two were in the vertebrobasilar

territory and were associated with coexistent basilar stenosis, while the rest were hemispheric and frequently due to carotid endarterectomy surgeries. The death rate was quite high, estimated at 40 deaths (41.7%). However, most deaths (52.5%) were cardiac related and only 8 (20%) were stroke related. The observed 5-year survival rate was 60% compared to 87% in a matched normal population. The authors conclude that vertebral artery origin lesions are associated with a low rate of brainstem infarction.

New England Posterior Circulation Registry

The New England Posterior Circulation Registry followed 407 consecutive patients with signs and symptoms of posterior circulation ischemia seen at New England Medical Center, Boston, MA.[8] Of these patients, 80 (20%) had severe stenosis or occlusion of the V1 segment. However, occlusive disease of the V1 segment was also associated with other potential mechanisms of stroke leading the authors to conclude that occlusive disease of the V1 segment is the primary mechanism in 9% of patients with vertebrobasilar ischemic strokes.[13] These patients had a high rate of stroke risk factors, including hypertension (70%), cigarette smoking (61%), coronary disease (54%), and diabetes mellitus (34%).

The study found that patients with V1 segment stenosis or occlusions also had a high rate of other potential mechanisms of stroke, such as intracranial stenosis or cardioembolism. Artery-to-artery embolism from V1 lesions was slightly more frequent than a hemodynamic mechanism. The study divided patients with extracranial vertebral artery disease ($n = 80$) into five groups.[13,18] The largest group (Group A) had 22 patients (27.5%) who likely had incidental extracranial vertebral artery stenosis, as they also had severe intracranial steno-occlusive disease that was felt to be more likely the cause of their ischemic stroke. Group B had 19 patients (24%) who likely had intra-arterial embolism from the extracranial vertebral artery stenosis. Group C had 20 patients (25%) who had multiple possible causes of the ischemic stroke including extracranial vertebral artery stenosis, cardiac source and/or intracranial branch disease. Group D had 13 patients (16%) who had hemodynamic mechanisms of brain ischemia and had multifocal steno-occlusive disease of both vertebral arteries and/or intracranial vessels. Group E consisted of six patients (7.5%) who had dissections of the V1 segment.

In Group B, symptomatic V1 lesions included mostly occlusions and very high-grade stenosis. Sites of emboli included most commonly the PICA (10 [53%] of 19 patients), followed by superior cerebellar artery (7 [37%] of 19 patients) and posterior cerebral artery (6 [32%] of 19 patients). Early outcomes were good with almost 90% of patients having no deficit or minor deficit on hospital discharge.[13,18]

Medical management

Randomized controlled clinical trials of best medical therapy specifically for symptomatic extracranial vertebral artery stenosis have not been performed. Recommendations have been extrapolated from stroke prevention treatment trials for non-cardioembolic sources of stroke and include antiplatelet agents, statins, antihypertensives, and other vascular risk factor interventions such as smoking cessation, glucose control, weight loss, exercise, and diet.[19]

Endovascular treatment of atherosclerotic lesions of the extracranial vertebral artery

Surgical reconstruction of V1 segment lesions has been associated with a high surgical morbidity in early reports of up to 20%.[4,20,21] Angioplasty and/or stent placement have been associated with a lower morbidity. We found 29 published reports (see Table 7.1) of extracranial vertebral artery angioplasty with or without stent placement and found a 30-day peri-procedure any stroke or death of 2.3% (16 out of 700 cases). However, these data are subject to publication bias since most are extrapolated from case series. Recurrent stroke and death rates at 1 year are inconsistently reported in the published case series so could not be compiled.

Primary angioplasty of the vertebral artery origin was the first described endovascular technique, but has been complicated by high rates of early vessel recoil and restenosis. Stent placement of the vertebral artery origin with balloon expandable stents has generally replaced angioplasty as the technique of choice because it achieves better immediate post-procedure lumen diameters (see Fig. 7.3). Although stents have reduced the rate of restenosis compared to primary angioplasty in the coronary literature,[22–24] this has not yet been shown in a convincing manner for the vertebral artery ostium. Stent placement of the vertebral artery ostium has been reported to have high rates of restenosis of 50% or greater, or up to 43% in one series.[25] Taylor et al. analyzed risk factors for restenosis in a cohort of 44 patients who underwent vertebral ostium stenting and also had angiographic follow-up.[26] They found that, similar to the coronary literature, the type of stent used affected the restenosis rates. The cobalt chromium stent (Vision, Abbott Vascular) had lower rates of restenosis than stainless steel stents (e.g., S670, Medtronic Vascular, Santa Rosa, CA). In addition, cigarette smoking was associated with a higher rate of restenosis. Drug-eluting stents are being investigated for use at the vertebral ostium to help reduce the high restenosis rates.

Embolic protection

Embolic strokes from vertebral artery angioplasty and stent placement procedures are relatively uncommon when compared to extracranial carotid artery stent placement. However, embolic signals may be detected on transcranial Doppler (TCD) monitoring during these procedures. In one study, 12 consecutive patients undergoing percutaneous transluminal angioplasty for subclavian and vertebral artery stenosis of atherosclerotic origin were studied using TCD monitoring before, during, and after angioplasty for 30 minutes at each time.[27] No embolic signals were detected in any patient before angioplasty.

During angioplasty, one embolic signal was detected immediately after balloon deflation in 1 of 12 patients. Several embolic signals were detected immediately after the procedure in 6 of 12 patients. These signals were detected despite the routine administration of antiplatelets and heparin. The clinical significance of these embolic signals is not fully understood.

A prospective study assessed the prevalence of asymptomatic microemboli in 52 consecutive patients with acute or recent vertebrobasilar ischemia within 48 hours after admission. TCD monitoring was performed according to established criteria for 20 minutes on each posterior cerebral artery.[15] Microembolic high-intensity transient signals characteristic of emboli were detected in ten patients (19%).

One study described 12 cases of vertebral origin stenting using distal protection (Filter EX; Boston Scientific).[28] Technical success of deployment of the device occurred in 11 cases. No strokes were seen in the 1 month peri-procedural period. The authors describe finding macroscopically visible debris in eight cases (large amounts in three devices and small amounts in five devices). However, retrieval of the embolic device may be difficult as the catheter may get trapped within the proximal margins of the stent as it hangs out into the subclavian artery. Despite these results, the use of embolic protection for vertebral origin stent placement is still not routine.

Technical aspects of endovascular treatment of vertebral artery disease
Patient selection

Stent placement is considered for patients with symptomatic vertebral artery origin stenosis of 50% or greater in severity. Previous investigators have recommended stent placement for vertebral artery stenosis in patients with ischemic symptoms refractory to antiplatelet treatment, or where recurrent stroke risk is considered increased due to either an incomplete circle of Willis, hypoplastic contralateral vertebral artery, or an anomalous vertebral artery circulation.[29,30] The severity of stenosis is similar to the criteria used for determining eligibility in the Stenting of Symptomatic Atherosclerotic Lesions in the Vertebral or Intracranial Arteries (SSYLVIA) trial.[31] The results of the study resulted in approval of NeuroLink stent (Guidant, Santa Clara, CA) for treatment of atherosclerotic disease of vertebral artery origin and intracranial stenosis under humanitarian use.

The percutaneous approach

A stable access to the extracranial vertebral artery can be difficult particularly with right vertebral artery procedures. The angulation between the vertebral artery origin and parent subclavian artery can also pose a difficult trajectory for entry of microwire and stent delivery devices. Therefore, the operator must decide between using a femoral or radial approach based on tortuosity of aorta and proximal vessels and angulation of the vertebral artery origin. For right

Table 7.1. Published reports of patients treated with angioplasty with or without stent placement at the VI vertebral artery segment

Series et al.	Study design	No of cases	Mean age (range)	Intervention	Type of stents	1 month any stroke/ death	Mean follow-up months	Stroke/ death at 1 year	Patients with recurrent TIA at 1 year	Restenosis rates
Motarjeme[32] 1982	Case series	11		Angioplasty	–	0	30	0	0	
Kachel[33] 1991	Case series	15	54	Angioplasty	–	0	58	0	0	
Higashida[34] 1993	Case series	33	NA	Angioplasty	–	0	12	1	0	1
Sampei[35] 1995	Case series	3	65(56–73)	Angioplasty	–	0		0	0	0
Storey[36] 1996	Case series	3	63(51–75)	Stent placement	BM	0	12	0	0	0
Fessler[4] 1998	Case series	5	63(45–76)	Stent placement	BM	0	9	0	0	0
Malek[37] 1999	Case series	13	65(47–82)	Stent placement	BM	2 (15%)	21	0	4	1
Chastain[38] 1999	Case series	50	63(23–86)	Stent placement	BM	2 (4%)	25	1	1	5
Mukherjee[39] 2001	Case series	12	72(63–81)	Stent placement	BM	0	6	0	0	1
Jenkins[40] 2001	Case series	32	67(38–85)	Stent placement	BM	0	11	0	1	1
Chiras[41] 2002	Case series	11	NA	PTA only = 2 Stent placement = 9	BM	0	12	0	1	1
Albuquerque[25] 2003	Case series	33	64 (49–81)	Stent placement	BM	1 (3%)	16	1	3	13
Cloud[42] 2003	Case series	14	56(39–71)	PTA only = 4 Stent placement = 10	BM	0	14	6	2	5
SSYLVIA[31] 2004	Non-randomized clinical trial	18	63(37–80)	Stent placement	BM	0	12	2	0	6
Janssens[43] 2004	Case series	16	53(38–70)	Angioplasty		0	30	0	1	3

Study	Type	N	Age	Treatment						
Hauth[44] 2004	Case series	12	62(49–74)	PTA only = 9 Stent placement = 3	BM	0	6	1	0	1
Ko[45] 2004	Case series	21	56(41–71)	Stent placement	BM = 20 DE = 1	0	25	3	0	3
Boulos[46] 2005	Case series	6	65(36–83)	Stent placement	BM	0	3	0	0	0
Hatano[47] 2005	Case series	101	71(46–84)	Stent placement	BM	0	3	0	2	8
Weber[48] 2005	Case series	36	61(44–75)	Stent placement	BM	0	11	2	1	10
Kantarci[49] 2005	Case series	12	62(48–77)	Stent placement	BM	2 (17%)	23	0	1	4
Qureshi[28] 2006	Case series	12	68(52–88)	Stent placement	BM = 10 DE = 3	0	1	0	0	0
Lin[50] 2006	Case series	80	72(54–91)	Stent placement	BM	3 (4%)	38	0	1	11
Dabus[51] 2006	Case series	25	67(57–84)	PTA only = 2 Stent placement = 23	BM	2 (8%)	24	0	5	5
Eberhardt[52] 2006	Case series	11	65	Stent placement	BM	0	13	0	1	1
(CAVATAS)[53] 2007	Randomized clinical trial	8	64(57–71)	PTA only = 2 Stent placement = 6	BM	0	54	3	2	3
Zavala-Alarcon[54] 2007	Case series	18	64(54–87)	Stent placement	BM = 6 DE = 18	0	14	3	3	1
Akins[55] 2008	Case series	12	64(44–80)	Stent placement	BM = 7 DE = 5	0	30	2	2	3
Siddiq[56] 2006	Case series	77	62(32–87)	Stent placement	BM	4 (5%)	9	2	12	19

Abbreviations used: PTA = Percutaneous transluminal angioplasty, BM = Bare metal, DE = Drug eluting.

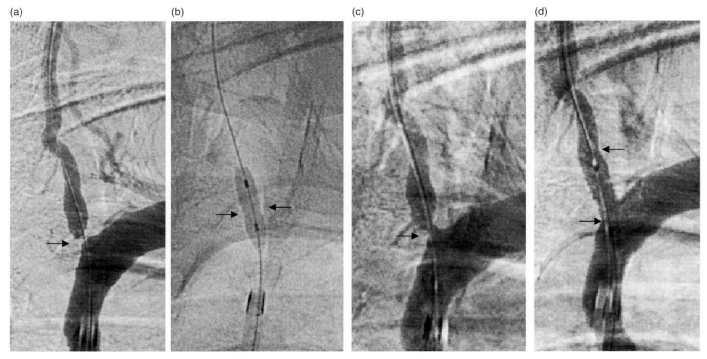

Fig. 7.3. Vessel recoil. A 51-year-old man with a history of chest radiation for Hodgkin's lymphoma had a left posterior inferior cerebellar artery infarction on medical therapy and was found to have a severe left vertebral ostium stenosis on angiography (a, arrow). Angioplasty with a Maverick 3.5 mm × 9 mm balloon was performed (b). The site of stenosis can be seen as mild waisting of the balloon (b, arrows). Post-angioplasty angiography shows significant recoil of the stenosis with persistent narrowing of greater than 50% (c). Stent placement using a Vision 4 mm × 12 mm balloon expandable stent was performed (proximal and distal stent margins demarked by arrows) (d). Immediate post-stent placement angiography shows no significant residual stenosis (d).

extracranial vertebral artery lesions, a serious consideration must be given to a radial approach.

Guidecatheter placement

Representative cases are presented in Figs. 7.3 to 7.8 highlighting various technical aspects of the procedure. Most extracranial vertebral artery procedures can be performed using a 6F guidecatheter. The guidecatheter can be introduced into the subclavian artery using a 0.035 inch guidewire in most circumstances but may require co-axial placement using a 5F 120 cm Simmons I catheter or advancement over an exchange length guidewire placed in position using a diagnostic catheter. The stability of the guidecatheter may be an issue because the distal end of the guidecatheter may have to be placed in the very proximal portion of the subclavian artery to allow access to the vertebral artery origin (which may originate from the proximal most portion of the subclavian artery). A 0.018 inch microwire that is advanced into the axillary artery through the guidecatheter may be used to create a support platform without compromising the lumen space to prevent concurrent passage of other devices. Another approach requires a long guide sheath that engages the origin of the subclavian artery to support guidecatheter placement through its lumen.

Morphological assessment of the vertebral artery origin

Most vertebral arteries originate from the posterior and medial aspect of the parent subclavian arteries. Adequate visualization of the point of origin may require complex projection and may not be possible in some patients. Therefore, the operator must carefully assess the value of various projections to determine the projection to use for traversing the origin. Vertebral artery origin can be tortuous, and a careful assessment of the tortuosity is required to decide on the segments that require to be covered with a stent.

Morphological assessment of the lesion

Most lesions in the vertebral artery origin are atherosclerotic in nature. However, dissections can also occur at similar locations. Certain aspects of the procedure may differ depending upon the underlying substrate (atherosclerosis vs dissection) such as the use of balloon angioplasty and choice of stents. The operator must review the demographic and clinical characteristics of the patient and supplement it with angiographic data. A lesion that extends beyond 10 mm after the origin of the vertebral artery or involves multiple segments distal to the origin lesion is unlikely to be atherosclerotic. Involvement of other extracranial vessels and lesion appearances may also provide diagnostic information. Therefore, careful visualization of other extracranial vessels need to be considered prior to performing the procedure.

Traversing the lesion

The microwire is used to engage the origin of the vertebral artery and advanced into the distal extracranial vertebral artery to provide adequate support for advancing the balloon catheter or stent delivery device across the lesion. The vertebral artery origin angulation can pose a challenge for engaging the origin with a microwire. A microcatheter with an angulated distal end may be required to facilitate the engagement of the vertebral origin. In difficult cases, a 4 F 120 cm angulated diagnostic catheter (e.g., Headhunter catheter) may be required to facilitate the engagement of the vertebral origin. The second challenge may be in advancing the microwire in the distal tortuous extracranial segments and may require microcatheter support to facilitate navigation.

Straightening the lesion segment

The stent delivery device or even the angioplasty balloon catheter may not traverse the lesion if the origin of the vertebral artery is very tortuous. The operator must decide on special strategies, preferably on initial angiographic assessment or following intra-procedural device failure, to straighten the initial vertebral artery segment for the procedure. There are two methods: (1) exchange the existing microwire for a stiffer 0.014 inch microwire using a microcatheter. The current balloon angioplasty catheter and stent delivery catheters require a microwire no greater than 0.014 inches; (2) place a support 0.018 inch microwire parallel to the existing microwire. The second microwire should be retracted prior to deployment of the stent to avoid entrapment between the stent and the vessel wall.

Placement of distal protection device

The value of placing a distal protection device in the vertebral artery during the procedure is not known. However, we have reported that the distal protection device (Filter EX™, Boston Scientific Corporation, Natick, MA) can be introduced through the lesion and deployed into the distal cervical segment of the vertebral artery. The deployment site must be in a segment of the vertebral artery that has a diameter large enough to allow adequate unfolding and relatively straight to allow proper alignment. After treatment of the stenosis, the distal protection device is retrieved using a 4-F angiographic catheter (MPA1-Tempo™4, length 125 cm, inner diameter 0.038 inch, Cordis Corporation, Miami, FL) in a contained format. This strategy was adopted after initial failure of using the retriever catheter provided by the manufacturers.

Choice of stent and stent sizes

The largest diameter of the vertebral artery that requires opposition of the stent is measured. The nominal diameter of the stent must exceed the vessel diameter. In our current practice, we use balloon expandable stents for treatment of vertebral artery origin stenosis. The choice is based on the large experience that exists with balloon expandable stents for this indication (see Table 7.2) and relatively precise deployment (that avoids excessive stent length overhanging in the subclavian artery). For vessels requiring a stent diameter of 3.5 mm or less, we prefer a drug-eluting stent such as either CYPHER® Sirolimus-eluting coronary stent (Cordis Corporation, Miami, FL), TAXUS® Express²™ Paclitaxel-eluting coronary stent (Boston Scientific Corporation, Natick, MA), ENDEAVOR® Zotarolimus-eluting coronary stent (Medtronic, Minneapolis, MN), or XIENCE®V Everolimus-eluting coronary stent (Abbott Vascular). According to the multi-society advisory panel, drug eluting stents should be avoided in patients who are undergoing preparation for percutaneous coronary intervention and are likely to require invasive or surgical procedures within the next 12 months. A consideration should be given to implantation of a bare-metal stent. For vessels requiring a stent diameter greater than 3.5 mm, we use a Multilink Vision coronary stent (Abbott Vascular), which is one of cobalt chromium stents (see Table 7.2). The ENDEAVOR® and XIENCE® stents are drug-eluting stents on a cobalt chromium stent platform that come in sizes larger than 3.5 mm, and may be an alternative. For adequately covering the proximal portion of the lesion, the proximal end of the stent may extend past the origin of the vertebral artery into the subclavian artery. An attempt must be made to limit the extent of the inevitable overhanging of the stent into the subclavian artery. The length of the stent must be selected to: (1) adequately cover the lesion; (2) consider the position of the distal end to avoid angulated or unopposed placement due to tortuosity or post-stenotic dilatation; and (3) adequately cover the proximal aspect of the lesion completely, possibly with some overhanging into the subclavian artery. Pre- or post-stent angioplasty is only performed in selected situations to provide the most optimal results. Primary angioplasty alone is avoided due to the high risk of recoil and dissections.

Choice of stent and stent sizes in stenosis related to dissections

An attempt should be made to determine if the dissection is acute or chronic based on the clinical presentation, magnetic resonance findings of thrombus within the wall (observed in acute dissections), or angiographic findings such as pseudo-aneurysm (observed in chronic dissections). Any angioplasty should be avoided in acute dissections if possible and self expanding stents alone can result in adequate expansion. Chronic dissections may require a concomitant angioplasty with self expanding stent for adequate results. Drug-eluting stents should be avoided in dissections because the drug will interfere with the natural recovery within the vessel wall. The procedure is described in more detail in Chapter 9.

Post-procedural management

A complete neurological examination is performed immediately as well as 24 hours after the procedure. Aspirin (325 mg daily) and clopidogrel (75 mg daily) are prescribed at discharge. The multi-society advisory panel stresses the

Table 7.2. Profiles of types of stents that may be used for treating vertebral ostium lesions

Stents (manufacturer)	Stent material, eluting drug	Minimum ID guide catheter	Diameters	Lengths*	Stent nominal pressure	Rated burst pressure
Multilink Vision® (Abbott Vascular)	Cobalt-chromium, non-drug eluting	0.056 inch (1.42 mm)	2.75 mm, 3.0 mm, 3.5 mm, 4.0 mm	8 mm, 12 mm,15 mm, 18 mm, 23 mm, 28 mm	9 atm	16 atm
Multi-Link Ultra® (Abbott Vascular)	Cobalt-chromium, non-drug eluting	0.066 inch (1.68 mm), 0.075 inch (1.91 mm) for 5.0 mm stent	4.5 mm, 5.0 mm	13 mm, 18 mm, 28 mm	9 atm	14 atm
Liberté® (Boston Scientific)	Stainless steel, non-drug eluting	0.058 inch (1.47 mm) or 0.066 inch for larger sizes	2.75 mm, 3.0 mm, 3.5 mm, 4.0 mm, 4.5 mm, 5.0 mm	8 mm, 12 mm,16 mm, 20 mm, 24 mm, 28 mm, 32 mm	9 atm	16–18 atm
Taxus® Express²™ (Boston Scientific)	Stainless steel, Paclitaxel	0.058 inch (1.47 mm) or 0.066 inch for larger sizes	2.25 mm, 2.5 mm, 2.75 mm, 3.0 mm, 3.5 mm	8 mm, 12 mm,16 mm, 20 mm, 24 mm, 28 mm, 32 mm	9 atm	18 atm
Cypher® Stent (Cordis)	Stainless steel, Sirolimus	0.056 inch, (1.42 mm)	2.5 mm, 2.75 mm, 3.0 mm, 3.5 mm	8 mm, 13 mm, 18 mm, 23 mm, 28 mm, 33 mm	11 atm	16 atm
Endeavor® (Medtronic)	Cobalt chromium, Zotarolimus	1.4 mm	2.25 mm, 2.5 mm, 2.75 mm, 3.0 mm, 3.5 mm, 4.0 mm	8–9 mm, 12 mm, 14–15 mm, 18 mm, 24 mm, 30 mm	9 atm	15–16 atm
Xience® V (Abbott Vascular)	Cobalt chromium, low-dose Everolimus	0.056 inch (1.42 mm)	2.5 mm, 2.75 mm, 3.0 mm, 3.5 mm, 4.0 mm	8 mm, 12 mm,15 mm, 18 mm, 23 mm, 28 mm	8–9 atm	16 atm

*not all lengths are necessarily available for each diameter size stent.

importance of 12 months of dual antiplatelet therapy after placement of a drug-eluting stent and educating the patient and healthcare providers about hazards of premature discontinuation. The panel also recommends postponing elective surgery for 1 year, and if surgery cannot be deferred, considering the continuation of aspirin during the perioperative period in high-risk patients with drug-eluting stents.

Dissections and other abnormalities

Extracranial vertebral artery dissections are more common in the V2 or V3 segment than the V1 segment. In the New England Posterior Circulation Registry, only four out of 407 (1%) patients had a dissection of the V1 segment as the suspected cause of the stroke. Current recommendations for the treatment of vertebral dissections include either antiplatelet agents or anticoagulation. Some authors have advocated anticoagulation for the treatment of acute vertebral artery occlusions to prevent stump emboli. Endovascular treatment

of vertebral artery dissection may be considered for patients who fail medical therapy, have hypoperfusion as the cause of their symptoms and other potentially high risk angiographic features (see chapter on dissections). Stents placed in the V2 vertebral artery segment are susceptible to external compression of the vertebral bodies and foramen during neck rotations. Therefore, it is best to avoid balloon-expandable stents in this location because external compression may permanently bend the stent inward. Instead, self-expandable stents maintain constant radial force and will return to their previous configuration after transient external compression (see Fig. 7.4).

Recommendations from professional societies

The American Stroke Association/American Heart Association Guidelines for the prevention of ischemic stroke and transient ischemic attack recommend that endovascular treatment of

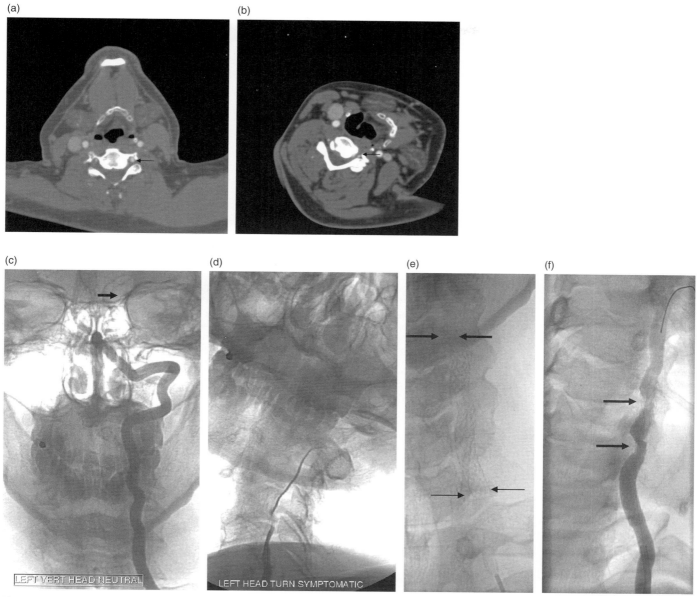

Fig. 7.4. A 40-year-old man after a motor vehicle accident presented with recurrent episodes of lightheadedness associated with head turning to the left that gradually increased in severity over 3 years. The more severe episodes were associated with ataxia followed by loss of consciousness. Computed tomographic (CT) angiography of the neck with the head in the neutral position (a) demonstrates a dominant left vertebral artery (arrow). After head turning to the left (b), the left vertebral artery is reduced in caliber (arrow) suggestive of external compression of this artery with head turning. Left vertebral artery injection with the head in the neutral position demonstrates a widely patent left vertebral artery (c). Repeat injection of the left vertebral artery with head turning to the left demonstrates occlusion of the left vertebral artery at the V2 segment (d). Overlapping self-expandable Xpert® stents (Abbott) were placed at the site of suspected external compression (e) thick arrows denote the distal stent margin and thin arrows denote the proximal stent margin. Injection of the left vertebral artery after stent placement with the head turned to the left demonstrates some external compression of the stent ((f) thick arrows) but improved flow to the distal vertebral artery. With the head back in the neutral position, the stents maintain their tubular shape and are not permanently altered by the external compression (not shown). The patient's symptoms improved and he has not required surgical decompression of the left vertebral artery, which may still be performed if needed. (Images courtesy of Dr. Ramu Tummula, Univeristy of Minnesota, Department of Neurosurgery.)

patients with symptomatic extracranial vertebral artery stenosis may be considered when patients are having symptoms despite medical therapies (antithrombotics, statins, and other treatments for risk factors) (Class IIb – usefulness/efficacy is less well established by evidence or opinion, Level C – expert opinion or case studies).[19] This is the same class/level of evidence status as the endovascular treatment of intracranial arterial disease. These guidelines also state that long-term follow-up data are limited, and further randomized studies are needed.

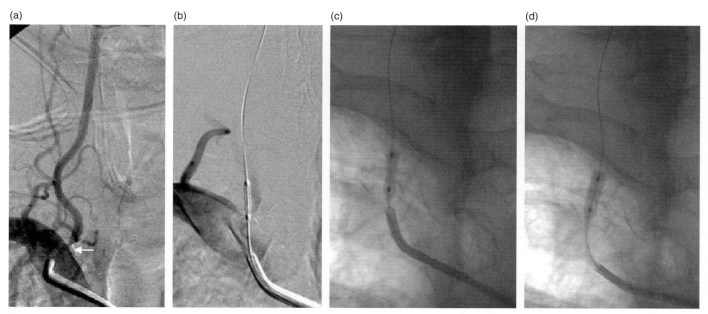

Fig. 7.5. Technical aspects of vertebral ostium stenting. Angiography over the neck with the catheter in the right subclavian artery shows a severe right vertebral ostium stenosis ((a) arrow)). Through a 5 French MPD envoy, a Synchro 0.014 inch wire and J-shaped Prowler 14 microcatheter were used to cross the right vertebral ostium lesion. A Luge 0.014 inch exchange length wire was left across the stenosis and a Vision 3 mm × 8 mm balloon expandable stent was positioned at the site of the stenosis (b). The stent was pulled a bit more proximally and the balloon was gradually inflated. The stent is seen midway in expansion (c). The marker bands mark the proximal and distal ends of the stent and the balloon can be seen to inflate a few millimeters beyond the stent margins (c) and (d). Full expansion of the balloon and stent at nominal pressure is shown (d). The balloon was deflated and removed from the catheter.

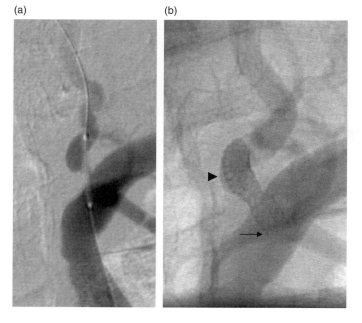

Fig. 7.6. Stent overhang. A focal left vertebral ostium stenosis was crossed with a 0.014 inch wire and a Vision 3.5 mm × 15 mm balloon expandable stent was positioned at the site of the stenosis (a). There is some post-stenotic dilatation and distal tortuosity of the vertebral artery which the exchange wire has partially straightened out (b). After deployment of the stent, significant stent overhang into the left subclavian artery is seen (arrow) and a gap between the stent and vessel wall is also seen (arrowhead). This demonstrates that choosing a stent that is too long for the lesion may lead to excessive stent overhang into the subclavian artery. Stent overhang will lead to difficulties catheterizing the vessel again if needed in the future, but the long-term clinical effect is still unknown. Deploying too long of a stent within the tortuous segment of the vertebral artery can potentially lead to vessel kinking.

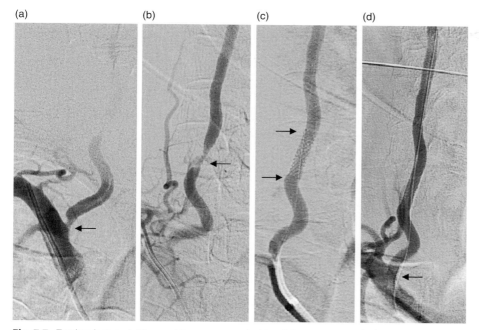

Fig. 7.7. Tandem lesions. A 58-year-old man presented with a right posterior cerebral artery watershed stroke in the setting of a chronic right internal carotid artery occlusion and left vertebral artery occlusion. Angiography shows a right vertebral ostium stenosis in the early phase ((a) arrow) followed by a distal V1 segment tandem severe stenosis ((b) arrow). After pre-dilation angioplasty of both lesions, a Driver® (Medtronic) 4 mm × 15 mm balloon-expandable stent was deployed at the distal lesion first ((c) arrows demarcate the stent). This stent was chosen for ease of trackability of the stent to the lesion compared to other balloon-expandable stents. The distal lesion is treated first in order to avoid difficulty passing one stent through the more proximal stent, especially if there would be problems with stent overhang into the subclavian artery. A Liberté® (Boston Scientific) 4 mm × 8 mm balloon expandable stent was then deployed at the ostium lesion ((d) arrow). Final angiographic images demonstrate no significant stenosis of either lesion (d).

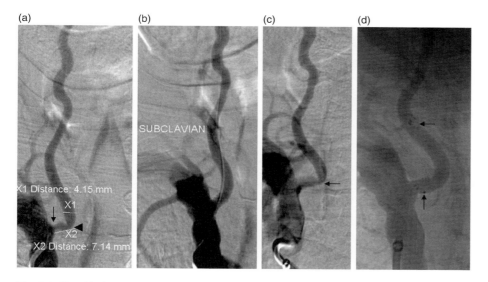

Fig. 7.8. Vessel kinking. A 62-year-old woman presented with a right parietal watershed stroke and was found to have a chronic right internal carotid artery occlusion with primary collaterals to the right hemisphere across the right posterior communicating artery. Both vertebral arteries had lesions with severe stenosis. Computed tomographic perfusion with diamox challenge demonstrated limited cerebral reserve in the left hemisphere. It was felt the cause of the stroke was hemodynamic compromise and the patient underwent stent placement in a right vertebral artery ostium lesion. Contrast injection of the right subclavian artery demonstrates a right vertebral ostium stenosis ((a) arrow) followed by a vessel kink ((a) arrowhead). A Vision 4 mm × 8 mm balloon expandable stent was deployed at the site of stenosis with apparent resolution of the stenosis and kink (b). However, after removal of the exchange wire the vessel is shown to develop the kink again ((c) arrow). The right vertebral artery was reselected with the wire and a Neuroform 4.5 mm × 20 mm self-expandable stent was deployed across the kink with resolution of the kink after the exchange wire was removed (d). The proximal and distal marker bands of the Neuroform stent are shown with arrows.

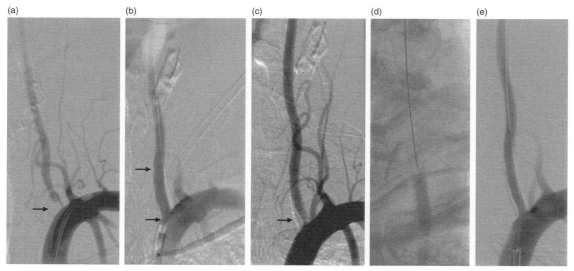

Fig. 7.9. In-stent restenosis. A 49-year-old man presented with acute dizziness, nausea, vomiting, and neck pain. Magnetic resonance (MR) imaging showed bilateral cerebellar strokes and MR angiography was suggestive for vertebral artery ostium stenosis. Cerebral angiogram showed a hypoplastic right vertebral artery and a high-grade stenosis of the left vertebral artery ostium (a). Due to the high-grade nature of this lesion and hypoplastic contralateral vertebral artery, it was decided to treat this lesion Pre-dilation angioplasty was performed with a 2.5 mm × 9 mm coronary balloon, followed by placement of a Vision 4 mm × 15 mm balloon-expandable stent (b). Six-month routine follow-up angiogram showed severe in-stent stenosis at the vessel origin (c). This lesion was then treated with an Angiosculpt 3.5 mm × 10 mm balloon (AngioScore, Inc, Fremont, CA), which was inflated to nominal pressure (d). Immediate post-angioplasty run shows significant improvement in the lumen diameter (e). The Angiosculpt balloon has a nitinol scoring element on the surface of a semi-compliant balloon that is supposed to facilitate uniform dilation of the plaque at lower inflation pressures with lower rates of vessel dissection. Other types of balloons that may be used for in-stent restenosis at this location include a high-pressure non-compliant coronary balloon, such as Powersail® (Guidant Corp), or a cutting balloon, which has 3–4 blades that protrude slightly out of the confines of the balloon to facilitate the angioplasty.

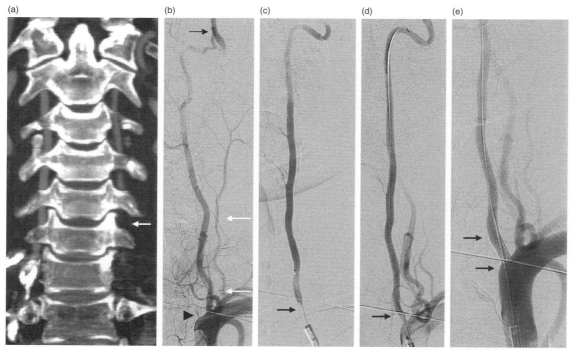

Fig. 7.10. Vertebral artery occlusion. A 52-year-old man presented with left-sided neck pain followed by a basilar artery embolism that was successfully lysed with intra-arterial thrombolytic treatment. He was found to have a left vertebral artery occlusion and was placed on anticoagulation and aspirin. He subsequently had another posterior circulation ischemic stroke event 5 days later. Computed tomographic (CT) angiogram (a) of the neck demonstrates contrast filling the left vertebral artery above the C5 vertebral body (arrow), but not below this level. Angiography from the left subclavian artery injection (b) demonstrates a left vertebral artery occlusion with reconstitution of the vessel via deep cervical artery collaterals (arrow). The left vertebral artery ostium is seen as a small whisp of flow ((b) arrowhead). The left vertebral artery was successfully catheterized with a Transcend EX 0.014 inch wire and SL-10 microcatheter. The microcatheter was placed just past the ostium and a microcatheter injection was performed demonstrating a normal V1 segment except for a focal ostium stenosis (c). After angioplasty of the vertebral ostium, a run from the left subclavian artery now demonstrates flow to the left vertebral artery (d). An Endeavor® (Medtronic) 4 mm × 9 mm drug-eluting stent was placed at the ostium and a final run demonstrates normal flow through the previously occluded left vertebral artery (e). Six-month follow-up angiogram showed no restenosis (not shown).

References

1. Fisher CM. Occlusion of the vertebral arteries causing transient basilar symptoms. *Arch Neurol* 1970;**22**:13–19.

2. Motarjeme A, Keifer JW, Zuska AJ. Percutaneous transluminal angioplasty of the vertebral arteries. *Radiology* 1981;**139**:715–17.

3. Schutz H, Yeung HP, Chiu MC, *et al.* Dilatation of vertebral-artery stenosis. *N Engl J Med* 1981;**304**:732.

4. Fessler RD, Wakhloo AK, Lanzino G, *et al.* Stent placement for vertebral artery occlusive disease: preliminary clinical experience. *Neurosurg Focus* 1998;**5**:e15.

5. Fisher CM, Gore L, Okabe N, White PD. Atherosclerosis of the carotid and vertebral arteries-extracranial and intracranial. *J Neuropathol Exp Neurol* 1965;**24**:455–76.

6. Newton TH, Mani RL. The vertebral artery. In: Newton TH, Potts DG, eds. *Radiology of the Skull and Brain.* Vol. **2**. Saint Louis: Mosby, 1974:1659–709.

7. Savitz SI, Caplan LR. Vertebrobasilar disease. *N Engl J Med* 2005;**352**:2618–26.

8. Caplan LR, Wityk RJ, Glass TA, *et al.* New England Medical Center Posterior Circulation registry. *Ann Neurol* 2004;**56**:389–98.

9. Bogousslavsky J, Van Melle G, Regli F. The Lausanne Stroke Registry: analysis of 1,000 consecutive patients with first stroke. *Stroke.* 1988;**19**:1083–92.

10. Moulin T, Tatu L, Vuillier F, *et al.* Role of a stroke data bank in evaluating cerebral infarction subtypes: patterns and outcome of 1,776 consecutive patients from the Besancon stroke registry. *Cerebrovasc Dis* 2000;**10**:261–71.

11. Vemmos KN, Takis CE, Georgilis K, *et al.* The Athens stroke registry: results of a five-year hospital-based study. *Cerebrovasc Dis* 2000;**10**:133–41.

12. Broderick J, Brott T, Kothari R, *et al.* The Greater Cincinnati/Northern Kentucky Stroke Study: preliminary first-ever and total incidence rates of stroke among blacks. *Stroke* 1998;**29**:415–21.

13. Wityk RJ, Chang HM, Rosengart A, *et al.* Proximal extracranial vertebral artery disease in the New England Medical Center Posterior Circulation Registry. *Arch Neurol* 1998;**55**:470–8.

14. Nedeltchev K, Remonda L, Do DD, *et al.* Acute stenting and thromboaspiration in basilar artery occlusions due to embolism from the dominating vertebral artery. *Neuroradiology* 2004;**46**:686–91.

15. Koennecke HC, Mast H, Trocio SS, Jr., *et al.* Microemboli in patients with vertebrobasilar ischemia: association with vertebrobasilar and cardiac lesions. *Stroke* 1997;**28**:593–6.

16. Hass WK, Fields WS, North RR, *et al.* Joint study of extracranial arterial occlusion. *II. Arteriography, techniques, sites, and complications. JAMA* 1968;**203**:961–8.

17. Moufarrij NA, Little JR, Furlan AJ, *et al.* Vertebral artery stenosis: long-term follow-up. *Stroke* 1984;**15**:260–3.

18. Caplan L. Posterior circulation disease: clinical findings, diagnosis and management. *Blackwell Science,* 1996:198–230.

19. Sacco RL, Adams R, Albers G *et al.* Guidelines for prevention of stroke in patients with ischemic stroke or transient ischemic attack: a statement for healthcare professionals from the American Heart Association/American Stroke Association Council on Stroke: co-sponsored by the Council on Cardiovascular Radiology and Intervention: the American Academy of Neurology affirms the value of this guideline. *Stroke* 2006;**37**:577–617.

20. Thevenet A, Ruotolo C. Surgical repair of vertebral artery stenoses. *J Cardiovasc Surg (Torino).* 1984;**25**:101–10.

21. Berguer R, Flynn LM, Kline RA, Caplan L. Surgical reconstruction of the extracranial vertebral artery: management and outcome. *J Vasc Surg* 2000;**31**:9–18.

22. Macaya C, Serruys PW, Ruygrok P, *et al.* Continued benefit of coronary stenting versus balloon angioplasty: one-year clinical follow-up of Benestent trial. Benestent Study Group. *J Am Coll Cardiol* 1996;**27**:255–61.

23. Serruys PW, de Jaegere P, Kiemeneij F, *et al.* A comparison of balloon-expandable-stent implantation with balloon angioplasty in patients with coronary artery disease. Benestent Study Group. *N Engl J Med* 1994; **331**:489–95.

24. Fischman DL, Leon MB, Baim DS, *et al.* A randomized comparison of coronary-stent placement and balloon angioplasty in the treatment of coronary artery disease. Stent Restenosis Study Investigators. *N Engl J Med* 1994; **331**:496–501.

25. Albuquerque FC, Fiorella D, Han P, *et al.* A reappraisal of angioplasty and stenting for the treatment of vertebral origin stenosis. *Neurosurgery* 2003;**53**:607–14.

26. Taylor RA, Siddiq F, Suri MF, *et al.* Risk factors for in-stent restenosis after vertebral ostium stenting. *J Endovasc Ther* 2008;**15**:203–12.

27. Sawada M, Hashimoto N, Nishi S, Akiyama Y. Detection of embolic signals during and after percutaneous transluminal angioplasty of subclavian and vertebral arteries using transcranial Doppler ultrasonography. *Neurosurgery.* 1997;**41**:535–40.

28. Qureshi AI, Kirmani JF, Harris-Lane P, *et al.* Vertebral artery origin stent placement with distal protection: technical and clinical results. *Am J Neuroradiol* 2006;**27**:1140–5.

29. Caplan LR. Atherosclerotic vertebral artery disease in the neck. *Curr Treatment Options in Cardiovasc Med* 2003;**5**:251–6.

30. Qureshi AI. Ten years of advances in neuroendovascular procedures. *J Endovasc Ther* 2004;**11** Suppl 2:II1–4.

31. Stenting of Symptomatic Atherosclerotic Lesions in the Vertebral or Intracranial Arteries (SSYLVIA): study results. *Stroke* 2004;**35**:1388–92.

32. Motarjeme A, Keifer JW, Zuska AJ. Percutaneous transluminal angioplasty of the brachiocephalic arteries. *Am J Roentgenol* 1982;**138**:457–62.

33. Kachel R, Basche S, Heerklotz I, *et al.* Percutaneous transluminal angioplasty (PTA) of supra-aortic arteries especially the internal carotid artery. *Neuroradiology* 1991;**33**:191–4.

34. Higashida RT, Tsai FY, Halbach VV, *et al.* Transluminal angioplasty for atherosclerotic disease of the vertebral and basilar arteries. *J Neurosurg* 1993;**78**:192–8.

35. Sampei K, Hashimoto N, Kazekawa K, Yoshimura S. Autoperfusion balloon catheter for treatment of vertebral artery stenosis. *Neuroradiology* 1995;**37**:561–3.

36. Storey GS, Marks MP, Dake M, *et al.* Vertebral artery stenting following percutaneous transluminal angioplasty. Technical note. *J Neurosurg* 1996; **84**:883–7.

37. Malek AM, Higashida RT, Phatouros CC, *et al.* Treatment of posterior

circulation ischemia with extracranial percutaneous balloon angioplasty and stent placement. *Stroke* 1999;**30**:2073–85.

38. Chastain HD, 2nd, Campbell MS, Iyer S, *et al.* Extracranial vertebral artery stent placement: in-hospital and follow-up results. *J Neurosurg* 1999;**91**:547–52.

39. Mukherjee D, Roffi M, Kapadia SR, *et al.* Percutaneous intervention for symptomatic vertebral artery stenosis using coronary stents. *J Invasive Cardiol* 2001;**13**:363–6.

40. Jenkins JS, White CJ, Ramee SR, *et al.* Vertebral artery stenting. *Catheter Cardiovasc Interv* 2001;**54**:1–5.

41. Chiras J, Vallee JN, Spelle L, *et al.* [Endoluminal dilatations and stenosis of symptomatic vertebral arteries]. *Rev Neurol (Paris)* 2002;**158**:51–7.

42. Cloud GC, Crawley F, Clifton A, *et al.* Vertebral artery origin angioplasty and primary stenting: safety and restenosis rates in a prospective series. *J Neurol Neurosurg Psychiatry* 2003;**74**:586–90.

43. Janssens E, Leclerc X, Gautier C, *et al.* Percutaneous transluminal angioplasty of proximal vertebral artery stenosis: long-term clinical follow-up of 16 consecutive patients. *Neuroradiology* 2004;**46**:81–4.

44. Hauth EA, Gissler HM, Drescher R et al. Angioplasty or stenting of extra- and intracranial vertebral artery stenoses. *Cardiovasc Intervent Radiol* 2004;**27**:51–7.

45. Ko YG, Park S, Kim JY, *et al.* Percutaneous interventional treatment of extracranial vertebral artery stenosis with coronary stents. *Yonsei Med J* 2004;**45**:629–34.

46. Boulos AS, Agner C, Deshaies EM. Preliminary evidence supporting the safety of drug-eluting stents in neurovascular disease. *Neurol Res* 2005;**27** Suppl 1:S95–102.

47. Hatano TT, OginoE, AoyamaT, Nakakuki T, *Murakami,. M. Stenting of vertebrobasilar artery stenosis. Acta Neurochir (Suppl).* 2005; **94**:137–41.

48. Weber W, Mayer TE, Henkes H, *et al.* Efficacy of stent angioplasty for symptomatic stenoses of the proximal vertebral artery. *Eur J Radiol* 2005; **56**:240–7.

49. Kantarci F, Mihmanli I, Albayram MS, *et al.* Follow-up of extracranial vertebral artery stents with Doppler sonography. *Am J Roentgenol* 2006;**187**:779–87.

50. Lin YH, Liu YC, Tseng WY, *et al.* The impact of lesion length on angiographic restenosis after vertebral artery origin stenting. *Eur J Vasc Endovasc Surg* 2006;**32**:379–85.

51. Dabus G, Gerstle RJ, Derdeyn CP, *et al.* Endovascular treatment of the vertebral artery origin in patients with symptoms of vertebrobasilar ischemia. *Neuroradiology* 2006;**48**:917–23.

52. Eberhardt O, Naegele T, Raygrotzki S, *et al.* Stenting of vertebrobasilar arteries in symptomatic atherosclerotic disease and acute occlusion: case series and review of the literature. *J Vasc Surg* 2006;**43**:1145–54.

53. Coward LJ, McCabe DJ, Ederle J, *et al.* Long-term outcome after angioplasty and stenting for symptomatic vertebral artery stenosis compared with medical treatment in the Carotid And Vertebral Artery Transluminal Angioplasty Study (CAVATAS): a randomized trial. *Stroke* 2007;**38**:1526–30.

54. Zavala-Alarcon E, Emmans L, Cecena F, *et al.* Percutaneous vertebral artery intervention: a necessary tool in every interventional cardiologist armamentarium. *Cardiovasc Revasc Med* 2007;**8**:107–13.

55. Akins PT, Kerber CW, Pakbaz RS. Stenting of vertebral artery origin atherosclerosis in high-risk patients: bare or coated? A single-center consecutive case series. *J Invas Cardiol.* 2008;**20**:14–20.

56. Siddiq F, Taylor R, Lee K, *et al.* Cobalt chromium stenting for the ostium of vertebral artery stenosis. *Congress of Neurological Surgeons Meeting.* 2006; Chicago, IL.

Intracranial stenosis

Farhan Siddiq MD, Muhammad Z. Memon MD, Adnan I. Qureshi MD and Camilo R. Gomez MD

Intracranial stenosis affects the proximal segments of the vessels that form the circle of Willis as well as the basilar and vertebral arteries and the petrous and cavernous segments of the internal carotid artery (ICA). Distal intracranial stenosis is encountered less commonly.

Incidence and prevalence

Population-based autopsy series have shown an average rate of atherosclerosis in the circle of Willis of 36%–47% among subjects in the fourth decade of life which increases to 75%–97% in the sixth decade.[1–4] Thirty percent of patients may have atherosclerotic changes in the intracranial vessels as early as in their second decade of life.[1] Using transcranial Doppler (TCD) ultrasound, Wong et al.[5] found that 13% of patients with one vascular risk factor had middle cerebral artery (MCA) stenosis. The prevalence increased up to four-fold among patients with more vascular risk factors. The Northern Manhattan Stroke Study, a large population-based analysis, indicated that intracranial atherosclerotic disease may underlie up to 8%–10% of all strokes.[6] Other large hospital-based studies have reported rates of symptomatic intracranial disease of 5%–8% among patients with ischemic stroke.[7,8]

Pathology of atherosclerotic lesions: quantification, characterization, vessel size determinations

Intracranial stenosis is a term used interchangeably with intracranial atherosclerosis. Intracranial atherosclerosis consists of atherosis (intra and extra-cellular lipid deposition) and sclerosis (fibrosis, reduced compliance, and endothelial dysfunction) of the vessel wall.[9,10] However, it should be noted that lumen narrowing (i.e., stenosis) may have other underlying pathology. Stenotic lesions have been described in the absence of cardiovascular risk factors in young patients[11] and also in patients with sickle cell disease and Moya Moya syndrome.[12,13] It remains unclear whether predominantly fibrotic narrowing of the vessel is the underlying cause of such lesions.

The conventional method of quantitating the severity of intracranial stenosis requires measurement of the lumen diameter at the site of maximal stenosis and expressing it as a ratio to the proximal vessel diameter.[14] Hemodynamically significant intracranial stenosis is defined as the presence of an atherosclerotic lesion that results in angiographically visible lumen reduction of 50% or more according to the method described above. However, percent area stenosis may be more clinically relevant.[15] This can be measured using a densitometric technique,[16] which is currently under investigation.

Mori et al.[17] first described the characteristics of various intracranial lesions based on catheter angiography (Table 8.1). They further suggested that therapeutic options and clinical as well as radiographic outcomes may differ among various lesion types.

Pathophysiology of ischemic stroke related to intracranial atherosclerosis

Several mechanisms have been proposed for ischemic stroke caused by intracranial atherosclerotic disease: hemodynamic restriction, thrombotic occlusion, and distal embolization. Hemodynamic restriction of the regional cerebral blood flow (rCBF) accounts for a large number of ischemic events attributed to intracranial stenosis.[18,19] Naritomi et al.[20] found normal rCBF in patients with less than 50% stenosis involving the MCA. Patients with 50%–74% stenosis had decreased flow on conventional angiography but rCBF was found to be normal by ^{133}Xe inhalation computed tomographic (CT) scan. Significant restriction of the rCBF detected with catheter angiography and ^{133}Xe CT scan was observed in patients with stenosis of 75% or greater. These patients also had larger areas of ischemic strokes in border-zone (subcortical and cortical) and cortical regions. Mazighi et al.[21] demonstrated that there was significant association between hemodynamically significant stenosis and recurrent stroke and transient ischemic attack in the territory of the stenotic artery.

Thrombotic occlusion at the site of stenosis, due to plaque rupture and direct occlusion of penetrating vessels by overlying

Table 8.1. Types of lesions in the intracranial arteries[17]

Type A	Type B	Type C
• Discrete, < 5 mm length	• Tubular, 5–10 mm length	• Diffuse, > 1 cm length
• Concentric	• Eccentric (≥ 90% diameter stenosis)	• Excessive tortuosity of proximal segment
• Eccentric (> 70%, < 90% diameter stenosis)	• Moderate tortuosity of proximal segment	• Extremely angulated segment ≥ 90°
• Readily accessible	• Moderately angulated segment ≥ 45°, < 90°	• Total occlusion > 3 months
• Smooth contour	• Irregular contour	• Inability to protect major side branches
• Little or no calcification	• Moderate to heavy calcification	
• Less than totally occlusive	• Total occlusion < 3 months	
• No major branch involvement	• Bifurcation lesions requiring double guide-wires	
• Absence of thrombus	• Some thrombus present	
• Nonangulated segment <45°		

plaque, also causes ischemic stroke in the distribution of the affected artery.[22–24] In situ thrombosis followed by acute artery-to-artery embolic phenomena is another mechanism causing ischemic stroke related to intracranial stenosis. Segura et al.[7] reported the results of transcranial Doppler scans performed in 387 patients with acute stroke. Microembolic signals were detected in 36% of the patients in the vascular distribution of symptomatic intracranial atherosclerotic disease patients during the acute phase. The prevalence of microemboli was very low in the chronic phase and microemboli were not detected in asymptomatic intracranial atherosclerosis patients.

Risk factors for intracranial atherosclerosis

Both frequency and severity of intracranial atherosclerosis increases with advancing age.[1] Race and ethnicity are significant risk factors for intracranial atherosclerotic disease.[1] The prevalence of intracranial stenosis is higher in Asians, African-Americans, and Hispanics.[8,25,26] Hypertension, diabetes mellitus, hypercholesterolemia, and cigarette smoking have also been identified as independent risk factors for intracranial stenosis.[6,27–30] Elevated blood pressure and hyperlipidemia are associated with an increased risk of stroke and other major vascular events in patients with symptomatic intracranial stenosis.[31] Socioeconomic factors may also play a role. In one autopsy series, women residing in indigent areas and men residing in urban areas had higher prevalence of intracranial stenosis.[32]

Natural history of intracranial stenosis

Several studies have identified a high rate of recurrent stroke and death among medically treated patients with symptomatic intracranial stenosis. Among the 164 patients enrolled in the Extracranial–Intracranial (EC–IC) Bypass Study treated medically, recurrent stroke or transient ischemic attack (TIA) occurred at a rate of 12% per year during the 42-month follow-up period.[33] The ipsilateral recurrent stroke rate was 8% per year among patients with middle cerebral artery stenosis.[24] In the retrospective Warfarin vs. Aspirin in Symptomatic Intracranial Disease (WASID) study,[34] an ipsilateral recurrent stroke rate of 8% and 18% per year for ipsilateral strokes was observed in patients treated with warfarin and aspirin, respectively. Thijs et al.[35] reported on 52 patients with symptomatic intracranial stenosis of whom 29 patients (56%) had an ischemic event while receiving either an antiplatelet agent (n = 16), warfarin (n = 9), or heparin (n = 4). In the multivariate model, older age was an independent factor associated with recurrent ischemic events. Recurrent TIAs, non-fatal or fatal stroke, or death occurred in 15 of 29 patients (52%) who failed antithrombotic treatment. The median time to recurrent TIA, stroke, or death was 36 days. Akins et al.[36] reported on 21 patients with 45 intracranial stenoses who were followed up for an average duration of 27 months. Progression of stenosis (increase of 10% or more in severity) was observed in 20% of intracranial ICA lesions and in 61% of anterior, middle, and posterior cerebral artery lesions. In the follow-up period, 4 TIAs and 1 intracerebral hemorrhage were observed. Qureshi et al.[37] reported a stroke free survival rate of 48% over 5 years among 102 patients with symptomatic stenosis located in the intracranial vertebral or basilar artery.

Subsequent prospective studies have confirmed the high rates of ischemic stroke or death associated with symptomatic intracranial stenosis. In the prospective double-blinded, multi-center WASID trial,[34] 569 patients with 50 to 99% symptomatic stenosis of a major intracranial artery were randomized to receive warfarin or aspirin. During a mean follow-up period of 1.8 years, the primary end point (ischemic stroke, intracranial hemorrhage, or vascular death) occurred in 22% of the patients in the aspirin-treated group and 22% in the warfarin-treated group. Among patients with intracranial stenosis with severity of 70% or greater,[38] the risk of recurrent ipsilateral stroke was 23% and 25% for 1 and 2 years post-randomization, respectively. The results from a European, multicenter, prospectively maintained GESICA registry[21] (Groupe d'Etude des Sténoses Intra-Crâniennes Athéromateuses symptomatiques) evaluated the rate of recurrent cerebral ischemic events among 102 patients with symptomatic intracranial stenosis followed over a mean period of 23 months. During the follow-up period, 38% of patients experienced an ipsilateral stroke or TIA; the rate of recurrent events was 61% among patients with a hemodynamically significant stenosis and 32% among those without a hemodynamically significant stenosis.

The highest risk of recurrent ischemic stroke appears to be within the first 2 weeks after the first event associated with intracranial stenosis. In the post-hoc analysis of the WASID trial,[38] the risk of ipsilateral stroke was highest in patients enrolled early ($\leq$ 17 days) after the qualifying event. In the Oxford Vascular Study and the Oxfordshire Community Stroke Project,[39] the highest risk of early recurrence was among patients with large vessel atherosclerosis including intracranial stenosis. The odds of recurrent events at 7 days (odds ratio [OR] = 3.3), 30 days (OR = 2.9), and 3 months (OR = 2.9) was higher than any other etiological subtype. This highlights the importance of early evaluation and treatment of such patients.

The high recurrent stroke and death rates in medically treated patients highlight the importance of developing new treatment modalities, such as endovascular therapy, for intracranial stenosis.

Pre-treatment evaluation and screening

A patient with suspected intracranial stenosis should ideally be evaluated by an experienced stroke neurologist prior to revascularization, in order to appropriately attribute the patient's neurological deficits to the target intracranial lesion and exclude other potential causes of cerebral ischemic symptoms. Almost all patients with ischemic stroke or TIA undergo non-invasive testing including magnetic resonance angiography (MRA), computed tomographic angiography (CTA), or transcranial Dopper ultrasound (TCD) for detection of possible intracranial steno-occlusive disease followed by conventional four-vessel catheter angiography for accurate characterization of the lesion. Currently, there are no accepted recommendations for screening of asymptomatic patients or population-based screening for intracranial stenosis.

A recent prospective multi-center trial[40] demonstrated that TCD and MRA can reliably exclude the presence of intracranial stenosis. However, confirmatory catheter angiography is required for identification and characterization of the lesions. Since MRA may overestimate the severity of intracranial stenosis, its use should be limited to screening until this technology becomes more reliable. With improvement in

three-dimensional CTA, there is potential for identification and characterization of intracranial steno-occlusive disease using a non-invasive test. Bash et al.[41] demonstrated that the sensitivity and positive predictive value of CTA may be better than that of MRA (98/93% and 70/65%, respectively), especially in the presence of slow flow through the affected arterial segment.

Further stratification based on the effect of intracranial stenosis on rCBF and vasodilatory reserve may be considered to identify patients at highest risk for ischemic events. Measurements of the cerebral mean transit time, cerebral blood volume, and rCBF can be obtained by various methods, including inhalation or intravenous injection of ^{133}Xe, single photon emission CT (SPECT), Xe^{133}-CT scan, positron emission tomography (PET), and CT or magnetic resonance (MR) perfusion studies. The choice of investigation varies by institution and treating physician. Patients with impaired vasodilatory capacity in response to a vasodilator stimulus, within the distribution of the stenosed vessel, maybe at a higher risk for ischemic events.[42] An rCBF measurement is obtained before and after an acetazolamide injection or carbon dioxide inhalation. Similar evaluation can also be performed measuring mean flow velocities using transcranial Doppler ultrasound before and after vasodilatory stimuli.[42,43] Impaired vasodilatory capacity is considered a marker of pre-existing maximal vasodilation in response to chronic hypoperfusion and inadequate compensatory collateral circulation.

Intravascular ultrasonography (IVUS) has been shown to be a safe and useful technique for assessing severity of stenosis and plaque morphology, and for serial assessment to detect plaque progression or regression in the coronary arteries.[44,45] There has been increasing interest in using IVUS for characterizing intracranial atherosclerosis.[46,47] IVUS provides accurate real-time dynamic measurements of artery morphology, histology of the plaque, and inflammation with in the plaque.[15] This may be a useful adjunct for selecting the size of the stent and assessing the extent of stent expansion in relation to the surrounding artery. The use of IVUS in intracranial vasculature is currently limited due to difficulties in navigating the IVUS catheter to the target vessel.

Pharmacology and role of antiplatelets and anticoagulation

Antiplatelet therapy

In the EC–IC bypass trial,[33] the medical treatment group consisted of patients who were treated with aggressive risk factor management and 1300 mg of aspirin daily. The annual mortality and stroke rate associated with aspirin treatment was 8%–10%. Results derived from more recent prospective studies evaluating the use of aspirin (WASID study) are described in the previous section.

Cilostazol, a phosphodiesterase III inhibitor, has been studied in a randomized, double-blinded, placebo controlled trial for its efficacy in symptomatic intracranial disease patients.[48] One hundred and thirty-five patients with acute symptomatic intracranial atherosclerosis were randomized to receive cilostazol or placebo for a period of 6 months. The primary outcome measure was increase in severity of stenosis detected by MRA. Recurrent stroke and progression of stenosis on TCD (defined by elevated velocities at the site of stenosis) were the secondary outcome measures. The rate of progression of intracranial stenosis in the cilostazol group (3 of 67 patients) was significantly lower than that observed in the placebo group (15 of 68). Further confirmatory studies are required because of limitations of severity quantification by MRA and relatively short follow-up.

Other antiplatelet agents including clopidogrel, extended-release dipyridamol plus low dose aspirin, and ticlodipine, do not have sufficient data to support their use in primary or secondary stroke prevention for the patients with intracranial stenosis. The European Stroke Prevention Study 2 (ESPS2)[49] and the European/Australasian Stroke Prevention in Reversible Ischaemia Trial (ESPRIT),[50] demonstrated the benefit of aspirin in combination with dipyridamole for secondary stroke prevention over aspirin alone. Neither study performed any subgroup analysis comparing risk reduction between aspirin and aspirin–dipyridamole combination among patients with symptomatic intracranial stenosis. Therefore, we do not have any data to support the preferential use of aspirin-dipyridamole combination in patients with intracranial stenosis. Similarly, other acute stroke trials were not designed to evaluate the efficacy of antiplatelets as secondary prevention for symptomatic intracranial atherosclerosis.[51,52]

Anticoagulation

Millikan et al.,[53] in 1955, first proposed the use of anticoagulation for patients with atherosclerotic disease in the basilar arteries. The effect of warfarin in comparison with aspirin has been studied in two large multi-center trials. The first trial was a retrospective, multi-center study of 151 patients with symptomatic intracranial atherosclerosis.[34] Eighty-eight of these patients were treated with warfarin and 68 treated with aspirin. During the mean follow-up period of 14.7 months, the warfarin-treated patients had an 8% rate of stroke and death and the aspirin treated patients had an 18% rate (mean follow-up time of 19 months). A Kaplan–Meier analysis revealed a significantly higher rate of major vascular ischemic stroke in patients treated with aspirin compared to warfarin ($P = 0.01$).

Based on the results of the first retrospective trial, a second larger NIH funded, multi-center, double-blinded, randomized trial was conducted between 1998 and 2003. The WASID trial[14] determined the safety and efficacy of warfarin compared to aspirin in patients with recent TIA or minor ischemic stroke related to intracranial disease. Patients with stenosis of greater than 50% diagnosed by conventional angiography were randomized to receive either warfarin (international

normalized ratio, 2.0 to 3.0) or aspirin (1300 mg per day). The trial was prematurely halted due to a concerning safety profile of the warfarin treated group (higher rate of hemorrhages), after randomizing 569 patients. The rates of ipsilateral ischemic stroke for the aspirin and warfarin treated groups were 12% and 11%, respectively, during a mean follow-up period of 1.8 years. The rates of death in the aspirin- and warfarin-treated patients were 4% and 10%, respectively ($P = 0.01$), and the rates of major hemorrhagic complication were 3% and 8%, respectively ($P = 0.02$). The study was unable to demonstrate any difference in the rates of ipsilateral ischemic stroke between the two treatments among patients with symptomatic intracranial stenosis, but the warfarin-treated group had higher morbidity and mortality.

Other medical therapies

Aggressive medical management of hypertension, diabetes mellitus, body mass index, and hyperlipidemia, and cessation of cigarette smoking are recommended as important components of optimal medical management. A subgroup analysis of the WASID study patients revealed that the risk of ischemic stroke increases with higher blood pressure.[54] High-dose statins have been shown to induce plaque regression in coronary arteries[55] but this therapeutic effect has not been studied in cerebral vascular disease, and the use of high dose statins has yet to be explored in patients with intracranial atherosclerotic disease.[55,56] The Stroke Prevention by Aggressive Reduction in Cholesterol Levels Trial (SPARCL)[57] demonstrated that 80 mg of atorvastatin per day reduces the overall incidence of strokes despite a small increase in the incidence of hemorrhagic stroke, in patients with recent ischemic stroke and TIA. Subgroup analysis of patients with intracranial stenosis was not performed in this study.

Surgical management

Donaghy and Yasargil,[58] in 1967, described a new surgical procedure involving a bypass from the extracranial circulation (superficial temporal artery) to the intracranial circulation (middle cerebral artery) to restore rCBF in patients with an occluded internal carotid or middle cerebral artery. Subsequently, other reports suggested the safety and feasibility of this intervention.[59] A large prospective, multi-center, randomized, controlled trial was performed to study the effect of extracranial-intracranial (EC–IC) bypass for patients with internal carotid or middle cerebral artery occlusion.[33] A total of 1377 patients with TIA, small hemispheric stroke, retinal infarction, or occlusive disease of the carotid artery or middle cerebral artery were randomized to EC–IC bypass surgery ($n = 663$) or best medical management ($n = 714$). After a mean follow-up of 56 months, fatal and non-fatal strokes occurred more frequently and earlier in the surgical group. Analyses of different subgroups based on angiographic lesion locations failed to demonstrate any benefit of EC–IC bypass surgery.

Patients with severe middle cerebral artery stenosis and persistent ischemic symptoms after internal carotid occlusion had worse outcomes in the surgical group. Since publication of these results, surgery has been largely abandoned for the treatment of intracranial stenosis.

After the negative results of the EC–IC bypass study, several investigators have attempted to identify a subset of patients with ICA stenosis or occlusion who could benefit from EC–IC bypass. During the last decade there has been a revival of interest in cerebral revascularization with the introduction of newer surgical techniques. Yamashita et al.[60] demonstrated that EC–IC bypass surgery may not have any effect on baseline rCBF but may improve vasodilatory capacity in a study of 15 patients with intracranial stenosis and occlusion. Murata et al.[61] showed that EC–IC bypass surgery may be able to maintain cerebral blood oxygenation immediately after surgery or gradually within 1 year when the pre-operative rCBF is below 24.5 to 25 ml/100 g/min.

Various types of operation for both high-flow and low-flow EC–IC bypass procedures are available. The superficial temporal artery is usually preferred as the donor vessel in the external carotid circulation. For high-flow bypass, the distal part of the internal carotid artery or M1 segment of the middle cerebral artery serve as recipient arteries, and for low-flow bypass, the recipient is the second or the third segment of the middle cerebral artery.[62,63] Van der Zwan et al.[64] was able to demonstrate that high-flow EC–IC bypass may be able to establish a larger (up to 3.7-fold higher) increase of rCBF compared with low-flow bypass.

Endovascular treatment of intracranial stenosis

Patient selection

There are no clear guidelines for identifying the appropriate patients with intracranial stenosis who could benefit from endovascular treatment. The criteria for selecting patients for endovascular treatment of intracranial stenosis in our practice are as follows.

1. Age greater than 18 years.
2. Ischemic events referable to the artery with the stenosis.
3. Ischemic symptoms despite antiplatelet therapy, defined by regular use of aspirin 81 mg or higher, clopidogrel 75 mg every day, or ticlopidine 250 mg twice daily; or anticoagulation defined 25 intravenous heparin (with activated partial thromboplastin time >1.5 times control) or oral warfarin (with an international normalized ratio greater than 2.0).
4. Intracranial stenosis involving the arteries within the cranium or those encased by the cranial bones, including the petrous and cavernous segments of the internal carotid artery and the intradural segment of the vertebral artery.
5. Presence of an atherosclerotic lesion with angiographically visible reduction (greater than 50% stenosis) of the lumen of the affected artery. The magnitude of stenosis is determined by measuring the narrowest segment visualized within the stenosis as a ratio to the proximal reference vessel.
6. After publication of the WASID trial, the eligibility criteria have been extended to include patients with angiographic stenosis of 70% or greater without medication failure, considering that such patients had a greater risk of ischemic events despite treatment with medication.[38]

Procedure selection

There is presently insufficient evidence to determine whether angioplasty or stent placement for intracranial stenosis, or a combination of these, should be preferred. Often, treatment paradigms are based solely on operator preference and experience. Various factors play a role in deciding primary angioplasty versus stent placement for the treatment of medically refractory symptomatic intracranial stenosis. After the development of more flexible and new generation stents for example, the Wingspan™ stent delivery system, stent placement may have been a preferred choice for selected patients based on experience at specific centers. In general, primary angioplasty is preferred for small vessels (< 2 mm in diameter); long lesions which would require long or multiple stents (> 12 mm); very tortuous proximal vessels (two or more acute curves that would be difficult to traverse as judged by experience); limited vessel length available distal to the lesion to allow stable placement of the microwire (e.g., basilar stenosis with hypoplastic or aplastic posterior cerebral arteries); lesions located in the anterior cerebral or posterior cerebral artery or M2 segment of the middle cerebral artery; or if the guide catheter can not be placed in the distal vertebral or internal carotid artery.

Technique of intracranial stenosis treatment
The percutaneous approach

Almost all intracranial angioplasty and/or stent procedures can be performed through the femoral route. A 6-French introducer sheath is placed in the femoral artery using percutaneous access. A stable access to the right vertebral artery can be difficult due to the angulation between the vertebral artery origin and parent subclavian artery. Therefore, serious consideration must be given to a radial approach if guide catheter placement is required in the right vertebral artery.

Guide catheter placement

Most intracranial procedures can be performed using a 6F (or even a 5F) guide catheter. The guide catheter can be introduced into the internal carotid or vertebral artery using a 0.035 inch guidewire in most circumstances but may require co-axial placement using a 5F 120 cm Simmons I catheter or advancement over an exchange length guidewire placed in position using a diagnostic catheter. The positioning of the guide catheter may be an issue, because the distal end of the guidewire may have to be placed in the distal portion of the cervical internal carotid artery or vertebral artery. There is risk of causing vasospasm or dissection because of tortuosity and relatively small diameter of these segments. Therefore, it is recommended that the guide catheter be advanced slowly into the distal segment and angiographic images be acquired after positioning for early detection of vasospasm or dissection. In certain situations, the guide catheter may be advanced over the shaft of the stent delivery device or balloon catheter to the target segment. The retropulsion created by forward movement of the stent delivery system or the balloon angioplasty catheter may result in proximal displacement of the guide catheter. A 0.018 inch microwire that is advanced into the cervical internal carotid or vertebral artery through the guide catheter creates a support platform without compromising the lumen space to prevent concurrent passage of other devices. Another approach requires a long guide sheath that engages the origin of the supra-aortic vessels to support guide catheter placement through its lumen. Despite these techniques, proximal tortuosity or small diameter of the vertebral artery may mandate using a 5F guide catheter or performing the procedure from a guide catheter in the subclavian artery.

Morphological assessment of the vessels proximal and distal to the target lesion

In general, the tortuosity of the anterior circulation poses a greater challenge than the posterior circulation for advancing an angioplasty balloon catheter and stent delivery system. The tortuosity of the cavernous segment of the internal carotid artery may prevent passage of the angioplasty balloon catheter and stent delivery system either at the petrous-cavernous junction or the supra-clinoid segment. The vertebro-basilar junction can be uniquely tortuous in some patients, posing similar challenges. The presence of proximal atherosclerotic disease limits the relative straightening of the vessels with the microwire, which is essential for the passage of these devices. In the presence of considerable proximal tortuosity, the operator may choose to perform only primary angioplasty or to place a microwire in the distal-most vessel segment (M3 segment of middle cerebral artery or P3 segment of posterior cerebral artery) using a microcatheter prior to advancing any devices. Microwire placement in distal segments allows availability of a relatively stiffer segment of the microwire to be available for advancing the device across the target lesion. However, not all distal segments are conducive to placement of microwires due to either tandem disease or hypoplasia/aplasia (particularly in the distal basilar artery). This information should be recorded on the initial angiographic images. If a good assessment of the distal vessel is not possible due to near occlusive lesions, traversing the lesion using a microcatheter and acquiring images using microcatheter contrast injections is recommended.

Morphological assessment of the lesion

Most lesions in the intracranial circulation are thought to be atherosclerotic in nature. However, dissections can also occur

at similar locations. In addition, lesions in the supra-clinoid segments of the internal carotid artery with or without involvement of the middle and anterior cerebral arteries in young individuals maybe have a non-atherosclerotic substrate. Certain aspects of the treatment procedure may differ depending upon the underlying substrate (atherosclerosis versus dissection) such as the use of balloon angioplasty and choice of stents. The operator must review the demographic and clinical characteristics of the patient and supplement that information with angiographic data. Involvement of other extracranial vessels and the appearance of the lesion may also provide diagnostic information. Therefore, careful visualization of other extracranial and intracranial vessels needs to be performed prior to the procedure. A lesion that involves a segment more than 15 mm or involves multiple segments proximal and distal to the primary lesion poses a unique challenge for stent placement, and a multi-segmented primary angioplasty may be preferred.

Traversing the lesion

A microwire is used to traverse the lesion and is then advanced into the distal segments to provide adequate support for advancing the balloon catheter or stent delivery device across the lesion. In rare circumstances, the microwire may traverse a lesion through a false lumen. Therefore, the trajectory of the microwire passage should be compared with the initially visualized lumen. It should be noted that some straightening of the vessel occurs after microwire passage and comparison of observed and expected trajectories should account for this straightening. A second challenge may be in advancing the microwire into distal tortuous segments, perhaps requiring microcatheter support to facilitate navigation. For lesions with severe stenosis, it is not unusual that placement of an angioplasty balloon catheter or stent device may be completely occlusive and prevent distal flow and image acquisition. This phenomenon should be anticipated and adequate images acquired prior to traversing the lesion.

Choice of angioplasty balloons and balloon sizes

A balloon angioplasty is almost always required prior to placing a self-expanding stent. A predilation is also helpful in patients with severe stenosis even if a balloon expandable stent is used because it may facilitate the passage of the device through the lesion.[65] The diameters of the intracranial artery proximal and distal to the lesion are measured. The following should be noted about the inflation pressure: nominal pressure (pressure at which label diameter is achieved), burst pressure (pressure at which half of the balloons will rupture), and semi-compliant pressure range (range in which incremental pressure results in incremental diameter of balloon). The semi-compliant pressure range is usually small because relatively non-compliant balloons are used for angioplasty. It is important to ensure that the diameter of the inflated balloon does not exceed the diameter of the normal vessel. The diameter of the balloon under various inflation pressures should be carefully

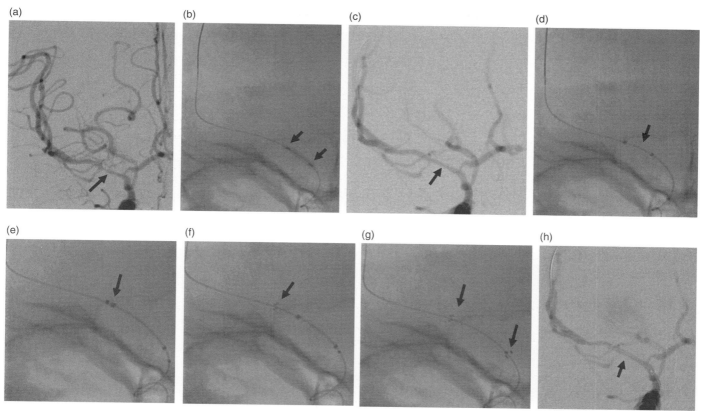

Fig. 8.1. Patient with high-grade symptomatic stenosis of the middle cerebral artery: (a) Antero-posterior view of the middle cerebral artery stenosis (arrow); (b) Angioplasty of the stenosis with radio-opaque markers of the balloon identified (arrows); (c) Post-angioplasty appearance (arrow); (d) A self-expanding stent positioned across the lesion (arrow); (e) Deployment of the stent initiated (arrow); (f) Distal portion of the stent deployed (arrow); (g) Complete deployment of the stent with radio-opaque markers identified at both ends (arrows); (h) Post-stent deployment appearance of the lesion with near complete resolution (arrow).

studied prior to insertion. Ideally, a single inflation of the angioplasty balloon must adequately dilate the lesion with some overlap in the normal segments on both sides of the lesion. However, multiple inflations may be required for longer lesions, and multiple inflations of varying diameters and pressures may be required if there are varying diameters proximal and distal to the lesion. A slow inflation over 30 to 60 seconds is recommended to reduce the risk of dissection or rupture. If multiple inflations at varying diameters and pressures are required, a balloon with a relatively large semi-compliant range should be selected.

Choice of stent and stent sizes

The largest diameter of the intracranial artery that requires opposition of the stent is measured. The nominal diameter of the stent must exceed the vessel diameter. The length of the stent must be selected to adequately cover the lesion with overlap over normal segments on both ends, and account for the position of the distal and proximal end to avoid angulated or unopposed placement due to tortuosity or post-stenotic dilation.

The interstitial spaces between the struts of a stent allow blood flow through the transverse axis of the stent. Therefore, the stent may be placed across the ostium of a medium-sized

artery (such as the anterior cerebral or vertebral artery) without any compromise to the flow. However, in the rare circumstance that endovascular access to the branch artery is anticipated, a stent should not be placed. A stent can also be safely placed across the ostium of small perforating vessels unless previous ischemic strokes have occurred in these distributions.

Post-stent angioplasty is only performed in select situations to provide optimal results. In our current practice, we use self-expanding stents (Wingspan,™ Boston Scientific Corporation, Natick, MA) for treatment of intracranial stenosis after angioplasty. The steps involved in a typical self-expanding stent deployment are shown in Figs. 8.1 and 8.2. The choice is based on comparative ease of delivery in the absence of any evidence of differential benefit between self-expanding and balloon expandable stents. Balloon expandable stents are still used for select lesions with high recoil. The steps involved in the deployment of a typical balloon expandable stent are shown in Fig. 8.3. For vessels requiring a stent after symptomatic restenosis following angioplasty, we consider a drug-eluting stent such as either the CYPHER® Sirolimus-eluting coronary stent (Cordis Corporation, Miami, FL), or the TAXUS® Express2™ Paclitaxel-eluting coronary stent (Boston Scientific Corporation, Natick, MA). However, according to a multi-society advisory panel, drug-eluting stents should be avoided in

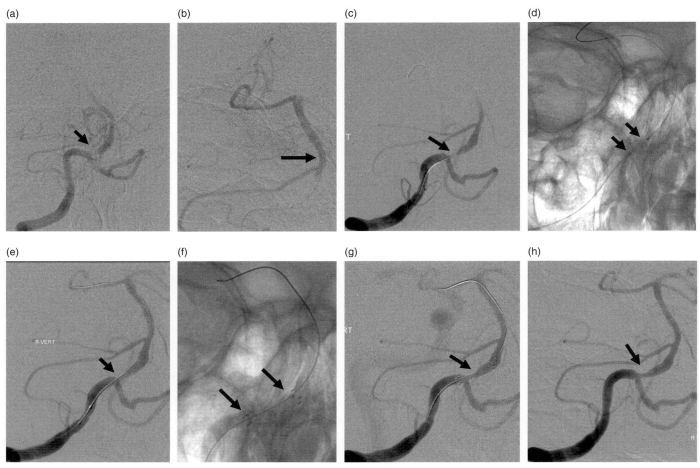

Fig. 8.2. Patient with high grade symptomatic stenosis of the vertebro-basilar junction: (a) Antero-posterior view of the vertebro-basilar artery junction stenosis (arrow). Notice poor visualization of the distal basilar artery and its branches; (b) Microcatheter placed distal to the lesion and contrast injection performed to visualize the status of the basilar artery (arrow); (c) A microwire is placed across the lesion through the microcatheter (arrow); (d) Angioplasty of the stenosis with radio-opaque markers of the balloon identified (arrows); (e) Post-angioplasty appearance (arrow); (f) Complete deployment of the stent with radio-opaque markers identified at both ends (arrows); (g) Post-stent deployment appearance of the lesion with significant resolution (arrow); (h) Post-stent deployment appearance of the lesion with significant resolution after removal of the microwire (arrow). Notice the opacification of the distal basilar artery and its branches not seen prior to the procedure.

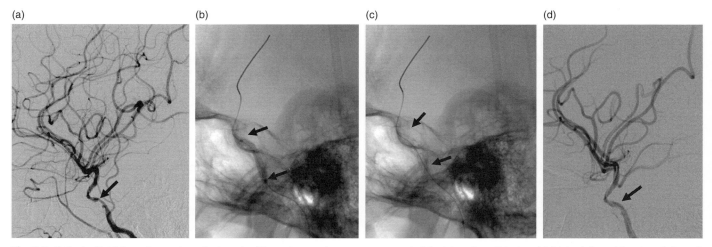

Fig. 8.3. Patient with high grade symptomatic stenosis of the petrous and cavernous segment of the internal carotid artery: (a) A lateral view of the stenosis (arrow); (b) A balloon expandable stent being deployed across the lesion and radio-opaque markers of the balloon identified (arrows); (c) Silhouette of the stent after deployment (arrows); (d) Resolution of the stenosis after deployment of the stent (arrow).

Table 8.2. Biomechanics of angioplasty catheters and stent devices

Stent (and manufacturer)	Material	Minimum ID guide catheter (mm)	Diameters (mm)	Lengths (mm)	Stent nominal pressure (atm)	Rated burst pressure (atm)	FDA Approval (HDE)
Wingspan™ (Boston Scientific)	Stainless steel	1.63	2.5–4.5	9–20	NA	NA	HDE
Pharos™ (Micrus)	Cobalt chromium	0.81	2.0–4.0	9–28	9	16	In Europe*
Taxus® Express2™ (Boston Scientific)	Paclitaxel-eluting	0.91	2.4–3.5	9–32	9	16–18	Off label
Cypher® (Cordis)	Sirolimus-eluting	0.85	2.5–3.5	8–33	11	16	Off label
Neuroform® (Boston Scientific)	Nitinol	1.27	2.5–4.5	10–30	NA	NA	HDE for aneurysms
Apollo® (MicroPort)	Stainless Steel	0.9	2.0–4.0	8–13	6	12	No
Maverick® (Boston Scientific)	Balloon (over-the-wire)	1.08	1.5–4.0	9–20	6	12–14	Off label
Gateway® (Boston Scientific)	Balloon (over-the-wire)	1.08	1.5–4.0	9–20	6	13–15	HDE

*for use in Europe only.
FDA: US Food and Drug Administration.
HDE: Humanitarian Device Exemption.
NA: Not applicable.

patients who are undergoing preparation for percutaneous coronary intervention and are likely to require invasive or surgical procedures within the next 12 months.[66] The biomechanics of angioplasty and stent devices are given in Table 8.2.

Choice of stent in stenosis related to dissection

An attempt should be made to determine if the dissection is acute or chronic based on the clinical presentation, magnetic resonance findings of thrombus within the wall (observed in acute dissections), or angiographic findings such as pseudoaneurysm (observed in chronic dissections). Any angioplasty should be avoided in acute dissections if possible and self-expanding stents alone can achieve adequate expansion. Chronic dissections may require concomitant angioplasty with a self-expanding stent for adequate results. Drug eluting stents should be avoided in dissections because the drug will interfere with the natural recovery within the vessel wall. The procedure is described in more detail in Chapter 9.

Peri-procedural management

Pre-operative medication, started 3 days prior to the procedure, should include a combination of aspirin (325 mg daily) and clopidogrel (75 mg daily).[67] If clopidogrel cannot be initiated 3 days prior to the procedure, a loading dose of 300 mg is used. Patients undergo laboratory testing for platelet, hematocrit, and electrolyte levels, and a coagulation profile is obtained before the procedure. Administration of warfarin is discontinued 3 days before the procedure in patients who were taking

that medication on a long-term basis, and these patients should have a repeat coagulation profile performed on the morning of the procedure.

Oxygen saturation, heart rate, blood pressure, urine output, and neurological status are monitored throughout the revascularization procedure. Most procedures can be performed under conscious sedation allowing regular evaluation of neurological status. General anesthesia may be required if adequate patient cooperation during the procedure is not anticipated. Heparin is intravenously administered as a bolus dose of 70 U/kg to achieve an activated coagulation time in the range of 300 to 350 seconds.[68] Routine use of intravenous glycoprotein IIB/IIIA inhibitors is not recommended due to the risk of intracranial hemorrhage. However, intravenous glycoprotein IIB/IIIA inhibitors maybe considered if intravascular thrombosis or dissection is observed during the procedure.[68] A lower dose of concomitant heparin is recommended to avoid systemic or intracranial hemorrhage.

Post-procedural management

A complete neurological examination is performed immediately as well as 24 hours after the procedure. Aspirin (325 mg daily) and clopidogrel (75 mg daily) are prescribed at discharge. Dual antiplatelet medications are continued for 1 month following primary angioplasty. If a bare metal stent is placed, it remains controversial whether dual antiplatelet treatment should be continued for 1 or 3 months. The multi-society advisory stresses the importance of 12 months of dual antiplatelet therapy after placement of a drug-eluting stent and of educating the patient and healthcare providers about the hazards of premature discontinuation.[66] It also recommends postponing elective surgery for 1 year, and if surgery cannot be deferred, considering the continuation of aspirin during the peri-operative period in high-risk patients with drug-eluting stents. Aggressive medical management of hypertension, diabetes mellitus, body mass index, and hyperlipidemia, and cessation of cigarette smoking cessation are recommended as important components of optimal adjunct management. Based on the subgroup analysis from WASID,[54] we recommend lowering of systemic blood pressure to below 140/90 mmHg and initiation of high dose atorvastatin (80 mg per day) if serum LDL cholesterol is 100mg/dl or higher (SPARCL study)[57] after the procedure.

Results of clinical studies evaluating endovascular treatment for intracranial stenosis

Three endpoints are considered in reports evaluating endovascular treatment for intracranial stenosis: (1) technical success, defined as the ability to either perform the angioplasty or deploy the stent with a residual stenosis of less than 30%, (2) one month (peri-procedural) rate of stroke or death; and (3) Prevention of ispsilateral stroke over a follow-up duration of at least one year. Currently, abundant data pertaining to technical success and 1 month rate of stroke and death are available for primary angioplasty and stent placement but there is paucity of long-term effectiveness data.

The incidence of peri-procedural neurologic events ranges from 5% to 33% in various reports.[69–82] The technical success rates are increasing and peri-procedural complications are decreasing over time with advancement in endovascular technology[37,67,70,83] and greater experience of the operators. Technical feasibility with success[70,80–82] rates greater than 90% has been reported in numerous series.[69–82] However, the rates of procedure-related complications vary greatly among different studies indicating that these procedures may be highly operator-dependent in terms of both success and complications (complication rates 0%–20%).[17,68,71–78,84–87] The overall stroke-free survival for the first year in patients treated with intracranial angioplasty with or without stent placement ranges from 88% to 93% in the preliminary studies.[67] Overall stroke-free survival at 36 months was estimated as 79%, and the ipsilateral stroke-prevention rate was estimated to be 87%.[67] The results of specific procedures are described below.

Primary angioplasty

Primary angioplasty is technically less challenging than placing an intracranial stent. However, the rates of immediate lesion recoil, acute dissections, and subacute re-stenosis may be higher. The exact clinical significance of the differential rates of these angiographic findings in the intracranial circulation is not completely understood. Mori and colleagues[85] initially reported on patients treated with primary intracranial angioplasty. They observed a 25% re-stenosis rate 3 months after angioplasty. In an attempt to find out the ideal time for angiographic follow-up to detect re-stenosis, the same group reported a series of 35 patients.[17] They performed follow-up studies for these patients at 3 months and 12 months. The rate of re-stenosis was 30% at 3 months. Patients without re-stenosis at 3 months were also free of recurrent disease at 12 months. They also recognized that lesions smaller than 5 mm in size, with little or no calcification and with smooth surface contours, were associated with higher success rate in terms of low morbidity and low rates of re-stenosis. Gress et al.[71] reported on 25 patients who were treated with intracranial angioplasty for medically refractory vertebral (intracranial segment) and basilar artery stenosis. They were able to show that primary angioplasty resulted in reduction of severity of stenosis by more than 40%. The reported risk of stroke and death in the peri-procedural period was 28% and disabling stroke and death was 16%. No further comments on long-term clinical outcome could be made from this report.

The rates of peri-procedural stroke and death in more recent reports have improved presumably because of using submaximal and slow dilatations during angioplasty and peri-procedural use of appropriate antiplatelet medications. Connors et al.[84] published a series of 70 patients with intracranial atherosclerotic disease treated by primary angioplasty. They reported the results derived from 50 patients in the "current period" treated with newer techniques of slow inflation and undersized balloons who had no abrupt vessel occlusion or strokes. Forty-nine out of 50 patients (98%) achieved good angiographic and short-term clinical outcome, defined as stable or improved neurologic status. The rate of asymptomatic re-stenosis at 3–12 months was 8% (4/49). Marks et al.[70] reported immediate and long-term outcomes in 23 patients who underwent intracranial angioplasty. The procedure success rate was 91% (1 death after procedure) and the annual rate of ipsilateral hemispheric stroke was 3% with mean follow-up period of 35 months. Marks et al.[79] subsequently reported results of primary angioplasty in 120 patients with 124 intracranial stenoses from multiple centers. The severity of stenosis at the time of treatment varied from 50% to 95% (mean severity of 82%). Post-treatment stenoses varied from 0% to 90% (mean severity of 36%). The combined peri-procedural (30 days post-procedure) rate of stroke and death was 6% (3 strokes and 4 deaths). During the follow-up period (mean 42 months), there were 11 strokes and 10 deaths. Six strokes were in the territory of the treated vessel, whereas five strokes occured in another vessel territory. The reported annual rates of stroke and ipsilateral stroke were 4% and 3%, respectively. The study suggested that intracranial angioplasty could be performed with a high degree of technical success and a low risk of complications. Long-term clinical follow-up suggests that stroke prevention following the procedure compares favorably with the expected rates among patients receiving medical therapy.

In 2006, Wojak et al.[79] reported on 60 consecutive patients with 71 intracranial lesions (67 symptomatic and 4 asymptomatic) who were treated with 62 primary angioplasty procedures and 22 angioplasty followed by stent procedures. A high rate of technical success was observed (in 91% of the procedures). There was a 5% rate of peri-procedural stroke and death; and 23 lesions had angiographic evidence of re-stenosis during a mean follow-up period of 4.6 months. Long term clinical outcome was available for all 60 patients. Over a period of 224 patient–years, there were four strokes and no deaths due to neurologic complications; four other patients died due to non-neurological causes. The annual rate of ipsilateral stroke was 2% and the overall annual stroke and death rate was 3%.

Intracranial stent placement

Some authors have proposed theoretical advantages of stent placement (over primary angioplasty) which include preventing early elastic recoil and negative remodeling.[86,87] However, this must be balanced against the technical challenges of achieving success (see Table 8.3).

Terada et al.[87] compared angioplasty and stent placement for symptomatic intracranial stenosis in 24 patients and suggested that stent placement may have improved early and late lumen gain. With the introduction of GFX (Arterial Vascular Engineering, Santa Rosa, CA) and Multi-Link (Abbott Vascular, Santa Clara, CA) coronary stents, which had good flexibility and wider strut spaces, intracranial lesions were finally made more amenable to stent placement. The wider struts enabled the stents to be placed without the complication of occluding smaller perforating vessels.

In 2000, Mori et al.[72] published the short term angiographic and clinical outcomes of intracranial angioplasty followed by stent placement. Stent placement was attempted in 10 patients with 12 lesions. The procedure was successful in 8 patients (two lesions were inaccessible). Pre-treatment stenosis of 80% was reduced to 7% in ten treated lesions, and no angiographic re-stenosis was seen at 3 months. No neurological events were reported after a mean follow-up of 11 months. After this successful deployment of stents in intracranial vasculature, many other reports followed demonstrating the safety and efficacy of intracranial stent placement using coronary stents. Lylyk et al.[74] published a series with stent placement in 34 patients with intracranial atherosclerotic disease or dissection ($\geq$ 50% lumen narrowing) with good angiographic outcomes (stenosis reduced to less than 30%). The peri-procedure mortality was 6%. There was no re-stenosis detected at 6-month angiographic follow-up in any patient. None of the patients died during the follow-up period. The overall morbidity (mean follow-up of 5 months) was 18% and neurological morbidity was 6%. Subsequently, Gupta et al.[75] and Kim et al.[76] reported higher procedural morbidity and mortality rates (28%/17% and 33%/8%, respectively). These variations are presumably related to patient selection and methodology of defining and ascertaining endpoints.

Table 8.3. Determinants of technical success following attempted stent placement

Probability of technical success	Determinants of results
High probability (95% or greater)	Absence of factors identified below
Moderate probability (75%–94%)	• Inability to place guide catheter up to base of skull OR • Segment of severe proximal tortuosity (defined as an angle of less than 90 degrees in any axis) OR • Segment of proximal intracranial atherosclerotic disease (defined as segment greater than 5 mm in length) OR • Required stent length for adequate lesion coverage >10 mm
Low probability ($\leq$75%)	Combination of above mentioned factors or multiple segments of proximal severe tortuosity or proximal intracranial atherosclerotic disease.

To reduce the risk of thrombotic complications, de Rochemont et al.[78] evaluated the use of undersized stent placement in 18 patients with symptomatic intracranial atherosclerosis and reported a 30-day combined stroke and death rate of 6%; there was one event related to reperfusion injury in the region of pre-existing stroke. It is important to note that, in 3 patients, complete apposition of the stent did not occur and that one stent dislodged from the intracranial vertebral artery into the basilar artery, without any neurological consequences. While the exact proportion of under-sizing is debated, most operators avoid over-sizing the balloon expandable stent to avoid vessel injury. A more recent study by Jiang et al.[77] reported a low rate of morbidity (10%) and mortality (3%) with new techniques. Jiang et al.[88] also demonstrated that the risk of stroke and intracerebral hemorrhage for stent treated intracranial stenosis did not worsen with the severity of stenosis. Failure to place a stent was the only predictor associated with target vessel territory stroke or hemorrhage in multivariate analysis.

However, whether stent placement provides additional clinical benefit compared with primary angioplasty has not been clearly demonstrated. Siddiq et al.[89] reported the clinical and angiographic follow-up of 187 patients with symptomatic intracranial stenosis treated with angioplasty and stent placement in the target vessel (94 angioplasties, 96 stent placements). After adjusting for age, gender and center, there was no difference seen in the rate of stroke and/or death for both groups.

Bare metal stent placement

In 2004, the Stenting in Symptomatic atherosclerotic Lesions of Vertebral and Intracranial Arteries (SSYLVIA) trial[69]

published data on the safety and efficacy of a new balloon catheter and stent (Neurolink,™ Guidant Corp., Menlo Park, CA) in 43 patients with symptomatic intracranial stenosis and 18 patients with extracranial vertebral artery stenosis. The technical success rate was 95% with a peri-procedural stroke rate of 7%. Forty-two patients completed a 12-month clinical follow-up. Four patients had new strokes after 30 days in the target lesion territory. Angiographic re-stenosis was observed in 35% of patients and was symptomatic in a third of these patients. Based on this finding, the FDA granted HDE[90] approval for the device to treat patients with significant intracranial atherosclerotic disease.

A recent prospective study was conducted to evaluate the efficacy and feasibility of the Apollo stent system (MicroPort Medical, Shanghai, China).[80] This system consists of a semi-compliant balloon, a stainless steel stent, and a delivery catheter. Forty-six patients with 48 symptomatic intracranial lesions had stent placement attempted with a 92% success rate. Three patients (7%) had minor strokes within 30 days. One patient (2%) suffered a minor stroke in the territory of the treated vessel. Angiographic follow-up performed in 25 patients detected seven re-stenoses (28%), but only one of them was symptomatic. The rate of new stroke was estimated to be 4 per 100 patient years.

Friorella et al.[82] reported a technical success rate of 95.7% in patients with symptomatic vertebrobasilar intracranial atheromatous disease treated with balloon-mounted bare metal stents. The peri-procedural morbidity and mortality was 26.1%. The average stenosis was reduced from 82.5% to 10%. They also demonstrated that mean intracranial vessel blood flow velocities, measured by TCD, were reduced from 127.7 cm/second to 54.0 cm/second immediately after stent placement. In-stent re-stenosis was observed in 12.5% of treated vessels at the time of follow-up and was associated with TIAs.

Drug-eluting stents

Drug-eluting stents using anti-proliferative drugs have shown encouraging results in clinical trials for prevention of re-stenosis after percutaneous coronary intervention.[91] The two approved drug-eluting stents are either Sirolimus-eluting or Paclitaxel-eluting coronary stents. Sirolimus is the generic name for rapamycin.[92] Although sirolimus was introduced as an antifungal agent, subsequent studies revealed antimitotic and immunosuppressive activities.[92] Paclitaxel is an antineoplastic medication used to treat metastatic breast and ovarian cancer, and Kaposi's sarcoma. In clinical trials, stents eluting the paclitaxel derivative 7-hexanolytaxol, or paclitaxel without a polymer, delay rather than prevent re-stenosis.[92–94] Slowing the release of paclitaxel with a polymer base in the TAXUS [paclitaxel]-eluting stent, has resulted in reduced re-stenosis rates at 12 and 18 months, indicating that polymer-based paclitaxel has longer effectiveness. There is a differential molecular mechanism of sirolimus and paclitaxel towards proliferation and migration.[92–94]

Qureshi et al.[95] reported technical success (defined as reduction of target lesion stenosis to < 30%) of 100% and a peri-procedure stroke rate of 6% (no deaths) in 18 patients treated with either Sirolimus- or Paclitaxel-eluting stents. At 6 month follow-up, no major stroke or death was observed. The estimated major stroke-free survival was 86% at 12 months following the procedure. Symptomatic angiographic re-stenosis was observed in one lesion (5.5%) during the follow-up period. Gupta et al.[96] reported a 3% peri-procedural complication rate and a 5% in-stent re-stenosis rate at a median follow-up period of 4 months in 59 patients treated with drug-eluting stent placement for symptomatic intracranial atherosclerosis.

Self-expanding stents

The Wingspan™ stent system is a self-expanding, nitinol stent sheathed in a delivery catheter. The Wingspan HDE Safety Study was conducted at 12 sites in Europe and Asia[81]. Forty-five patients with medically refractory symptomatic intracranial atherosclerosis ($\geq$50% stenosis) were enrolled in the study, out of which 44 subsequently underwent stent placement. The procedural success rate was 98%, and a 4% ($n = 2$) rate of death or ipsilateral stroke was reported at 30 days post-procedure. Forty-three patients completed the 6-month follow-up with a 7% ($n = 3$) rate of death and ipsilateral stroke. Further lesion reduction was observed in 24 of the 40 patients (mean severity 28%) who had 6-month angiographic follow-up. Based on the results of this study, the FDA granted HDE approval for the Wingspan™ Stent System with Gateway™ PTA Balloon Catheter in 2007.

A US multicenter study published the peri-procedural results of 78 patients with 82 symptomatic intracranial lesions treated with the Wingspan Stent System[97]. The success rate was 99% (one failure related to a tortuous carotid artery). Five patients (6%) suffered major neurological complications in the peri-procedural period, four of which were fatal. A recently published NIH registry on the use of the Wingspan stent[98] enrolled 129 patients with symptomatic intracranial stenoses (range 70%–99%) from 16 medical centers and demonstrated a technical success rate of 97%. The rate of stroke and death within the peri-procedural period was 14%. The rate of re-stenosis in 52 patients with angiographic follow-up was 25%.

Comparison of primary angioplasty and stent placement

In a single center study,[107] no difference in time to major stroke or death, and time to major stroke, repeat procedure, or death was observed with primary angioplasty (reserved for more complex lesions) compared with stent placement (concurrent unmatched controls). At 12 months, major stroke-free survival was 95% ($\pm$standard error of 4%) for the stent-treated patients and 93% ($\pm$7%) for the angioplasty-treated patients. In a subsequent multicenter review,[89] there was no difference in follow-up survival (stroke or stroke-and/or-death) between the 95 angioplasty treated versus the 98 stent treated groups, respectively, after adjusting for age, gender and center. The stroke and/or death-free survival at 2 years for the angioplasty group and the stent treated group was 92 ± 4% and 89 ± 5% respectively. Significant restenosis-free survival at 12 months was 68% for the 66 angioplasty treated group and 64% for the 68 stent treated group with DSA follow-up.

In a systematic review[108] of 69 studies (33 primary angioplasty studies, 1,027 patients and 36 stent placement studies, 1291 patients), there were a total of 91 stroke and deaths reported in the angioplasty treated group compared with 104 in the stent treated group during the 1-month period [$p = 0.5$]. The 1-year stroke and death in patients treated with angioplasty was 20% compared with 14% in the stent treated patients ($p = 0.009$). The pooled restenosis rate was 14% in the angioplasty treated group compared with 11% in the stent treated group ($p = 0.04$). There was no effect of the publication year of the studies on the risk of stroke and death.

Comparison of endovascular treatment with best medical treatment

A comparison[98] between matched 254 patients recruited in the WASID trial and 158 entered in the NIH Wingspan multi-center stent registry determined the differential rates primary outcome of stroke or death within 30 days or ipsilateral stroke beyond 30 days within subgroups having 50–69% and 70–99% stenosis. The patients in the stent registry had significantly higher severity of stenosis (mean stenosis of 78% vs. 68%) and shorter duration from qualifying event to enrollment (median 9.5 vs. 18 days). The frequency of the primary outcome at 1 and 6 months in WASID patients with 70–99% stenosis was 7% and 16%, respectively; the comparable rates at 1 and 6 months in stent treated were 10% and 13%, respectively, suggesting a possible benefit. The frequency of the primary outcome at 1 and 6 months in WASID patients with 50–69% stenosis was 4% and 7%, respectively; the comparable rates at 1 and 6 months in stent treated patients was 4% and 14%, respectively, suggesting no clear benefit due to the low event rates in the medically treated patients.

Complications

The potential adverse events associated with angioplasty and stent placement include the following:

1. Cerebral ischemia
2. Stent thrombosis
3. Death
4. Embolic stroke
5. Intimal dissection
6. Intracerebral/intracranial hemorrhage
7. Post-procedure bleeding
8. Stent migration
9. Vasospasm
10. Vessel perforation
11. Vessel thrombosis
12. Hyperperfusion injury

There may be other systemic and local side effects at the site of vascular access, and contrast-related nephrotoxicity can also occur. We discuss some of the specific adverse events associated with intracranial angioplasty and stent placement.

1. *In-stent thrombosis.* Stent thrombosis and occlusion have been observed secondary to mechanical plaque disruption, intimal injury and thrombogenicity of the stent.[76,99–102] The highest risk of stent thrombosis is within the first 24 hours after placement and the risk decreases substantially after the first 72 hours. Platelet glycoprotein IIb/IIIa inhibitors including abciximab, eptifibatide, and tirofiban may be used to treat in-stent thrombosis. Intra-arterial thrombolysis may also be used to treat parent vessel occlusion. If treatment is initiated early, cerebral ischemia can be prevented. Patients must be pre-treated with dual antiplatelets, (aspirin and clopidogrel), prior to attempting stent placement to prevent in-stent thrombosis. The use of distal protection devices in the treatment of intracranial stenosis to prevent distal emboli has not yet been developed.

2. *Intimal dissection.* Intimal dissection may occur during angioplasty or stent placement. If dissection is observed, the operator must decide whether it is flow limiting. Flow-limiting dissections can be treated by placing a second stent. If the intimal flap is not flow limiting but is associated with thrombosis, short-term use of intravenous anticoagulation or platelet glycoprotein IIB/IIIA inhibitors and follow-up angiography may be required. Dissections with small flaps (intimal irregularities) which are asymptomatic may require observation only.

3. *Vessel perforation.* Vessel perforation may cause fatal subarachnoid hemorrhage. Unfortunately, there are no reasonable therapeutic options available in case of this catastrophic event. Rapid reversal of intravenous heparin using protamine and platelet transfusion for reversing platelet inhibition by antiplatelet agents should be considered.

4. *Reperfusion hemorrhage.* A patient with a recent large ischemic stroke is particularly at risk of intracranial hemorrhage after revascularization. The hemorrhage is presumably related to restoration of rCBF in maximally dilated blood vessels (pre-existing due to long-standing hypoperfusion) and anticoagulation and antiplatelet treatment. Treatment should be preferably delayed in patients with large ischemic strokes. Strict blood pressure

control may help to avoid this potentially devastating complication. In rare, severe cases, surgical evacuation may be indicated.

5. *Vasospasm*. Catheter manipulation or microwire placement may result in vasospasm of the intracranial vessels. Almost all vasospasm is transient and resolves as soon as the devices are withdrawn. If distinction between vasospasm and dissection is required without losing access to the distal vessel, a microcatheter maybe placed over the microwire with subsequent removal of the microwire. This maneuver relieves some of the distortional stress on the vessel wall while preserving distal access. Follow-up angiography after 5–10 minutes may be performed to confirm resolution of vasospasm. If vasospasm persists, an intra-arterial calcium channel blocker, magnesium, or papaverine may be utilized with varying success.

Re-stenosis

Re-stenosis in intracranial arteries is frequently observed after endovascular treatment regardless of the procedure used (primary angioplasty, bare metal stent placement, drug-eluting stent placement, or self expanding stent placement). Re-stenosis results from a combination of elastic recoil of the artery, neo-intimal hyperplasia, and vascular remodeling.[91,93 109,110] The process involves stimulation of smooth muscle cell migration and proliferation and activation of endothelial cells at injury sites.[93,103] Re-stenosis is further categorized as intra-stent or peri-stent depending on the location of the re-stenosis in relationship to the previously placed stent.

Mori et al.[17,85] reported 25%–29.6% re-stenosis at 3 months in their series of angioplasty-treated patients. Patients without re-stenosis at 3 months were also free of recurrent disease at 12 months. Connors et al.[84] reported a re-stenosis rate of 8% (4/49) at 3–12 months after angioplasty of intracranial stenosis. The re-stenosis rate in the SSYLVIA trial[69] was 35% and was symptomatic in a third of these. The Apollo stent trial[80] reported a 28% re-stenosis rate in 25 patients who had angiographic follow-up at 6 months. Qureshi et al.[95] reported that only one out of 18 patients (5.5%) treated with drug-eluting stents had symptomatic angiographic re-stenosis during the follow-up period (median: 6 months). Siddiq et al.[89] reported a re-stenosis rate of 35% in 134 angioplasty- and stent-treated patients at 9-month angiographic follow-up. The rate of re-stenosis did not differ between angioplasty- and stent-treated groups. Levy et al.[99] reported imaging follow-up on 84 patients treated with Wingspan™ stent placement. Twenty five treated lesions (30%) had significant re-stenosis at a mean follow-up of 6 months. Zaidat et al.[98] reported a re-stenosis rate of 25% in 52 patients treated with Wingspan™ stent placement and subsequent angiographic follow-up.

No preventive treatment strategy has been identified. If severe re-stenosis (particularly if symptomatic) occurs, re-treatment may be necessary. Re-treatment usually consists of angioplasty within a previously placed stent or stent placement if primary angioplasty was the first procedure.

Recommended indications from professional organizations

The American Society of Interventional and Therapeutic Neuroradiology, the Society of Interventional Radiology, and the American Society of Neuroradiology[104] agree that sufficient evidence now exists to recommend that intracranial angioplasty, with or without stent placement, be offered to symptomatic patients with intracranial stenoses >50% demonstrated on catheter angiography, who have failed medical therapy. Patient benefit from revascularization for symptomatic intracranial arterial stenosis is critically dependent on a low peri-procedural stroke and death rate and should therefore be performed at experienced endovascular centers. Patients with asymptomatic intracranial arterial stenosis should first be counseled regarding optimal medical therapy. Due to the lack of sufficient evidence, endovascular therapy is not recommended in asymptomatic patients with severe intracranial atherosclerosis. They should be counseled regarding the nature and extent of the disease, monitored for new neurological symptoms, and have periodic imaging at regular intervals of 6 to 12 months (MRA or CTA initially and then cerebral angiography if warranted). Optimal prophylactic medical therapy should be instituted, which may include antiplatelet and/or statin therapy.

The Brain Attack Coalition[105] recognizes the lack of data from large, prospective randomized trials. Intracranial angioplasty and stent placement for cerebrovascular disease is considered an optional component for a comprehensive stroke center, although there are selected cases in which such techniques may be useful. If a center does offer this procedure, it is recommended that cases be entered into a registry to track outcomes. It is recommended that, if a comprehensive stroke center does not offer extracranial and intracranial angioplasty/ stenting, referral arrangements to transfer select patients to another facility that does offer these interventions should be in place.

The American Heart Association and American Stroke Association[106] guidelines state that the usefulness of endovascular therapy (angioplasty and/or stent placement) for patients with hemodynamically significant intracranial stenosis who have symptoms despite medical therapies (antithrombotics, statins, and other treatments for risk factors), is uncertain and is considered investigational (Class IIb, Level of Evidence C). A summary of indications and recommendations for different treatment options are given in Table 8.4.

The consensus conference on intracranial atherosclerosis[109,110] identified principles of management, and research priorities in various aspects upon which leading experts could

Table 8.4. A summary of indications used for treating intracranial atherosclerosis in various studies with quality of evidence

Treatment	Indications	Safety and effectiveness	Recommendations
Aspirin	Symptomatic intracranial atherosclerosis	Level II●[33,69]	Grade C
Warfarin	Symptomatic intracranial atherosclerosis refractory to initial medical management	Level II[69]	Grade C
Surgery	Symptomatic intracranial atherosclerosis not amenable to endovascular therapy	Level II[33]	Grade C
Angioplasty	Symptomatic intracranial atherosclerosis refractory to medical management	Level III[71,73,79,84,85]	Grade C[106]
Stent placement	Symptomatic intracranial atherosclerosis refractory to medical management	Level II–III[72,74,88]	Grade C[106]
Bare metal stents	Symptomatic intracranial atherosclerosis refractory to medical management	Level II–III[69,80]	Grade C[106]
Drug-eluting stents	Symptomatic intracranial atherosclerosis refractory to medical management	Level II–III[95]	Grade C[106]
Self-expandable stents	Symptomatic intracranial atherosclerosis refractory to medical management	Level II–III[81,97]	Grade C[106]

●Level I – Derived from multiple randomized controlled trials.
Level II – Derived from a single randomized trial of nonrandomized studies.
Level III – Consensus opinion of experts.

agree (using "Delphi" method). Consensus statements were catalogued under 9 broad categories, corresponding roughly to the topics presented at the conference. There were 64 statements in the original list. Statements receiving an average vote of less than 8.0 on a scale of 10 possible points were removed; yielding 49 consensus statements (see Table 8.5). The proceedings stated that intracranial angioplasty with or without stent placement has evolved as a therapeutic option for patients with symptomatic intracranial atherosclerosis particularly those with high grade stenosis with recurrent ischemic symptoms and/or medication failure. A matched comparison between medical treated patients in the WASID study and stent treated patients in the National Institutes of Health intracranial stent registry concluded that stent placement may offer benefit in patients with 70–99% stenosis.

Regulatory approvals – Food and Drug Administration, Center of Medicare and Medicaid Services

Two stents are approved under the provision for humanitarian use devices by the FDA (see Table 8.5). Effective January 1, 2006, the American Medical Association issued specific CPT® Codes (61630 and 61635) for intracranial angioplasty and stenting procedures. Effective November 6, 2006, the Centers for Medicare and Medicaid Services (CMS) decided to allow national Medicare coverage of intracranial angioplasty and stent placement as part of certain investigational

device exemption (IDE) clinical trials. Currently, however, procedures which involve the Wingspan Stent System and Gateway PTA Balloon Catheter for the HDE-approved indication remain a non-covered service under Medicare. Other health insurers who choose to cover intracranial angioplasty and stent placement cases will reimburse hospitals for inpatient care using a variety of mechanisms including per diems, diagnosis related groups (DRGs), case rates, or percentage of billed charges.

Future directions

Randomized controlled trials are warranted to clearly establish the role of intracranial angioplasty and stent placement for symptomatic intracranial artery disease. The best medical therapy is not established at this time for comparison. Various advances in stent delivery systems are anticipated to alter the course of in-stent stenosis and improve access to tortuous vessels. The NIH-funded, randomized, open-label, Stent Placement versus Aggressive Medical Management for the Prevention of Recurrent stroke in Intracranial Stenosis (SAMMPRIS)[98] trial will be able to answer some of these questions. All 40- to 80-year-old patients who meet the following criteria will be enrolled in this trial: TIA or non-severe stroke within 30 days of enrollment attributed to 70%–99% stenosis of a major intracranial artery, modified Rankin score of 3 or less, target area of stenosis in an intracranial artery that has a normal diameter of 2.0 mm to 4.5 mm, and target area of stenosis ≤14 mm. The two arms of the

Table 8.5. Pertinent consensus statement derived from the Consensus conference on intracranial atherosclerotic disease[109,110]

Diagnosis and Quantitation of Intracranial Stenosis

- Due to the high negative predictive value, non-invasive tests are important in evaluation of patients with suspected intracranial stenosis (ICAS) primarily by excluding the presence of disease.

- If accurate categorization of a lesion detected on non-invasive testing is needed for clinical decision making or recruitment in clinical trials, complete digital subtraction angiogram (DSA) is recommended.

- Complete digital subtraction angiogram and other appropriate testing is recommended to distinguish atherosclerotic disease from non-atherosclerotic vasculopathies.

- There appears to be a difference in the reliability of imaging study results derived from single- and multicenter studies. This difference is likely due to the vulnerability of single centers to un-blinded assessment, small sample size, and verification bias. Therefore, caution is recommended prior to applying the results of single-center studies to broader perspective.

- The value of three-dimensional reconstructed images in assessing the severity of stenosis and characterizing plaque remains unestablished. It is recommended to use source images in assessing both.

- In preliminary studies, it appears that intracranial atherosclerotic disease (ICAD) in different arteries and segments (e.g., the petrous segment of the internal carotid artery) may provide different negative and positive predictive values. It is recommended that future studies account for these differences.

- Combining multiple non-invasive imaging modalities should be explored as a means to better select patients for conventional DSA.

- The role of non-invasive tests such as transcranial Doppler ultrasound (TCD), magnetic resonance angiography (MRA), and computed tomographic angiography (CTA) in detecting in-stent restenosis is not established. DSA remains the most accurate modality for determining in-stent restenosis.

Medical Treatment of Patients with ICAD

- In general, patient management should be based on best available evidence, and can be reasonably extrapolated from published guidelines regarding secondary prevention of stroke. However, some issues regarding medical management cannot be addressed by randomized clinical trials due to practical and logistical considerations.

- Progression (or regression) of an intracranial lesion may occur, with some heterogeneity depending upon the location. Such dynamicity is the result of various processes, including superimposed thrombus formation, intraplaque hemorrhage, and actual increase in atherosclerotic growth. These processes imply a need for surveillance and medical intervention.

- Best medical management must be targeted to antithrombotic treatment, plaque stabilization and regression, and global risk management.

- Best medical management is recommended as complementary to any intervention, and not as a comparative treatment.

- Aspirin is recommended for most patients based on results of randomized clinical trials to prevent recurrent ischemic events because it has a better safety profile than anticoagulation. However, anticoagulation may still be a consideration in select patients, such as those refractory to antiplatelet therapy, those in whom endovascular treatment is not an option, and those with intraluminal thrombotic, non-atherosclerotic lesions.

- Management of cardiovascular risk factors, including hypertension, hyperlipidemia, diabetes and cigarette smoking, are strongly advised in accord with standing secondary prevention guidelines. The targets for these treatments are derived from studies conducted in patients with ischemic stroke or transient ischemic attack regardless of etiology. The target for blood pressure is systolic blood pressure (SBP) <140 mm Hg; for cholesterol, LDL < 70 mg/dl; and for diabetes, HbA1c < 7%.

- Aggressive antihypertensive treatment may not be possible in patients with suspected hemodynamically significant lesions. Therefore, in patients with severe ICAS, assessment of perfusion distal to the stenosis is advised to determine vulnerability to blood pressure reduction.

- While current strategies have been directed towards cardiovascular risk factors, no studies exist to verify the precipitating factors for ischemic events in patients with intracranial atherosclerosis. Studies of specific precipitating factors may provide novel preventive strategies.

- One study demonstrated the benefit of phosphodiesterase inhibitors in reducing progression of ICAS. However, clinical benefit has not been established. Therefore, further evaluation of these agents is required prior to recommending routine use.

The Evolution and Role of Endovascular Therapy for the Treatment of ICAD

- In patients being considered for endovascular treatment, special caution is advised for patients with age less than 50 years and those with supraclinoid internal carotid artery stenosis (due to suspected high rate of restenosis).

- No validated criteria exist for selecting patients for intracranial stenting. However, symptomatic patients with ≥ 70% ICAS are at high risk for recurrent ischemic events. Similarly, patients with ischemic symptoms that can be attributed to hemodynamic changes appear

Table 8.5. (*cont.*)

to have a disproportionately high rate of recurrent ischemic events. Therefore, it is reasonable to consider these patients for endovascular treatment, clinical studies and institutional protocols.

- No clear data are available to support the effectiveness of primary angioplasty over stent placement for treatment of ICAS. Both primary angioplasty alone and angioplasty with a self-expanding stent have been evaluated in a non-randomized trial with high technical success, and with recurrent ischemic events no worse than the natural history of lesions treated with medical management alone.

- Balloon expandable stents may have value for lesions with high recoil. Utility of these stents is limited by the technical difficulty in placing them.

- No clear data exist regarding the relationship between residual stenosis and the risk of subsequent ischemic events. Further studies are required to determine a target for immediate post-procedure residual stenosis.

- Ischemic strokes can occur post-procedure in the distribution of a vessel treated with a stent. Common mechanisms include early in-stent restenosis, early antiplatelet termination, and other undefined mechanisms. Prevention of these outcomes should be a priority for research and development.

- The rate of angiographic restenosis is relatively high after primary angioplasty in the intracranial circulation (compared to those defined in coronary intervention). However, the clinical significance, natural history and treatment of asymptomatic restenosis remain unknown.

- Angiographic restenosis is best detected by DSA. Although no uniform definition exists for restenosis, constriction of lumen $\geq$50% relative to the reference vessel, and a relative constriction of $\geq$20% compared with the immediate pre-procedure angiogram, is acceptable.

- Further studies are required to determine the predictors of angiographic restenosis, including etiology, location of lesion, size of vessel, and patient age.

Periprocedural Management of Patients with Endovascular Treatment of ICAD

- There is no clear advantage to performing an angioplasty procedure and DSA in one setting versus two separate settings, and this paradigm should be individualized to the preference of the operator.

- Dual antiplatelet treatment is mandatory for performing angioplasty, preferably beginning at least 72 hours prior to the procedure. The benefit of dual antiplatelet agents is in preventing acute stent thrombosis. No conclusive evidence is available regarding the effect on restenosis. If clopidogrel is not initiated 72 hours prior to the procedure, a bolus of at least 300 mg is recommended. There are some data that a higher dose (450–600 mg) may lead to higher levels of platelet inhibition.

- Data regarding periprocedural management, particularly antiplatelet treatment, are derived from trials of coronary intervention. Most of the principles of peri-procedural management can be extrapolated to intracerebral intervention; however, several factors must be considered on a case-by-case basis, such as the lesion characteristics, extent of angioplasty and stent placement, and comorbid conditions.

- The required duration of dual antiplatelet treatment following optimal stent placement is not known. Dual antiplatelet agents should be used for at least 1 month in any case, and at least 6 months if drug eluting stents are used.

- Therapeutic platelet inhibition with clopidogrel is not always achieved despite standard doses of oral administration. This is observed more frequently with patients administered clopidogrel within 6 hours of a procedure. Further studies are required to calibrate the appropriate clinical correlates of effective dosing.

- The value of routine platelet function testing during a procedure is unproved. Further research in this area is recommended because routine testing could be of value in identifying compliance and resistance.

- High blood pressure in the post-procedure period may be related to hyperperfusion, although a cause-effect relationship is not established. Multiple distributions, flow limiting lesions may increase the risk. Blood pressure <140/90 mmHg is recommended if it can be tolerated in the post-procedure period, although caution is advised in the presence of multiple flow limiting lesions. A rapid, uncontrolled drop in pressure should be avoided, so intravenous titration is the preferred modality for control. Hyperperfusion is relatively infrequent but may occur with carotid angioplasty and stent placement.

- Intra-procedural heparin should be administered to maintain ACT > 250 seconds. Routine use of GPIIbIIIa inhibitors is not recommended and should be used only in selected patients. Post-procedural heparin has not been demonstrated to be of value in coronary intervention, and by extension is not recommended for intracranial interventions.

Research Priorities for ICAD

- New methods need to be explored for describing severity of stenosis, such as percent area of stenosis.

- New endovascular imaging modalities for identifying vulnerable plaques such as intravascular ultrasound, thermography and palpography should be explored with technical improvements to ensure feasibility and reliability of these techniques.

Table 8.5. (*cont.*)

- Further studies are required for validation of plaque regression as a surrogate endpoint, and treatment strategies directed towards inducing plaque regression need to be explored.

- Further studies are required to study agents that promate angiogenesis in patients who are candidates for revascularization. Local administration of adenovirus containing vascular endothelial growth factor (VEGF) is an option, considering the encouraging results observed in patients with refractory angina.

- Antiproliferative therapies for preventing plaque formation should be explored.

trial consist of an experimental stent treatment arm (Wingspan™ stent and best medical management) and an experimental medical arm (management of blood pressure, lipids, and other risk factors for vascular events). The purpose of the trial is to determine whether intracranial stent placement with intensive medical therapy is superior to the medical therapy alone for preventing a second stroke in high-risk patients with symptomatic stenosis of a major intracranial artery. This trial started enrollment in February 2008 and is estimated to end by February 2013.

References

1. Baker AB, Resch JA, Loewenson RB. Cerebral atherosclerosis in European populations: a preliminary report. *Stroke* 1973;4:898–903.

2. World Health Organization: Special subjects – vascular lesions affecting central nervous system. *World Health Stat Rep* 2: **481–509** (No 9) 1969.

3. Baker AB, Iannone A, Kinnard J. Cerebrovascular disease. 5. A comparative study of an American and a Norwegian population. *World Neurol* 1960;1:127–36.

4. Baker AB, Refsum S, Dahl E. Cerebrovascular disease. IV. A study of a Norwegian population. *Neurology* 1960;10:525–9.

5. Wong KS, Ng PW, Tang A, Liu R, Yeung V, Tomlinson B. Prevalence of asymptomatic intracranial atherosclerosis in high-risk patients. *Neurology* 2007;**68**:2035–8.

6. Sacco RL, Kargman DE, Gu Q, Zamanillo MC. Race-ethnicity and determinants of intracranial atherosclerotic cerebral infarction. The Northern Manhattan Stroke Study. *Stroke; a journal of cerebral circulation* 1995;**26**:14–20.

7. Segura T, Serena J, Castellanos M, Teruel J, Vilar C, Davalos A. Embolism in acute middle cerebral artery stenosis. *Neurology* 2001;56:497–501.

8. Wityk RJ, Lehman D, Klag M, Coresh J, Ahn H, Litt B. Race and sex differences in the distribution of cerebral atherosclerosis. *Stroke* 1996;27:1974–80.

9. Chen XY, Wong KS, Lam WW, Zhao HL, Ng HK. Middle cerebral artery atherosclerosis: histological comparison between plaques associated with and not associated with infarct in a postmortem study. *Cerebrovascular diseases (Basel, Switzerland)* 2008; **25**:74–80.

10. Kolodgie FD, Nakazawa G, Sangiorgi G, Ladich E, Burke AP, Virmani R. Pathology of atherosclerosis and stenting. *Neuroimaging Clin N Am* 2007;17:285–301, vii.

11. Qureshi AI, Siddiq F, Suri MFK, Taylor RA, Chaloupka JC. Intracranial stenosis in the young patients is a distinct syndrome. *A multicenter review. AAN abstract.* In American Academy of Neurology. Chicago, IL; 2008.

12. Rothman SM, Fulling KH, Nelson JS. Sickle cell anemia and central nervous system infarction: a neuropathological study. *Ann Neurol* 1986;**20**: 684–90.

13. Yamashita M, Oka K, Tanaka K. Histopathology of the brain vascular network in moyamoya disease. *Stroke* 1983;**14**:50–8.

14. Chimowitz MI, Lynn MJ, Howlett-Smith H, *et al.* Comparison of warfarin and aspirin for symptomatic intracranial arterial stenosis. *The New England journal of medicine* 2005;352:1305–16.

15. Suri MFK, Hoffman KR, Qureshi AI. Intracranial atherosclerotic disease: Medical, Biomechanical, Imaging, and Flow Dynamic perspective. *Journal of Neuroimaging* 2008(In press).

16. Simons MA, Kruger RA, Power RL. Cross-sectional area measurements by digital subtraction videodensitometry. *Invest Radiol* 1986;21:637–44.

17. Mori T, Mori K, Fukuoka M, Arisawa M, Honda S. Percutaneous transluminal cerebral angioplasty: serial angiographic follow-up after successful dilatation. *Neuroradiology* 1997;**39**:111–16.

18. Derdeyn CP, Grubb RL, Jr., Powers WJ. Cerebral hemodynamic impairment: methods of measurement and association with stroke risk. *Neurology* 1999;53:251–9.

19. Grubb RL, Jr., Derdeyn CP, Fritsch SM, *et al.* Importance of hemodynamic factors in the prognosis of symptomatic carotid occlusion. *Jama* 1998;**280**:1055–60.

20. Naritomi H, Sawada T, Kuriyama Y, Kinugawa H, Kaneko T, Takamiya M. Effect of chronic middle cerebral artery stenosis on the local cerebral hemodynamics. *Stroke; a journal of cerebral circulation* 1985;**16**:214–19.

21. Mazighi M, Tanasescu R, Ducrocq X, *et al.* Prospective study of symptomatic atherothrombotic intracranial stenoses: the GESICA study. *Neurology* 2006;**66**:1187–91.

22. Constantinides P. Pathogenesis of cerebral artery thrombosis in man. *Arch Pathol* 1967;**83**:422–8.

23. Caplan LR. Intracranial branch atheromatous disease: a neglected, understudied, and underused concept. *Neurology* 1989;**39**:1246–50.

24. Bogousslavsky J, Barnett HJ, Fox AJ, Hachinski VC, Taylor W. Atherosclerotic disease of the middle cerebral artery. *Stroke* 1986; **17**:1112–20.

25. Caplan LR, Gorelick PB, Hier DB. Race, sex and occlusive cerebrovascular

disease: a review. *Stroke; a journal of cerebral circulation* 1986;**17**:648–55.

26. Craig DR, Meguro K, Watridge C, Robertson JT, Barnett HJ, Fox AJ. Intracranial internal carotid artery stenosis. *Stroke* 1982;**13**:825–8.

27. Ingall TJ, Homer D, Baker HL, Jr., Kottke BA, O'Fallon WM, Whisnant JP. Predictors of intracranial carotid artery atherosclerosis. Duration of cigarette smoking and hypertension are more powerful than serum lipid levels. *Arch Neurol* 1991;**48**:687–91.

28. Inzitari D, Hachinski VC, Taylor DW, Barnett HJ. Racial differences in the anterior circulation in cerebrovascular disease. How much can be explained by risk factors? *Arch Neurol* 1990;**47**:1080–4.

29. Fisher CM. Cerebral arterial occlusion-remarks on pathology, pathophysiology, and diagnosis. *Clini neurosurg* 1963; **9**:88–105.

30. Baker AB, Resch JA, Loewenson RB. Hypertension and cerebral atherosclerosis. *Circulation* 1969;**39**:701–10.

31. Chaturvedi S, Turan TN, Lynn MJ, *et al.* Risk factor status and vascular events in patients with symptomatic intracranial stenosis. *Neurology* 2007;**69**:2063–8.

32. Loewenson RB, Flora GC, Baker AB. The role of socioeconomic factors in cerebral atherosclerosis. *Stroke* 1971;**2**:378–82.

33. Failure of extracranial-intracranial arterial bypass to reduce the risk of ischemic stroke. Results of an international randomized trial. The EC/IC Bypass Study Group. *N Engl J med* 1985;**313**:1191–200.

34. Chimowitz MI, Kokkinos J, Strong J, *et al.* The Warfarin-Aspirin Symptomatic Intracranial Disease Study. *Neurology* 1995;**45**:1488–93.

35. Thijs VN, Albers GW. Symptomatic intracranial atherosclerosis: outcome of patients who fail antithrombotic therapy. *Neurology* 2000;**55**:490–7.

36. Akins PT, Pilgram TK, Cross DT, 3rd, Moran CJ. Natural history of stenosis from intracranial atherosclerosis by serial angiography. *Stroke* 1998; **29**:433–8.

37. Qureshi AI, Ziai WC, Yahia AM, *et al.* Stroke-free survival and its determinants in patients with symptomatic vertebrobasilar stenosis:

a multicenter study. *Neurosurgery* 2003;**52**:1033–9; discussion 9–40.

38. Kasner SE, Chimowitz MI, Lynn MJ, *et al.* Predictors of ischemic stroke in the territory of a symptomatic intracranial arterial stenosis. *Circulation* 2006;**113**:555–63.

39. Lovett JK, Coull AJ, Rothwell PM. Early risk of recurrence by subtype of ischemic stroke in population-based incidence studies. *Neurology* 2004; **62**:569–73.

40. Feldmann E, Wilterdink JL, Kosinski A, *et al.* The Stroke Outcomes and Neuroimaging of Intracranial Atherosclerosis (SONIA) trial. *Neurology* 2007;**68**:2099–106.

41. Bash S, Villablanca JP, Jahan R, *et al.* Intracranial vascular stenosis and occlusive disease: evaluation with CT angiography, MR angiography, and digital subtraction angiography. *Ajnr* 2005;**26**:1012–21.

42. Marshall RS, Rundek T, Sproule DM, Fitzsimmons BF, Schwartz S, Lazar RM. Monitoring of cerebral vasodilatory capacity with transcranial Doppler carbon dioxide inhalation in patients with severe carotid artery disease. *Stroke* 2003;**34**:945–9.

43. Karnik R, Valentin A, Ammerer HP, Donath P, Slany J. Evaluation of vasomotor reactivity by transcranial Doppler and acetazolamide test before and after extracranial-intracranial bypass in patients with internal carotid artery occlusion. *Stroke* 1992;**23**:812–17.

44. Reid DB, Diethrich EB, Marx P, Wrasper R. Intravascular ultrasound assessment in carotid interventions. *J Endovasc Surg* 1996;**3**:203–10.

45. Fuessl RT, Hoepp HW, Sechtem U. Intravascular ultrasonography in the evaluation of results of coronary angioplasty and stenting. *Curr Opin Cardiol* 1999;**14**:471–9.

46. Ravalli S, LiMandri G, Di Tullio MR, *et al.* Intravascular ultrasound imaging of human cerebral arteries. *J Neuroimaging* 1996;**6**:71–5.

47. Wehman JC, Holmes DR, Jr., Hanel RA, Levy EI, Hopkins LN. Intravascular ultrasound for intracranial angioplasty and stent placement: technical case report. *Neurosurgery* 2006;**59**:ONSE481–3; discussion ONSE3.

48. Kwon SU, Cho YJ, Koo JS, *et al.* Cilostazol prevents the progression of the symptomatic intracranial arterial stenosis: the multicenter double-blind placebo-controlled trial of cilostazol in symptomatic intracranial arterial stenosis. *Stroke* 2005;**36**:782–6.

49. Diener HC, Cunha L, Forbes C, Sivenius J, Smets P, Lowenthal A. European Stroke Prevention Study. 2. Dipyridamole and acetylsalicylic acid in the secondary prevention of stroke. *J Neurol Sci* 1996;**143**:1–13.

50. Halkes PH, van Gijn J, Kappelle LJ, Koudstaal PJ, Algra A. Aspirin plus dipyridamole versus aspirin alone after cerebral ischaemia of arterial origin (ESPRIT): randomised controlled trial. *Lancet* 2006;**367**:1665–73.

51. CAST: randomised placebo-controlled trial of early aspirin use in 20,000 patients with acute ischaemic stroke. CAST (Chinese Acute Stroke Trial) Collaborative Group. *Lancet* 1997;**349**:1641–9.

52. The International Stroke Trial (IST): a randomised trial of aspirin, subcutaneous heparin, both, or neither among 19435 patients with acute ischaemic stroke. International Stroke Trial Collaborative Group. *Lancet* 1997;**349**:1569–81.

53. Millikan CH, Siekert RG, Shick RM. The use of anticoagulant drugs in the treatment of intermittent insufficiency and thrombosis within the basilar arterial system. *Trans Ame Neurol Assoc* 1955:132–4.

54. Turan TN, Cotsonis G, Lynn MJ, Chaturvedi S, Chimowitz M. Relationship between blood pressure and stroke recurrence in patients with intracranial arterial stenosis. *Circulation* 2007;**115**:2969–75.

55. Nissen SE, Nicholls SJ, Sipahi I, *et al.* Effect of very high-intensity statin therapy on regression of coronary atherosclerosis: the ASTEROID trial. *JAMA* 2006;**295**:1556–65.

56. Schoenhagen P, Tuzcu EM, Apperson-Hansen C, *et al.* Determinants of arterial wall remodeling during lipid-lowering therapy: serial intravascular ultrasound observations from the Reversal of Atherosclerosis with Aggressive Lipid Lowering Therapy (REVERSAL) trial. *Circulation* 2006;**113**:2826–34.

57. Amarenco P, Bogousslavsky J, Callahan A, 3rd, et al. High-dose atorvastatin after stroke or transient ischemic attack. *The New England journal of medicine* 2006;**355**:549–59.

58. Donaghy RMPYM. *Microvascular Surgery*: St. Louis, MO: Georg Thieme Verlag.

59. Sundt TM, Jr., Siekert RG, Piepgras DG, Sharbrough FW, Houser OW. Bypass surgery for vascular disease of the carotid system. *Mayo Clinic Proc* 1976;**51**:677–92.

60. Yamashita T, Kashiwagi S, Nakano S, et al. The effect of EC-IC bypass surgery on resting cerebral blood flow and cerebrovascular reserve capacity studied with stable XE-CT and acetazolamide test. *Neuroradiology* 1991;**33**:217–22.

61. Murata Y, Katayama Y, Sakatani K, Fukaya C, Kano T. Evaluation of extracranial-intracranial arterial bypass function by using near-infrared spectroscopy. *J Neurosurg* 2003;**99**:304–10.

62. Klijn CJ, Kappelle LJ, van der Grond J, van Gijn J, Tulleken CA. A new type of extracranial/intracranial bypass for recurrent haemodynamic transient ischaemic attacks. *Cerebrovasc Dis* (Basel, Switzerland) 1998;**8**:184–7.

63. Klijn CJ, Kappelle LJ, van der Zwan A, van Gijn J, Tulleken CA. Excimer laser-assisted high-flow extracranial/intracranial bypass in patients with symptomatic carotid artery occlusion at high risk of recurrent cerebral ischemia: safety and long-term outcome. *Stroke* 2002;**33**:2451–8.

64. van der Zwan A, Tulleken CA, Hillen B. Flow quantification of the non-occlusive excimer laser-assisted EC-IC bypass. *Acta neurochirurgica* 2001;**143**:647–54.

65. Lylyk P, Vila JF, Miranda C, et al. Endovascular reconstruction by means of stent placement in symptomatic intracranial atherosclerotic stenosis. *Neurol Res* 2005;**27** Suppl 1:S84–8.

66. Pinto Slottow TL, Waksman R. Overview of the 2006 Food and Drug Administration Circulatory System Devices Panel meeting on drug-eluting stent thrombosis. *Catheter Cardiovasc Interv* 2007;**69**:1064–74.

67. Qureshi AI, Suri MF, Siddiqui AM, et al. Clinical and angiographic results of dilatation procedures for symptomatic intracranial atherosclerotic disease. *J Neuroimaging* 2005;**15**:240–9.

68. Qureshi AI, Luft AR, Sharma M, Guterman LR, Hopkins LN. Prevention and treatment of thromboembolic and ischemic complications associated with endovascular procedures: Part II–Clinical aspects and recommendations. *Neurosurgery* 2000;**46**:1360–75; discussion 75–6.

69. Stenting of Symptomatic Atherosclerotic Lesions in the Vertebral or Intracranial Arteries (SSYLVIA): study results. *Stroke* 2004;**35**:1388–92.

70. Marks MP, Marcellus M, Norbash AM, Steinberg GK, Tong D, Albers GW. Outcome of angioplasty for atherosclerotic intracranial stenosis. *Stroke* 1999;**30**:1065–9.

71. Gress DR, Smith WS, Dowd CF, Van Halbach V, Finley RJ, Higashida RT. Angioplasty for intracranial symptomatic vertebrobasilar ischemia. *Neurosurgery* 2002;**51**:23–7; discussion 7–9.

72. Mori T, Kazita K, Chokyu K, Mima T, Mori K. Short-term arteriographic and clinical outcome after cerebral angioplasty and stenting for intracranial vertebrobasilar and carotid atherosclerotic occlusive disease. *Am J Neuroradiol* 2000;**21**:249–54.

73. Wojak JC, Dunlap DC, Hargrave KR, DeAlvare LA, Culbertson HS, Connors JJ, 3rd. Intracranial angioplasty and stenting: long-term results from a single center. *Am J Neuroradiol* 2006;**27**:1882–92.

74. Lylyk P, Cohen JE, Ceratto R, Ferrario A, Miranda C. Angioplasty and stent placement in intracranial atherosclerotic stenoses and dissections. *Am J Neuroradiol* 2002;**23**:430–6.

75. Gupta R, Schumacher HC, Mangla S, et al. Urgent endovascular revascularization for symptomatic intracranial atherosclerotic stenosis. *Neurology* 2003;**61**:1729–35.

76. Kim JK, Ahn JY, Lee BH, et al. Elective stenting for symptomatic middle cerebral artery stenosis presenting as transient ischaemic deficits or stroke attacks: short term arteriographical and clinical outcome. *J Neurol Neurosurg Psychiatry* 2004;**75**:847–51.

77. Jiang WJ, Wang YJ, Du B, et al. Stenting of symptomatic M1 stenosis of middle cerebral artery: an initial experience of 40 patients. *Stroke* 2004;**35**:1375–80.

78. de Rochemont Rdu M, Turowski B, Buchkremer M, Sitzer M, Zanella FE, Berkefeld J. Recurrent symptomatic high-grade intracranial stenoses: safety and efficacy of undersized stents–initial experience. *Radiology* 2004;**231**:45–9.

79. Marks MP, Wojak JC, Al-Ali F, et al. Angioplasty for symptomatic intracranial stenosis: clinical outcome. *Stroke* 2006;**37**:1016–20.

80. Jiang WJ, Xu XT, Jin M, Du B, Dong KH, Dai JP. Apollo stent for symptomatic atherosclerotic intracranial stenosis: study results. *Am J Neuroradiol* 2007;**28**:830–4.

81. Bose A, Hartmann M, Henkes H, et al. A novel, self-expanding, nitinol stent in medically refractory intracranial atherosclerotic stenoses: the Wingspan study. *Stroke* 2007;**38**:1531–7.

82. Fiorella D, Chow MM, Anderson M, Woo H, Rasmussen PA, Masaryk TJ. A 7-year experience with balloon-mounted coronary stents for the treatment of symptomatic vertebrobasilar intracranial atheromatous disease. *Neurosurgery* 2007;**61**:236–42; discussion 42–3.

83. Qureshi AI. Endovascular treatment of cerebrovascular diseases and intracranial neoplasms. *Lancet* 2004;**363**:804–13.

84. Connors JJ, 3rd, Wojak JC. Percutaneous transluminal angioplasty for intracranial atherosclerotic lesions: evolution of technique and short-term results. *J Neurosurg* 1999;**91**:415–23.

85. Mori T, Arisawa M, Honda S, Fukuoka M, Kurisaka M, Mori K. [Three months angiographic follow-up after successful percutaneous transluminal angioplasty]. *No Shinkei Geka* 1993;**21**:141–6.

86. Taylor RA, Kasner SE. Treatment of intracranial arterial stenosis. *Expert Rev neurother* 2006;**6**:1685–94.

87. Terada T, Tsuura M, Matsumoto H, et al. Endovascular therapy for stenosis of the petrous or cavernous portion of the internal carotid artery: percutaneous transluminal angioplasty compared with stent placement. *J Neurosurg* 2003;**98**:491–7.

88. Jiang WJ, Xu XT, Du B, et al. Comparison of elective stenting of severe vs moderate intracranial atherosclerotic stenosis. *Neurology* 2007;**68**:420–6.

89. Siddiq F, Vazquez G, Memon MZ, *et al.* Comparison of primary angioplasty with stent placement for treating symptomatic intracranial atherosclerotic disease: a Multi-center Study. *Stroke* 2008; **39**: 2505–10.

90. Qureshi AI. Ten years of advances in neuroendovascular procedures. *J Endovasc Ther* 2004;**11** Suppl 2:II1–4.

91. Garas SM, Huber P, Scott NA. Overview of therapies for prevention of restenosis after coronary interventions. *Pharmacol Ther* 2001;**92**:165–78.

92. Sehgal SN. Sirolimus: its discovery, biological properties, and mechanism of action. *Transpl Proc* 2003;**35**:7S–14S.

93. Doggrell SA. Sirolimus- or paclitaxel-eluting stents to prevent coronary artery restenosis. *Expert Opin Pharmacother* 2004;**5**:2209–20.

94. Liuzzo JP, Ambrose JA, Coppola JT. Sirolimus- and taxol-eluting stents differ towards intimal hyperplasia and re-endothelialization. *J Invas Cardiol* 2005;**17**:497–502.

95. Qureshi AI, Kirmani JF, Hussein HM, *et al.* Early and intermediate-term outcomes with drug-eluting stents in high-risk patients with symptomatic intracranial stenosis. *Neurosurgery* 2006;**59**:1044–51; discussion 51.

96. Gupta R, Al-Ali F, Thomas AJ, *et al.* Safety, feasibility, and short-term follow-up of drug-eluting stent placement in the intracranial and extracranial circulation. *Stroke* 2006;**37**:2562–6.

97. Fiorella D, Levy EI, Turk AS, *et al.* US multicenter experience with the wingspan stent system for the treatment of intracranial atheromatous disease: periprocedural results. *Stroke* 2007; **38**:881–7.

98. Zaidat OO, Klucznik R, Alexander MJ, et al. The NIH registry on use of the Wingspan stent for symptomatic 70–99% intracranial arterial stenosis. *Neurology* 2008;**70**:1518–24.

99. Levy EI, Turk AS, Albuquerque FC, *et al.* Wingspan in-stent restenosis and thrombosis: incidence, clinical presentation, and management. *Neurosurgery* 2007;**61**:644–50; discussion 50–1.

100. Kim DJ, Lee BH, Kim DI, Shim WH, Jeon P, Lee TH. Stent-assisted angioplasty of symptomatic intracranial vertebrobasilar artery stenosis: feasibility and follow-up results. *Ajnr* 2005;**26**: 1381–8.

101. Chaturvedi S, Yadav JS. The role of antiplatelet therapy in carotid stenting for ischemic stroke prevention. *Stroke* 2006;**37**:1572–7.

102. Wholey MH, Eles G, Toursakissian B, Bailey S, Jarmolowski C, Tan WA. Evaluation of glycoprotein IIb/IIIa inhibitors in carotid angioplasty and stenting. *J Endovasc Ther* 2003; **10**:33–41.

103. Holmes DR, Jr., Vlietstra RE, Smith HC, *et al.* Restenosis after percutaneous transluminal coronary angioplasty (PTCA): a report from the PTCA Registry of the National Heart, Lung, and Blood Institute. *Am J Cardiol* 1984;**53**:77C–81C.

104. Higashida RT, Meyers PM, Connors JJ, *et al.* Intracranial angioplasty & stenting for cerebral atherosclerosis: a position statement of the American Society of Interventional and Therapeutic Neuroradiology, Society of Interventional Radiology, and the American Society of Neuroradiology. *J Vasc Interv Radiol* 2005;**16**:1281–5.

105. Alberts MJ, Latchaw RE, Selman WR, *et al.* Recommendations for comprehensive stroke centers: a consensus statement from the Brain Attack Coalition. *Stroke* 2005;**36**:1597–616.

106. Sacco RL, Adams R, Albers G, *et al.* Guidelines for prevention of stroke in patients with ischemic stroke or transient ischemic attack: a statement for healthcare professionals from the American Heart Association/American Stroke Association Council on Stroke: co-sponsored by the Council on Cardiovascular Radiology and Intervention: the American Academy of Neurology affirms the value of this guideline. *Stroke* 2006;**37**:577–617.

107. Qureshi AI, Hussein HM, El-Gengaihy A, Abdelmoula M, Suri MF. Concurrent comparison of outcomes of primary angioplasty and of stent placement in high-risk patients with symptomatic intracranial stenosis. *Neurosurgery* 2008;**62**:1053–1060; discussion 1060–60.

108. Siddiq F, Memon MZ, Vazquez G, Safdar A, Qureshi AI. Comparison between primary angioplasty and stent placement for symptomatic intracranial atherosclerotic disease: meta-analysis of case series. *Neurosurgery* 2009;**65**:1024–33; discussion 1033–4.

109. Qureshi AI, Feldmann E, Gomez CR, *et al.* Consensus conference on intracranial atherosclerotic disease: rationale, methodology, and results. *J Neuroimaging* 2009;**19** Suppl 1: 1S–10S.

110. Qureshi AI, Feldmann E, Gomez CR, *et al.* Intracranial atherosclerotic disease: an update. *Ann Neurol* 2009;**66**:730–8.

Extracranial and intracranial arterial dissections

YihLin Nien MD, José Rafael Romero MD, Thanh N. Nguyen MD and Adnan I. Qureshi MD

Introduction

Cervical artery dissection (CAD) was first reported in an autopsy study by Pratt-Thomas in 1947.[1] CAD occurs when a tear in the intima allows blood to enter between the layers of the vessel wall, thus forming an intramural hematoma. Exposure of the intima and the presence of an intimal flap lead to increased thrombogenicity and stroke may result from embolization or flow-limiting stenosis of the vessel's true lumen. Early detection and treatment are important as the recurrence of stroke is highest during the first month following the event. Over the past years, increased awareness and advances in diagnostic imaging have led to increased detection of CAD with or without associated ischemic events. CAD is now recognized as one of the most common causes of stroke in the young, accounting for up to 30% of cases.[2,3] CAD is commonly preceded by direct or indirect neck trauma (traumatic CAD, discussed in chapter 10). In the present chapter we will focus on spontaneous (i.e. not trauma-related) CAD and we will discuss clinical features, diagnosis, and available treatment options.

Epidemiology

Spontaneous CAD accounts for 2% of all ischemic strokes.[4] Although CAD affects all age groups, there is a predilection for younger individuals. In a previous report, CAD accounted for 25%–30% of all the strokes in patients younger than 45 years.[2] The higher incidence of traumatic injuries and the early manifestation of hereditary and autoimmune disorders may lead to the higher prevalence in the young population. In one study, the mean age of patients at the time of diagnosis of dissection was 46 years,[3] with a peak incidence in the fifth decade of life, with similar rates observed in men and women. In a population-based study, the annual incidence of spontaneous CAD was estimated to be 3 per 100 000 persons. The incidence of internal carotid artery dissection ranged from 2.6 to 2.9 per 100 000 persons and incidence of dissection vertebral artery from 0.97 to 1.12 per 100 000 persons.[5] The study also found that the incidence of CAD has increased significantly within

the last decade, presumably due to improvement in detection rather than an actual increase in occurrence.[6] The recurrence rate of stroke following CAD is estimated to be < 0.3% per year unless there is a family history of arterial dissection.[7] Recurrent dissection is uncommon, with a reported risk of 2% during the first month, followed by an annual risk of 1% afterwards.[8] In contrast, familial cases of CAD have a reported cumulative recurrence rate of 55% over 10 years.[9] The occurrence of CAD among patients with connective tissue disease may be as high as 20%.[10] Still, only a minority of patients with spontaneous CAD is currently diagnosed with a definitive connective tissue disorder.

Pathogenesis and pathophysiology

The mechanism of arterial injury is usually multifactorial. Neck trauma is the most common setting in which CAD is observed. Direct trauma to the artery, a torsional or stretching force that induces shear stress to the intima, or injury against surrounding bony structures may be the causative factors. When a tear in the intimal lining is created, it allows blood to fill into and dissect an intramural layer (Fig. 9.1(a)). A subintimal dissection causes formation of an intramural hematoma, which can progress to the point of occluding the true lumen (Fig. 9.1(b)) thereby impairing blood flow to the brain. In other instances, the intramural hematoma can re-enter the main circulatory flow via a second tear distally, creating a "double vessel lumen" (Fig. 9.1(c)).

Exposure of the subintima to the flowing blood triggers platelet activation, aggregation, and the coagulation cascade, promoting local thrombosis with the possibility of embolism or arterial occlusion. The dissection can also occur in a plane between the media and adventitia, creating an aneurysmal outpouching devoid of muscular wall, called pseudoaneurysm. Histopathological studies have demonstrated structural differences between intracranial and extracranial arteries. The thinner layer of adventitia, the presence of collagenous fibers in the adventitial coat, and the absence of external elastic lamina of the intracranial arteries may predispose to pseudoaneurysm

Textbook of Interventional Neurology, ed. Adnan I. Qureshi. Published by Cambridge University Press. © Cambridge University Press 2011.

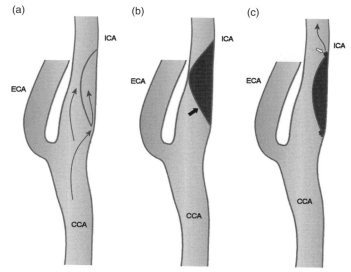

Fig. 9.1. (a) A tear in the intimal layer allows blood to fill in and create a "double lumen." (b) Expansion of the intramural hematoma may cause occlusion of the parent artery (black arrow). (c) The intramural hematoma can re-enter the main circulatory flow through a distal tear leading to embolic events (white arrow). ECA: external carotid artery; ICA: internal carotid artery; CCA: common carotid artery.

formation and subarachnoid hemorrhage in the intracranial circulation.[11]

In several reports, spontaneous CAD has been related to minor events, such as sneezing, coughing, vomiting, flexion/extension/rotation movements of the neck (as in chiropractic manipulation or endotracheal intubation), swimming, or yoga.[1,12–14] It is estimated that CAD occurs in 1 out of 20 000 neck manipulations. The higher susceptibility to trauma of some arterial segments may be explained by their relation to adjacent bony structures. CAD is more common in the extracranial than in the intracranial vessels, possibly due to the higher mobility and greater vulnerability of extracranial arteries to torsional stress. The internal carotid artery is mobile from its origin at the bifurcation to its entrance in the skull. Its most vulnerable region is at the junction between the mobile (cervical) and relatively fixed (petrous) segments where susceptibility to torsion stress is increased. In the vertebral arteries, the segment after the exit from the vertebral transverse foramina between the C1 and C2 levels and prior to entering the skull base (V3 segment) is mobile and highly prone to stretch injury.

Another factor predisposing to CAD are inherent defects of the arterial wall. Brandt et al.[15] analyzed the connective tissue of skin biopsies in patients with spontaneous CAD, and noted that despite the absence of clinical signs, there were ultrastructural abnormalities in the morphology of the connective tissue such as elastic fiber fragmentation, or medial degeneration in 50%–60% of studied patients[15] similar to the findings observed in hereditary connective tissue diseases. Diseases such as Marfan's syndrome, Ehlers–Danlos syndrome type IV, fibromuscular dysplasia, cystic medial necrosis, alpha 1 antitrypsin deficiency, polycystic kidney disease, osteogenesis imperfecta type I among others are associated with higher occurrence of CAD. In addition, elevation of homocysteine levels may be a risk factor for spontaneous CAD and ischemic stroke, but the mechanism for this relationship is unknown.[16] The search for gene mutations in patients with spontaneous CAD has had low yield. In a study of seven families with familial CAD, a mis-sense mutation in the COL3A1 gene, which encodes for type III pro-collagen and causes Ehlers–Danlos type IV, was detected in two members from one family. Two patients from another family carried a polymorphism in COL5A1 and one carried a variant in COL5A2.[17] Other studies, however, have failed to establish an association between CAD and gene mutations. Such studies are limited by a small sample size due to the low incidence of these disorders. More recently a systematic review of all published data on genetic determinants of CAD showed no evidence for an underlying monogenic disease in sporadic CAD. Only three studies showed positive association with MTHFR 677TT genotype.[18]

Clinical manifestations

A summary of clinical presentations associated with CAD is presented in Table 9.1. Pain, either isolated or in association with focal neurological deficits, is the most common symptom. Ipsilateral or sometimes bilateral neck pain, often radiating to the face and head, are the most common patterns. Isolated contralateral neck pain is infrequent.[19,20] Arterial dissection can produce ischemic stroke or transient ischemic attack (TIA) by different mechanisms: embolism from the intramural hematoma, thrombosis at the site of intimal tear, or arterial occlusion secondary to intramural hematoma expansion or progression of thrombosis. Recurrent hemispheric TIAs or transient monocular visual deficits can occur and lead to cerebral/retinal infarction and permanent deficits. Repetitive neurological deficits localized to the same arterial territory, or postural exacerbation, suggests a hemodynamic mechanism with cerebral hypoperfusion of an occluded or severely compromised carotid lumen.

Carotid dissection can be misdiagnosed as migraine, especially in the absence of focal neurological findings. The headache is often unilateral, throbbing, but can involve the entire head, often accompanied with jaw pain and pulsatile tinnitus. Head or neck pain associated with Horner's syndrome (usually partial, consisting of ptosis and miosis) is highly suggestive of extracranial carotid dissection. Lower cranial nerve palsies involving the IX through XII cranial nerves have been described causing dysphagia, hoarseness and tongue deviation, secondary to nerve ischemia related to impairment of blood flow in the ascending pharyngeal artery, or by mechanical compression or stretching of the cranial nerves at the jugular foramen by the dissected internal carotid artery.[13,21] Pulsatile tinnitus is thought to be secondary to the mass effect of the dissected artery as it courses near the inner ear.[22]

Table 9.1. Clinical manifestations of arterial dissection

Asymptomatic

Pain

Headache, neck pain, jaw pain

Carotid circulation

Hemiparesis, hemisensory loss, aphasia, Horner's syndrome, pulsatile tinnitus

Vertebro-basilar system

Dysarthria, dysphagia, vertigo, diplopia, dysmetria, hemidnopsia, impaired consciousness, Wallenberg's syndrome, tetraparesis, coma

Ophthalmologic

Retinal infarct, amaurosis fugax

Cranial neuropathies

IX, X, XII

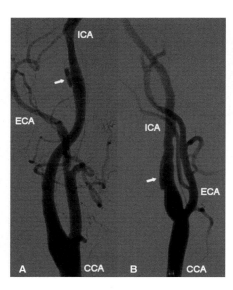

Fig. 9.2. Digital subtraction angiography: contrast injection of the common carotid artery reveals a false lumen at the cervical portion of the ICA (white arrows). ECA: external carotid artery; ICA: internal carotid artery; CCA: common carotid artery.

Cervical vertebral dissection produces ipsilateral neck pain posteriorly, often radiating to the occipital region and/or shoulder area. Neurological manifestations include posterior circulation TIAs and ischemic stroke. Symptoms can include dizziness, diplopia, vertigo, dysarthria, ataxia, and gait instability. Brainstem involvement usually occurs in the medulla and posterior inferior cerebellar artery (PICA) territory.[13] Homonymous hemianopsias or quadrantanopsias due to infarction of the posterior cerebral artery territories must be differentiated from the monocular visual loss in carotid dissection. Loss of consciousness can occur in severe cases where vertebral dissection extends intracranially to occlude the basilar artery.[23]

Diagnosis

Patients can be asymptomatic, or present several hours, days, or even weeks after the onset, regardless of whether trauma is identifiable or not. Even though digital subtraction angiography (DSA) remains the gold standard, non-invasive imaging tests such as computed tomography angiography (CTA), magnetic resonance imaging (MRI), magnetic resonance angiography (MRA) and Doppler sonography have largely replaced the need for catheter angiogrphy in most instances. In addition to confirming the diagnosis of arterial dissection, associated findings may reveal clues to the underlying etiology.

Digital subtraction angiography (DSA) (Fig. 9.2)

DSA is considered the "gold standard" for diagnosis allowing good visualization of the vasculature, particularly in the presence of delayed filling of affected vessels and in differentiating

hypoplasia from dissection in the vertebral arteries. In contrast to atherosclerotic disease, carotid dissection usually does not affect the origin of the carotid bulb, but occurs 1.5 to 2 cm distal to the carotid bulb origin. The anatomical site, multisegmented involvement, and findings such as tapering occlusion, or concomitant occurrence of narrowing and dilatation are suggestive of the diagnosis of dissection. A "string sign" can be observed as the lumen is being compressed by the intramural hematoma or distal flow may be entirely absent. Segmental dilatation associated with pseudoaneurysms is better visualized with DSA. Less common findings include an intimal flap and a double lumen sign. A luminal filling defect suggestive of intravascular thrombus may be infrequently seen on angiographic images.

Computed tomography angiography (CTA) (Fig. 9.3)

CTA has the advantage of being a non-invasive study with good sensitivity to detect flow disruption. In a small series comparing CTA, MRA, US and DSA in diagnosing >70% carotid artery stenosis, the sensitivity of CTA was 81%–93%, specificity was 91%–100%, and diagnostic accuracy was 90%–98%. However, CTA showed an underestimation rate of 7.5% when compared to DSA.[24–26] CTA may also reveal a linear lucency within the vessel, which corresponds to the flap separating the true and false lumen. CTA also allows visualization of stenosis and aneurysmal dilatation. It has a complementary role in the evaluation of CAD and in some instances it provides additional information not obtained with MRI.[27–29] In a retrospective study of 18 patients with cervical artery dissection who underwent both CTA and MRA, two neuroradiologists rated each vessel on the basis of whether the imaging findings (stroke, luminal narrowing, vessel irregularity, wall thickening/ hematoma, pseudoaneurysm, intimal flap)

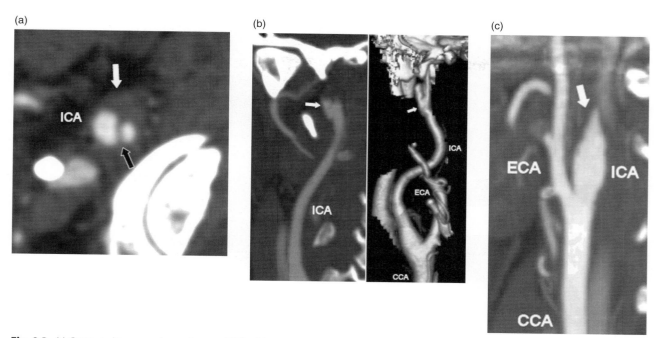

Fig. 9.3. (a) Computed tomography angiogram (CTA) of the ICA showing a mural thrombus (white arrow), and an intimal flap separating the true and false lumen (black arrow). (b) Coronal view of the neck CTA (left) demonstrating dilatation of the distal cervical ICA (white arrow), and 3D-CTA reconstruction (right). (c) Lateral view of neck CTA showing tapering of the ICA after its bifurcation in a "flame-shape" pattern (arrow). ECA: external carotid artery; ICA: internal carotid artery; CCA: common carotid artery.

were better visualized with one modality compared to the other. Overall, CT/CTA was preferred for diagnosis, particularly for vertebral artery dissection, whereas both modalities were similar for ICA dissection.[30]

Magnetic resonance imaging (MRI) and magnetic resonance angiography (MRA) (Fig. 9.4)

MRI T1W axial sequences with fat saturation allow high resolution visualization of the arterial wall by suppressing high signals from the perivascular fat. A crescent-shaped, band-like, eccentric lesion corresponding to an intramural hematoma is highly suggestive of the diagnosis. An increase in the external luminal diameter has a high specificity for carotid dissection.[31–33] The imaging characteristics of the mural hematoma may help identify the timing of CAD onset. In the acute phase, the intramural hematoma may be isointense or slightly hyperintense on T1 and T2 weighted images due to the lack of methemoglobin; in the subacute period, the hematoma is hyperintense on T1 weighted images followed by T2 hyperintensity. Chronic hematomas remain hyperintense on T1 for approximately 2 months and by 6 months hematomas become isointense on T1 and T2 weighted images and may be unrecognizable. It is also possible to detect an intimal flap separating the true and false lumen.

MRA three-dimensional reconstructions in conjunction with phase contrast technique allow direct visualization of the hematoma and aneurysmal dilatation.[32,33] Levy *et al.*

compared the yield of DSA and MR techniques, reporting high sensitivity and specificity for MRA in detecting carotid artery dissection (95% and 99%, respectively), but low accuracy in detecting vertebral artery dissection (20% and 100%, respectively).[31] One explanation is that vertebral arteries are smaller in diameter with broad variation in caliber and thus more difficult to visualize and evaluate. MRI was inferior to MRA in detecting carotid artery dissection (sensitivity 84%, specificity 99%), but superior in detecting vertebral artery dissection (60% and 98%, respectively).

Doppler ultrasound (Fig. 9.5)

Doppler ultrasonography is limited because only a segment of the extracranial portion of ICA or vertebral artery can be visualized. Previous studies reported sensitivities in the range from 80%–96% in the carotid artery and 70%–92% in the vertebrobasilar territory for detection of dissections. The specificity is 92%–94% in the carotid arteries.[21,34–37] The most specific signs such as an echogenic intimal flap or a double lumen are infrequently detected. The yield is even lower in low-grade stenosis and in patients without ischemic events.[21] Combination of extracranial and transcranial Doppler examination can improve the detection of indirect signs of hemodynamic compromise secondary to CAD. Changes in velocities can be seen as part of compensatory hemodynamics in cases of severe stenosis or occlusion. Decreased velocities in the ipsilateral MCA in carotid dissection, and increased contralateral velocities in vertebral occlusion have been reported.

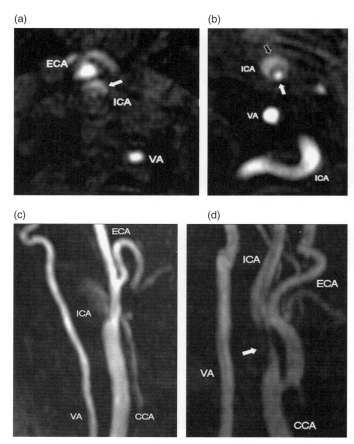

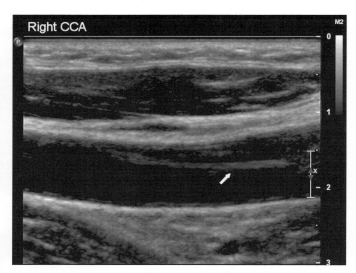

Fig. 9.5. Duplex ultrasound of the mid portion of the CCA reveals an intimal flap separating the true lumen (bottom) from the false lumen (top). CCA: common carotid artery.

Fig. 9.4. (a) and (b) Axial images of neck magnetic resonance angiography (MRA) showing a crescent shaped lumen (white arrow) in a dissected ICA. (b) True lumen (white arrow) surrounded by a less hyperintense signal corresponding to the false lumen (black arrow). (c) and (d) MRA (MIP) reconstruction of the carotid artery showing loss of flow in the ICA after its bifurcation (c), and flow-void signal causing a "string sign" representing the residual lumen (d), white arrow. ECA: external carotid artery; ICA: internal carotid artery; CCA: common carotid artery; VA: vertebral artery; MIP: maximum intensity projection.

Natural history and predictors of outcome

The risk of recurrent stroke after cervical artery dissection is low. Most patients are treated with anticoagulant or antiplatelet therapy, therefore the natural history without medical therapy is not well known. A smaller number of patients are treated by endovascular or surgical means. All interventional options have risks, which must be balanced against natural history on medical therapy.

In a study of 130 patients with angiographically proven dissection of a cervical artery, 4 patients died (3%), and 126 patients were followed for 3906 person/years.[38] Of these, only 17 patients (13%) had symptoms, including 6 strokes and 11 TIAs. Treatment with either anticoagulation or aspirin was used at the discretion of the treating physician. Recurrent ischemic stroke occurred in six patients (4.8%) within the first 2 weeks. While the number of events was small, no difference was found between patients treated with aspirin versus those treated with anticoagulation.

In another study, 27 patients with extracranial cervical dissection (22 spontaneous, 5 traumatic) were treated with anticoagulantion ($n = 18$) or antiplatelet therapy ($n = 9$), and followed for a mean period of 58 months. Of the 27 patients, 23 (85%) had no disability or minor sequelae (modified Rankin score 0 to 1), and four patients had moderate deficits (modified Rankin score 2 to 3).[39] Two patients had a recurrent ischemic stroke, one unrelated to recurrent dissection, and the other following balloon angioplasty and stent placement for treatment of a persistent vertebral artery pseudoaneurysm. Recanalization and improvement in lumen diameter is seen in the majority of patients. In a previous study of angiographically proven arterial dissection, 68% of cases had gradual recanalization after an average of 51 days.[40]

There is limited data that identifies patients at high risk for primary or recurrent ischemic complications after spontaneous dissections. Baumgartner et al. reviewed 200 cases of extracranial carotid dissections and found that patients with ischemic events had a higher prevalence of high-grade stenosis (>80%) and occlusion secondary to the CAD than those without ischemic events. Of note, patients without ischemic events had a higher prevalence of ipsilateral Horner's syndrome and lower cranial nerve palsies.[36] Another study[41] analyzed 69 consecutive medically-treated patients admitted with spontaneous cervico-cranial dissections during a 7-year period and evaluated the effect of demographics (age, gender), vascular risk factors, and angiographic findings (vascular features, percentage of stenosis, presence of pseudoaneurysm, and fibromuscular dysplasia findings) on subsequent neurological events. A total of 11(16%) patients experienced neurological deterioration in the hospital, ten with TIA and ischemic stroke, and one death. An additional four patients developed neurological deterioration between discharge and follow-up at 1 year; three with TIA and ischemic stroke and one death.

Overall, a total of 15 (22%) patients experienced deterioration within one year. Women and those with involvement of both vertebral arteries are at high risk for neurological deterioration.

CAD and aneurysm formation

The natural history of aneurysmal cervical artery dissection was studied among 71 patients with cervical artery dissection. Thirty-five patients (49%) had a total of 42 aneurysms.[42] An aneurysm was defined as an extraluminal pouch (saccular aneurysm) or a segmental dilatation of the lumen (fusiform aneurysm). Thirty aneurysms were located on a symptomatic artery (internal carotid artery 23, vertebral artery 7), and 12 on an asymptomatic artery (internal carotid artery 10, vertebral artery 2). Patients with aneurysms more often had multiple dissections and arterial redundancy. There was a trend towards higher frequency of migraine and cigarette smoking in patients with aneurysmal dilatations. During a mean follow-up of three years, no patient had cerebral ischemia, local compression, or rupture. Forty-six percent of the aneurysms involving the symptomatic ICA remained unchanged, 36% were completely resolved, and 18% had decreased in size. Resolution was more common for vertebral artery than for ICA aneurysms (83% vs. 36%). The authors concluded that, while aneurysms due to CAD frequently persist, there is a very low risk of clinical sequelae, which should be kept in mind before treatment is contemplated.

Treatment

During the first month following an arterial dissection, the risk of recurrent ischemic stroke is highest, and subsequently declines. Treatment options include medical treatment and/or surgical or endovascular intervention.

Medical management

At present, there are no randomized controlled studies comparing the use of antiplatelet with anticoagulant agents. Both have been used to prevent further ischemic complications, whether there is arterial occlusion or stenosis, and with or without associated thromboembolic events.[43] Some clinicians opt to use short-term anticoagulation until there is recanalization on a subsequent follow-up imaging study. The recommended duration of anticoagulation with warfarin (target INR between 2.0 and 3.0) ranges from 6 weeks to 6 months. There is no consensus regarding the use of intravenous heparin for immediate treatment. A follow-up vessel imaging study is usually performed at 3 months. If there is persistence of luminal irregularities, or stenosis, some advocate continuation of anticoagulation until good flow through the affected area is visualized, with subsequent use of antiplatelet agents if the irregularities persist.

Rarely, progression and delayed occlusion after dissection treated with anticoagulants has been reported.[44] Although the pathophysiology is unknown, it is speculated that anticoagulation can in rare cases exacerbate intramural bleeding and intramural clot expansion with subsequent occlusion of a stenotic segment. In addition, in patients with evidence of large cerebral infarction, the likelihood of hemorrhagic complications including symptomatic intraparenchymal hemorrhage with anticoagulation is higher than with antiplatelet therapy.

A previous Cochrane systematic review found that aspirin is likely to be effective and is probably safer than anticoagulation, acknowledging the need for further studies due to lack of strong evidence.[45] Menon et al. reported a meta-analysis of patients who received antiplatelets or anticoagulation therapy for dissection; there was no significant difference in mortality (1.8% vs. 1.8%) or rate of ipsilateral stroke (1.9% vs. 2%, respectively). For the combined endpoint of TIA and stroke, the incidence was 7% in those treated with antiplatelet agents and 3.8% with anticoagulation, but this difference was not statistically significant and was not adjusted for differences in patient characteristics.[43] In a prospective study of 298 consecutive patients with spontaneous cervical carotid artery dissection, 202 patients were treated with anticoagulation and 96 were treated with aspirin. Prospective follow-up was obtained at 3 months by neurological exam (97%) or telephone interview. Ischemic events were rare (0.3% stroke, TIA 3.4%, retinal ischemia 1%), and there was no significant difference in events between those treated with anticoagulation as opposed to those treated with aspirin. Hemorrhagic adverse events were also similar between the two groups (anticoagulants 2%, aspirin 1%). Recurrent ischemic events were more frequent in patients with ischemic events at onset than in patients with local symptoms or those who were asymptomatic.[46]

Current practice guidelines from the American Heart Association/American Stroke Association Council on Stroke state that: "for patients with ischemic stroke or TIA and extracranial arterial dissection, use of warfarin for 3 to 6 months or use of antiplatelet agents is reasonable (Class IIa, Level of Evidence B). Beyond 3 to 6 months, long-term antiplatelet therapy is reasonable for most stroke or TIA patients. Anticoagulant therapy beyond 3 to 6 months may be considered among patients with recurrent ischemic events (Class IIb, Level of Evidence C)."[47] In patients with intracranial dissection anticoagulation is contraindicated given the higher risk of pseudoaneurysm formation and SAH.[11]

Thrombolysis

Intra-arterial thrombolysis with urokinase and t-PA have been used and described in retrospective reports. In patients presenting with acute occlusion related to dissection, a local thrombotic component is invariably present. The results of thrombolysis may depend upon the thrombus burden or on the presence of distal embolization. Despite theoretical concerns about extension of intramural hematoma with progression of intraluminal stenosis, pseudoaneurysm formation, or vessel rupture, current data does not support significant progression of local signs or symptoms or higher rate of adverse events among patients with ICA dissection treated with thrombolysis. The rate of asymptomatic hemorrhagic transformation in the brain has been reported to be around 8%, whereas symptomatic hemorrhagic transformation was seen in only 2%–3% of patients.[43,48,49] Only a few case reports exist on the use of intra-arterial thrombolysis for vertebral artery dissection complicated by basilar occlusion.[23,50] Due to the small number of patients included in these studies, data are insufficient to draw conclusions and provide recommendations. The inherent complications from the procedure itself need to be balanced against potential benefits on a case-by-case basis.

Surgical management

Surgery is rarely used in the treatment of CAD. Available surgical options include ICA ligation and aneurysm resection with carotid reconstruction with interposition of a saphenous vein graft. In distal extracranial ICA lesions near the base of the skull, a cervical to intracranial ICA bypass surgery has been utilized.[51] The American Heart Association/American Stroke Association Council on Stroke recommends consideration of surgical treatment for patients who fail or are not candidates for endovascular therapy (Class IIb, Level of Evidence C).[47]

Endovascular approach

Once endovascular treatment is decided, careful assessment of the angiographic characteristics of the dissection and clinical judgment are required.

In the following section we present details of procedural considerations for the treatment of CAD and intracranial dissections.

Selection of patients

No uniformly accepted criteria exist for selecting patients with dissection who should undergo endovascular treatment. Most practitioners advocate recurrent ischemic symptoms despite antiplatelet or anticoagulant medications as an indication for endovascular treatment. The American Heart Association/American Stroke Association Council on Stroke[47] recommends consideration of endovascular therapy for patients who have definite recurrent ischemic events despite adequate antithrombotic therapy (Class IIb, Level of Evidence C). However, the recurrent ischemic event may be a major ischemic stroke with high rate of disability or death despite medical treatment. Therefore, recent efforts have focused on the early identification of patients at risk for recurrent ischemic events and on intervention prior to deterioration. Angiographic characteristics such as occlusion or high grade stenosis (80% or greater) without presence of robust angiographic collaterals maybe used for selecting patients prior to deterioration. Other measures of collateral failure such as

impairment of vasodilatory reserve on perfusion studies may be used for selecting patients for early intervention. The details about measurement and interpretation of vasodilatory reserve have been described in Chapter 6. The existence of significant hypoperfusion or a large penumbra on MR diffusion and perfusion is another criterion that has been proposed for selecting patients for endovascular treatment.[52] Recent studies have suggested that patients with bilateral vertebral artery dissection may have a higher risk of refractory ischemia and should may be considered for early endovascular treatment.

Morphological assessment of the lesion

Most dissections of the ICA start in the high cervical region and continue into the petrous segment. The clinician must review the demographic and clinical characteristics of the patient and supplement it with angiographic data. A lesion that extends beyond 20 mm after the origin of the ICA or involves multiple segments distal to the origin is unlikely to be atherosclerotic. The vertebral artery has multiple segments of vulnerability to dissection. It travels inside the vertebral foramen from either C5 or C6 to C2 (V2 segment). The junctions (mobile–fixed interface) with segments proximal (V1) and distal (V3) are prone to dissections. The junction between extra- and intracranial artery is also prone to dissections. The vertebral artery may be involved in multiple segments; therefore, assessment of all segments is necessary. Involvement of other extracranial vessels may also provide diagnostic information. Therefore, careful visualization of other extracranial vessels is required (a thorough review of angiographic images or other non-invasive tests performed as part of diagnostic evaluation) prior to performing any endovascular procedure. In addition, study of the renal arteries may help diagnose fibromuscular dysplasia.

An attempt should be made to determine if the dissection is acute or chronic based on the clinical presentation and/or imaging characteristics; for instance, magnetic resonance findings of thrombus within the wall (observed in acute dissections), or angiographic findings such as pseudoaneurysm (observed in chronic dissections). In acute dissections, angioplasty should be avoided if possible and self-expanding stents alone can result in adequate vessel lumen expansion. In chronic dissections, the intervention may require a concomitant angioplasty with self-expanding stent for adequate results.

Pertinent angiographic characteristics of dissection

The initial angiographic images must be carefully reviewed to identify the "dissected segment" as evidenced by irregularity, occlusion, ectatic dilation, or stenosis. The extent of the dissected segment must be defined at both proximal and distal ends within the vessel "normal segment." It should be noted that the "diseased segment" may extend beyond the segment with angiographic abnormalities in one projection. Therefore, the identification of the "dissected segment" requires review of images acquired from multiple projections. The distal extent of the "dissected segment" may be hard to visualize because of poor contrast opacification in the presence of a flow limiting lesion and requires a microcatheter injection distal to the initially visualized "dissected segment." The diameter of the artery in adjacent normal segments should be measured to appropriately size the stent. Distal vessel visualization for measurement may only be possible from a microcatheter injection after traversing the lesion. Alternatively, use of a CT angiogram may provide more accurate measurements.

In the event near occlusion or occlusion of the dissected segment is visualized, an effort must be made to assess the segment distal to the diseased segment for accurate estimation of the extent of dissection and vessel patency. Such visualization can occur by retrograde filling from collateral vessels (from contralateral vertebral artery into distal ipsilateral vertebral artery) or by distal reconstitution from anastomotic artery (filling of cavernous segment of internal carotid artery via retrograde filling of ophthalmic artery). Distal arterial occlusion subsequent to embolization from a dissected segment is not uncommon and may undermine the value of proximal revascularization. Such occlusion may be identified during contrast filling of ipsilateral middle cerebral artery from contralateral anterior circulation or basilar artery branches from contralateral vertebral artery. The overall pattern of blood supply to the distribution of the artery with the "dissected segment" must be understood. The presence of collateral supply from other blood vessels must be identified by selective contrast injections from other pertinent arteries.

Traversing the lesion

A sheath is placed typically in the common femoral artery. A guide catheter is then positioned in the ipsilateral vertebral or carotid artery proximal to the lesion (see Figs. 9.6 and 9.7). The size of the guide catheter must be appropriate to accommodate the stent system. The lesion is traversed with a microwire (shaped in J configuration) and preferably a large microcatheter (2.3F) under roadmap or smart mask fluoroscopic guidance with careful attention not to enter the dissected lumen, which carries the risk of thrombus dislodgment and embolization. The microcatheter is placed distal to the injured segment and contrast is injected to visualize the distal vessel. It is important to confirm that the microcatheter is within the true lumen of the artery to verify the patency of the distal segment. The microwire should be placed as distal as possible with the help of the microcatheter to ensure adequate support for advancing the stent. If the microwire cannot traverse the lesion, proximal administration of thrombolytics or vasodilators may assist in resolution of thrombosis or spasm with subsequent visualization of residual lumen. The distinction between "true" and "false" lumen can be challenging and the term "available" lumen may more accurately reflect the presence of an arterial channel that connects intact proximal and distal arterial segments.

Stent placement

The microcatheter is removed, the microwire is left in position, and the stent is advanced over the microwire. Adequate positioning of the stent should be confirmed using contrast injections and bony landmarks identified from previously

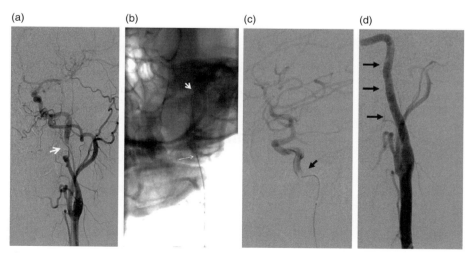

Fig. 9.6. A 39-year-old woman presented with lightheadedness upon standing and blurred vision in the left eye. Cerebral angiography demonstrated bilateral carotid artery dissection. Subsequently, treatment of the symptomatic left internal carotid artery (LICA) dissection was performed using stent placement. (a) Left common carotid artery injection, antero-posterior (AP) projection. The arrow points at the severely narrowed LICA lumen. (b) Unsubtracted oblique view of the cervical region. The thick arrow points to the tip of the microwire which has been given a "J" shape. The "J" shape is used when traversing a dissection in order to avoid entering the false lumen. The thin wire points to the proximal marker of the microwire. (c) Microcatheter injection, lateral projection, performed to verify microcatheter placement in the true lumen. The arrow points at the microcatheter tip. (d) Left common carotid artery injection, AP projection post stent placement. The internal carotid fills normally (arrows).

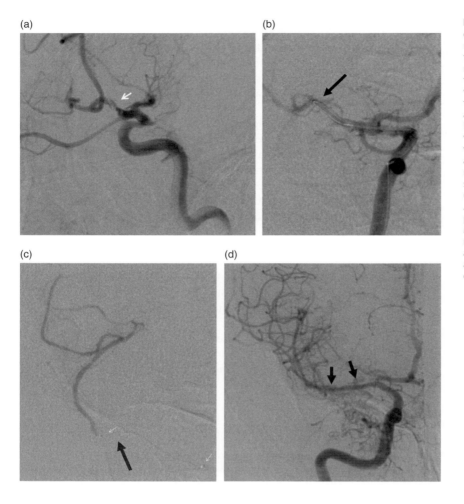

(a)

(b)

(c)

(d)

Fig. 9.7. A 31-year-old man presented with a sudden onset of a severe right-sided headache. Magnetic resonance imaging and angiography demonstrated a right temporal parietal infarct and suggestion of intracranial middle cerebral artery (MCA) dissection. He was admitted to the hospital. The next day, the patient developed worsening of his previous symptoms and was taken to the angiography suite for intervention. (a) Cerebral angiography, subtracted oblique view of the right internal carotid artery. The middle cerebral artery is visualized and demonstrates a filling defect consistent with an intimal flap (arrow). (b) Cerebral angiography, anterior–posterior cranial view. Note the tip of the microwire in the M1 segment of the right MCA, with a "J" shape that was used to traverse the area of dissection. (c) Cerebral angiography, subtracted lateral view. A microcatheter run is performed to demonstrate its position in the true lumen, the superior division of the right MCA is visualized. Arrows point at the markers of the microcatheter. (d) Cerebral angiography, subtracted anterior–posterior view of the right internal carotid artery after stent placement. Note patency of the M1 segment of the MCA (arrows) and its superior and inferior divisions.

acquired angiographic images. The stent is deployed either by inflation of the balloon (balloon mounted) or withdrawal of the outer sheath (self-expanding). Self-expanding stents are preferred to avoid further injury to the dissected segment because they have less radial force. Prominent improvement in lumen diameter may be observed after placement of a self-expanding stent without any angioplasty. Drug-eluting stents are avoided to allow endothelization without interference by anti-mitotic drugs. Rarely, submaximal (2.0–3.0 mm) angioplasty may be required to create luminal space to facilitate stent delivery. The largest diameter of the target segments that requires opposition of the stent is measured. The nominal diameter of the stent must exceed the vessel diameter. The length of the stent must be selected to: (1) adequately cover the lesion; (2) consider the position of the distal end to avoid angulated or unopposed placement due to tortuosity or post-stenotic dilatation; and (3) estimate the consequences of deployment into the distal internal carotid artery (size mismatch). The distal aspect of the stent is usually placed in the petrous segment of the internal carotid artery. Such self-expanding stents are currently available for intracranial use. The proximal aspect of the stent may require partial placement in the common carotid artery. Since the stent required for

common carotid artery requires a 6 F guide sheath instead of 6 F guide catheter, early anticipation of such proximal deployment may lead to consideration of a guide sheath placement. The vessel diameter of the distal internal carotid artery may be much smaller than the diameter of the proximal internal or common carotid artery. However, stents of differing diameters are sequentially deployed with overlap, to address the mismatch.

Placement of multiple stents

Multiple stent placements may be required to adequately cover the entire length of the diseased segment and/or address the distal to proximal size mismatch. The rule is that the distal-most segment of the dissection should be covered first. Such distal-to-proximal serial stent placement avoids resistance to passage of stent delivery devices through proximally placed stents. Furthermore, mechanical manipulation of proximally placed stents may lead to stent displacement or dislodgement. After the stent is deployed, angiographic images are acquired and carefully reviewed to assess the need for additional stents or coil placement outside the stents to ensure adequate resolution of the lesion. The stents should overlap in order to avoid leaving uncovered arterial segments. Uncovered segments are more prone to restenosis or further dissection. Sometimes, there may be resistance to passage of a second stent through the proximal section of the first stent. The resistance is usually a result of sharp angulation encountered by the relatively inflexible distal end of the stent delivery device as it enters the relatively straight vessel with limited compliance due to the proximal part of the first stent. Changing the angle of entry by advancing the microwire further distally or advancing the guide catheter/sheath further may be helpful. External manipulation of the neck may also change the angulation. If the resistance is secondary to small diameter within the first stent, an angioplasty may be necessary prior to re-attempting to place the second stent.

Adjuvant use of thrombolytics, antiplatelets, and anticoagulants

Thromboembolic phenomena resulting from arterial dissections due to thrombogenicity induced by stasis and subintimal exposure are frequent. Intra-arterial thrombolysis may be required concomitantly with stent placement to treat thrombosis in, or distal embolization from, the dissected segment. Thrombolysis may be initiated after the microcatheter traverses the original lesion and distal occlusion is visualized.

Patients are administered aspirin (325 mg daily) and clopidogrel (75 mg daily) prior to, and intravenous heparin during, the procedure to reduce the risk of thrombo-embolism associated with the procedure. Clopidogrel may be administered as a bolus of 300 mg to 600 mg if daily doses have not been initiated 3 days prior to procedure to achieve optimal antiplatelet effect. Activated coagulation time is used to monitor the level of anticoagulation during the procedure. The level of anti-coagulation is controversial, but lower doses (30–50 U/kg) are preferable in the presence of new ischemic lesions. Intravenous antiplatelet agents (platelet glycoprotein IIB/IIIA inhibitors) including abciximab, and eptifibatide have rarely been used as adjunctive treatment with intravenous heparin during the procedure. Currently, the use of glycoprotein IIB/IIIA inhibitors is restricted to patients with intravascular thrombus or new neurological deficits during the procedure (rescue treatment). It should be noted that if glycoprotein IIB/IIIA inhibitors are to be used, heparin dose should be reduced to maintain activated coagulation time below 200 seconds.

Intracranial dissections and pseudoaneurysms

The treatment strategy for intracranial dissections presenting with ischemic deficits is very similar to the strategy outlined above for extracranial carotid and vertebral artery lesions (see Figs. 9.6 and 9.7). The choice of stents is different and adjusted to match unique needs for deliverability, flexibility, and size. Self-expanding stents are used preferentially to avoid injury to the diseased artery. The treatment of

pseudoaneurysms is described in both the chapters on traumatic vascular injury and intracranial aneurysms.

Follow-up

Aspirin (325 mg daily) and clopidogrel (75 mg daily) are prescribed at discharge and continued for a period of 1 to 3 months. Subsequently, aspirin is continued indefinitely. A detailed account of the peri-procedural management is presented in Chapter 4. The usual clinic follow-ups are scheduled at 1 month, 6 months, and 1 year and then subsequently at yearly intervals. Routine screening of all patients who have undergone stent placement for dissection cannot be recommended based on the low prevalence of restenosis and late strokes. Non-invasive testing may be helpful in patients who had complete occlusion secondary to dissection due to the possibility of spontaneous partial recanalization or distal reconstitution via collaterals. It is an acceptable practice to perform a conventional angiogram at 6 months to detect any ectasia or pseudoaneurysm formation at the site of stent placement or dissection. Carotid Doppler ultrasound as a follow-up study may be inadequate because it offers limited visualization of high cervical segments. Similarly, CTA and MRA may be limited by stent artifact.

Experience with stent placement for dissections

There are several case series and reports on stent placement for dissection, most of which were implemented in the setting of failed, or contraindication to, anticoagulation therapy, hemodynamically significant stenosis, and MRI perfusion demonstrating significant mismatch.[52–57] In general, in these series, significant improvement in recanalization of the lumen was achieved to less than 25% residual diameter, and good outcome was achieved in most patients.

In one series of nine patients with cervical or intracranial dissection refractory to medical management, the self-expanding Neuroform stent was deployed (Boston Scientific, Fremont, CA), with three patients undergoing stent-assisted coil embolization.[58] There were no procedure-related complications, but two patients died as a result of the initial sequelae of vertebral-basilar artery thrombosis. In follow-up, delayed in-stent stenosis was seen in two patients, and all surviving patients demonstrated clinical improvement or resolution of symptoms.

Another series of ten patients with traumatic carotid artery dissection and hemodynamically significant hemispheric hypoperfusion, or in whom anticoagulation was contraindicated, or failed medical management, stenting was used.[59] Mean stenosis was reduced from 69% to 8%. During a mean follow-up of 16 months, patients remained free of ischemic events and none had in-stent stenosis by ultrasound. The same authors reported on a patient with bilateral extracranial vertebral artery dissection, multiple embolic infarctions precluding anticoagulation and a right vertebral artery with intraluminal thrombi. The dominant left vertebral artery was reconstructed with multiple tandem balloon-mounted stents, and the contralateral vertebral artery was occluded with coils.[56] The addition of emboli protection device has also been reported for symptomatic vertebral artery dissection treated with stent angioplasty.[55]

Another study[60] reported the immediate and long-term clinical and angiographic outcomes of high risk patients presenting with ischemic symptoms undergoing stent placement for spontaneous cervico-cranial dissections.

A total of 14 patients were treated with stent placement for dissection located in the following sites: intracranial internal carotid artery ($n = 2$), proximal middle cerebral artery ($n = 1$), extracranial internal carotid ($n = 6$), intracranial vertebral artery ($n = 4$). Clinical follow-up ranged from 26–900 days (mean period of 355 days). There was one TIA (7%) and one minor ischemic stroke (7%), and no deaths observed during follow-up. Stroke-free survival was 93% at 1 month after the procedure. Two of 14 patients were treated for pseudoaneurysm. For 12 patients treated for severe stenosis, post-procedure there was complete resolution of stenosis in all but two

patients. Angiographic follow-up was available in nine patients ranging from 26–612 days (mean period 245 days). There was no change in within-stent or per-stent lumen diameter on follow-up angiography.

Conclusions

Cervical artery dissection is a common cause for cerebral ischemic events in young adults with ischemic stroke, with increasing detection with common use of current non-invasive imaging. Trauma, connective tissue disorders are common underlying predispositions to the development of carotid or vertebral artery dissection. The clinical manifestations of cervical artery dissection display a wide spectrum, from asymptomatic to isolated pain and large hemispheric stroke. While no randomized controlled trials exist, medical therapy with antiplatelet or anticoagulant treatment is first-line therapy, with the majority of patients demonstrating no recurrent ischemic symptoms and healing of the artery on follow-up. Endovascular therapy with stenting has been reported in several small case series, and is generally considered for patients who fail medical therapy.

References

1. Schievink WI. Spontaneous dissection of the carotid and vertebral arteries. *N Engl J Med* 2001;**344**:898–906.

2. Ducrocq X, Lacour JC, Debouverie M, Bracard S, Girard F, Weber M. [Cerebral ischemic accidents in young subjects. A prospective study of 296 patients aged 16 to 45 years]. *Rev Neurol (Paris)* 1999;**155**:575–82.

3. Pratt-Thomas HR, Switzer PK. Sicklemia; its pathological and clinical significance. *South Med J* 1949;**42**:376–84.

4. Giroud M, Fayolle H, Andre N, *et al.* Incidence of internal carotid artery dissection in the community of Dijon. *J Neurol Neurosurg Psychiatry* 1994; **57**:1443.

5. Lee VH, Brown RD, Jr., Mandrekar JN, Mokri B. Incidence and outcome of cervical artery dissection: a population-based study. *Neurology* 2006;**67**:1809–12.

6. Hufnagel A, Hammers A, Schonle PW, Bohm KD, Leonhardt G. Stroke following chiropractic manipulation of the cervical spine. *J Neurol* 1999; **246**:683–8.

7. Touze E, Gauvrit JY, Moulin T, Meder JF, Bracard S, Mas JL. Risk of stroke and recurrent dissection after a cervical artery dissection: a multicenter study. *Neurology* 2003;**61**:1347–51.

8. Schievink WI, Mokri B, O'Fallon WM. Recurrent spontaneous cervical-artery dissection. *N Engl J Med* 1994; **330**:393–7.

9. Schievink WI, Mokri B, Piepgras DG, Kuiper JD. Recurrent spontaneous arterial dissections: risk in familial versus nonfamilial disease. *Stroke* 1996;**27**:622–4.

10. Schievink WI, Wijdicks EF, Michels VV, Vockley J, Godfrey M. Heritable connective tissue disorders in cervical artery dissections: a prospective study. *Neurology* 1998;**50**:1166–9.

11. Wilkinson IM. The vertebral artery. Extracranial and intracranial structure. *Arch Neurol* 1972;**27**:392–6.

12. Norris JW, Beletsky V, Nadareishvili ZG. Sudden neck movement and cervical artery dissection. The Canadian Stroke Consortium. *Cmaj* 2000;**163**:38–40.

13. Caplan LR, Zarins CK, Hemmati M. Spontaneous dissection of the extracranial vertebral arteries. *Stroke* 1985;**16**:1030–8.

14. Fisher CM, Ojemann RG, Roberson GH. Spontaneous dissection of cervico-cerebral arteries. *Can J Neurol Sci* 1978; **5**:9–19.

15. Brandt T, Morcher M, Hausser I. Association of cervical artery dissection with connective tissue abnormalities in

skin and arteries. *Front Neurol Neurosci* 2005;**20**:16–29.

16. Benninger DH, Herrmann FR, Georgiadis D, *et al.* Increased prevalence of hyperhomocysteinemia in cervical artery dissection causing stroke: a case-control study. *Cerebrovasc Dis* 2009;**27**:241–6.

17. Martin JJ, Hausser I, Lyrer P, *et al.* Familial cervical artery dissections: clinical, morphologic, and genetic studies. *Stroke* 2006;**37**:2924–9.

18. Debette S, Markus HS. The genetics of cervical artery dissection. A Systematic Review. Stroke 2009;**40**:e459–66.

19. Biousse V, D'Anglejan-Chatillon J, Massiou H, Bousser MG. Head pain in non-traumatic carotid artery dissection: a series of 65 patients. *Cephalalgia* 1994;**14**:33–6.

20. Sturzenegger M. Headache and neck pain: the warning symptoms of vertebral artery dissection. *Headache* 1994;**34**:187–93.

21. Sturzenegger M, Huber P. Cranial nerve palsies in spontaneous carotid artery dissection. *J Neurol Neurosurg Psychiatry* 1993;**56**:1191–9.

22. Liess BD, Lollar KW, Christiansen SG, Vaslow D. Pulsatile tinnitus: a harbinger of a greater ill? *Head Neck* 2009;**31**:269–73.

23. Cerrato P, Berardino M, Bottacchi E, *et al.* Vertebral artery dissection complicated by basilar artery occlusion successfully treated with intra-arterial thrombolysis: three case reports. *Neurol Sci* 2008;**29**:51–5.

24. Magarelli N, Scarabino T, Simeone AL, *et al.* Carotid stenosis: a comparison between MR and spiral CT angiography. *Neuroradiology* 1998;**40**:367–73.

25. Simeone A, Carriero A, Armillotta M, *et al.* Spiral CT angiography in the study of the carotid stenoses. *J Neuroradiol* 1997;**24**:18–22.

26. Sameshima T, Futami S, Morita Y, *et al.* Clinical usefulness of and problems with three-dimensional CT angiography for the evaluation of arteriosclerotic stenosis of the carotid artery: comparison with conventional angiography, MRA, and ultrasound sonography. *Surg Neurol* 1999;**51**: 301–8; discussion 308–9.

27. Elijovich L, Kazmi K, Gauvrit JY, Law M. The emerging role of multidetector row CT angiography in the diagnosis of cervical arterial dissection: preliminary study. *Neuroradiology* 2006;**48**:606–12.

28. Egelhof T, Jansen O, Winter R, Sartor K. [CT angiography in dissections of the internal carotid artery. Value of a new examination technique in comparison with DSA and Doppler ultrasound]. *Radiologe* 1996;**36**:850–4.

29. Leclerc X, Godefroy O, Salhi A, Lucas C, Leys D, Pruvo JP. Helical CT for the diagnosis of extracranial internal carotid artery dissection. *Stroke* 1996;**27**:461–6.

30. Vertinsky AT, Schwartz NE, Fischbein NJ, Rosenberg J, Albers GW, Zaharchuk G. Comparison of multidetector CT angiography and MR imaging of cervical artery dissection. *Am J Neuroradiol* 2008;**29**:1753–60.

31. Levy C, Laissy JP, Raveau V, *et al.* Carotid and vertebral artery dissections: three-dimensional time-of-flight MR angiography and MR imaging versus conventional angiography. *Radiology* 1994;**190**:97–103.

32. Kitanaka C, Tanaka J, Kuwahara M, Teraoka A. Magnetic resonance imaging study of intracranial vertebrobasilar artery dissections. *Stroke* 1994;**25**:571–5.

33. Provenzale JM. Dissection of the internal carotid and vertebral arteries: imaging features. *Am J Roentgenol* 1995;**165**:1099–104.

34. Benninger DH, Georgiadis D, Gandjour J, Baumgartner RW. Accuracy of color duplex ultrasound diagnosis of spontaneous carotid dissection causing ischemia. *Stroke* 2006;**37**:377–81.

35. Dittrich R, Dziewas R, Ritter MA, *et al.* Negative ultrasound findings in patients with cervical artery dissection. Negative ultrasound in CAD. *J Neurol* 2006; **253**:424–33.

36. Baumgartner RW, Arnold M, Baumgartner I, *et al.* Carotid dissection with and without ischemic events: local symptoms and cerebral artery findings. *Neurology* 2001;**57**:827–32.

37. Nebelsieck J, Sengelhoff C, Nassenstein I, *et al.* Sensitivity of neurovascular ultrasound for the detection of spontaneous cervical artery dissection. *J Clin Neurosci* 2009;**16**:79–82.

38. Arauz A, Hoyos L, Espinoza C, Cantu C, Barinagarrementeria F, Roman G. Dissection of cervical arteries: long-term follow-up study of 130 consecutive cases. *Cerebrovasc Dis* 2006;**22**:150–4.

39. Gonzales-Portillo F, Bruno A, Biller J. Outcome of extracranial cervicocephalic arterial dissections: a follow-up study. *Neurol Res* 2002;**24**:395–8.

40. Steinke W, Rautenberg W, Schwartz A, Hennerici M. Noninvasive monitoring of internal carotid artery dissection. *Stroke* 1994;**25**:998–1005.

41. Ameer E Hassan MFS, Adnan I Qureshi *et al.* Clinical and radiological predictors of neurological deterioration in spontaneous cervico-carotid dissections. *Abstract submitted in the International Stroke Conference* **2010** San Antonio, TX 2009.

42. Touze E, Randoux B, Meary E, Arquizan C, Meder JF, Mas JL. Aneurysmal forms of cervical artery dissection: associated factors and outcome. *Stroke* 2001;**32**:418–23.

43. Menon R, Kerry S, Norris JW, Markus HS. Treatment of cervical artery dissection: a systematic review and meta-analysis. *J Neurol Neurosurg Psychiatry* 2008;**79**:1122–7.

44. Dreier JP, Lurtzing F, Kappmeier M, *et al.* Delayed occlusion after internal carotid artery dissection under heparin. *Cerebrovasc Dis* 2004;**18**: 296–303.

45. Lyrer P, Engelter S. Antithrombotic drugs for carotid artery dissection. *Cochrane Database Syst Rev* 2003: CD000255.

46. Georgiadis D, Arnold M, von Buedingen HC, *et al.* Aspirin vs anticoagulation in carotid artery dissection: a study of 298 patients. *Neurology* 2009;**72**:1810–5.

47. Sacco RL, Adams R, Albers G, *et al.* Guidelines for prevention of stroke in patients with ischemic stroke or transient ischemic attack: a statement for healthcare professionals from the American Heart Association/American Stroke Association Council on Stroke: co-sponsored by the Council on Cardiovascular Radiology and Intervention: the American Academy of Neurology affirms the value of this guideline. *Circulation* 2006;**113**:e409–49.

48. Georgiadis D, Lanczik O, Schwab S, *et al.* IV thrombolysis in patients with acute stroke due to spontaneous carotid dissection. *Neurology* 2005;**64**:1612–14.

49. Arnold M, Nedeltchev K, Sturzenegger M, *et al.* Thrombolysis in patients with acute stroke caused by cervical artery dissection: analysis of 9 patients and review of the literature. *Arch Neurol* 2002;**59**:549–53.

50. Price RF, Sellar R, Leung C, O'Sullivan MJ. Traumatic vertebral arterial dissection and vertebrobasilar arterial thrombosis successfully treated with endovascular thrombolysis and stenting. *AJNR Am J Neuroradiol* 1998;**19**:1677–80.

51. Schievink WI, Piepgras DG, McCaffrey TV, Mokri B. Surgical treatment of extracranial internal carotid artery dissecting aneurysms. *Neurosurgery* 1994;**35**:809–15; discussion 815–16.

52. Cohen JE, Leker RR, Gotkine M, Gomori M, Ben-Hur T. Emergent stenting to treat patients with carotid artery dissection: clinically and radiologically directed therapeutic decision making. *Stroke* 2003;**34**:e254–7.

53. Ansari SA, Thompson BG, Gemmete JJ, Gandhi D. Endovascular Treatment of Distal Cervical and Intracranial Dissections with the Neuroform Stent. *Neurosurgery* 2008; **62**(3): 636–46.

54. Malek AM, Higashida RT, Phatouros CC, *et al.* Endovascular management of extracranial carotid artery dissection achieved using stent angioplasty. *AJNR Am J Neuroradiol* 2000;**21**:1280–92.

55. Cohen JE, Gomori JM, Umansky F. Endovascular management of symptomatic vertebral artery dissection achieved using stent angioplasty and

emboli protection device. *Neurol Res* 2003;**25**:418–22.

56. Cohen JE, Gomori JM, Umansky F. Endovascular management of spontaneous bilateral symptomatic vertebral artery dissections. *AJNR Am J Neuroradiol* 2003;**24**:2052–6.

57. Abboud H, Houdart E, Meseguer E, Amarenco P. Stent assisted endovascular thrombolysis of internal carotid artery dissection. *J Neurol*

Neurosurg Psychiatry 2005;**76**: 292–3.

58. Ansari SA, Thompson BG, Gemmete JJ, Gandhi D. Endovascular treatment of distal cervical and intracranial dissections with the neuroform stent. *Neurosurgery* 2008;**62**:636–46; discussion 646.

59. Cohen JE, Ben-Hur T, Rajz G, Umansky F, Gomori JM. Endovascular stent-assisted angioplasty in the management of traumatic internal

carotid artery dissections. *Stroke* 2005;**36**:e45–7.

60. Ameer E Hassan GJR, Nauman Tariq, Gabriela Vazquez, M Fareed Suri, Adnan I Qureshi. Long-term clinical and angiographic outcomes in patients with spontaneous cervico-cranial dissections treated with stent placement. *Abstract submitted in the International Stroke Conference* San Antonio TX 2010 2009.

Chapter 10

Traumatic vascular injury

Jefferson T. Miley MD, Qaisar A. Shah MD and Adnan I. Qureshi MD

Introduction

Improvement and development of new endovascular devices have allowed the use of endovascular techniques as yet another treatment modality for traumatic vascular injuries.

The history of traumatic vascular injuries begins nearly 500 years ago, when Ambrose Pare (1510–1590) in 1552 performed the first carotid artery ligation in a French soldier who suffered a penetrating vascular injury from a bayonet[1] and later Verneuil reported the first treatment of blunt carotid artery injury in 1872.[2]

For many years, the treatment of traumatic vascular injuries was either surgical or medical. In 1964, Fedor Serbinenko first performed an endovascular balloon occlusion of the internal carotid artery.[3] Later Charles Dotter in 1969 introduced the concept of endovascular stent-grafts.[4] Endovascular repair with stent grafts in neurovascular trauma was accomplished in the 1990s,[5,6] initiating the use of endovascular treatment for traumatic vascular injuries.

Classification

Multiple classifications have been used to describe vascular injuries. A common and acceptable scheme is based on the underlying mechanism of injury. Blunt trauma is defined as a serious injury caused by a blunt object or collision with a blunt surface (as in a vehicle accident or fall from a building). Penetrating trauma is defined as an injury incurred when an object (such as a knife, bullet or shrapnel) penetrates into the vessel.

Other classifications commonly used are based on the angiographic appearance[7] (Table 10.1), morphology of vascular injury[8] (Table 10.2), and anatomical location of the injury. For the purpose of this chapter, anatomical locations will be classified as intracranial and cervical.

Penetrating injuries to the neck are classified into three zones where the anatomical limits are skull base, sternal notch, clavicles and sternocleidomastoid muscles.[9,10] The vascular contents found on each zone are compiled in Table 10.3.

Table 10.1. Angiographic classification of vascular injuries

Grade I	Luminal irregularity or dissection with <25% luminal narrowing
Grade II	Dissection or intramural thrombus with >25% luminal narrowing, intraluminal thrombus, or raised intimal flap
Grade III	Pseudoaneurysm
Grade IV	Occlusion
Grade V	Transection with free extravasation

Table 10.2. Morphological classification of vascular injuries

Simple lacerations
Laceration with partial wall loss
Transection
Simple contusion
Contusion with elevated intimal flap and thrombosis
Contusion with true aneurysm
Contusion with spasm
Contusion with subintimal hematoma
False aneurysm
Arteriovenous fistula
Extrinsic compression

Zone I originates at the clavicles and sternal notch, and extends into the cricoid cartilage. The non-vascular structures in this zone are the lungs, esophagus, trachea, and the thoracic duct. Zone II extends from the cricoid cartilage to the angle of the mandible and includes the larynx and hypopharynx. Zone III originates in the angle of the mandible and extends to the base of the skull and contains hypopharynx as the only non-vascular structure.

Textbook of Interventional Neurology, ed. Adnan I. Qureshi. Published by Cambridge University Press. © Cambridge University Press 2011.

Histology of intracranial arteries

Intracranial arteries have a different histological appearance compared to extracranial vessels (Fig. 10.1). When arteries become intradural, the adventitia and medial muscular layers become thinner. A reduction of the elastic fibers is seen, the internal elastic lamina becomes prominent, and the external elastic lamina disappears. The tunica intima is the only layer that remains unchanged. These changes can be seen within 5 mm before the attachment of the dura.[11,12]

Incidence
Blunt cervical vascular trauma

The incidence of blunt cervical vascular injuries (BCVI) has varied with sensitivity of diagnostic technology. In the past, blunt carotid artery injuries (BCAI) and blunt vertebral artery injuries (BVAI) were considered uncommon conditions accounting for a few case reports and small case series.[13–20] These patients would be frequently diagnosed when a neurologic deficit occurred.

Table 10.3. Vascular contents of the neck, by zone

Zone I
Subclavian vessels
Brachiocephalic veins
Common carotid arteries
Aortic arch
Jugular veins
Zone II
Carotid arteries
Vertebral arteries
Jugular veins
Zone III
Carotid arteries
Jugular veins

Prior to 1996, the incidence of BCAI in trauma victims was 0.08%–0.33%.[21–24] Since, the reported incidence of BCAI and BVAI has increased to 0.5%–0.86%[21,25–27] and 0.4%–1.11%,[25–29] respectively. An explanation for this increase is that, since 1996 awareness among medical professionals has increased, with higher availability of non-invasive imaging in trauma victims higher proportion of the asymptomatic cases are detected with improving imaging technology.[23,26,27,30] Since 1996, the overall incidence of BCVI is 0.92%–1.55%.[25,27,30–32]

Common places where blunt vascular injuries can occur are at transition segments, such as where the cervical arteries enter the skull (petrous segment of internal carotid and V3 segment of vertebral artery) or where the vertebral artery enters or exits the transverse processes. The internal carotid artery can also sustain injuries at its origin and the vertebral arteries can be injured when an adjacent vertebral fracture occurs.

Penetrating cervical vascular trauma

Penetrating injuries to the neck are seen in approximately 5%–10% of all civilian trauma victims.[33] In 14.4%–36.9%[34–38] of the cases, concurrent vascular injuries are seen.

The size of a vascular structure (radius and length) is directly proportional to the risk of vascular injury in penetrating neck injuries. For this reason, when the penetrating artifact crosses the midline the risk of vascular injury increases.[38,39] Vessels commonly injured are the common carotid artery, internal jugular vein, internal carotid artery, and external carotid artery.[34,35,40–42]

In the civilian population, since zone II is the most exposed area of the neck, injuries are more common in zone II than zone I and III combined.[34–36,41,43]

The incidence of penetrating neck injuries related to a war has varied through history. Some factors that have contributed to the variable incidence are the development of offensive and protective military technology. The incidence in soldiers from the present conflict in Iraq and Afganistan that were evaluated in Landstuhl Regional Medical Center (Germany) was 21%.[44] Vascular trauma was seen in 33% of the soldiers evaluated at Walter Reed Army Medical Center.[45]

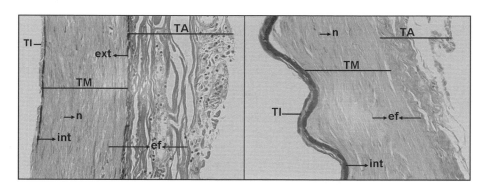

Fig. 10.1. Photomicrography of a coronary artery (left) and intracranial internal carotid artery (right) using identical magnification (Verhoeff-Van Gieson). ef = elastic fiber, ext = external elastic membrane, int = internal elastic membrane, n = nuclei of smooth muscle cells, TA = tunica adventitia, TI = tunica intima, TM = tunica media. Courtesy of H.B.Clark MD, PhD. Director of Neuropathology. University of Minnesota. See plate section.

Intracranial vascular trauma

Penetrating or blunt trauma can result in intracranial vascular injuries. These include aneurysm, dissection, and fistula formation (Chapters 9, 11, and 14).

Aneurysms can be classified into true and false aneurysms. True aneurysms have disruption of the intima, internal elastic lamina, and media layers. The adventitial layer is intact. In false aneurysms, a disruption of all vessel layers with a hematoma in surrounding tissue is found. This is the most common form of traumatic intracranial aneurysms (TICA)[46] or pseudoaneurysms.

Trauma is the responsible mechanism in less than 1% of intracranial aneurysms.[47,48] Most of these aneurysms occur in patients younger than 18 years.[49,50] The incidence of TICA in penetrating injuries is reported to be as low as 0.1%,[51] but in other reports the incidence range from 3.2%–12%.[52–56]

The penetrating arterial injuries, occur when the missile fragment or sharp object enters through the temporal, parietal or frontal bone.[54,55,57] The reported cases of TICA have almost exclusively involved the anterior circulation,[46,53–55,57–59] and rarely the posterior circulation.[54,58] Most of the aneurysms are found in the distal portion of the missile trajectory.[46]

Blunt TICA can occur in almost any intracranial vessel. These are commonly found where the vascular structure attaches or travels adjacent to the dura mater, in sharp surfaces of the skull like the sphenoid ridge or even adjacent skull fractures.[60–71] An observed predilection for distal cerebral vessels has also been suggested for both blunt[72] and penetrating injuries.[53]

There are few reliable estimates of traumatic intracranial dissections. These occur mainly in young people and blunt trauma is considered to be the principal mechanism. In 22%–60% of the victims, a history of trauma can be obtained, but the severity of the trauma may be trivial.[73,74]

Dissection of intracranial vessels occurs when the internal elastic lamina and the tunica media are disrupted along with the development of an intramural hematoma with an intact adventitia. Involvement of the adventitia can result in subarachnoid hemorrhage (SAH).[75,76] Dissection can cause stenosis, vessel occlusion or even pseudoaneurysms.[73,74,77] No clear distinction has been established in the literature regarding the difference between TICA and pseudoaneurysms.

The vessels reported to be injured include the vertebral artery,[74,78,79] internal carotid artery,[65,74,80] posterior inferior cerebellar artery,[64] anterior cerebral artery,[61,73,74,81,82] middle meningeal artery,[66–68] and middle cerebral artery.[62,73,74,77,81,82]

Stroke rate and mortality

Blunt cervical vascular trauma

Trauma victims with BCVI are at risk for stroke and death. Rates for both of these events are higher when the internal carotid arteries are injured when compared with the vertebral arteries.

The rate of stroke varies between studies. Factors such as medical treatment and time interval used for screening of asymptomatic vascular injury contribute to this variability. In BCAI the rate is 6.8%–64%,[21,25,26,83] and in BVAI is 2.6%–26%.[25,26,28,83]

The mortality attributed to vascular injury is 11%–15%,[21,25,26] 4%–7.9%,[25,26,28] and 9.5%–27%[25,27,30,32,83] for BCAI, BVAI, and all BCVI, respectively. Arterial transection carry the highest immediate mortality among vascular injuries.

Penetrating cervical vascular trauma

Victims of penetrating neck trauma can have vascular and nonvascular injuries. Unfortunately, most of these injuries result in stroke or even death prior to hospital arrival.[40]

The rate of stroke in penetrating neck injuries ranges between 3% and 28%.[36,41,43] The in-hospital mortality ranges between 9% and 22%,[34,36,41,43,84,85] and mortality related to vascular injury ranges between 1.5% and 18.5%.[34,35,41,86,87] The common causes of death are exsanguination or neurological deficits.[41,43,86,88] Gun shot wounds are more likely to result in vascular trauma when compared with other penetrating injuries.[38]

Vascular injuries to zones I and III carry a high mortality. Surgical access to the thorax or to the skull base can be difficult contributing to the likelihood of death. The treatment is targeted at achieving hemostasis control of zone III proximally and zone I distally.[35,43]

The mortality from wartime penetrating neck injuries has varied. These variations are influenced by warfare technology but also by medical attention protocols. In World War I the mortality was 11%[89] and this decreased to 4.5% in World War II.[90] In World War II, the concept was introduced that all penetrating neck injuries should be explored surgically. With the development of a Mobile Army Surgical Hospital (MASH) the mortality decreased to 2.5% in Korea.[90] Later, in Vietnam, it increased to 8% as result of improved offensive military equipment.[91] Recently, the Task Force Ranger presence in Somalia[91] and the war in Iraq/Afghanistan[45] reported a mortality of 7% and 3.2%, respectively.

Intracranial vascular trauma

Little is known about stroke risk related to intracranial vascular injuries. In case series of patients with known TICA, the risk of hemorrhage is 19%–36%.[47,52] The mortality related to TICA rupture is reported to be as high as 50%.[92–94] Mortality from traumatic dissections is not known but in cases of spontaneous dissection, it can be up to 75%.[76,95]

Pathophysiology

Blunt injuries

Blunt neurovascular injuries can occur from direct blows to the neck or sudden acceleration/decelerations resulting in

Table 10.4. Causes of blunt vascular injury[25,26,28,29,79,83,96–98]

Motor vehicle accidents
Falls
Assaults
Pedestrian struck
Motorcycle crash
Near hangings
Sports related injuries
Iatrogenic
Endotracheal intubation
Chiropractic manipulation

Table 10.5. Imaging screening for high risk patients[25,28,29,83,99,100]

Fractures
Skull base
Carotid canal
Vertebral fractures
Subluxation
Foramen transversarium
Cervical vertebrae
Displaced midface or complex mandibular fracture
Near hanging or seat belt abrasion in the neck

hyperextension, hyperflexion, or rotation of head and neck. Two mechanisms of vascular injury have been proposed.[76,96]

1. Rotation–extension: Cervical rotation with extension can result in intimal tear of the posterior wall of the internal carotid artery by compression from the transverse processes of the C-2 and C-3 vertebrae. The vertebral artery is also prone to injury at C1–C2 vertebral levels during cervical rotation.
2. Flexion: During flexion of neck, the internal carotid artery can be compressed between the cervical vertebra and angle of mandible resulting in intimal tear.

The common causes of vascular blunt injuries are secondary to motor vehicle accidents, falls and assaults (Table 10.4).

Where vessels travel adjacent to bone structures they are most susceptible to injuries. Vertebral and carotid artery injuries should always be suspected when vertebral fractures and skull base fractures are identified. Screening guidelines to detect vascular injuries have been published by multiple centers (Table 10.5).

The two proposed mechanisms of ischemic stroke following traumatic vascular injury are as follows.[101]

1. *Hemodynamic restriction:* When intimal injury occurs, initiation of coagulation cascade and platelet aggregation resulting in development of a focal thrombus within the

Table 10.6. Causes of penetrating vascular injuries

Trauma
Projectile (e.g., bullet, shrapnel, flying glass)
Sharp object (e.g., knife)
Iatrogenic[98,103–108]
Spine surgery[105]
Vascular access[104]
Tonsillectomy[103]
Skull base surgery[108]

dissected segment that may expand, resulting in vessel stenosis or thrombosis.
2. *Embolism:* The development of a non-occlusive thrombus at the site of intimal injury can result in a distal embolism. In most cases, both mechanisms may contribute to ischemic events.

Penetrating vascular injuries

Penetrating vascular injuries are commonly secondary to projectiles or sharp objects. Missile injuries are frequently caused by bullets or shrapnel artifacts traveling at high velocities. Sharp object injuries are seen in assaults or trauma, but can also be iatrogenic (Table 10.6).

Vascular injury can occur by direct or indirect mechanisms.[102]

1. *Direct:* The fragment trajectory impacts directly the vascular structure resulting in perforation. This is the principal mechanism of penetrating injuries. Such injury can also be seen in projectile injuries.
2. *Indirect:* The fragment trajectory passes close by the vascular structure, but tissue expansion created by the missile results in vascular trauma from the creation of a temporary cavity. This is only seen in high velocity projectile injuries. The temporary cavity is developed by the release of energy by the missile, which is transmitted into the tissue producing an explosive effect. This cavity is directly proportional to the mass and velocity of the projectile.

The likelihood of vascular injury is directly proportional to its proximity in reference to the missile trajectory. Some microscopic changes can be seen in all the arterial layers as a result of missile injury. The intimal layer is usually disrupted at the site where the internal elastica is also disrupted. The tunica media can undergo disruption and develop intrinsic hemorrhages with thrombi formation. Hemorrhages can also be seen in the adventitia.[102]

Diagnosis of neurovascular injuries
Clinical

In all trauma victims, the history, injury mechanism, clinical examination, and the findings on initial imaging dictate the treatment and diagnostic confirmation tests.

The spectrum of neurovascular injury is wide. Clinical presentations associated with dissections can be divided into signs and symptoms related to intrinsic vessel injury and those related to cerebral perfusion from stenosis, occlusion or even embolism.

Signs and symptoms of intrinsic vascular injury are Horner's syndrome, cranial nerve palsy (hypoglossal, glosso-pharyngeal, and facial), headache, neck pain, pulsatile tinnitus, and neck hematoma.

Headache is the most common symptom in both extracranial and intracranial dissections. In internal carotid artery dissections, the headache can be constant or throbbing, frontal or frontoparietal, and ipsilateral to the lesion. Neck pain can occur but it is less common. Headaches are also the most common symptom in vertebral artery dissections. These headaches have a throbbing or pressure quality, and the headache or neck pain has a tendency to radiate into the occipital area unilaterally or bilaterally.[109–113] Cranial nerve palsies are seen more frequently in blunt trauma victims than in cases of penetrating injuries.[41]

Clinical findings related to cerebral hypoperfusion can present as transient deficits or as a stroke. These include weakness, sensory loss, visual effects, balance disturbances, and reduced level of consciousness.

Patients with traumatic intracranial aneurysms have a presentation different from dissections. They present with intracranial hemorrhages (epidural, subdural, intraparenchymal, or subarachnoid) delayed by hours to days from the onset of trauma. Other presentations include Maurer's triad (head trauma, monocular blindness and epistaxis),[114] life-threatening epistaxis,[65,70,71,115–118] enlarging skull fractures,[119] cranial neuropathy,[65,120,121] throbbing tinnitus, and otalgia.[117]

Imaging

With improving technology and resolution of cross-sectional imaging methods, non-invasive imaging has become the modality of choice for the initial evaluation of suspected traumatic neurovascular injuries.

Computed tomography

Computed tomography (CT) is the primary imaging modality for evaluation of trauma victims. When neurovascular injury is suspected, computed tomographic angiography (CTA) can be performed in a relatively short time during the initial imaging evaluation. CTA provides valuable angiographic information that can be used to determine a treatment strategy. CTA can also provide information on the integrity of brain tissue, facial bones, skull base, vertebral elements, neck structures, and the penetrating injury trajectory. The disadvantages are the susceptibility to artifact related to movement, metal, beam hardening, and adverse effects from contrast media.

In studies where CTA was used as a screening tool for blunt vascular injuries, the 4-slice Multi-Detector Computed Tomography (MDCT) was considered to be suboptimal[122,123], but the 16-slice MDCT was able to detect all the clinical significant vascular injuries.[27,124,125] CTA is also an acceptable screening tool in the evaluation of clinically stable patients with penetrating injuries,[126,127] but has not yet replaced the need for conventional angiography.

Magnetic resonance

Magnetic resonance imaging (MRI) can provide images in great detail, but the prolonged duration of the study and the need to establish magnetic compatibility (absence of pacemaker or implanted metal) makes MRI less appropriate in the immediate evaluation of trauma victims.

Once patients are stable, MRI can be used to assess the brain for changes of ischemia and also detect vessel wall morphological features of the dissection when black blood T1 and fat suppression T2 techniques are used.[128] The low sensitivity and variable specificity of magnetic resonance angiography (MRA) to detect arterial dissections has turned this into a less attractive imaging modality.[122,123]

Digital substraction angiography

Conventional cerebral digital subtraction angiography (DSA) is still considered the confirmatory gold standard imaging modality for vascular injuries.

The invasive nature of this test, and the increased risk of complications in emergent angiography when compared to elective angiography[129,130] require attention. In penetrating neck injury victims, the risk of complications can range from 0.16%–3%.[26,38,127,131,132]

Since all non-invasive imaging modalities are considered screening tools, and multiple vascular injuries can be seen in up to 41% of blunt trauma victims[21,25,122] and 45% in penetrating injuries,[34,35,41] a four- or six-vessel cerebral angiogram should be performed as a confirmatory test in those suspected of neurovascular injury.

The use of angiography in the evaluation of zone II penetrating injuries has been controversial since surgical exploration is not always indicated, but in zone I and zone III angiography is always indicated. Injuries in these two zones are uncommon, but can result in high mortality as a result of exsanguination. Angiography in these injuries will not only be diagnostic but also therapeutic as endovascular repair can be achieved in the same setting.

During angiography of head and neck, the arterial, capillary, and venous phases should be visualized, to avoid missing venous injury.

The pathognomonic sign of dissection is visualization of a double lumen that corresponds to the true lumen and an intramural lumen. The most accepted angiographic classification to date consist of five grades[7] (Table 10.1), but other angiographic characteristics have been used. Angiographic images referring to the five grade system are presented through Figs. 10.2–10.10. DSA can reveal both dynamic and morphologic characteristics of the lesion.

(a)

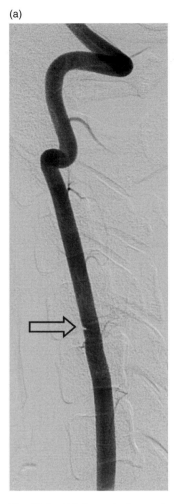

(b)

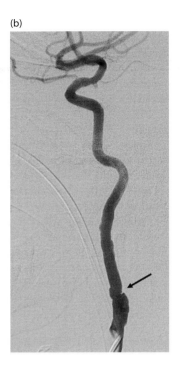

(c)

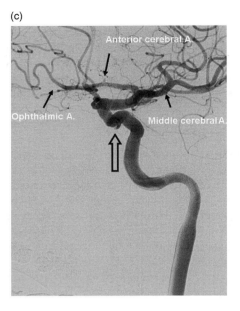

Fig. 10.2. (a) Left vertebral artery, lateral view. There is vessel irregularity with minimal luminal stenosis (arrow) at the level of C4-C5 vertebral body (Grade I). (b) Left internal carotid artery, lateral view. There is vessel dissection 2 cm distal to the origin of left internal carotid artery (arrow) with vessel irregularity (Grade I). (c) Left internal carotid artery, anterior oblique view. There is dissection of the distal cavernous segment (broad arrow) with a prominent vessel flap; no narrowing of the parent vessel is seen (Grade I).

- Dynamic abnormalities are seen when the contrast flow becomes slow or pools in a single vessel, while contrast in other vessels has already reached the capillary or venous phase.
- Morphologic angiographic abnormalities: refer to the image patterns observed during angiography described below:[76]
  1. String sign
  2. Tapering occlusion (flame shape)
  3. Smooth or scalloped narrowing with distal normalization
  4. Pseudoaneurysm

Medical treatment

The management of penetrating injuries has long been a topic of discussion for emergency department physicians and trauma surgeons. It is unclear what medical therapeutic approach should be followed when vascular injury is detected, considering that data from large case studies is available.

Most of the literature regarding the medical treatment for traumatic vascular injuries refers to blunt trauma victims. The medical options are the use of antiplatelets (aspirin or clopidogrel), anticoagulation (heparin, low molecular heparin, or warfarin), or observation.

Many case series have shown a reduction in neurological morbidity and overall mortality if antiplatelet therapy or anticoagulation with heparin was used for one week to maintain a partial thromboplastin time between 40–50 seconds, followed by warfarin with a target INR between 1.5 and 1.8 among patients with blunt vascular injury.[23,25,26,122] Fabian, in 1996, presented the first results of neurologic outcomes at discharge using heparin as the only medical therapy: 4.3% (2/47) of the patients in the treatment group, experienced neurological deterioration prior to discharge, compared to 13.3% (3/15) in the control group.[23]

(a)

(b)

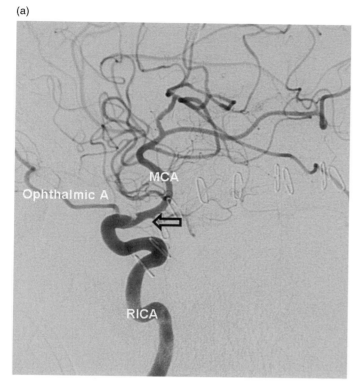
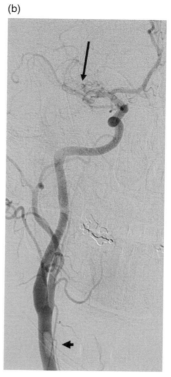

Fig. 10.3. (a)Right internal carotid artery, lateral view. There is dissection with luminal narrowing greater than 25% in the proximal supraclinoid segment of internal carotid artery (arrow), (Grade II). (b) Right common carotid artery, anteroposterior (AP) view. There is dissection of the distal common carotid artery, with underlying intramural thrombus and vessel narrowing of greater than 25% (arrow head). There is partial occlusion of right middle cerebral artery secondary to distal emboli (arrow), (Grade II).

Case series have shown a consistent trend with results favoring the use of heparin over aspirin. Antithrombotic (anticoagulation or antiplatelets) should always be considered in all patients, since the rate of stroke without medical therapy can be as high as 64% (Table 10.7).[25,26,122]

The complications associated with heparin should always be considered and if heparin is contraindicated, antiplatelets should be used. The common complications are those related to surgical or traumatic wounds and gastrointestinal hemorrhages. When a large ischemic stroke is discovered (i.e., over 2/3 on the middle cerebral artery territory) heparin should be avoided or used with caution due to the risk of hemorrhagic transformation.

Another controversial topic is the medical management of intracranial dissections. If anticoagulation is chosen, a theoretical risk is that dissection can later evolve into a subarachnoid hemorrhage. For this reason many practitioners have favored antiplatelets over anticoagulation in the treatment of intracranial dissections.

Natural history

Little is known about the angiographic natural history of blunt vascular injuries. In Table 10.8, the results are presented from publications of blunt injuries with follow-up angiography from 7 days through 125 days.

When anticoagulation is used in grade I and II dissections, 56% or more are expected to heal, but 24% can later progress to pseudoaneurysms, therefore follow up angiography should be considered. Arterial occlusions are uncommon occurrences.

If pseudoaneurysms are detected, 75%–87% of them remain unchanged with medical therapy favoring endovascular treatment if reduction in size is necessary.

Vascular occlusions tend to remain occluded despite medical therapy, but a concern is if recanalization occurs (rarely), a underlying lesion can potentially lead to embolism subsequent to antereograde flow resulting in stroke.

Overall, for grade I and II arterial injuries, medical management is acceptable but a close angiographic follow-up should be performed as early as 7–10 days. Even a third follow-up may be considered since management can change if these lesions progress to pseudoaneurysms.

All pseudoaneurysms should be secured surgically or endovascularly because the majority do not improve with medical therapy.

The management of grade IV injuries (occlusions) can be of debate since most vessels remain occluded with either anticoagulation or no therapy at all. Because recanalization can occur, vessel occlusion (surgery or endovascular) with sustained results can be considered.

The natural course of TICA is controversial, but gradual growth and aneurysm expansion can occur. These aneurysms

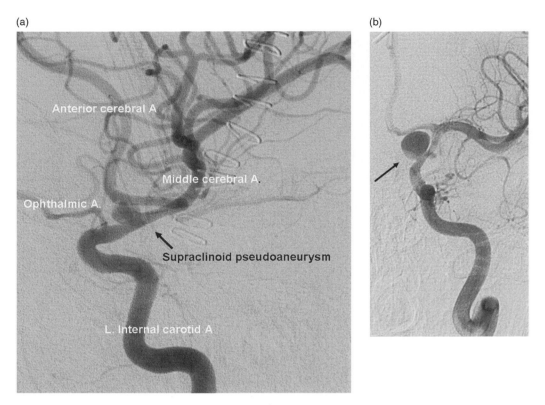

Fig. 10.4. (a) Left internal carotid artery, lateral view. There is an irregular pseudoaneurysm (arrow) originating from the proximal supraclinoid segment (Grade III). (b) Left internal carotid artery, antero-posterior (AP) view. There is a large pseudoaneurysm (arrow) with underlying luminal narrowing in the supraclinoid segment (Grade III).

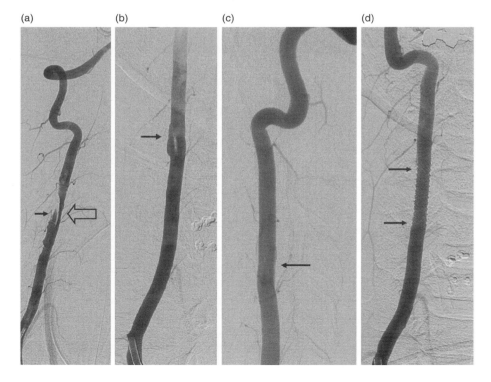

Fig. 10.5. (a) Right vertebral artery, AP view. There is dissection with luminal narrowing (large arrow) at the C5 and C6 vertebral bodies, with pseudoaneurysm formation (small arrow) at the level of C5 (Grade III). (b), (c) Right vertebral artery, AP and lateral views. Six months later the dissection and narrowing has healed with persistent pseudoaneurysm (arrow) at the level of C5 vertebral body. It is important to note that the pseudoaneurysm is not well visualized in lateral images. (d) Right vertebral artery, AP view. Endovascular stent placement (Jo-Stent Graftmaster), with complete obliteration of the pseudoaneurysm.

(a)

(b)

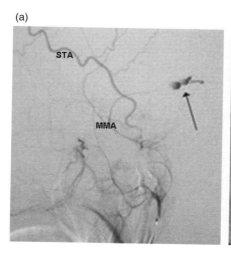

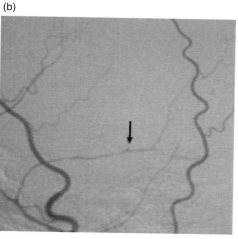

Fig. 10.6. (a), (b) Left external carotid artery, lateral view. There is an irregular pseudoaneurysm (Grade III) originating from the posterior division of left middle meningeal artery (arrow). A repeat angiogram (right) demonstrated spontaneous resolution of the pseudoaneurysm within 1 month (arrow).

(a)

(b)

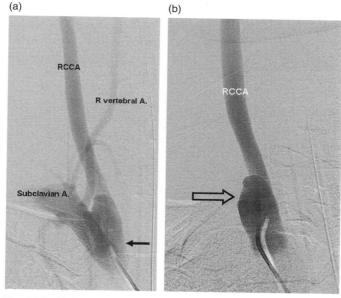

Fig. 10.7. (a), (b) Brachiocephalic artery, AP view. There is an irregular pseudoaneurysm at the origin of right common carotid artery (arrows), with underlying luminal narrowing (Grade III).

Table 10.9): (1) bleeding from the site of the vessel injury; (2) anticipated surgical exploration and manipulation increasing the chance of bleeding; and (3) occlusion or stenosis of the vessel with consequent regional ischemia to the brain. For the first two indications, acute therapeutic occlusion of the injured blood vessel at both proximal and distal ends is recommended. For regional ischemia, revascularization and reconstruction of the artery using stents is recommended. (Fig. 10.11(a)–(g))

Intervention may be required at a later interval for vascular injury for three indications: (1) development of pseudoaneurysm with compression of surrounding structures or consequent thromboembolism because of turbulent flow; (2) high grade stenosis due to fibrosis leading to regional ischemia to the brain; and (3) embolic events from occlusion or stenosis of the injured artery. For the first two indications, stent or stent-graft placement is recommended. For pseudoaneurysms, further embolization through the struts of the stent may be required for adequate obliteration of the pseudoaneurysm. For the last indication, stent placement to restore the lumen of the vessel or therapeutic occlusion (if stent placement is not possible) is recommended.

Acute intervention may also be required for injury to the branches of the external carotid artery. In the presence of active or recurrent bleeding, embolization of selected branches of the external carotid artery may be necessary to achieve hemostasis.

Technical aspects of various procedures

Therapeutic occlusion of the injured carotid or vertebral artery

The initial angiographic images must be carefully reviewed to identify the "injured segment" by angiographically defined occlusion or extravasation. The extent of the injured segment must be defined at both proximal and distal ends within the vessel and subsequently the "normal segment" is delineated. The normal segment should be reviewed to identify the "vital normal segment". These segments may provide origin to branches or serve as the conduit for a collateral supply. Examples include a vertebral artery segment that gives origin to the posterior inferior

can become symptomatic and later present with intracranial hemorrhage in 19%–36% of cases.[47,52] Aneurysmal rupture is most likely to occur between day 10 and 6 weeks following the initial trauma,[46,47,54,57,61,65,133,134] but it can occur even in the first 24 hours or even after a year.[54,58,62,66] Spontaneous healing or disappearance of traumatic intracranial aneurysms has been reported in victims where surgery was not an option.[53,54]

Endovascular treatment

Indications for acute neuroendovascular procedures

There are three indications for acute intervention for vascular injury in the cervical carotid or vertebral artery (see

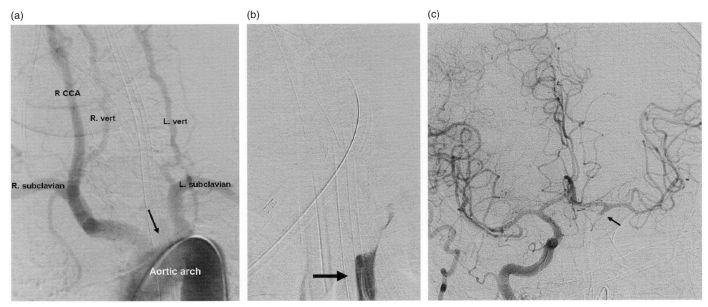

(a) R CCA
R. vert
L. vert
R. subclavian
L. subclavian
Aortic arch

Fig. 10.8. (a) Aortic arch, anterior oblique view. There is complete occlusion at the origin of left common carotid artery (arrow) secondary to dissection (Grade IV) (b) Left common carotid artery, AP view. Careful selective catheterization of the left common carotid artery demonstrates complete occlusion (arrow) a few centimeters distal to the origin. (c) Right common carotid artery, AP view. There is cross filling through a patent anterior communicating artery into the anterior and middle cerebral artery distributions with retrograde filling of left supraclinoid segment (arrow).

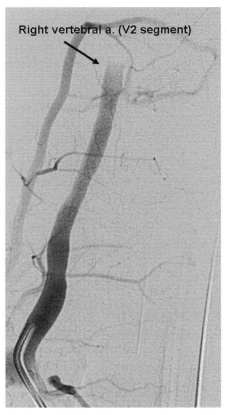

Right vertebral a. (V2 segment)

Fig. 10.9. Right vertebral artery, AP view, showing complete occlusion of the right vertebral artery (arrow), at the C5 vertebral body (Grade IV).

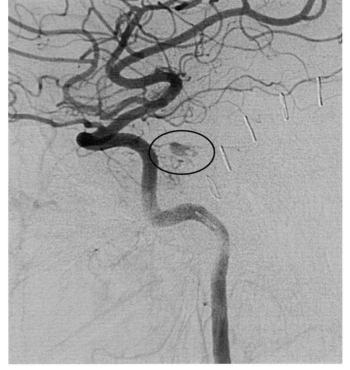

Fig. 10.10. Left internal carotid artery, lateral view. There is transection of the cavernous segment of the left internal carotid artery, with a small focus of extravasation (circle) secondary to an adventitial tear (Grade V).

cerebral artery or the segment where anastomosis of the ascending cervical branch of the thyrocervical trunk occurs distal to the occlusion. The diameter of the artery in adjacent "normal segments" should be measured to appropriately select the coils.

The overall pattern of blood supply to the distribution of the artery with the "injured segment" must be understood. The presence of collateral supply from other blood vessels must be identified by selective contrast injections from other pertinent

Table 10.7. Stroke rates by medical therapy in patients with vascular trauma

Author, year and arterial injury	Heparin	Aspirin	Aspirin or heparin	No therapy
Miller 2001[26]				
Carotid artery injury	n/a	n/a	6.8%	64%
Vertebral artery injury	n/a	n/a	2.6%	54%
Biffl 2002[25]				
Carotid and vertebral artery injury	1%	9%	n/a	n/a
Miller 2002[122]				
Carotid artery injury	11%	17%	n/a	n/a

arteries. The therapeutic occlusion should spare the "vital normal segments" of the artery.

A guide catheter is placed through femoral artery or (rarely) radial artery access. The guide catheter is placed in the ipsilateral vertebral or carotid artery proximal to the lesion. If active bleeding is occurring, a guide catheter with a balloon at its distal end should be considered. Placing the guide catheter in the affected vessel with subsequent inflation of the balloon ensures flow arrest. The artery should be carefully visualized to identify the "injured segment" and "occlusion target segment." The injured segment is identified by angiographically defined irregularity, occlusion, extravasation, or stenosis. The "occlusion target segment" is the segment adjacent to "injured segment" with no angiographically demonstrable abnormalities. A microcatheter is

Table 10.8. Angiographic progression of vascular blunt injuries based on medical intervention[23,25,26,31,135]

Angiographic progression	Initial vascular injury		
	Grade I and II Intimal tear	Grade III Pseudoaneurysm	Grade IV Occlusion
Anticoagulation			
Healed	85 (56.29%)	2 (6.06%)	0 (0.00%)
Grade I-II	36 (23.84%)	0 (0.00%)	2 (16.67%)
Grade III	29 (19.21%)	29 (87.88%)	0 (0.00%)
Grade IV	1 (0.66%)	2 (6.06%)	10 (83.33%)
Total	151 (100%)	33 (100%)	12 (100%)
Antiplatelets			
Healed	12 (46.15%)	1 (25.00%)	0 (0.00%)
Grade I-II	12 (46.15%)	0 (0.00%)	0 (0.00%)
Grade III	2 (7.69%)	3 (75.00%)	0 (0.00%)
Grade IV	0 (0.00%)	0 (0.00%)	0 (0.00%)
Total	26 (100%)	4 (100%)	0 (0%)
No medical therapy			
Healed	23 (60.53%)	0 (0.00%)	0 (0.00%)
Grade I-II	11 (28.95%)	0 (0.00%)	0 (0.00%)
Grade III	4 (10.53%)	1 (100.00%)	0 (0.00%)
Grade IV	0 (0.00%)	0 (0.00%)	0 (0.00%)
Total	38 (100%)	1 (100%)	0 (100%)
Therapy details not disclosed in the observational period			
Healed	4 (23.53%)	1 (5.88%)	0 (0.00%)
Grade I–II	7 (41.18%)	0 (0.00%)	1 (11.11%)
Grade III	3 (17.65%)	15 (88.24%)	0 (0.00%)
Grade IV	3 (17.65%)	1 (5.88%)	8 (88.89%)
Total	17 (100%)	17 (100%)	9 (100%)
Total 308	232	55	21

Table 10.9 Indications for acute endovascular procedures in cervical arterial injuries

Procedures	Devices	Indications
Both-end occlusion	Coils, detachable balloons	Bleeding or risk of bleeding from injured large or medium sized artery
One-end occlusion	Coils, detachable balloons	Embolic events due to stenosis or near occlusion of large or medium sized artery
Non-porous arterial reconstruction	Covered stents or stent assisted coil placement	Bleeding or risk of bleeding from injured large or medium sized artery; or pseudoaneurysm
Porous arterial reconstruction	Self expanding stent	Dissection with near occlusion or occlusion of large or medium sized artery and ischemia
Vascular bed obliteration	Embolic particles	Diffuse small arterial injury with active bleeding

advanced to the occlusion target segment of the artery. In some cases, the target segment for occlusion is determined by the need to preserve certain branches such as posterior inferior cerebellar artery. Coils are delivered and deployed in the target segment. A configuration that involves a smaller area would require a smaller number of coils to achieve an occlusion. Hydrogel covered coils ensure a tight occlusive seal at the proximal and distal end of the injured artery. Coils should be deployed until no angiographic flow is visualized in the target segment. Subsequently, the contralateral vertebral or carotid artery is catheterized and the distal end of the injured vessel is catheterized in a retrograde manner. The microcatheter is advanced to the occlusion target segment and coils are deployed until no flow is visualized angiographically in the target segment.

Stent or covered stent placement in the injured artery

The initial angiographic images must be carefully reviewed to identify the "injured segment" as evidenced by irregularity, occlusion, extravasation, or stenosis. The extent of the injured segment must be defined at both proximal and distal ends within the vessel. It should be noted that the "injured segment" may extend beyond the segment with angiographic abnormalities in one projection. Therefore, the identification of the "injured segment" requires review of images acquired from multiple projections. The distal extent of the "injured segment" may be hard to visualize because of poor contrast opacification in the presence of a flow-limiting lesion and requires a microcatheter injection distal to the initially visualized "injured segment." The diameter of the artery in adjacent normal segments should be measured to appropriately size the stent. The overall pattern of blood supply to the distribution of the artery with the "injured segment" must be understood. The presence of collateral supply from other blood vessels must be identified by selective contrast injections from other pertinent arteries.

A guide catheter is placed through femoral artery or (rarely) radial artery access. The guide catheter is placed in the ipsilateral vertebral or carotid artery proximal to the lesion. The size of the guide catheter must be appropriate to accommodate the covered stent system if use is anticipated. It should be noted that the covered stent grafts have an inner and outer diameter and the outer diameter determines the radial force applied to the surrounding vessel. The lesion is traversed using a microwire and preferably a microcatheter. The microcatheter is placed distal to the injured segment and contrast is injected to visualize the distal vessel. It is important to confirm that the microcatheter is within the true lumen of the artery and to verify the patency of the distal segment. The microwire should be placed as distal as possible with the help of the microcatheter to ensure adequate support for advancing the stent. The microcatheter is removed, the microwire is left in position, and the stent is advanced over the microwire. Adequate positioning of the stent should be confirmed using contrast injections and bony landmarks identified from previously acquired angiographic images. The stent is deployed either by inflation of the balloon (balloon mounted) or withdrawal of the outer sheath (self-expanding). After the stent is deployed, angiographic images are acquired and carefully reviewed to assess the need for additional stents or coil placement outside the stents to ensure adequate resolution of the lesion.

There are different types of covered stents available. One commonly used is the Jo-Stent Graftmaster (Abbott Vascular, Rancho Cordova, California). The device comes in a pre-mounted delivery system with a semi-compliant balloon catheter. The stent is made of stainless steel and a thin layer of expandable graft material, polytetrafluoroethylene (PTFE) which is between the two layers of the stent. This stent can be placed in a vessel ranging from 3.0–5.0 mm and requires a 7 French delivery system. Another system, the Fluency® Plus (Bard Peripheral Vascular, Tempe, Arizona) is a self-expanding nitinol stent. There is a single nitinol skeleton which is encapsulated within two ultrathin layers of PTFE. It requires an 8–9 French delivery system. Other stent systems e.g., Viabahn (W.L. Gore and Assoc., Flagstaff, Arizona), and Wallgraft (Boston Scientific, Natick, MA), are also available. The point to remember is that all these stent systems are approved for cardiac, peripheral vascular, or tracheobronchial applications and to use them for off-label purposes (intracranial or cervical vessels) may require institutional review board (IRB) approval.

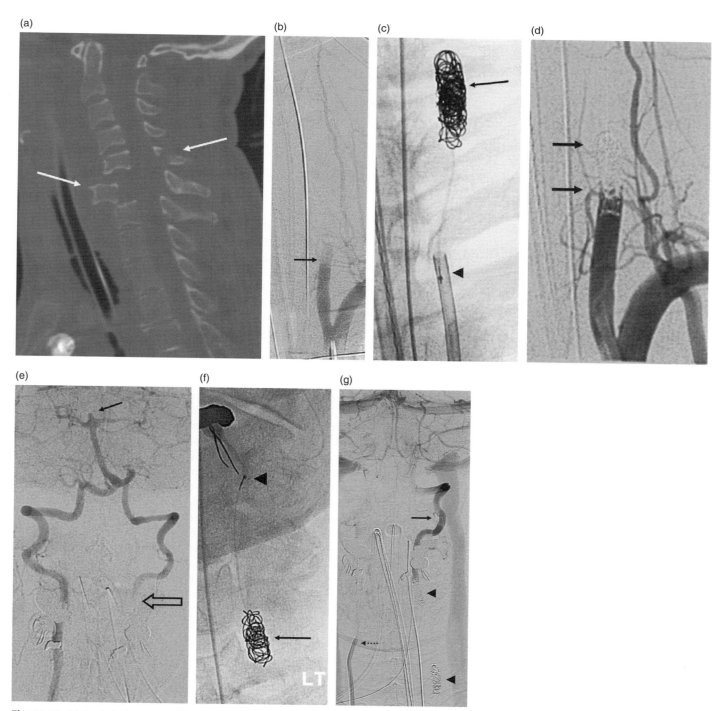

Fig. 10.11. (a) Cervical spine computed tomographic (CT) scan with sagittal reconstruction. The C5 vertebra has a left lamina fracture (right arrow) with a left transverse process and a right lamina fracture (not seen). The C6 vertebra has a grade 4 anterior dislocation (left arrow) and a comminuted fracture involving bilateral transverse processes (not seen). (b) Left vertebral artery, AP view. There is complete occlusion of left vertebral artery (arrow) at the junction of V1 and V2 segment (Grade IV). (c) Left vertebral artery, AP unsubtracted view. Endovascular coil embolization from both proximal and distal segment was performed in order to reduce the risk of surgical bleeding during cervical spine reconstruction. Arrow head demonstrates position of the distal end of the microcatheter. Arrow points to the coil deployed proximal to the occlusion. (d) Left vertebral artery, AP view, post coil embolization. (e) Right vertebral artery, AP view. There is retrograde filling into left vertebral artery up to mid V2 segment (bold arrow). There is an incidental unruptured basilar tip aneurysm (arrow). (f) Endovascular coil embolization of distal left vertebral artery (arrow) via microcatheter (arrow head) positioned in a retrograde fashion through right vertebral artery. (g) Right vertebral artery. AP view late arterial phase demonstrating the coil mass above and below the level of injury (arrow heads). Guide catheter in right vertebral artery (dashed arrow), retrograde filling of left vertebral artery (arrow). Coil mass is seen in both proximal and distal segment of left vertebral artery (arrow heads).

Table 10.10. Risk stratification for bleeding related to anticoagulant or antiplatelet medication in patients with vascular trauma

	Low risk	Moderate risk	High risk
Mechanism of injury	Blunt	Penetrating	Penetrating with active bleeding
Superficial or musculoskeletal injuries	None or compressible sites	Active bleeding	Active bleeding secondary to major arterial injury; e.g., femoral artery
Intracranial injury	None	Diffuse injury	Intracranial hemorrhage or focal contusion
Internal injuries	None	No active bleeding or bleeding site secured	Active bleeding or unsecured bleeding site or bleeding due to major arterial injury; e.g., abdominal or thoracic aorta

Embolization of small arteries

In patients with craniofacial trauma, multiple small arteries may be transected due to direct injury or shear injury secondary to fractures and dislocations. The bleeding is diffuse and obliteration of a single medium size artery is inadequate. These networks of small sized arteries derive blood supply from multiple medium sized arteries. Even if angiographic images suggest a single arterial supply, the external carotid artery can form extensive collaterals leading to immediate supply from another medium sized artery in the event of occlusion of the parent artery. Therefore, the occlusion must occur in the small sized arteries for adequate hemostasis. Presence of local swelling and location of hematomas on computed tomographic scans can identify the general location of the bleeding vessels. An initial angiogram is performed to identify the vascular site of bleeding (target region) and the arterial supply/supplies (conduits) to the target region. The target region is characterized by a network of small arteries with multiple constrictions and dilations (due to spasm and thrombosis) and contrast extravasation (due to active bleeding).

Each of the supplying medium sized arteries (usually branches of the external carotid artery) are selectively catheterized with a microcatheter. Selective microcatheter injections confirm the presence of vascular injury in the distal distribution of the catheterized artery. The microcatheter is placed at a position where injection of embolic material can only flow towards the injured arteries. Subsequently, embolic material (particles of 250–700 microns) mixed with diluted contrast are injected through the microcatheter. The transient opacification during injection of embolic particles confirms the flow of embolic material in the correct vessels. Adequate obliteration is identified with accumulation and sluggish flow of contrast. Microcatheter and guide catheter injections are required to confirm the obliteration of the target vessels.

Adjuvant medications for interventional procedures

Endovascular devices introduce a state of local thrombogenicity at the site of deployment. This exacerbates the existing thrombogenicity that exists due to arterial injury with exposure of the thrombogenic subintima and secondary thrombosis. However, both anticoagulant and antiplatelet agents increase the risk of bleeding. Therefore, prior to the procedure, stratification for bleeding risk associated with antiplatelet or anticoagulant medication is necessary in patients with trauma. There are three risk strata for bleeding risk as demonstrated in Table 10.10. An understanding of these risk strata can help the decision making process for adjuvant antiplatelet or anticoagulant medication during the procedure.

In almost all traumatic vascular injury cases, premedication with antiplatelet medication is not possible. In patients for whom therapeutic occlusion of the vessel is planned, intravenous heparin during the procedure is recommended. An activated coagulation time ranging between 250 and 350 seconds is recommended. In rare cases, post-procedure heparin infusion may be necessary if there is any radiological or clinical evidence of thrombus propagation or embolism. In patients for whom stent placement is required, antiplatelet medications are necessary to prevent stent thrombosis. A single dose of aspirin (325 mg) and a bolus of clopidogrel (300–600 mg) via a nasogastric tube is advisable. Intravenous heparin is used during the procedure as mentioned above. Since there is delay (approximately 6 hours) between administration and therapeutic activity for both aspirin and clopidogrel, an intravenous platelet glycoprotein inhibitor may be necessary to prevent acute stent thrombosis. The benefit has to be weighed against the risk of new bleeding from the injured vessel or another source in cases of multiple organ injury. If the person is at high risk for bleeding, the use of these agents should be limited to situations with radiological or clinical evidence of thrombus propagation or embolism. A provision for platelet transfusions in the event of major bleeding to reverse the antiplatelet activity must be available.

Summary

Traumatic vascular injury in the cervical and intracranial compartment can be readily diagnosed with new non-invasive imaging modalities. A detailed understanding of the natural history and indications for endovascular procedures is essential for recommending the best treatment option for the patient. Future studies are required to understand the long-term outcomes following endovascular treatment for traumatic vascular injury.

References

1. Key G: *The Apologie and Treatise of Ambroise Pare Containing the Voyages Made Into Divers Places With Many Writings Upon Surgery.* London U: Falcon Education Books, 1957.

2. Verneuil AAS. *Contusions mulfiples; délire violent; hémiplégie a droite sdccBAN,* 1872;**36**:46–56. M.

3. Serbinenko FA. Balloon catheterization and occlusion of major cerebral vessels. *J Neurosurg* 1964;**41**:125–45.

4. Dotter CT. Transluminally-placed coilspring endarterial tube grafts. Long-term patency in canine popliteal artery. *Invest Radiol* 1969;**4**:329–32.

5. Parodi JC. Endovascular repair of abdominal aortic aneurysms and other arterial lesions. *J Vasc Surg* 1995;**21**:549–555; discussion 556–7.

6. Marks MP, Dake MD, Steinberg GK, Norbash AM, Lane B. Stent placement for arterial and venous cerebrovascular disease: preliminary experience. *Radiology* 1994;**191**:441–6.

7. Biffl WL, Moore EE, Offner PJ, Brega KE, Franciose RJ, Burch JM. *Blunt carotid arterial injuries: Implications of a new grading scale.* 1999.

8. Frykberg ER. Vascular trauma iCA In Ernst CB (eds). *Vascular Surgery: Theory and Practice.* New York: McGraw-Hill, 1995, p. 992.

9. Monson DO, Saletta JD, Freeark RJ. Carotid vertebral trauma. *J Trauma* 1969;**9**:987–99.

10. Roon AJ, Christensen N. Evaluation and treatment of penetrating cervical injuries. *J Trauma* 1979;**19**:391–7.

11. Wilkinson IM. The vertebral artery. Extracranial and intracranial structure. *Arch Neurol* 1972;**27**:392–6.

12. Ratinov G. Extradural intracranial portion of carotid artery; a clinicopathologic study. *Arch Neurol* 1964;**10**:66–73.

13. Krajewski LP, Hertzer NR. Blunt carotid artery trauma: report of two cases and review of the literature. *Ann Surg.* 1980;**191**:341–6.

14. Perry MO, Snyder WH, Thal ER. Carotid artery injuries caused by blunt trauma. *Ann Surg* 1980;**192**:74–7.

15. Yamada S, Kindt GW, Youmans JR. Carotid artery occlusion due to nonpenetrating injury. *J Trauma* 1967;**7**:333–42.

16. Crissey MM, Bernstein EF. Delayed presentation of carotid intimal tear following blunt craniocervical trauma. *Surgery* 1974;**75**:543–9.

17. Kobernick M, Carmody R. Vertebral artery transection from blunt trauma treated by embolization. *J Trauma* 1984;**24**:854–6.

18. Six EG, Stringer WL, Cowley AR, Davis CH, Jr. Posttraumatic bilateral vertebral artery occlusion: Case report. *J Neurosurg* 1981;**54**:814–17.

19. Golueke P, Sclafani S, Phillips T, Goldstein A, Scalea T, Duncan A. Vertebral artery injury–diagnosis and management. *J Trauma* 1987;**27**:856–65.

20. Hilton-Jones D, Warlow CP. Non-penetrating arterial trauma and cerebral infarction in the young. *Lancet* 1985;**1**:1435–8.

21. Biffl WL, Moore EE, Ryu RK, *et al.* The unrecognized epidemic of blunt carotid arterial injuries: early diagnosis improves neurologic outcome. *Ann Surg.* 1998;**228**:462–70.

22. Davis JW, Holbrook TL, Hoyt DB, Mackersie RC, Field TO, Jr., Shackford SR. Blunt carotid artery dissection: Incidence, associated injuries, screening, and treatment. *J Trauma* 1990;**30**:1514–17.

23. Fabian TC, Patton JH, Jr., Croce MA, Minard G, Kudsk KA, Pritchard FE. Blunt carotid injury. Importance of early diagnosis and anticoagulant therapy. *Ann Surg* 1996;**223**:513–522; discussion 522–5.

24. Carrillo EH, Osborne DL, Spain DA, Miller FB, Senler SO, Richardson JD. Blunt carotid artery injuries: Difficulties with the diagnosis prior to neurologic event. *J Trauma* 1999;**46**:1120–5.

25. Biffl WL, Ray CE, Jr., Moore EE, *et al.* Treatment-related outcomes from blunt cerebrovascular injuries: Importance of routine follow-up arteriography. *Ann Surg* 2002;**235**:699–706; discussion 706–7.

26. Miller PR, Fabian TC, Bee TK, *et al.* Blunt cerebrovascular injuries: Diagnosis and treatment. *J Trauma* 2001;**51**:279–85; discussion 285–6.

27. Berne JD, Reuland KS, Villarreal DH, McGovern TM, Rowe SA, Norwood SH. Sixteen-slice multi-detector computed tomographic angiography improves the accuracy of screening for blunt cerebrovascular injury. *J Trauma.* 2006;**60**:1204–9; discussion 1209–10.

28. Biffl WL, Moore EE, Elliott JP, *et al.* The devastating potential of blunt vertebral arterial injuries. *Ann Surg* 2000;**231**:672–81.

29. Cothren CC, Moore EE, Biffl WL, *et al.* Cervical spine fracture patterns predictive of blunt vertebral artery injury. *J Trauma* 2003;**55**:811–13.

30. Kerwin AJ, Bynoe RP, Murray J, *et al.* Liberalized screening for blunt carotid and vertebral artery injuries is justified. *J Trauma* 2001;**51**:308–14.

31. McKinney A, Ott F, Short J, McKinney Z, Truwit C. Angiographic frequency of blunt cerebrovascular injury in patients with carotid canal or vertebral foramen fractures on multidetector ct. *Eur J Radiol* 2007;**62**:385–93.

32. Schneidereit NP, Simons R, Nicolaou S, *et al.* Utility of screening for blunt vascular neck injuries with computed tomography angiography. *J Trauma* 2006;**60**:209–15; discussion 215–16.

33. Thal ER, Meyer DM. Penetrating neck trauma. *Curr Probl Surg* 1992;**29**:1–56.

34. Rao PM, Ivatury RR, Sharma P, Vinzons AT, Nassoura Z, Stahl WM. Cervical vascular injuries: a trauma center experience. *Surgery* 1993;**114**:527–31.

35. Mittal VK, Paulson TJ, Colaiuta E, *et al.* Carotid artery injuries and their management. *J Cardiovasc Surg (Torino)* 2000;**41**:423–31.

36. Bell RB, Osborn T, Dierks EJ, Potter BE, Long WB. Management of penetrating neck injuries: A new paradigm for civilian trauma. *J Oral Maxillofac Surg* 2007;**65**:691–705.

37. Sclafani AP, Sclafani SJ. Angiography and transcatheter arterial embolization of vascular injuries of the face and neck. *Laryngoscope* 1996;**106**:168–73.

38. Demetriades D, Theodorou D, Cornwell E, *et al.* Evaluation of penetrating injuries of the neck: Prospective study of 223 patients. *World J Surg* 1997;**21**:41–7; discussion 47–8.

39. Demetriades D, Asensio JA, Velmahos G, Thal E. Complex problems in penetrating neck trauma. *Surg Clin North Am* 1996;**76**:661–83.

40. Demetriades D, Skalkides J, Sofianos C, Melissas J, Franklin J. Carotid artery

injuries: Experience with 124 cases. *J Trauma* 1989;**29**:91–4.

41. Ramadan F, Rutledge R, Oller D, Howell P, Baker C, Keagy B. Carotid artery trauma: a review of contemporary trauma center experiences. *J Vasc Surg* 1995;**21**:46–55; discussion 55–6.

42. Feliciano DV, Bitondo CG, Mattox KL, *et al.* Civilian trauma in the 1980s. A 1-year experience with 456 vascular and cardiac injuries. *Ann Surg* 1984;**199**:717–24.

43. du Toit DF, van Schalkwyk GD, Wadee SA, Warren BL. Neurologic outcome after penetrating extracranial arterial trauma. *J Vasc Surg* 2003;**38**:257–62.

44. Xydakis MS, Fravell MD, Nasser KE, Casler JD. Analysis of battlefield head and neck injuries in iraq and afghanistan. *Otolaryngol Head Neck Surg* 2005;**133**:497–504.

45. Fox CJ, Gillespie DL, Weber MA, *et al.* Delayed evaluation of combat-related penetrating neck trauma. *J Vasc Surg* 2006;**44**:86–93.

46. Haddad FS, Haddad GF, Taha J. Traumatic intracranial aneurysms caused by missiles: Their presentation and management. *Neurosurgery* 1991;**28**:1–7.

47. Asari S, Nakamura S, Yamada O, Beck H, Sugatani H. Traumatic aneurysm of peripheral cerebral arteries. Report of two cases. *J Neurosurg* 1977;**46**:795–803.

48. Benoit BG, Wortzman G. Traumatic cerebral aneurysms. Clinical features and natural history. *J Neurol Neurosurg Psychiatry.* 1973;**36**:127–38.

49. Buckingham MJ, Crone KR, Ball WS, Tomsick TA, Berger TS, Tew JM, Jr. Traumatic intracranial aneurysms in childhood: two cases and a review of the literature. *Neurosurgery* 1988;**22**:398–408.

50. Ventureyra EC, Higgins MJ. Traumatic intracranial aneurysms in childhood and adolescence. Case reports and review of the literature. *Childs Nerv Syst* 1994;**10**:361–79.

51. Ferry DJ, Jr., Kempe LG. False aneurysm secondary to penetration of the brain through orbitofacial wounds. Report of two cases. *J Neurosurg* 1972;**36**:503–6.

52. Kieck CF, de Villiers JC. Vascular lesions due to transcranial stab wounds. *J Neurosurg* 1984;**60**:42–6.

53. du Trevou MD, van Dellen JR. Penetrating stab wounds to the brain: The timing of angiography in patients presenting with the weapon already removed. *Neurosurgery* 1992;**31**:905–11; discussion 911–12.

54. Amirjamshidi A, Rahmat H, Abbassioun K. Traumatic aneurysms and arteriovenous fistulas of intracranial vessels associated with penetrating head injuries occurring during war: Principles and pitfalls in diagnosis and management. A survey of 31 cases and review of the literature. *J Neurosurg* 1996;**84**:769–80.

55. Aarabi B. Traumatic aneurysms of brain due to high velocity missile head wounds. *Neurosurgery* 1988;**22**:1056–63.

56. Levy ML, Rezai A, Masri LS, *et al.* The significance of subarachnoid hemorrhage after penetrating craniocerebral injury: correlations with angiography and outcome in a civilian population. *Neurosurgery* 1993;**32**:532–40.

57. Alvarez JA, Bambakidis N, Takaoka Y. Delayed rupture of traumatic intracranial pseudoaneurysm in a child following gunshot wound to the head. *J Craniomaxillofac Trauma* 1999;**5**:39–44

58. Horowitz MB, Kopitnik TA, Landreneau F, *et al.* Multidisciplinary approach to traumatic intracranial aneurysms secondary to shotgun and handgun wounds. *Surg Neurol* 1999;**51**:31–41; discussion 41–2.

59. Cohen JE, Rajz G, Itshayek E, Shoshan Y, Umansky F, Gomori JM. Endovascular management of traumatic and iatrogenic aneurysms of the pericallosal artery. Report of two cases. *J Neurosurg* 2005;**102**:555–7.

60. Levine NB, Tanaka T, Jones BV, Crone KR. Minimally invasive management of a traumatic artery aneurysm resulting from shaken baby syndrome. *Pediatr Neurosurg* 2004;**40**:128–31.

61. Nakstad P, Nornes H, Hauge HN. Traumatic aneurysms of the pericallosal arteries. *Neuroradiology* 1986;**28**:335–8.

62. Ohta M, Matsuno H. Proximal m2 false aneurysm after head trauma–case report. *Neurol Med Chir (Tokyo)* 2001;**41**:131–4.

63. Quintana F, Diez C, Gutierrez A, Diez ML, Austin O, Vazquez A. Traumatic aneurysm of the basilar artery. *Am J Neuroradiol.* 1996;**17**:283–5.

64. Schuster JM, Santiago P, Elliott JP, Grady MS, Newell DW, Winn HR.

Acute traumatic posteroinferior cerebellar artery aneurysms: Report of three cases. *Neurosurgery* 1999;**45**:1465–1467; discussion 1467–8.

65. Hern JD, Coley SC, Hollis LJ, Jayaraj SM. Delayed massive epistaxis due to traumatic intracavernous carotid artery pseudoaneurysm. *J Laryngol Otol* 1998;**112**:396–8.

66. Singh M, Ahmad FU, Mahapatra AK. Traumatic middle meningeal artery aneurysm causing intracerebral hematoma: a case report and review of literature. *Surg Neurol* 2006;**66**:321–3; discussion 323.

67. Bruneau M, Gustin T, Zekhnini K, Gilliard C. Traumatic false aneurysm of the middle meningeal artery causing an intracerebral hemorrhage: Case report and literature review. *Surg Neurol* 2002;**57**:174–8; discussion 178.

68. Garza-Mercado R, Rangel RA. Extradural hematoma associated with traumatic middle meningeal artery pseudoaneurysm: Report of two cases. *Neurosurgery* 1979;**5**:500–3.

69. Rumbaugh CL, Bergeron RT, Kurze T. Intracranial vascular damage associated with skull fractures. Radiographic aspects. *Radiology* 1972;**104**:81–7.

70. Bhatoe HS, Suryanarayana KV, Gill HS. Recurrent massive epistaxis due to traumatic intracavernous internal carotid artery aneurysm. *J Laryngol Otol* 1995;**109**:650–2.

71. Mahmoud NA. Traumatic aneurysm of the internal carotid artery and epistaxis. (review of literature and report of a case). *J Laryngol Otol* 1979;**93**:629–56.

72. Jackson FGJ, Janon E: The traumatic cranial and intracranial aneurysms. In Vinken P, Bruyn G:, eds. *Handbook of Clinical Neurology.* New York: Elsevier, 1976, p. 381.

73. Lin CH, Jeng JS, Yip PK. Middle cerebral artery dissections: Differences between isolated and extended dissections of internal carotid artery. *J Neurol Sci* 2005;**235**:37–44.

74. Pelkonen O, Tikkakoski T, Leinonen S, Pyhtinen J, Sotaniemi K. Intracranial arterial dissection. *Neuroradiology* 1998;**40**:442–7.

75. Yonas H, Agamanolis D, Takaoka Y, White RJ. Dissecting intracranial aneurysms. *Surg Neurol* 1977;**8**:407–15.

76. Hart RG, Easton JD. Dissections of cervical and cerebral arteries. *Neurol Clin* 1983;**1**:155–82.

77. Miyata M, Yamasaki S, Hirayama A, Tamaki N. [traumatic middle cerebral artery occlusion]. *No Shinkei Geka* 1994;**22**:253–7.

78. Malek AM, Halbach VV, Phatouros CC, Meyers PM, Dowd CF, Higashida RT. Endovascular treatment of a ruptured intracranial dissecting vertebral aneurysm in a kickboxer. *J Trauma* 2000;**48**:143–5.

79. McCrory P. Vertebral artery dissection causing stroke in sport. *J Clin Neurosci* 2000;**7**:298–300.

80. Joseph T, Kandiyil N, Beale D, Tiivas C, Imray CH. A novel treatment for symptomatic carotid dissection. *Postgrad Med J* 2005;**81**:**e6**.

81. Amagasa M, Sato S, Otabe K. Posttraumatic dissecting aneurysm of the anterior cerebral artery: Case report. *Neurosurgery* 1988;**23**:221–5.

82. Schmitt HP, Miltner E. Dissection of the anterior and middle cerebral artery with fatal ischemia following kicks to the head. *Forensic Sci Int* 1991;**49**:113–20.

83. McKevitt EC, Kirkpatrick AW, Vertesi L, Granger R, Simons RK. Blunt vascular neck injuries: Diagnosis and outcomes of extracranial vessel injury. *J Trauma* 2002;**53**:472–6.

84. Bumpous JM, Whitt PD, Ganzel TM, McClane SD. Penetrating injuries of the visceral compartment of the neck. *Am J Otolaryngol* 2000;**21**:190–4.

85. Hersman G, Barker P, Bowley DM, Boffard KD. The management of penetrating neck injuries. *Int Surg* 2001;**86**:82–9.

86. Nason RW, Assuras GN, Gray PR, Lipschitz J, Burns CM. Penetrating neck injuries: analysis of experience from a canadian trauma centre. *Can J Surg* 2001;**44**:122–6.

87. Sclafani SJ, Scalea TM, Wetzel W, *et al.* Internal carotid artery gunshot wounds. *J Trauma* 1996;**40**:751–7.

88. McConnell DB, Trunkey DD. Management of penetrating trauma to the neck. *Adv Surg* 1994;**27**:97–127.

89. *Medical Department of the United States Army in the World War.* Vol2. Washington D, US Government Printing Office, 1927, p. 68.

90. Chipps JE, Canham RG, Makel HP. Intermediate treatment of maxillofacial injuries. *US Armed Forces Med J.* 1953;**4**:951–76.

91. Mabry RL, Holcomb JB, Baker AM, *et al.* United states army rangers in somalia: An analysis of combat casualties on an urban battlefield. *J Trauma* 2000;**49**:515–528; discussion 528–9.

92. Holmes B, Harbaugh RE. Traumatic intracranial aneurysms: a contemporary review. *J Trauma* 1993;**35**:855–60.

93. Parkinson D, West M. Traumatic intracranial aneurysms. *J Neurosurg* 1980;**52**:11–20.

94. Voelker JL, Ortiz O. Delayed deterioration after head trauma due to traumatic aneurysm. *W V Med J* 1997;**93**:317–19.

95. Schievink WI, Mokri B, Piepgras DG. Spontaneous dissections of cervicocephalic arteries in childhood and adolescence. *Neurology* 1994;**44**:1607–12.

96. Zelenock GB, Kazmers A, Whitehouse WM, Jr., *et al.* Extracranial internal carotid artery dissections: noniatrogenic traumatic lesions. *Arch Surg* 1982;**117**:425–32.

97. Saeed AB, Shuaib A, Al-Sulaiti G, Emery D. Vertebral artery dissection: Warning symptoms, clinical features and prognosis in 26 patients. *Can J Neurol Sci* 2000;**27**:292–6.

98. Gould DB, Cunningham K. Internal carotid artery dissection after remote surgery. Iatrogenic complications of anesthesia. *Stroke* 1994;**25**:1276–8.

99. Biffl WL, Moore EE, Offner PJ, *et al.* Optimizing screening for blunt cerebrovascular injuries. *Am J Surg* 1999;**178**:517–22.

100. Cothren CC, Moore EE, Ray CE, Jr., Johnson JL, Moore JB, Burch JM. Cervical spine fracture patterns mandating screening to rule out blunt cerebrovascular injury. *Surgery* 2007;**141**:76–82.

101. Benninger DH, Georgiadis D, Kremer C, Studer A, Nedeltchev K, Baumgartner RW. Mechanism of ischemic infarct in spontaneous carotid dissection. *Stroke* 2004;**35**:482–5.

102. Amato JJ, Billy LJ, Gruber RP, Lawson NS, Rich NM. Vascular injuries. An experimental study of high and low velocity missile wounds. *Arch Surg* 1970;**101**:167–74.

103. Carvalho KS, Edwards-Brown M, Golomb MR. Carotid dissection and stroke after tonsillectomy and adenoidectomy. *Pediatr Neurol* 2007;**37**:127–9.

104. Reuber M, Dunkley LA, Turton EP, Bell MD, Bamford JM. Stroke after internal jugular venous cannulation. *Acta Neurol Scand* 2002;**105**:235–9.

105. Burke JP, Gerszten PC, Welch WC. Iatrogenic vertebral artery injury during anterior cervical spine surgery. *Spine J.* 2005;**5**:508–14; discussion 514.

106. Inamasu J, Guiot BH. Vascular injury and complication in neurosurgical spine surgery. *Acta Neurochir (Wien)* 2006;**148**:375–87.

107. Inamasu J, Guiot BH. Iatrogenic vertebral artery injury. *Acta Neurol Scand* 2005;**112**:349–57.

108. Raymond J, Hardy J, Czepko R, Roy D. Arterial injuries in transsphenoidal surgery for pituitary adenoma; the role of angiography and endovascular treatment. *Am J Neuroradiol* 1997;**18**:655–65.

109. Munari LM, Belloni G, Moschini L, Mauro A, Pezzuoli G, Porta M. Carotid pain during percutaneous angioplasty (pta). Pathophysiology and clinical features. *Cephalalgia* 1994;**14**:127–31.

110. Arnold M, Cumurciuc R, Stapf C, Favrole P, Berthet K, Bousser MG. Pain as the only symptom of cervical artery dissection. *J Neurol Neurosurg Psychiatry* 2006;**77**:1021–4.

111. Silbert PL, Mokri B, Schievink WI. Headache and neck pain in spontaneous internal carotid and vertebral artery dissections. *Neurology* 1995;**45**:1517–22.

112. Bogousslavsky J, Despland PA, Regli F. Spontaneous carotid dissection with acute stroke. *Arch Neurol* 1987;**44**:137–40.

113. Baumgartner RW, Bogousslavsky J. Clinical manifestations of carotid dissection. *Front Neurol Neurosci* 2005;**20**:70–6.

114. Maurer JJ, Mills M, German WJ. Triad of unilateral blindness, orbital fractures and massive epistaxis after head injury. *J Neurosurg* 1961;**18**:837–40.

115. Han MH, Sung MW, Chang KH, Min YG, Han DH, Han MC. Traumatic pseudoaneurysm of the intracavernous ica presenting with massive epistaxis:

Imaging diagnosis and endovascular treatment. *Laryngoscope* 1994;**104**:370–7.

116. Chen D, Concus AP, Halbach VV, Cheung SW. Epistaxis originating from traumatic pseudoaneurysm of the internal carotid artery: Diagnosis and endovascular therapy. *Laryngoscope* 1998;**108**:326–31.

117. Banfield GK, Brasher PF, Deans JA, Barker PG, Taylor WJ. Intrapetrous carotid artery aneurysm presenting as epistaxis and otalgia. *J Laryngol Otol* 1995;**109**:865–7.

118. Chambers EF, Rosenbaum AE, Norman D, Newton TH. Traumatic aneurysms of cavernous internal carotid artery with secondary epistaxis. *Am J Neuroradiol* 1981;**2**:405–9.

119. Endo S, Takaku A, Aihara H, Suzuki J. Traumatic cerebral aneurysm associated with widening skull fracture. Report of two infancy cases. *Childs Brain* 1980;**6**:131–9.

120. Abad JM, Alvarez F, Blazquez MG. An unrecognized neurological syndrome: Sixth-nerve palsy and horner's syndrome due to traumatic intracavernous carotid aneurysm. *Surg Neurol* 1981;**16**:140–4.

121. Wang AN, Winfield JA, Gucer G. Traumatic internal carotid artery aneurysm with rupture into the sphenoid sinus. *Surg Neurol* 1986;**25**:77–81.

122. Miller PR, Fabian TC, Croce MA, *et al.* Prospective screening for blunt cerebrovascular injuries: analysis of diagnostic modalities and outcomes. *Ann Surg* 2002;**236**:386–393; discussion 393–5.

123. Biffl WL, Ray CE, Jr., Moore EE, Mestek M, Johnson JL, Burch JM. Noninvasive diagnosis of blunt cerebrovascular injuries: a preliminary report. *J Trauma* 2002;**53**:850–6.

124. Biffl WL, Egglin T, Benedetto B, Gibbs F, Cioffi WG. Sixteen-slice computed tomographic angiography is a reliable noninvasive screening test for clinically significant blunt cerebrovascular injuries. *J Trauma* 2006;**60**:745–751; discussion 751–2.

125. Eastman AL, Chason DP, Perez CL, McAnulty AL, Minei JP. Computed tomographic angiography for the diagnosis of blunt cervical vascular injury: Is it ready for primetime? *J Trauma* 2006;**60**:925–929; discussion 929.

126. Munera F, Soto JA, Palacio DM, *et al.* Penetrating neck injuries: Helical ct angiography for initial evaluation. *Radiology* 2002;**224**:366–72.

127. Gracias VH, Reilly PM, Philpott J, *et al.* Computed tomography in the evaluation of penetrating neck trauma: a preliminary study. *Arch Surg* 2001;**136**:1231–5.

128. Bachmann R, Nassenstein I, Kooijman H, *et al.* High-resolution magnetic resonance imaging (mri) at 3.0 tesla in the short-term follow-up of patients with proven cervical artery dissection. *Invest Radiol* 2007;**42**:460–6.

129. Heiserman JE, Dean BL, Hodak JA, *et al.* Neurologic complications of cerebral angiography. *Am J Neuroradiol* 1994;**15**:1401–7; discussion 1408–11.

130. Willinsky RA, Taylor SM, TerBrugge K, Farb RI, Tomlinson G, Montanera W. Neurologic complications of cerebral angiography: Prospective analysis of 2,899 procedures and review of the literature. *Radiology* 2003;**227**:522–8.

131. Jarvik JG, Philips GR, 3rd, Schwab CW, Schwartz JS, Grossman RI. Penetrating neck trauma: sensitivity of clinical examination and cost-effectiveness of angiography. *Am J Neuroradiol* 1995;**16**:647–54.

132. Rivers SP, Patel Y, Delany HM, Veith FJ. Limited role of arteriography in penetrating neck trauma. *J Vasc Surg* 1988;**8**:112–16.

133. Baratham G, Dennyson WG. Delayed traumatic intracerebral haemorrhage. *J Neurol Neurosurg Psychiatry* 1972;**35**:698–706.

134. Fleischer AS, Patton JM, Tindall GT. Cerebral aneurysms of traumatic origin. *Surg Neurol* 1975;**4**:233–9.

135. Mokri B. Traumatic and spontaneous extracranial internal carotid artery dissections. *J Neurol* 1990;**237**:356–61.

Intracranial aneurysms

Alexandros L. Georgiadis, Matthew D. Ford, David A. Steinman, Nauman Tariq and Adnan I. Qureshi

Introduction
Overview

Intracranial aneurysms are focal dilatations originating from medium-sized arteries as a result of congenital and acquired defects of the media[1] and exposure to factors that promote degenerative changes in the arterial wall such as hypertension and cigarette smoking.[2,3] In autopsy series the reported frequency of intracranial aneurysms has varied widely from 0.2% to 9.9% of the population (mean frequency 5%).[4] Based on the estimated mean frequency, the number of people in the US that harbor intracranial aneurysms should exceed 10 million. In a review of the existing literature up to 1996 comprising 56 304 patients, Rinkel and colleagues[5] found a prevalence of 0.4% (retrospective autopsy studies) to 6% (prospective angiographic studies). The overall prevalence for adults with no risk factors was 2.3%. Patients with polycystic kidney disease, familial predisposition, and atherosclerosis were identified as having an increased risk (relative risk of 4.4, 4.0, and 2.3, respectively).

Enlargement and rupture of aneurysms results from the interplay between hemodynamic factors and the factors that initiated the development of the aneurysm. Pathologically, a major rupture may be preceded by fibrinous and leukocytic infiltration of the wall, bleb formation, and minor hemorrhage.[2,3] From a natural history standpoint, intracranial aneurysms can be divided into two groups:[156] (1) aneurysms that rupture early in the course of development and are commonly detected as small ruptured aneurysms (early vulnerability); and (2) aneurysms that rupture late in the course of development and are commonly detected in the unruptured stage rupturing only after growing to a critical size (late vulnerability). The factors that differentiate the two groups are unclear.

The rupture of intracranial aneurysms results in subarachnoid hemorrhage (SAH) sometimes accompanied by intra-parenchymal and/or intra-ventricular hemorrhage. In a meta-analysis of 18 studies, Linn et al.[6] found an incidence for SAH of 8 to 21 per 100 000 person–years (women: men, 1.6 : 1).

SAH is associated with high morbidity and mortality.[7] The lifetime cost for the care of the annual cases of patients hospitalized with SAH in the US has been estimated at $1 755 600 000.[5]

Natural history

The International Study of Unruptured Intracranial Aneurysms (ISUIA) evaluated the natural history of unruptured intracranial aneurysms in 1449 patients with 1937 aneurysms.[8] Group 1 consisted of 727 patients with no previous history of SAH, and group 2 of 722 patients with a history of SAH from a different aneurysm that was successfully obliterated. Of the 1449 patients, 32 had confirmed aneurismal rupture during follow-up (66% were fatal), and in 28 of the 32, the rupture occurred within the first 7.5 years of follow-up. The cumulative risk of rupture for patients in group 1 was 0.05% per year for aneurysms <10 mm and <1% per year for aneurysms ≥10 mm. Giant aneurysms (≥25 mm) had a 6% rupture risk in the first year. In group 2, the risk of rupture for aneurysm with diameter <10mm was significantly higher at 0.5% per year. The rupture rate of larger aneurysms was 1% per year.

Wiebers et al. reported on the natural history of unruptured intracranial aneurysms in 1692 patients with 2686 aneurysms (mean follow-up 4.1 years).[9] Among patients who did not have a history of SAH with aneurysms of the anterior circulation, the cumulative 5-year rupture rates were 0%, 2.6%, 14.5%, and 40% for aneurysms less than 7 mm, 7–12 mm, 13–24 mm, and 25 mm or greater, respectively. Posterior circulation aneurysms (including the posterior communicating artery) had rupture rates of 2.5%, 14.5%, 18.4%, and 50%, respectively, for the same size categories. In patients with prior history of SAH, the 5-year cumulative rupture rates for anterior circulation aneurysms less than 7mm was 1.5% compared to 3.4% for the same size posterior circulation aneurysms.

Juvela et al.[10] reported on 142 patients with 181 unruptured aneurysms that were followed for a median period of 20 years (range 1–39 years). Six patients had a symptomatic aneurysm, five had an incidentally discovered aneurysm, and

Table 11.1. Overview of surgical and endovascular treatments for intracranial aneurysms. (Adapted from Qureshi *et al. Lancet Neurol* 2007: **6**: 616–25)

Surgical treatments	Endovascular treatments
Direct clipping (clips vary based on strength, shape, and size)	Detachable coil placement (coils vary based on strength, shape, and size)
Direct clipping with decompression of aneurysmal sac (may include thrombectomy)	Detachable coil placement with temporary balloon assistance
Direct clipping with neuroprotection using barbiturate anesthesia or hypothermia	Placement of an intravascular stent followed by coil embolization
Proximal ligation (abrupt or gradual) or trapping with or without use of bypass	Liquid embolic agent injection with intravascular balloon or stent assistance
Wrapping or coating	Occlusion of parent vessel
Direct clipping of remnant aneurysm following endovascular treatment	Detachable coil placement in remnant aneurysm following surgical treatment

131 had multiple aneurysms, of which the ruptured aneurysm was surgically treated at the beginning of the follow-up study. During 2575 person-years of follow-up, there were 33 first-time episodes of hemorrhage from previously unruptured aneurysms, for an average annual incidence of 1.3%. The cumulative rate of rupture among these 142 patients with unruptured intracranial aneurysms was 10.5% at 10 years, and 30.3% at 30 years.

Regarding the rate of re-rupture, Jane *et al.*[11] reported data derived from experience collected at the Atkinson Morley's Hospital, Wimbledon, UK, and Cooperative Aneurysm Study, The International Cooperative Study on the Timing of Aneurysm Surgery, and an analysis of incidental aneurysms in Charlottesville, VA. In patients with ruptured aneurysms, the rate of re-bleeding within the first 6 months is 50%. After the first 6 months, the rate of re-bleeding is 3% per year.

The indications and effectiveness of treatment options will be discussed in following sections.

The evolution of obliteratve treatment

The goal of obliterative treatment is to prevent primary or recurrent SAH. In 1937, Walter Dandy performed the first surgical treatment of an aneurysm using a vascular clip designed by Harvey Cushing.[12,13] Since that time, advancements in neurosurgical technique, including the use of operating microscopes, microsurgical instruments, new and improved clip design, neuroanesthesia, and perioperative management for complications such as hydrocephalus and symptomatic vasospasm, have allowed the neurosurgeons to be able to offer treatment for the majority of intracranial aneurysms. For almost four decades, surgical treatment was the predominant treatment for intracranial aneurysms. Placement of iron particles, detachable balloons, and pushable platinum coils had been attempted through the endovascular route.[14] Such treatment was successful in appropriate cases but limited in applicability due to the relatively high rates of aneurysm rupture, balloon deflations, and migrating particles. In the late 1980s, soft platinum coils soldered to a stainless steel delivery wire

that could be introduced through a microcatheter into the aneurysm sac were developed.[15] Protection against rupture resulted from the coil mass "buffering" the hemodymamic stress against the fundus of the aneurysm.[16,17] The development and subsequent approval of Guglielmi detachable coils (GDC, Target Therapeutics, Fremont, CA) by the Food and Drug Administration in 1995 initiated a reassessment of intracranial aneurysm treatment.

Initially endovascular treatment was utilized in patients considered to be poor candidates for surgical treatment.[14,18] Those were patients of advanced age, poor clinical grade, posterior circulation or cavernous segment of the internal carotid artery aneurysms, presentation between 3 and 10 days after symptom onset, or active cerebral vasospasm. Over the last decade, treatment paradigms for intracranial aneurysms have rapidly evolved as new endovascular techniques such as balloon- and stent-assisted coil embolization were introduced and with the advent of newer generation coil systems. These paradigms vary considerably among institutions and practitioners in spite of the efforts of national organizations and medical institutions to ensure uniform and evidence-based adaptation of the new techniques. Due to widespread availability, the importance of the issue is far greater now than 5 years ago when endovascular treatment was only available in selected centers. Table 11.1 offers an overview of available surgical and endovascular techniques.

Biomechanics of aneurysms
Overview of hemodynamic forces that govern aneurysms

When a blood vessel wall is exposed to high hemodynamic forces, it attempts to remodel itself, so as to bring those forces back to baseline.[19] In this section, we will define these forces and then discuss their role in aneurysm formation, growth and rupture.

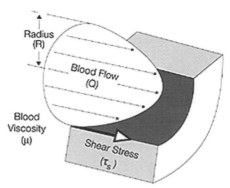

Fig. 11.1. Cross-sectional schematic of a blood vessel illustrating hemodynamic shear stress, τ_s, the frictional force per unit area acting on the inner vessel wall and on the luminal surface of the endothelium as a result of the flow of viscous blood. (From Malek et al., 1999, ". Hemodynamic shear stress and its role in atherosclerosis," JAMA) with permission.

Poiseuille's Law $\quad \tau_s = \dfrac{4\mu Q}{\pi R^3}$

It should be noted that, beyond hemodynamics, there are a number of factors that influence the life cycle of an aneurysm including genetics, the structural and mechanical properties of the wall, cigarette smoking, hypertension and alcohol consumption.[20]

Intra-aneurysmal pressure

The force that the aneurysmal wall is exposed to (intra-aneurysmal pressure) is the sum of intra-arterial pressure (*static* pressure) and forces exerted by the flowing blood (*dynamic* pressure). Intra-arterial pressure can be thought of in the same manner as the perpendicular force that air inside a balloon applies to the balloon walls, thus maintaining its structural stability. Dynamic pressure results from the impingement of blood flow on the vessel wall which creates a stagnation point and an associated area of high pressure. The dynamic pressure contributes $\approx 5\%$ to the total intra-aneurysmal pressure and is therefore not likely to play a significant role in aneurysm rupture.[21,22] However, although dynamic pressure may not be the primary cause of aneurysm formation, growth or rupture, it may contribute to secondary effects that lead the vessel to initiate the remodeling process and hence increase its vulnerability. Remodeling of arteries is known to lead to plaque formation and is implicated in the formation and growth of aneurysms.

Wall shear stress

Flowing blood exerts a frictional force on to the vessel wall which is known as Wall Shear Stress (WSS). WSS acts tangentially to the aneurysm wall and is proportional to the viscosity of the blood and to the rate of change of blood flow velocity near the wall (Fig. 11.1). Since WSS is typically even lower than dynamic pressure, its importance is not necessarily in its direct action on the vessel wall, but in the reaction of the vessel wall to abnormalities or gradients in WSS values that are outside the normal range.[23] It is not only the instantaneous magnitude of WSS that is important, but also how its directionality and magnitude change over the cardiac cycle. These two phenomena are commonly referred to as the wall shear stress gradient (WSSG) and oscillatory shear index (OSI). Extremes in WSS,[24] WSSG and OSI can induce remodeling of the arterial wall.

Unsteady and turbulent flow

Unsteady or turbulent flows are flows that are aperiodic and flows that vary within the cardiac cycle or exhibit vortex shedding (creation and subsequent periodic release of vortices). These flows not only lead to rapid changes in dynamic pressure and WSS (which could impact the behavior and integrity of red blood cells and platelets), but may also lead to vibrations in the aneurysm wall.[25] Early work by Ferguson[26] showed that bruits were present in a large percentage of aneurysms, leading to the conclusion that unsteady or turbulent flow is the norm and not the exception in aneurysms.

Assessing hemodynamic forces in aneurysms

Present day research has focused on understanding the origin of hemodynamic forces and their role in the life cycle of aneurysms. Three main techniques can be used to assess intra-aneurysmal hemodynamics: in vivo imaging, experimental modeling, and computational modeling. All three methods are concerned with the effect that local pressure distribution, shear stress patterns, and flow dynamics have on the rate of growth and the risk of rupture of aneurysms.

In vivo imaging

Recent advances in medical imaging allow high-quality, three-dimensional reconstructions of aneurysms and associated vasculature. However, in terms of hemodynamics, in vivo imaging (angiography or Doppler ultrasound) can only provide limited information. For that reason, much of what we know of aneurysm hemodynamics is based upon experimental and/or computational studies.

Experimental (in vitro) modeling

In vitro modeling was first used in combination with idealized aneurysm models constructed nominally of transparent material (glass, silicone, etc.) to understand intra-aneurysmal flow, pressure and forces as well as the effect of variable boundary conditions.[27,28] Unfortunately, idealized models are limited in their usefulness due to their simplistic geometric shape as compared with in vivo aneurysms. Therefore, efforts have been made to create "patient-specific" models. Early models were based on post-mortem casts,[29,30] while, more recently, advances in medical imaging have made the non-invasive construction of "patient-specific" aneurysm phantoms possible.[31,32] These advances have furthered our understanding of blood flow and have allowed to test endovascular devices in anatomically realistic models in the laboratory.[33] In vitro experiments are, however, limited by the need for specialized infrastructure.

Computational modeling

In the last 5 years, the combination of high-resolution in vivo imaging and computational fluid dynamics (CFD) has offered the possibility of large-scale "patient-specific studies."[34,36] Early CFD modeling used idealized models of aneurysm geometry to understand the general hemodynamic and shear stress patterns along with the local pressure distributions,[37] while later work has focused on understanding these phenomena in anatomically realistic models.[34,35,38]

CFD applies the principles of numerical methods to solve the equations that govern fluid flow which cannot be solved analytically over complex domains. Instead, these complex domains are broken up into smaller, regular shapes known as finite elements or finite volumes, which are more densely concentrated in regions of complex flow. Computational effort depends on the number of elements, so there is always a trade-off between accuracy and speed. Even today, CFD simulations of an individual case can take several hours on powerful desktop workstations. A distinct advantage of CFD is the ease with which any hemodynamic parameter can be extracted from the three-dimensional velocity and dynamic pressure fields. On the other hand, CFD has two main limitations. First, for practical purposes, a number of simplifications are usually made, including rigid walls, constant blood viscosity, fixed resting heart and flow rates. Second, the accuracy of the data depends on the proper choice of the inlet and outlet boundary conditions[39,40] and on the quality and extent of the geometric reconstruction from the patient data set.[41,42] Since this reconstruction from the patient data set cannot be entirely accurate owing to the various modeling assumptions and sources of uncertainty, it is suggested that the term "patient specific" be replaced by "anatomically realistic." Because of those limitations, it remains essential that CFD data be validated against accurate in vivo data or carefully obtained in vitro data whenever possible.[43,44]

The effects of endovascular treatment on biomechanics

As previously mentioned, aneurysms form as a consequence of remodeling and weakening of the vessel wall. Aneurysms are continuously changing their geometry in an attempt to return the forces experienced by the vessel wall back to baseline. As geometry changes, the location and magnitude of the forces acting on the vessel wall also change, and thus the remodeling process continues until equilibrium is reached or the aneurysm ruptures. Recent work has suggested that aneurysms grow in areas with low WSS.[34,45] Cebral and colleagues have also demonstrated that ruptured aneurysms experience more confined inflow jets, smaller impingement zones and unsteady flow patterns as compared to unruptured intracranial aneurysms.[35] This observation suggests that aneurysms prone to rupture are forced to undertake greater remodeling in the areas of hemodynamic extremes and thus, in the instance of rupture, the forces on the aneurysm exceed the strength of the remodeled wall.

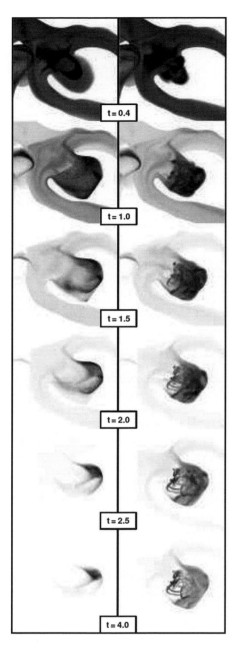

Fig. 11.2. Virtual angiograms of aneurysm before coil placement (left column) and aneurysm with 10cm coil (right column). Times given are relative to the period of the cardiac cycle. (From: Cebral et al., 2005, "Efficient simulation of blood flow past complex endovascular devices using an adaptive embedding technique," *IEEE Trans Med Imaging* with permission.)

t = 0.4

t = 1.0

t = 1.5

t = 2.0

t = 2.5

t = 4.0

It is obvious from the above that treatment of aneurysms should be aimed at isolating them from the intra-arterial hemodynamics. The goal of endovascular therapy is to disturb intra-aneurysmal hemodynamics enough, so as to cause thrombosis of the aneurysmal sac. It was initially thought that the small electric current used to detach the coils would stimulate thrombosis.[15] However, it is now recognized that the main effect of the coils is to induce flow retardation and stagnation, which eventually leads to thrombosis. The coils that cross the neck of the aneurysm are, thereby, the most important, since they retard the flow of blood entering the aneurysm (Fig. 11.2). More recently, stents have been used in the treatment of aneurysms. As stents are placed across the neck of the aneurysm, they prevent coil loops from herniating into the parent vessel. Also, as demonstrated by Lieber *et al.* stents retard the flow of blood into the aneurysm, much in the same way as coils that cross the neck of the aneurysm do, thus reducing hemodynamic stress.[21] Endovascular stenting may not be as effective when there is direct impingement of blood flow onto the stent (Fig. 11.3).[46] In such cases, as well as in cases involving wide-necked aneurysms, the combination of coil-embolization and stent placement is likely to be more effective (Fig. 11.4).[47]

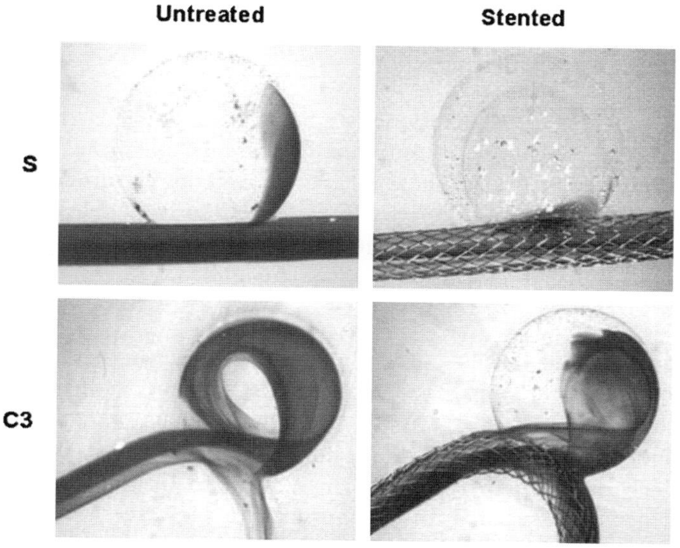

Untreated	Stented

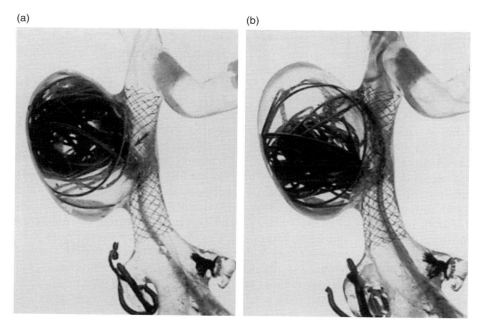

Fig. 11.3. Dye visualizations showing how parent artery curvature may reduce the effectiveness of stents for blocking flow into the aneurysm sac. (From: Meng *et al.* 2006 Saccular aneurysms on straight and curved vessels are subject to different hemodynamics: implications of intravascular stenting. AJNR, 1861–5 with permission.)

Practical applications of CFD
Predicting thrombosis and coil compaction

Current research using CFD is focused on understanding the impact that implantation of endovascular devices has on local hemodynamics and the forces experienced by the devices themselves.[48,49] Understanding the effect of endovascular devices on local hemodynamics carries the obvious benefit of assessing the level of occlusion required to induce thrombosis and is also helpful in perfecting the design of future devices. Knowledge of the forces that act on devices helps assess the potential for thrombus formation on stent struts, the potential for coil compaction and possibly even aneurysm regrowth. Coil compaction may be associated with strong jet-impact zones,[38] which can be predicted by CFD. Unfortunately, the calculation of those forces comes at a very high computational cost. There is approximately a 10-fold length scale disparity between the diameter of the parent vessel and that of the wires that form the stent mesh. In order to accurately capture the forces exerted on the endovascular device it is essential that this scale disparity be accurately modeled (Fig. 11.5).[49]

Predicting rupture

Perhaps the "holy grail" of aneurysm research is the ability to predict rupture. Presently, the only available method would be combining information on aneurysm size,[9] geometric aneurysmal abnormalities, and clinical experience. Due to the difficulties involved in visualizing and understanding intra-aneurysmal hemodynamics on a patient-specific basis, current research is focused on determining markers which can be used to infer the risk of rupture of an aneurysm. Many different avenues are being pursued, including quantification of the effects of WSS and dynamic pressure on rupture,[22,34,38,50] and studying the effects of local hemodynamics and in

(a)　　　　(b)

Fig. 11.4. Impact of coil placement on slipstream flow in a wide-necked basilar artery aneurysm. (From: Imbesi *et al.* 2001 Analysis of slipstream flow in a wide-necked basilar artery aneurysm: evaluation of potential treatment regimens. AJNR 721–4 with permission.)

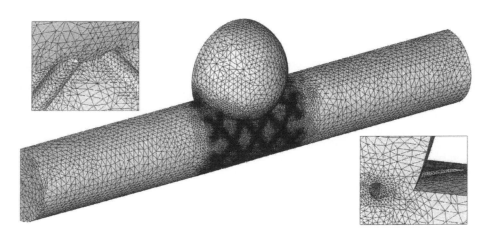

Fig. 11.5. Mesh densities required to resolve wall shear stresses at a sidewall aneurysm CFD model with stent in position. (From: Stuhne et al. 2004 Finite-element modeling of the hemodynamics of stented aneurysms. J. Biomech Eng. 382–7, with permission).

particular disturbed local hemodynamics[35] on the propensity of aneurysms to rupture. Other researchers are looking to use geometric factors and shape indices to predict the likelihood of rupture[51,53] and hemodynamic information to determine specific geometric markers predictive of a particular flow phenotype.[54] Ultimately, of course, it would be desirable to know not only the mechanical stresses to which an individual aneurysm is exposed, but also its mechanical strength and possible focal defects; however, the latter remain difficult to characterize non-invasively.

Conclusions

Image-derived CFD-models can provide substantial hemodynamic information that may be useful for planning aneurysm treatment. These models are however not yet routinely available in clinical practice. Alternatively, geometric markers (determined based upon the general flow patterns associated with specific geometric conditions) may provide the means to identify those aneurysms that are prone to rupture or to treatment complications, thus eliminating the need to perform CFD simulations on every patient who requires treatment.

Endovascular vs. surgical treatment
Comparison of patient outcomes

We will provide an objective assessment of available evidence comparing endovascular and surgical treatments for intracranial aneurysms using data derived from single center studies ($n = 10$), multicenter studies with ($n = 2$) and without ($n = 4$) independent outcome ascertainment, and randomized clinical trials ($n = 3$). Surgery and endovascular intervention were compared among patients with ruptured and unruptured aneurysms who were candidates for either or both types of treatment. Among patients with ruptured intracranial aneurysms, the rates of aneurismal obliteration were higher, and early rebleeding and requirement for second treatment were lower among patients treated surgically. However, discharge outcome, 2–6-month outcome, 1-year outcome, and late survival were superior among patients treated endovascularly (derived from observational studies and randomized trials). Among patients with unruptured intracranial aneurysms, discharge outcomes and hospital charges were lower with endovascular treatment (derived from observational studies). No clear difference was identified in 1-year outcomes and late rebleeding, although available data are limited.

Single-center studies

Several single-center comparisons have been reported in the literature (see Table 11.2).[55,65] The value of these studies is that they provide an estimate of the number of patients treated with each modality in various settings and also information on outcomes associated with each procedure. However, the comparative value of these studies is limited due to prominent heterogeneity in the criteria used for patient selection and imbalances between the two treatment groups. Some of these studies suggested higher rates of incomplete obliteration with endovascular treatment,[61,62] but without an increased risk of early rebleeding.[57,61] Thus, the effect of incomplete obliteration on the overall outcome of the patients treated endovascularly appears to be small. Studies that have reported better outcomes with surgical treatment also reported a higher rate of unfavorable baseline characteristics among endovascularly treated patients. Among studies where endovascular intervention was the treatment of choice, a large proportion of patients was deemed unsuitable for endovascular treatment and subsequently underwent surgery.

An adjusted comparison was provided in one study. Johnston et al.[66] performed a blinded review of the outcome of 130 patients with unruptured intracranial aneurysms treated with surgery ($n = 62$) or endovascular procedures ($n = 68$). All of the 130 aneurysms were considered treatable by either surgery or endovascular approach by a panel of neurointerventionalists and neurosurgeons. A significantly higher frequency of postprocedural disability (modified Rankin scale [mRS] ≥ 2) was observed in patients who underwent surgical treatment compared with those who underwent endovascular treatment (25% vs. 8%). The total length of stay, intensive care days, and hospital charges were higher in the surgical patients. There

Table 11.2. Summary of the characteristics and outcome comparisons between surgical and endovascular treatments derived from single center comparisons. Good outcome was defined variably among studies. (Adapted from Qureshi et al.[156] with permission.)

Study	Treated aneurysms		Endovascular treatment			Surgical treatment			Imbalance between treatment groups	Conclusions
			Number of cases		Good outcome (%)	Number of cases		Good outcome (%)		
Gruber DP et al.[57]	R UR	26 15	R UR	11 10	90%	R UR	15 5	65%	The endovascular group had worse baseline characteristics	Endovascular treatment was associated with better clinical outcome
Gruber A et al.[56]	R	156	R	45	35%	R	111	48%	Groups were not matched for Hunt and Hess Grade and aneurysm location	The incidence of delayed ischemic infarction was higher in the endovascular group. GOS was similar in both groups
Kahara et al.[59]	R UR	130 20	R UR	29 15	93%	R UR	101 5	85%	None documented	The difference in outcome was not significant
Kaku et al.[65]	R UR	79 40	R UR	47 28	R 81% UR NA	R UR	32 12	R 78% UR NA	None documented	A case-by-case evaluation of the individual characteristics of each aneurysm by a combined neurosurgical-endovascular team is essential
Helland et al.[64]	R	286	R	83	66%	UR	203	48%	None documented	Endovascular treatment was associated with better clinical outcome
Taha et al.[63]	R UR	53 80	R UR	28 43	R 62% UR 93%	R UR	25 37	R 44% UR 81%	Endovascular group had worse baseline characteristics	Surgery had better outcome at discharge and lower mortality in good grade patients but had no effect on symptomatic vasospasm in good or poor grade patients
Kato et al.[60]	R	179	R	59	44%	R	120	69%	Endovascular group had worse baseline characteristics	Surgery had better outcomes in poor grade patients
Hoh et al.[58]	R	515	R	102	33%	R	413	55%	Endovascular group had worse baseline characteristics	Surgery had better outcome at discharge and lower mortality in good grade patients but had no effect on symptomatic vasospasm in good or poor grade patients
Bairstow et al.[55]	R	22	R	10	NA	R	12	NA	None documented	Endovascular treatment was associated with better functional outcomes
Johnston et al.[66]	UR	130	UR	62	92%	UR	68	75%	None documented	Endovascular treatment has higher rates of favorable outcomes among patients with unruptured aneurysms

Table 11.2. (*cont.*)

Study	Treated aneurysms	Endovascular treatment		Surgical treatment		Imbalance between treatment groups	Conclusions
		Number of cases	Good outcome (%)	Number of cases	Good outcome (%)		
Raftopoulos et al.[62]	R 59 UR 68	64	87%	63	94%	Endovascular treatment was the treatment of choice. Surgery was performed in patients who were ineligible for endovascular treatment	Surgery was associated with better outcomes
Lot et al.[61]	R 280 UR 115	293	92%	102	85%	Endovascular treatment was the treatment of choice. Surgery was performed in patients who were ineligible for endovascular treatment	With appropriate patient selection, endovascular treatment is a good alternative to surgery

Abbreviations: GOS, Glasgow Outcome Scale; NA, not available; R, ruptured; UR, unruptured.

were three delayed subarachnoid or intracranial hemorrhages in the endovascular group and one in the surgical group after a follow-up of 3.9 years per patient.

Multicenter studies

Observational studies using multicenter databases consistently demonstrate lower rates of in-hospital death and disability among patients treated endovascularly. In the absence of complete knowledge of the baseline patient characteristics that affect outcome, superiority of any procedure cannot be inferred. However, lower length of stay and hospitalization cost in addition to better clinical outcomes support the use of endovascular treatment in existing paradigms. Johnston et al.[67] compared complications of surgical and endovascular treatment for unruptured intracranial aneurysms at 60 University Health System Consortium hospitals between 1994 and 1997. Adverse outcomes defined as in-hospital death or transfer to a nursing home or rehabilitation hospital at discharge were more common among the 2357 surgical cases (19%) than among the 255 endovascular cases (11%). In-hospital mortality was higher in surgical cases (2.3% vs. 0.4%) but the difference was not significant in the multivariate model. Lengths of stay and hospital charges were greater for surgical cases after adjusting for confounding factors.

A further review of 2069 patients with unruptured intracranial aneurysms used a statewide database of hospital discharges in California.[68] Adverse outcomes defined as in-hospital death or discharge to nursing home or rehabilitation hospital were more frequent in the 1069 patients treated with surgery (25%) than in those with endovascular therapy (10%). In-hospital death occurred in 3.5% of surgical cases and 0.5% of endovascular cases. Total lengths of stay and hospital charges were greater in surgical cases. Adverse outcomes declined significantly for endovascular therapy (1991 vs. 1998, 26% vs. 4%) but not for surgery (26% vs. 21%).

Berman et al.[69] evaluated the impact of hospital characteristics on outcome following the treatment of 2200 ruptured and 3763 unruptured cerebral aneurysm patients in New York State from 1995 through 2000. With every increment of 10% in the number of patients treated endovascularly, adverse outcomes (death or discharge to a rehabilitation hospital or long-term facility) declined. Hospital procedure volume and the propensity of a hospital to use endovascular therapy were both independently associated with better outcome.

A prospective multicenter study (ATENA)[70] was conducted to determine clinical outcome and risks of endovascular treatment in 649 patients with a total of 1100 aneurysms from 27 Canadian and French neurointerventional centers treated by endovascular coil embolization. Of these, 739 unruptured intracranial aneurysms were treated during 700 procedures. Aneurysms were treated electively in the majority of cases (98.4%). Embolizations were carried out with coils alone (54.5%), the balloon remodeling technique (37.3%), and stent-assisted coil placement (7.8%). Endovascular treatment failed in 32 aneurysms (4.3%). Technical adverse events with or without clinical impact were encountered in 15.4% of patients and included thromboembolic complications (7.1%), intraoperative rupture (2.6%), and device-related problems (2.9%). Adverse events associated with transient or permanent neurological deficit or deaths were encountered in 5.4% of cases. The 1-month morbidity and mortality rates were 1.7% and 1.4%, respectively.

Multicenter observational studies with independent outcome ascertainment

Multicenter observational studies with independent outcome ascertainment highlight the differences in peri-procedural morbidity and mortality according to procedure type and patient characteristics. The rates of peri-procedural morbidity and mortality were higher than those shown in self-reported studies (see Table 11.2) suggesting the presence of important reporting bias in the latter. The results also suggest that the higher rates of second treatment observed following endovascular treatment do not impact patients' clinical outcome. The ISUIA[9] enrolled patients with at least one unruptured untreated intracranial aneurysm. Prospective assessment of cognitive status and other forms of neurologic disability before and after aneurysm treatment were performed and end points were centrally adjudicated. When analyzing the ISUIA data regarding treatment, one should keep in mind that the study was not designed for comparison between treatment modalities. The endovascular treatment cohort was found to be a higher-risk group than those receiving surgery because of increased patient age, increased aneurysmal size, and more aneurysms in the posterior circulation. Operative morbidity and mortality was 12% and 10% for 1917 patients undergoing surgical treatment and 451 undergoing endovascular treatments, respectively. Importantly, patient age did not affect outcome in endovascularly treated patients to the same extent as seen with surgery.

In an ambidirectional cohort study,[71] all patients with ruptured intracranial aneurysms at any of nine participating institutions (with recognized expertise in endovascular and surgical treatment) were followed up for early and delayed (>1 year) re-rupture, and re-treatment. A total of 1010 patients (711 surgically treated, and 299 treated with endovascular therapy) were included. Rebleeding during the first month after treatment occurred in 2.7% of the endovascular treatment group and in 1.0% of the surgical patients. After the first year, the annual rate of rebleeding of the index aneurysm was very low in both treatment groups: 0.1% in the endovascular group (904 person–years of follow-up) and 0% in the surgical group (2666 person–years). Aneurysm re-treatment after 1 year was more frequent in the endovascular group, but major complications were rare during re-treatment. The investigators concluded that late events are unlikely to influence early differences between procedures at 1-year follow-up.

Randomized studies

A prospective randomized trial[72,73] compared endovascular and surgical treatment within 72 hours of SAH. The study evaluated the angiographic outcome, and 3- and 12-month clinical outcome (including neuropsychiatric evaluation) in 109 patients suitable for both endovascular and surgical therapy. Significantly better angiographic outcomes were achieved after surgery in patients with anterior cerebral artery aneurysms and after endovascular treatment in those with posterior circulation aneurysms. Early rebleeding was observed in one patient following endovascular treatment. The technique-related mortality was 2% and 4% in the endovascular and surgical group, respectively. The composite endpoint of rebleeding, stroke, and death was observed in 6 of 52 patients who underwent endovascular treatment and 3 of 57 patients who were treated by surgery. Good or moderate recovery by Glasgow Outcome Scale (GOS) was observed in 79% of the endovascular and 75% of the surgical treated groups. Neuropsychiatric tests performed at 3 and 12 months did not reveal any significant differences between the groups. Crossover from endovascular to surgical treatment ($n = 12$) was significantly more common than crossover from surgical to endovascular treatment ($n = 4$).

The randomized, multi-center phase III International Subarachnoid Aneurysm Trial (ISAT)[74] compared the efficacy of endovascular treatment to surgery in 2143 patients with ruptured aneurysms suitable for either treatment. The study question was: Can endovascular treatment reduce the rate of death or disability (defined by modified Rankin scale (mRS) score of 3–6) by 25% or more at 1 year among patients with ruptured intracranial aneurysms for whom both endovascular and surgical treatments were acceptable options. A total of 1070 and 1073 patients were randomly assigned to surgical and endovascular treatment, respectively. Recruitment was prematurely stopped after a planned interim analysis showed reduced disability in the endovascular treatment group. A higher proportion of patients allocated to surgery (31% of 793) were dependent or dead at 1 year compared with patients allocated to endovascular treatment (24% of 801). However, the requirement for a second procedure was higher among patients treated endovascularly. The risk of rebleeding from the ruptured aneurysm after 1 year was two per 1276 and zero per 1081 patient-years for patients allocated to endovascular and surgical treatment, respectively.

The study also assessed survival and long-term outcome by reviewing the certified causes of death, and the case record forms, the clinical records, and post-mortem details, when available. Follow-up data were sought at 1 year and annually thereafter by mailing a questionnaire to known surviving patients.[75] The early survival advantage with endovascular treatment was maintained for up to 7 years and was significant (log rank $P = 0.03$). The risk of epilepsy was substantially lower in patients allocated to endovascular treatment, but the risk of late rebleeding was higher. Nine patients (seven allocated to endovascular and two allocated to neurosurgical treatment) had confirmed rebleeding from the target aneurysm after 1 year. A follow-up study of the patients treated in ISAT was performed to compare the frequency and timing of aneurysm recurrence requiring retreatment.[76] Retreatment was performed in 191 of 1096 (17.4%) patients after endovascular treatment and in 39 of 1012 patients (3.8%) after surgical treatment. There was a difference in the rate of follow-up angiography which was performed in 88% and 46% of the patients treated with endovascular and surgical treatment, respectively. Late treatment (after 3 months of index procedure) was performed in 87 patients in the absence of rebleeding following endovascular treatment. Although late retreatment was 6.9 times more likely after endovascular treatment, no permanent complications were reported with the late retreatment. The mean time to retreatment was 21 months and 6 months after endovascular and surgical treatment, respectively, suggesting that recurrences can occur after delayed periods in endovascular patients. However, as retreatment was associated with low peri-procedural complications it did not offset the benefit of endovascular treatment on long-term survival.

In 2009 long-term follow-up results from the ISAT patients were published.[77] The authors assessed the long-term risks of death, disability, and re-bleeding. Annual follow-up was performed for 6 to 14 years (mean of 9 years). A total of 24 re-bleeds had occurred more than 1 year after treatment; 13 were from the treated aneurysm (10 and 3 in the endovascular and surgical groups, respectively). Four re-bleeds occurred from a pre-existing aneurysm and six from new aneurysms. At 5 years, 11% and 14% of the patients in the endovascular and surgical group had died ($P = 0.03$). The proportion of survivors at 5 years who were independent did not differ between the two groups: endovascular 83% and neurosurgical 82%. Overall, there was an increased risk of recurrent bleeding from an endovascularly treated aneurysm compared with a surgically treated aneurysm, but the risk was small.

A metanalysis[78] of three randomized trials comparing endovascular and surgical treatment in 2272 patients with SAH reported the following results. After one year of follow-up, the relative risk of poor outcome for endovascular treatment versus surgical treatment was 0.76 (95% confidence interval (CI) 0.67 to 0.88). The absolute risk reduction was 7% (95% CI, 4% to 11%). For patients with anterior circulation aneurysms, the relative risk of poor outcome was 0.78 (95% CI 0.68 to 0.90) and the absolute risk decrease was 7%. For those with a posterior circulation aneurysm, the relative risk was 0.41 (95% CI 0.19 to 0.92) and the absolute decrease in risk was 27%. The analysis concluded that for patients in good clinical condition with ruptured aneurysms of either the anterior or posterior circulation (considered suitable for both surgical and endovascular treatment), endovascular treatment is associated with a better outcome.

Endovascular versus surgical treatment: cost-effectiveness

As new and potentially more expensive technology is introduced, it is important to determine whether the difference in outcomes compensates for the cost difference. Bairstow et al.[55]

compared the cost and outcome of endovascular ($n = 10$) and surgical treatments ($n = 12$) of ruptured intracranial aneurysms. Although the cost of endovascular procedures was higher, staffing costs and overall length and hospitalization cost were lower. Following endovascular treatment, patients tended to return to normal activity and paid employment sooner and have more favorable functional outcomes. This was not accounted for in the cost-comparison. Another study[79] compared the cost-effectiveness of the two treatments among 62 patients recruited in the ISAT. There were no significant differences in the total cost of treatment (related to the inpatient stay) between the endovascular ($n = 30$) and the surgical ($n = 32$) treated patients. The benefits of decrease in length of hospital stay in the endovascularly treated patients were offset by higher procedural costs. There were no significant differences in clinical outcomes at 2 months and at 1 year.

Cost-utility analysis[80] in which benefits of an intervention are quantified in terms of quality-adjusted life-years (QALYs) has now become the standard for cost-effectiveness analysis. An incremental cost-effectiveness ratio below about $20 000 per additional QALY is exceptionally beneficial. Incremental cost-effectiveness ratios between $20 000 and about $40 000 per additional QALY are acceptable. Incremental cost effectiveness ratios between about $60 000 and $100 000 per additional QALY are higher than most currently accepted programs, and ratios above $100 000 are not desirable.

A cost-utility analysis[81] compared surgical and endovascular treatment with no treatment for unruptured aneurysms. The net benefit in QALYs and cost per QALY of each therapy and deferred treatment were estimated in a hypothetical cohort of 50-year-old women over their projected lifetime. For an asymptomatic unruptured aneurysm less than 10 mm in diameter in patients with no history of SAH from a different aneurysm, both procedures resulted in a net loss in QALYs (surgical treatment, loss of 1.6 QALY; endovascular treatment, loss of 0.6 QALY). For larger aneurysms ($\geq$10 mm), those producing symptoms by compressing neighboring nerves and brain structures, or in patients with a history of SAH from a different aneurysm, treatment was cost-effective. Endovascular treatment appeared more cost-effective than surgical treatment but these differences depended on relatively uncertain model parameters. For surgical treatment, cost-utility ratios ranged from $11 000/QALY to $38 000/QALY. For endovascular treatment, cost-utility ratios ranged from $5 000/QALY to $42 000/QALY. The investigators concluded that both treatments appeared to be cost-effective for aneurysms that are $\geq$10 mm or symptomatic, and in patients with a history of SAH.

The existing data supports that the higher cost of endovascular procedures is counter-balanced by cost saved in reduced length of hospitalization. The studies are limited to comparison over a relatively short-term follow-up and do not account for lost productivity. Another important and yet unaddressed issue is the cost-effectiveness of new and more expensive endovascular technology over existing endovascular techniques.

Maud *et al.*[82] carried out a comparison of cost-effectiveness in patients with ruptured intracranial aneurysms who were eligible to undergo either type of treatment using data from ISAT, Premier Perspective Comparative Database, data from long-term care in stroke patients, and relevant literature. Incremental cost-effectiveness ratios (ICERs) were estimated during a 1-year period. The median estimated costs of endovascular and neurosurgical treatments (in US dollars) were $45 493 (95th percentile range $44 693–$46 365) and $41 769 (95th percentile range $41 094–$42 518), respectively. The overall QALYs in the endovascular group were 0.69, and 0.64 in the neurosurgical group. The cost per QALY in the endovascular group was $65 424 (95th percentile range $64 178–$66 772), and in the neurosurgical group it was $64 824 (95th percentile range $63 679–$66 086). The median estimated ICER at 1 year for endovascular treatment vs. neurosurgical treatment was $72 872 (95th percentile range $50 344–$98 335) per QALY gained. Therefore, the authors concluded that endovascular treatment is more costly but is associated with better outcomes than the neurosurgical alternative among patients with ruptured intracranial aneurysms that can be treated with either procedure. With accrual of additional years with a better outcome status, the ICER for endovascular treatment would be expected to progressively decrease and eventually reverse.

Endovascular versus surgical treatment: quality of life and functional measures

Brilstra *et al.*[83] in a prospective multi-center observational study measured the impact of surgical and endovascular treatment of unruptured aneurysms on functional health, quality of life, and the level of anxiety and depression. In the surgical group ($n = 32$), 4 patients (12%) had a permanent complication; 36 of 37 aneurysms (97%) were successfully treated. At 3 months post-surgery quality of life was worse than pre-treatment, and at 12 months post-surgery the quality of life had improved but had not completely returned to baseline. In the endovascular group ($n = 19$), no complications with permanent deficits occurred; 16 of 19 aneurysms (84%) were occluded by 90% or greater. One patient died from subsequent rupture of the treated aneurysm. In the others, quality of life after 3 months and after 1 year was similar to that before treatment. In the short term, surgical treatment (but not endovascular treatment) of patients with an unruptured aneurysm has a considerable impact on functional health and quality of life.

Recommendations from professional and regulatory organizations

Endovascular treatment of intracranial aneurysms was initiated after the Food and Drug Administration (FDA) approved the use of GDC in September 1995, for treatment of high-risk or inoperable ruptured and unruptured brain aneurysms.[84]

In August 2003, the FDA approved the use of endovascular treatment for all brain aneurysms.

In 1997, aneurysmal SAH guidelines from the Canadian Neurosurgical Society[85] recommended early surgery for aneurysm treatment, unless the aneurysm location or size rendered treatment technically difficult. Open microsurgery and clip placement was recommended as the first line of treatment. Other treatment options mentioned included proximal parent artery occlusion, "trapping" of the aneurysmal segment of the artery, and embolization of the aneurysm using endovascular techniques.

In 2000, the Stroke Council of the American Heart Association[86] recognized endovascular treatment as a treatment option for unruptured intracranial aneurysms. Although the technique was being used with increasing frequency, the Council considered it premature to judge the effectiveness or efficacy of endovascular treatment for unruptured intracranial aneurysms without a case-controlled, randomized prospective trial.

In 2002, the Committee on Cerebrovascular Imaging of the American Heart Association Council on Cardiovascular Radiology[18] recommended endovascular treatment as an option for the treatment of ruptured and unruptured intracranial aneurysms. Special consideration for endovascular treatment was recommended in patients where surgery is not feasible or is associated with high risk, as is the case with posterior circulation aneurysms.

In 2003, after the results of ISAT were published, the American Society of Interventional and Therapeutic Neuroradiology and the American Society of Neuroradiology[87] recommended that endovascular therapy must be considered as a treatment option for every patient with a ruptured intracranial aneurysm. A consultation with a neuroendovascular specialist should take place. If one treatment method is recommended over another, the reasons for this decision should be documented in accordance with the usual standards for informed consent. Patients who have aneurysms unsuitable for endovascular treatment should be treated surgically if that option is considered appropriate by a vascular neurosurgeon.

In 2003, the German Society of Neurosurgery[88] in their position statement reiterated that the outcome after a specific treatment (surgical or endovascular) of ruptured intracranial aneurysms is determined by both the peri-procedural complication rate and the success of preventing re-bleeding from the treated aneurysm. Endovascular treatment was deemed a safe method associated with fewer complications than surgical treatment in experienced hands. At the same time, it was stressed that the success of complete obliteration is higher after surgery, that incompletely occluded aneurysms have a higher rate of re-rupture, and that the definitive long-term re-rupture rate following endovascular intervention still remained unknown.

The National Institute of Clinical Excellence (NICE) stated in 2003[89] that current evidence suggested that endovascular treatment is efficacious in obliterating unruptured intracranial aneurysms and that its safety is similar to that of surgical treatments. However, the risks of treating unruptured intracranial aneurysms by any procedure may exceed the annual risk of rupture without treatment. The NICE statement regarding ruptured intracranial aneurysms in the same year was similar, stating that current evidence on the safety and efficacy appears adequate to support the use of endovascular treatment, provided that normal arrangements are in place for consent, audit, and clinical governance.

The Brain Attack Coalition stated in the 2005 guidelines for comprehensive stroke centers[90] that endovascular treatment of aneurysms is a safe and effective alternative to surgery in selected patients (grade IA). Therefore, a comprehensive stroke center is required to have the capability to perform surgical and endovascular treatments. If a comprehensive stroke center is temporarily unable to offer this therapy, it is recommended that protocols be developed for the rapid transfer of patients in need of endovascular treatment to a nearby facility that can offer it.

The special writing group of the Stroke Council of the American Heart Association in 2009[91] issued the following statements and recommendations:

- Surgical or endovascular treatment should be performed to reduce the rate of rebleeding after aneurysmal SAH (Class I, Level of Evidence B). Further points were:
- Complete obliteration is to be performed whenever possible (Class I, Level of evidence B). Aneurysms that have been wrapped, coated, or incompletely treated have an increased risk of hemorrhage compared to those that have been completely obliterated and therefore require long-term angiographic follow-up.
- For patients with ruptured aneurysms judged by an experienced team of cerebrovascular surgeons and endovascular practitioners to be candidates for both treatments, endovascular treatment can be beneficial (Class I, Level of Evidence B).
- The individual characteristics of the patient and the aneurysm should be taken into consideration when deciding the best means of repair. Management of patients in centers offering both treatments is probably indicated (Class IIa, Level of Evidence B).
- Early aneurysm treatment is reasonable and probably indicated in the majority of cases (Class IIa, Level of Evidence B).

A careful review of the existing literature (see Table 11.3) and the above-mentioned guidelines suggests the following:

1. Availability of both endovascular and surgical treatment options is essential for any center that treats patients with intracranial aneurysms.
2. There is reasonable evidence to support considering endovascular treatment as an initial treatment option for all ruptured and unruptured intracranial aneurysms. It should be noted that only part of this evidence is derived

from randomized controlled trials and the need for new studies still exists.

3. It should be understood that certain aneurysms are better treated surgically. Physicians with endovascular expertise must be familiar with the pros and cons of both treatment modalities so as to be able to recommend the best option to each patient.
4. While significant emphasis has been placed on selecting the appropriate treatment, it should be recognized that conservative management may be the best option for certain patients. Therefore, the physicians involved in the care of patients with aneurysms must possess a thorough understanding of the natural history of intracranial aneurysms in various settings.
5. As more technologically advanced and expensive devices are introduced into practice, practicing physicians and treating institutions are encouraged to consider cost-effectiveness prior to incorporating new technology in their practice.

Shortcomings of current clinical practice

It has been estimated that a treatment that would increase the rate of discharge home among SAH patients by 6% would lead to annual savings of $11.4 million if applied to 20% of patients and $28.6 million if applied to 50% of patients.[92] However, current evidence suggests that a significant proportion of eligible patients is not treated at all. In a previous study[7], we observed that one-third and one-half of the patients admitted with SAH or unruptured intracranial aneurysms underwent either surgical or endovascular treatment during hospitalization in the US. Cross et al.[93] reported that 34% of 16 399 admissions for SAH in 18 states from 1998 to 2000 resulted in treatment for intracranial aneurysms using either surgical (29%) or endovascular (5%) techniques. These numbers fall short of the estimated 60% that represents the proportion of SAH patients who were found to be eligible for treatment by Fogelholm et al. among a cohort in Finland.[94]

Impact of the emergence of endovascular treatment on patient outcomes

We evaluated changes in morbidity and mortality rates in adult patients who were hospitalized for ruptured and unruptured intracranial aneurysms in the US using National Hospital Discharge Survey data.[7] All the variables pertaining to hospitalization were compared for three time periods: 1986–1990, 1991–1995, and 1996–2001. Mortality rates for hospitalizations related to SAH demonstrated no significant change between those periods (27.6%, 24.6%, and 26.3%, respectively). There was an overall trend ($P = 0.07$) toward reduced in-hospital mortality for unruptured intracranial aneurysms (5.9%, 6.3%, and 1.4%, respectively).

Another study reviewed the trend in treatment modalities and clinical outcomes among 1609 patients with SAH admitted

Table 11.3. A summary of available evidence comparing endovascular to surgical treatment for intracranial aneurysms. (Adapted from Qureshi *et al.*)[156] with permission

Variables	Ruptured intracranial aneurysms		Unruptured intracranial aneurysms	
	Candidates for any treatment**	**Candidates for either treatment**	**Candidates for any treatment****	**Candidates for either treatment**
Angiographic obliteration	Higher with surgical treatment (SCS)[56,59]	Higher with surgical treatment (RCT)[76]	Higher with surgical treatment (SCS)[56,59]	N/A
Cerebral vasospasm	Higher with endovascular treatment*(SCS)[55]	N/A	N/A	N/A
Discharge outcome	Superior with endovascular treatment*(SCS)[59]	N/A	Superior with endovascular treatment (MOS)[68,69]	Superior with endovascular treatment (SCS)[57]
Hospital charges	No significant difference (SCS)[60]	No significant difference (SCS)[76]	Lower with endovascular treatment (MOS)[68,69]	Lower with endovascular treatment (SCS)[57]
2–6 month outcome	N/A	Superior with endovascular treatment (RCT)[76]	N/A	N/A
1 year outcome	N/A	Superior with endovascular treatment (RCT)[76]	No significant difference (MOSI)[11]	N/A
Neuropsychiatric outcome	N/A	No difference (RCT)[75]	Non-significantly lower with endovascular treatment (MOSI)[11]	N/A
Peri-operative and long-term risk of seizures	N/A	Lower with endovascular treatment (RCT)[75]	N/A	N/A
Quality of life (short term 1-year outcome)	N/A	N/A	Superior with endovascular treatment (MOS)[84]	N/A
Early rebleeding	N/A	Non-significantly higher with endovascular treatment (RCT)[76]	N/A	N/A
Late rebleeding	No significant difference (MOSI)[72]	No significant difference (RCT)[75]	N/A	No significant difference (SCS)[57]
Need for second treatment	Higher with endovascular treatment (MOSI)[72]	Higher with endovascular treatment (RCT)[76]	N/A	N/A
Late survival	N/A	Superior with endovascular treatment (RCT)[75]	N/A	N/A

Symbols used: *, not consistently demonstrated; **, endovascular treatment preferentially used patients with poor clinical and angiographic characteristics.
Abbreviations used: SCS, single center study; MOS, multicenter observational study; MOSI, multicenter observational study with independent outcome ascertainment; RCT, randomized controlled trial; N/A, not available.

over 9 years (1990 to 1998) in a single center in the UK.[95] The rate of surgery fell from 66% to 35% (overall 54%), while the rate of endovascular treatment increased from 0.6% to 18% (overall 8%). The rate of conservative management increased from 28% to 46% (overall 38%). The decrease in use of surgery was attributed to improvements in endovascular technique and higher rates of admission of patients in poor clinical condition.

The higher proportion of poor grade patients was also partly accountable for an increase in mortality rates from 18% to 32%.

The benefits of endovascular treatment can be obscured in SAH patients due to preferential treatment of poor grade patients in whom outcome is predominantly determined by their initial clinical condition. Similarly, endovascular treatment has also increased the proportion of treated elderly patients with unruptured or ruptured aneurysms in whom long-term survival is influenced by other co morbidities.

Impact of the International Subarachnoid Aneurysm Trial

The ISAT study was criticized for the low mean age of the enrolled patients. Indeed, this is easily confirmed by comparing the characteristics of patients hospitalized for SAH in the US[7] with those of the patients randomized in the ISAT.[74] Therefore, the overall in-hospital mortality was only 6% in ISAT compared with 26%, which is the average rate for SAH in the US. The overall mortality reported in Japan is similar at 22% (data from the Japanese Standard Stroke Registry Study; treatment performed in 63% of all SAH cases, 59% surgical, 3% endovascular).[96] These observations suggest that the patients treated in the ISAT had more favorable baseline clinical characteristics compared with those of the general population and thus raise questions about the general validity of the study results. To answer this criticism, a center that participated in the ISAT study[97] evaluated the treatment and outcomes of patients not recruited into ISAT (72% of all admissions). Their findings supported the validity of the ISAT. Nine patients were treated conservatively, 67 underwent surgery, and 46 underwent endovascular treatment. At 12 months, a good grade (mRS 0–2) was achieved in 72% of endovascular and 49% of surgical patients.

A report from a single neurosurgical unit in the UK[98] showed that the proportion of patients undergoing surgery decreased from 51% to 31% while endovascular treatment of aneurysms increased from 35% to 68% following the publication of the ISAT results. Over the same time period, there was a non-significant trend towards better outcomes at 6-month follow-up and a decrease in the mean total duration of hospital stay. Another study[99] analyzed the therapeutic decision-making process and outcome in 100 consecutive patients with SAH treated since the publication of the ISAT. Forty-seven patients underwent direct surgical clip application, 41 underwent endovascular treatment, and 12 a combination of the two procedures. Good functional outcome (mRS 0 to 2) after 6 months was achieved in 71% of patients. The study suggested that in routine clinical practice, excellent functional results could be seen with complementary surgical and endovascular treatments using the data from ISAT to assign treatment.

Overview of endovascular techniques

Diagnostic angiography

The initial diagnostic images are essential for the correct planning and execution of the embolization. The assessment includes:

1. Aneurysm morphology (spheroidal, ellipsoidal single-sac, ellipsoidal multiple sac), which is important in selecting the ideal strategy for micro-catheter placement and coil delivery.

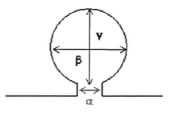

Fig. 11.6. Aneurysm measurements

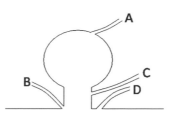

Fig. 11.7. Possible relationships between aneurysms and arterial branches. In case A coli embolization is preferably avoided.

2. Aneurysm size. The largest dimensions on both planes are used to select the size of the coils (see Fig. 11.6).
3. Relationship between the aneurysm neck, the parent vessel, and surrounding arteries. The aneurysm is examined from different angles, preferably using three-dimensional reconstruction images, in order to achieve optimal visualization of the sac and the neck, so that their size can be measured accurately. A roadmap, derived from the projection that best shows the relationship of the neck to the parent vessel and adjacent arteries (see Fig. 11.7), is used for navigating the micro-catheter/micro-wire system into the aneurysm.
4. Neck size, neck-to-dome ratio (see Fig. 11.6). Broad neck aneurysms will require assisted coil placement (either by balloon or by stent). They are defined as aneurysms with a neck of > 0.4 mm or a neck-to-dome ratio of > 0.5.
5. Relationship of the aneurysm to surrounding structures. Coil embolization increases weight and sometimes volume of the aneurysmal sac. This can lead to compression of the brainstem or cranial nerves.

Intervention

Guide-catheter placement

Based on the aneurysm characteristics, the procedure is planned with or without balloon/stent assistance. A sheath and guide-catheter are chosen so as to accommodate the micro-catheter and potential balloon- or stent- delivery catheters. The guide-catheter is positioned in the cervical vessel that allows access to the aneurysm. In the case of posterior circulation aneurysms, the vertebral artery with the wider diameter and less tortuosity is preferred. Distal catheter placement offers superior system stability (needed especially if stent placement is anticipated) at a cost of a higher incidence of dissection and vasospasm.

Micro-catheter placement

The micro-catheters used for coil-embolization have two radio-opaque markers at their distal end. In general, micro-catheters and micro-wires of smaller diameter are used for smaller aneurysms. The micro-catheter/micro-wire system is advanced through the guide-catheter until it is seen protruding out of its distal end. A high-magnification roadmap is obtained and the micro-wire is advanced into the intracranial vessels, followed after short segments by the micro-catheter. Serial roadmaps may be required until the system reaches the aneurysm. At that time, reproducing the 3-D angiography settings that clarified the relationship of structures and best showed the aneurysm neck, a roadmap is created at maximal magnification. With the roadmap displayed on one plane, the other plane is used to visualize as long as possible a segment of the parent vessel proximal to the aneurysmal neck so as to monitor micro-catheter stability. The micro-catheter and micro-wire should approach the aneurysm neck in minimal steps so as to avoid inadvertent system propulsion. A large distance between the micro-wire and the micro-catheter tip (free micro-wire) should be avoided for the same reason. It is preferable to enter ruptured aneurysms with the micro-catheter leading the entry. This can be achieved by gently pulling the micro-wire back into the micro-catheter tip, thus creating some forward momentum of the micro-catheter. The micro-catheter should be positioned centrally inside the sac. Too close proximity to the wall is best avoided. Withdrawal of the micro-wire under fluoroscopy is important to ensure that the micro-catheter retains its position.

Coil structure and function

Coils are made of platinum and are available with and without bioactive coating. They are attached to a delivery micro-wire via a detachment junction and the whole system is contained within a micro-catheter. By pushing the delivery micro-wire, the coil is extruded and it assumes a pre-determined shape and size. Only the coil and a distal marker of the delivery micro-wire are radio-opaque. The mechanism of detachment at the junction varies depending on the type of coil. Table 11.4 provides an overview of the specifications of some of the available coils.

Placement of the first coil

With the first coil, the aim is to construct a frame ("cage"), which will contain all the subsequent coils. Choice of the optimal initial coil, both in terms of size and of configuration, is therefore of great importance. In ruptured aneurysms, the first coil is usually slightly undersized so as to avoid creating additional tension upon the wall. In unruptured aneurysms, the dimensions of the coil should match or even slightly exceed those of the aneurysm, so as to ensure firm adherence to the wall. For spheroidal aneurysms, complex-shaped coils, such as three-dimensional coils are preferred. For ellipsoidal coils, other forms, such as helical-shaped coils may be more suitable.

If the aneurysm has multiple sacs, depending on their size and spatial relationship, they may be dealt with as separate aneurysms. In this case, the distal sac is embolized first and the catheter is then withdrawn for embolization of the proximal sac. After the coil is placed, its configuration must be carefully studied prior to deployment. Protrusion of a loop into the parent vessel must be ruled out. The coil must be spread across the sac as evenly as possible. If the result is not satisfactory, the coil can be partially or completely retrieved and re-extruded, or it can be replaced by a different coil if it is felt that the choice of coil was wrong.

Coil deployment

Coils can be deployed only when the distal marker of the delivery micro-wire has crossed the proximal micro-catheter marker. Once the coil is detached, the delivery micro-wire is carefully withdrawn.

After the first coil has been deployed, coils of less complex shapes are used to fill the spaces within the meshwork created by the initial coil. At the same time, coils with reduced width and length are chosen in a stepwise fashion. If a coil encounters excessive resistance, then further downsizing may be required. Using "soft" or "ultrasoft" coils is another possible alternative. Roadmaps without contrast injection ("blank roadmaps") or unsubtracted fluoroscopic images may be the best way to assess the position and orientation of the new coils prior to detachment. As the coils are extruded, the position of the proximal micro-catheter marker must be carefully monitored, since the distal marker is commonly obscured by coil loops. Retrograde movement of the proximal marker may be the only visible sign of retropulsion of the micro-catheter tip inside the aneurysm.

Embolization continues until placement of additional coils meets too much resistance or radiographic obliteration of the aneurysm is achieved. If further coil deployment is not possible, but there is significant residual opacification of the aneurysm or a small pocket within it, repositioning of the micro-catheter can be considered. If there is prolapse of the micro-catheter out of the sac, the operator has to weigh the necessity for further embolization against the technical difficulty and potential risk of re-introducing the micro-catheter. If the prolapse occurs during introduction of a coil, simultaneous retraction of the coil and slight forward push to the micro-catheter may be enough to re-introduce the micro-catheter. Should this fail, the coil must be withdrawn and the micro-wire should be re-introduced to guide the micro-catheter back into the sac. After the embolization has been completed, the micro-catheter is withdrawn under fluoroscopy with care to not interfere with the coil meshwork. In case there is any resistance to micro-catheter movement, indicating that the tip may be entangled in the coils, a micro-wire should be introduced so as to straighten the tip and disentangle the micro-catheter prior to removing it. Fig. 11.8 shows a case of coil-embolization of a narrow-neck aneurysm.

Table 11.4. Features of some available coil types for embolization of intracranial aneuryms

Cerebral coils						
Company	Product	Material	Coil types	Detachment method	Key benefits	FDA market cleared
Boston Scientific Corporation	GDC Matrix	Bare platinum Matrix coating	Standard, 3D, 360, Soft, Soft SR, Ultrasoft Firm, 3D, 360, Soft, SR, Ultrasoft	Electrolytic	Durable aneurysm occlusion Healing mechanisms with Matrix biopolymer coating	Yes
Cordman Neurovascular	Trufill DCSOrbit Detachable Coils	Bare platinum	Complex Fill, Complex Standard, Mini Complex Fill, Helical Fill, Tight Distal Loop Technology	Hydraulic	Conformability and concentric filling for outstanding packing density	Yes
ev3 Inc.	Axium Detachable Coils	Bare Platinum	Framing, filling, finishing	Linear release	Stretch-resistance, optimal balance of softness, stability and volume for increased packing density	Yes
MicroVention Terumo	HydroCoil MicroPlex	Bare platinum, platinum hydrogel coating	MicroPlex coil system (compass/complex for framing, helical coils for filling, HyperSoft for finishing), HydroCoil and HydroSoft embolic systems, combine platinum coils and hydrogel technology (HydroSoft for filling/finishing)	V-Grip detachment controller, self-contained integrated power supply, rapid coil detachment: 0.75 seconds	Hydrogel provides increased filling and greater mechanical stability; platinum coils provide versatile framework, stability and conformability	Yes
Micrus Endovascular Corp	Micrus Endovascular Microcoil System	Bare platinum, Cerecyte-PGA	Microsphere, Presidio, and Cashmere 3D Coils; Helipaq, Ultipaq, and Interpaq 2D Coils	Mechanical detachment using resistive heating	Frontline framing and filling coils; conformability with increased packing volume; cerecyte line of enhanced embolic coils	Yes

Balloon-assisted embolization

Balloon-assisted embolization was developed for treating broad-necked aneurysms. The concept involves positioning of a balloon across the neck of the aneurysm during placement of the coils so as to prevent prolapse of the coils into the parent artery. The length of the balloon should exceed the dimensions of the aneurysm neck and the diameter should match the diameter of the vessel proximal and distal to the aneurysm origin. The balloon is temporarily inflated during the placement of coils and deflated prior to detachment to detect any prolapse while retaining the ability to retract the coil. In aneurysms located in small and/or tortuous arteries, a micro-catheter can be placed across the neck of the aneurysm instead of a balloon to provide temporary support for coil deployment. Balloon-assisted embolization is being replaced by stent-assisted embolization because the platform provided by the stent is permanent. Fig. 11.9 shows a case of balloon-assisted coil-embolization.

Stent-assisted embolization

Stent-assisted embolization is a procedure analogous to balloon-assisted embolization, also used for treating broad-neck aneurysms. Positioning of the stent follows the same principles as described above. However, a few additional issues need to be taken into consideration. A careful review of several projections is necessary to identify the normal proximal and distal vessel segments in case the parent artery is diseased. The length of the stent should allow the proximal and distal ends of the stent (at least 3 mm on each end) to be placed across normal vessel segments. The stent diameter must exceed the diameter of the largest diameter of the vessel (proximal or distal). After the stent is placed, a micro-catheter and micro-wire are used to enter the sac of the aneurysm through the struts of the stent. There is a risk of moving a freshly placed stent during entry of the micro-wire or micro-catheter. This risk can be minimized by using longer stents that allow considerable overlap between the struts and the parent vessel. If movement of the stent is

(a) (b)

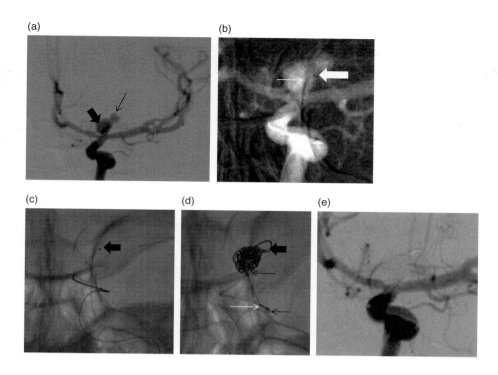

(c) (d) (e)

Fig. 11.8. *Background:* A 48-year-old man presented with severe headache and somnolence and was diagnosed with SAH at an outside institution. Computed tomographic (CT) angiography CTA showed a left internal carotid artery (ICA) terminus aneurysm. He was transferred for endovascular treatment. Diagnostic angiography (a): ICA injection, AP projection. The thick black arrow shows an aneurysm at the ICA bifurcation with a daughter sac (small black arrow). The aneurysm measured 6 mm × 6 mm, with a neck of 3 mm. The daughter sac measured 3 mm at its largest dimension. Procedure 8, (b)–(d): Under roadmap guidance, a micro-catheter was advanced over a Transend 14 micro-wire into the distal ICA. The aneurysm was entered with the micro-catheter leading (8(b), roadmap; the thick arrow points at the tip of the micro-catheter, the thin arrow points at the tip of the micro-wire). (c) (Unsubtracted image) shows the microcatheter in position (arrow) as the first coil is being advanced. (d) Unsubtracted image obtained prior to coil deployment. The position of the micro-catheter markers is indicated by the thin black arrows. The coil marker (white arrow) has crossed the proximal micro-catheter marker. Two coil loops are filling the daughter sac (thick black arrow). Coils used: Cosmos Complex 10, 6 mm × 18 cm, 5 mm × 22 cm, 4 mm × 12 cm; Microplex 10, 3 mm × 8 cm, 2 mm × 4 cm. Post-procedure angiography (e): There is good flow into the anterior and middle cerebral arteries. There is no residual filling of the aneurysm.

(a) (b) (c)

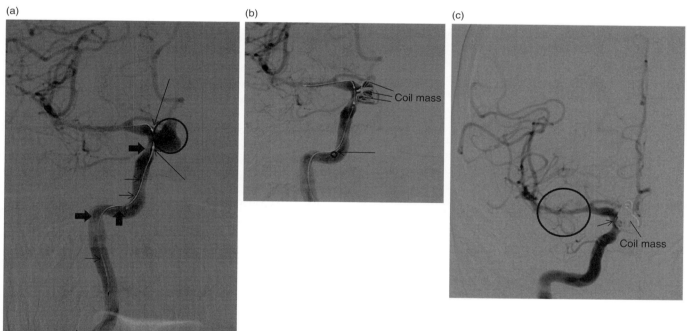

Coil mass

Coil mass

Fig. 11.9. *Background:* A 54-year-old woman presented with a 4-day history of headache. Diagnostic angiography revealed an intracranial bi-lobed, irregular ICA aneurysm measuring 11 mm × 10 mm with a 4 mm neck ((a), circle). *Procedure (a), (b):* Through a 7-F sheath, a 7-F straight guide-catheter was placed in the distal extracranial internal carotid artery (ICA) (block arrow in (a) points at the guide-catheter tip). A Nautica micro-catheter ((a), thick arrows) was positioned inside the aneurysm sac over a Transend 14 micro-wire. A Hyper glide 4 × 7 mm balloon catheter ((a), small thin arrows) was then advanced into the ICA and placed across the neck of the aneurysm ((a), long thin arrows point at the balloon markers). The following Cashmere 14 coils were deployed during temporary balloon inflation: 11 mm × 27 cm (1), 9 mm × 22 cm (1), 7 mm × 17 cm (1), 6 mm × 15 cm (2). A final 5 mm × 12 cm coil could not be positioned satisfactorily inside the sac due to herniation and was therefore removed. The arrow in (b) points at the coil marker that has just crossed the proximal micro-catheter marker (circle). *Post-procedure angiography (c):* There is no significant residual aneurysm filling, no contrast extravasation and no distal embolism. A single coil loop (arrow) protruded into the ICA lumen. Due to slight worsening of the pre-existing middle cerebral artery vasospasm (circle), 5 mg of IA nicardipine were administered prior to removal of the micro-catheter. All images are AP projections following ICA injection.

213

observed, allowing the stent to endothelialize over 4 weeks prior to further manipulation may be considered. If such a delay is not possible, using a softer micro-catheter or deploying a second larger stent are further options. Coils are placed under direct fluoroscopic guidance to ensure that all the loops of the coils are placed inside the sac and are not prolapsing through the struts. There are currently two self-expanding stents available for stent-assisted embolization: Neuroform (Boston Scientific) and Enterprise (Cordis Corporation). Fig. 11.10 shows a case of stent-assisted coil-embolization.

Adjuvant medications

Endovascular coils induce a state of local thrombogenicity at the site of deployment. This exacerbates the already increased clotting tendency that SAH patients exhibit. However, both anticoagulants and antiplatelet agents can increase the risk of bleeding in those patients and should be used with caution. Intravenous heparin is used to achieve an activated clotting time (ACT) of 250–300 seconds. Instead of administering the heparin bolus after guide-catheter positioning, some practitioners will wait until the first coil has been placed in the aneurysmal sac. Should stent placement be required, 325 mg of aspirin and 300–600 mg of clopidogrel must be administered via a nasogastric tube. Since there is a latent period of approximately 6 hours until the onset of action of both drugs occurs, use of an intravenous antiplatelet agent should be considered so as to prevent acute in-stent thrombosis. The risk of thrombosis should be weighed against the risk of rebleeding from the aneurysm. Again, some practitioners choose to defer the administration of intravenous antiplatelets until the aneurysm has been partially secured through the placement of the first coil.

Patients with unruptured aneurysms can be pre-treated with 325 mg of aspirin and 75 mg of clopidogrel daily for 3–5 days prior to the procedure if stent placement is anticipated. The goal ACT is again 250–300 seconds. Following stent placement, dual antiplatelet therapy is continued for 4 to 6 weeks, at which time clopidogrel can be discontinued. Aspirin is to be taken idefinitely.

Management of intra-procedural complications

Risk factors and situations that predispose to complications are summarized in Table 11.5.

Coil prolapse or migration

A coil loop can protrude out of the aneurysm neck, thus creating a risk of parent vessel thrombosis. In one study, coil herniation was seen in nine of the 216 consecutive patients treated by endovascular coil embolization.[100] The causes of coil herniation appeared to be coil instability after detachment ($n = 6$), excessive embolization ($n = 1$), microcatheter-related problems ($n = 1$), and interaction between coils ($n = 1$). There was one instance of coil migration.

If the coil has not yet been detached, it can be retracted and re-introduced. If the coil has been deployed, the available options include observation, infusion of intravenous antiplatelets over a few hours potentially followed by oral antiplatelets, coil removal with a coil retrieval device,[101] and placing a stent across the aneurysm neck so as to trap the protruding loop between the vessel wall and the struts of the stent.[100,102] The extent of the prolapse, the presence of hemodynamic consequences, and the observation of active thrombosis should be factored into the decision making. In the event that multiple coils are prolapsing or that the coil in question is enmeshed, coil retrieval is not recommended. Small coils can dislodge from the sac and migrate into the distal parent vessel. Using a coil retrieval device is recommended in this setting. Clinical consequences of coil herniation without hemodynamic compromise or active thrombosis are uncommon.

Thrombosis of normal adjacent arteries

Vessel occlusion can occur during or shortly after endovascular procedures as a result of local thrombosis or distal embolization. Both coils and stents invoke thrombogenic responses when placed in vessels.[103,104] The coils most commonly used in endovascular procedures are platinum detachable coils.[15] Platinum is three to four times more thrombogenic than stainless steel. Although the initial thrombotic reaction after coil placement is important for aneurysm obliteration, fresh thrombus in the aneurysmal sac can embolize distally. The table presents the risk factors for thrombosis during or immediately after embolization of aneurysms. If thrombosis is observed, it is divided into four categories: (1) filling defect without any hemodynamic consequences; (2) filling defect with delay in distal flow or distal embolization; (3) vessel occlusion filling of distal vessels from collateral circulation; (4) vessel occlusion with no or poor flow in distal vessels. The indication to actively intervene is greater in the latter categories and has to be counterbalanced with the risk of bleeding from a recently ruptured aneurysm.

In a systematic review of 1547 patients who underwent GDC embolization,[105] thromboembolic events were observed in 127 (8.2%). Twelve patients had asymptomatic events, 29 patients had transient ischemic attacks, and 86 patients had a stroke. The outcome among the 86 patients who had a stroke was as follows: full recovery ($n = 15$), good recovery ($n = 27$), partial recovery ($n = 19$), no recovery ($n = 11$), death ($n = 12$), and undetermined ($n = 2$).

Derdeyn and colleagues reported that thrombus protruding into the parent artery was noted during six of 159 embolization procedures,[106] resulting in a clinical deficit in one patient. Seven additional events occurred within 24 hours of the procedure and three events occurred after 24 hours. Aneurysm diameter and protruding coils were significant independent predictors of post-procedure ischemic events. The actuarial risk of stroke was 4%.

In another series, Ries *et al.*[107] observed thromboembolic incidents during embolization of 48 out of 515 aneurysms

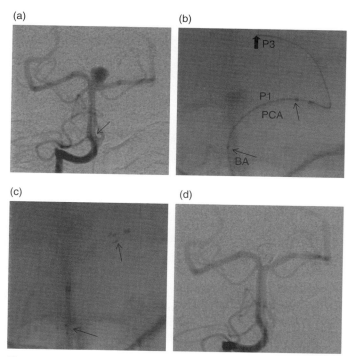

(a) (b)

P3

P1

PCA

BA

(c) (d)

Fig. 11.10. *Background:* A 64-year-old man presented with essential tremor. Neuroimaging revealed an incidental basilar artery tip aneurysm. *Diagnostic angiography (A)*: This AP projection following a right vertebral artery (VA) injection shows the wide-neck aneurysm. The neck extends onto the proximal left P-1 segment of the posterior cerebral artery (PCA). It measures 7 mm × 5 mm. The basilar artery is fenestrated (arrow). *Procedure (b), (c)*: A 6-F MPD guide-catheter was positioned in the right extracranial VA. A 3.5 × 20 mm Neuroform stent was then advanced over a Synchro 2 micro-wire (b), thick arrow points at the micro-wire tip) into the left PCA. The proximal stent remained in the distal basilar artery (b), the thin arrows point at the stent markers). After control angiography (not shown) showed good patency of all vessels the stent was deployed (c), the arrows point at the markers post deployment). A Prowler 14 LP ES 45 degree micro-catheter was then navigated through the struts of the stent into the sac over a Synchro 2 micro-wire. A total of six coils were deployed sequentially starting with a 7 mm × 17 cm Cashmere coil. *Post-procedure angiography (10D)*: There is minimal residual filling and no complications. All images are AP projections. All injections were into the right VA.

Table 11.5. *Overview of factors that predispose to intra-procedural complications*

Factors that predispose to intra-procedural complications	
Pre-existing factors	Procedure characteristics and complications
Aneurysm diameter >25 mm	Thrombus formation
Broad-neck aneurysms	Dissection
Radiologically visible intra-aneurysmal thrombus	Flow abnormality related to coil protrusion or prolapse
Suspected aneurysm-related embolic event	Stent-assisted procedure
Atherosclerosis proximal to the aneurysm	Balloon-assisted procedure

range, 450 000 to 1 300 000 IU; infusion rate, 20 000 IU/min). Partial recanalization was observed in nine patients. The authors observed that recanalization was best achieved when mechanical fragmentation of the thrombus and superselective drug infusion were possible. Nine of ten patients who had complete recanalization experienced good recovery, whereas only five of nine patients who had partial recanalization experienced good recovery. Intracerebral hemorrhage (ICH) occurred in one patient, and aneurysm rupture with SAH occurred in two patients.

Hähnel et al.[109] described nine patients who suffered thromboembolic complications during neuroendovascular procedures. These patients were treated by intra-arterial thrombolysis with the use of rt-PA (maximum dose of 0.9 mg/kg). Successful recanalization was achieved in four of nine patients. All nine patients suffered cerebral ischemic infarctions, and none of the patients developed ICH. The ischemic stroke was fatal in two patients, four patients remained moderately disabled, and three patients were severely disabled 3 months after thrombolysis.

Platelet activation and aggregation are important components of processes occurring at the surface of endovascular devices and site of intimal injury within the arteries.[104] It is possible that thrombus formation related to endovascular procedures may be platelet-rich and therefore more resistant to thrombolytic therapy and more amenable to platelet glycoprotein (GP) II B/IIIA inhibitors.

In the above-mentioned series, Ries et al.[107] treated 42 of the 48 patients with either intra-arterial or intravenous abciximab using a standard bolus of 0.25 mg/kg. Complete recanalization at procedure termination was achieved in 6/42 (14.3%) cases. Partial recanalization was seen in 25/42 cases (59.5%). No effect of treatment was detected in the remaining cases. No infarction on follow-up CT was detected in 29/42 (69.0%) patients. Combining their 42 patients with the 90 previously published cases that had been treated with intra-arterial or intravenous abciximab, they reported that complete

treated consecutively at their institution. A thromboembolic event was defined as any event with complete or partial occlusion of arteries at the site of the aneurysm (proximal thrombus) or distal to the vascular territory where the endovascular procedure was performed (distal thrombus). Proximal thrombus formation at the coil/parent vessel interface was detected in 25 cases and distal thromboembolism was present in the remaining 23 cases.

Intra-arterial thrombolysis is an attractive treatment for such occlusions because expedient local delivery of thrombolytics is possible as a result of existing arterial access. Cronqvist et al.[108] reviewed 19 cases of thromboembolic events that occurred during endovascular treatment of aneurysms. Embolisms associated with the procedure were observed in the middle cerebral artery in 14 patients, the anterior cerebral artery in three, and the basilar trunk in two. Complete recanalization was observed in ten of the 19 patients after intra-arterial administration of urokinase (mean dose, 975 000 IU;

Table 11.6. Recommendations for management of transtentorial herniation (Brain Code).[112] (Adapted from Qureshi *et al.*[112])

Emergent intubation if the patient is not intubated. Manual hyperventiiation using ventilation bag connected to the endotracheal tube. Attempt is made to maintain $PaCo_2$ between 25 and 30 mmHg by ventilating at a rate between 30 and 40 breaths/min.

Intravenous administration of mannitol in doses of 0.5–1 g/kg over 5 mins. Rapid bolus can lead to lysis of red blood cells in the venous system. Intravenous administration of thiopental if mean arterial pressure >150 mmHg, with dose titrated to keep mean arterial pressure between 90 mmHg and 140 mmHg.

Intravenous bolus of phenylephrine (1–2 µg/kg, repeated if no response) if mean arterial pressure is <90 mm Hg.

Intravenous bolus of 500 ml of isotonic crystalloid or colloid attire same time. Phenylephrine infusion is continued if hypotension does not resolve with treatment of mass effect, intravenous dopamine is another alternative particularly if bradycardia develops, either as a response to vagotonic effects of phenylephrine or Kocher-Cushings phenomenon.

If no clinical response (defined as resolution of pupillary dilatation with or without improvement in level of consciousness) after hyperventiiation and mannitol, a bolus of 30 ml of 23.4% sodium chloride is administered over 15 mins. A second dose of 30 mL can be repeated if there is no response after the first 30 ml.

Emergent non-contrast computed tomographic scan of the head. Based on the computed tomographic scan results, pentobarbital infusion or surgical decompression is considered.

or partial recanalization had been achieved in 114 of 132 cases. Among the 76 patients who had follow-up CT scan, infarction was seen in 20. Bleeding complications clearly attributable to the use of the GP IIb/IIIa inhibitor occurred at an estimated rate of 2%.

Based on equivalent results to thrombolytics in regards to recanalization and better safety profile, our current practice involves using intra-arterial small boluses of platelet GP IIB/IIIA inhibitors until recanalization is achieved followed by intravenous infusion for 12–24 hours.

Intra-procedural aneurysm rupture

Intra-procedural rupture can occur during angiography, microcatheter placement, or coil placement. A rupture is suspected based on movement of microcatheter or coil beyond the angiographically delineated limits of the aneurysm sac. The clinical manifestations are consistent with acute elevation with intracranial pressure and include acute change in level of consciousness, posturing, and seizures. These manifestations are obscured in many situations because the procedure is performed during general anesthesia. Rapid alterations in systemic blood pressure and heart rate and increase in intracranial pressure (if a monitor is in position) occur concomitantly. A contrast injection demonstrates extravasation in the vicinity of the aneurysm and spasm of the surrounding arteries. A delayed contrast transit suggestive of elevated regional intracranial pressure may also be observed.

A meta-analysis of the results from 17 published retrospective reports on complications of embolization therapy[110] reported the rates of perforation and associated morbidity and mortality in ruptured and unruptured aneurysms. The risk of intra-procedural perforation was significantly higher in patients with ruptured aneurysms (4%) compared with patients with unruptured aneurysms (0.5%). The combined risk of permanent neurologic disability and death associated with intra-procedural aneurysm perforation was 38% for

ruptured aneurysms and 29% for unruptured aneurysms. The morbidity and mortality rates with perforations caused by coils (39%) and microcatheters (33%) were higher than those caused by microguidewire perforations (0%).

Intra-procedural rupture occurred in 14.6% of 1010 patients (299 coiled, 711 clipped) analyzed in the Cerebral Aneurysm Rerupture After Treatment (CARAT) study.[111] The rates were 19% and 5% with surgical and endovascular treatment, respectively. Among the endovascularly treated patients, 63% with intra-procedural rupture had periprocedural death or disability compared to 15% without intra-procedural rupture. Independent predictors of intra-procedural rupture included Asian race, black race, chronic obstructive pulmonary disease, and lower initial Hunt and Hess Grade.

Once an intra-procedural rupture is recognized, immediate steps need to be undertaken. These include possible repositioning of the coil, reversal of heparin using intravenous protamine, temporary hyperventilation and administration of intravenous bolus of mannitol. If the patient is not intubated, the procedure needs to be interrupted for emergent intubation and mechanical ventilation. The following steps need to be considered (see also Table 11.6)[112]: (1) emergent intubation, if the patient is not intubated; (2) manual hyperventilation with a ventilation bag. An attempt should be made to maintain $PaCO_2$ between 25 mmHg and 30 mmHg by ventilating at a rate between 30 and 40 breaths/min; (3) administration of an osmotic agent, usually mannitol (0.5–1 gm/kg) intravenously. Thiopental or propofol can be used in case of a pronounced hypertensive response (defined as mean arterial pressure >150 mm Hg) accompanying the episode; (4) Administration of vasopressors and fluid boluses, if required, to keep mean arterial pressure >90 mmHg; (5) administration of a second osmotic agent, hypertonic saline, if adequate response is not observed with the first osmotic agent after 10 mins. A maintenance infusion of hypertonic saline may be started in selected patients to achieve serum sodium between 145–155 mmol/L.

Emergent ventriculostomy placement is important in cases of elevated intracranial pressure (ICP) if not in place already.[113] Intraventricular catheters enable drainage of cerebrospinal fluid and thus reduction of ICP, and also ICP monitoring. Continued aneurysm packing with coils is possible and recommended in most patients.[114,115] Once the patient has been stabilized, further coil placement may be pursued to achieve complete obliteration of the aneurysm. Rarely, surgical decompression and clip placement may be required. Prolonged systemic hypertension, persistent dye extravasation after deployment of the first GDC, and persistent prolongation of contrast dye transit time (suggesting ongoing ICP elevation), correlate with poor outcomes.[113]

Coil compaction

Recurrence of intracranial aneurysms treated by endovascular treatment is another issue that requires discussion. A classification has been proposed to grade the angiographic obliteration after completion of the procedure and during follow-up angiography.[116,117] Class 1 result means complete obliteration, including the neck. A residual neck (class 2) is defined as the persistence of any portion of the original defect of the arterial wall as seen on any single projection but without opacification of the aneurysmal sac. Any opacification of the sac is classified as residual aneurysm (class 3). A recurrence is defined as any increase in the size of the remnant. The recurrence is qualified as major if it was saccular and its size would theoretically permit re-treatment with coils. Raymond et al.[117] performed follow-up angiography for 383 aneurysms in 356 patients from a total of 501 treated aneurysms in 466 patients. Approximately half of the lesions (54.1%) were acutely ruptured at the time of treatment. The location of aneurysms was as follows: basilar bifurcation (28%), ophthalmic carotid (18%), anterior (14%), posterior communicating artery (11%), and middle cerebral arteries (7%). Short-term ($\leq$1 year) follow-up angiograms were available in 353 aneurysms (70.5%) and long-term (>1 year) follow-up angiograms, in 277 (55%). Recurrences using the above-mentioned classification were found in 34% of treated aneurysms and appeared at a mean$\pm$SD time of 12 $\pm$ 11 months after treatment. Major recurrences presented in 21%. Patients with major recurrences were most often re-treated with coil placement (39/79, or 49%). Another study[118] evaluated the relationship between packing, complex coils, and angiographic recurrence of 255 aneurysms in 223 patients. The follow-up angiographic results were dichotomized into presence or absence of recurrence. Recurrence was observed in 29% of aneurysms at a mean follow-up of 12 months; 6% were amenable to re-treatment. There was no significant difference in percentage of complex coils, aneurysm location, or multiplicity of aneurysms and recurrence. Previous studies have identified aneurysm size $\geq$10 mm, treatment during the acute phase of rupture, incomplete initial occlusions, and duration of follow-up as risk factors for recurrence of aneurysm.[117,119]

A systematic review reported on 17 studies that included data on retreatments, which was defined as follow-up treatment of an aneurysm, which occurred at a minimum of 1 month after the first treatment.[120] A total of 249 patients required a second treatment of the 4640 patients in these studies. Of these, 33 were patients who had been surgically treated (1% of clipped patients), and 216 had been endovascularly embolized (10%). In the ISAT study, retreatment was performed in 191 of 1096 (17%) patients after primary endovascular embolization and in 39 of 1012 patients (4%) after neurosurgical treatment.[76] After excluding early retreatment, nine patients undergoing surgical treatment were retreated and 94 patients undergoing embolization were retreated. The mean time to late retreatment was 20 months. Late retreatments were performed in 87 patients who were initially treated without rebleeding for angiographic demonstration of reopening or regrowth. Procedural complications occurred in 6% and resulted in transient neurological symptoms only. Late retreatments were performed in seven (0.6%) patients after rebleeding. In two patients, "de novo" aneurysm was reported in continuity with the treated aneurysm. One patient died 12 months after endovascular retreatment after another episode of rebleeding. No procedural complications were recorded. The predictors of retreatment included age, lumen size, and incomplete occlusion. No significant influence of gender, aneurysm location, or neck size was observed.

Overview of devices
Coils

In the following section we will provide a brief review of currently available coils. Table 11.7[121,134] summarizes the findings of pertinent studies.

Guglielmi Detachable Coils (GDC)

GDC coils are manufactured from a platinum I tungsten alloy wire which is wound into a primary or main coil. Depending upon the desired final configuration, the coil is either formed into a secondary helical shape (standard and Stretch Resistant GDC), vortex shape (GDC-18 Fibered VortX), or tertiary shape (3D GDC). GDC coils are attached to a delivery wire, which consists of a ground stainless-steel core wire with a platinum coil welded at the distal end and a Teflon outer jacket introduced through infusion catheters with two tip markers. The GDC is detached by electrolytically dissolving a small portion of the delivery wire upon desired placement of the coil in the aneurysm. Detachment of the occlusion coil from the delivery wire is accomplished by means of an electrolytic reaction in which the anode, or positive, electrode is the GDC stainless-steel delivery wire, and the cathode, or negative, electrode is a patient return electrode. GDC coils are available in a range of sizes for use with either Boston Scientific Target's –10 or –18.

Table 11.7. Overview of studies of aneurysm embolization with a single coil type. Outcome parameters were defined variably in different studies. An effort was made to present results as homogeneously as possible

Coil type	Study type	Number of aneurysms		Posterior circulation	Satisfactory angiographic obliteration[a]	Peri-procedural		Thrombo-embolism	Aneurysm perforation	Recurrence
						Morbidity	Mortality			
GDC[134]	MC	R	403	57%	35%–71%*	8.9%	1.7%	2%**	0.7%**	N/A
GDC[122]	MC	R UR	83 67	100%	R 75% UR 76%	N/A†	R 4.8% UR 0%	R 9%§ UR 5%§	0%	R 22% UR 19%
GDC[124]	MC	R	705	12%	97.6%	8.6%	1.4%	5.2%	3.6%	4.7%
Matrix[128]	SC	R UR	53 65	22%	75%	R 7.5% UR 0%	0.9%	1.7%	3.4%	19.5%
Matrix[129,131]	MC	R UR	138[b] 98[b]	7%	69%	4.3%	R 1.4% UR 0%	R 14%[c] UR 11%[c]	2.1%	25.7%
Trufill DCS Orbit[125]	MC	R UR	130[b] 161[b]	20%	81.3%	6.2%	0%	4.7%	1%	16.2%
Radioactive[132]	SC	R UR	17[b] 24[b]	45%	75%	5%	0%	7%	0%	31%
Micrus[130]	MC	R UR	50 30	11%	96%	1.3%	1.3%	5%	0%	N/A
Cerecyte[133]	SC	R UR	58 31	17%	97%	1.2%	0%	1.2%	0%	6.7%
Hydrocoil[126]	MC	R UR	32 48	10%	92.5%	19.7%[d]	0%	2.6%	0%	11%
Hydrocoil[123]	MC	R UR	31 19	38%	94%	2%	0%	2%	2%	17%
Hydrocoil[121]	MC	R UR	71 120	N/A	92%	3.3%	N/A	8.1%	R 2.8% UR 0%	N/A
Onyx[127]	MC	R UR	10 90	7%	98%	13.4%	2%	7.2%	2%	10%

*9 cases equivocal; c: unrelated to the procedure, d: 20 cases of transient deficits, 16 cases of permanent deficits.

[a]Complete or near-complete obliteration, variably defined.

[b]Number of patients.

[c]Most cases clinically silent.

[d]Mostly aseptic meningitis.

*Depending on aneurysm size.

**By the time of discharge complication rates were: perforation 2.7%, thrombo-embolism 5.5%.

†The study lists peri- and post-procedure complications combined.

§Symptomatic thromboembolism.

Abbreviations used: R, ruptured; UR, unruptured; N/A, not available; MC, multi-center; SC, single-center; GDC, Guglielmi Detachable Coil.

Matrix detachable coils

Matrix detachable coils are comprised of a platinum-tungsten alloy coil which is coated with a biocompatible absorbable polymer. The coil is coated with polyglycolic–polylactic acid (PGPLA) designed to stimulate an inflammatory reaction within the aneurysm that induces an accelerated organization of thrombus and ultimately fibrosis and subsequently elicits a faster and more complete neointimal overgrowth of the aneurysm neck. The device is loaded into an introducer sheath and is then placed in a dispenser coil contained within a foil pouch. Matrix Detachable Coils are detached using Boston Scientific's GDCW Power Supply.[136]

Micrus MicroCoil Systems

Micrus MicroCoils are available in both bare platinum implants and stretch resistant implants containing either absorbable suture (PGA) or non-absorbable suture (polypropylene). Micrus Cerecyte MicroCoils are fabricated from a platinum alloy wire, which is first wound into a primary coil (containing an absorbable polymer suture inside the wind) and then formed into a secondary helical or spherical shape. Micrus MicroCoils are also available in both 10 and 18 sizes and in spherical and helical shapes in a variety of lengths and diameters. The Micrus Modified MicroCoil (Cerecyte) consists of an embolic coil ("MicroCoil") attached to a Device Positioning Unit (DPU) (single use, sterile). The Cerecyte System is compatible with commercially available 2-tip marker microcatheters which have internal lumen diameters between 0.017″ and 0.021″. The coils are available in helical and spherical shapes and are available in various lengths ranging from 4 to 30 centimeters and diameters range from 2 to 20 millimeters.[136]

Hydrogel-coated coils

The MicroPlex® Coil System (MCS) and HydroCoil Embolic System (HES, Fig. 11.11) consist of an implantable coil attached to a delivery system called a V-TRAK™ Delivery Pusher. The hydrogel-coated coils are coated with a desiccated hydrogel that absorbs water and swells considerably upon introduction into the blood environment. The –10, –14, and –18 size hydrocoils swell to five, seven, and 11 times the volume of the standard "platinum–10" sized coils. The Delivery Pusher is a variable stiffness, stainless steel and tapered mandrel. Two silver electrical leads run along the outside of the mandrel from the proximal to the distal end. Platinum and stainless steel wires are wound around the distal end of the mandrel to form the electrical heater and provide kink-resistance. Two outer layers of PET tubing cover the distal end of the pusher assembly. A layer of polyimide tubing covers the proximal end. The proximal end of the HES coils incorporates a platinum coupler for attachment to the Delivery Pusher. A polyolefin elastomer filament is attached to the proximal end of the coil. This filament runs through the inner

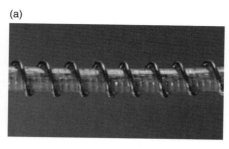

(a)

(b)

Fig. 11.11. Pre- and post-expansion states of the HydroCoil system (MicroVention, Aliso Viejo, CA). Reprinted with permission from: Suri MF, Memon ZM, Qureshi AI. Journal of Vascular and Interventional Neurology 2008;1(2):42–45.

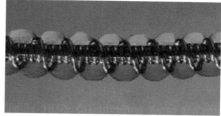

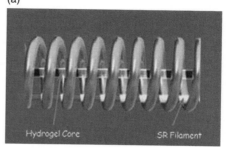

(a)

Hydrogel Core   SR Filament

(b)

Fig. 11.12. Pre- and post-expansion states of the HydroSoft coil. Reprinted with permission from: Suri MF, Memon ZM, Qureshi AI. *Journal of Vascular and Interventional Neurology* 2008;1(2):42–45.

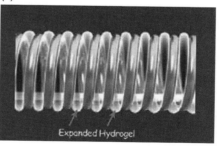

Expanded Hydrogel

lumen of the coil coupler and is attached to the distal end of the Delivery Pusher.[137]

Recently, a new design of hydrogel-coated coils has become available. The HydroSoft coil (Fig. 11.12) is constructed as a platinum coil with an inner core of hydrogel and a stretch-resistant filament. The outer diameter of the platinum coil is 0.012 inches. When exposed to blood, the hydrogel swells to its maximal diameter of 0.013 inches in approximately 20 minutes. The idea behind the HydroSoft coils was to improve upon the limitations of the HydroCoil by being relatively less stiff.

Fig. 11.13 shows some cases of embolization with hydrogel-coated coils.

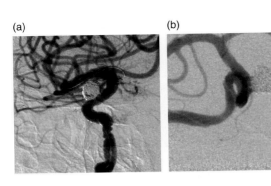

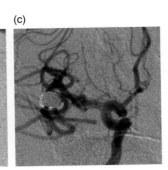

Fig. 11.13. Post-procedure angiography in three cases of coil-embolization with hydrogel-coated platinum coils. Patient characteristics and procedure results are summarized in the table bellow. Reprinted with permission from: Suri MF, Memon ZM, Qureshi AI. *Journal of Vascular and Interventional Neurology* 2008;1(2):42–45.

Trufill DCS Orbit detachable coils

The Trufill DCS and Trufill DCS Orbit detachable coils are each an embolic coil system that consists of a platinum detachable coil, a delivery system (delivery tube and coil introducer), and a syringe. Each system has been designed to deliver, position and detach embolic coils in order to embolize intracranial aneurysms. The detachment mechanism is hydraulic. The coils are available as Helical Fill (2 mm–12 mm in diameter, 2 cm–30 cm in length), Complex Standard (6 mm–20 mm in diameter, 15 cm–30 cm in length), and Complex Mini (2 mm–12 mm in diameter, 1.5 cm – 30 cm in length). The Trufill DCS system consists of a 0.012-inch bare platinum coil with a 0.018-inch detachment zone. The detachment zone is a polymer gripper, which is mounted to the coil delivery system.[138] The delivery system is a metallic hypotube with a hub at the proximal end. The hub is attached to a saline-filled syringe, and under hydraulic pressure the gripper releases the coil. The coils are placed through a 2.1F outer diameter (OD) microcatheter (Prowler Plus, Cordis Neurovascular).

The Trufill DCS Orbit represents the second generation of the Trufill DCS system. Although no changes to the coil were made, the profile of the detachment zone has been reduced to 0.014 inches, which allows coil placement through a smaller microcatheter (1.8F OD; Prowler 14, Cordis Neurovascular). Orbit coils are the evolution of the Trufill Detachable Coil System (Cordis) with a reduced detachment system profile to allow compatibility with 0.014-inch microcatheters. Orbit complex coils are shaped in a complex 3-D configuration and have a wire thickness of 0.012 inches. The complex shape has been developed to increase packing attenuation in the same way that the GDC 360° does. According to the company, the complex shape assures "random coil loops and breaks that seek out the true periphery of the aneurysm." Available size range is 2–20 mm.

Comparison between bioactive or coated coils and bare platinum coils

White and Raymond[139] performed a systematic review of the literature from 2002 to 2007 to identify the literature on bioactive coils including hydrogel-coated coil (HydroCoil), polyglycolic acid (PGA) coated coils (Cerecyte), polyglycolactic acid (PGLA) coated coils (Matrix and Nexus), and fibered coil (Sapphire coils). Of the studies identified, 15 were on Matrix (PGLA-coated coils from Boston Scientific, Natick, Mass), 11 were on hydrogel-coated coils (HydroCoil embolic system; MicroVention, Aliso Viejo, CA), one was on both hydrogel and Matrix, two were on Sapphire fibered coils (ev3, Irvine, CA), and three were on Cerecyte (PGA-coated coils; Micrus, Sunnyvale, CA). The morbidity/mortality rates in these studies ranged from 2.9% to 5.4%, but none of the differences were statistically significant by the prespecified definition for the systematic review. There was no significant difference in the proportion of aneurysms incompletely obliterated on angiographic control between hydrogel-coated coils (17%) and PGA-coated coils (10%). There was a significant difference in incomplete obliteration rates between hydrogel (17%) and PGLA (25%) ($P = 0.001$) and also between PGA-coated (10%) and PGLA-coated coils (25%). There was a significant difference between retreatment rates in hydrogel-coated (5%) and PGLA-coated coils (13%) but not between hydrogel-coated (5%) and PGA-coated coils (2%); the significance of the difference between PGA- and PGLA-coated coils was borderline.

Two large randomized trials have compared the outcomes between bioactive coils and bare platinum coils. The HELPS trial[140] randomized 499 patients with either ruptured (55%) or unruptured (45%) aneurysm to either hydrogel coated ($n = 249$) or bare platinum ($n = 250$) coils. The procedure-related morbidity was similar between the two groups (8% vs. 9%). The rate of thrombo-embolic complications (6% vs. 10%) and aneurysmal rupture (3% vs. 3%) was similar between those treated with hydrogel-coated and bare platinum coils. The rate of major remnant/recurrence was higher among those treated with bare platinum compared with those treated with hydrogel-coated coils (37% vs. 27%) over a mean follow-up period of 17 months.

The Cerecyte trial[141] randomized 500 patients with aneurysms ranging in size between 2 mm and 18 mm to either Cerocyte or bare platinum coils. The randomized patients include those treated for ruptured (47%) and unruptured aneurysms (53%). The aneurysms were located in the anterior (84%) or posterior (16%) circulation. The procedure-related morbidity and mortality in the overall study have been 7% and 1%, respectively. Thromboembolic complications and aneurysm rupture have been reported in 3% and 4% of the treated patients, respectively. The comparative results between the two treatment groups have not been reported.

A comparison was performed between 401 patients treated in the CLARITY trial with bare platinum coils and 377 patients treated in the Matrix study with Matrix coils in multiple centers in France.[142] Embolization failure occurred with 2% and 4% of patients treated with bare platinum and Matrix coils, respectively. Thrombo-embolic events occurred in 14% and 13% of patients treated with bare platinum and Matrix coils, respectively. Intra-procedural rupture occurred in 4% and 4% in each of the patient groups.

An analysis compared the combined procedural and clinical outcomes observed in the HELPS and Cerecyte trial (n = 490) with 837 matched patients in the ISAT trial.[143] The analysis compared the outcomes with bioactive coils with bare platinum coils (used in ISAT) for patients with ruptured intracranial aneurysms. The proportion of patients with aneurysms sized ≥10 mm was higher in the bioactive coil treated patients (15% vs. 7%). The proportion of patients with mRS 0–2 was higher among patients treated with bioactive coils compared with those treated with bare platinum coils (87% vs. 79%) with a similar death rate (5% vs. 4%). The rate of retreatment within 1 year in the ISAT was higher than retreatment within 18 months in the HELPS and Cerecyte trials (13% vs. 4%).

Intravascular stents

The Neuroform 2 microdelivery stent system

The system consists of several components: the 3F Microdelivery Catheter used to deliver the Stent to the treatment site; the 2F Stabilizer Catheter used within the 3F Microdelivery Catheter to hold the Stent stationary and enable deployment; the Peelable Sheath used to facilitate guidewire backloading into the 3F Microdelivery Catheter and through the preloaded Stent. The neuroform stent has a tubular mesh with 4, 6, or 8 distinct sections along its length, depending on the overall length of the stent. Sections are joined by interconnecting struts. The stent has four radiopaque markerbands at each end. The Microdelivery catheter is a single lumen, over-the-wire microcatheter with three distinct stiffness regions: proximal, middle, and distal. The proximal end has a strain relief and a standard female luer fitting. The Microdelivery catheter is hydrophilically coated and is provided sterile with the stent and peelable sheath preloaded. The shaft has an overall length of 135 cm. The stabilizer catheter contains a proximal hub, polymer tubing, and a radiopaque marker band at the distal tip. It is also provided sterile and has an overall length of 161.5 cm. The stent is available in five diameters (2.5, 3.0, 3.5, 4.0, and 4.5 mm) and four lengths (10, 15, 20, and 30 mm) in order to allow a minimum of 4 mm on each side of the aneurysm neck along the parent vessel. The Neuroform 2 Microdelivery Stent System is an upgrade of the original Neuroform Microdelivery Stent System and is used to reduce the likelihood of rupture. The following design elements have been changed.

- The 3F Microdelivery catheter has been replaced with the licensed Renegade catheter
- Manufacturing improvements were made to the stabilizer catheter
- Chamfering (rounding) of the marker bands

A European clinical study was conducted to evaluate the safety and effectiveness of the Neuroform 2 microdelivery stent system in patients with wide neck (ruptured or unruptured), saccular, intracranial aneurysms or aneurysms on the level of the skull base. Thirty-nine stents were implanted in 29 patients (30 aneurysms) that met the inclusion criteria. Twenty patients had one stent implanted, eight patients had two stents, and one patient had three stents. The stents implanted ranged from 3.5 mm to 4.5 mm. One patient required a secondary endovascular procedure to place a second stent in the correct location because the original stent was inadvertently not deployed at the aneurysm site; this counts for two of the stents. One patient had the original stent successfully deployed but the stent was dislodged during the embolic coil placement procedure when the clinical study investigator attempted to snare the errant coil loop and dislodged the stent. A replacement stent was implanted in its place, and this counts for two of the stents. For seven patients, multiple stents were used to treat one aneurysm in cases where (1) the endovascular procedure left the tail of an embolic coil in the vessel or (2) the neck of aneurysm was estimated at an incorrect width and a second or third stent was necessary to cover the neck of the aneurysm. Stents implanted ranged in diameter from 3.5 mm to 4.5 mm. Previous attempts had been made to treat 17 of the 30 aneurysms using other devices. With regard to patient accounting, 31 patients were originally entered into the study; however, two did not receive the stent. Of the 29 patients implanted with the stent, 22 patients exhibited adverse events, all of which occurred prior to or by the time of discharge, including one death immediately post-procedure. There were 12 serious adverse events and 21 other adverse events. No adverse events occurred between discharge and the 6-month follow-up. There was no stent stenosis or migration. There were no embolic coil migrations, parent vessel thrombosis, occlusions, or dissections. All patients exhibited angiographic aneurysm occlusion of 95%–99% both at discharge and the 6-month follow-up. A 100% occlusion was observed in 59% and 69% of the treated patients at discharge and at 6 months, respectively. Additional long-term follow-up data (20–27 months) was provided for 14 patients and did not indicate any device- or procedure-related adverse events.

A survey of physicians at six US centres was also conducted to determine post-market experience with the Neuroform microdelivery stent system. Information provided included the clinical outcomes through discharge for aneurysm neck size, dome size, and occlusion success rate of the 30 aneurysms studied above and 137 others from the post-market data collection. Occlusion success rate (at immediate post-procedure) was 86% for all aneurysms.[144]

A retrospective study of 42 patients with wide-necked cerebral aneurysms treated with the Neuroform stent with coil placement was performed. Clinical and angiographic follow-up was available in 38 patients (90.5%). The overall follow-up time ranged from 6 months to 5 years (mean, 42 months). Successful deployment of 41 stents (97%) was obtained. Permanent procedural morbidity was observed in only one patient (2.4%). Long-term complete aneurysmal occlusion was obtained in 27 patients (71%). Aneurysmal regrowth was observed in four patients (9.5%) on the first control angiogram. After the first control angiogram, no delayed recanalization or regrowth was observed. During the follow-up period, there were no hemorrhagic events, no delayed thrombosis, and no stent displacement.[145]

Another study reported upon 64 patients with 74 aneurysms treated with 86 Neuroform stents. Of 64 patients, 16 (25%) were treated in the context of SAH (eight acute, seven subacute, one remote). Indications for stent use included broad aneurysm neck diameter ($n = 51$ stents; average neck diameter, 5.1 mm; aneurysm size, 8.2 mm), fusiform/dissecting morphology ($n = 17$), salvage/bailout for coils prolapsed into the parent vessel ($n = 7$), and giant aneurysm ($n = 11$). Sixty-one aneurysms underwent stent and coil placement with complete or near complete (>95%) occlusion in 28 patients (45.9%) and partial occlusion (<95%) in 33 patients (54%). Follow-up angiographic ($n = 43$) or magnetic resonance angiographic ($n = 5$) data (average follow-up, 4.6 mo) for 48 aneurysms (46 patients) after stent-supported coil embolization demonstrated progressive thrombosis in 25 patients (52%), recanalization in 11 patients (23%) (eight of whom were retreated), and no change in 12 patients (25%). Follow-up angiography in 5 additional patients with dissecting aneurysms treated with stents alone demonstrated interval vascular remodeling with decreased aneurysm size in all patients. Delayed, severe, in-stent stenosis was observed in three patients, one of whom was symptomatic and required angioplasty and subsequently superficial temporal artery-to-middle cerebral artery bypass surgery. Using the second-generation Neuroform2 delivery system (n = 53), very few technical problems with stent delivery and deployment have been encountered ($n = 2$).[146]

Another report provided data on 56 patients with wide-necked intracranial aneurysms suitable for stent-assisted coil placement. A total of 49 aneurysms in 48 patients were treated with this procedure. In eight cases, stent deployment failed. Forty-one of the aneurysms were initially treated stent, followed by coil placement. Six aneurysms were with stent only, and one aneurysm was initially embolized, followed by stent placement. There were five deaths (8.9%), one of which occurred secondary to a stroke after the procedure (1.8%). Four patients (7%) experienced thromboembolic events, three of which were considered to have been secondary to the procedure (5.3%). In addition, there were two femoral pseudoaneurysms. The overall complication rate was 10.7%.[147]

The Cordis Enterprise™ vascular reconstruction device and delivery system

The Cordis Enterprise™ vascular reconstruction device and delivery system is a self-expanding, neurovascular stent and delivery system consisting of Vascular Reconstruction Device (VRD/stent) and delivery system. The stent has a tubular mesh structure laser cut from Nitinol. The ends of the stent are flared and feature four radiopaque tantalum markers at each end. The stent-marker assembly is covered with an insulating polymer. The stent is available in one diameter (4.5 mm) and four lengths (14 mm, 22 mm, 28 mm, and 37 mm). The delivery system is composed of an introducer and delivery wire. The introducer consists of a polymer tube with a distal tapered end. It protects the stent and distal segment of the delivery wire from damage and creates an uninterrupted passage for the stent to be transferred to the microcatheter. The delivery wire is a ground nitinol corewire that tapers down from the proximal to distal end, providing different stiffness zones. The distal section of the delivery wire has three radiopaque markers with gaps between them, which serve different purposes. The delivery wire facilitates navigation into the distal neurovasculature. The delivery system is provided sterile with the stent pre-loaded in the introducer.

Twenty-seven of 28 subjects entered into the initial study received the Cordis Enterprise™ vascular reconstruction device (VRD/stent) and were followed for 6 months. One subject died post-operatively. Two subjects received two stents. Successful stent placement with satisfactory coil mass position immediately post-procedure was 100%. Successful stent placement was defined as stable stent placement with complete coverage across the aneurysm neck and parent artery patency, while satisfactory coil mass position was defined as the stent maintaining coil position within the sac with preservation of parent artery patency. Maintenance of coil mass position was 96% at 6 months. Fifty-seven adverse events that were considered to be at least possibly procedure or device related occurred in 20 subjects. The majority (68.4%) of these events occurred by 30 days. Serious adverse events occurred in seven of 28 patients and included intracerebral hemorrhage ($n = 2$, one fatal), aneurysm recanalization ($n = 2$), transient ischlmic attack ($n = 2$), ischemic stroke ($n = 1$), cranial nerve deficit ($n = 2$), and groin hematoma ($n = 1$).[148]

A prospective clinical study reported upon 31 saccular, wide-necked intracranial aneurysms in 30 patients treated with the Enterprise stent. Stent deployment was successful in all procedures. Additional coil embolization was performed in all aneurysms. Initial complete angiographic occlusion was achieved in six aneurysms, a neck remnant was left in 18 aneurysms and there were seven residual aneurysms. Angiographic follow-up examinations of 30 lesions after 6 months demonstrated 15 complete occlusions, eight neck remnants and seven residual aneurysms. One patient refused the 6-month angiographic follow-up. Spontaneous occlusion of the aneurysm had occurred in 14 patients, and six aneurysms showed recanalization. Four of these residual aneurysms were retreated. At the 6-month follow-up, 29 parent arteries were unaffected, whereas two parent vessels demonstrated minor asymptomatic narrowing at the stent site. Two patients experienced one or more possible or probable device-related serious adverse events during the 6-month follow-up period. There was no procedural morbidity or mortality at 6 months after the procedure.[149]

A collaborative registry across ten institutions reported initial experience in using the Enterprise in real-world practice. A total of 141 patients (119 women) with 142 aneurysms underwent 143 attempted stent deployments. The use of Enterprise assistance with coil placement was associated with a 76% rate of ≥90% occlusion. An inability to navigate or deploy the stent was experienced in 3% of cases, as well as a 2% occurrence of inaccurate deployment. Procedural data demonstrated a 6% temporary morbidity, 2.8% permanent morbidity, and 2% mortality (0.8% unruptured, 12% ruptured). The overall morbidity and mortality rates were low; however, caution should be exercised when considering Enterprise deployment in patients with SAH as the authors' experience demonstrated a high rate of associated hemorrhagic complications leading to death.[150]

Solitaire™ AB neurovascular remodeling device

The Solitaire AB system is a new, fully retrievable, self-expanding neurovascular stent, which has a high radial force and delivered through a standard 0.021″ or 0.027″ micro catheter on a 0.016″ pushwire.[151] The ev3 Rebar microcatheter is recommended for the delivery of the Solitaire™AB stent. Distal and proximal markers ensure that the exact position of Solitaire AB is always known. Solitaire AB has a radial force that allows for flexibility and optimal coil mass support due to closed cell design and high cell deformation resistance and is combined with coil or Onyx embolization for the treatment of wide-necked aneurysms. The stent is available in 4 mm and 6 mm diameters and in lengths of 26, 31, and 41mm. The Solitaire closed cell design provides optimum scaffolding to prevent coil herniation into the parent artery.

Fifteen patients with 18 wide-necked intracranial aneurysms were treated using the SOLO stent system and detachable platinum coils. Eleven aneurysms were small, six were large, and one was giant. Only one of these aneurysms was in the acute stage of SAH; balloon remodeling alone failed to keep the coils in the aneurysm sac. Only one stent required retrieving and repositioning after it had been fully deployed, and retrieval was easy and successful. No thromboembolic complication, dissection/rupture, or vasospasm occured during stent placement. Follow-up angiograms obtained at 6 months post-treatment in the 18 aneurysms demonstrated that all stents were patent with no evidence of intimal hyperplasia or stenosis. In all cases but one, 100% aneurysm occlusion was observed at the 6-month angiographic examination. Only one aneurysm had recanalized.[152]

Low porosity stents for sole or combined treatment

Low porosity stents have been introduced for placement across the entry point of the aneurysm to reduce inflow and promote thrombosis within the aneurysm. The SILK system (Balk Extrusion) is a stent with high density 48 wire braiding that promotes hemodynamic changes within the aneurysm. The sliding cells of braided wire technology ensure high opposition and conformability. There are four radio-opaque longitudinal markers for visibility and positioning. A registry collected data from 18 centers using the SILK flow diverter.[153] A total of 55 aneurysms were treated with SILK alone and 15 were treated with a combination of coils and SILK. Poor deployment was reported in 14 (20%) of the procedures. Clinical worsening was observed in seven of the 68 patients at 30 days after the procedure. There were three new neurological deficits and two transient symptoms after aneurysm thrombosis. Follow-up imaging demonstrated in 38 patients demonstrated initial complete occlusion in seven (18%) and delayed complete occlusion in 19 (50%) of the treated aneurysms. There were seven arterial occlusions and two in-stent stenoses.

Another flow director that is introduced is Pipeline which is a self-expanding stent made of chromo-cobalt alloy with a 48 wire braided design that can be introduced through a 2.7F microcatheter. A total of 84 patients with 110 aneurysms located in proximity to internal carotid artery bifurcation or vertebrobasilar junction were treated.[154] Embolization using coils was performed either previously ($n = 15$) or during the procedure ($n = 6$). The reconstruction was adequate at 3 months in 58%, 93% at 6 months, and 96% at 12 months. In another study, 19 aneurysms in 18 patients were treated.[155] The device was used alone in ten patients and with additional coils in nine patients. Immediate complete occlusion was seen in four patients. One patient died from rupture of a coexisting aneurysm. Complete aneurysm occlusion was seen in 17 of 18 aneurysms with angiographic follow-up. There was no difference in occlusion rates among aneurysms treated with Pipeline alone or in combination with coils. A total of 27 side branches were covered. One immediate and two late ophthalmic artery occlusions occurred.

Comparison between plain coil-embolization and remodeling techniques for intracranial aneurysms

An analysis from the ATENA study compared outcomes between 325 patients who were treated with coils alone and 222 patients were treated with the remodeling technique (stent or balloon assisted).[70] The overall rate of adverse events related to the treatment was 10.8% (35 of 325) for treatment with coils alone and 11.7% (26 of 222) for the remodeling technique. Thromboembolic events, intra-procedural rupture, and device-related problems were encountered in 6%, 2%, and 3% of 325 patients treated with coils and in 5%, 3%, and 3% of 222 patients in the remodeling technique group, respectively. The morbidity and mortality rates were not different: 2% and 0.9% in the coil alone group and 2% and 1% in the remodeling technique group, respectively.

Onyx liquid embolic agent

Onyx is a non-adhesive liquid embolic agent comprising EVOH (ethylene vinyl alcohol) copolymer dissolved in DMSO (dimethyl sulfoxide), and suspended micronized tantalum powder to provide contrast for visualization under fluoroscopy. The Onyx Liquid Embolic System (LESTM) consists of a 1.5 ml vial of Onyx, a 1.5 ml vial of DMSO, and three 1 ml Onyx delivery syringes. A DMSO compatible delivery micro catheter that is indicated for use in the neuro vasculature (e.g. MarathonTM, RebarTM or UltraFlowTM HPC catheters) is used to access the embolization site. Onyx is available in two product formulations, Onyx 18 (6% EVOH) and Onyx 34 (8% EVOH). Onyx 18 will travel more distally and penetrate deeper into the nidus due to its lower viscosity compared to Onyx 34. Final solidification occurs within 5 minutes for both product formulations.

Onyx is delivered by slow controlled injection through a micro catheter into the aneurysm under fluoroscopic control. The DMSO solvent dissipates into the blood, causing the EVOH copolymer and suspended tantalum to precipitate in situ into a spongy, coherent embolus. Onyx immediately forms a skin as the polymeric embolus solidifies from the outside to the inside, while traveling more distally in the lesion.

Summary

Endovascular treatment was initially introduced in the treatment of SAH for patients who are poor candidates for surgical treatment. Since then, a crescent body of literature and the results of ISAT support endovascular treatment as a valid alternative for patients with intracranial aneurysms who are candidates for both surgical or endovascular treatment (see Table 11.3). However, the definition of these patients is somewhat arbitrary and depends upon individual concepts and expertise. Endovascular treatment for unruptured intracranial aneurysms is based on observational studies with treatment choices determined by individual concepts and expertise in local institutions. A better understanding of the long-term risk of rupture and peri-procedural results and complications associated with available procedures is helping determine whether any therapeutic intervention is warranted in the case of unruptured intracranial aneurysms. The research priorities include a comparison between treatments for unruptured intracranial aneurysms that can be treated by either surgical or endovascular treatment and a comparison between effectiveness of treatments for ruptured intracranial aneurysms in patient populations not included in ISAT using randomized clinical trials and prospective multicenter registry with independent outcome ascertainment. As physicians, we should use the available data to guide our decisions in a case by case basis, keeping in perspective that selection of appropriate patients for each therapeutic method can improve the overall results.

References

1. Abruzzo T, Shengelaia GG, Dawson RC3rd, et al. Histologic and morphologic comparison of experimental aneurysms with human intracranial aneurysms. Am J Neuroradiol 1998;**19**:1309–14.

2. Ferguson GG. Physical factors in the initiation, growth, and rupture of human intracranial saccular aneurysms. J Neurosurg 1972;**37**:666–77.

3. Sekhar LN, Heros RC. Origin, growth, and rupture of saccular aneurysms: a review. Neurosurgery 1981;**8**:248–60.

4. Wiebers DO, Torner JC, Meissner I. Impact of unruptured intracranial aneurysms on public health in the United States. Stroke 1992;**23**:1416–19.

5. Rinkel GJ, Djibuti M, Algra A, van Gijn J. Prevalence and risk of rupture of intracranial aneurysms: a systematic review. Stroke 1998;**29**:251–6.

6. Linn FH, Rinkel GJ, Algra A, van Gijn J. Incidence of subarachnoid hemorrhage: role of region, year, and rate of computed tomography: a meta-analysis. Stroke 1996;**27**:625–9.

7. Qureshi AI, Suri MF, Nasar A, et al. Trends in hospitalization and mortality for subarachnoid hemorrhage and unruptured aneurysms in the United States. Neuro surgery 2005;**57**:1–8.

8. International Study of Unruptured Intracranial Aneurysms Investigators. Unruptured intracranial aneurysms – risk of rupture and risks of surgical intervention. N Engl J Med 1998;**339**:1725–33.

9. Wiebers DO, Whisnant JP, Huston J 3rd, et al. Unruptured intracranial aneurysms: natural history, clinical outcome, and risks of surgical and endovascular treatment. Stroke 2003;**362**:103–10.

10. Juvela S, Porras M, Poussa K. Natural history of unruptured intracranial aneurysms: probability and risk factors for aneurysm rupture. Neurosurg Focus 2000;**8**:Preview 1.

11. Jane JA, Kassell NF, Torner JC, Winn HR. The natural history of aneurysms and arteriovenous malformations. J Neurosurg 1985;**62**:321–3.

12. Louw DF, Asfora WT, Sutherland GR. A brief history of aneurysm clips. Neurosurg Focus 2001;**11**:E4.

13. Cohen-Gadol AA, Spencer DD. Harvey W. Cushing and cerebrovascular surgery: Part I, Aneurysms 2004;**101**:547–52.

14. Qureshi AI. Endovascular treatment of cerebrovascular diseases and intracranial neoplasms. Lancet 2004;**363**:804–13.

15. Guglielmi G, Vinuela F, Sepetka I, Macellari V. Electrothrombosis of saccular aneurysms via endovascular approach. Part 1: Electrochemical basis, technique, and experimental results. J Neurosurg 1991;**75**:1–7.

16. Stiver SI, Porter PJ, Willinsky RA, Wallace MC. Acute human histopathology of an intracranial aneurysm treated using Guglielmi detachable coils: case report and review of the literature. Neurosurgery 1998;**43**:1203–8.

17. Macdonald RL, Mojtahedi S, Johns L, Kowalczuk A. Randomized comparison of Guglielmi detachable coils and

cellulose acetate polymer for treatment of aneurysms in dogs. *Stroke* 1998;**29**:478–85; discussion 485–6.

18. Johnston SC, Higashida RT, Barrow DL, *et al.* Recommendations for the endovascular treatment of intracranial aneurysms: a statement for healthcare professionals from the Committee on Cerebrovascular Imaging of the American Heart Association Council on Cardiovasc Radiol *Stroke* 2002;**33**:2536–44.

19. Humphrey JD Canham, PB. Structure, mechanical properties, and mechanics of intracranial saccular aneurysms. *J Elast* 2000;**61**:49–81.

20. Brisman JL, Song JK, Newell DW. Cerebral aneurysms. *N Engl J Med* 2006;**355**:928–39.

21. Lieber BB, Gounis MJ. The physics of endoluminal stenting in the treatment of cerebrovascular aneurysms. *Neurol Res* 2002;**24**:S33–42.

22. Shojima M, Oshima M, Takagi K, *et al.* Role of the bloodstream impacting force and the local pressure elevation in the rupture of cerebral aneurysms. *Stroke* 2005;**36**:1933–8.

23. Malek AM, Alper SL, Izumo S. Hemodynamic shear stress and its role in atherosclerosis. *J Am Med Assoc* 1999;**282**:2035–42.

24. Ku DN, Giddens DP, Zarins CK, Glagov S. Pulsatile flow and atherosclerosis in the human carotid bifurcation. Positive correlation between plaque location and low oscillating shear stress. *Arteriosclerosis* 1985;**5**:293–302.

25. Ishida F, Ogawa H, Simizu T, Kojima T, Taki W. Visualizing the dynamics of cerebral aneurysms with four-dimensional computed tomographic angiography. *Neurosurgery* 2005;**57**:460–71; discussion 460–71.

26. Ferguson GG. Turbulence in human intracranial saccular aneurysms. *J Neurosurg* 1970; **33**:485–97.

27. Steiger HJ, Poll A, Liepsch D, Reulen HJ. Basic flow structure in saccular aneurysms: a flow visualization study. *Heart Vessels* 1987;**3**:55–65.

28. Steiger HJ, Liepsch DW, Poll A, Reulen HJ. Hemodynamic stress in terminal saccular aneurysms: a laser-Doppler study. *Heart Vessels* 1988;**4**:162–9.

29. Kerber CW, Imbesi SG, Knox K. Flow dynamics in a lethal anterior communicating artery aneurysm. *Am J Neuroradiol* 1999;**20**:2000–3.

30. Imbesi SG, Kerber CW. Analysis of slipstream flow in two ruptured intracranial cerebral aneurysms. *Am J Neuroradiol* 1999;**20**:1703–5.

31. Knox K, Kerber CW, Singel SA, Bailey MJ, Imbesi SG. Stereolithographic vascular replicas from CT scans: choosing treatment strategies, teaching, and research from live patient scan data. *Am J Neuroradiol* 2005;**26**:1428–31.

32. Wetzel SG, Ohta M, Handa A, *et al.* From patient to model: stereolithographic modeling of the cerebral vasculature based on rotational angiography. *Am J Neuroradiol* 2005;**26**:1425–7.

33. Imbesi SG, Kerber CW. Analysis of slipstream flow in a wide-necked basilar artery aneurysm: evaluation of potential treatment regimens. *Am J Neuroradiol.* 2001;**22**:721–4.

34. Shojima M, Oshima M, Takagi K, *et al.* Magnitude and role of wall shear stress on cerebral aneurysm: computational fluid dynamic study of 20 middle cerebral artery aneurysms. *Stroke* 2004;**35**:2500–5.

35. Cebral JR, Castro MA, Burgess JE, *et al.* Characterization of cerebral aneurysms for assessing risk of rupture by using patient-specific computational hemodynamics models. *Am J Neuroradiol* 2005;**26**:2550–9.

36. Hassan T, Timofeev EV, Saito T, *et al.* A proposed parent vessel geometry-based categorization of saccular intracranial aneurysms: computational flow dynamics analysis of the risk factors for lesion rupture. *J Neurosurg* 2005;**103**:662–80.

37. Burleson AC, Strother CM, Turitto VT. Computer modeling of intracranial saccular and lateral aneurysms for the study of their hemodynamics. *Neurosurgery* 1995;**37**:774–82; discussion 782–4.

38. Steinman DA, Milner JS, Norley CJ, Lownie SP, Holdsworth DW. Image-based computational simulation of flow dynamics in a giant intracranial aneurysm. *Am J Neuroradiol* 2003;**24**:559–66.

39. Venugopal P, Valentino D, Schmitt H, et al. Sensitivity of patient-specific numerical simulation of cerebal aneurysm hemodynamics to inflow boundary conditions. *J Neurosurg* 2007;**106**:1051–60.

40. Castro MA, Putman CM, Cebral JR. Patient-specific computational fluid dynamics modeling of anterior communicating artery aneurysms: a study of the sensitivity of intra-aneurysmal flow patterns to flow conditions in the carotid arteries. *Am J Neuroradiol* 2006;**27**:2061–8.

41. Cebral JR, Castro MA, Appanaboyina S, *et al.* Efficient pipeline for image-based patient-specific analysis of cerebral aneurysm hemodynamics: technique and sensitivity. *IEEE Trans Med Imaging.* 2005;**24**:457–67.

42. Castro MA, Putman CM, Cebral JR. Computational fluid dynamics modeling of intracranial aneurysms: effects of parent artery segmentation on intra-aneurysmal hemodynamics. *Am J Neuroradiol* 2006;**27**:1703–9.

43. Rayz VL, Boussel L, Acevedo-Bolton G, *et al.* Numerical simulations of flow in cerebral aneurysms: comparison of CFD results and in vivo MRI measurements. *J Biomech Eng.* 2008;**130**:**051011**.

44. Ford MD, Nikolov HN, Milner JS, *et al.* PIV-measured versus CFD-predicted flow dynamics in anatomically realistic cerebral aneurysm models. *J Biomech Eng* 2008;**130**:**021015**.

45. Boussel L, Rayz V, McCulloch C, *et al.* Aneurysm growth occurs at region of low wall shear stress: patient-specific correlation of hemodynamics and growth in a longitudinal study. *Stroke* 2008;**39**:2997–3002.

46. Meng H, Wang Z, Kim M, Ecker RD, Hopkins LN. Saccular aneurysms on straight and curved vessels are subject to different hemodynamics: implications of intravascular stenting. *Am J Neuroradiol* 2006;**27**:1861–5.

47. Imbesi SG, Kerber CW. Analysis of slipstream flow in a wide-necked basilar artery aneurysm: evaluation of potential treatment regimens. *Am J Neuroradiol* 2001;**22**:721–4.

48. Cebral JR, Lohner R. Efficient simulation of blood flow past complex endovascular devices using an adaptive embedding technique. *IEE Trans Med Imaging* 2005;**24**:468–76.

49. Stuhne GR, Steinman DA. Finite-element modeling of the hemodynamics of stented aneurysms. *J Biomech Eng* 2004;**126**:382–7.

50. Jou LD, Quick CM, Young WL, *et al.* Computational approach to quantifying hemodynamic forces in giant cerebral aneurysms. *Am J Neuroradiol* 2003;**24**:1804–10.

51. Ma B, Harbaugh RE, Raghavan ML. Three-dimensional geometrical characterization of cerebral aneurysms. *Am Biomed Eng* 2004;**32**:264–73.

52. Raghavan ML, Ma B, Harbaugh RE. Quantified aneurysm shape and rupture risk *J Neurosurg* 2005;**102**:355–62.

53. Ujiie H, Tamano Y, Sasaki K, Hori T. Is the aspect ratio a reliable index for predicting the rupture of a saccular aneurysm? *Neurosurgery* 2001;**48**:495–502; discussion 502–3.

54. Ford MD, Lee SW, Lownie SP, Holdsworth DW, Steinman DA. On the effect of parent-aneurysm angle on flow patterns in basilar tip aneurysms: towards a surrogate geometric marker of intra-aneurismal hemodynamics. *J Biomech* 2008;**41**:241–8.

55. Bairstow P, Dodgson A, Linto J, Khangure M. Comparison of cost and outcome of endovascular and neurosurgical procedures in the treatment of ruptured intracranial aneurysms. *Australas Radiol* 2002;**46**:249–51.

56. Gruber A, Ungersbock K, Reinprecht A, *et al.* Evaluation of cerebral vasospasm after early surgical and endovascular treatment of ruptured intracranial aneurysms. *Neurosurgery* 1998;**42**:258–67; discussion 267–8.

57. Gruber DP, Zimmerman GA, Tomsick TA, *et al.* A comparison between endovascular and surgical management of basilar artery apex aneurysms. *J Neurosurg* 1999;**90**:868–74.

58. Hoh BL, Topcuoglu MA, Singhal AB, *et al.* Effect of clipping, craniotomy, or intravascular coiling on cerebral vasospasm and patient outcome after aneurysmal subarachnoid hemorrhage. *Neurosurgery* 2004;**55**:779–86; discussion 786–9.

59. Kahara VJ, Seppanen SK, Kuurne T, Laasonen EM. Patient outcome after endovascular treatment of intracranial aneurysms with reference to microsurgical clipping. *Acta Neurol Scand* 1999;**99**:284–90.

60. Kato Y, Sano H, Dong PT, *et al.* The effect of clipping and coiling in acute severe subarachnoid hemorrhage after international subarachnoid aneurysmal trial (ISAT) results. *Aminim Invasive Neurosurg* 2005;**48**:224–7.

61. Lot G, Houdart E, Cophignon J, Casasco A, George B. Combined management of intracranial aneurysms by surgical and endovascular treatment. Modalities and results from a series of 395 cases. *Acta Neurochir (Wien)* 1999;**141**:557–62.

62. Raftopoulos C, Mathurin P, Boscherini D, *et al.* Prospective analysis of aneurysm treatment in a series of 103 consecutive patients when endovascular embolization is considered the first option. *J Neurosurg* 2000;**93**:175–82.

63. Taha MM, Nakahara I, Higashi T, *et al.* Endovascular embolization vs surgical clipping in treatment of cerebral aneurysms: morbidity and mortality with short-term outcome. *Surg Neurol* 2006;**66**:277–84; discussion 284.

64. Helland CA, Krakenes J, Moen G, Wester K. A population-based study of neurosurgical and endovascular treatment of ruptured, intracranial aneurysms in a small neurosurgical unit. *Neurosurgery* 2006;**59**:1168–75; discussion 1175–6.

65. Kaku Y, Watarai H, Kokuzawa J, Tanaka T, Andoh T. Cerebral aneurysms: conventional microsurgical technique and endovascular method. *Surg Technol Int* 2007;**16**:228–35.

66. Johnston SC, Wilson CB, Halbach VV, *et al.* Endovascular and surgical treatment of unruptured cerebral aneurysms: comparison of risks. *Ann Neurol* 2000;**48**:11–19.

67. Johnston SC, Dudley RA, Gress DR, Ono L. Surgical and endovascular treatment of unruptured cerebral aneurysms at university hospitals. *Neurology* 1999;**52**:1799–805.

68. Johnston SC, Zhao S, Dudley RA, Berman MF, Gress DR. Treatment of unruptured cerebral aneurysms in California. *Stroke* 2001;**32**:597–605.

69. Berman MF, Solomon RA, Mayer SA, Johnston SC, Yung PP. Impact of hospital-related factors on outcome after treatment of cerebral aneurysms. *Stroke* 2003;**34**:2200–7.

70. Pierot L, Spelle L, Vitry F. Immediate clinical outcome of patients harboring unruptured intracranial aneurysms treated by endovascular approach: results of the ATENA study. *Stroke* 2008;**39**:2497–504.

71. Rates of delayed rebleeding from intracranial aneurysms are low after surgical and endovascular treatment. *Stroke* 2006;**37**:1437–42.

72. Koivisto T, Vanninen R, Hurskainen H, *et al.* Outcomes of early endovascular versus surgical treatment of ruptured cerebral aneurysms. A prospective randomized study. *Stroke* 2000;**31**:2369–77.

73. Vanninen R, Koivisto T, Saari T, Hernesniemi J, Vapalahti M. Ruptured intracranial aneurysms: acute endovascular treatment with electrolytically detachable coils–a prospective randomized study. *Radiology* 1999;**211**:325–36.

74. Molyneux A, Kerr R, Stratton I, *et al.* International Subarachnoid Aneurysm Trial (ISAT) of neurosurgical clipping versus endovascular coiling in 2143 patients with ruptured intracranial aneurysms: a randomised trial. *Lancet* 2002;**360**:1267–74.

75. Molyneux AJ, Kerr RS, Yu LM, *et al.* International subarachnoid aneurysm trial (ISAT) of neurosurgical clipping versus endovascular coiling in 2143 patients with ruptured intracranial aneurysms: a randomised comparison of effects on survival, dependency, seizures, rebleeding, subgroups, and aneurysm occlusion. *Lancet* 2005;**366**:809–17.

76. Campi A, Ramzi N, Molyneux AJ, *et al.* Retreatment of ruptured cerebral aneurysms in patients randomized by coiling or clipping in the International Subarachnoid Aneurysm Trial (ISAT). *Stroke* 2007;**38**:1538–44.

77. Molyneux AJ, Kerr RS, Birks J, *et al.* Risk of recurrent subarachnoid haemorrhage, death, or dependence and standardised mortality ratios after clipping or coiling of an intracranial aneurysm in the International Subarachnoid Aneurysm Trial (ISAT): long-term follow-up. *Lancet Neurol* 2009;**8**:427–33.

78. van der Schaaf I, Algra A, Wermer M, *et al.* Endovascular coiling versus neurosurgical clipping for patients with aneurysmal subarachnoid haemorrhage. *Cochrane Database Syst Rev* 2005:CD003085.

79. Javadpour M, Jain H, Wallace MC, *et al.* Analysis of cost related to clinical and angiographic outcomes of aneurysm patients enrolled in the international subarachnoid aneurysm trial in a North

American setting. *Neurosurgery* 2005;**56**:886–94; discussion 886–94.

80. Rasanen P, Roine E, Sintonen H, *et al*. Use of quality-adjusted life years for the estimation of effectiveness of health care: a systematic literature review. *Int J Technol Assen Health Care* 2006;**22**:235–41.

81. Johnston SC, Gress DR, Kahn JG. Which unruptured cerebral aneurysms should be treated? A cost-utility analysis. *Neurology* 1999;**52**:1806–15.

82. Maud A, Lakshminarayan K, Suri MF, *et al*. Cost-effectiveness analysis of endovascular versus neurosurgical treatment for ruptured intracranial aneurysms in the United States. *J Neurosurg* 2009;**110**:880–6.

83. Brilstra EH, Rinkel GJ, van der Graaf Y, *et al*. Quality of life after treatment of unruptured intracranial aneurysms by neurosurgical clipping or by embolisation with coils. A prospective, observational study. *Cerebrovasc Dis* 2004;**17**:44–52.

84. Qureshi AI. Ten years of advances in neuroendovascular procedures. *J Endovasc Ther* 2004;**11** Suppl 2:II1–4.

85. Findlay JM. Current management of aneurysmal subarachnoid hemorrhage guidelines from the Canadian Neurosurgical Society. *Can J Neurol Soc* 1997;**24**:161–70.

86. Bederson JB, Awad IA, Wiebers DO, *et al*. Recommendations for the management of patients with unruptured intracranial aneurysms: A Statement for healthcare professionals from the Stroke Council of the American Heart Association. *Stroke* 2000;**31**:2742–50.

87. Derdeyn CP, Barr JD, Berenstein A, *et al*. The International Subarachnoid Aneurysm Trial (ISAT): a position statement from the Executive Committee of the American Society of Interventional and Therapeutic Neuroradiology and the American Society of Neuroradiology. *Am J Neuroradiol* 2003;**24**:1404–8.

88. Raabe A, Schmiedek P, Seifert V, Stolke D. German Society of Neurosurgery Section on Vascular Neurosurgery: Position Statement on the International Subarachnoid Hemorrhage Trial (ISAT). *Zentraibl Neurochir* 2003;**64**:99–103.

89. National Institutes for Clinical Excellence. Coil embolization of unruptured intracranial aneurysms. Interventional procedure guidance 106. London, UK. NICE. 2003.; Jan 10, 2006; http://www.nice.org.uk/page.aspx?o=240344.

90. Alberts MJ, Latchaw RE, Selman WR, et al. Recommendations for comprehensive stroke centers: a consensus statement from the Brain Attack Coalition. *Stroke* 2005;**36**:1597–616.

91. Bederson JB, Connolly ESJ, Batjer HH, *et al*. Guidelines for the management of aneurysmal subarachnoid hemorrhage: a statement for healthcare professionals from a special writing group of the Stroke Council, American Heart Association. *Stroke* 2009;**40**:994–1025.

92. Qureshi AI, Hopkins LN. Comparison between endovascular and surgical treatment for intracranial aneurysms: challenges for clinical trials. 29th International Stroke Conference; San Diego, CA:February 5–7, 2004.

93. Cross DT, 3rd, Tirschwell DL, Clark MA, *et al*. Mortality rates after subarachnoid hemorrhage: variations according to hospital case volume in 18 states. *J Neurosurg* 2003;**99**:810–17.

94. Fogelholm R, Hernesniemi J, Vapalahti M. Impact of early surgery on outcome after aneurysmal subarachnoid hemorrhage. A population-based study. *Stroke* 1993;**24**:1649–54.

95. Ogungbo B, Gregson BA, Blackburn A, Mendelow AD. Trends over time in the management of subarachnoid haemorrhage in Newcastle: review of 1609 patients. *Br J Neurosurg* 2001;**15**:388–95.

96. Ikawa F, Ohbayashi N, Imada Y, *et al*. Analysis of subarachnoid hemorrhage according to the Japanese Standard Stroke Registry Study – incidence, outcome, and comparison with the International Subarachnoid Aneurysm Trial. *Neurol Med Chir (Tokyo)* 2004;**44**:275–6.

97. Flett LM, Chandler CS, Giddings D, Gholkar A. Aneurysmal subarachnoid hemorrhage: management strategies and clinical outcomes in a regional neuroscience center. *Am J Neuroradiol* 2005;**26**:367–72.

98. Gnanalingham KK, Apostolopoulos V, Barazi S, O'Neill K. The impact of the international subarachnoid aneurysm trial (ISAT) on the management of aneurysmal subarachnoid haemorrhage in a neurosurgical unit in the UK. *Clin Neurol Neurosurg* 2006;**108**:117–23.

99. Lanzino G, Fraser K, Kanaan Y, Wagenbach A. Treatment of ruptured intracranial aneurysms since the International Subarachnoid Aneurysm Trial: practice utilizing clip ligation and coil embolization as individual or complementary therapies. *J Neurosurg* 2006;**104**:344–9.

100. Luo CB, Chang FC, Teng MM, Guo WY, Chang CY. Stent management of coil herniation in embolization of internal carotid aneurysms. *Am J Neuroradiol* 2008;**29**:1951–5.

101. Dinc H, Kuzeyli K, Kosucu P, Sari A, Cekirge S. Retrieval of prolapsed coils during endovascular treatment of cerebral aneurysms. *Neuroradiology* 2006;**48**:269–72.

102. Lavine SD, Larsen DW, Giannotta SL, Teitelbaum GP. Parent vessel Guglielmi detachable coil herniation during wide-necked aneurysm embolization: treatment with intracranial stent placement: two technical case reports. *Neurosurgery* 2000;**46**:1013–17.

103. Qureshi AI, Luft AR, Sharma M, Guterman LR, Hopkins LN. Prevention and treatment of thromboembolic and ischemic complications associated with endovascular procedures: Part I – Pathophysiological and pharmacological features. *Neurosurgery* 2000;**46**:1344–59.

104. Qureshi AI, Saad M, Zaidat OO, *et al*. Intracerebral hemorrhages associated with neurointerventional procedures using a combination of antithrombotic agents including abciximab. *Stroke* 2002;**33**:1916–19.

105. Qureshi AI, Luft AR, Sharma M, Guterman LR, Hopkins LN. Prevention and treatment of thromboembolic and ischemic complications associated with endovascular procedures: Part II– Clinical aspects and recommendations. *Neurosurgery* 2000;**46**:1360–75; discussion 1375–6.

106. Derdeyn CP, Cross DT 3rd, Moran CJ, *et al*. Postprocedure ischemic events after treatment of intracranial aneurysms with Guglielmi detachable coils. *J Neurosurg* 2002;**96**:837–43.

107. Ries T, Siemonsen S, Grzyska U, Zeumer H, Fiehler J. Abciximab is a safe rescue therapy in thromboembolic

events complicating cerebral aneurysm coil embolization: single center experience in 42 cases and review of the literature. *Stroke* 2009;**40**:1750–7.

108. Cronqvist M, Pierot L, Boulin A, *et al.* Local intraarterial fibrinolysis of thromboemboli occurring during endovascular treatment of intracerebral aneurysm: a comparison of anatomic results and clinical outcome. *Am J Neuroradiol* 1998;**19**:157–65.

109. Hähnel S, Schellinger PD, Gutschalk A, *et al.* Local intra-arterial fibrinolysis of thromboemboli occurring during neuroendovascular procedures with recombinant tissue plasminogen activator. *Stroke* 2003;**34**:1723–8.

110. Cloft HJ, Kallmes DF. Cerebral aneurysm perforations complicating therapy with Guglielmi detachable coils: a meta-analysis. *Am J Neuroradiol* 2002;**23**:1706–9.

111. Elijovich L, Higashida RT, Lawton MT, *et al.* Predictors and outcomes of intraprocedural rupture in patients treated for ruptured intracranial aneurysms: the CARAT study. *Stroke* 2008;**39**:1501–6.

112. Qureshi AI, Geocadin RG, Suarez JI, Ulatowski JA. Long-term outcome after medical reversal of transtentorial herniation in patients with supratentorial mass lesions. *Crit Carc Med* 2000;**28**:1556–64.

113. Tummala RP, Chu RM, Madison MT, *et al.* Outcomes after aneurysm rupture during endovascular coil embolization. *Neurosurgery* 2001;**49**:1059–66; discussion 1066–7.

114. Doerfler A, Wanke I, Egelhof T, *et al.* Aneurysmal rupture during embolization with Guglielmi detachable coils: causes, management, and outcome. *Am J Neuroradiol* 2001;**22**:1825–32.

115. Li MH, Gao BL, Fang C, *et al.* Prevention and management of intraprocedural rupture of intracranial aneurysm with detachable coils during embolization. *Neuroradiology* 2006;**48**:907–15.

116. Roy D, Milot G, Raymond J. Endovascular treatment of unruptured aneurysms. *Stroke* 2001;**32**:1998–2004.

117. Raymond J, Guilbert F, Weill A, *et al.* Long-term angiographic recurrences after selective endovascular treatment of aneurysms with detachable coils. *Stroke* 2003;**34**:1398–403.

118. Piotin M, Spelle L, Mounayer C, *et al.* Intracranial aneurysms: treatment with bare platinum coils–aneurysm packing, complex coils, and angiographic recurrence. *Radiology* 2007;**243**:500–8.

119. Tamatani S, Ito Y, Abe H, *et al.* Evaluation of the stability of aneurysms after embolization using detachable coils: correlation between stability of aneurysms and embolized volume of aneurysms. *Am J Neuroradiol* 2002;**23**:762–7.

120. Raja PV, Huang J, Germanwala AV, *et al.* Microsurgical clipping and endovascular coiling of intracranial aneurysms: a critical review of the literature. *Neurosurgery* 2008;**62**:1187–202; discussion 1202–3.

121. Cloft HJ. HydroCoil for Endovascular Aneurysm Occlusion (HEAL) study: periprocedural results. *Am J Neuroradiol* 2006;**27**:289–92.

122. Eskridge JM, Song JK. Endovascular embolization of 150 basilar tip aneurysms with Guglielmi detachable coils: results of the Food and Drug Administration multicenter clinical trial. *J Neurosurg* 1998;**89**:81–6.

123. Gaba RC, Ansari SA, Roy SS, *et al.* Embolization of intracranial aneurysms with hydrogel-coated coils versus inert platinum coils: effects on packing density, coil length and quantity, procedure performance, cost, length of hospital stay, and durability of therapy. *Stroke* 2006;**37**:1443–50.

124. Gallas S, Pasco A, Cottier JP, *et al.* A multicenter study of 705 ruptured intracranial aneurysms treated with Guglielmi detachable coils. *Am J Neuroradiol* 2005;**26**:1723–31.

125. Hirsch JA, Bendok BR, Paulsen RD, *et al.* Midterm clinical experience with a complex-shaped detachable platinum coil system for the treatment of cerebral aneurysms: Trufill DCS Orbit detachable coil system registry interim results. *J Vasc Interv Radiol* 2007;**18**:1487–94.

126. Kang HS, Han MH, Lee TH, *et al.* Embolization of intracranial aneurysms with hydrogel-coated coils: result of a Korean multicenter trial. *Neurosurgery* 2007;**61**:51–8; discussion 58–9.

127. Molyneux AJ, Cekirge S, Saatci I, Gal G. Cerebral Aneurysm Multicenter European Onyx (CAMEO) trial: results of a prospective observational study in 20 European centers. *Am J Neuroradiol* 2004;**25**:39–51.

128. Murayama Y, Vinuela F, Ishii A, *et al.* Initial clinical experience with matrix detachable coils for the treatment of intracranial aneurysms. *J Neurosurg* 2006;**105**:192–9.

129. Pierot L, Bonafe A, Bracard S, Leclerc X. Endovascular treatment of intracranial aneurysms with matrix detachable coils: immediate posttreatment results from a prospective multicenter registry. *Am J Neuroradiol* 2006;**27**:1693–9.

130. Pierot L, Flandroy P, Turjman F, *et al.* Selective endovascular treatment of intracranial aneurysms using micrus microcoils: preliminary results in a series of 78 patients. *J Neuroradiol* 2002;**29**:114–21.

131. Pierot L, Leclerc X, Bonafe A, Bracard S. Endovascular treatment of intracranial aneurysms with matrix detachable coils: midterm anatomic follow-up from a prospective multicenter registry. *Am J Neuroradiol* 2008;**29**:57–61.

132. Raymond J, Roy D, Leblanc P, *et al.* Endovascular treatment of intracranial aneurysms with radioactive coils: initial clinical experience. *Stroke* 2003;**34**:2801–6.

133. Veznedaroglu E, Koebbe CJ, Siddiqui A, Rosenwasser RH. Initial experience with bioactive cerecyte detachable coils: impact on reducing recurrence rates. *Neurosurgery* 2008;**62**:799–805; discussion 805–6.

134. Vinuela F, Duckwiler G, Mawad M. Guglielmi detachable coil embolization of acute intracranial aneurysm: perioperative anatomical and clinical outcome in 403 patients. *J Neurosurg* 1997;**86**:475–82.

135. www.accessdata.fda.gov/cdrh_docs/pdf3/K031168.pdf.

136. http://www.accessdata.fda.gov/cdrh_docs/pdf5/K053160.pdf.

137. http://www.accessdata.fda.gov/cdrh_docs/pdf5/K050954.pdf.

138. Wakhloo AK, Gounis MJ, Sandhu JS, *et al.* Complex-shaped platinum coils for brain aneurysms: higher packing density, improved biomechanical stability, and midterm angiographic outcome. *Am J Neuroradiol* 2007;**28**:1395–400.

139. White PM, Raymond J. Endovascular coiling of cerebral aneurysms using "bioactive" or coated-coil technologies: a systematic review of the literature. 2009;30:219–26.

140. White P. HELPS. Update on clinical trial results. *Interventional Neuroradiol* 2009;15 (suppl 1): 24.

141. Cekirge S. Cerecyte. Update on clinical trial results. *Interventional Neuroradiol* 2009;15 (suppl 1): 24.

142. Cognard C PL RF AR. Clinical results of aneurysm embolization with GDC and Matrix coils in clarity study. *Interventional Neuroradiol* 2009;15 (suppl 1): 86.

143. White PM MAJ MZ LS SM FL. Clinical and procedural outcomes in patients with ruptured cerebral aneurysms in the HELPS & Cerecyte randomized trials: a meta-analysis and comparison with matched dataset from ISAT. *Interventional Neuroradiol* 2009;15 (suppl 1): 48.

144. http://www.accessdata.fda.gov/cdrh_docs/pdf2/H020002b.pdf.

145. Sedat J, Chau Y, Mondot L, *et al.* Endovascular occlusion of intracranial wide-necked aneurysms with stenting (Neuroform) and coiling: mid-term and long-term results. *Neuroradiology* 2009;51:401–409.

146. Fiorella D, Albuquerque FC, Deshmukh VR, McDougall CG. Usefulness of the Neuroform stent for the treatment of cerebral aneurysms: results at initial (3–6-mo) follow-up. *Neurosurgery* 2005;56:1191–201; discussion 1201–2.

147. Benitez RP, Silva MT, Klem J, Veznedaroglu E, Rosenwasser RH. Endovascular occlusion of wide-necked aneurysms with a new intracranial microstent (Neuroform) and detachable coils. *Neurosurgery* 2004;54:1359–67; discussion 1368.

148. http://www.accessdata.fda.gov/cdrh_docs/pdf6/H060001b.pdf.

149. Weber W, Bendszus M, Kis B, *et al.* A new self-expanding nitinol stent (Enterprise) for the treatment of wide-necked intracranial aneurysms: initial clinical and angiographic results in 31 aneurysms. *Neuroradiology* 2007;49:555–61.

150. Mocco J, Snyder KV, Albuquerque FC, *et al.* Treatment of intracranial aneurysms with the Enterprise stent: a multicenter registry. *J Neurosurg* 2009;110:35–9.

151. http://www.ev3.net/assets/006/5638.pdf.

152. Yavuz K, Geyik S, Pamuk AG, *et al.* Immediate and midterm follow-up results of using an electrodetachable, fully retrievable SOLO coil system in the endovascular coil occlusion of wide-necked cerebral aneurysms. *J Neurosurg* 2007;107:49–55.

153. Byrne JBRYJ. The SILK registry: intracranial aneurysm treatment with a new flow diverter. *Interventional Neuroradiol* 2009;15(Suppl 1): 112–13.

154. Lylyk P LJ FA CR SE PB. Intracranial endovascular reconstruction in brain aneurysms with a flow divertor device Pipeline: initial experience and mid-term follow-up. *Interventional Neuroradiol* 2009;15 (Suppl 1:46).

155. Szikora I NP BA BZ MM KZ VZ LW GI. The efficacy of flow modification in the treatment of aneurysms: follow-up results on aneurysms treated by the Pipline Embolization Device. *Interventional Neuroradiol* 2009;15 (Suppl 1:113).

156. Qureshi AI, Janerdhan V, Hanel RA, Lanzino G. Coiling of aneurysms. *Lancet Neurol* 2007;6:616–25.

Chapter 12

Cerebral vasospasm

Adnan I. Qureshi, Mushtaq H. Qureshi, Jefferson T. Miley, Nauman Tariq and Giuseppe Lanzino

Introduction

Cerebral vasospasm is a major cause of delayed morbidity and death in patients with subarachnoid hemorrhage (SAH).[1,2] Angiographic vasospasm can be demonstrated in up to 70%, and neurological deterioration secondary to vasospasm in 30 to 35%[3] of patients with aneurysmal SAH. About half the patients who develop symptomatic vasospasm either die or suffer neurologic disability as a direct result of ischemia. With the widespread adoption of early surgical and endovascular treatment of ruptured aneurysms to prevent rebleeding, delayed ischemia has become the leading cause of death and disability in patients with SAH.[4] The peak incidence of vasospasm is 4 to 14 days after onset of SAH.[5]

A variety of therapies have been used to prevent and treat vasospasm including pharmacological agents and volume expansion to increase cerebral perfusion. Patient outcome has improved with the use of calcium channel antagonists such as nimodipine and hypervolemic, hypertensive therapy. After the institution of a standardized protocol focused on early surgery and intravascular volume expansion at Columbia-Presbyterian Medical Center in 1986, 30-day mortality among Hunt–Hess Grade 1 to 3 patients fell from 35% to 4%.[6] However, up to 16% of all patients who have symptomatic vasospasm continue to deteriorate despite intensive hemo-dynamic management.[7–9] In addition, despite careful hemo-dynamic monitoring, pulmonary edema has been reported in up to 26% of SAH patients treated with hypervolemic therapy.[8,10]

In recent studies, cerebral vasospasm by transcranial Doppler (TCD) criteria is found in 40% to 55% of patients and 23% to 32% of the patients develop ischemic symptoms related to vasospasm.[11–14] In the Clazosentan to Overcome Neurological Ischemia and Infarction Occurring After Subarachnoid Hemorrhage (CONSCIOUS-1) trial,[15] moderate or severe angiographic vasospasm occurred in 66% of the 96 placebo-treated patients and 24% of the placebo-treated patients required rescue therapy with endovascular treatment. In the Balloon Prophylaxis for Aneurysmal Vasospasm (BPAV) Study, 46 (54%) of the 85 patients in the control group developed vasospasm demonstrated by TCD and 22 (26%) of these patients developed ischemic symptoms refractory to medical treatment requiring endovascular treatment.[14]

In recent years, there have been some advances in management and prevention of vasospasm secondary to SAH using endovascular treatment. The purpose of this discussion is to review the use of these new endovascular modalities.

Pathogenesis of vasospasm

Understanding of the pathogenic mechanism underlying vasospasm is necessary to gain insight into various therapeutic modalities for its prevention and treatment. The following section discusses the spasmogenic properties of the blood clot and the role of free radicals and endothelium-dependent factors in the occurrence of cerebral vasospasm.

Spasmogenic effect of blood products

Based on animal and human work,[16,17] it is now recognized that persistence of a large blood clot in the subarachnoid space is responsible for vasospasm. Many investigators have assayed the vasoactivity of incubated and aged mixtures of whole blood and blood components with dog and cat basilar arteries in vitro and found that lysed red blood cells have significant vasoactivity, whereas fresh, intact red blood cells are inert.[18–22] Further studies in vitro revealed that hemoglobin stimulates contraction of smooth muscles and cerebral arteries of several different species.[23–25] In a randomized and controlled study of 40 monkeys, 23 were given multiple intrathecal injections of oxyhemoglobin, methemoglobin, bilirubin, and mock cerebrospinal fluid (CSF) for 6 days. Significant vasospasm of middle cerebral artery developed in animals injected with oxyhemoglobin and hemoglobin. Pure methemoglobin produced no significant arterial narrowing. Furthermore, Ohta *et al.*[26] found that vasospasm correlated with concentrations of oxyhemoglobin in periarterial hematomas after SAH. Thus, based on in vitro and in vivo evidence, oxyhemoglobin is considered to be the principal spasminogen in SAH.

Textbook of Interventional Neurology, ed. Adnan I. Qureshi. Published by Cambridge University Press. © Cambridge University Press 2011.

Role of free radicals in vasospasm:

Recent experiments have revealed that an inflammatory reaction in the perivascular space is capable of producing vasospasm.[27] Inflammation in SAH is thought to be mediated through activation of non-enzymatic lipid peroxidation[28] by blood clot degeneration products. Oxyhemoglobin spontaneously auto-oxidizes to methemoglobin releasing superoxide anion radical.[29,30] In conjunction with the iron in hemoglobin, superoxide anion radical has been postulated to initiate and propagate lipid peroxidation[27–31] in the vascular and cerebral compartments. Elevated levels of metabolites of the lipo-oxygenases pathway have been reported in cisternal CSF in patients with SAH.[32–34] These compounds are capable of inducing vasospasm in human and animal models of SAH.[35,36]

Role of endothelium-dependent factors

Endothelium-dependent relaxation is impaired in cerebral arteries from humans and experimental models of SAH.[37–41] This may be mediated through impairment of the nitric oxide (NO) pathway and an increase in endothelial production. Active binding of hemoglobin to NO may prevent entry of NO into the smooth muscle.[16] Additionally, hemoglobin can destroy NO by generation of superoxide anion. Hemoglobin can induce gene expression leading to the synthesis of endothelin, a potent and long lasting vasoconstrictor peptide produced by endothelium,[42,43] as reflected by elevated endothelin levels in the basilar arteries and CSF after SAH.[44,45] Phosphoramidon, an inhibitor of endothelin converting enzyme, may reduce the magnitude of vasospasm after SAH.[46] The safety and tolerability of the novel endothelin A (ETA) receptor antagonist clazosentan has been evaluated in patients with SAH. In Phase IIa multicenter study,[47] clazosentan reduced the frequency and severity of cerebral vasospasm following severe aneurysmal SAH with an incidence and severity of adverse events comparable to that of placebo. In another randomized, double-blind, placebo-controlled, dose-finding study[15] the efficacy and safety of 1, 5, and 15 mg/h intravenous clazosentan was assessed in 413 patients. Clazosentan significantly decreased moderate and severe vasospasm in a dose-dependent manner and showed a trend for reduction of vasospasm-related morbidity/mortality in patients with aneurysmal SAH. A Phase III clinical trial (CONSCIOUS-2) will compare the clinical outcomes in patients with SAH treated with either placebo or clazosentan.

Pathologic correlate of vasospasm

Acutely, vasospasm is primarily due to active smooth muscle contraction[48] mediated by oxyhemoglobin, derivatives of arachidonic acid, and lipid hydroperoxides. However, these substances do not have a prolonged effect on cerebral vascular smooth muscles because of insufficient concentrations in CSF and their short half-life.[49] Recent data suggest that not only a physiological change, but also a structural change occurs in the vessel wall after SAH. The most prominent histological changes comprise subintimal cellular proliferation and necrotic changes.[50–52] In addition, collagen fiber deposition increases in cerebral arteries after human and experimental SAH[53,54] along with proliferation of myofibroblasts. CSF from patients with SAH can stimulate re-arrangement of collagen by myofibroblasts in experimental models and henceforth produce vascular constriction.[55] Histological changes are most prominent after severe degrees of arterial constriction with large doses of epinephrine, suggesting that the duration and severity of vasospasm may be important in determining the histology.[56] These histological changes may be initiated by mechanical or anoxic damage to the vessel wall. The morphological changes are responsible for the resistance of vasospastic arteries to conventional vasodilator drugs and lack of reconstriction after transluminal balloon angioplasty.

Based on the above evidence, early and effective removal of the clot from the subarachnoid space prior to maximal release of erythrocyte breakdown products may prevent vasospasm. However, once vasospasm occurs, pharmacological or mechanical dilation of the involved arteries may be necessary. Later in the course of vasospasm, permanent structural changes may appear in the vessel wall, after which the benefits of pharmacological vasodilation are limited.

Additional pathophysiological mechanisms for cerebral vasospasm
Microvascular changes

Induced SAH in the canine model produces a significant impairment in regional cerebral blood flow (rCBF) irrespective of the degree of vasospasm of large cerebral vessels. The findings support the presumptive role of the microvasculature in regard to delayed cerebral ischemia after SAH.[57] Other studies have demonstrated functional and structural changes in microcirculation in experimental studies in a rat model of SAH with associated with acute ischemia.[58] In another experimental model of SAH, abnormal cerebral pial microcirculation was found resulting from spasm of microvessels, decreased blood flow, and agglutination of red blood cells.[59] Impaired CBF autoregulation during vasospasm is probably related to impaired capacity of distal vessels to dilate in response to reduced local perfusion pressure because of maximal vasodilation due to low perfusion pressure distal to large arteries in spasm.[60] Regional cerebral blood volume (CBV), CBF, and oxygen extraction fraction in regions with and without angiographic vasospasm obtained from 29 positron tomography studies performed after intracranial aneurysm rupture were compared with data from 19 normal volunteers and five patients with carotid artery occlusion. Regional CBF was reduced compared to normal in regions from SAH patients with and without vasospasm as well as with ipsilateral carotid occlusion ($P < 0.0001$). Regional oxygen extraction fraction was higher during vasospasm and distal to carotid occlusion than both normal and SAH without vasospasm. Regional CBV was reduced compared to normal in regions with and without spasm, whereas it was increased ipsilateral to carotid occlusion. These findings of paradoxically reduced regional CBV in patients with vasospasm under conditions of hypoperfusion that produce increased CBV in patients with carotid occlusion suggest that arterioles distal to arteries with angiographic spasm after SAH have impaired autoregulatory vasodilation. A qualitative and quantitative analysis of the cortical microcirculation after SAH[61] was undertaken by means of orthogonal polarization spectral imaging, during aneurysm surgery in three patients with an incidental intracerebral aneurysm and ten patients with SAH. Vessel diameters, red blood cell velocity, and functional capillary density were analyzed before and after surgical treatment of aneurysms. In patients with SAH, mono- and multisegmental microvasospasms in arterioles were observed, with a reduction of vessel diameters up to 75.1%. In patients with SAH, capillary density is significantly decreased and small arteries and arterioles of the cortical surface exhibit vasospasm that cannot be detected by angiography or transcranial Doppler sonography.

Microvascular thrombosis

Cerebral ischemia associated with SAH is considered to be caused by vasospasm. However, not all patients with cerebral ischemid associated with SAH have vasospasm. Inversely, not all patients with vasospasm develop clinical symptoms and signs of ischemia. A detailed review[62] found evidence that cerebral ischemia cannot always be attributed to vasospasm. An in-depth analysis of clinical and autopsy studies suggested the role of microthrombosis in the pathogenesis of cerebral ischemia. Clinical studies show that ischemia is associated with an activation of the coagulation cascade within a few days after SAH, preceding the time window during which vasospasm occurs. Furthermore, impaired fibrinolytic activity, inflammatory and endothelium-related processes lead to the formation of microthrombi, which ultimately result in ischemia. The presence of microthrombi is confirmed by autopsy studies. Crompton[63], in an autopsy study, found evidence of cerebral infarctions for 119 of 159 patients who died as a result of aneurysmal rupture. The author attributed one infarction to thromboembolism originating from the aneurysmal sac. Sutherland et al.[168] observed active platelet deposition within the aneurysmal sac for 6 of the 10 patients with unruptured aneurysms but not for any of the three patients with ruptured aneurysms. Previous studies suggested that the size of the aneurysm is important in determining the risk of in situ thrombosis. Schunk[64] reviewed autopsy results for 110 patients to determine the incidence and predisposing factors for thrombosis within the aneurysmal sac. The author found that larger aneurysms were associated with a higher frequency of thrombosis. Black and German[65] demonstrated, in an experimental model, that large-volume aneurysmal sacs with smaller orifices were predisposed to sluggish flow, with a higher risk of thrombosis. However, a clear relationship between aneurysm size and distal embolization has not been established.

A transcranial Doppler (TCD) study[66] determined the frequency and characteristics of microembolic signals (MES) in 23 patients with subarachnoid hemorrhage (SAH). Each middle cerebral artery was monitored for 30 minutes three times each week. Eleven individuals without SAH or other cerebrovascular diseases who were treated in the same unit served as control subjects. MES were detected in 16 of 23 patients (70%) and 44 of 138 patient vessels (32%) monitored, compared with 2 of 11 control subjects (18%) and 2 of 22 control vessels (9%). MES were observed in 83% of patients with clinical vasospasm and 54% of those without clinical vasospasm. Aneurysms proximal to the monitored artery were identified in 38 of 138 vessels, of which 34% exhibited MES, which is similar to the frequency for vessels without proximal aneurysms (31%). Endovascular and surgically treated and unsecured aneurysms exhibited similar frequencies of MES.

Acute treatment of vasospasm
Transluminal balloon angioplasty

In recent years, endovascular treatment of vasospasm with balloon angioplasty, i.e., mechanical dilation of the stenotic arteries through a microballoon catheter under fluoroscopic guidance has been performed in select patients (see Fig. 12.1 and 12.2). Balloon angioplasty is effective in reversing vessel constriction. Balloon dilation of arteries leads to a transient alteration in myocyte structure.[67] However, the long lasting effect is caused by disruption of the normal architecture of the collagen lattice in the arterial wall.[68] The results from clinical trials using balloon angioplasty are summarized in Table 12.1.[69–80] Significant and sustained neurological improvement was seen in the majority of treated cases and recurrence was very infrequent on follow-up angiogram. One of the potential limitations of balloon angioplasty is that despite successful dilation of vasospastic arteries in all cases, the clinical outcome may not improve in one third of the patients. Zubkov et al[69] found that improvement was always most prominent in patients who presented with Hunt–Hess Grade 1 or 2 and subsequently deteriorated (all 13 patients improved). Among SAH patients in Hunt–Hess Grade 3 at presentation, 85% improved with balloon angioplasty compared with 40% improvement in Grades 4 and 5. Eskridge et al.[70] found that balloon angioplasty was most successful if done within 12 hours of onset of symptoms (presumably before ischemic tissue underwent infarction).

Most studies excluded patients who had computerized tomography (CT) evidence of cerebral infarction. Coyne et al.[73] included patients with cerebral infarction on CT scan and found no cases of hemorrhagic transformation after balloon angioplasty. However, despite complete resolution of angiographic vasospasm, clinical improvement was seen in

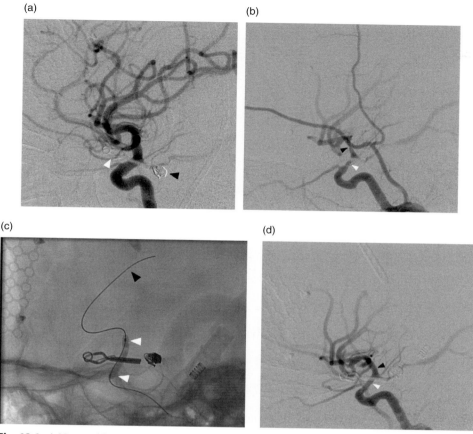

Fig. 12.1. A 35-year-old woman with aneurysmal subarachnoid hemorrhage (Hunt and Hess Grade III and Fischer Grade 3), underwent left posterior communicating artery aneurysm clipping and right posterior communicating artery aneurysm embolization. On hospital day 7, a routine transcranial Doppler demonstrated increased left middle cerebral artery velocities. **(a) Left internal carotid artery (ICA) angiography. Lateral view.** Angiography demonstrates native left ICA and left middle cerebral artery (MCA) vessel caliber following right posterior communicating artery aneurysm embolization (black arrowhead). Surgical clip artifact (white arrow head) in the left posterior communicating artery aneurysm is also visualized. **(b) Left common carotid artery angiography. Lateral view.** Angiography demonstrates severe vasospasm of the intracranial distal left ICA (white arrowhead) and Left MCA M1 segment (black arrowhead). **(c) Left ICA and MCA balloon angioplasty. Single Frame.** Distal left internal carotid artery and left MCA M1 segment Gateway 2.25 × 9 mm balloon angioplasty (white arrowheads) over a Synchro 2 microwire (black arrowhead). **(d) Left ICA angiography. Lateral view.** Follow up angiography after balloon angioplasty demonstrated interval vasospasm improvement of left ICA (white arrowhead) and left M1 segment (black arrowhead).

only one third of cases. These findings suggest that the maximum benefit with balloon angioplasty may be seen in patients with good clinical status on admission with subsequent acute deterioration due to vasospasm unresponsive to intensive medical therapy. There may be a window for intervention extending up to 12 hours, although most physicians' bias is to intercede much earlier if aggressive hypervolemic, hypertensive therapy does not result in rapid clinical improvement.

Although rare, the main complication of balloon angioplasty is rupture or occlusion of the vessel on which angioplasty is performed.[70,81,82] Patients with balloon angioplasty proximal to an unclipped aneurysm may be at risk for rupture of the aneurysm.[70,76] Therefore, surgical clipping or endovascular treatment of aneurysms prior to balloon angioplasty has been recommended for patients with unsecured ruptured aneurysms.[83] Balloon angioplasty is ineffective for vasospasm in distal arteries that are inaccessible to the balloon catheter as well as for diffuse vasospasm. Recent efforts have been directed toward the development of new catheters,[84] and the use of

vasodilating agents as an adjunct to balloon angioplasty.[85] Despite these limitations, balloon angioplasty may represent an effective modality to reverse vasospasm resistant to medical therapy.

Intra-arterial infusion of vasodilators

Intra-arterial vasodilators have been used for treating vasospasm in arteries that are not amenable to primary balloon angioplasty. Other indications include severe vasospasm with lumen restriction that prevents the balloon catheter from traversing the lesion as a precursor to angioplasty. However, the response in regards to magnitude and duration of vasodilation is variable. The hypothesis of a vasodilator-resistant phase of vasospasm does not seem consistent with the data, as a number of patients continue to improve with infusion as many as 19 days after SAH. Table 12.2 summarizes some data on the intra-arterial vasodilators that have been used for treatment of cerebral vasospasm.

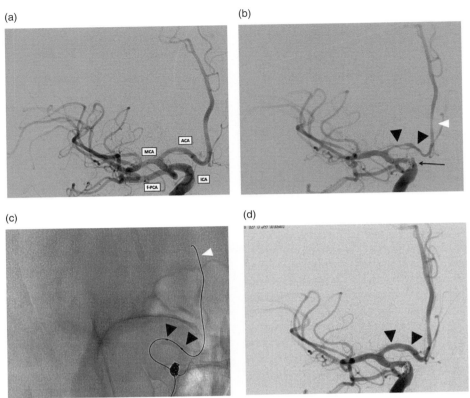

(a)   (b)

(c)   (d)

Fig. 12.2. 52-year old woman with a ruptured basilar tip aneurysm (Hunt/Hess grade III and Fischer grade 3). On day 6 post-subarachnoid hemorrhage, the patient developed bilateral lower extremity weakness. **(a) Right internal carotid artery (ICA) angiography prior to aneurysm coil embolization. Right anterior oblique projection**. Angiography demonstrates normal caliber of the right ICA, fetal posterior cerebral (f-PCA), middle cerebral (MCA) and anterior cerebral arteries (ACA). **(b) Right ICA angiography. Right anterior oblique projection**. Angiography demonstrates coil artifact (black arrow), severe vasospasm in the right anterior cerebral artery A1 segment (black arrowheads) and moderate vasospasm in the A2 segment (white arrowhead). **(c) Balloon angioplasty. Single frame during inflation. Right anterior oblique projection**. Intra-arterial nicardipine (5 mg) was infused prior to balloon angioplasty. An X-pedion microwire was positioned in the distal right ACA (white arrowhead) and angioplasty was performed using a HyperGlide 4 mm × 10 mm balloon (black arrowheads). **(d) Right ICA angiography. Follow up after angioplasty. Right anterior oblique projection**. Angiography demonstrates interval improvement of right anterior cerebral artery (black arrowheads) A1 segment vessel caliber following angioplasty.

The initial approaches used intra-arterial papaverine for inducing vasodilation of cerebral arteries with vasospasm. Papaverine is an opium alkaloid that causes vasodilation of cerebral arteries through direct action on smooth muscle. It also prevents the constriction of smooth muscle secondary to a wide variety of stimuli. The mechanism of action is uncertain but may be related to inhibition of cyclic adenosine monophosphate (cAMP) and cyclic guanosine 3,5′ monophosphate (cGMP) activity in smooth muscles and an increase in intracellular cAMP and cGMP turnover.[86,87] In order to achieve therapeutic levels of papaverine in cerebral vessels, it is essential to infuse the drug just proximal to the spastic arterial segments. Other routes of administration, such as intrathecal administration in animal models, have been unsuccessful for the treatment of vasospasm.[88,89] The doses of papaverine required for intravenous administration, are large and can lead to systemic hypotension. Theoretically, the timing of papaverine infusion is also important because papaverine may be less effective for dilating vasospastic arteries after 3 to 5 days when collagen remodeling starts taking place in the arterial wall.[90]

Several clinical series[91–93] have evaluated the effect of selective intra-arterial papaverine in the treatment of vasospasm (Table 12.3).[91–96] The benefit was most prominent in patients who underwent balloon angioplasty along with intra-arterial papaverine administration[92] for symptomatic vasospasm in vascular territories not accessible to balloon angioplasty. The doses of papaverine in these patients were selected empirically and ranged from 6 to 600 mg administered as boluses or continuous infusion. Kassell et al.,[91] after administering various doses, concluded that papaverine in doses of 300 mg/100 ml saline was adequate and safe in most cases. Interestingly, in several patients, no appreciable change in the arterial diameter was noted over the first 30 to 60 minutes of infusion, but then fairly dramatic dilation occurred in the last 30 minutes. All three studies excluded patients with cerebral infarction on CT scan.

Recurrence rates of up to 20% were seen in patients who received only intra-arterial papaverine. In the series published by Kassell et al.,[91] vasospasm recurred in two patients 5 days after the first infusion. Both of these patients improved markedly after a second infusion of papaverine, Delay in initiation of papaverine treatment, inadequate dosing, and inadequate

Table 12.1. Results of balloon angioplasty for cerebral vasospasm in patients with subarachnoid hemorrhage

Series	No. of patients and characteristics	Timing of angioplasty	Angiographic results	Clinical results	Recurrence	Complications	Comments
Zubkov et al.[69]	89 All grades of vasospasm	51 pts pre-op 16 pts post-op 14 pts in sub-acute phase	100% improved	71.9% improved	0% at 5–7d	3 pts arterial rupture 1 pt TIA 1 pt worsened	Improvement most prominent in pts with admit H-H <3
Eskridge et al.[70]	48 1 Recent onset of symptoms 2-Not reversed by standard treatment	Within 18 hours of DIND	100% improved	66% improved	0%	2 pts arterial rupture 2 rebleeds from unclipped aneurysms 1 thrombosis after 6 weeks	Improvement most prominent within 12 hours of onset of ischemia
Higashida et al.[71]	13 1 Failure of standard treatment 2- No evidence of infarction on CT		100% improved	69% improved	0%	1 pt hemorrhagic infarct	No improvement in pts with admission H-H >3
Konishi et al.[74]	8 1 Admit H-H <3 with deterioration 2. No response to HV and HTN	5–12 d after	100% improved	62.5% improved	0%	1 pt ruptured unclipped aneurysms	Angioplasty effective
Bracard et al.[72]	5 No response to nimodipine	Post-op	100% improved	100% improved	0%	none	Angioplasty effective in early period of symptom onset
Coyne et al.[73]	13 1 No response to HV and HTN 2- Included pts with infarct on CT	<48 hours of DIND	100% improved	31% improved		none	Angioplasty poor outcome if poor grade at time of angioplasty
Takahashi et al.[76]	20 1 No response to medical therapy 2. No evidence of infarct on CT		100% improved	70% improved	0%	1 pt ruptured aneurysm	Better results with early angioplasty (<6 hours)
Nemoto et al.[75]	10 No response to medical therapy		60% improved	40% improved			Minimal benefit in pts with infarction and brain swelling

Table 12.1. (cont.)

Series	No. of patients and characteristics	Timing of angioplasty	Angiographic results	Clinical results	Recurrence	Complications	Comments
Terry et al.[80]	75 underwent 85 balloon angioplasty procedures;mean Hunt and Hess grade was III	Mean 8 days, range 3–24 days (after SAH)	100% in distal ICA 94% in M1 73% in VA 88% in BA 34% in A1		Follow-up angiography was performed in 38 of the 75 patients out of which 10 had a recurrence	Thromboembolism (n=1), retro-peritoneal hematoma (n=1), hypotension during the procedure (n=1) early sheath dislodgement (n=1) excessive bleeding at puncture site (n=1)	Balloon angioplasty success rate of greater than 90% in the distal ICA and the M1 segment. However, proximal ACA remains a technical challenge, with a treatment success rate of only 34%
Bejjani et al.[77]	31 5 pts with H-H=4, 15 pts with H-H=3, 7 pts with H-H=2, 4 pts with H-H=1	Mean 6–9 days, range 1–14 days after SAH		72%	1 pt at 7 days after angioplasty	2 pts had femoral hematoma 1 pt had retroperitoneal hematoma	Significant improvement in patients with earlier angioplasty
Eskridge et al.[78]	50 27 pts with H-H= 1–2, 23 pts with H-H= 3–5	47 pts 4–14 days after SAH 3 pts 2 weeks after SAH	98%	61% improved within 72 hours	0%	none	The longer the vessel has been in spasm, the more difficult it is to perform angioplasty
Firlik et al[79]	14 H-H ranged from 2–4 8 of 14 pts were infused with papaverine for recurrent vasospasm.	Range between 6 and 12 days	100% in 3 cases. Atleast some degree of vasospasm persisited in the remaining cases	92%	0%	1 pt developed ICH and in 1 pt angioplasty was not technically possible because catheter positioning within the left M1 segment was too unstable to attempt balloon inflation.	Using intra-arterial papaverine infusion in addition to angioplasty provided no benefit to some of these patients and perhaps a minimal benefit to others.

Recurrence depicts angiographic recurrence when follow up angiogram was done.

Abbreviations used: pt(s), patient(s); pre-op, pre operative; post-op, postoperative; TIA, transient Ischemic Attack; H-H, Hunt-Hess grades; DIND, delayed ischemic neurologic deficit; CT computed tomographic scan. HV, hypervolemia; HTN, hypertensive Therapy,; ICH Intracerebral Hemorrhage; d, day; SAH, subarachnoid hemorrhage; ICA, internal carotid artery; VA, vertebral artery; ACA, anterior cerebral artery.

Modified from Qureshi AI, Recent advances in the management of vasospasm in patients with subarachnoid hemorrhage. *The Neurologist* 1996. With permission from Walter Kluwers Publishers.

Table 12.2. Various vasodilators used intra-arterially to treat cerebral vasospasm in patients with subarachnoid hemorrhage

Agent	Mechanism of action	Minimum and maximum dose	Side effects
Papaverine[100,111,115,117,118,121]	Potent vasodilator believed to inhibit cAMP and cGMP phosphodiesterases in smooth muscle to increase intracellular levels of cAMP and cGMP.	300 mg administered at a rate of 3 ml/minute. Min dose 200 mg max dose 400 mg	Increase in ICP, transient neurological deficits (including mydriasis and brainstem depression, monocular blindness, seizures), thrombocytopenia, precipitation of crystal emboli during infusion, and paradoxical exacerbation of vasospasm leading to cerebral infarction. Selective gray matter changes in MRI scan
Nimodipine[110,149]	Inhibition of Ca influx in to cerebral vascular smooth muscle causing vasodilation.	0.8 to 3.2 mg	Hypotension
Verapamil[102,113]	Ca ion influx inhibitor in smooth muscle.	2 to 120 mg	Hypotension, bradycardia
Nicardipine[104–106,114,116]	Selective smooth muscle vasodilation.	0.5 to 40 mg	Raised intracranial pressure
Milirinone[109,112,119]	Phosphodiestereases III inhibition having smooth muscle vasodilation and inotropic properties.	2.5–24 mg	Hypotension, hypokalemia
Colforsin[120]	Directly stimulates adenylate cyclase, which in turn causes vasorelaxation via elevated intracellular concentrations of cyclic adenosine monophosphate.	3 mg	Tried in two patients; no side effects observed
Magnesium[104]	Inhibits the pre-synaptic release of excitatory amino acids and is a non-competitive antagonist to postsynaptic N-methyl D-aspartic acid (NMDA) receptors.	250 mg to 1000 mg	None reported

Abbreviations used: ICP, intracranial pressure; MRI, magnetic resonance imaging.

duration of treatment have been suggested as possible mechanisms.[91,97] Papaverine was the agent of choice for a long time, but its side effects, including seizures and neurotoxicity have recently limited its use.[98,99] Recent reports of adverse events have also included transient mental status changes, ophthalmic complications, and increases in heart rate and intracranial pressure. Intra-arterial delivery of papaverine preserved with chlorobutanol into vasospastic anterior cerebral arteries may result in marked neurological deterioration with selective gray matter changes on MRI imaging. This effect is consistent with a permanent toxic effect to human brain.[100] Analogs of papaverine have been shown to deposit in the corneal epithelium due to their high lipophilic properties.[101]

Intra-arterial infusion of calcium channel blockers like verapamil and nicardipine has recently gained more popularity due to better safety profiles.[102–104] Several investigators have published their experience with intra-arterial nicardipine as a preferred vasodilator therapy with prolonged angiographic dilation and improved clinical outcome without major adverse effects (see Table 12.4).[104–106] Nicardipine is a dihydropyridine voltage-sensitive Ca^{2+} channel antagonist, which exerts its effect by local vasodilatory actions with increase in regional CBF and blockade of calcium entry into the ischemic brain cells.[107,108] We recently reported results from a study[104] involving administering magnesium sulfate, along with nicardipine intra-arterially through the microcatheter during endovascular treatment of vasospasm to augment the effect of nicardipine. Intra-arterial magnesium sulfate (250–1000 mg) was administered via a microcatheter in the affected vessels in combination with a vasodilator (nicardipine 2.5–20.0 mg). A total of 58 vessels were treated in 14 patients; 40 vessels (69%) had immediate angiographic improvement with intra-arterial nicardipine and magnesium sulfate alone and 18 vessels (31%) required concomitant balloon angioplasty with complete reversal of the vasospasm. Re-treatment was required in 13 vessels (22%) and the median time for retreatment was 2 days (range 1–13 days). Nicardipine treatment resulted in the reduction of MAP (12.3 mmHg, standard error [SE] 1.34) without any significant change in ICP. Magnesium sulfate infusion was not associated with change in MAP or ICP. Among 31 procedures, immediate neurological improvement was observed in 22 (71%) procedures. In 12 (86%) patients, there were no infarctions in the follow-up CT scan acquired between 24 and 48 h (see Table 12.2).[100,102–104,106,109–122]

A comparison between the three case series that used intra-arterial nicardipine for vasospasm treatment in SAH

Table 12.3. Results of intra-arterial papaverine for vasospasm cerebral vasospasm in patients with subarachnoid hemorrhage

Series	No. of patients and characteristics	Dosage and timing of papaverine	Angiographic results	Clinical results	Recurrence	Complications	Comments
Kassell et al.[91]	12 candidates for balloon angioplasty	100–300 mg by infusion	66% improved	33% improved	17%	1 pt transient mental status and hemiparesis 1 pt transient mydriasis	3 pts responded changes after 10 d of SAH onset
Kaku et al.[92]	14 1-new ischemic deficit unresponsive to medical therapy 2-no evidence of infarct on CT	6–20 mg in repeated doses with angioplasty and IA nicardipine	92% improved	80% improved	0%	Tachycardia	Papaverine has long-lasting effect
Cloustan et al.[93]	10 1-new ischemic deficit unresponsive to medical therapy 2-no evidence of infarct on CT scan	150–600 mg by manual injection <48 h after DIND	93% improved	50% improved	21%	1 pt permanent monocular blindness; 1 pt arterial rupture without neurologic decline	Angiographic results do not correlate with clinical outcome
Morgan et al.[95]	84 1-five underwent balloon angioplasty. 2-twelve were treated with barbiturate	Daily administration of papaverine until vasospasm resolved.	94% improved	65% improved	20%	26% developed vasospasm, 17% underwent papaverine angioplasty. 6% were entered in barbiturate coma.	5.5% mortality and no difference in outcome of pts who developed angiographic vasospasm and those who did not.
Schuknecht et al.[96]	30 Papaverine given in 66 arteries and angioplasty in 15 arteries	300 mg/100 ml saline over 20 min/territory by manual injection	96% improved	73% improved	23%	1 pt developed transient hemiparesis	Papaverine has better outcome with PTA in both symptomatic and asymptomatic vasospasm after SAH
Katoh et al.[94]	14 4 with clinical vasospasm and 10 with angiographic vasospasm	40–160 mg by slow IA infusion in therapeutic group (4pts)	35%	25%	16%	36% decrease LOC, 14% elevated BP, 1% decerebrate posture, 1% conjugate deviation, hemiparesis, tachycardia	PTA is superior to IA papaverine for treatment of vasospasm after SAH

Pt(s), patients; SAH, subarachnoid hemorrhage; CT, computed tomography; IA, intra-arterial; DIND, delayed ischemic neurologic deficit; PTA, percutaneous transluminal angioplasty; d, day; LOC, level of consciousness; BP, blood pressure.

Modified from Qureshi AI, Recent advances in the management of vasospasm in patients with subarachnoid hemorrhage. *The Neurologist* 1996. With permission from Walter Kluwers Publishers.

patients was reported (see Table 12.4).[104–106] Badjatia et al.[105] reported their initial experience of using intra-arterial nicardipine in 18 subarachnoid hemorrhage patients. The doses ranged from 2.5 to 20 mg per procedure. Similarly, Tejada et al.[106] published their series of 11 patients who were administered high dose intra-arterial nicardipine infusions. The dosages they used ranged from 10 mg to 40 mg per procedure. There was no statistically significant difference in the rates of immediate angiographic and clinical improvement between the two published case series with nicardipine alone and series of patients with combination of magnesium and nicardipine. The rates of cerebral infarction on follow-up CT scan appeared lower in combination series compared to the rates reported by Tejada et al.[106], but did not reach statistical significance. Similarly, the re-treatment rates were prominently high in Tejada et al.[106] compared to combination

Table 12.4. Comparison of demographic, angiographic and clinical characteristics of patients treated with nicardipine and magnesium sulfate with published case series that used nicardipine only

	Shah et al.[104]	Badjatia et al.[105]	Tejada et al.[106]	P-value
Demographics				
No. of patients	14	18	11	<0.01
Mean age (range)	42 (24–57)	50 (28–67)	57 (43–76)	Ns
Women	11 (79%)	13 (72%)	10 (91%)	
No. of procedures	31	24	20	
No. of vessels	58	48	34	
Clinical characteristics				
Mean Hunt and Hess grade (range)	3 (1–5)	4 (1–5)	3 (1–4)	Ns
Coil embolization for aneurysm treatment	12 (86%)	–	9 (82%)	
Intra-arterial vasodilator	Nicardipine + magnesium sulfate	Nicardipine only	Nicardipine only	
Median nicardipine dose/ procedure, mg (range)	7.5 (2.5–20)	5 (2.5–15)	25 (10–40)	
Angiographic and clinical outcomes				
Procedures with angiographic improvement	31 (100%)	24 (100%)	20 (100%)	Ns
Patients with clinical improvement	11 (79%)	8 (44%)	10 (83%)	Ns
Patients with cerebral infarction on follow-up CT	2 (14%)	–	3 (25%)	Ns
Re-treatment				
Patients received re-treatment	8 (57%)	–	7 (64%)	0.06
Vessels undergoing re-treatment	13 (22%)	–	14 (14%)	0.05

Ns = not significant; CT, computed tomography.

(taken with permission from Neurocritical care published in 2009 by Springer Link).

treatment series (41% vs. 22%), but not statistically significant. Badjatia et al.[105] did not report cerebral infarctions on follow-up CT and none of their procedures were re-treatment.

Comparison between primary balloon angioplasty and intra-arterial vasodilators

Current evidence suggests that balloon angioplasty results in a more pronounced and sustained effect on vasospastic arteries, thus reducing the need for re-treatment. Balloon angioplasty was compared with papaverine infusion for the treatment of proximal anterior circulation vasospasm following SAH.[123] Between 1989 and 1995, 125 vasospastic distal internal carotid artery- or proximal middle cerebral artery-vessel segments were treated in 52 patients with balloon angioplasty or papaverine infusion. Balloon angioplasty alone was performed in 101 vessel segments (81%) in 39 patients (75%), whereas papaverine infusion alone was used in 24 vessel segments (19%) in 13 patients (25%). Repeated treatment after balloon angioplasty was needed in only one vessel segment, whereas repeated treatment following papaverine infusion was required in 10 vessel segments (42%) in six patients because of recurrent

vasospasm. Seven vessel segments (29%) with recurrent spasm following papaverine infusion were treated with balloon angioplasty. Although vessel segments treated with papaverine demonstrated a 20% mean decrease in blood flow velocity by TCD on post-treatment Day 1, velocities were not significantly lower than pre-treatment levels by post-treatment Day 2. Balloon angioplasty resulted in a 45% mean decrease in TCD velocity to a normal level following treatment, a decrease that was sustained. In another study 25 patients[124] were treated by, balloon angioplasty intra-arterial papaverine infusion. Balloon angioplasty was performed for proximal vasospasm located in the main arterial trunk and intra-arterial papaverine infusion was chosen for distal vasospasm. In the proximal vasospasm group, all patients achieved good outcome or moderate disability. In the distal vasospasm group, eight patients had an outcome categorized as good or were moderately disabled, and four patients were severely disabled. Diffuse vasospasm revealed a high mortality rate in spite of endovascular therapy.

In a systematic review of clinical series,[125] balloon angioplasty produced clinical improvement in 62% of patients, significantly improved mean TCD velocities, significantly improved regional CBF in 85% of patients (studied by xenon techniques and serial single photon emission computerized

Table 12.5. Different parameters showing treatment benefit on surrogate markers with either angioplasty and/or intra-arterial vasodilators

Study	Angioplasty performed	IA-vasodilators used	TCD velocity	rCBF by SPECT	Cerebral metabolism by PET scan	Others
Morgan et al.[95]	Yes	Papaverine				
Eskridge et al.[78]	Yes	Nimodipine	Improved		Improved	
Ohkawa et al.[144]	Yes					Altered myocytes on histology
Firlik et al.[79]	Yes	Papaverine		Improved	Improved	
Beck et al.[137]						
Schuknecht et al.[96]	Yes	Papaverine	Improved			
Fandino et al.[139]	Yes	Papaverine	Improved	Improved		
Milburn et al.[142]	Yes	Papaverine				
Firlik et al.[111]	Yes	Papaverine		Improved (Xe-CT)		
Zubkov et al.[163]	Yes	Papaverine	Improved			
Oskouian et al.[145]	Yes	Papaverine	Improved	Improved		
Majoie et al.[141]	Yes	Papaverine			Improved (CTP)	
Terry et al.[80]	Yes	Papaverine				
Murai et al.[143]	Yes	Papaverine	Improved			
Lewis et al.[140]	Yes	Papaverine	Improved	Improved		

Abbreviations used: rCBF, regional Cerebral Blood Flow; TCD, Transcranial Doppler. Study; SPECT, Single Positron Emission Computed Tomography.

tomography),[133] and was associated with a 5% complication rate and 1% vessel rupture. Intra-arterial papaverine therapy produced clinical improvement in 43% of patients but only transiently, requiring multiple treatment sessions (1.7 treatments per patient); significantly improved mean TCD velocities but only for less than 48 hours; improved CBF in 60% of patients but only for less than 12 hours; and was associated with increases in intracranial pressure and a complication rate of 9.9%. Intra-arterial nicardipine therapy produced clinical improvement in 42% of patients, significantly improved mean TCD velocities for 4 days, and was associated with no complications in small series.

The rate of short-term neurological improvement of 69 patients undergoing endovascular treatment for symptomatic cerebral vasospasm was determined in a subset of patients enrolled in the multicenter North American Trial of Tirilazad in SAH.[126] Thirty-one patients were treated with intra-arterial administration of papaverine. Fourteen patients were only treated with TBA, and 24 patients received a combination of balloon angioplasty and papaverine. Daily clinical staging with the modified Glasgow Coma Scale (GCS) and every-other-day TCD measurements allowed for a close monitoring of the clinical course. Although TCD studies demonstrated a decrease in flow velocities (dv) in the middle cerebral artery in both treatment groups, indicating a vasodilating effect of

both treatment modalities (d$v = -18.4$ cm/second for papaverine, d$v = -26.04$ cm/second for balloon angioplasty), there was no significant difference in clinical improvement at Days 1 and 4 post-procedure. Neither of the two treatment forms showed an effect of therapy timing on neurological outcome.

Comparison of percutaneous treatment with best medical treatment for cerebral vasospasm

Both balloon angioplasty and intra-arterial vasodilators have been incorporated into the management of patients with subarachnoid hemorrhage who develop vasospasm.[138] Different parameters showing treatment benefit on surrogate markers with either angioplasty and/or intra-arterial vasodilators are summarized in Table 12.5. However, the evidence for superior clinical outcomes for such procedures is based on practitioners experience, case–control studies, and analysis from administrative datasets. A study compared outcomes between endovascular treatment (balloon angioplasty and intra-arterial papaverine infusion) in 44 patients with another 40 patients treated with standard medical therapy (including hypervolemic and hypertensive hemodilution) for cerebral vasospasm.[94] The outcome tended to be better for patients treated with balloon angioplasty, but not for those treated with papaverine infusion, than for those treated conservatively. Recurrence of vasospasm was more frequent after papaverine infusion than after balloon angioplasty. Balloon angioplasty appeared to be superior to conservative management for treatment of vasospasm. Another study[127] assessed the effect of institutional factors in the outcomes of patients treated for cerebral aneurysms in the academic medical centers of the University Health Systems Consortium. Institutional availability of balloon angioplasty for vasospasm was identified by a single case of subarachnoid hemorrhage with treatment code *ICD-9* 39.50 during the study period. Among the 9534 ruptured aneurysm cases treated at 70 centers, patients treated at institutions that used balloon angioplasty for vasospasm had a 16% reduction in risk of in-hospital death compared with patients treated at other institutions. This effect was independent of institutional volume and use of coil embolization.

Jestaedt *et al.*[128] reported on 38 patients with angiographically confirmed severe vasospasm (>70% vessel narrowing). A total of 118 vessels with severe vasospasm in the anterior circulation including the middle cerebral artery and ICA were treated with balloon angioplasty; the anterior cerebral artery was not treated. The frequency of infarction in the distribution of vessels undergoing angioplasty was significantly lower than in vessels not undergoing angioplasty; infarction after balloon angioplasty occurred in four middle cerebral artery territories (four out of 57 [7%]), whereas the infarction rate was 23 out of 61 (38%) in the anterior cerebral artery territories not subjected to balloon angioplasty. Three procedure-related complications occurred during angioplasty (dissection, $n = 1$; temporary vessel occlusions, $n = 2$). One of these remained asymptomatic, whereas this may have contributed to the development of infarction on follow-up computed tomographic scans in two cases.

Prophylactic balloon angioplasty for prevention of cerebral vasospasm

The effect of prophylactic in vivo transluminal balloon angioplasty was studied in a canine model of hemorrhagic cerebral vasospasm of the high cervical internal carotid artery (ICA).[129] Balloon angioplasty resulted in immediate angiographic enlargement of the ICA lumen that was still evident 7 days later, despite the placement of clotted blood around the artery. Scanning and transmission electron microscopy demonstrated flattening of the intima and internal elastic lamina in these dilated arteries, associated with patchy losses of endothelial cells. In contrast, ICAs that had been exposed to clotted blood but had not undergone prior angioplasty developed consistent angiographic and morphological vasospasm. Subsequently, a pilot trial of balloon angioplasty[130] within 3 days of onset in 13 patients Fisher Grade 3 SAH who had a very high probability of developing vasospasm was conducted. In all patients, regardless of the site of the ruptured aneurysm, target vessels for prophylactic balloon angioplasty were as follows: the internal carotid artery, A1 segment, M1 segment, and P1 segment bilaterally; the basilar artery; and one vertebral artery.

Prophylactic balloon angioplasty was considered satisfactory when it could be performed in at least two of the three parts of the intracranial circulation (right and/or left carotid system and/or vertebrobasilar system), and included the aneurysm-bearing part of the circulation. Of the 13 patients, none developed symptomatic vasospasm or more than mild vasospasm according to TCD criteria. At 3 months post-treatment, eight patients had made a good recovery, two were moderately disabled, and three had died; one patient died because of a vessel rupture during transluminal angioplasty (TBA) and two elderly individuals died of medical complications associated with poor clinical condition on admission.

A phase II multicenter randomized clinical trial[14] enrolled 178 patients with Fisher grade III subarachnoid hemorrhage if their aneurysm was satisfactorily secured by surgical or endovascular treatment and if they could be treated with prophylactic balloon angioplasty within 96 hours of SAH. Patients were excluded if vasospasm occurred before randomization or an unsecured aneurysm was present in the location where the balloon angioplasty procedure would be performed. Target vessels for the anterior circulation were the A1 segment of each anterior cerebral artery, the M1 segment of the middle cerebral artery, and the supraclinoid segment of the internal carotid artery. The posterior circulation target vessels were the P1 segment of each posterior cerebral artery, the basilar artery, and the intradural segment of the dominant vertebral artery. During the study, the protocol was revised to exclude the A1 and P1 segments because of perceived safety issues. Balloons were inflated to the vessel diameter until apposition of the balloon to the vessel wall was identified fluoroscopically. Target arteries were treated along their entire length, with 5-second duration for each inflation and a slight overlap of each segment on sequential inflations, whenever possible. Balloon angioplasty was considered satisfactory when it could be performed in at least two of the three parts of the intracranial circulation (right and/or left carotid system and/or vertebrobasilar system) and included the aneurysm-bearing part of the circulation. Eighty-five patients were randomized to prophylactic balloon angioplasty and 85 were randomized to the control group. A total of 483 vessel segments were treated with balloon angioplasty. Four patients were randomized to receive percutaneous transluminal angioplasty (pTBA) but were not treated. Of the 81 patients treated with pTBA, at least 4 vessel segments (of the possible six) were successfully treated by balloon angioplasty in 71 patients, at least three vessel segments in 74 patients, and at least two vessel segments in 78 patients. Three patients underwent treatment of only one vessel segment, i.e., fewer than dictated by the study protocol. Twenty-six percent of patients in the control group and 12% of patients in the pTBA group required endovascular treatment for medically refractory vasospasm, a statistically significant difference. Overall pTBA resulted in an absolute risk reduction of 6% and a relative risk reduction of 10% for unfavorable outcome. Outcome analysis as per the dichotomized GOS revealed a trend toward GOS higher rates of favorable outcomes in the treatment group, but the differences were not statistically significant. Sixty-six patients with good Hunt–Hess grades (i.e., 1 or 2) were analyzed separately. pTBA resulted in an absolute risk reduction of unfavorable outcome of 10% and a relative risk reduction of 29%. Compared with patients with good Hunt–Hess grades (i.e., 1 or 2), poor grade patients (Hunt–Hess grades 3, 4, or 5) showed no improvement from pTBA. Length of stay in intensive care unit and hospital was similar in both groups. Four patients had a procedure-related vessel perforation, of which three patients died. Four patients had study-related adverse events, resulting in a procedure-related complication rate of 5%, or an approximate risk of 1% per treated vessel segment. In two patients, this involved arterial perforation by a guidewire and in two patients, arterial rupture during balloon inflation.

Combined endovascular treatment of aneurysms and vasospasm

Patients with active cerebral vasospasm are at high risk for complications following surgical treatment. In such patients, a combined procedure may be required to secure the aneurysm and prevent ischemic events related to vasospasm. As mentioned above, balloon angioplasty in the vicinity of an unsecured ruptured aneurysm may precipitate rebleeding. Therefore, the aneurysm should be secured prior to performance of balloon angioplasty. If severe vasospasm is observed and precludes safe access to the aneurysm, intra-arterial vasodilators may be used to facilitate embolization. In other cases, the vasospasm can get exacerbated during the manipulation required for embolization and may require intra-arterial vasodilators.[131] Murayama et al.[131] reported the results of combined embolization and balloon angioplasty in a single session for the treatment of ruptured aneurysms associated with symptomatic vasospasm in 12 patients. The patients underwent aneurysm occlusion and balloon angioplasty ($n = 6$), intra-arterial papaverine infusion ($n = 2$), or both ($n = 4$) in a single session. In nine patients, aneurysm obliteration was performed first. In all patients, angiographic improvement of vasospasm was obtained. In one patient, a thromboembolic complication occurred and was treated with urokinase. Clinical outcomes at discharge were good recovery in six, moderate disability in two, severe disability in three, and death in one.[131]

Technical aspects of the procedure
Patient selection

Endovascular treatment is currently reserved for patients with cerebral vasospasm who develop ischemic symptoms and do not improve after institution of hypertensive and hypervolemic treatment. Several definitions have been used to define symptomatic vasospasm. The BPAV trial defined symptomatic vasospasm when all of the following criteria were met: (1) onset between days 3 and 14 after SAH; (2) classic clinical symptoms, including worsening of headache, stiff neck, insidious onset of

confusion, disorientation and/or decline in level of consciousness, or focal deficit, which may fluctuate in severity; (3) in comatose patients, a decline of at least 2 points from the previous GCS score; (4) a head CT scan that excluded other causes of neurologic worsening, such as rebleeding or hydrocephalus; (5) exclusion of other systemic cause for worsening, such as fever, hyponatremia, hypo-oxygenation, or infection; and (6) confirmation of vasospasm by TCD, angiography, or CT angiography. Moderate TCD vasospasm was diagnosed when the mean velocity was > 120 m/s, in the presence of a Lindegaard index of ≥ 3, and severe vasospasm was diagnosed when the mean velocity was > 200 m/s. Patients who developed clinical cerebral ischemia were treated with vasopressors to induce hypertension with the goal of maintaining a mean arterial pressure of 100 to 120 mm Hg. When the ischemia persisted despite hypertensive and hypervolemic therapy, a cerebral angiogram was obtained, and when feasible, therapeutic TBA and/or infusion of vasodilators were performed. Therapeutic hypervolemia (central venous pressure, 8–12 mmHg) and therapeutic hypertension (mean arterial pressure, 120–140 mmHg) have been used to define maximal medical treatment.[132]

In the Clazosentan to Overcome Neurological Ischemia and Infarction Occurring after Subarachnoid Hemorrhage,[15] symptomatic vasospasm was defined as focal vasospasm on DSA or TCD associated with neurological worsening lasting for at least 2 hours. Neurological worsening was defined as a decline of at least 2 points in the modified GCS or an increase of at least 2 points in the abbreviated National Institutes of Health Stroke Scale. When patients could not be assessed neurologically, ischemia was defined as clinical signs of vasospasm (e.g., unexplained fever, new neurological deficit) with vasospasm on DSA or TCD or a new hypodensity on a postprocedure CT scan. TCD criteria for vasospasm were a Lindegaard ratio ≥ 3, a mean middle or anterior cerebral artery flow velocity > 200 cm/s, or an increase > 50 cm/s per 24 hours. Other causes of neurological worsening had to be excluded.

Computed tomographic perfusion (CTP) imaging provides data about CBF, CBV, and time to peak (TTP). Perfusion CT has been introduced as a method of assessing perfusion abnormalities in the acute setting of vasospasm and in patients with poor neurological examination. A perfusion study indicating diminished CBF or extended TTP has been used an indication for performing cerebral angiogram to confirm and treat cerebral vasospasm.[133] TTP is defined as the time delay (in seconds) between the first arrival of the contrast bolus within major arteries included in the section imaged and the local bolus peak in the brain tissue. A regional TTP value greater than 8 to 9 seconds suggests cerebral ischemia and may be used to select patients for endovascular treatment. Another study[134] reviewed the CTP mean transit time (MTT), CBF, and CBV maps independently; they evaluated five anatomical regions (frontal, temporal, parietal, occipital/thalami, and basal ganglia/insula) and graded them for abnormality (0 if normal, 1 if abnormal in $< 50\%$ of the region, and 2 if abnormal in $\geq 50\%$ of the region). MTT (R(2) = 0.939) and CBF (R(2) = 0.907) scores correlated best with DSA scores. In another study,[135] assessment of CBV, CBF, MTT and time to peak (TTP) for eight predefined regions of interest demonstrated prominent asymmetry among patients with symptomatic vasospasm. Optimal threshold values distinguishing between patients with and without cerebral ischemia were 0.77 for CBV and 0.72 for CBF ratios, and 0.87 seconds for MTT and 1.0 second for TTP differences.[134] The study demonstrated that MTT considered alone represented the most sensitive parameter for identification of vasospasm. A cortical CBF value ≤ 39.3 $(mL \times 100\,g^{-1} \times min^{-1})$ represented the most accurate (95%) indicator for selection of patients for endovascular therapy.

Perfusion-weighted magnetic resonance imaging (pwMRI) provides the possibility of detecting tissue at risk for infarction. The areas of perfusion changes in pwMRI correlated well with the neurological deficits of the patients and were larger than the areas of changed diffusion in diffusion-weighted MRI performed at the same time.[136] However, difficulties in acquiring MR images in patients in critical condition prevent widespread use of this technique.

The percutaneous approach and guidecatheter placement

For almost all procedures, a femoral approach is adequate. The guidecatheter is placed in the ipsilateral cervical vertebral or internal carotid artery. The size of the guidecatheter must be appropriate to accommodate the anticipated microcatheter and concomitant balloon catheter (if angioplasty is anticipated). Most procedures are performed using a 6F guide catheter.

Angiographic assessment

Cerebral vasospasm is a process that involves multiple arteries of varying diameter within the same distribution. If the distribution of ischemic deficits is easily identifiable, it is reasonable to access the target proximal artery with a guidecatheter and acquire angiographic images followed by treatment. In the event the ischemic symptoms are poorly localized, angiographic images of all possible involved arteries maybe required prior to deciding an intervention plan. The angiographic severity of vasospasm may be the predominant factor for selecting the arteries to treat if clear clinical localization is not possible.

Angiographic quantification of severity of vasospasm lacks clear standardization. Several methods have been proposed based on expressing the minimum lumen diameter (segment affected by vasospasm) as a fraction of lumen diameter of a corresponding segment prior to occurrence of vasospasm (baseline angiographic images) (see Table 12.6). Quantitating severity of lumen narrowing does not provide an assessment of vasospasm in small arteries and arterioles. Measuring the time required for opacification of a pre-specified arterial

segment and venous segment after a fixed dose of contrast can assess the time required for transit of contrast through the small arteries and arterioles (see Table 12.7). Rapid acquisition of angiographic images (3–15 frames per second) is required to assess the time that contrast requires to reach various anatomical points in regions of interest. Both measures have been used in patients with subarachnoid hemorrhage (see Table 12.5).[77–80,95,96,111,122,137–145]

Ohkuma et al.[146] found that, in patients with severe angiographic vasospasm, rCBF was significantly lower than that in the patients with moderate or none/mild vasospasm. However, there was no statistical difference in rCBF between patients with moderate vasospasm and patients with none or wild vasospasm. Overall, there was correlation between arterial diameter and rCBF predominantly in the presence of severe vasospasm. The contrast transit time showed an inverse correlation with rCBF. The inverse correlation was seen in patients with severe, moderate, and mild/none vasospasm. In another study,[147] longer contrast transit time correlated with severity of angiographic vasospasm and subsequently with occurrence of ischemic deficits. It should be noted that angiographic severity of vasospasm does not appear to correlate with long-term functional outcome presumably because it does not provide assessment of collateral flow and distal microvasculature.[148]

Hanggi et al.[149] used a combination of arterial diameter and contrast transit time to determine the effect endovascular treatment has on vasospasm. Early positive angiographic effect was classified as "minor," "moderate," or "major" improvement. "Minor" changes were classified angiographically by observation of the reduced circulation time only, "moderate" changes consisted of reduced circulation time and reduction of the arterial narrowing, and a "major" response included a complete angiographic reversal of the cerebral vasospasm. The vasospasm usually involves multiple segments along the length of each artery, thereby complicating the assessment of the normal segment (reference artery) diameter. The difficulty in assessing the normal diameter of the target arteries has implications in both quantification of severity of vasospasm and selection of balloon sizes for treatment. A more practical algorithm for quantifying the severity of vasospasm is presented in Table 12.6.[93,101–104] Estimating the diameter of the artery prior to occurrence of vasospasm may require measurement of: (1) artery diameters from initial angiographic images acquired at the time of admission; (2) corresponding contralateral arteries if unaffected; and/or (3) expected approximate normal diameters of affected arteries from historical controls. A conservative approach (underestimation) is recommended if accurate assessment of arterial diameter prior to occurrence of vasospasm is not possible.

A special consideration is required for the tortuosity of the target and surrounding arteries. There is inevitable straightening of arteries with placement of microwires and balloon catheters. This straightening and manipulation may lead to temporary worsening of vasospasm. Such worsening is

Table 12.6. Methods of quantitating severity of angiographic vasospasm in various studies

Study	Reference study	Grading method	Mild	Moderate	Severe	Diffuse
Nicardipine and Tirilazad studies	Baseline angiogram	Image analysis system	minimal	25–50%	> 50%	
Petruk et al.[164]	Baseline angiogram		10–30%	30–50%	> 50%	> 1 vascular distribution
CONSCIOUS-1[15]	Baseline angiogram	Absolute diameter of vessels measured	0–33%	34–66%	67–100%	
Weidauer et al.[165]	Baseline angiogram	Absolute values and ratio of absolute values to extradural ICA or VA	11–33%	34–66%	67–100%	> 50% of the segment length involved in at least one vessel segment
Ohkuma et al.[146]	Pre-operative angiogram	Average of minimum diameters in pre-specified segments of MCA and ICA	< 25%	25–50%	> 50%	
Ko et al.[166]	Normal vessel caliber	Determined by visual estimate	< 30%	30–60%	61–99%	

Abbreviations used: ICA, internal carotid artery; MCA, middle cerebral artery; VA, vertebral artery.

Table 12.7. Methods of quantitating contrast transit through angiographic images in various studies

Study	Method
Weidauer et al.[165]	Time period between intradural arterial inflow of the contrast medium bolus at the level of the carotid siphon and the contrast enhancement of the bridging veins
Ohkuma et al.[146]	Difference in MTT in ICA and rolandic vein expressed as a ratio to extraparenchymal large arteries; ROI set in the vertical intracavernous portion of the ICA, the cortical segment of the rolandic artery, and the rolandic vein on the images of lateral projection
Udoetuk et al.[167]	Contrast dye transit time from the arterial to the venous phase was measured (supraclinoid ICA to parietal cortical veins)
Iwabuchi et al.[162]	Time to peak measured at contrast opacification of proximal portion of the middle cerebral artery in the early arterial phase, the distal portion of the middle cerebral artery in the late arterial phase, and the transverse sinus in the venous phase.
Okada et al.[147]	Difference between the time showing peak optical density at the carotid and the venous portion

Abbreviations used: MTT, mean transit time; ICA, internal carotid artery; ROI, region of interest.

frequent during balloon angioplasty of the proximal and distal anterior cerebral artery. The distal extent of the vasospasm should be carefully identified. The diameter and tortuosity of the arteries that form the distal area of vasospasm helps in deciding whether primary balloon angioplasty alone or a combination of primary balloon angioplasty and intra-arterial vasodilators may be required. For most instances, a combination of both modalities is required.

Primary angioplasty

Primary balloon angioplasty should be performed whenever possible for treating cerebral vasospasm. The process requires the placement of a microwire through the affected segments and advancing the balloon catheter over the microwire across the affected segments (see Figs. 12.1 and 12.2). The low profile and flexibility of the current balloon catheters permit advancing the microwire with balloon catheters as the primary step in traversing the target arteries. Rarely, an exchange length microwire may need to be placed with the assistance of a microcatheter distal to and through the target arteries, and subsequently the balloon catheter may be advanced over a stable microwire platform. Multiple balloon angioplasty procedures may be required along the length of arteries sequentially to treat the entire vasospastic segment. If a relatively non-compliant balloon is used, the diameter and insufflation pressure of the balloon must be selected to avoid overinflation. An inflation that targets 80% of the normal arterial diameter is considered adequate. The diameter differences between proximal and distal affected arteries may require insufflation of increasing pressures (and diameter) with the same balloon starting from the distal segment and proceeding to proximal segments by stepwise inflation, deflation, and retraction of the balloon catheter. After the balloon catheter is adequately repositioned proximally, the cycle of inflation, deflation, and repositioning is repeated. The mismatch between diameters of distal and proximal arteries may require changing the balloon cathethers to a larger size for the same distribution (i.e., proximal middle cerebral artery and supraclinoid internal carotid artery).

Over-inflation is a lesser consideration for a compliant balloons because the radial force is low thus limiting the chance of arterial injury. The same balloon can be used starting distally and retracted proximally in the manner described above. During the procedure, a careful review of the angiography images to visualize the site of balloon angioplasty and the distal portion of the guidecatheter are necessary to identify any iatrogenic dissections. If a dissection is flow limiting, emergent stent placement maybe necessary as discussed in Chapter 9.

Characteristics of angioplasty balloon catheters

The balloon catheters used for the treatment of cerebral vasospasm can be classified by their degree of compliance (Fig. 12.3). At present, the most commonly used balloons include Maverick (Boston Scientific), Gateway (Boston Scientific), Hyperglide (EV3) and Hyperform balloons. A summary of these devices is seen in Table 12.8.

In order to obtain appropriate and safe results, special attention should be paid to the balloon nominal pressure value (value at which the balloon achieves its stated diameter) and the rated burst pressure value (value at which half the balloons will rupture) of the balloon. For intracranial procedures, a high contrast-to-saline ratio is recommended (70% contrast and 30% saline) to improve radio-opacity and visualization during insufflation. However, the operator should be aware that due to increase in the viscosity of the mixture (inversely proportional to the contrast concentration), the speed of deflation is reduced.

Maverick and Gateway balloon catheters are non-compliant balloons and considered to be identical devices. The Gateway balloon is a semi-compliant balloon designed for low pressure inflation, modeled after the Maverick balloon (Boston Scientific), with the addition of hydrophilic coating. Both are advanced over a 0.014-inch microwire and have two ports (wire-flush port and balloon port). The balloons have two radiopaque balloon markers to identify the boundaries of the balloon, except for 1.5 mm balloons which use a single balloon marker. A monorail system is only available in Maverick, but this is not recommended for intracranial use since the lack of a continuous flush port compromises device navigability (Fig. 12.4). Once the balloon is positioned in the segment of interest, an insufflation device with a manometer in atmospheres is connected to the balloon port. Both balloons achieve their nominal diameters at 6 atmospheres, regardless of the diameter or length of the balloon (Fig. 12.5). Another advantage of these balloons over the compliant balloons (see below) is that medications can be infused though the wire flush port.

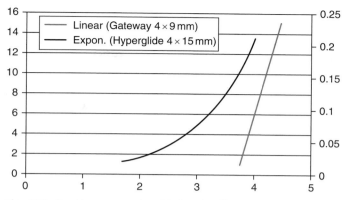

Fig. 12.3. Graphic representation of balloon insufflation comparing non-compliant[38] (blue line) and compliant balloons.[36] Notice that non-compliant balloons increase their diameter in a linear fashion compared to compliant balloons (exponential).

Hyperglide and Hyperform balloon catheters are compliant balloons primarily used for the treatment of wide neck aneurysms (balloon-assisted coiling). The Hyperform is rarely used as an angioplasty balloon. These balloons differ in their shape (Fig. 12.6), but the device preparation is identical. Both balloons are advanced over a 0.010-inch microwire, consist of a single lumen through which the wire is advanced, and the insufflation is performed using the side port. Hyperglide is only available in a fixed 4 mm diameter but with variable lengths (10 mm, 15 mm, 20 mm, and 30 mm) and Hyperform is available in 4 mm and 7 mm diameters with a fixed length (7 mm). These balloons can tolerate large volumes of fluid with small changes in pressure. Therefore, a predetermined inflation volume is used rather than pressure during balloon insufflations to achieve the desired balloon diameter (Fig. 12.7). For example, when using a hyperglide (4 mm × 15 mm) balloon for the treatment of vasospasm in a native 3 mm vessel, the balloon should be insufflated using the recommended predetermined volume (0.06 mL^3). The balloons should be prepared outside of the body by first introducing the wire into the single lumen until seen at the balloon catheter tip followed by a contrast infusion. During the insufflation, the wire should always be kept "crossing" both balloon markers. If air is visualized in the balloon, the wire should be withdrawn and contrast infused again to "flush out" the air. This exercise should be repeated until air is no longer visualized. The wire should always be kept past the tip of the device and beyond both balloon markers to avoid retrograde filling of the lumen and balloon impairing both insufflation and visualization. A 1 cm^3 syringe with contrast is used to infuse the determined volume to achieve the desired balloon diameter.

There are no randomized studies comparing the performance of compliant and non-compliant balloons in the treatment of cerebral vasospasm. Therefore, the balloon selection is based on operator's choice. Recently, Tariq et al.[150] presented results comparing outcomes in 30 patients with cerebral vasospasm from subarachnoid hemorrhage who were treated with compliant (34 vessels) and non-compliant (50 vessels) balloons. The rate of recurrent vasospasm was not significantly different

Table 12.8. Characteristics of balloon catheters used for treatment of cerebral vasospasm

	Maverick[1]	Gateway[2]	Hyperglide [3]	Hyperform[4]
Manufacturer	Boston Scientific	Boston Scientific	EV3	EV3
Class	Non-compliant	Non-compliant	Compliant	Compliant
Diameter	1.5–4.0 mm	1.5–4.0 mm	4 mm	4.0 mm and 7.0 mm
Length	9 mm 15 mm 20 mm	9 mm 15 mm 20 mm	10 mm 15 mm 20 mm 30 mm	7 mm only
Balloon markers	All balloons have two markers, except 1.5 mm (single balloon marker)	All balloons have two markers, except 1.5 mm (single balloon marker)	Two	Two
Nominal	6 atmospheres	6 atmospheres	Variable volume	Variable volume
Outer diameter	3.2 French	3.2 French	0.040 inches	0.040 inches
Wire	0.014 inches	0.014 inches	0.010 inches	0.010 inches
Over the wire	Yes; available in monorail (OD 2.6 French)	Yes	Yes	Yes
Medication infusion possible	Yes	Yes	No	No

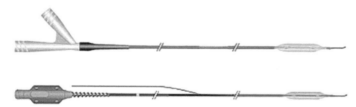

Fig. 12.4. Maverick over the wire (above), Maverick monorail (below). See plate section.

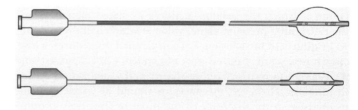

Fig. 12.6. Compliant balloons. Hyperform balloon (below), Hyperglide balloon (above).

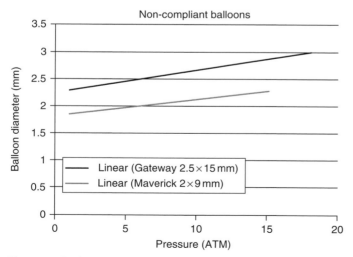

Fig. 12.5. Graphic comparison between the relative change in diameter and pressure for non-compliant (Gateway and Maverick) balloons. Notice that the balloon diameter increases in linear fashion as the pressure increases (atmospheres).

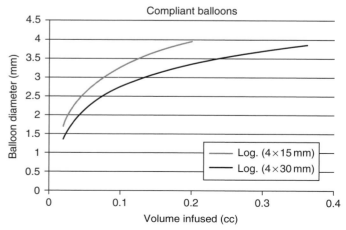

Fig. 12.7. Graphic comparison of two compliant balloons (Hyperglide-3).

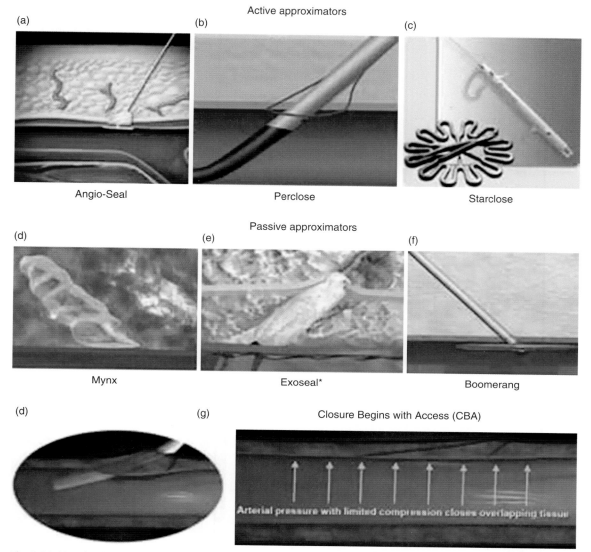

Active approximators

(a)

Angio-Seal

(b)

Perclose

(c)

Starclose

Passive approximators

(d)

Mynx

(e)

Exoseal*

(f)

Boomerang

(d)

(g) Closure Begins with Access (CBA)

Arterial pressure with limited compression closes overlapping tissue

Fig. 2.10. Vascular closure devices by mechanism of action (a)–(f). In the bottom row, cartoons (g), (h) depict the effects of Arstasis* access and closure. On the left (g), the sheath has been placed across a shallow diagonal entry path. A small "pilot" track was used for access for the Arstasis device. On the right (h), the sheath has been pulled from the diagonal track, which has sealed. Devices including SuperStitch (Sutura, Fountain Valley,CA), X-Site (St. Jude), and FemoSeal* (St. Jude). Other passive approximation devices include VasoSeal/On-Site (St. Jude) and Duett (Vascular Solutions). Other CBA: FISH (Femoral Introducer Sheath and Hemostasis, Morris Innovative Research, Bloomington, IN). (*Investigational device).

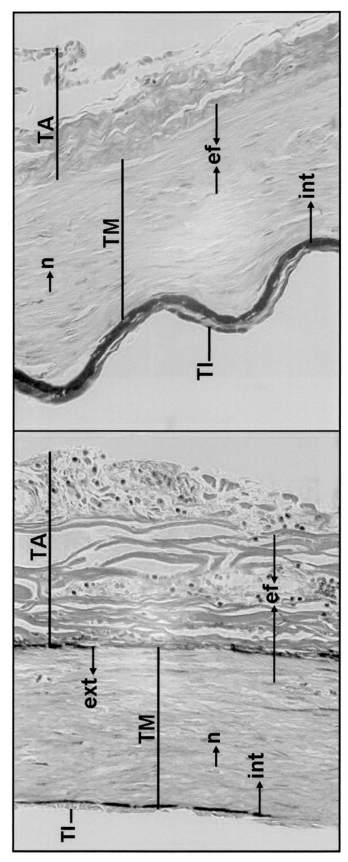

Fig. 10.1. Photomicrography of a coronary artery (left) and intracranial internal carotid artery (right) using identical magnification (Verhoeff-Van Gieson). ef = elastic fiber, ext = external elastic membrane, int = internal elastic membrane, n = nuclei of smooth muscle cells, TA = tunica adventitia, TI = tunica intima, TM = tunica media. Courtesy of H.B.Clark MD, PhD. Director of Neuropathology. University of Minnesota.

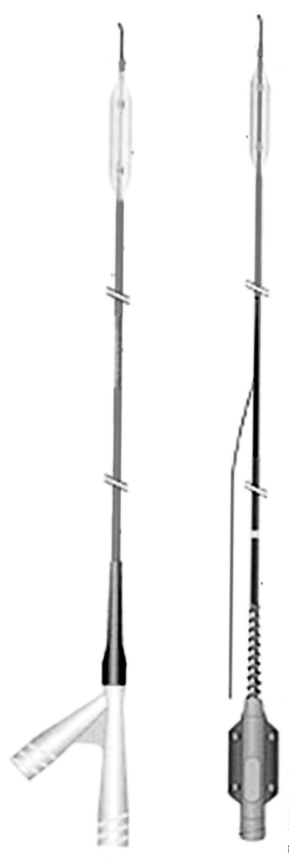

Fig. 12.4. Maverick over the wire (above), Maverick monorail (below).

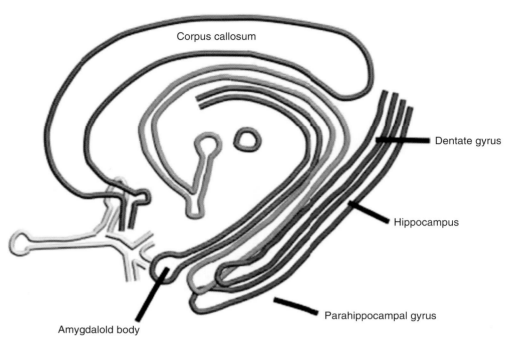

Corpus callosum

Dentate gyrus

Hippocampus

Parahippocampal gyrus

Amygdalold body

Fig. 17.1. Pituitary venous drainage.

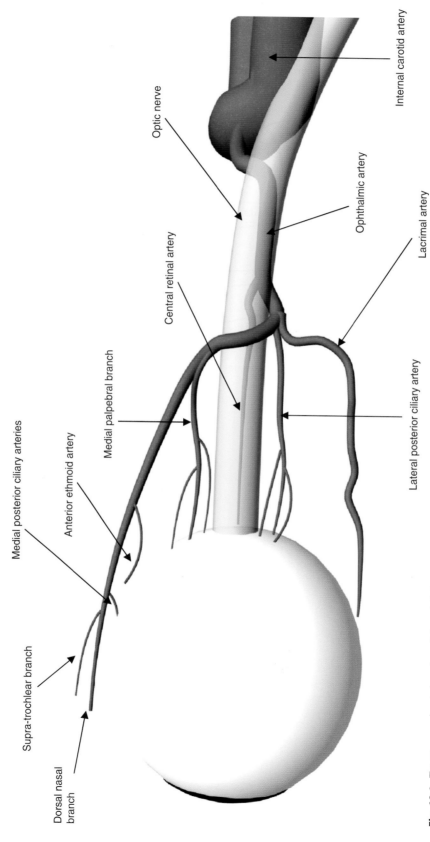

Fig. 19.1. The course and main branches of the ophthalmic artery.

Internal carotid artery

Optic nerve

Ophthalmic artery

Lacrimal artery

Central retinal artery

Lateral posterior ciliary artery

Medial palpebral branch

Medial posterior ciliary arteries

Anterior ethmoid artery

Supra-trochlear branch

Dorsal nasal branch

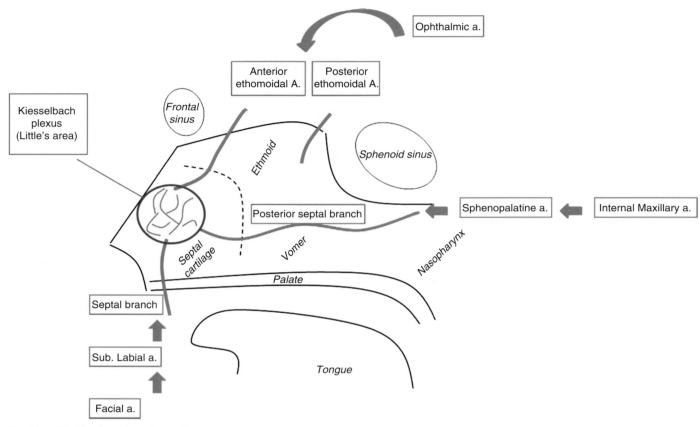

Fig. 20.1. The blood supply to the nasal septum.

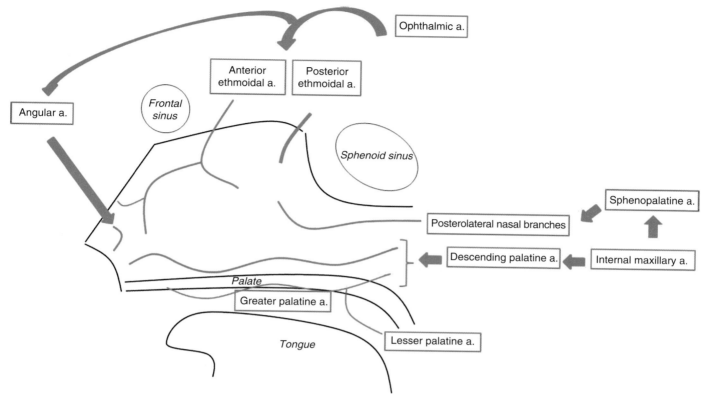

Fig. 20.2. Blood supply to the lateral nasal walls.

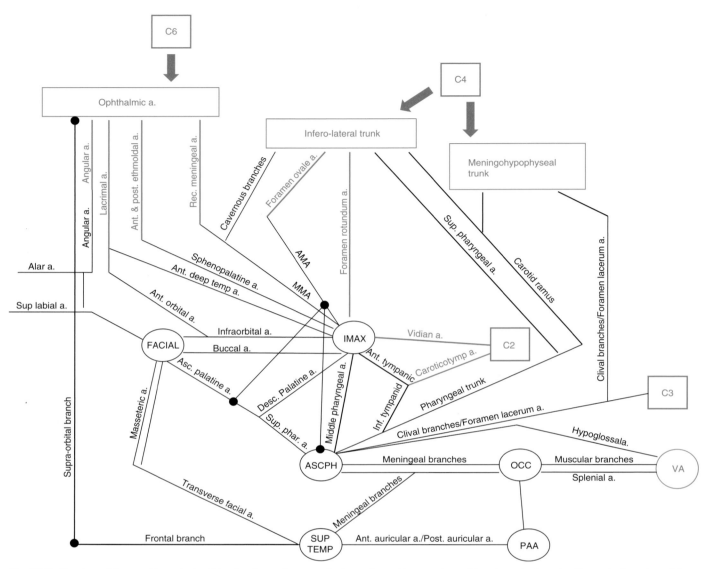

Fig. 20.4. Overview of the most important collateral pathways between the internal carotid, external carotid, and vertebral arteries. First-order branches of the external carotid artery are encircled. First-order branches of the internal carotid artery are highlighted in boxes. Black lines represent external carotid artery branches; Gray lines represent internal carotid artery branches. The names of internal carotid artery branches are shown in red. Abbreviations used: a, artery; AMA, accessory meningeal artery; MMA, middle meningeal artery; Ant, anterior; Post, posterior; Asc, ascending; Desc, descending; Sup, superior; Occ, occipital artery; IMAX, internal maxillary artery; ASC PH, ascending pharyngeal artery; SUP TEMP, superior temporal artery; PAA, C2-C6, internal carotid artery divisions; VA, vertebral artery.

in patients treated with compliant balloons when compared with non-compliant (32% vs. 53%) balloons suggesting that neither one is superior for this indication.

Intra-arterial vasodilators

Intra-arterial vasodilators have been used for treating vasospasm in arteries that are not amenable to primary angioplasty. Other indications include severe vasospasm with lumen restriction that prevents the balloon catheter from traversing the lesion in which case, vasodilators are used as a precursor to angioplasty. It is preferable to perform balloon angioplasty prior to vasodilator administration whenever possible. Vasodilators artificially modify the lumen diameter resulting in improper sized balloon selection. Furthermore, a dilated artery with altered compliance may be less responsive to the radial force of the inflated balloon. Another potential indication for primary vasodilator administration are arteries with preexisting dissection or an unsecured aneurysm which increases the risk associated with primary angioplasty.

A microcatheter is placed proximal to the target arteries using standard techniques. A larger microcatheter (2.3 F) is preferred to facilitate infusion of vasodilators. An angiographic image prior to infusion using contrast injection from the microcatheter is helpful to identify the pattern of flow of the vasodilators after injection. Efforts should be made to advance the microcatheter in a position that prevents filling of the normal arteries by injected contrast or vasodilators because any liquid will preferentially distribute in arteries of low outflow resistance (normal arteries). On a similar basis, superselective placement of the microcatheter in the affected artery facilitates adequate delivery of vasodilators to the target arteries. Injections prior to the origin of the ophthalmic artery should be avoided to prevent excessive vasodilation of retinal arteries. Table 12.2 summarizes the intra-arterial vasodilators with doses used for treatment of cerebral vasospasm.

In our studies, nicardipine (Cardene IV; ESP Pharma, Inc.; Edison, NJ) 5 mg (2 mL) is diluted in 23 mL of 0.9% sodium chloride to acquire a concentration of 0.2 mg/mL administered via microcatheter. A dose ranging from 2.5 g to 20.0 mg per vessel is administered. The dose is titrated to angiographic effect on the vessel and hemodynamic response of the patient, but limited to the acceptable safe dose known from the published reports.[105,106] Hemodynamic parameters such as oxygen saturation, heart rate, systolic, and diastolic blood pressures are strictly monitored throughout the infusion. Magnesium sulfate 1 g (2 mL) solution is diluted in 28 mL of 0.9% sodium chloride to yield a concentration of 33.3 mg/mL and administered intra-arterially through the microcatheter. The dose ranges from 0.25 g to 1 g in each vessel. This dose selection was derived from the known safety and tolerability parameters for intravenous magnesium sulfate.[151,152] Similar hemodynamic parameters are monitored as during the infusion of nicardipine. Another dose-limiting factor is the dose-dependent adverse effect on intracranial pressure during

infusion of vasodilators. If elevated intracranial pressure is observed prior to a satisfactory angiographic response, temporary measures to reduce intracranial pressure such as hyperventilation, cerebrospinal fluid drainage, and/or administration of mannitol or hypertonic saline may be indicated. The angiographic increase in lumen diameter is used as the index of effectiveness.[142,153] Transit time defined as the time interval from angiographic opacification of an artery to opacification of the respective venous sinus may be useful to assess the effect on microvascular flow.[154] The value of this measure is predominantly as a serial measure (pre- and post-treatment) and requires image acquisition at multiple frames (16 to 32 frames per second).

Post-procedure management

A follow-up angiography to detect recurrence is usually considered between 24 and 48 hours, particularly if vasodilators are used. An earlier follow-up with retreatment may be indicated if symptoms recur or worsen. A CT scan in the interval period may be helpful to identify any areas of infarction in the territories of arteries with vasospasm. Other etiologies may need to be considered if clinical improvement does not correspond to the angiographic improvement.

Aspects of clinical response following endovascular treatment

Predictors of response

Several factors have been identified that predict outcome after endovascular treatment of cerebral vasospasm (see Table 12.9).[124,155–157] A better understanding of these factors is essential for appropriate patient selection and allocation of resources.

Angiographic–clinical response mismatch

Several studies have identified that immediate and long-term clinical outcomes are not improved in a proportion of patients who undergo endovascular procedures despite angiographic improvement in vasospasm. Several reasons have been proposed for the observed angiographic–clinical response mismatch. In some patients, the initial poor clinical condition prior to onset of vasospasm obscures the benefit of vasospasm treatment. The transient nature of the benefit of intra-arterial vasodilators may prevent sustained clinical benefit. In some patients, neurological deterioration maybe related to other factors such as seizures or hydrocephalus and therefore, the benefit of vasospasm treatment is limited.

Polin et al.[158] analyzed data from 38 patients enrolled as part of the North American Trial of Tirilazad in Aneurysmal SAH who underwent balloon angioplasty for symptomatic cerebral vasospasm. Fifty-three percent of these patients showed good recovery or moderate disability based on their 3-month Glasgow Outcome Scale score. Among the 38 patients who

Table 12.9. Predictors of clinical response following endovascular treatment

Advanced age[156]
Poor clinical status on admission[156]
Vasospasm involves multiple arterial territories[124,155]
Sustained ICP elevation following intra-arterial vasodilators[155]
Distal arterial vasospasm[124]
Delay (>2 hours after symptom onset) in instituting endovascular procedure [157]
Presence of infarction on CT scan[73]

Abbreviations used: CT, computed tomography; ICP, intracranial pressure.

underwent balloon angioplasty, the severity and type of vasospasm, use of papaverine in addition to balloon angioplasty, timing of treatment, and dose of study drug did not have an effect on outcome. A comparison of outcomes of these patients with individuals matched for age, sex, dose of study drug, admission neurological grade, and modified GCS score at the time of angioplasty did not demonstrate a clear benefit on rates of favorable outcomes. A second analysis by Polin et al.[158] examined 31 patients undergoing papaverine infusion for the treatment of symptomatic vasospasm enrolled in the North American Trial of Tirilizad for Aneurysmal Subarachnoid Hemorrhage. These individuals were matched with patients from the same trial who exhibited similar clinical characteristics (including the degree of vasospasm and the modified GCS scores measured at the time of admission and on the day of papaverine infusion) but received medical management alone. No statistical difference in the 3-month Glasgow Outcome Scale scores between patients receiving papaverine and control subjects (58% favorable outcomes for control subjects versus 45% for patients receiving papaverine) was found. The authors concluded that alterations in the timing of or indications for drug treatment might produce beneficial effects.

Rosenwasser et al.[157] evaluated the relationship between the time interval from symptom onset to treatment and clinical outcomes in 93 patients who underwent endovascular management of clinical vasospasm; 84 of the 93 patients had a 6-month follow-up available. All patients were treated using a combination of angioplasty and intra-arterial papaverine. Of these, 51 patients underwent endovascular management within a 2-hour window, and 33 patients underwent treatment more than 2 hours after the symptom onset. Compared with the group treated more than 2 hours after neurological decline, the group that underwent endovascular management within a 2-hour window after the development of symptoms demonstrated sustained clinical improvement. The results indicate that a 2-hour window may exist for restoration of blood flow to ultimately improve the patient's outcome. However, symptom onset can be difficult to detect in some patients. In one study, the time course of symptom onset was divided into rapid (onset within 4 h) or insidious (progressive deterioration

for > 4 h). Rapid onset was seen in only 42 of the 70 patients with symptomatic vasospasm.[132]

Guidelines from professional societies

The Special Writing Group of the Stroke Council, American Heart Association advocates volume expansion, induction of hypertension, and hemodilution (triple-H therapy) as a reasonable approach to symptomatic cerebral vasospasm (Class IIb, Level of Evidence B). Alternatively, cerebral balloon angioplasty and/or selective intra-arterial vasodilator therapy may be reasonable after, together with, or in the place of medical therapy, depending on the clinical scenario (Class IIb, Level of Evidence B). The Brain Attack Coalition guidelines for comprehensive stroke center state that although balloon angioplasty for vasospasm has not been subjected to rigorous clinical study, it is considered very effective and is a standard therapy for severe vasospasm. Because the other therapeutic options for symptomatic vasospasm are limited and often ineffective, the ability to perform intracranial balloon angioplasty or IA infusions of vasodilators is recommended for a comprehensive stroke center (CSC). If a CSC is temporarily unable to offer this therapy, it is recommended that protocols be developed for the rapid transfer of patients needing these treatments to a nearby facility that does offer this therapy. The German professional society guidelines state that despite the lack of data supporting standards (grade A) or guidelines (grade B), avoidance and rigorous treatment of hypotension and hypovolemia remain the mainstay in the prophylaxis and treatment of a delayed ischemic neurological deficit (DIND). Therapeutic hypertensive hypervolemic hemodilution is recommended as a treatment of symptomatic vasospasm but no prospective studies are available (grade C recommendation). Suggested target values for moderate triple-H therapy are CPP 80–120 mmHg (MAP 90–130), CVP > 7 mmHg and Hk 0.25–0.40. Balloon angioplasty should be considered for treatment of DIND caused by focal, proximal cerebral vasospasm. Clinical data indicate that current prophylaxis and treatment of cerebral vasospasm is still insufficient and aggressive triple-H therapy is associated with an increased incidence of complications.

Vasospasm in other disease entities
Cerebral vasospasm in traumatic brain injury

A review of all admissions was performed on patients with neurotrauma and a diagnostic cerebral angiogram.[159] The decision to proceed to digital subtraction angiography was initially based on a penetrating fragment traversing areas of known vessel concentration (pterional, transorbital, etc.), CT evidence of SAH, and known cerebral vessel occlusion or sacrifice before admission. Later the indication was expanded to include: (1) blast injury in a patient with a presenting GCS score lower than 8, (2) TCD evidence of vasospasm, (3) known surgically treated intracranial pseudoaneurysm before admission, (4) spontaneous decrease in the partial pressure of brain-tissue oxygen or cerebral blood flow, and (5) lack of improvement in GCS without other known causes. Fifty-seven out of 119 neurosurgical consults were evaluated. Of these, 47% had traumatic vasospasm. For those with traumatic vasospasm, the average duration of spasm was 14 days (range, 6–30 days). Within this group, 10 (37%) patients received best medical management, including hypertensive, hypervolemic, hemodilution therapy, whereas 17 (63%) received best medical treatment and early endovascular interventions including microballoon angioplasty. In the vasospasm group, angioplasty with microballoon significantly lowered middle cerebral artery and basilar blood-flow velocities. The mortality was significantly lower among patients treated with endovascular treatment compared with those treated with medical treatment alone (6% vs. 30%).

Cerebral vasospasm in eclampsia

Significantly higher middle cerebral artery (MCA) velocities in eclamptic, but not pre-eclamptic, women compared with those in normotensive pregnant women suggests that moderate to severe vasospasm is associated with eclampsia.[160] A case of a 27-year-old woman was reported who presented 10 days postpartum with severe mental status changes and left arm and bilateral leg weakness that were refractory to magnesium therapy. Cerebral angiography demonstrated diffuse severe vasospasm and she was treated with balloon angioplasty of the bilateral middle and posterior cerebral arteries, basilar artery, and bilateral internal carotid arteries. Balloon angioplasty resulted in excellent angiographic improvement. The patient immediately became responsive and appropriate with improved strength in all extremities. She continued to improve throughout her hospital stay and was discharged 10 days post-angioplasty.[161]

Cerebral vasospasm in AVMs

A report[122] presented the results of using intra-arterial papaverine and balloon angioplasty in two patients with severe, symptomatic cerebral vasospasm who suffered ruptured arteriovenous malformations (AVMs). In both cases, the AVMs were located in the superior vermis and there was minimal subarachnoid hemorrhage. The first patient underwent removal of the AVM before the period of cerebral vasospasm and the second patient underwent removal of the AVM after the cerebral vasospasm had resolved. Another two cases of treatment by intra-arterial papaverine of cerebral vasospasm complicating the resection of an AVM were reported.[122] Both cases had successful reversal of vasospasm documented on angiography. In the first case, sustained neurological improvement occurred resulting in a normal outcome by the time of discharge. In the second case, neurological deterioration occurred with the development of cerebral edema. This complication was thought to be due to normal perfusion pressure breakthrough, on the basis of angiographic arterial vasodilation and increased cerebral blood flow.

Cerebral vasospasm in other conditions

Intra-arterial vasodilators have been used in anecdotal cases with idiopathic reversible vasospasm and with intraparenchymal hemorrhage[162] with high tolerability and reversal of angiographic vasospasm.

These new approaches for the treatment of vasospasm secondary to SAH may reduce the high morbidity and mortality associated with SAH. Attempts should be directed toward easy and early access for patients with SAH to centers that specialize in these procedures.

References

1. Fisher CM, Ojemann RG. Basal rupture of saccular aneurysm. A pathological case report. *J Neurosurg* 1978; **48**:642–4.

2. Hills E, Dunstan CR, Wong SY, Evans RA. Bone histology in young adult osteoporosis. *J Clin Pathol* 1989;**42**:391–7.

3. Adams HP, Jr. Prevention of brain ischemia after aneurysmal subarachnoid hemorrhage. *Neurol Clin* 1992;**10**:251–68.

4. Kassell NF, Torner JC, Haley EC, Jr., Jane JA, Adams HP, Kongable GL. The international cooperative study on the timing of aneurysm surgery. Part 1: Overall management results. *J Neurosurg* 1990;**73**:18–36.

5. Kindt GWMJ, Pritz M, Giammota S. Hypertension and hypervolemia as therapy for patients with vasospasm. *Proceedings of the Second International Workshop*, 1979:659.

6. SA M. Fluid management in sah. *Neurologist*. 1995;**1**:71–85.

7. Awad IA, Carter LP, Spetzler RF, Medina M, Williams FC, Jr. Clinical vasospasm after subarachnoid hemorrhage: Response to hypervolemic hemodilution and arterial hypertension. *Stroke* 1987;**18**:365–72.

8. Kassell NF, Peerless SJ, Durward QJ, Beck DW, Drake CG, Adams HP. Treatment of ischemic deficits from vasospasm with intravascular volume expansion and induced arterial hypertension. *Neurosurgery* 1982;**11**:337–43.

9. Nakajima K, Okuda OHN, Maeda M. Hypervolemic hemodilution therapy for symptomatic cerebral vasospasm. In: Sano k tk, Kassell NF, Sasaki T, eds. *Cerebral Vasospasm*. Tokyo: University of Tokyo Press; 1990:352–3.

10. Medlock MD, Dulebohn SC, Elwood PW. Prophylactic hypervolemia without calcium channel blockers in early aneurysm surgery. *Neurosurgery* 1992;**30**:12–16.

11. Tseng MY, Hutchinson PJ, Richards HK, *et al*. Acute systemic erythropoietin therapy to reduce delayed ischemic deficits following aneurysmal subarachnoid hemorrhage: a phase ii randomized, double-blind, placebo-controlled trial. Clinical article. *J Neurosurg* 2009;**111**:171–80.

12. McGirt MJ, Garces Ambrossi GL, Huang J, Tamargo RJ. Simvastatin for the prevention of symptomatic cerebral vasospasm following aneurysmal subarachnoid hemorrhage: a single-institution prospective cohort study. *J Neurosurg* 2009;**110**:968–74.

13. de Oliveira JG, Beck J, Ulrich C, Rathert J, Raabe A, Seifert V. Comparison between clipping and coiling on the incidence of cerebral vasospasm after aneurysmal subarachnoid hemorrhage: a systematic review and meta-analysis. *Neurosurg Rev* 2007;**30**:22–30; discussion 30–21.

14. Zwienenberg-Lee M, Hartman J, Rudisill N, *et al*. Effect of prophylactic transluminal balloon angioplasty on cerebral vasospasm and outcome in patients with Fisher Grade iii subarachnoid hemorrhage: results of a phase ii multicenter, randomized, clinical trial. *Stroke* 2008;**39**:1759–65.

15. Macdonald RL, Kassell NF, Mayer S, *et al*. Clazosentan to overcome neurological ischemia and infarction occurring after subarachnoid hemorrhage (conscious-1): randomized, double-blind, placebo-controlled phase 2 dose-finding trial. *Stroke* 2008;**39**:3015–21.

16. Macdonald RL, Weir BK. A review of hemoglobin and the pathogenesis of cerebral vasospasm. *Stroke* 1991;**22**:971–82.

17. Fisher CM, Kistler JP, Davis JM. Relation of cerebral vasospasm to subarachnoid hemorrhage visualized by computerized tomographic scanning. *Neurosurgery* 1980;**6**:1–9.

18. White RP, Hagen AA, Morgan H, Dawson WN, Robertson JT. Experimental study on the genesis of cerebral vasospasm. *Stroke* 1975;**6**:52–7.

19. Osaka K. Prolonged vasospasm produced by the breakdown products of erythrocytes. *J Neurosurg* 1977;**47**:403–11.

20. Miyaoka M, Nonaka T, Watanabe H, Chigasaki H, Ishi S. [etiology and treatment of prolonged vasospasm – experimental and clinical studies – (author's transl)]. *Neurol Med Chir (Tokyo)* 1976;**16**:103–14.

21. Sonobe M, Suzuki J. Vasospasmogenic substance produced following subarachnoid haemorrhage, and its fate. *Acta Neurochir (Wien)* 1978;**44**:97–106.

22. Okwuasaba F, Cook D, Weir B. Changes in vasoactive properties of blood products with time and attempted identification of the spasmogens. *Stroke* 1981;**12**:775–80.

23. Toda N. Mechanisms of contracting action of oxyhemoglobin in isolated monkey and dog cerebral arteries. *Am J Physiol* 1990;**258**:H57–63.

24. Fujii S, Fujitsu K. Experimental vasospasm in cultured arterial smooth-muscle cells. Part 1: Contractile and ultrastructural changes caused by oxyhemoglobin. *J Neurosurg* 1988;**69**:92–7.

25. Zaza A, Kline RP, Rosen MR. Effects of alpha-adrenergic stimulation on intracellular sodium activity and automaticity in canine purkinje fibers. *Circ Res* 1990;**66**:416–26.

26. Ohta t kh, Famatsu N, Yoshikawa Y, Someda K. Cerebral vasospasm and its relaxation response to vasodilation. Proceedings of the Second International Workshop. 1979

27. Peterson JW, Kwun BD, Hackett JD, Zervas NT. The role of inflammation in experimental cerebral vasospasm. *J Neurosurg* 1990;**72**:767–74.

28. Asano TWT, Tkakura K, Sano K, Shimizu T. Activation of lipooxygenase pathway following sub-arachnoid hemorrage; its relevance to cerebral vasospasm. New York: Raven Press; 1988.

29. Dupont JR, Van Wart CA, Kraintz L. The clearance of major components of whole blood from cerebrospinal fluid following simulated subarachnoid hemorrhage. *J Neuropathol Exp Neurol* 1961;**20**:450–5.

30. Wahlgren NG, Bergstrom K. Determination of haem derivatives in the cerebrospinal fluid – a semi-quantitative method. *J Neurol Neurosurg Psychiatry* 1983;**46**:653–8.

31. Sasaki T, Tanishima T, Asano T, Mayanagi Y, Sano K. Significance of lipid peroxidation in the genesis of chronic vasospasm following rupture of an intracranial aneurysm. *Acta Neurochir Suppl (Wien)* 1979;**28**:536–40.

32. Walker V, Pickard JD, Smythe P, Eastwood S, Perry S. Effects of subarachnoid haemorrhage on intracranial prostaglandins. *J Neurol Neurosurg Psychiatry* 1983;**46**:119–25.

33. Rodriguez y Baena R, Gaetani P, Grignani G, *et al*. Role of arachidonate metabolites in the genesis of cerebral vasospasm. *Adv Prostaglandin Thromboxane Leukot Res* 1987;**17B**:938–42.

34. Paoletti P, Gaetani P, Grignani G, Pacchiarini L, Silvani V, Rodriguez y Baena R. Csf leukotriene c4 following subarachnoid hemorrhage. *J Neurosurg* 1988;**69**:488–93.

35. White RP. Vasospasm 1 Experimental Findings. In Fox JL, ed. *Intra-cramial Aneurysms*, Vol I New York: Springer-Verlag; 1983, pp. 218–49.

36. Boullin DJ, Bunting S, Blaso WP, Hunt TM, Moncada S. Responses of human and baboon arteries to prostaglandin endoperoxides and biologically generated and synthetic prostacyclin: Their relevance to cerebral arterial spasm in man. *Br J Clin Pharmacol* 1979;**7**:139–47.

37. Paul KS, Whalley ET, Forster C, Lye R, Dutton J. Prostacylin and cerebral vessel relaxation. *J Neurosurg* 1982;**57**:334–40.

38. Onoue H, Kaito N, Akiyama M, Tomii M, Tokudome S, Abe T. Altered reactivity of human cerebral arteries after subarachnoid hemorrhage. *J Neurosurg* 1995;**83**:510–15.

39. Kim P, Lorenz RR, Sundt TM, Jr., Vanhoutte PM. Release of endothelium-derived relaxing factor after subarachnoid hemorrhage. *J Neurosurg* 1989;**70**:108–14.

40. Kim P, Schini VB, Sundt TM, Jr., Vanhoutte PM. Reduced production of cgmp underlies the loss of endothelium-dependent relaxations in the canine basilar artery after subarachnoid hemorrhage. *Circ Res* 1992;**70**:248–56.

41. Kim P, Sundt TM, Jr., Vanhoutte PM. Alterations in endothelium-dependent responsiveness of the canine basilar artery subarachnoid hemorrhage. *J Neurosurg* 1988;**69**:239–46.

42. Ohlstein EH, Storer BL. Oxyhemoglobin stimulation of endothelin production in cultured endothelial cells. *J Neurosurg* 1992;**77**:274–8.

43. Hamann GF, del Zoppo GJ. Leukocyte involvement in vasomotor reactivity of the cerebral vasculature. *Stroke* 1994;**25**:2117–19.

44. Fujimori A, Yanagisawa M, Saito A, *et al*. Endothelin in plasma and cerebrospinal fluid of patients with subarachnoid haemorrhage. *Lancet* 1990;**336**:633.

45. Kraus GE, Bucholz RD, Yoon KW, Knuepfer MM, Smith KR, Jr. Cerebrospinal fluid endothelin-1 and endothelin-3 levels in normal and neurosurgical patients: a clinical study

and literature review. *Surg Neurol* 1991;**35**:20–9.

46. Matsumura Y, Ikegawa R, Suzuki Y, *et al.* Phosphoramidon prevents cerebral vasospasm following subarachnoid hemorrhage in dogs: the relationship to endothelin-1 levels in the cerebrospinal fluid. *Life Sci* 1991;**49**:841–8.

47. Vajkoczy P, Meyer B, Weidauer S, *et al.* Clazosentan (axv-034343), a selective endothelin a receptor antagonist, in the prevention of cerebral vasospasm following severe aneurysmal subarachnoid hemorrhage: results of a randomized, double-blind, placebo-controlled, multicenter phase iia study. *J Neurosurg* 2005;**103**:9–17.

48. Weir B, MacDonald L. Cerebral vasospasm. *Clin Neurosurg* 1993;**40**:40–55.

49. Wilkins RH, Levitt P. Intracranial arterial spasm in the dog. A chronic experimental model. *J Neurosurg* 1970;**33**:260–9.

50. Conway LW, McDonald LW. Structural changes of the intradural arteries following subarachnoid hemorrhage. *J Neurosurg* 1972;**37**:715–23.

51. Peerless SJKN, Komatsu K, Hunter IG. Cerebral vasospam, acute proliferative vasculopathy?. *Proceeding of the Second International Workshop.* 1979;88–96.

52. Smith RR, Clower BR, Grotendorst GM, Yabuno N, Cruse JM. Arterial wall changes in early human vasospasm. *Neurosurgery* 1985;**16**:171–6.

53. Tanabe Y, Sakata K, Yamada H, Ito T, Takada M. Cerebral vasospasm and ultrastructural changes in cerebral arterial wall. An experimental study. *J Neurosurg* 1978;**49**:229–38.

54. Yamashima T, Hayashi M, Sato K, Hayase H, YamamotoS. [pathology of myonecrosis following cerebral vasospasm]. *Neurol Med Chir (Tokyo).* 1984;**24**:335–42.

55. Yamamoto Y, Bernanke DH, Smith RR. Accelerated non-muscle contraction after subarachnoid hemorrhage: cerebrospinal fluid testing in a culture model. *Neurosurgery* 1990;**27**:921–8.

56. Alksne JF, Greenhoot JH. Experimental catecholamine-induced chronic cerebral vasospasm. Myonecrosis in vessel wall. *J Neurosurg* 1974;**41**:440–5.

57. Bassiouni H, Schulz R, Dorge H, Stolke D, Heusch G. The impact of subarachnoid hemorrhage on regional cerebral blood flow and large-vessel diameter in the canine model of chronic vasospasm. *J Stroke Cerebrovasc Dis* 2007;**16**:45–51.

58. Kozniewska E, Michalik R, Rafalowska J, *et al.* Mechanisms of vascular dysfunction after subarachnoid hemorrhage. *J Physiol Pharmacol* 2006;**57** Suppl 11:145–60.

59. Sun BL, Zheng CB, Yang MF, Yuan H, Zhang SM, Wang LX. Dynamic alterations of cerebral pial microcirculation during experimental subarachnoid hemorrhage. *Cell Mol Neurobiol* 2009;**29**:235–41.

60. Yundt KD, Grubb RL, Jr., Diringer MN, Powers WJ. Autoregulatory vasodilation of parenchymal vessels is impaired during cerebral vasospasm. *J Cereb Blood Flow Metab* 1998;**18**:419–24.

61. Uhl E, Lehmberg J, Steiger HJ, Messmer K. Intraoperative detection of early microvasospasm in patients with subarachnoid hemorrhage by using orthogonal polarization spectral imaging. *Neurosurgery* 2003;**52**:1307–15; discussion 1315–17.

62. Vergouwen MD, Vermeulen M, Coert BA, Stroes ES, Roos YB. Microthrombosis after aneurysmal subarachnoid hemorrhage: An additional explanation for delayed cerebral ischemia. *J Cereb Blood Flow Metab* 2008;**28**:1761–70.

63. Crompton MR. The pathogenesis of cerebral infarction following the rupture of cerebral berry aneurysms. *Brain* 1964;**87**:491–510.

64. Schunk H. Spontaneous thrombosis of intracranial aneurysms. *Am J roentgenol* 1964;**91**:1327–38.

65. Black SPWGW. Observations on the relationship between the volume and the size of the orifice of experimental aneurysms. *J Neurosurg* 1960;**17**.

66. Romano JG, Forteza AM, Concha M, Koch S, Heros RC, Morcos JJ, Babikian VL. Detection of microemboli by transcranial doppler ultrasonography in aneurysmal subarachnoid hemorrhage. *Neurosurgery* 2002;**50**:1026–30; discussion 1030–1.

67. Chavez L, Takahashi A, Yoshimoto T, Su CC, Sugawara T, Fujii Y. Morphological changes in normal canine basilar arteries after transluminal angioplasty. *Neurol Res* 1990;**12**:12–16.

68. Yamamoto Y, Smith RR, Bernanke DH. Mechanism of action of balloon angioplasty in cerebral vasospasm. *Neurosurgery* 1992;**30**:1–5; discussion 5–6.

69. Zubkov YN, Alexander LF, Smith RR, Benashvili GM, Semenyutin V, Bernanke D. Angioplasty of vasospasm: is it reasonable? *Neurol Res* 1994;**16**:9–11.

70. Eskridge JM, Newell DW, Pendleton GA. Transluminal angioplasty for treatment of vasospasm. *Neurosurg Clin N Am* 1990;**1**:387–99.

71. Higashida RT, Halbach VV, Cahan LD, *et al.* Transluminal angioplasty for treatment of intracranial arterial vasospasm. *J Neurosurg* 1989;**71**:648–53.

72. Bracard S, Picard L, Marchal JC, *et al.* Role of angioplasty in the treatment of symptomatic vascular spasm occurring in the post-operative course of intracranial ruptured aneurysms. *J Neuroradiol* 1990;**17**:6–19.

73. Coyne TJ, Montanera WJ, Macdonald RL, Wallace MC. Percutaneous transluminal angioplasty for cerebral vasospasm after subarachnoid hemorrhage. *Can J Surg* 1994;**37**:391–6.

74. Konishi Y TM, Sata E. *Pta for vasospasm after sah.* Tokyo: University of Tokyo Press; 1990.

75. Nemoto S AT, Tanaka H, Sakamotot, Aruga T, Takakura K. *Percutaneous Transluminal Angioplasty for Cerebral Vasospasm Following Sub-arachnoid Hemorrhage.* Tokyo: University of Tokyo Press; 1990.

76. Takahashi A Yt, Mizoi K, Sugawara T, Fujii Y. *Transluminal Balloon Angioplasty for Cerebral Vasospasm after Sub-arachnoid Hemorrage.* Tokyo: University of Tokyo Press; 1990.

77. Bejjani GK, Bank WO, Olan WJ, Sekhar LN. The efficacy and safety of angioplasty for cerebral vasospasm after subarachnoid hemorrhage. *Neurosurgery* 1998;**42**:979–86; discussion 986–7.

78. Eskridge JM, McAuliffe W, Song JK, *et al.* Balloon angioplasty for the treatment of vasospasm: Results of first 50 cases. *Neurosurgery* 1998;**42**:510–16; discussion 516–17.

79. Firlik AD, Kaufmann AM, Jungreis CA, Yonas H. Effect of transluminal angioplasty on cerebral blood flow in the management of symptomatic vasospasm following aneurysmal subarachnoid hemorrhage. *J Neurosurg* 1997;**86**:830–9.

80. Terry A, Zipfel G, Milner E, et al. Safety and technical efficacy of over-the-wire balloons for the treatment of subarachnoid hemorrhage-induced cerebral vasospasm. Neurosurg Focus 2006;21:E14.

81. Newell DW, Eskridge J, Mayberg M, Grady MS, Lewis D, Winn HR. Endovascular treatment of intracranial aneurysms and cerebral vasospasm. Clin Neurosurg 1992;39:348–60.

82. Linskey ME, Horton JA, Rao GR, Yonas H. Fatal rupture of the intracranial carotid artery during transluminal angioplasty for vasospasm induced by subarachnoid hemorrhage. Case report. J Neurosurg 1991; 74:985–90.

83. Le Roux PD, Newell DW, Eskridge J, Mayberg MR, Winn HR. Severe symptomatic vasospasm: the role of immediate postoperative angioplasty. J Neurosurg 1994;80:224–9.

84. Terada T, Nakamura Y, Yoshida N, et al. Percutaneous transluminal angioplasty for the m2 portion vasospasm following sah: development of the new microballoon and report of cases. Surg Neurol 1993;39:13–17.

85. Livingston K, Guterman LR, Hopkins LN. Intraarterial papaverine as an adjunct to transluminal angioplasty for vasospasm induced by subarachnoid hemorrhage. Am J Neuroradiol. 1993;14:346–7.

86. Bolton TB. Mechanisms of action of transmitters and other substances on smooth muscle. Physiol Rev 1979;59:606–718.

87. Miyamoto M, Takayanagi I, Ohkubo H, Takagi K. Actions of papaverine on intestinal smooth muscle and its inhibition of cyclic amp and cyclic gmp phosphodiesterases. Jpn J Pharmacol. 1976:114–17.

88. Ogata MMB, Longhead WM. Observation on the effect of intrathecal papaverine on symptomatic vasospasm. J Neurosurg 1975;38.

89. Segawa HSi, Okada T, Nagayama I, Kitamura K, Sano K. Efficacy of Intracisternal Papaverine on Symptomatic Vasospasm. New York: Raven Press; 1988.

90. Vorkapic P, Bevan RD, Bevan JA. Longitudinal time course of reversible and irreversible components of chronic cerebrovasospasm of the rabbit basilar artery. J Neurosurg 1991;74:951–5.

91. Kassell NF, Helm G, Simmons N, Phillips CD, Cail WS. Treatment of cerebral vasospasm with intra-arterial papaverine. J Neurosurg. 1992;77:848–52.

92. Kaku Y, Yonekawa Y, Tsukahara T, Kazekawa K. Superselective intra-arterial infusion of papaverine for the treatment of cerebral vasospasm after subarachnoid hemorrhage. J Neurosurg. 1992;77:842–7.

93. Clouston JE, Numaguchi Y, Zoarski GH, Aldrich EF, Simard JM, Zitnay KM. Intraarterial papaverine infusion for cerebral vasospasm after subarachnoid hemorrhage. Am J Neuroradiol 1995;16:27–38.

94. Katoh H, Shima K, Shimizu A, et al. Clinical evaluation of the effect of percutaneous transluminal angioplasty and intra-arterial papaverine infusion for the treatment of vasospasm following aneurysmal subarachnoid hemorrhage. Neurol Res 1999;21: 195–203.

95. Morgan MK, Jonker B, Finfer S, Harrington T, Dorsch NW. Aggressive management of aneurysmal subarachnoid haemorrhage based on a papaverine angioplasty protocol. J Clin Neurosci 2000;7:305–8.

96. Schuknecht B, Fandino J, Yuksel C, Yonekawa Y, Valavanis A. Endovascular treatment of cerebral vasospasm: Assessment of treatment effect by cerebral angiography and transcranial colour doppler sonography. Neuroradiology 1999;41:453–62.

97. Marks MP, Steinberg GK, Lane B. Intraarterial papaverine for the treatment of vasospasm. Am J Neuroradiol 1993;14:822–6.

98. Mathis JM, Jensen ME, Dion JE. Technical considerations on intra-arterial papaverine hydrochloride for cerebral vasospasm. Neuroradiology 1997;39:90–8.

99. Carhuapoma JR, Qureshi AI, Tamargo RJ, Mathis JM, Hanley DF. Intra-arterial papaverine-induced seizures: Case report and review of the literature. Surg Neurol 2001;56:159–63.

100. Smith WS, Dowd CF, Johnston SC, et al. Neurotoxicity of intra-arterial papaverine preserved with chlorobutanol used for the treatment of cerebral vasospasm after aneurysmal subarachnoid hemorrhage. Stroke 2004;35:2518–22.

101. Becker U, Ehrhardt C, Schaefer UF, et al. Tissue distribution of moxaverine-hydrochloride in the rabbit eye and plasma. J Ocul Pharmacol Ther 2005;21:210–16.

102. Feng L, Fitzsimmons BF, Young WL, et al. Intraarterially administered verapamil as adjunct therapy for cerebral vasospasm: Safety and 2-year experience. Am J Neuroradiol. 2002;23:1284–90.

103. Shah QA, Georgiadis A, Suri MF, Rodriguez G, Qureshi AI. Preliminary experience with intra-arterial nicardipine in patients with acute ischemic stroke. Neurocrit Care 2007;7:53–7.

104. Shah QA, Memon MZ, Suri MF, et al. Super-selective intra-arterial magnesium sulfate in combination with nicardipine for the treatment of cerebral vasospasm in patients with subarachnoid hemorrhage. Neurocrit Care 2009; 11(2): 190–8.

105. Badjatia N, Topcuoglu MA, Pryor JC, et al. Preliminary experience with intra-arterial nicardipine as a treatment for cerebral vasospasm. Am J Neuroradiol. 2004;25:819–26.

106. Tejada JG, Taylor RA, Ugurel MS, Hayakawa M, Lee SK, Chaloupka JC. Safety and feasibility of intra-arterial nicardipine for the treatment of subarachnoid hemorrhage-associated vasospasm: Initial clinical experience with high-dose infusions. Am J Neuroradiol. 2007;28:844–8.

107. Amenta F, Tomassoni D. Treatment with nicardipine protects brain in an animal model of hypertension-induced damage. Clin Exp Hypertens 2004;26:351–61.

108. Kittaka M, Giannotta SL, Zelman V, et al. Attenuation of brain injury and reduction of neuron-specific enolase by nicardipine in systemic circulation following focal ischemia and reperfusion in a rat model. J Neurosurg. 1997;87:731–7.

109. Arakawa Y, Kikuta K, Hojo M, Goto Y, Ishii A, Yamagata S. Milrinone for the treatment of cerebral vasospasm after subarachnoid hemorrhage: Report of seven cases. Neurosurgery 2001;48: 723–8; discussion 728–30.

110. Conti A, Angileri FF, Longo M, Pitrone A, Granata F, La Rosa G. Intra-arterial nimodipine to treat symptomatic cerebral vasospasm following traumatic subarachnoid haemorrhage. Technical

case report. *Acta Neurochir (Wien)* 2008;**150**:1197–202; discussion 1202.

111. Firlik KS, Kaufmann AM, Firlik AD, Jungreis CA, Yonas H. Intra-arterial papaverine for the treatment of cerebral vasospasm following aneurysmal subarachnoid hemorrhage. *Surg Neurol* 1999;**51**:66–74.

112. Fraticelli AT, Cholley BP, Losser MR, Saint Maurice JP, Payen D. Milrinone for the treatment of cerebral vasospasm after aneurysmal subarachnoid hemorrhage. *Stroke* 2008;**39**:893–8.

113. Keuskamp J, Murali R, Chao KH. High-dose intraarterial verapamil in the treatment of cerebral vasospasm after aneurysmal subarachnoid hemorrhage. *J Neurosurg* 2008;**108**:458–63.

114. Linfante I, Delgado-Mederos R, Andreone V, Gounis M, Hendricks L, Wakhloo AK. Angiographic and hemodynamic effect of high concentration of intra-arterial nicardipine in cerebral vasospasm. *Neurosurgery* 2008;**63**:1080–6; discussion 1086–7.

115. Liu JK, Couldwell WT. Intra-arterial papaverine infusions for the treatment of cerebral vasospasm induced by aneurysmal subarachnoid hemorrhage. *Neurocrit Care* 2005;**2**:124–32.

116. Nogueira RG, Lev MH, Roccatagliata L, *et al.* Intra-arterial nicardipine infusion improves ct perfusion-measured cerebral blood flow in patients with subarachnoid hemorrhage-induced vasospasm. *Am J Neuroradiol* 2009;**30**:160–4.

117. Numaguchi Y, Zoarski GH. Intra-arterial papaverine treatment for cerebral vasospasm: Our experience and review of the literature. *Neurol Med Chir (Tokyo)* 1998;**38**:189–95.

118. Polin RS, Hansen CA, German P, Chadduck JB, Kassell NF. Intra-arterially administered papaverine for the treatment of symptomatic cerebral vasospasm. *Neurosurgery* 1998;**42**:1256–64; discussion 1264–7.

119. Romero CM, Morales D, Reccius A, *et al.* Milrinone as a rescue therapy for symptomatic refractory cerebral vasospasm in aneurysmal subarachnoid hemorrhage. *Neurocrit Care* 2008; **11** (2): 165–71.

120. Suzuki S, Ito O, Sayama T, Yamaguchi S, Goto K, Sasaki T. Intraarterial injection of colforsin daropate hydrochloride for the treatment of vasospasm after aneurysmal subarachnoid hemorrhage: Preliminary report of two cases. *Neuroradiology* 2006;**48**:50–3.

121. Tsurushima H, Hyodo A, Yoshii Y. Papaverine and vasospasm. *J Neurosurg* 2000;**92**:509–11.

122. Zubkov AY, Lewis AI, Scalzo D. Transluminal angioplasty and intra-arterial papaverine for the treatment of cerebral vasospasm after ruptured arteriovenous malformations. *Surg Neurol* 1999;**51**:75–9; discussion 80.

123. Elliott JP, Newell DW, Lam DJ, *et al.* Comparison of balloon angioplasty and papaverine infusion for the treatment of vasospasm following aneurysmal subarachnoid hemorrhage. *J Neurosurg* 1998;**88**:277–84.

124. Terada T, Kinoshita Y, Yokote H, *et al.* The effect of endovascular therapy for cerebral arterial spasm, its limitation and pitfalls. *Acta Neurochir (Wien)* 1997;**139**:227–34.

125. Hoh BL, Ogilvy CS. Endovascular treatment of cerebral vasospasm: Transluminal balloon angioplasty, intra-arterial papaverine, and intra-arterial nicardipine. *Neurosurg Clin N Am* 2005;**16**:501–16.

126. Coenen VA, Hansen CA, Kassell NF, Polin RS. Endovascular treatment for symptomatic cerebral vasospasm after subarachnoid hemorrhage: Transluminal balloon angioplasty compared with intraarterial papaverine. *Neurosurg Focus* 1998;**5**:e6.

127. Johnston SC. Effect of endovascular services and hospital volume on cerebral aneurysm treatment outcomes. *Stroke* 2000;**31**:111–17.

128. Jestaedt L, Pham M, Bartsch AJ, *et al.* The impact of balloon angioplasty on the evolution of vasospasm-related infarction after aneurysmal subarachnoid hemorrhage. *Neurosurgery* 2008;**62**:610–17; discussion 610–17.

129. Megyesi JF, Findlay JM, Vollrath B, Cook DA, Chen MH. In vivo angioplasty prevents the development of vasospasm in canine carotid arteries. Pharmacological and morphological analyses. *Stroke* 1997;**28**:1216–24.

130. Muizelaar JP, Zwienenberg M, Rudisill NA, Hecht ST. The prophylactic use of transluminal balloon angioplasty in patients with fisher grade 3 subarachnoid hemorrhage: a pilot study. *J Neurosurg* 1999;**91**:51–8.

131. Murayama Y, Song JK, Uda K, *et al.* Combined endovascular treatment for both intracranial aneurysm and symptomatic vasospasm. *Am J Neuroradiol* 2003;**24**:133–9.

132. Qureshi AI, Suarez JI, Bhardwaj A, Yahia AM, Tamargo RJ, Ulatowski JA. Early predictors of outcome in patients receiving hypervolemic and hypertensive therapy for symptomatic vasospasm after subarachnoid hemorrhage. *Crit Care Med* 2000;**28**:824–9.

133. Harrigan MR, Magnano CR, Guterman LR, Hopkins LN. Computed tomographic perfusion in the management of aneurysmal subarachnoid hemorrhage: new application of an existent technique. *Neurosurgery* 2005;**56**:304–17; discussion 317.

134. Wintermark M, Dillon WP, Smith WS, *et al.* Visual grading system for vasospasm based on perfusion ct imaging: comparisons with conventional angiography and quantitative perfusion ct. *Cerebrovasc Dis* 2008;**26**:163–70.

135. van der Schaaf I, Wermer MJ, van der Graaf Y, Hoff RG, Rinkel GJ, Velthuis BK. Ct after subarachnoid hemorrhage: Relation of cerebral perfusion to delayed cerebral ischemia. *Neurology* 2006;**66**:1533–8.

136. Hertel F, Walter C, Bettag M, Morsdorf M. Perfusion-weighted magnetic resonance imaging in patients with vasospasm: a useful new tool in the management of patients with subarachnoid hemorrhage. *Neurosurgery* 2005;**56**:28–35; discussion 35.

137. Beck J, Raabe A, Lanfermann H, *et al.* Effects of balloon angioplasty on perfusion- and diffusion-weighted magnetic resonance imaging results and outcome in patients with cerebral vasospasm. *J Neurosurg* 2006;**105**:220–7.

138. Chaturvedi S, St Pierre ME, Bertasio B. Cerebral angioplasty practice at major medical centers in the United States. *Neuroradiology* 2000;**42**:218–20.

139. Fandino J, Kaku Y, Schuknecht B, Valavanis A, Yonekawa Y. Improvement of cerebral oxygenation patterns and metabolic validation of superselective intraarterial infusion of papaverine for the treatment of cerebral vasospasm. *J Neurosurg* 1998;**89**:93–100.

140. Lewis DH, Paul Elliott J, Newell DW, Eskridge JM, Richard Winn H.

Interventional endovascular therapy: Spect cerebral blood flow imaging compared with transcranial doppler monitoring of ballon angioplasty and intraarterial papaverine for cerebral vasospasm. *J Stroke Cerebrovasc Dis* 1999;**8**:71–5.

141. Majoie CB, van Boven LJ, van de Beek D, Venema HW, van Rooij WJ. Perfusion ct to evaluate the effect of transluminal angioplasty on cerebral perfusion in the treatment of vasospasm after subarachnoid hemorrhage. *Neurocrit Care* 2007;**6**:40–4.

142. Milburn JM, Moran CJ, Cross DT, 3rd, Diringer MN, Pilgram TK, Dacey RG, Jr. Increase in diameters of vasospastic intracranial arteries by intraarterial papaverine administration. *J Neurosurg* 1998;**88**:38–42.

143. Murai Y, Kominami S, Kobayashi S, Mizunari T, Teramoto A. The long-term effects of transluminal balloon angioplasty for vasospasms after subarachnoid hemorrhage: analyses of cerebral blood flow and reactivity. *Surg Neurol* 2005;**64**:122–6; discussion 127.

144. Ohkawa M, Fujiwara N, Tanabe M, *et al.* Cerebral vasospastic vessels: Histologic changes after percutaneous transluminal angioplasty. *Radiology* 1996;**198**:179–84.

145. Oskouian RJ, Jr., Martin NA, Lee JH, *et al.* Multimodal quantitation of the effects of endovascular therapy for vasospasm on cerebral blood flow, transcranial doppler ultrasonographic velocities, and cerebral artery diameters. *Neurosurgery* 2002;**51**:30–41; discussion 41–3.

146. Ohkuma H, Manabe H, Tanaka M, Suzuki S. Impact of cerebral microcirculatory changes on cerebral blood flow during cerebral vasospasm after aneurysmal subarachnoid hemorrhage. *Stroke* 2000;**31**:1621–7.

147. Okada Y, Shima T, Nishida M, *et al.* [evaluation of angiographic delayed vasospasm due to ruptured aneurysm in comparison with cerebral circulation time measured by ia-dsa]. *No Shinkei Geka* 1994;**22**:439–45.

148. Frontera JA, Fernandez A, Schmidt JM, *et al.* Defining vasospasm after subarachnoid hemorrhage: what is the most clinically relevant definition? *Stroke* 2009;**40**:1963–8.

149. Hanggi D, Turowski B, Beseoglu K, Yong M, Steiger HJ. Intra-arterial nimodipine for severe cerebral vasospasm after aneurysmal subarachnoid hemorrhage: Influence on clinical course and cerebral perfusion. *Am J Neuroradiol* 2008;**29**:1053–60.

150. Tariq N, Qureshi MN, Suri MFK, *et al.* Compliant versus non-compliant balloons for endovascular treatment of vasospasm after subarachnoid hemorrhage. *American Academy of Neurology 61st Annual Meeting.* 2009.

151. Schmid-Elsaesser R, Kunz M, Zausinger S, Prueckner S, Briegel J, Steiger HJ. Intravenous magnesium versus nimodipine in the treatment of patients with aneurysmal subarachnoid hemorrhage: a randomized study. *Neurosurgery* 2006;**58**:1054–65; discussion 1054–65.

152. Boet R, Mee E. Magnesium sulfate in the management of patients with fisher grade 3 subarachnoid hemorrhage: a pilot study. *Neurosurgery* 2000;**47**:602–6; discussion 606–7.

153. Milburn JM, Moran CJ, Cross DT, 3rd, Diringer MN, Pilgram TK, Dacey RG, Jr. Effect of intraarterial papaverine on cerebral circulation time. *Am J Neuroradiol* 1997;**18**:1081–5.

154. Liu JK, Tenner MS, Gottfried ON, *et al.* Efficacy of multiple intraarterial papaverine infusions for improvement in cerebral circulation time in patients with recurrent cerebral vasospasm. *J Neurosurg* 2004;**100**:414–21.

155. Andaluz N, Tomsick TA, Tew JM, Jr., van Loveren HR, Yeh HS, Zuccarello M. Indications for endovascular therapy for refractory vasospasm after aneurysmal subarachnoid hemorrhage: experience at the university of cincinnati. *Surg Neurol* 2002;**58**:131–8; discussion 138.

156. Rabinstein AA, Friedman JA, Nichols DA, *et al.* Predictors of outcome after endovascular treatment of cerebral vasospasm. *Am J Neuroradiol* 2004;**25**:1778–82.

157. Rosenwasser RH, Armonda RA, Thomas JE, Benitez RP, Gannon PM, Harrop J. Therapeutic modalities for the management of cerebral vasospasm: timing of endovascular options. *Neurosurgery* 1999;**44**:975–9; discussion 979–80.

158. Polin RS, Coenen VA, Hansen CA, *et al.* Efficacy of transluminal angioplasty for the management of symptomatic cerebral vasospasm following aneurysmal subarachnoid hemorrhage. *J Neurosurg* 2000;**92**:284–90.

159. Armonda RA, Bell RS, Vo AH, *et al.* Wartime traumatic cerebral vasospasm: Recent review of combat casualties. *Neurosurgery* 2006;**59**:1215–25; discussion 1225.

160. Qureshi AI, Frankel MR, Ottenlips JR, Stern BJ. Cerebral hemodynamics in preeclampsia and eclampsia. *Arch Neurol* 1996;**53**:1226–31.

161. Ringer AJ, Qureshi AI, Kim SH, Fessler RD, Guterman LR, Hopkins LN. Angioplasty for cerebral vasospasm from eclampsia. *Surg Neurol* 2001;**56**:373–8; discussion 378–9.

162. IA K. Cerebral vasospasm in intracerebral hemorrhage-case report. *J Vasc and Interventional Neurol* 2009;**2**:139–41.

163. Zubkov AY, Lewis AI, Scalzo D, Bernanke DH, Harkey HL. Morphological changes after percutaneous transluminal angioplasty. *Surg Neurol* 1999; **51**:399–403.

164. Petruk KC, West M, Mohr G, *et al.* Nimodipine treatment in poor-grade aneurysm patients. Results of a multicenter double-blind placebo-controlled trial. *J Neurosurg* 1988;**68**:505–17.

165. Weidauer S, Lanfermann H, Raabe A, Zanella F, Seifert V, Beck J. Impairment of cerebral perfusion and infarct patterns attributable to vasospasm after aneurysmal subarachnoid hemorrhage: a prospective mri and dsa study. *Stroke* 2007;**38**:1831–6.

166. Ko NU, Rajendran P, Kim H, *et al.* Endothelial nitric oxide synthase polymorphism (-786t->c) and increased risk of angiographic vasospasm after aneurysmal subarachnoid hemorrhage. *Stroke* 2008;**39**:1103–8.

167. Udoetuk JD, Stiefel MF, Hurst RW, Weigele JB, LeRoux PD. Admission angiographic cerebral circulation time may predict subsequent angiographic vasospasm after aneurysmal subarachnoid hemorrhage. *Neurosurgery* 2007;**61**:1152–9; discussion 1159–61.

168. Sutherland GR, King ME, Peerless SJ, Vezina WC, Brown GW, Chamberlain MJ. Platelet interaction within giant intracranial gneurgsms. *J Neurosurg* 1982;**56**(1):53–61.

Intracranial arteriovenous malformations

Dorothea Strozyk MD, Carlos E. Baccin MD, Johnny C. Pryor MD and Raul G. Nogueira MD

Introduction

Arteriovenous malformations (AVMs) are relatively uncommon, but increasingly recognized lesions than can cause serious neurological symptoms or death.[1,2] AVMs are highly complex vascular lesions that resemble tortuous agglomerations of abnormally dilated arteries and veins in the brain. They are typically supplied by one or more feeding arteries, and drain into deep veins, superficial veins, or both. In their core region or nidus, the AVMs lack a capillary bed, thereby allowing high-flow AV shunting.

AVMs typically present in young adults and have a variety of clinical manifestations including hemorrhage, seizures, headaches, and progressive neurological deterioration with or without focal signs. Although AVMs most commonly present with intracranial hemorrhage (ICH), since the advent of contemporary brain imaging techniques, an increasing number of AVMs are detected before they rupture. Indeed, the number of AVMs identified before rupture/hemorrhage is now twice those identified after rupture. This has led to new considerations and modifications of interdisciplinary AVM management strategies.[3]

Over the last decade, there have been significant developments in the management of AVMs including novel and optimized endovascular as well as microsurgical and radiosurgical techniques. The most common and compelling reason for treatment is the prevention of hemorrhage. Existing data indicate that only complete eradication of the lesion provides protection from future ICH, whereas partial treatment is not helpful and may, in fact, increase the rate of future hemorrhage.[4–6]

To a greater extent than any of the other vascular lesions of the central nervous system, the treatment of intracranial AVMs requires a multimethod and multidisciplinary approach. The available options for treatment include endovascular embolization, microsurgical resection, radiosurgery, medical management or a combination of these treatment modalities.

The most critical step in the successful management of any patient's AVM is the formulation of a treatment strategy designed to optimize the risk-to-benefit ratio. This is predicated on an understanding of the natural history of the lesion, as well as the morbidity and mortality associated with various treatments.

The following chapter will discuss the epidemiology, etiology, classification, and clinical presentation of brain AVMs in adults. Further, it will provide a detailed review of various endovascular treatment options.

Epidemiology

The incidence and prevalence of intracranial AVMs are not known with certainty, although there are data available from autopsy series and retrospective population-based studies on the incidence of AVMs. In the Cooperative Study of Subarachnoid hemorrhage, still the largest such series to date, symptomatic AVMs were found in 549 of 6368 cases, representing an incidence of 8.6% of all non-traumatic subarachnoid hemorrhages (SAH).[7] Because SAH accounts for roughly 10% of strokes, AVMs make up approximately 1% of all strokes.

During the era before non-invasive brain imaging, one autopsy study detected 196 AVMs among 4530 consecutive autopsies, yielding an incidence of 4.3%.[8] Although not derived from a population-based study, these data are of interest because they represent a careful autopsy-based effort to determine the prevalence of AVMs, both symptomatic and asymptomatic. Only 24 of the 196 patients (12.2%) in this study had experienced AVM-related symptoms. This figure yields a symptomatic AVM incidence of 0.53% in this population that underwent autopsy, which is in the range of the 1% prevalence derived from clinical studies. Among the 24 patients with symptomatic AVMs, 21 had suffered ICH, and the remaining three had seizures or focal neurological signs. Calculated estimates from hospital based autopsy data may be unreliable as the data might be affected by the frequency of imaging tests that were performed searching for such lesions, the age and cause of death of the patient, and the presence of neurological symptoms.

In the Netherlands Antilles between 1980 and 1990, an annual incidence of 1.1 symptomatic AVMs per 100 000 people was identified.[9] Of the 17 patients identified, 16 presented with ICH. In this fairly isolated and homogenous population, however, an unusually high proportion of the patients had multiple brain AVMs (25%), and hereditary hemorrhagic teleangiectasia (Rendu–Osler–Weber disease) (35%), making it difficult to compare the findings with those described in other populations. In a retrospective, population-based study conducted over 27 years in Olmsted County, MN, the incidence of symptomatic ICH due to any type of intracranial vascular malformations was 0.8 per 100 000.[10,11] Of the 20 patients recorded, 17 (85%) had an underlying brain AVM. No separate incidence for AVM hemorrhage was calculated.

The New York Island AVM Hemorrhage Study is an ongoing prospective population-based survey determining the incidence of AVM hemorrhage and associated morbidity and mortality rates in a population of over 9 million people located in New York. Initial results calculated an AVM detection rate of 1.34 per 100 000 person years, and a first-ever acute AVM hemorrhage rate of 0.51 per 100 000 person–years.[12] These rates reflect increased use of MRI due to low threshold for imaging. Many AVMs were discovered before hemorrhage in this study.

Etiology and pathogenesis

Whether AVMs are present at birth, are acquired during infancy, or grow in size during childhood are questions of debate, but most reports assume that these lesions are primarily congenital. Growing insights into the development of the human cerebrovasculature system have fostered theories on the etiology of arteriovenous malformations.[2]

The introduction of fetal ultrasound screening has offered an opportunity to study vascular malformations during gestation, and a few patients have also been studied by prenatal magnetic resonance imaging.[13] Due to these studies an increasing number of vascular malformations has been detected, i.e., vein of Galen malformations, but comparable detection rates of fetal AVMs have not been described.[14] The lack of observed cases in which a brain AVM was detected at earlier fetal stages challenges the widespread assumption that these lesions arise from an embryonic disturbance at the time of the vessel formation.

Arteries, veins, and capillaries do not exist per se in the earliest stages of fetal development. Initially, all embryonic cerebral vessels are simple endothelial tubes. As heart function develops and intracranial blood flow commences, some of these primitive vascular channels normally evolve into arterial vessels, whereas others become venous. It has been hypothesized that retention of the primordial, direct vascular connections between the future arterial and venous circulations combined with agenesis or poor development of the capillary network may lead to AVMs.[15]

A number of pathological changes underlie the structure of brain AVMs including (1) clusters of abnormally muscularized arteries, which may display changes in the elastica layer varying from destruction to duplication and fibrosis of the media as well as focal thinning of the wall; (2) arterialized veins of different sizes and wall thickness; (3) ambiguous vessels showing both arterial and venous characteristics or formed by fibrous tissue; and (4) intervening gliotic neural parenchyma.

The exact pathogenetic mechanisms leading to the lack of capillaries in the AVM nidus remain as yet unclear. The capillary density – that is, the number of capillaries in a given volume of brain tissue – remains stable after the fourth month of gestation, whereas the relative capillary volume in the cortex increases in a linear fashion from the end of the first trimester throughout infancy.[16] A higher endothelial turnover in the AVM vasculature may suggest the presence of active angiogenesis or ongoing vascular remodeling through early childhood.[17] Much effort is currently being devoted to defining predisposing factors at the molecular level that modulate the development of brain vasculature. In regards to AVMs, several candidate proteins are currently under investigation, including endothelial angiopoeitin receptor Tie-2,[18,19] basic fibroblast growth factor (FGF-2),[20] nitric oxidase synthase (NOS),[21] transforming growth factor beta (TGF-β),[22,23] vascular endothelial growth factor (VEGF),[21,24] and endoglin.[25]

Once the initial lesion has emerged, the permanent intraluminal stress arising from abnormal flow and pressure may lead to so-called secondary angiopathy, a non-reversible abnormal remodeling process in otherwise normal neighboring vessels. Whether any of the suggested molecular factors may play a role in the biologic mechanisms that eventually lead to AVM growth, to secondary angiopathy, and to phenomena such as spontaneous obliteration[26] and recurrence after successful therapy[27] has yet to be determined. AVM recurrences have been almost exclusively described in patients under 20 years of age, which implies the propensity of recurrence of cerebral AVMs in immature brain vasculature,[27,28] and supports the notion that angiogenesis may play a major role in the etiology of AVMs.

The presumably congenital nature of AVMs might be expected to yield many cases with a family history, but the familial incidence appears to be quite rare.[29–32] Only 20 families have been reported in the literature (44 cases).[33] The mode of inheritance is uncertain. AVMs usually occur in isolation, unrelated to other disease states, but a few have been associated with Rendu–Osler–Weber disease (hereditary hemorrhagic teleangiectasia), most of them small.[34,35] AVMs have also been described in the Wyburn–Mason syndrome, von Hippel Lindau disease, and Sturge–Weber disease.[33,35–37]

Clinical presentation

Intracranial AVMs are occasionally seen in the elderly, but are typically diagnosed before the patient has reached the age of 40 years (mean 35 years ± standard deviation 18).[12] There is no gender predilection.

ICH is the initial manifestation of AVMs in at least 50% of cases, although the exact numbers depend on whether the series has been collected in a referral center for neurological or neurosurgical diseases.[10,12,38,39] Parenchymal hemorrhage occurs more commonly, although SAH and intraventricular hemorrhage can also occur. Unlike SAH related to intracranial aneurysms, AVM related hemorrhages into the subarachnoid space are generally confined to local subarachnoid spaces and do not spread widely into the large cisterns. Severe vasospasm from AVM-related hemorrhage is distinctly uncommon, but it has been occasionally noted.[40]

The next most common presentation is seizure, which occurs in about 20%–50% of cases, often alerting the physician to the presence of an AVM before it ruptures.[41–43] The available literature documents a remarkable variation in incidence of seizures associated with AVMs. In general, seizures are believed to be the initial manifestation in about one-third of cases. Inconsistent data from reports precludes accurate determination of the relationship between seizures and subsequent risk of ICH. Several types of attacks labeled as seizures occur, and the type of seizure is often unreported in studies. Seizures can be either focal or generalized and may be an indicator of the location of the lesion. The role of anatomic location in seizure occurrence has received limited study, but suggestions have been made of a correlation of seizures with AVMs at the cortical surface. Several studies found seizures to be associated with AVMs of the cerebral surface but not with deep AVMs.[7,44–46] Whether the character of the seizure differs when it is associated with a hematoma is not certain.

Headache is the presenting symptom in about 15% of AVM patients. Because headaches are a common complaint in the population at large, it has been difficult to determine whether the headaches associated with AVMs are unique to the condition. In contrast to early assumptions, the headaches in AVMs are of no distinctive type, frequency, persistence or severity. Migraine headaches with and without aura have been documented in the literature,[47] and there are reports that migraine headaches may be associated with AVMs in the occipital region presenting with hemianopic deficits always on the same side, and the hemianopia following rather than preceding the headache.[48,49] Very little evidence supports the claim that recurrent unilateral headaches should arouse suspicion of an ipsilateral AVM. The yield for AVMs in evaluation for headache is low; in one study, only 0.2% of patients with normal neurologic findings who underwent neuroimaging for headache were diagnosed with AVM.[50]

The post-operative disappearance of migraine headaches is not unusual and may occur after any type of operation. The question raised is whether all patients with migraine should be evaluated for an AVM. We recommend neuroimaging for any patient with new onset migraines, focal signs, or unusual features.

Focal neurological signs without hemorrhage are very rare. Slowly progressing neurological deficits, which were once considered very common, are part of the presentation in only few patients (4% to 8%).[51–55] Insidiously developing neurological deficits can be focal or more general, in the form of cognitive dysfuntion.[56] Shunting through a low resistance AVM results in hypoperfusion of the surrounding normal brain tissue, a phenomenon known as vascular "steal"; however, evidence for a causal link with ischemic symptoms is lacking.[41] Venous hypertension and mass effect of the nidus offer alternative explanations for progressing focal neurological deficits.[57] An exceptional manifestation of AVMs is cranial nerve dysfunction, such as pulsatile tinnitus and hemifacial spasm, through pressure by a dilated draining vein.[58]

Natural history

The natural history of AVMs is variable depending upon several clinical and angiographic characteristics. The studies assessing the natural history of AVMs are limited by variations in patient characteristics, duration of follow-up, treatments used, and ascertainment of endpoints. Most series have retrospectively collected data, usually with limited follow-up periods, often lacking consistent angiographic assessment, and focusing on non-operable lesions causing a bias towards AVMs that are larger, deeper, or located in "eloquent" areas of the brain.

Notwithstanding these short-comings, a reasonable overall estimate is an annual risk of bleeding of 2% to 4%.[43,59–61] Several studies have addressed the difference in baseline characteristics of AVMs presenting with hemorrhage and AVMs with other clinical manifestations, and a single study followed two such groups for an average period of 10 months.[62] Among those patients who presented with symptoms other than hemorrhage, the annual risk for hemorrhage was 2.2% (3.3% per year for men and 1.3% per year for women).

If one assumes an annual hemorrhage risk among people with previously unruptured AVMs of 2% to 4% per year, the lifetime risk of ICH in a person with an AVM is approximated by the following formula:[63,64]

Lifetime risk (%) = 105–the patient's age in years

In the year immediately after a symptomatic hemorrhage, the re-hemorrhage risk is generally thought to be considerably higher, on the order of 6%[65,66] to 18%[62,67] per year, gradually returning toward the 2% to 4% baseline with time.[61,68]

Graf *et al.* reviewed the records of 191 patients with AVMs with a mean period of follow-up of two to five years.[65] They found a high rate of initial ICH in the age group 11 to 35 years old, and the rate of rebleeding was about 2% per year. Smaller lesions were more prone to ICH, and approximately 13% of the patients died as a result of the hemorrhage.

The risk of recurrent hemorrhage may be even higher in the first year after the second hemorrhage and has been reported to be 25% during that year.[66] However, the increased rate in the first year after initial hemorrhage has not been noted consistently.[59] Asymptomatic hemorrhages may not come to medical attention leading to underreporting in bleeding rates. One study has shown that approximately 15% of operated AVMs show evidence of prior asymptomatic hemorrhage.[69]

Risk factors for hemorrhage identified by more than one study, and therefore not likely to represent a chance finding, include: history of prior hemorrhage,[62,70] exclusive deep venous drainage,[71–73] presence of a single draining vein,[70,74] high intranidal pressures,[72,75,76] and the presence of intranidal aneurysms.[77,78] The relevance of these risk factors was recently reported by Stapf *et al.* These authors analyzed follow-up data on 622 consecutive patients from the prospective Columbia AVM database, limited to the period between initial AVM diagnosis and the start of treatment (i.e., any endovascular, surgical, or radiation therapy). The mean pretreatment follow-up was 829 days (median: 102 days), during which 39 (6%) patients experienced AVM hemorrhage. Increasing age (hazard ratio [HR] 1.05, 95% CI 1.03 to 1.08), initial hemorrhagic AVM presentation (HR 5.38, 95% CI 2.64 to 10.96), deep brain location (HR 3.25, 95% CI 1.30 to 8.16), and exclusive deep venous drainage (HR 3.25, 95% CI 1.01 to 5.67) were independent predictors of subsequent hemorrhage. Annual hemorrhage rates on follow-up ranged from 0.9% for patients without hemorrhagic AVM presentation, deep AVM location, or deep venous drainage to as high as 34.4% for those harboring all three risk factors.[79] The impact of other patient characteristics such as gender or history of hypertension has not been consistently identified as risk factors for hemorrhage.

The mortality from the first hemorrhage is between 10% and 25%,[43,59] although some data suggest the mortality rate may be even lower.[80] An estimated 10% to 30% of survivors have long-term disability.[68]

Diagnosis

Intracranial AVMs may be diagnosed with a variety of diagnostic imaging studies. Computed tomography (CT) without contrast has a low sensitivity, but calcification and hypointensities may be noted alerting the physician to pursue more detailed imaging; enhancement is seen within the AVM nidus after contrast administration.[81] CT angiography (Fig. 13.1(a), 13.1(b)) has become a valuable adjunct in the diagnosis and therapeutic planning of cerebral AVMs and may even allow for the identification of the rupture site in some situations (Fig. 13.2(a)).[82]

Magnetic resonance imaging (MRI) is very sensitive, showing inhomogenous signal void T1- and T2-weighted sequences, commonly with hemosiderin suggesting prior hemorrhage.[83,84] MRI can also provide information detailing the localization and topography of an AVM if intervention is being considered. Non-invasive conventional and functional MRI techniques are playing an increasing role in the interventional management because they facilitate localization of the nidus in relation to the brain and further identify functionally important brain areas adjacent to the nidus.[85,86]

In addition, magnetic resonance (MR) angiography can provide further data. Indeed, new MR techniques combining highly temporally resolved and highly spatially resolved MR angiography have allowed for non-invasive assessment of not only the vascular anatomy but also the hemodynamics of cerebral AVMs.[87] Nevertheless, the detailed AVM characteristics such as presence of intranidal or feeding artery aneurysms, comprehensive data on venous drainage patterns, or subtle AVM nidus characterization are better delineated with cerebral angiography.[88]

Catheter angiography remains the gold standard for defining the arterial and venous anatomy. Common international guidelines for diagnosing brain AVMs have not as yet been established. Confidence in the diagnosis of AVMs is crucial in planning the appropriate therapy. Brain AVMs must be separated from other intracranial AV fistulas, which at times have similar morphologic features on conventional imaging studies. These lesions, however, differ in terms of pathogenesis, natural course, and treatment strategies.

On the basis of available information, it is recommended that an MRI study and a four-vessel angiogram be obtained to delineate the anatomy of the AVM.

The angiographic evaluation of a cerebral AVM is usually performed in two steps: (1) selective angiographic investigation of the AVM itself and the remainder of the cerebral vasculature, and (2) superselective angiographic investigation of the AVM nidus with microcatheters. The diagnostic images are acquired and reviewed to identify the important aspects of AVMS outlined in Table 13.1.[89]

A selective, technically complete, diagnostic angiogram studying an AVM should provide detailed information regarding the individual feeding arteries and their vascular territories as well as delineate the venous drainage. Assessment of the nidus and identification of flow-related angiopathy, both arterial and venous, should be performed. The angiographic images should be evaluated carefully for the presence of aneurysms. Because of their propensity for hemorrhage, flow-related aneurysms proximal to the nidus and nidal aneurysms should generally be addressed before the remainder of the lesion. The venous phase images represent another critical component of the angiographic evaluation. The visualization of draining veins can vary with the parent vessel injected because different parts of the nidus are opacified and are associated with patterns of contrast washout. The presence of any pre-existing venous outflow stenoses should be noted because inadvertent occlusion of venous efflux during embolization represents one of the most dangerous complications that may be encountered. In many cases, the specific arterial branches supplying the lesion can be difficult to identify before superselective angiography. However, the vascular distributions involved and the approximate number and size of feeding arterial vessels can be ascertained. This information is usually sufficient to estimate the number of stages that will be required for adequate presurgical embolization. In addition, superselective angiography with microcatheters should provide more extensive and detailed information, including angiopathic changes in the feeding arteries, delineation of the nidus, and outlet obstruction or ectasias in the draining venous system. Superselective angiography is often combined with endovascular treatment of these lesions.

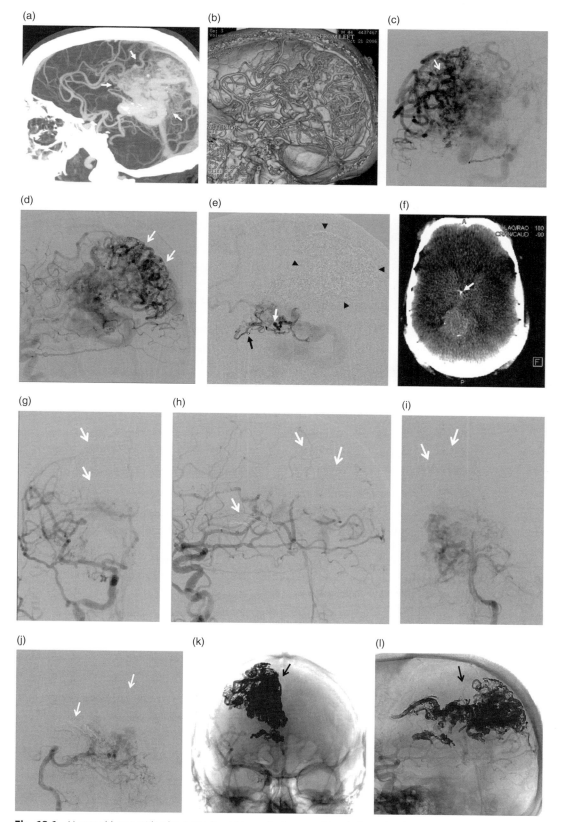

Fig. 13.1. 44 year-old man with a long-standing history of seizures and headaches related to an inoperable right parieto-occipital AVM who presented with an intraventricular hemorrhage (IVH). Pre-radiosurgical embolization was then carried out in multiple sessions. (a),(b). Maximum Intensity Projection (a) and 3-D Volume Rendering (b) CT Angiography images demonstrate a large parieto-occipital AVM supplied by branches of the right anterior, middle, and posterior cerebral arteries. (c),(d). Pre-treatment right common carotid angiography showing the anterior circulation supply to the AVM. Pre-treatment angiography of the posterior circulation is not shown. (e). Superselective angiography of the medial posterior chroidal artery showing supply to the AVM with filling of an intranidal aneurysm (white arrow), which was thought to represent the source of the patient's hemorrhage. Black arrowheads: subtracted Onyx cast from the previous four embolizations; Black arrow: microcatheter tip. (f). Intra-procedural Dyna-CT demonstrating the location of the microcatheter tip (as seen in (e)) in relation to the brain parenchyma and AVM. Intra-arterial injection of Amytal (50 mg) and Lidocaine (20 mg) was subsequently performed from this site while the patient was awake. The provocative testing was deemed negative. Therefore embolization of that pedicle was performed. This resulted in obliteration of the deeper AVM compartment, including the intranidal aneurysm. (g),(h). Post-treatment right common carotid angiography showing near complete obliteration of the anterior circulation supply to the AVM. (i),(j). Post-treatment left vertebral angiography showing the residual posterior circulation supply to the AVM. The patient was then referred to radiosurgery. (k),(l). Post-treatment (6 stages) native images showing the Onyx cast.

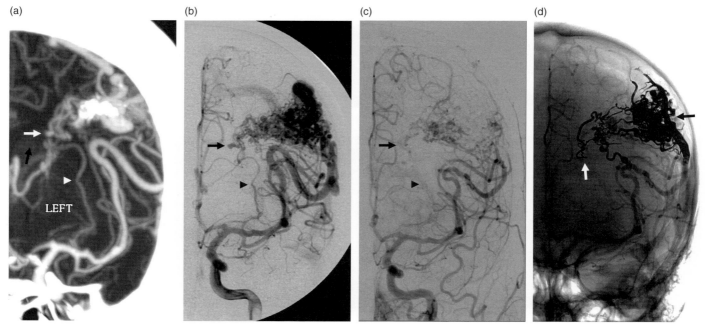

Fig. 13.2. 49 year-old female presenting with an IVH in the setting of a left frontoparietal AVM. (a). Head CT angiography demonstrates an intranidal aneurysm (white arrow) supplied by an enlarged and tortuous lateral lenticulostriate artery (white arrowhead). This was thought to be the source of the patient's IVH (black arrow). (b). Pre-treatment left internal carotid angiography showing the intranidal aneurysm (black arrow) supplied by an enlarged lateral lenticulostriate artery (black arrowhead). (c). Post-treatment left internal carotid angiography showing complete conclusion of the intranidal aneurysm (black arrow) as well as of the distal lateral lenticulostriate artery (black arrowhead). (d). Post-treatment native images showing the final Onyx cast. The lenticulostriate artery was not amenable to microcatheterization given its tortuousity and the patient was embolized from a distal left MCA pedicle (black arrow). Note the remote transnidal deposition of Onyx into the distal lenticulostriate artery (white arrow).

The mean transit time (MTT) of feeding arteries and draining veins has been measured with the use of time-density curves obtained by digital subtraction angiography. In one study,[90] there was a significant difference in the mean number of draining veins, the MTT of the feeding artery, and the ratio of the MTT of the draining to the feeding vessels between ruptured and unruptured AVMs. The Ethiodol droplet DSA method can provide accurate transit time measurements and precise, detailed, and dynamic AVM visualization. In one study,[91] standard contrast medium was superselectively injected into each target pedicle, followed by infusion of 20 µL of insoluble Ethiodol microdroplets before enbucrilate embolization of 24 AVM feeding pedicles in 13 patients. Transport of contrast material was assessed using high-speed biplane pulsed digital subtraction angiography (DSA) operating at 15 frames per second. The mean blood flow transit times through AVMs after administration of Ethiodol were found to be approximately half as long as in those measured after injection of soluble contrast materials. The discrete Ethiodol microdroplets travel more closely approximated the dynamic behavior of enbucrilate, allowing the AVM structure to be traced with high spatial and temporal resolution. High arterial input pressure (FMAP) may be quantifiable and a risk predictor for hemorrhagic AVM presentation. The influence of feeding mean arterial pressure (FMAP) measured during superselective angiography in conjunction with other morphological or clinical risk factors in determining the probability of

hemorrhagic presentation was determined in patients with brain AVMs.[72] In the 129 patients that had FMAP measurements, only exclusively deep venous drainage and FMAP were independent predictors of hemorrhagic presentation; size, location, and the presence of aneurysms were not independent predictors.

Classification

AVMs vary in size from tiny malformations to massive anomalies that encompass multiple cerebral lobes. The arterial supply also varies, from the extremes of all major vessels including cortical, brainstem, or cerebellar arterial systems, to a single artery. The feeding arteries in the larger malformations frequently are abnormally enlarged and ectatic. Deep arterial feeders such as lenticulostriate, choroidal, or thalamoperforating arteries often feed the malformation after passing through healthy tissues (Fig. 13.2(a),(b)). The venous drainage of AVMs eventually reaches recognizable venous channels, usually appearing abnormally distended because of the large volumes of blood that flow through the shunt. The veins follow two basic routes, the more common being superficial drainage coursing over the cortex directly to the major sinuses. The other route is through the deep venous system. In the larger lesions, there is often a dual venous network of drainage comprising both superficial and deep veins.

Table 13.1. Summary of brain arteriovenous malformation attributes[89]

A.	General definitions
A.1.	Clinical presentation
A.2.	Date of presentation (DOP)
A.3.	Imaging source and date (IS&D)
B.	Location and size
B.1.	Lesion side
B.2.	Handedness
B.3.	BAVM size
B.4.	BAVM location
B.5.	BAVM eloquence
B.6.	BAVM border with adjacent brain
B.7.	BAVM hemorrhage
B.7.1.	Evidence of new BAVM hemorrhage
B.7.2.	Age of new BAVM hemorrhage
B.7.3.	Is new BAVM hemorrhage symptomatic?
B.7.4.	Evidence of old BAVM hemorrhage
B.7.5.	Age of old BAVM hemorrhage
B.7.6.	Was old BAVM hemorrhage symptomatic?
B.7.7.	Hemorrhage location
B.7.8.	Hemorrhage size
C.	Venous drainage
C.1.	Superficial vs. deep venous drainage
C.2.	Periventricular drainage
C.3.	Number of draining veins leaving nidus
C.4.	Number of veins reaching sinus
C.5.	Venous stenosis/occlusion
C.6.	Venous ectasia (dilatation)
C.7.	Venous reflux
C.8.	Sinus thrombosis/occlusion
D.	Arterial supply
D.1.	Feeding arteries
D.2.	Arterial aneurysms
D.2.1.	Number of arterial aneurysms
D.2.2.	Arterial aneurysms location
D.2.3.	Arterial aneurysms hemorrhagic history
D.2.4.	Arterial aneurysms hemorrhagic date
D.3.	Number of vessels to be embolized
D.4.	Moyamoya-type changes
D.5.	Pial-to-pial collateralization
D.6.	Intravascular pressure measurements

Taken with permission from Stroke.

Hemodynamic effects due to shunting cause an opening of collateral vessels in territories adjacent to but not primarily involved in the AVM. Collateral vessels that are enlarged because of hemodynamic effects can be prominently seen during angiography and can be easily misinterpreted as being part of the nidus. Such collateral vessels are sometimes referred to as areas of angiomatous change.[92] It is important during angiographic analysis of an AVM to differentiate the tortuous, often bizarre appearance of such collateral vessels from the primary nidus. Additionally, a dysplastic appearance is frequently seen in the angiographic behavior of feeding pedicles in an AVM. This morphologic change is termed flow-induced angiopathy.[93] AVMs are most commonly wedge-shaped with the apex of the wedge directed toward the ventricular system (Fig. 13.1(k),(l)). They may also assume cylindrical or globoid forms in the white matter.

Careful volumetric studies suggest that there is no special predilection for AVMs in any part of the brain. The locations encountered seem simply to reflect the relative volume of the brain represented by a given region. The frontal lobe, occupying 30% of the brain volume, is shown to harbor 30% of the AVMs. The posterior fossa, forming 12% of brain volume, harbors 12% to 14% of the malformations; thus most AVMs are located in the cerebral hemispheres. Depending on their location, cerebral AVMs are classified as superficial or deep. The ratio of superficial (convexity) to deep AVMs is approximately 2:1 to 3:1.[94,95] Fifty percent of AVMs appear to straddle or are located near the arterial border-zone territories. Only 2% of the AVMs are multiple.

Grading

A widely used method to predict the risk of morbidity and mortality attending the operative treatment of AVMs is the Spetzler–Martin grading system (Table 13.2, Table 13.3). The total grade reflects the sum of points assigned for nidus size (<3 cm, 3–6 cm, >6 cm), eloquence of adjacent brain, and

Table 13.2. Classification of arteriovenous malformations (AVM) proposed by Spetzler and Martin (Spetzler 1986)

AVM characteristics	Grading
Size of the AVM	
• Small (<3cm)	**1** point
• Medium (3–6cm)	**2** points
• Large (>6cm)	**3** points
Localization of the AVM	
• Non-eloquent	**0** point
• Eloquent	**1** point
Venous drainage	
• Only superficial	**0** point
• Deep	**1** point

Table 13.3. Proposed data elements[89] for BAVM description

A. General definitions

A.1. Clinical presentation

Choose all applicable (yes/no):

- Incidental
- Hemorrhage
- Seizure
- Focal neurological deficit
- Headache
- Other

A.2. Date of presentation *(date)*

A.3. Imaging source and date *(date)*

B. Location and size

B.1. Lesion side

- Right
- Left
- Midline

B.2. Handedness

- Right
- Left
- Ambidextrous

B.3. BAVM size *(integer; mm)*

B.4. BAVM location

Choose all applicable:

- Cortical
- Subcortical
- Ventricular
- Corpus callosum
- Frontal
- Temporal
- Parietal
- Occipital

- Basal ganglia
- Internal capsule
- Intraventricular
- Cerebellar hemisphere
- Vermian (paramedian)
- Deep cerebellar nuclei
- Brainstem

B.5. BAVM eloquence

Choose all applicable:

- NOT eloquent
- Sensorimotor cortex
- Visual cortex
- Language cortex

- Internal capsule
- Cerebellar peduncle
- Deep cerebellar nuclei
- Brain stem

- Thalamus/hypothalamus/basal ganglia

- Other eloquence

B.6. BAVM border with adjacent brain

- Compact (sharp)
- Diffuse

B.7. BAVM hemorrhage

B.7.1. Evidence of NEW BAVM hemorrhage *(yes/no)*

B.7.2. Age of NEW BAVM hemorrhage *(integer; day)*

B.7.3. Is NEW BAVM hemorrhage symptomatic? *(yes/no)*

B.7.4. Evidence of OLD BAVM hemorrhage *(yes/no)*

B.7.5. Age of OLD BAVM hemorrhage *(mo)*

B.7.6. Was OLD BAVM hemorrhage symptomatic? *(yes/no)*

B.7.7. Hemorrhage location

Choose all applicable:

- Ventricular
- Parenchymal
- Subarachnoid

B.7.8. Hemorrhage size *(mm)*

C. Venous drainage

C.1. Superficial vs deep venous drainage

- Both superficial and deep
- Superficial only
- Deep only

C.2. Periventricular drainage *(yes/no)*

C.3. Number of draining veins leaving nidus *(count)*

C.4. Number of veins reaching sinus *(count)*

C.5. Venous stenosis/occlusion *(integer; percentage, where 100% = occlusion)*

C.6. Venous ectasia (dilatation) *(yes/no)*

C.7. Venous reflux *(yes/no)*

C.8. Sinus thrombosis/occlusion *(integer; percentage, where 100% = occlusion)*

D. Arterial supply

D.1. Feeding arteries

Table 13.3. (*cont.*)

Choose all applicable:

- Anterior choroidal a.
- Posterior choroidal a.
- Anterior cerebral a. cortical branches
- Superior cerebellar a.
- Anterior cerebral a. penetrators
- Anterior inferior cerebellar a.
- Middle cerebral a. cortical branches
- Posterior inferior cerebellar a.
- Middle cerebral a. penetrators
- External carotid a. branches
- Other internal carotid a. branches
- Basilar a. penetrators
- Internal carotid a. penetrators
- Vertebral a. branches
- Posterior cerebral a. cortical branches
- Vertebral a. penetrators
- Posterior cerebral a. penetrators
- Other a.

D.2. Arterial aneurysms

D.2.1. Number of arterial aneurysms (count)

D.2.2. Arterial aneurysms location

Pick all applicable to any aneurysm:

- Flow-related
- Proximal
- Not flow-related
- Distal
- Nidal

D.2.3. Arterial aneurysms hemorrhagic history (yes/no)

D.2.4. Arterial aneurysms hemorrhagic (date)

D.3. Number of vessels to be embolized (count)

D.4. Moyamoya-type changes (yes/no)

D.5. Pial-to-pial collateralization

Choose all applicable

- Same territory
- Between territories
- None

D.6. Intravascular pressure measurements (mm Hg)

Taken with permission from Stroke.

pattern of venous drainage (deep vs. superficial). Spetzler–Martin grades range from 1 to 5 summing the points for each category. A separate grade 6 is reserved for inoperable lesions.

The Spetzler–Martin grading system was originally developed to predict the peri-operative and post-surgical outcome, and as such has shown a reliable correlation with surgical outcome.[96] Although many other grading scales have been proposed,[64,97–99] all of which focus on anatomic, hemodynamic, and physiological properties of the AVM, the Spetzler–Martin grading scale has become the scale most often used by treating physicians.

In general, Spetzler–Martin AVM grades 1, 2, or 3 were found to have low treatment-associated morbidity (1% to 3%) but much higher morbidity rates were observed for grade 4 and 5 lesions, reaching 31% and 50%, respectively, in the early post-operative period. In addition, the rate for permanent deficit was 29.9% for grade 4 lesions and 16.7% for grade 5 lesions.[100] A similar relationship between Spetzler–Martin scale and outcome was observed by Heros *et al.*[101]

To date, these data form the foundation for most management decisions regarding AVM therapy. Operative morbidity and mortality rates for grade 1 and 2 AVMs are around 1%. These lesions are generally resected, because the risk of hemorrhage far outweighs the risk for surgical resection. In such lesions, pre-operative embolization is not frequently pursued, given that the risk of the embolization procedure may approach or even surpass the risk of surgery. In highly eloquent brain regions, stereotactic radiosurgery, rather than surgical resection, may be pursued. The role for curative embolization of these low-grade AVMs has yet to be evaluated in a systematic basis and compared with these surgical results.

The operative morbidity and mortality rate for a grade 3 AVM is 3%. This complex and heterogenous group requires an individualized assessment on a case-by-case basis. Most of these lesions are treated with either radiosurgery or preoperative embolization followed by surgical resection.

Some authors suggested to modify the Spetzler–Martin scale based on a subclassification derived from a series of 174 brain grade 3 AVMs.[102] Small-sized grade 3 AVMs carried a combined surgical morbidity and mortality risk of 2.9%. Medium-sized/deep grade 3 AVMs had a 7.1% surgical risk, and medium/eloquent grade 3 AVMs (size 2, venous drainage 0, eloquence 1) had a 14.8% surgical risk. No large-sized grade 3 AVMs were treated in the series reported. Based on these data, the authors recommended that small-sized grade 3 have a surgical risk similar to that of low-grade AVMs and can be safely treated with microsurgical resection. Medium-sized/deep grade 3 AVMs have intermediate surgical risks and should be judiciously selected for surgery. Medium-sized/eloquent grade 3 AVMs have a surgical risk approaching that of high-grade AVMs and are best managed conservatively, or with a multimodal approach.

The surgical resection of grade 4 and 5 AVMs is generally associated with a risk of operative morbidity and mortality that exceeds the risks associated with the natural history of the lesion.[6] In addition, in this group of patients partial AVM treatment substantially increased the yearly risk for hemorrhage. In accordance with these observations, surgical treatment for grade 4 and 5 AVMs is recommended only in patients with progressive neurological deficits attributable to repeated hemorrhage or disabling symptoms, such as intractable seizures.

Although the Spetzler–Martin grading scale was designed to predict surgical outcome, it has also been evaluated in the combined management of AVMs, including surgical resection, embolization followed by surgical resection, embolization alone, or radiosurgery.[103] Deterioration due to treatment was seen in 19% of patients with grade 1 and 2 AVMs, 35% of patients with grade 3 lesions, and 42% of patients with grade 4 and 5 lesions. The scale does not include characteristics such as associated aneurysms, venous stasis, or venous aneurysms that have been associated with hemorrhagic risk. There are no reliable data, in fact, correlating such features with treatment risk.

Treatment

Even if the presentation and the future risks of patients with AVMs were less heterogenous, balancing the pros and cons of the available treatment options would be difficult, for several reasons. First, our knowledge about the natural history of AVM has its limitations (see Natural history). A second problem is that the benefits and risks of any treatment can only be measured over many years, particularly if the lesion has not been completely obliterated and if the unwanted effects of treatment do not emerge until years later, such as with radiosurgery. A third factor that is difficult to quantify in decision analysis is the patient's psychological attitude to living with an unoperated or unsecured lesion in the brain that may bleed at an unpredictable time. Some patients show admirable easiness in coping with this knowledge, but in other cases the patient's life may turn out to be so dominated by the perceived danger that he or she may insist on intervention even when the balance of risks would seem to argue against such a course of action. Finally, the balance between benefits and risks for any form of treatment (surgical excision, endovascular embolization, or radiosurgery) has never been assessed in randomized controlled trials. Despite the heterogeneity of lesions, such trials, necessarily in the form of a multicenter effort, are the best possible way of therapeutic advancement in this area.[1]

For those stated reasons, therapeutic management of AVMs requires a careful multidisciplinary approach. All patients should be evaluated by physicians with expertise in endovascular embolization, surgical resection, and radiosurgery. After a careful consideration of the clinical data and AVM anatomy, a risk-to-benefit ratio for treatment can be estimated. As soon as a treatment plan is agreed on, all parties must have a clear understanding of their individual roles to facilitate successful treatment.

Recent North American multidisciplinary management guidelines have recommended the following approach.[104]

- Surgical excision is the single treatment of choice for Spetzler–Martin grade 1 and 2 brain AVMs.
- Radiosurgery is the preferred single treatment for small (less than 3 cm diameter) grade 1 and 2 brain AVMs if the anatomy is unsuitable for surgery.

- A combined approach to eradicate the brain AVM nidus using embolization – perhaps repeatedly – prior to surgery or radiosurgery is the treatment of choice for other suitable grade 2 to 5 lesions.
- Surgery alone is unsuitable for grade 4 and 5 brain AVMs.
- Palliative embolization (without complete brain AVM eradication) is beneficial when a reduced arterial inflow is required in view of venous outflow obstruction or true "steal."

Despite this apparent consensus, brain AVMs continue to pose a regular management problem because of the pace of development of surgical, endovascular, and radiation therapies. There is uncertainty about whether to treat patients at all, and if so, which intervention(s) to use. This uncertainty is reflected by the variation in current treatment practices within and between different countries. For example, the treatment of small, superficial brain AVMs may be equally appealing to neurosurgeons, neurointerventionalists, and radiation therapists, depending to some extent on the clinical history, location, and angioarchitecture of the brain AVM, but surgical excision is more likely to be used in North America, whilst there is a growing tendency in Europe to use endovascular techniques to treat such brain AVMs.

Neuroendovascular therapy

The role of neuroendovascular therapy in the management of brain AVMs depends ultimately on the overall treatment plan.[105] In general, the lesion can be monitored expectantly with the understanding that the patient would have some risk of hemorrhage or other neurological symptoms. Alternatively, intervention can be undertaken with the goal of complete AVM obliteration, because subtotal therapy does not confer protection from hemorrhage and may indeed increase its likelihood.

Five scenarios comprise the vast majority of rational endovascular management strategies (listed from the most to least common):[105]

1. Pre-operative: embolization as a precursor to complete curative surgical resection
2. Targeted therapy: embolization to eradicate a specific bleeding source
3. Pre-radiosurgery: embolization as a precursor to radiation therapy
4. Curative: embolization for attempted cure
5. Palliative: embolization to palliate symptoms attributed to shunting

Pre-operative embolization

AVM embolization is most commonly performed as a precursor to curative surgical resection. Studies comparing surgery with and without embolization do not exist in a prospectively controlled fashion, because the introduction of this technique was immediately believed to be advantageous, and subsequent randomization was deemed inappropriate. Advantages include diminished blood loss and shorter surgical times, the ability to occlude vessels deemed difficult to control by the operating surgeon, and the benefits of staging flow reduction in the nidus.[106–108]

The goals of presurgical embolization are to decrease the nidus size of the AVM and to attempt to occlude surgically inaccessible or deep arterial feeding vessels such as the lenticulostriates, choroidal vessels, or posterior cerebral arteries in order to facilitate surgical excision.

In a series of patients treated with combined endovascular and surgical interventions, morbidity resulting from preoperative endovascular embolization was classified as mild in 3.9% of the cases, moderate in 6.9%, and severe in 1.98%.[109] Morgan et al. described a 33% total complication rate in their predominantly surgical series, which included only 18% preoperative embolizations.[110] The data was not presented separately for ruptured and unruptured cases.

In the Columbia AVM series, 119 AVM patients were followed prospectively after treatment. Treatment-related non-disabling neurologic deficits were found in 50 patients (42%), resulting from surgery in 32%, from embolization in 6%, and from both treatment types in 4%. Another six patients had persistent disabling deficits (3% from surgery and 2% from embolization).[111] The most striking figures, however, are seen when treatment outcome is analyzed separately for ruptured and unruptured AVM cases. Among patients who initially presented with ICH, only 27% experienced new treatment-related deficits. By comparison, among patients diagnosed with an unruptured AVM, 58% experienced new treatment-related deficits. Hence, the risk of new treatment-related deficits in patients with a non-hemorrhagic presentation appear to be significantly higher than for patients after initial rupture. These observational data raise concerns that embolization of unruptured AVMs may increase the risk of both symptomatic ICH and the onset of an acute, disabling persisting clinical syndrome.

Hemorrhagic complication rates associated with embolization range from 2% to 4.7%. The sources of hemorrhagic complication include arterial perforation, intranidal aneurysm rupture, or venous occlusion. Mortality rates associated with embolization have been reported to be 2% or less, and neurological deficits 2% to 8.9% have been reported with the use of new-generation microcatheters.[106,107,112]

The efficacy of modern AVM embolization using n-butyl-cyanoacrylate (n-BCA) in converting high Spetzler–Martin grade lesions to lower-grade lesions, with a concurrent reduction in morbidity and mortality, has been demonstrated in several clinical studies.[108,113] One randomized controlled trial was intended to test equivalence between the embolic agents n-BCA and polyvinyl alcohol (PVA) particles for the preoperative embolization of brain AVMs.[114] The study was conducted to obtain US Food and Drug Administration (FDA) approval for the use of n-BCA. The method of randomization and single blinding were not described in the paper. Double

blinding would not have been possible because the central radiologist determining the degree of vascular occlusion was unblinded due to the fact that n-BCA is radiopaque. The primary outcome was the degree of vascular occlusion achieved as judged by the percent nidus reduction and number of feeding vessels treated on catheter angiography, and secondary outcomes were the duration of subsequent surgical resection and the number of transfusions required during surgery. The reduction of AVM dimensions (79.4% in the n-BCA group and 86.9% in the PVA group) and the mean number of vessels embolized (2.2 in the NBCA group and 2.1 in the PVA group) were similar in the two groups. There was no difference in secondary outcomes except for more post-resection ICHs in the PVA group ($p < 0.05$).

Targeted therapy

With few exceptions, all treatment strategies for AVM management should ultimately be directed toward the complete obliteration of the lesion. However, in some patients with grade 4 and 5 AVMs not suitable for surgical resection, partial treatment targeted to eliminate an identified bleeding source is undertaken. Similarly, targeted embolization can be performed to occlude high-risk lesions such as flow-related (Fig. 13.3(a)–(f)) or intra-nidal (Fig. 13.2(a)–(d)) aneurysms prior to surgical or radiosurgical treatments.

Aneurysms are identified in association with AVMs in 7% to 20% of cases.[73,78,115,116] These aneurysms may be located on vessels that are remote from the nidus, on a feeding vessel – so-called flow-related aneurysms – or within the nidus itself. In addition, intranidal pseudoaneurysms composed of an organized hematoma that communicates with the intravascular space, may form after AVM-related ICH. Both intra- and extranidal aneurysms are considered risk factors for ICH in patients with AVMs.[117] However, the increased risk for hemorrhage in the setting of an extranidal aneurysm may be attributed to aneurysm rupture rather than hemorrhage from the AVM nidus itself.[116] On conventional angiographic views, nidal aneurysms may be occasionally obscured by overlying vessels or other portions of the AVM nidus. Thus, when one or more AVM related hemorrhages are observed in patients with unresectable AVMs, endovascular exploration with superselective angiography represents a reasonable strategy. In these cases, if the AVM cannot be resected, a targeted embolization may be undertaken to eradicate the aneurysm either using a liquid embolic agent for a nidal aneurysm, or coils for flow-related and remote aneurysms.

Preradiosurgery embolization

The success of radiotherapy is inversely related to the size of the AVM nidus.[118] AVMs with a volume of less than 10 ml (diameter of less than 3 cm) are frequently suitable for radiosurgery, with estimated rates of cure at 2 years ranging between 80% and 88%.[119,120] The major disadvantage of radiation therapy is a persistent risk of ICH which may be as high as 10% until the lesion disappears and may persist even after obliteration of the AVM.[121,122] A multicenter analysis of 1255 patients treated with radiotherapy found that 8% of the patients developed a neurological deficit after radiation therapy.[123] Possible adverse effects include extended radiation necrosis, cyst formation, intracranial arterial stenosis, and cranial nerve injury and are more likely to occur with increasing radiation dose, in patients with deep AVM location, and those who experience AVM rupture.

Endovascular therapy used before radiosurgery has three potential goals (Fig. 13.1(a)–(l)): (1) to decrease the nidus diameter to less than 3 cm because smaller volumes have higher cure radiosurgical rates with less morbidity (2) target therapy for components predisposed to hemorrhage, such as aneurysms; and (3) to attempt to obliterate large arteriovenous fistulae that are typically more refractory to the effects of radiosurgery, and thereby reducing symptoms related to venous hypertension.

Gobin et al. described their experience with 125 patients who underwent embolization as a precursor to radiosurgery. Most embolizations were performed using durable cyanoacrylate polymers. Embolization produced total obliteration in 11.2% of AVMs and reduced 76% of AVMs enough to allow radiosurgery. Embolization and radiosurgery together produced total obliteration in 65% of the partially embolized AVMs.[124] More recently, Henkes et al. reported "total" obliteration in only 47% of patients undergoing combined embolization and radiosurgery. Most of the treated AVMs were of very high grade possibly explaining the lower "total" obliteration rates.[125] From the existing data, no compelling evidence exists to justify or refute the value of preradiotherapy embolization.

No ideal embolic material has been identified for preradiotherapy use. However, most centers recommend the use of more permanent agents such as cyanoacrylate polymers or Onyx, because of several reports that less durable agents may result in about 16% recanalization rates after radiosurgery.[126] However, there is also some evidence that the use of newer, more permanent agents may also result in a recanalization rate of 11.8%.[124] The late recanalization may be dependent on the concentration of acrylic deposited within the nidus.[124,127,128] Flow reduction alone without evidence of reduction of AVM volume may not provide any benefit before radiotherapy, and in fact, it may make it more difficult to determine a conformal dose plan at the time of radiotherapy planning.[126]

Curative embolization

AVMs can also be cured completely using embolization alone (Figs. 13.3 and 13.4). Although the reported rates vary, most estimates are in the range of 9.7% to 14%.[4,124,129,130] The chance of a cure appears to be inversely proportional to the AVM volume and the number of feeding pedicles. Wikholm et al. reported success being heavily dependent on the size of the AVM nidus with complete obliteration rates of 71% with AVMs smaller than 4 ml, and only 15% with AVMs ranging

from 4 to 8 ml.[4] Conversely, Valavanis and Christoforidis did not find that size or number of feeding pedicles significantly predicted the potential for endovascular cure. These authors reported a 40% cure rate in a series of 387 consecutive patients.[131] With improved techniques and growing experience, the proportions of AVMs that are successfully obliterated with embolizations are increasing. Recently, Yu et al. reported a 22% cure rate with cyanoacrylate in a series of 27 patients. In all patients with curative obliteration, the AVM nidus size was less than 3 cm, was fed by fewer than three pedicles, and was easily accessible with the tip of the microcatheter. There were no AVM recurrences during follow-up ranging from 17 to 32 months.

However, it is important to note that these estimates are based on series that predate the widespread application of Onyx. The introduction of Onyx as an embolic material for AVMs a few years ago has made embolization more successful in obliterating larger parts of the AVM and has resulted in complete obliteration rates as high as 18% to 49%.[132–135] The reason for this success lies in the nature of the material itself, which allows for prolonged and repeated injections resulting in deeper penetration into the AVM nidus. The material also allows the procedure to be carried out more safely due to better control of embolic material distribution.

Palliative embolization

Palliative embolization may be undertaken for patients who have large, inoperable AVMs and in patients presenting with seizures resistant to medical management or with progressive neurological deficit thought to be secondary to venous hypertension or arterial steal. It is believed that partial embolization reduces the severity of arterial shunting and thereby improves perfusion pressure in the surrounding functional brain parenchyma. Evidence for this strategy comes from a few small series.[76,136] Another study reported improvement in motor weakness after palliative embolization of large AVMs located in the rolandic motor cortex.[137] Partial embolization may be successful in reversing the patients' signs and symptoms; however, it is often only temporary, because collaterals develop rapidly, reducing the effectiveness of the therapy. In addition, there is evidence that indicates that partial treatment of large AVMs – with either embolization or surgery – increases the risk of subsequent ICH.[4–6] At present, there is no sufficient information to accurately identify patients who will benefit from partial treatment.

Staging

Depending on morphological characteristics of the AVM and the preferences of the neurointerventionalist, the number of embolization procedures varies for each patient. The main rationale for multiple staged procedures is to avoid hemorrhage related to normal perfusion pressure breakthrough (NPPB), which has been linked to overembolization of large AVMs. NPPB is thought to be secondary to the sudden

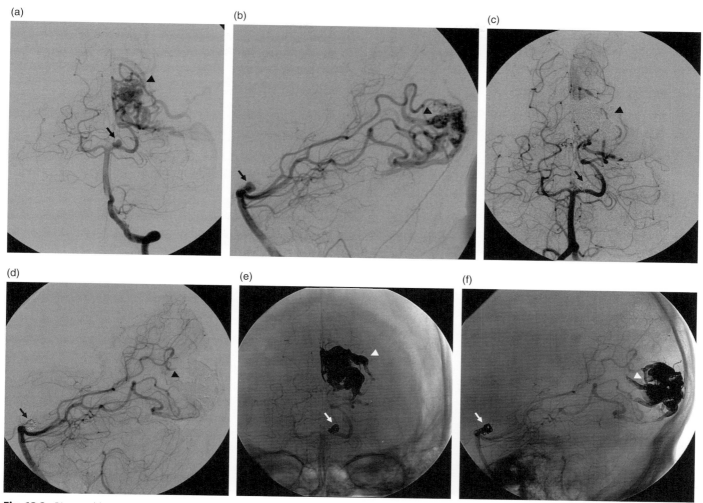

Fig. 13.3. 51 year-old man presenting with a Hunt-Hess Grade 4 SAH in the setting of a ruptured 7 mm flow-related left posterior cerebral artery (PCA) aneurysm and a left occipital AVM. He underwent coil embolization of the left PCA aneurysm in the acute setting. He made a full neurological recovery and his AVM was embolized to completion four months later in two stages. Follow-up angiography performed one year later demonstrated persistent complete occlusion of both the AVM and the aneurysm. (a),(b). Pre-treatment left vertebral angiography showing the flow-related left PCA aneurysm (arrow) and the left occipital AVM (arrowhead). (c),(d). Post-treatment left vertebral angiography showing complete occlusion of the aneurysm (arrow) and AVM (arrowhead). (e),(f). Post-treatment native images showing the coil mass (arrow) and the Onyx cast (arrowhead).

increase in perfusion pressure in the surrounding normal brain parenchyma, which suffers from chronically impaired autoregulation, after AVM embolization or resection. In general, several embolization procedures may be needed before surgery or radiotherapy to reduce the size of the AVM, particularly if the AVM is larger than 3 cm. If multiple vascular distributions provide supply to the lesion, some neurointerventionalists prefer embolizing feeders from only one vascular distribution during any given session. The decision on the number of stages and pedicles to embolize also depends on the choice of the embolysate. In procedures using n-BCA embolysate as many as five superselective catheterizations and embolizations may be performed per session. However with Onyx, much larger volumes of the embolic material can be injected from a single super-selective microcatheter placement, reducing the number of pedicles catheterized at any given session.

Embolysates
Liquid embolysates

Liquid embolysates are the most widely used and most effective agents for AVM embolization (Table 13.4). The most commonly used are the cyanoacrylate polymers (e.g., N-butyl 2-cyanoacrylate [n-BCA]), often referred to as glue. The second most commonly used is an ethylene vinyl alcohol copolymer dissolved in dimethyl sulfoxide (Onyx). Onyx is a liquid nonadhesive embolic agent that was only approved by the US Food and Drug Administration in July 2005 as an embolic agent for brain AVMs, but has been used in Europe prior to that. Finally, ethanol (ETOH), which has been used effectively to treat peripheral AVMs, has also been applied with some success for the treatment of central nervous system lesions.

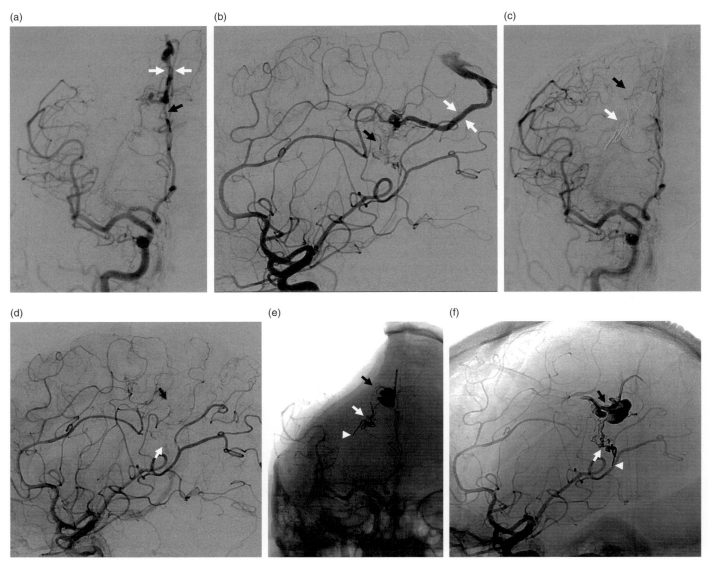

Fig. 13.4. 33 year-old male who suffered a large ICH related to a small right fronto-parietal AVM. He underwent surgical evacuation of the hematoma and hemicraniectomy in the acute setting. His AVM was embolized six months later in a single stage. (a),(b). Pre-treatment right internal carotid angiography showing the small right fronto-parietal AVM. The AVM had a fistuluous component (black arrow) supplied by the pericallosal artery (black arrowhead) and a plexiform component (white arrow) supplied by the anterior choroidal artery (white arrowhead), with drainage in a single superficial vein (opposing white arrowheads). (c),(d). Post-treatment right internal carotid angiography showing complete occlusion of both components of the AVM. (e),(f). Post-treatment native images showing the Onyx cast (arrows). Note the transnidal deposition of Onyx into the distal anterior choroidal artery (white arrowhead).

Liquid adhesive polymer agents offer several important advantages: (1) the potential for penetration deep into the AVM nidus; (2) permanent embolization with durable obliteration of the vessel or pedicle; (3) the ability to be delivered through small, flexible, flow-directed catheters that can be manipulated safely and atraumatically into the most distal locations within the cerebrovasculature; and (4) the ability to be delivered into the pedicle quickly.

Several disadvantages of the liquid adhesives have been reported. First, safe injection requires a high level of expertise to achieve adequate nidal penetration without allowing the agent to extend into the vein. Second, there is a risk of the liquid agents adhering to the catheter, making withdrawal traumatic or impossible.

N-butyl 2-cyanoacrylate (n-BCA)

n-BCA is a liquid embolic tissue-adhesive agent admixed with ethiodized oil, which was Food and Drug Administration approved for pre-surgical embolization of cerebral vascular malformations in 2000. n-BCA polymerizes to form a stable solid when it comes into contact with a solution containing anions, such as the hydroxyl groups in blood. The rate of polymerization and the rate of injection determine how far the agent will travel within the cerebral vasculature before

Table 13.4. Neurovascular liquid embolics

Company name	Product name	Materials used	Indication	Key benefits	FDA market cleared
Codman Neurovascular	Trufill n-BCA Liquid Embolic System	n-BCA	Embolization of cerebral AVMs when presurgical devascularization is desired	Trufill n-BCA is a clear, free-flowing liquid, which polymerizes quickly upon contact with body fluid or tissue; it offers convenient preparation and delivery, customized radiopacity for visualization, and effective penetration of AVMs	PMA device
ev3 Inc.	Onyx Liquid Embolic System: Onyx 18 and Onyx 34	EVOH, DMSO, Tantalum	US: presurgical embolization of brain AVMs; EU: embolization of vascular lesions	Onyx Liquid Embolic System is an EVOH copolymer that provides full penetration and complete packing for neurovascular disorders, obliterating vascular lesions	PMA device
	Onyx HD-500		US: treating intracranial, saccular, sidewall aneurysms that present with a wide neck ($\geq$4 mm) or with a dome-to-neck ratio <2 that are not amenable to treatment with surgical clipping; EU: embolization of intracranial aneurysms	Onyx HD-500 is a high-viscosity formulation liquid embolic for the treatment of intracranial wide-necked aneurysms that provides complete volumetric filling to reduce recanalization and retreatment	HDE device

Abbreviations for all charts: 2D, two-dimensional; 3D, three-dimensional; AVM, arteriovenous malformation; DMSO, dimethyl sulfoxide; EVOH, ethylene vinyl alcohol; HDE, humanitarian device exemption; HVT, hypervascular tumor; ID, inner diameter; n-BCA, nbutyl cyanoacrylate; PGA, polyglycolic acid; PGLA, poly (lactic-co-gylcolic acid); PMA, premarket approval.
Taken with permission from *Endovascular Today*, April 2009.

solidifying. The n-BCA itself is radiolucent and must be mixed with a radiopaque agent, typically ethiodized oil. Higher concentrations of ethiodized oil decrease the polymerization rate and increase the viscosity of the embolic material. Ratios used in the prospective, randomized clinical study of the n-BCA liquid embolic system varied from 10% to 70% n-BCA and 30% to 80% ethiodized oil by volume. The appropriate formulation of any additives is dependent upon the neurointerventionalist's evaluation of the relationship of anatomy, hemodynamics, and the catheter system. Typically, a 1:1.5 to 1:3 (n-BCA:oil) mixture is used for most embolizations. This translates into 2 to 7 seconds polymerization time. Glacial acetic acid may be added in low concentrations to delay polymerization and lead to increased penetration. Tantalum powder may be mixed with the n-BCA: oil mixture to provide greater radio-opacity.

n-BCA is, for all intents and purposes, a permanent embolic agent. After solidifying – provided a sufficient volume has been injected – n-BCA creates an immediate obliteration of the embolized pedicle. An intense inflammatory reaction follows that leads to fibrous ingrowth that, in turn, produces durable obliteration.[138] Although recanalization can occur, it is rare after an adequate embolization.

Ethylene-vinyl alcohol copolymer with dimethyl sulfoxide (Onyx)

Onyx is a non-adhesive liquid embolic agent with a lava-like flow pattern. Onyx is supplied in ready-to-use vials. Each vial contains ethylene-vinyl alcohol copolymer (EVOH), dimethyl sulfoxide (DMSO), and tantalum. EVOH is formed of 48 mol/L ethylene and 53 mol/L vinyl alcohol. The polymer is dissolved in the organic solvent DMSO and is prepared in three different concentrations: 6.0%, 6.5%, and 8.0%. Micronized tantalum powder (35% wt/vol) is added for radiopacity. The vials are kept on a shaker for at least 20 minutes to ensure proper mixing of the tantalum powder. The lower the concentration of the copolymer, the less viscous the agent and the more distal penetration can be achieved. Viscosity of Onyx at 6.0%, 6.5%, and 8.0% is 18, 20, and 34 cP, respectively. Onyx is manufactured as Onyx 18, Onyx 20 (not available in US), and Onyx 34. Generally, Onyx 18 and 20 are used for embolization of a plexiform nidus, and Onyx 34 is used for embolization of large arteriovenous shunts in the AVM. When the mixture contacts aqueous media, such as blood, DMSO rapidly diffuses away from the mixture, causing in-situ precipitation and solidification of the polymer, with formation of a spongy embolus. This solidification occurs more slowly than that of cyanoacrylates and since Onyx is non-adherent to the walls of the vessel or microcatheter, this material allows prolonged injection times while decreasing the chances of permanent microcatheter retention. If proximal microcatheter reflux is observed or unfavorable distal filling occurs, the injection is stopped and resumed after 30 seconds to 2 minutes (reflux-hold-reinjection technique).

Due to its properties and increased predictability, the use of Onyx may allow for more controlled injections with better distal nidus or fistula penetration when compared to cyanocrylate. In addition, control angiography can be performed during the embolization to assess the status of the AVM nidus and draining veins as well as to rule out non-target embolization. Another potential advantage of Onyx is the possibility of transnidal embolization of arterial feeders that are difficult, unsafe, or impossible to catheterize (Figs. 13.3 and 13.4). The main disadvantage of Onyx over n-BCA is the prolonged procedural and fluoroscopy times associated with the former agent.

Initially, animal studies demonstrated that the DMSO component of the mixture induced vasospasm and angionecrosis.[139,140] Subsequent investigations, however, indicated that these effects could largely be eliminated by reducing the volume of DMSO injected and limiting the rate at which it was introduced.[141] One clinicopathological study showed mild acute inflammation in the vessel walls of specimen resected 24 hours after embolization.[142] Angionecrosis was noted in two specimens, albeit without parenchymal hematoma and without destruction of the vessel wall integrity. It is important to note what is known as a typical sequence of histopathological events in embolized AVMs with n-BCA or solid particles: acute inflammation with mural angionecrosis occurs immediately followed by prominent chronic granulomatous vasculitis, which remains stable and is detectable for a very long time, even in AVMs with a maximum exposure time of more than 6 years.[143]

Although only limited long-term data is currently available for Onyx, Onyx is, like n-BCA, for all intents and purposes, a permanent agent. No recanalization was reported in a small number of patients imaged up to 32 months after embolization.[132,142,144]

Several studies have examined the feasibility and safety of Onyx in AVM embolization. Von Rooij et al. reported an average size reduction of 75% following Onyx embolization in 44 patients. Total obliteration was achieved in 16% of the treated patients (all of which were Spetzler–Martin grades 1 and 2) at the cost of mortality and permanent morbidity rates of 2.3% and 4.6%, respectively.[135] Weber et al. described a complete obliteration rate of 20% after Onyx embolization alone in 93 patients harboring 94 brain AVMs. Two angiographic recurrences were evident at 3 months' follow-up, resulting in a complete obliteration rate of 18%. The overall procedural complication rate was 12% (11 cases) including clinically significant deficits (modified Rankin Scale >2) in 5 patients (5%) and acute ICH in 2 patients (2%).[132,133]

Mounayer et al. reported their experience in the treatment of 94 brain AVM patients. A total of 210 embolizations were performed, with Onyx as the sole embolic agent in 88 procedures; Onyx and n-BCA in combination in 50 procedures, and n-BCA alone in 72 procedures. At the time of their report, angiographic cure was accomplished in 26 of the 53 patients (49%) in whom endovascular treatment had been completed. Procedure-related permanent neurologic deficits were observed in eight (8.5%, 8/94) patients and another three (3.2%, 3/94) patients died from procedure-related complications.[134] Katsaridis et al. described their experience with Onyx in the curative embolization of 101 brain AVM patients. At the time of their report, treatment had been concluded in 52 of the patients. Complete AVM obliteration was obtained in 28 patients (53.9% of the completely treated and 27.7% of all patients) and near-total occlusion was obtained in another 18 patients. The rates of permanent morbidity and mortality were 8% (8/101) and 3% (3/101), respectively.[132,133] Since Onyx approval by the FDA, we have performed 83 embolization sessions in 30 brain AVM patients. At this time, embolization treatment has been completed in 27 patients. Nine patients were cured after embolization (33.3%, 9/27) and another 14 after surgical resection (51.8%, 14/27). The remaining four patients were treated with radiosurgery. After embolization, two patients had new mild/non-disabling neurological deficits (minor morbidity rate: 2.4%/procedure; 6.7%/patient) and another three patients had new disabling neurological deficits (major morbidity rate: 3.6%/procedure; 10%/patient), which included one post-procedural PICA stroke (Fig. 13.5) and two post-procedural ICHs (Fig. 13.6). There have been no mortalities.

Ethanol (ETOH)

Embolization of brain AVMs with undiluted absolute ethyl alcohol (ETOH) (98% dehydrated alcohol injection) has been advocated on the basis of its success in eradicating peripheral vascular malformations. ETOH has a direct toxic effect on the endothelium resulting in acute thrombosis of the vessel. For the embolization procedure, ETOH is mixed with a contrast medium, most commonly ethiodized oil.

To date, only one group reported their results of brain AVM embolization with ETOH in 17 patients. They were able to cure seven patients with ETOH alone (42%). Despite this impressive cure rate, it is important to note that two patients with partially treated lesions died and eight patients experienced complications related to therapy.[145]

If large amounts of absolute alcohol enter the systemic circulation, toxic effects can occur, therefore Ethanol 1 mg/kg is the maximum amount that can be injected during a single session. High-dose ethanol has been found to induce pulmonary precapillary vasospasm leading to cardiopulmonary arrest. In addition, ETOH causes significant brain edema, necessitating treatment with high doses of steroids before and 2 weeks after treatment. Occasionally, mannitol therapy needed to be administered due to high intracranial pressures.

Given those risks and the relative widespread experience and comfort level with cyanoacrylates and now Onyx, there has been a general reluctance among most neurointerventionalists to use ETOH for the embolization of brain AVMs.

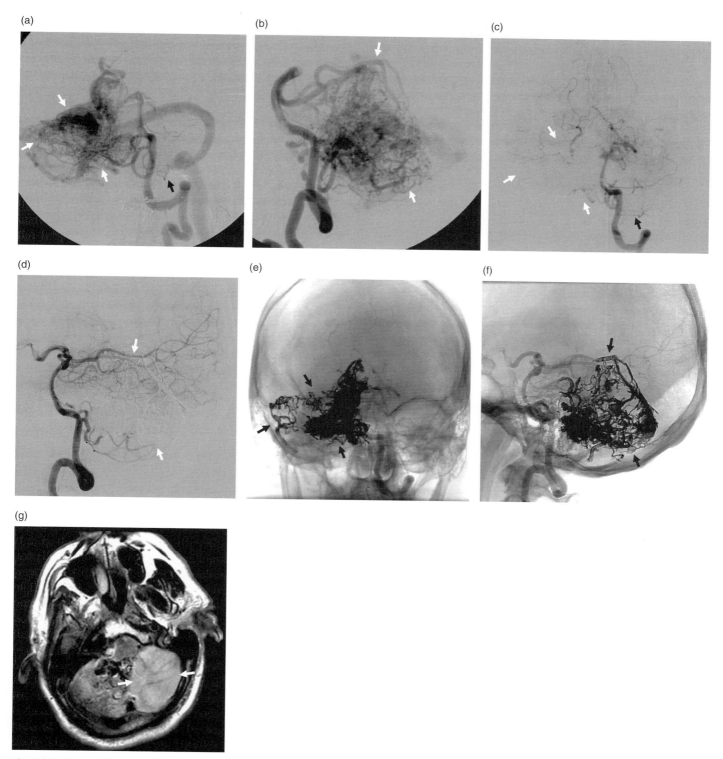

Fig. 13.5. 63 year-old male with history of multiple cerebellar hemorrhages in the past related to a large right cerebellar AVM which was refractory to previous radiosurgical treatment. Complete obliteration of the AVM was achieved after 4 stages of Onyx embolization. The last stage of the treatment was complicated by fracture of the distal portion of the microcatheter within the pedicle of the left PICA that supplied the AVM. The patient woke up well from the procedure; however, several hours later he started complaining of headaches and a new left dysmetria was noted on exam. Brain MRI revealed a large left PICA infarct. (a),(b). Pre-treatment left vertebral angiography showing the large right cerebellar AVM (white arrows). The AVM was supplied by the right superior cerebellar artery, right AICA, and right PICA as well as by a branch of the left PICA (black arrow). (c),(d). Post-treatment left vertebral angiography showing complete occlusion of the right cerebellar AVM (white arrows). Note that the left PICA remained patent on the immediate post-treatment angiography (black arrow). (e),(f). Post-treatment native images showing the Onyx cast (black arrows). (g) Brain MRI (FLAIR sequence) showing the left PICA infarct (white arrows).

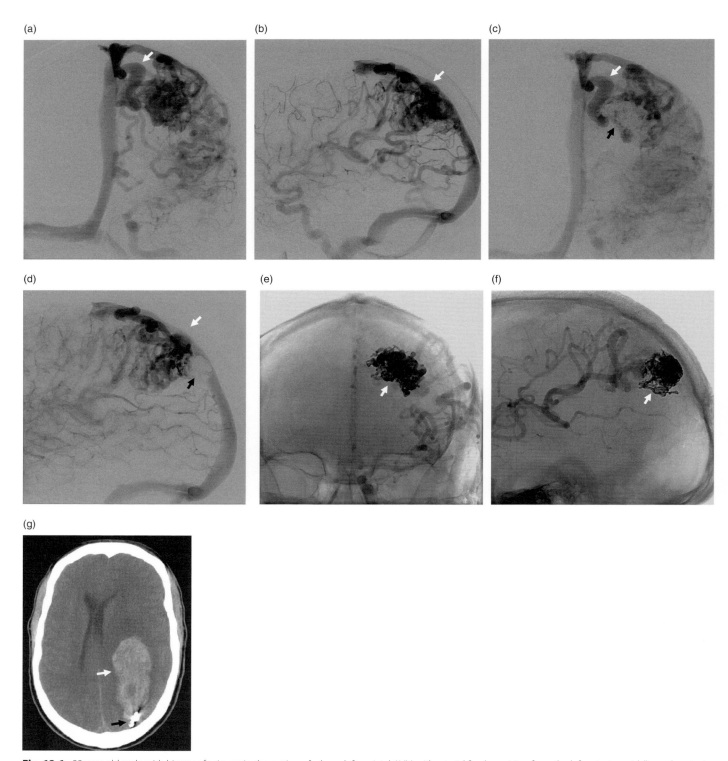

Fig. 13.6. 33 year-old male with history of seizures in the setting of a large left parietal AVM with arterial feeders arising from the left anterior, middle, and posterior cerebral arteries. Stage I Onyx embolization was performed without any immediate complications; however, two days after the procedure that patient had a seizure. A head CT showed a large ICH at the anterosuperior aspect of the AVM. The hematoma was successfully evacuated. Unfortunately, the patient had a bad neurological outcome (modified Ranki scale of 5). (a),(b). Pre-treatment left internal carotid angiography (later arterial phase) showing the large left parietal AVM. Note the predominant venous drainage into an enlarged superficial vein (white arrow) that drains into the superior sagittal sinus. (c),(d). Post-treatment left internal carotid angiography showing occlusion of the inferoposterior portion of the AVM. Note that the venous drainage of the residual AVM appears widely patent (white arrow). The black arrows point to the subtracted Onyx cast. (e),(f). Post-treatment native images showing the Onyx cast (white arrows). (g). Head CT showing the large ICH (white arrow) at the anterosuperior aspect of the AVM. The black arrow points to the Onyx cast.

Table 13.5. Embolization spheres

Embolic spheres						
Company	**Product name**	**Composition**	**Type**	**Sizes (μm)**	**Color coded**	**Indicated use**
AngioDynamics	LC Bead	Polyvinyl alcohol hydrogel microsphere	Calibrated sphere	100–300, 300–500, 500–700	Labels are color coded and the beads are tinted blue for better visualization	Embolization of HVTs and peripheral AVMs
BioSphere Medical	Embosphere Microspheres	Trisacryl crosslinked with gelatin	Spherical microsphere	40–120, 100–300, 300–500, 500–700, 700–900, 900–1200	Labels are color coded	Embolization of AVMs, HVTs, and symptomatic uterine fibroids
	EmboGold Microspheres					Embolization of HVTs and AVMs
	Quadrasphere	Super absorbent polymer	Expanding spherical microsphere	Dry sizes: 50–100, 100–150, 150–200		Embolization of HVTs and peripheral AVMs
Boston Scientific Corporation	Contour SE Microspheres	Spherical PVA	Sphere	100–300, 300–500, 500–700, 700–900, 900–1200	Packaging by size	Embolization of peripheral HVTs, including leiomyoma uteri and peripheral AVMs
CeloNova BioSciences, Inc.	Embozene Color-Advanced Microspheres	Hydrogel core with Polyzene-F coating	Sphere	40, 100, 250, 400, 500, 700, 900	Microspheres are dyed size-specific colors for definitive visualization and increased procedural safety, with corresponding color-coded syringes, labels, and boxes	Embolization of HVTs and AVMs
Terumo Interventional Systems	Bead Block	Acrylamido polyvinyl alcohol macromer	Sphere	100–300, 300–500, 500–700, 700–900, 900–1200	Spheres, syringe, and box by size	Embolization of HVTs and AVMs

Taken with permission from *Endovascular Today*, April 2009.

Particles

PVA

At the beginning of the 1990s, many authors reported results of pre-operative embolizations with polyvinyl alcohol (PVA) particles.[106,146,147] PVA particles come prepackaged by the manufacturer in different sizes 150 μm–1000 μm (Table 13.5). Various packages exist, some of them mix PVA with collagen fibers and 30% ETOH (e.g., Los Angeles mixture). There are many drawbacks related to PVA embolization: PVA particles do not afford long-term obliteration of embolized arteries and nidus, hence recanalization is more frequent. It has been reported on the order of 12% to 43%.[148,149]

Migration of particles in normal adjacent branches is much more likely because catheterization is less distal than with the flexible microcatheters used with liquid embolic agents. Further, different arteriovenous shunt sizes may be observed within the nidus, which carries the risk that the particles may reach the venous side in some instances and produce either no embolization efficacy or, on the contrary, inadvertent venous occlusion. To avoid migration, neurointerventionalists have first placed coils into large arteriovenous shunts in an attempt to prevent particles migrating into the pulmonary circulation. Finally, multiple injections are usually required to occlude one pedicle, which increases the procedural time to minutes rather than seconds as for n-BCA. PVA embolization also carries increased risks for hemorrhage after embolization.[114] In general, PVA embolization is now limited to pre-operative embolization in anticipation to complete resection of the AVM.

Coils

There are two different types of coils that can be used for embolization, the detachable (e.g., Guglielmi detachable coils) and the injectable Berenstein liquid coils. They are both useful for the obliteration of large arteriovenous fistulae within the AVM nidus. The coil is selected on the basis of the size of the feeding artery as estimated on superselective angiography or guide catheter angiography. Detachable coils can be manipulated within the feeding artery to achieve optimal positioning, and non-detachable coils can be visualized under fluoroscopy to provide some indication of their stability within the artery. After detachment, a second coil is immediately introduced, and this is repeated until a stable basket is formed. One or more liquid coils may then be deployed. Finally, after the coil pack has adequately slowed flow through the fistula, the pedicle may be occluded with injection of a liquid embolic agent.

When detachable coils are used, the over-the-wire manipulation of a microcatheter with two distal markers into the pedicle is necessary, introducing the potential for vascular perforation. The introduction of coils into friable arterial feeders of an AVM also presents a risk of perforation. Finally, if the coils are improperly sized, there is the potential for embolization through the fistula and into the venous system.

If the arterial pedicle supplying the fistula is small enough, embolization with injectable or small pushable coils can be chosen. Liquid coils may be introduced through the smaller internal diameter, flexible, flow-directed microcatheters, eliminating the need for an exclusively over-the-wire catheterization. After the introduction of the coils has sufficiently slowed transit through the fistula, occlusion can be once again achieved safely with a liquid embolic agent.

Anesthesia

The embolization is performed under general anesthesia or deep intravenous sedation in the angiography suite. There is no evidence that either general endotracheal anesthesia or intravenous sedation is associated with a lower rate of complications.[150] Both methods have their advantages and disadvantages. Arguments for embolization under general anesthesia include improved visualization of structures with the absence of patient movement, especially with temporary apnea or when the ventilator is synced with digital subtraction angiography contrast injection. Intravenous sedation trades off the potential for patient movement against the increased knowledge of the true functional anatomy of a given patient. However, this approach demands deep intravenous sedation to render the patient comfortable during catheter placement, and yet keep the patient appropriately responsive for selective neurological testing. There is no evidence one regimen is superior to any other; propofol and midazolam have been directly compared and found to be similarly efficacious.[151]

At the present time, most centers perform embolizations under general anesthesia, and some use neuroelectrophysiological monitoring (somatosensory evoked potentials and electroencephalography) to monitor neurological function during the procedure.

Recommendations for premedication with corticosteroids, anticonvulsants, aspirin, calcium channel blockers, and antibiotics have been made, but none has received rigorous support for its use. Direct transduction of arterial pressure is indicated for intracranial embolization procedures. The femoral artery introducer sheath is easily used to monitor arterial pressure. Intravascular pressures may also be monitored from the guiding catheter, as well as via the superselective catheter. Hypotension may be induced to slow the flow through the fistula and provide a more controlled deposition of embolic material, particularly if n-BCA is being used. Blood pressure reduction can be achieved with vasoactive agents, general anesthetics, or even by brief, adenosine-induced cardiac pause.[152]

In addition to the recommended monitoring parameters by the American Society of Anesthesiology, additional considerations include placement of an additional pulse oximeter on the foot of the leg that will receive the femoral introducer catheter as an early warning of femoral artery obstruction or distal thromboembolism and excessive external compression for achieving post-procedure hemostasis. Bladder catheters assist in fluid management as well as patient comfort. Supplemental oxygen should be given to all patients who have received sedative-hypnotic agents.

Procedures may be performed awake to allow provocative testing of the pedicles selected prior to permanent embolization. In this setting, superselective injection of Amytal (amobarbitol) or thiopental into the feeder vessel is performed prior to the AVM embolization (Fig. 13.1(e)).[153–155] Neurological examination as well as cognitive testing are then immediately performed. The evoked deficits resolve with dissipation of the injected agent within several minutes. Rauch *et al.* reported their experience with 147 embolizations of supratentorial AVMs following Amytal tests in 30 awake patients.[153–155] Two out of five embolizations performed after a positive Amytal test were followed by neurologic complications. Conversely, none of the 82 embolizations performed as single embolizations immediately after a negative Amytal test were associated with neurologic complications. The authors also highlighted the importance of concomitant EEG evaluation since many patients develop EEG changes in the absence of clinical symptoms. In addition, they emphasized that changes in hemodynamics related to the subsequent embolization make the Amytal test performed during the initial procedure no longer an accurate method for predicting the risk of future embolizations.

Complications during endovascular navigation of the cerebral vasculature can be rapid and dramatic and require interdisciplinary collaboration. The primary responsibility of the anesthesia team is to preserve cardiovascular function and gas exchange and, if indicated, secure the airway. If emergent endotracheal intubation is necessary, a thiopental and relaxant induction should be preferred to induce a transient decrease in perfusion pressure. Complications that may arise during AVM embolization are inadvertent vascular occlusion or hemorrhagic transformation. In the setting of vascular occlusion, the systemic blood pressure may be increased to drive adequate flow via collaterals to the area of ischemia as a temporizing measure.[156] Direct thrombolysis has been used to open up vessels.[157] In the setting of a hemorrhagic complication, immediate protamine reversal of heparin (if heparin was used during the procedure) should be done as rapidly as possible.[156]

Technique

Access is achieved through the femoral artery with placement of a 5 or 6 French sheath. Anticoagulation decisions for AVMs are made on a case-by-case basis but we typically do not advocate the use of systemic heparin. A 5 or 6 French guiding catheter and a flow-directed microcatheter are used for the embolization procedure. The guiding catheter is attached to continuous heparinized saline flush via a pressurized bag.

Pedicles targeted for embolization are identified on the initial angiographic images. If n-BCA is to be used, the vast majority of catheterizations are performed using a microcatheter over a microwire. The microcatheter is navigated primarily using a flow-directed technique. The microwire is generally maintained within the confines of the catheter functioning to add support to the proximal aspects of the catheter as it is advanced distally. After the microcatheter has been successfully manipulated into a perinidal position, a gentle injection of contrast is performed on a blank roadmap. If the fluoroscopic images demonstrate catheterization of a potential pedicle for embolization, a superselective digital subtraction angiographic image is acquired. A higher frame rate is sometimes helpful, particularly if the pedicle courses into a region with brisk arteriovenous shunting to identify contrast opacification distinctly in various stages.

The image acquired from microcatheter injection is then reviewed. Four primary considerations when evaluating the superselective injection images are as follows: (1) the identification of any normal parenchymal branches arising from the pedicle to be embolized; (2) the anatomy of the catheterized pedicle proximal to the catheter tip and AVM nidus – specifically the identification of, and localization of the origin of, any eloquent branches arising from the targeted pedicle that could be compromised by reflux; (3) the rate of transit of contrast through the nidus; and (4) the anatomy of the draining vein that appears first.[105]

The most important observation to be made is the identification of any parenchymal branches arising from the pedicle. These are vessels that course beside the nidus primarily to supply normal brain, but simultaneously give rise to multiple small side branches that extend into the nidus. With a few exceptions, pedicles that give rise to viable parenchymal branches should not be embolized. However, sometimes those branches may receive adequate leptomeningeal collateral flow to maintain the viability of any functional surrounding brain tissue in the region. Those decisions are made on a case-by-case basis.

The positioning of the microcatheter in terms of the orientation of the pedicle and the location of the nidus are critical. In at least one view, the neurointerventionalist should orient the image intensifier such that the microcatheter is elongated and proximally does not overlap with either the nidus or the draining vein. This orientation facilitates the early visualization of reflux, thus minimizing the risk of gluing the catheter in place or occluding proximal eloquent branches. This is also relevant for occlusion of a draining vein.

The rate of contrast transit through the AVM nidus provides data that can be helpful in the determination of the optimal composition of the n-BCA-to-ethiodized oil mixture. The anesthesiologist should be informed of an imminent n-BCA infusion, which may require a prolonged 90 seconds apnea to render the patient motionless. In addition, if brisk arteriovenous shunting is present, it may be helpful to reduce the systolic blood pressure to 90 mmHg.

After the microcatheter is purged with a solution of 5% dextrose in water, the n-BCA injection is performed with the patient apneic under blank fluoroscopic roadmap control. When the desired n-BCA cast is achieved, the microcatheter is gently aspirated and briskly removed from the patient. A control angiogram is then obtained to evaluate the status of the nidus, the draining veins, and any complications that may have occurred.

The technique and pace of an Onyx injection is very distinct from n-BCA and has been termed the "plug-and-push" technique. The main advantage of Onyx is that the injection of the embolic material can be delivered deliberately with the luxury of periodically being able to stop the infusion to assess the progress of the cast, the patency of the nidus and draining veins, and the status of parenchymal vessels. We strongly recommend the early formation of a short but dense plug proximal to the microcatheter tip prior to any antegrade Onyx injection. While this concept of early dense reflux sounds somewhat counterintuitive, it has allowed, in our experience, for much greater nidal depositions while ultimately minimizing the amount of reflux. The rationale for this technique is relatively simple. The older the Onyx deposition is, the more solid the embolus will be. Therefore, if one decides to adopt an early antegrade Onyx deposition technique, he/she will ultimately face reflux and much more reflux will be required to eventually break through the antegrade cast since this is an older, denser, and more solid embolus than the newer refluxed Onyx. With this idea in mind, we have adopted a technique where we purposefully avoid an initial antegrade deposition and try to promote reflux of the embolic agent during the initial phases of our injection. This early proximal plug can be more easily built with the initial use Onyx-34 for two reasons: (1) the higher concentration of the EVOH copolymer in Onyx-34 increases its viscosity which makes a proximal deposition/early reflux more likely, and (2) the lower concentration of DMSO in Onyx-34 leads to a faster precipitation and consequently to a denser early plug. In our experience, this technique of using

Onyx 34 for the initial injection has resulted in a more rapid creation of a denser proximal plug that subsequently facilitates an optimal antegrade deposition of Onyx-18 while minimizing the ultimate amount of reflux. We have used this technique in all of our AVMs regardless of their angioarchitecture (e.g., plexiform, fistulous, or mixed type).

We almost invariably use the combination of the Marathon microcatheter (ev3 Inc., Irvine, CA) with the X-pedion 0.010-inch microwire (ev3 Inc.) for the distal navigation into the AVM pedicles, typically using over-the-wire technique. We frequently perform a more proximal angiogram within the pedicle that will be embolized in order to establish the presence of normal brain-supplying branches and thus define the safety limits for reflux of the embolic material. We subsequently advance the microcatheter to an intra- or peri-nidal position, where a second microcatheter angiography is performed to further analyze the anatomy and flow dynamics of the AVM. While an optimal microcatheter position is essential for a good nidal deposition, we try to avoid positioning the microcatheter in very small caliber vessels, particularly if there is proximal tortuousity, since these factors are associated with more difficulty in microcatheter removal. We do not recommend a wedging microcatheter position for Onyx embolization. Once we are satisfied with the microcatheter position, we perform a final microcatheter angiography. This is followed by a guide-catheter angiography using the same projection and magnification. We then save reference images of both the microcatheter as well as of the guide-catheter angiograms on the early arterial, parenchymal, and late venous phases. These reference images can be quickly flipped back and forth during the Onyx injection and can be of extreme help in answering questions about where exactly the embolic agent is flowing. The microcatheter is subsequently flushed with 5 mL of saline. DMSO and Onyx-34 are prepared in two different 1-mL luerlock syringes. The deadspace of the microcatheter is then slowly filled with 0.24 mL of DMSO, and the microcatheter hub is bathed with DMSO forming a meniscus.

Onyx is slowly injected over 90 seconds to fill the microcatheter and replace the DMSO in the dead space. Fast injections of DMSO may result in vasospasm or even angionecrosis. Under continuous blank fluoroscopic roadmap control, the Onyx injection is then slowly carried out by using a "thumb-tapping" technique. We recommend starting fluoroscopy after 0.1–0.15 mL of Onyx has been injected, since inhomogeneousity of the DMSO-Onyx mixture within the microcatheter may result in Onyx deposition within the pedicle even before the entire deadspace of the microcatheter has been replaced by Onyx. The goal of this initial injection is to stay as proximal to the microcatheter as possible, and therefore the injection is halted if any antegrade deposition is observed. A waiting time of 30 to 90 seconds is typically allowed in this case. The initial objective is to form a dense Onyx cast around the tip of the microcatheter with minimal initial antegrade deposition. Once that is achieved, we promote reflux of Onyx over a short

distance (5–7 mm). We then keep injecting Onyx in the same region of the refluxed cast until a dense retrograde plug is formed. At that point, we start the antegrade Onyx injection. Onyx-18 is used for the remainder of the procedure, after the first 1 mL of Onyx-34 is injected. One should know that the process of breaking through this early plug may result in additional initial reflux and several injection pauses may be required before an antegrade deposition occurs. Extremely careful observation of the blank roadmap and native fluoroscopic images is essential during this phase of nidal deposition, preferably using biplane technology and with the assistance of a second operator who should focus on the appearance of new reflux. Injection pauses of 30 to 120 seconds are performed whenever unwanted reflux or flow into non-target areas (e.g., different arterial pedicles or venous outflow region) is observed. This seems to allow for precipitation of the Onyx at those areas, which results in diversion of the newly injected Onyx to other areas. We do not recommend pauses longer than 2 minutes, as they result in Onyx precipitation/solidification within the microcatheter with consequent termination of the embolization. Thus the operator should ensure that enough Onyx is periodically injected in order to avoid this problem. At times, it may be difficult to visualize small amounts of reflux. Breathing movement artifacts may give the false impression that small amounts of Onyx have been injected. We therefore recommend periodic visual inspection of the syringe to assess for small injection volumes. Angiography is occasionally performed through the guide catheter during the injection pauses to evaluate for residual flow to the AVM or non-target embolization. Using this technique it is not uncommon that very large volumes of Onyx are injected into the AVM nidus from one single microcatheter position. Therefore, we typically only perform embolization of one to two pedicles per session. The injection should be terminated under the following circumstances: (1) the targeted portion of the nidus has been embolized; (2) concerns about venous outflow obstruction and/or slowing of venous flow arise; (3) excess of reflux; (4) resistance to injection increases significantly as this may precede rupture of the microcatheter or vessel. The amount of tolerated reflux varies depending on several factors including: (1) the existence of proximal branches; (2) the caliber of the vessel being embolized; (3) the tortuousity of the proximal vessels; and (4) the density of the reflux. After the injection is completed, the syringe is aspirated gently and gentle traction is gradually applied to remove the microcatheter. There is a broad variation in the amount of time required for microcatheter removal depending on the length and density of the reflux as well as the proximal tortuousity and caliber of the vessels embolized. We have seen removal times ranging from almost immediate retrieval in some cases to longer than 90 minutes in some other cases. As in every other stage of Onyx embolization, patience is the essence. It is common for the Onyx cast to show some deflection while traction is being applied to the microcatheter. To better quantify the intensity of the phenomenon and titrate the

Table 13.6. Summary of clinical studies and comparative effectiveness

Trial	Patients	Technical/procedural adverse events	Angiographic obliteration	Clinical endpoints	Comments
n-BCA Trail Investigators[114]	54 n-BCA/Tantalum Powder/Ethiodol mixture and 52 Trufill PVA in 13 centers	27 of 54 (50%) and 28 of 52 (54%)	Reduction of AVM dimensions (79% in the n-BCA group and 87% in the PVA group)	ICH: 3 of 54 and 6 of 52; Death: 1 of 54 and 3 of 52; Stroke: 1 of 54 and 3 of 52	n-BCA and PVA are similar in percent of nidus reduction, number of pedicles embolized, surgical resection time, surgical blood loss, fluid replacement, and Glasgow Outcome Scale score
Onyx versus Cordis TRUFILL n-BCA[159]	54 n-BCA and 46 Onyx in 20 centers	17 of 54 (31%) and 14 of 46 (30%)	≥50% angiographic reduction in AVM nidus: 43 of 51(84%) and 41 of 42 (98%)	ICH: 8 of 54 and 6 of 46; Death: 0 of 54 and 2 of 46; Neurological deterioration: 5 of 54 and 7 of 46	Randomization to Onyx was associated with a higher angiographic success rate by ITT than n-BCA in multivariate analysis
BRAVO[160]	122 patients in 11 centers treated by Onyx	Pending	Pending	Pending	Pending

amount of additional traction to be applied, we typically obtain a blank fluoroscopic roadmap prior to applying any traction to the microcatheter. We also include the guide-catheter in the visualization field since the microcatheter traction can inadvertently move the guide-catheter forward and cause vasospasm or dissection. This can be easily prevented by holding the guide-catheter in place. We periodically increase the amount of traction on the microcatheter. This should be done under fluoroscopic guidance, while monitoring for additional deflection of the cast. Constant microcatheter traction should then be maintained for a few minutes before additional traction is applied. Attention should also be paid to the vital signs. Tachycardia and hypertension may reflect pain and need for additional analgesia. Bradycardia with or without hypotension may be occasionally seen during microcatheter retrieval from the posterior circulation. This should prompt immediate relief of any traction. The patient should then be treated with glycopyrrolate or atropine before additional attempts to remove the microcatheter. Finally, bradycardia and hypertension may represent a Cushing's response and should prompt angiographic evaluation to rule out the possibility of ICH secondary to AVM or vessel rupture. Neurophysiological monitoring, if applied, can obviously assist with difficult retrieval processes. It is not uncommon for some degree of stretching of the microcatheter to happen and we have seen cases where the final length of the microcatheter was increased by more than 10% of its original length. While stretching may promote thinning of the distal portion of the microcatheter and therefore facilitate its extraction, it may also translate into a higher chance of microcatheter fracture. If the microcatheter cannot be retrieved without excessive stress on the cast or vasculature, it should be left in place and cut off at its end at the groin.

Clinical studies and comparative effectiveness

Table 13.6 presents the results of important multicenter clinical studies regarding embolization of AVMs using various agents. In one study,[114] the number of stages was greater in the PVA group compared with n-BCA. Intent-to-treat analysis of fluoroscopy time showed no significant difference between groups. Recorded duration of fluoroscopy was greater in the PVA group (n = 43) than in the n-BCA group ($n = 41$) per protocol (109.6 vs. 93.8 min), with a 15.8-min (16.8%) difference. In another study[158] of 182 embolizations in 88 patients (n-BCA, 60 patients and 106 procedures; Onyx, 20 patients and 43 procedures; and 39 combined procedures), the mean fluoroscopy and procedure times were increased for Onyx (57 min; 2.6 h) compared with n-BCA (37 min; 2.1 h) embolizations. Cumulative mean procedure time was increased in the n-BCA/Onyx group (10.4 h) compared with n-BCA (3.7 h) and Onyx (5.4 h). Seventy patients (80%) underwent AVM resection. No significant differences in surgical blood loss or complication rates were observed among the cohorts.

Complications

Embolization of brain AVMs can be performed with a high degree of technical success and a relatively low rate of permanent neurologic complications. A recent large retrospective study reported overall permanent disabling complications or deaths occurring in only 1.6%.[161] In that study, 489 embolization procedures were performed in 192 patients. Of the 178 patients who were mRS 0–2 pre-embolization, 4 (2.3%) were dependent or dead (mRS >2) at follow-up. However, overall postprocedural neurological complications have been reported in 7%–39% of patients.

Microcatheter retention

Retention of the microcatheter tip in the nidus occurs in less than 3% of all embolizations. Retained catheters can be removed with AVM surgical resection soon after the embolization or even a few weeks after if there is no adhesion to the vessel wall. Straight microcatheters within the vessel lumen do not appear to cause thrombosis. However, some neurointerventionalists prefer a 3- to 6-month course of anticoagulation to prevent thrombosis if deemed safe for the patient.[162] In our series of 83 consecutive Onyx AVM embolization procedures, we have experienced two cases of microcatheter fracture/retention (2.4%).

Ischemic complications

Catheter-induced thrombo-emboli, non-target embolization, or reflux of embolic material into normal cerebral vessels are the most common causes of cerebral ischemia during AVM embolization (Fig. 13.5). Thrombotic emboli can be prevented with systemic heparinization and/or flush of all catheters with heparinized saline. Reflux of embolic material into normal parenchymal branches during embolization can be prevented with high-quality imaging systems, general anesthesia, optimal positioning of the microcatheter and the appropriate dilution of the liquid embolic agent to allow for desired polymerization times.[162]

Intracranial hemorrhage

Intracranial hemorrhage, during or after embolization, represents one of the most feared complications of AVM treatment. The possible etiologies are diverse but most frequently include: (1) vessel perforation during microcatheter navigation; (2) venous outflow obstruction related to either venous occlusion by the embolic material or late venous thrombosis due to abrupt venous flow reduction; (3) normal perfusion pressure breakthrough hemorrhage, which can be the sequelae of an abrupt reduction in arteriovenous shunting leading to sudden increase in the perfusion pressure of the adjacent normal brain parenchyma that has impaired autoregulatory capacity (Fig. 13.6).

The use of flow-directed catheters has significantly reduced the incidence of vessel perforations as they do not require metal guidewires beyond the tip to navigate into the AVM feeders.[162] The risk of venous outflow occlusion can be minimized using a dilute cyanoacrylate (25%)/ethiodol (75%) mixture.[162] NPPB tends to occur in patients with large high flow AVMs and multiple large feeding vessels. Reduction of the patient's mean arterial pressure 15% to 20% below the baseline during the first 24 hours after embolization and limiting embolization to 30% of the AVM nidus per session are strategies to reduce the risk of ICH due to NPPB. In one study, the predictors of intracranial hemorrhage following n-BCA embolization were identified in 195 consecutive patients with 26 patients experiencing ICHs.[163] The risk of post-procedural ICH was higher in the first week, and associated with increasing age, AVM borderzone location, and feeding artery aneurysms.

Hydrocephalus

Intraventricular hemorrhage may cause hydrocephalus. Hydrocephalus may require insertion of ventricular drainage catheters, which can also be used to monitor intracranial pressure. Compression of the aqueduct of Sylvius by large draining veins can also result in hydrocephalus.[104] Finally, choroidal AVMs may be associated with overproduction of CSF and hydrocephalus.

Seizures

Incidence of seizures may be reduced after AVM obliteration. There is an 8% incidence of new-onset seizures after AVM treatment and 83% of the patients are seizure free over a 2-year follow-up with no need for anticonvulsant medication in almost half of them. Intermittent seizures continue in 17% of patients after AVM treatment; however, improved seizure control is reported in some of these patients compared with before surgery.[164] Surgical or radiosurgical obliteration of an AVM will reduce the frequency of seizure activity.[104,165]

Post-procedural care

The recommendations for post-procedural care include neurological intensive care monitoring for at least 24 hours. Patients are preferably extubated after the procedure to allow for neurological exams to monitor the patient's condition.

Post-procedural heparinization should be considered for patients with sluggish venous outflow or compromise of an important component of the venous outflow system. Sluggish flow in the veins can lead to venous thrombosis with subsequent hemorrhage from the remaining nidus.

The arterial sheath is left in place if a second stage embolization procedure or intraoperative angiography is anticipated the following day. In general, a low systolic blood pressure (100–140 mmHg) is maintained after embolization procedures to avoid the theoretical possibility of NPPB hemorrhage. A nicardipine or labetalol drip is the preferred IV antihypertensive medication.

A new neurological deficit after embolization is usually investigated with a CT scan to rule out a new ICH or hydrocephalus. MRI scanning with diffusion-weighted imaging may be appropriate if an ischemic infarct is under consideration or in cases where a large Onyx cast may prevent adequate CT evaluation.

Conclusion

The ultimate goal of AVM therapy is the complete obliteration of the lesion, since any residual AVM might result in hemorrhage and partial treatment may indeed increase the chances of bleeding. Complete obliteration is more commonly achieved by multimodal therapy rather than by embolization alone. Thus, a multidisciplinary approach to any detected AVM is recommended. Neuroendovascular therapy continues to be a critical component of this multidisciplinary and multimodal approach. Although promising, it remains unclear at the present time how the development and introduction of newer embolization techniques and embolic agents will affect the treatment and complication rates associated with AVM treatment. While better techniques allow a much more aggressive embolization of the AVM nidus, it is likely that some portion of the complication risks previously carried by surgical resection may be transferred to the embolization procedure. In general, since the risk of rebleeding is high, and the main cause of disability in patients with AVMs is hemorrhage, early assessment and delineation of stepwise treatment plan is recommended for those who have experienced an AVM-related intracranial hemorrhage.

References

1. Warlow CP. *Stroke: A Practical Guide to Management*. 2nd edn: Wiley-Blackwell, 2000.

2. Mohr JP. *Stroke: Pathophysiology, Diagnosis, and Management*. 4th edn: Chuchill Livingstone, 2004.

3. Rinkel GJ. Intracranial aneurysm screening: indications and advice for practice. *Lancet Neurol* 2005;4:122–8.

4. Wikholm G, Lundqvist C, Svendsen P. Embolization of cerebral arteriovenous malformations: Part I – Technique, morphology, and complications. *Neurosurgery* 1996;39:448–57; discussion 57–9.

5. Miyamoto S, Hashimoto N, Nagata I, *et al.* Posttreatment sequelae of palliatively treated cerebral arteriovenous malformations. *Neurosurgery* 2000;46:589–94; discussion 594–5.

6. Han PP, Ponce FA, Spetzler RF. Intention-to-treat analysis of Spetzler–Martin grades IV and V arteriovenous malformations: natural history and treatment paradigm. *J Neurosurg* 2003;98:3–7.

7. Perret G, Nishioka H. Report on the cooperative study of intracranial aneurysms and subarachnoid hemorrhage. Section VI. Arteriovenous malformations. An analysis of 545 cases of cranio-cerebral arteriovenous malformations and fistulae reported to the cooperative study. *J Neurosurg* 1966;25:467–90.

8. McCormick WF, Rosenfield DB. Massive brain hemorrhage: a review of 144 cases and an examination of their causes. *Stroke* 1973;4:946–54.

9. Jessurun GA, Kamphuis DJ, van der Zande FH, Nossent JC. Cerebral arteriovenous malformations in The Netherlands Antilles. High prevalence of hereditary hemorrhagic telangiectasia-related single and multiple cerebral arteriovenous malformations. *Clin Neurol Neurosurg* 1993;95:193–8.

10. Brown RD, Jr., Wiebers DO, Torner JC, O'Fallon WM. Frequency of intracranial hemorrhage as a presenting symptom and subtype analysis: a population-based study of intracranial vascular malformations in Olmsted Country, Minnesota. *J Neurosurg* 1996;85:29–32.

11. Brown RD, Jr., Wiebers DO, Torner JC, O'Fallon WM. Incidence and prevalence of intracranial vascular malformations in Olmsted County, Minnesota, 1965 to 1992. *Neurology* 1996;46:949–52.

12. Stapf C, Mast H, Sciacca RR, *et al.* The New York Islands AVM Study: design, study progress, and initial results. *Stroke* 2003;34:e29–33.

13. Campi A, Scotti G, Filippi M, Gerevini S, Strigimi F, Lasjaunias P. Antenatal diagnosis of vein of Galen aneurysmal malformation: MR study of fetal brain and postnatal follow-up. *Neuroradiology* 1996;38:87–90.

14. Yuval Y, Lerner A, Lipitz S, Rotstein Z, Hegesh J, Achiron R. Prenatal diagnosis of vein of Galen aneurysmal malformation: report of two cases with proposal for prognostic indices. *Prenat Diagn* 1997;17:972–7.

15. Mullan S, Mojtahedi S, Johnson DL, Macdonald RL. Embryological basis of some aspects of cerebral vascular fistulas and malformations. *J Neurosurg* 1996;85:1–8.

16. Nelson MD, Jr., Gonzalez-Gomez I, Gilles FH. Dyke Award. The search for human telencephalic ventriculofugal arteries. *Am J Neuroradiol* 1991;12:215–22.

17. Hashimoto T, Mesa-Tejada R, Quick CM, *et al.* Evidence of increased endothelial cell turnover in brain arteriovenous malformations. *Neurosurgery* 2001;49:124–31; discussion 131–2.

18. Vikkula M, Boon LM, Carraway KL, 3rd, *et al.* Vascular dysmorphogenesis caused by an activating mutation in the receptor tyrosine kinase TIE2. *Cell* 1996;87:1181–90.

19. Hashimoto T, Lam T, Boudreau NJ, Bollen AW, Lawton MT, Young WL. Abnormal balance in the angiopoietin-tie2 system in human brain arteriovenous malformations. *Circ Res* 2001;89:111–13.

20. Rothbart D, Awad IA, Lee J, Kim J, Harbaugh R, Criscuolo GR. Expression of angiogenic factors and structural proteins in central nervous system vascular malformations. *Neurosurgery* 1996;38:915–24; discussion 924–5.

21. Hashimoto T, Emala CW, Joshi S, *et al.* Abnormal pattern of Tie-2 and vascular endothelial growth factor receptor expression in human cerebral arteriovenous malformations. *Neurosurgery* 2000;47:910–18; discussion 918–19.

22. Malik G, Abdulrauf S, Yang XY, Gutierrez JA, Rempel SA. Expression of transforming growth factor-beta complex in arteriovenous malformations. *Neurol Med Chir (Tokyo)* 1998;38 Suppl:161–4.

23. Hirschi KK, Rohovsky SA, D'Amore PA. PDGF, TGF-beta, and heterotypic cell–cell interactions mediate endothelial cell-induced recruitment of 10T1/2 cells and their differentiation to a smooth muscle fate. *J Cell Biol* 1998;141:805–14.

24. Sonstein WJ, Kader A, Michelsen WJ, Llena JF, Hirano A, Casper D. Expression of vascular endothelial growth factor in pediatric and adult cerebral arteriovenous malformations: an immunocytochemical study. *J Neurosurg* 1996;85:838–45.

25. Matsubara S, Bourdeau A, terBrugge KG, Wallace C, Letarte M. Analysis of endoglin expression in normal brain tissue and in cerebral arteriovenous malformations. *Stroke* 2000;31:2653–60.

26. Abdulrauf SI, Malik GM, Awad IA. Spontaneous angiographic obliteration of cerebral arteriovenous malformations. *Neurosurgery* 1999;44:280–7; discussion 287–8.

27. Kader A, Goodrich JT, Sonstein WJ, Stein BM, Carmel PW, Michelsen WJ.

Recurrent cerebral arteriovenous malformations after negative postoperative angiograms. *J Neurosurg* 1996;**85**:14–18.

28. Hashimoto N, Nozaki K. Do cerebral arteriovenous malformations recur after angiographically confirmed total extirpation? *Crit Rev Neurosurg* 1999;**9**:141–6.

29. Snead OC, 3rd, Acker JD, Morawetz R. Familial arteriovenous malformation. *Ann Neurol* 1979;**5**:585–7.

30. Gerosa MA, Cappellotto P, Licata C, Iraci G, Pardatscher K, Fiore DL. Cerebral arteriovenous malformations in children (56 cases). *Childs Brain* 1981;**8**:356–71.

31. Boyd MC, Steinbok P, Paty DW. Familial arteriovenous malformations. Report of four cases in one family. *J Neurosurg* 1985;**62**:597–9.

32. Barre RG, Suter CG, Rosenblum WI. Familial vascular malformation or chance occurrence? Case report of two affected family members. *Neurology* 1978;**28**:98–100.

33. Herzig R, Burval S, Vladyka V, *et al.* Familial occurrence of cerebral arteriovenous malformation in sisters: case report and review of the literature. *Eur J Neurol* 2000;**7**:95–100.

34. Putman CM, Chaloupka JC, Fulbright RK, Awad IA, White RI, Jr., Fayad PB. Exceptional multiplicity of cerebral arteriovenous malformations associated with hereditary hemorrhagic telangiectasia (Osler–Weber–Rendu syndrome). *Am J Neuroradiol* 1996;**17**:1733–42.

35. Kadoya C, Momota Y, Ikegami Y, Urasaki E, Wada S, Yokota A. Central nervous system arteriovenous malformations with hereditary hemorrhagic telangiectasia: report of a family with three cases. *Surg Neurol* 1994;**42**:234–9.

36. Willinsky RA, Lasjaunias P, Terbrugge K, Burrows P. Multiple cerebral arteriovenous malformations (AVMs). Review of our experience from 203 patients with cerebral vascular lesions. *Neuroradiology* 1990;**32**:207–10.

37. Ruigrok YM, Rinkel GJ, Wijmenga C. Genetics of intracranial aneurysms. *Lancet Neurol* 2005;**4**:179–89.

38. Kupersmith MJ, Vargas ME, Yashar A, *et al.* Occipital arteriovenous malformations: visual disturbances and presentation. *Neurology* 1996;**46**:953–7.

39. Lobato RD, Rivas JJ, Gomez PA, Cabrera A, Sarabia R, Lamas E. Comparison of the clinical presentation of symptomatic arteriovenous malformations (angiographically visualized) and occult vascular malformations. *Neurosurgery* 1992;**31**:391–6; discussion 396–7.

40. Maeda K, Kurita H, Nakamura T, *et al.* Occurrence of severe vasospasm following intraventricular hemorrhage from an arteriovenous malformation. Report of two cases. *J Neurosurg* 1997;**87**:436–9.

41. Mast H, Mohr JP, Osipov A, *et al.* 'Steal' is an unestablished mechanism for the clinical presentation of cerebral arteriovenous malformations. *Stroke* 1995;**26**:1215–20.

42. Wilkins RH. Natural history of intracranial vascular malformations: a review. *Neurosurgery* 1985;**16**:421–30.

43. Brown RD, Jr., Wiebers DO, Forbes G, *et al.* The natural history of unruptured intracranial arteriovenous malformations. *J Neurosurg* 1988;**68**:352–7.

44. Garrido E, Stein B. Removal of an arteriovenous malformation from the basal ganglion. *J Neurol Neurosurg Psychiatry* 1978;**41**:992–5.

45. Turjman F, Massoud TF, Sayre JW, Vinuela F, Guglielmi G, Duckwiler G. Epilepsy associated with cerebral arteriovenous malformations: a multivariate analysis of angioarchitectural characteristics. *Am J Neuroradiol* 1995;**16**:345–50.

46. Stapf C, Mohr JP, Sciacca RR, *et al.* Incident hemorrhage risk of brain arteriovenous malformations located in the arterial borderzones. *Stroke* 2000;**31**:2365–8.

47. Lees F. The migrainous symptoms of cerebral angiomata. *J Neurol Neurosurg Psychiatry* 1962;**25**:45–50.

48. Haas DC. Arteriovenous malformations and migraine: case reports and an analysis of the relationship. *Headache* 1991;**31**:509–13.

49. Bruyn GW. Intracranial arteriovenous malformation and migraine. *Cephalalgia* 1984;**4**:191–207.

50. Evans RW. Diagnostic testing for the evaluation of headaches. *Neurol Clin* 1996;**14**:1–26.

51. Hofmeister C, Stapf C, Hartmann A, *et al.* Demographic, morphological, and clinical characteristics of 1289 patients with brain arteriovenous malformation. *Stroke* 2000;**31**:1307–10.

52. Hillman J. Population-based analysis of arteriovenous malformation treatment. *J Neurosurg* 2001;**95**:633–7.

53. Simon HT, Reef H, Phadke RV, Popovic EA. A population-based study of brain arteriovenous malformation: long-term treatment outcomes. *Stroke* 2002;**33**:2794–800.

54. Khaw AV, Mohr JP, Sciacca RR, *et al.* Association of infratentorial brain arteriovenous malformations with hemorrhage at initial presentation. *Stroke* 2004;**35**:660–3.

55. Halim AX, Johnston SC, Singh V, *et al.* Longitudinal risk of intracranial hemorrhage in patients with arteriovenous malformation of the brain within a defined population. *Stroke* 2004;**35**:1697–702.

56. Jaillard AS, Peres B, Hommel M. Neuropsychological features of dementia due to dural arteriovenous malformation. *Cerebrovasc Dis* 1999;**9**:91–7.

57. Miyasaka Y, Kurata A, Tanaka R, *et al.* Mass effect caused by clinically unruptured cerebral arteriovenous malformations. *Neurosurgery* 1997;**41**:1060–3; discussion 1063–4.

58. Konan AV, Roy D, Raymond J. Endovascular treatment of hemifacial spasm associated with a cerebral arteriovenous malformation using transvenous embolization: case report. *Neurosurgery* 1999;**44**:663–6.

59. Ondra SL, Troupp H, George ED, Schwab K. The natural history of symptomatic arteriovenous malformations of the brain: a 24-year follow-up assessment. *J Neurosurg* 1990;**73**:387–91.

60. Aminoff MJ. Treatment of unruptured cerebral arteriovenous malformations. *Neurology* 1987;**37**:815–19.

61. Jane JA, Kassell NF, Torner JC, Winn HR. The natural history of aneurysms and arteriovenous malformations. *J Neurosurg* 1985;**62**:321–3.

62. Mast H, Young WL, Koennecke HC, *et al.* Risk of spontaneous haemorrhage after diagnosis of cerebral arteriovenous malformation. *Lancet* 1997;**350**:1065–8.

63. Kondziolka D, McLaughlin MR, Kestle JR. Simple risk predictions for arteriovenous malformation hemorrhage. *Neurosurgery* 1995;**37**:851–5.

64. Brown RD, Jr. Simple risk predictions for arteriovenous malformation hemorrhage. *Neurosurgery* 2000;**46**:1024.

65. Graf CJ, Perret GE, Torner JC. Bleeding from cerebral arteriovenous malformations as part of their natural history. *J Neurosurg* 1983;**58**:331–7.

66. Forster DM, Steiner L, Hakanson S. Arteriovenous malformations of the brain. A long-term clinical study. *J Neurosurg* 1972;**37**:562–70.

67. Fults D, Kelly DL, Jr. Natural history of arteriovenous malformations of the brain: a clinical study. *Neurosurgery* 1984;**15**:658–62.

68. Itoyama Y, Uemura S, Ushio Y, *et al.* Natural course of unoperated intracranial arteriovenous malformations: study of 50 cases. *J Neurosurg* 1989;**71**:805–9.

69. Krayenbuehl H, Siebenmann R. Small Vascular Malformations as a Cause of Primary Intracerebral Hemorrhage. *J Neurosurg* 1965;**22**:7–20.

70. Pollock BE, Flickinger JC, Lunsford LD, Bissonette DJ, Kondziolka D. Factors that predict the bleeding risk of cerebral arteriovenous malformations. *Stroke* 1996;**27**:1–6.

71. Langer DJ, Lasner TM, Hurst RW, Flamm ES, Zager EL, King JT, Jr. Hypertension, small size, and deep venous drainage are associated with risk of hemorrhagic presentation of cerebral arteriovenous malformations. *Neurosurgery* 1998;**42**:481–6; discussion 487–9.

72. Duong DH, Young WL, Vang MC, *et al.* Feeding artery pressure and venous drainage pattern are primary determinants of hemorrhage from cerebral arteriovenous malformations. *Stroke* 1998;**29**:1167–76.

73. Marks MP, Lane B, Steinberg GK, Chang PJ. Hemorrhage in intracerebral arteriovenous malformations: angiographic determinants. *Radiology* 1990;**176**:807–13.

74. Miyasaka Y, Yada K, Ohwada T, Kitahara T, Kurata A, Irikura K. An analysis of the venous drainage system as a factor in hemorrhage from arteriovenous malformations. *J Neurosurg* 1992;**76**:239–43.

75. Young WL, Prohovnik I, Ornstein E, *et al.* The effect of arteriovenous malformation resection on cerebrovascular reactivity to carbon dioxide. *Neurosurgery* 1990;**27**:257–66; discussion 266–7.

76. Kusske JA, Kelly WA. Embolization and reduction of the "steal" syndrome in cerebral arteriovenous malformations. *J Neurosurg* 1974;**40**:313–21.

77. Turjman F, Massoud TF, Vinuela F, Sayre JW, Guglielmi G, Duckwiler G. Correlation of the angioarchitectural features of cerebral arteriovenous malformations with clinical presentation of hemorrhage. *Neurosurgery* 1995;**37**:856–60; discussion 860–2.

78. Redekop G, TerBrugge K, Montanera W, Willinsky R. Arterial aneurysms associated with cerebral arteriovenous malformations: classification, incidence, and risk of hemorrhage. *J Neurosurg* 1998;**89**:539–46.

79. Stapf C, Mast H, Sciacca RR, *et al.* Predictors of hemorrhage in patients with untreated brain arteriovenous malformation. *Neurology* 2006;**66**:1350–5.

80. Hartmann A, Mast H, Mohr JP, *et al.* Morbidity of intracranial hemorrhage in patients with cerebral arteriovenous malformation. *Stroke* 1998;**29**:931–4.

81. Kumar AJ, Fox AJ, Vinuela F, Rosenbaum AE. Revisited old and new CT findings in unruptured larger arteriovenous malformations of the brain. *J Comput Assist Tomogr* 1984;**8**:648–55.

82. Tanaka H, Numaguchi Y, Konno S, Shrier DA, Shibata DK, Patel U. Initial experience with helical CT and 3D reconstruction in therapeutic planning of cerebral AVMs: comparison with 3D time-of-flight MRA and digital subtraction angiography. *J Comput Assist Tomogr* 1997;**21**:811–17.

83. Huston J, 3rd, Rufenacht DA, Ehman RL, Wiebers DO. Intracranial aneurysms and vascular malformations: comparison of time-of-flight and phase-contrast MR angiography. *Radiology* 1991;**181**:721–30.

84. Kucharczyk W, Lemme-Pleghos L, Uske A, Brant-Zawadzki M, Dooms G, Norman D. Intracranial vascular malformations: MR and CT imaging. *Radiology* 1985;**156**:383–9.

85. Schlosser MJ, McCarthy G, Fulbright RK, Gore JC, Awad IA. Cerebral vascular malformations adjacent to sensorimotor and visual cortex. Functional magnetic resonance imaging studies before and after therapeutic intervention. *Stroke* 1997;**28**:1130–7.

86. Latchaw RE, Hu X, Ugurbil K, Hall WA, Madison MT, Heros RC. Functional magnetic resonance imaging as a management tool for cerebral arteriovenous malformations. *Neurosurgery* 1995;**37**:619–25; discussion 625–6.

87. Saleh RS, Lohan DG, Villablanca JP, Duckwiler G, Kee ST, Finn JP. Assessment of craniospinal arteriovenous malformations at 3T with highly temporally and highly spatially resolved contrast-enhanced MR angiography. *Am J Neuroradiol* 2008;**29**:1024–31.

88. Turjman F, Massoud TF, Vinuela F, Sayre JW, Guglielmi G, Duckwiler G. Aneurysms related to cerebral arteriovenous malformations: superselective angiographic assessment in 58 patients. *Am J Neuroradiol* 1994;**15**:1601–5.

89. Reporting terminology for brain arteriovenous malformation clinical and radiographic features for use in clinical trials. *Stroke* 2001;**32**:1430–42.

90. Todaka T, Hamada J, Kai Y, Morioka M, Ushio Y. Analysis of mean transit time of contrast medium in ruptured and unruptured arteriovenous malformations: a digital subtraction angiographic study. *Stroke* 2003;**34**:2410–14.

91. Wakhloo AK, Lieber BB, Rudin S, Fronckowiak MD, Mericle RA, Hopkins LN. A novel approach to flow quantification in brain arteriovenous malformations prior to enbucrilate embolization: use of insoluble contrast (Ethiodol droplet) angiography. *J Neurosurg* 1998;**89**:395–404.

92. Morris P. *Practical Neuroangiography.* 2nd edn: Lippincott Williams & Wilkins; 2007.

93. Pile-Spellman JM, Baker KF, Liszczak TM, *et al.* High-flow angiopathy: cerebral blood vessel changes in experimental chronic arteriovenous fistula. *Am J Neuroradiol* 1986;**7**:811–15.

94. Valavanis A. The role of angiography in the evaluation of cerebral vascular malformations. *Neuroimaging Clin N Am* 1996;**6**:679–704.

95. Muller-Forell W, Valavanis A. How angioarchitecture of cerebral arteriovenous malformations should influence the therapeutic considerations. *Minim Invasive Neurosurg* 1995;**38**:32–40.

96. Spetzler RF, Martin NA. A proposed grading system for arteriovenous malformations. *J Neurosurg* 1986;**65**:476–83.

97. Tamaki N, Ehara K, Lin TK, *et al.* Cerebral arteriovenous malformations: factors influencing the surgical difficulty and outcome. *Neurosurgery* 1991;**29**:856–61; discussion 861–3.

98. Pertuiset B, Ancri D, Kinuta Y, *et al.* Classification of supratentorial arteriovenous malformations. A score system for evaluation of operability and surgical strategy based on an analysis of 66 cases. *Acta Neurochir (Wien)* 1991;**110**:6–16.

99. Shi YQ, Chen XC. A proposed scheme for grading intracranial arteriovenous malformations. *J Neurosurg* 1986;**65**:484–9.

100. Hamilton MG, Spetzler RF. The prospective application of a grading system for arteriovenous malformations. *Neurosurgery* 1994;**34**:2–6; discussion 7.

101. Heros RC, Korosue K, Diebold PM. Surgical excision of cerebral arteriovenous malformations: late results. *Neurosurgery* 1990;**26**:570–7; discussion 577–8.

102. Lawton MT. Spetzler-Martin Grade III arteriovenous malformations: surgical results and a modification of the grading scale. *Neurosurgery* 2003;**52**:740–8; discussion 748–9.

103. Spetzler RF, Hargraves RW, McCormick PW, Zabramski JM, Flom RA, Zimmerman RS. Relationship of perfusion pressure and size to risk of hemorrhage from arteriovenous malformations. *J Neurosurg* 1992;**76**:918–23.

104. Ogilvy CS, Stieg PE, Awad I, *et al.* Recommendations for the management of intracranial arteriovenous malformations: a statement for healthcare professionals from a special writing group of the Stroke Council, American Stroke Association. *Circulation* 2001;**103**:2644–57.

105. Fiorella D, Albuquerque FC, Woo HH, McDougall CG, Rasmussen PA. The role of neuroendovascular therapy for the treatment of brain arteriovenous malformations. *Neurosurgery* 2006;**59**:S163–77; discussion S3–13.

106. Purdy PD, Batjer HH, Risser RC, Samson D. Arteriovenous malformations of the brain: choosing embolic materials to enhance safety and ease of excision. *J Neurosurg* 1992;**77**:217–22.

107. Purdy PD, Batjer HH, Samson D, Risser RC, Bowman GW. Intraarterial sodium amytal administration to guide preoperative embolization of cerebral arteriovenous malformations. *J Neurosurg Anesthesiol* 1991;**3**:103–6.

108. Jafar JJ, Davis AJ, Berenstein A, Choi IS, Kupersmith MJ. The effect of embolization with N-butyl cyanoacrylate prior to surgical resection of cerebral arteriovenous malformations. *J Neurosurg* 1993;**78**:60–9.

109. Vinuela F, Dion JE, Duckwiler G, *et al.* Combined endovascular embolization and surgery in the management of cerebral arteriovenous malformations: experience with 101 cases. *J Neurosurg* 1991;**75**:856–64.

110. Morgan MK, Zurin AA, Harrington T, Little N. Changing role for preoperative embolisation in the management of arteriovenous malformations of the brain. *J Clin Neurosci* 2000;**7**:527–30.

111. Hartmann A, Mast H, Mohr JP, *et al.* Determinants of staged endovascular and surgical treatment outcome of brain arteriovenous malformations. *Stroke* 2005;**36**:2431–5.

112. Castel JP, Kantor G. [Postoperative morbidity and mortality after microsurgical exclusion of cerebral arteriovenous malformations. Current data and analysis of recent literature]. *Neurochirurgie* 2001;**47**:369–83.

113. DeMeritt JS, Pile-Spellman J, Mast H, *et al.* Outcome analysis of preoperative embolization with N-butyl cyanoacrylate in cerebral arteriovenous malformations. *Am J Neuroradiol* 1995;**16**:1801–7.

114. N-butyl cyanoacrylate embolization of cerebral arteriovenous malformations: results of a prospective, randomized, multi-center trial. *Am J Neuroradiol* 2002;**23**:748–55.

115. Lasjaunias P, Piske R, Terbrugge K, Willinsky R. Cerebral arteriovenous malformations (C. AVM) and associated arterial aneurysms (AA). Analysis of 101 C. AVM cases, with 37 AA in 23 patients. *Acta Neurochir (Wien)* 1988;**91**:29–36.

116. Kim EJ, Halim AX, Dowd CF, *et al.* The relationship of coexisting extranidal aneurysms to intracranial hemorrhage in patients harboring brain arteriovenous malformations. *Neurosurgery* 2004;**54**:1349–57; discussion 1357–8.

117. Brown RD, Jr., Wiebers DO, Forbes GS. Unruptured intracranial aneurysms and arteriovenous malformations: frequency of intracranial hemorrhage and relationship of lesions. *J Neurosurg* 1990;**73**:859–63.

118. Kwon Y, Jeon SR, Kim JH, *et al.* Analysis of the causes of treatment failure in gamma knife radiosurgery for intracranial arteriovenous malformations. *J Neurosurg* 2000;**93** Suppl 3:104–6.

119. Steiner L, Lindquist C, Adler JR, Torner JC, Alves W, Steiner M. Clinical outcome of radiosurgery for cerebral arteriovenous malformations. *J Neurosurg* 1992;**77**:1–8.

120. Lunsford LD, Kondziolka D, Flickinger JC, *et al.* Stereotactic radiosurgery for arteriovenous malformations of the brain. *J Neurosurg* 1991;**75**:512–24.

121. Maruyama K, Kawahara N, Shin M, *et al.* The risk of hemorrhage after radiosurgery for cerebral arteriovenous malformations. *N Engl J Med* 2005;**352**:146–53.

122. Pollock BE. Stereotactic radiosurgery for arteriovenous malformations. *Neurosurg Clin N Am* 1999;**10**:281–90.

123. Flickinger JC, Kondziolka D, Lunsford LD, *et al.* A multi-institutional analysis of complication outcomes after arteriovenous malformation radiosurgery. *Int J Radiat Oncol Biol Phys* 1999;**44**:67–74.

124. Gobin YP, Laurent A, Merienne L, *et al.* Treatment of brain arteriovenous malformations by embolization and radiosurgery. *J Neurosurg* 1996;**85**:19–28.

125. Henkes H, Nahser HC, Berg-Dammer E, Weber W, Lange S, Kuhne D.

Endovascular therapy of brain AVMs prior to radiosurgery. *Neurol Res* 1998;**20**:479–92.

126. Pollock BE, Kondziolka D, Lunsford LD, Bissonette D, Flickinger JC. Repeat stereotactic radiosurgery of arteriovenous malformations: factors associated with incomplete obliteration. *Neurosurgery* 1996;**38**:318–24.

127. Rao VR, Mandalam KR, Gupta AK, Kumar S, Joseph S. Dissolution of isobutyl 2-cyanoacrylate on long-term follow-up. *AJNR Am J Neuroradiol* 1989;**10**:135–41.

128. Fournier D, Terbrugge K, Rodesch G, Lasjaunias P. Revascularization of brain arteriovenous malformations after embolization with bucrylate. *Neuroradiology* 1990;**32**:497–501.

129. Fournier D, TerBrugge KG, Willinsky R, Lasjaunias P, Montanera W. Endovascular treatment of intracerebral arteriovenous malformations: experience in 49 cases. *J Neurosurg* 1991;**75**:228–33.

130. Vinuela F, Duckwiler G, Guglielmi G. Contribution of interventional neuroradiology in the therapeutic management of brain arteriovenous malformations. *J Stroke Cerebrovasc Dis* 1997;**6**:268–71.

131. Valavanis AC, G. Endovascular management of cerebral arteriovenous malformations. *Neurointenterventionist* 1999:34–40.

132. Weber W, Kis B, Siekmann R, Jans P, Laumer R, Kuhne D. Preoperative embolization of intracranial arteriovenous malformations with Onyx. *Neurosurgery* 2007;**61**:244–52; discussion 252–4.

133. Katsaridis V, Papagiannaki C, Aimar E. Curative embolization of cerebral arteriovenous malformations (AVMs) with Onyx in 101 patients. *Neuroradiology* 2008; **50** (7): 589–97.

134. Mounayer C, Hammami N, Piotin M, *et al.* Nidal embolization of brain arteriovenous malformations using Onyx in 94 patients. *Am J Neuroradiol* 2007;**28**:518–23.

135. van Rooij WJ, Sluzewski M, Beute GN. Brain AVM embolization with Onyx. *Am J Neuroradiol* 2007;**28**:172–7; discussion 178.

136. Luessenhop AJ, Mujica PH. Embolization of segments of the circle of Willis and adjacent branches for management of certain inoperable cerebral arteriovenous malformations. *J Neurosurg* 1981;**54**:573–82.

137. Fox AJ, Girvin JP, Vinuela F, Drake CG. Rolandic arteriovenous malformations: improvement in limb function by IBC embolization. *Am J Neuroradiol* 1985;**6**:575–82.

138. Wikholm G, Lundqvist C, Svendsen P. The Goteborg cohort of embolized cerebral arteriovenous malformations: a 6-year follow-up. *Neurosurgery* 2001;**49**:799–805; discussion 806.

139. Sampei K, Hashimoto N, Kazekawa K, Tsukahara T, Iwata H, Takaichi S. Histological changes in brain tissue and vasculature after intracarotid infusion of organic solvents in rats. *Neuroradiology* 1996;**38**:291–4.

140. Chaloupka JC, Vinuela F, Vinters HV, Robert J. Technical feasibility and histopathologic studies of ethylene vinyl copolymer (EVAL) using a swine endovascular embolization model. *Am J Neuroradiol* 1994;**15**:1107–15.

141. Murayama Y, Vinuela F, Ulhoa A, *et al.* Nonadhesive liquid embolic agent for cerebral arteriovenous malformations: preliminary histopathological studies in swine rete mirabile. *Neurosurgery* 1998;**43**:1164–75.

142. Jahan R, Murayama Y, Gobin YP, Duckwiler GR, Vinters HV, Vinuela F. Embolization of arteriovenous malformations with Onyx: clinicopathological experience in 23 patients. *Neurosurgery* 2001;**48**:984–95; discussion 995–7.

143. Mazal PR, Stichenwirth M, Gruber A, Sulzbacher I, Hainfellner JA. Tissue reactions induced by different embolising agents in cerebral arteriovenous malformations: a histopathological follow-up. *Pathology* 2006;**38**:28–32.

144. Yu SC, Chan MS, Lam JM, Tam PH, Poon WS. Complete obliteration of intracranial arteriovenous malformation with endovascular cyanoacrylate embolization: initial success and rate of permanent cure. *AJNR Am J Neuroradiol* 2004;**25**: 1139–43.

145. Yakes WF, Rossi P, Odink H. How I do it. Arteriovenous malformation management. *Cardiovasc Intervent Radiol* 1996;**19**:65–71.

146. Nakstad PH, Bakke SJ, Hald JK. Embolization of intracranial arteriovenous malformations and fistulas with polyvinyl alcohol particles and platinum fibre coils. *Neuroradiology* 1992;**34**:348–51.

147. Wakhloo AK, Juengling FD, Van Velthoven V, Schumacher M, Hennig J, Schwechheimer K. Extended preoperative polyvinyl alcohol microembolization of intracranial meningiomas: assessment of two embolization techniques. *Am J Neuroradiol* 1993;**14**:571–82.

148. Sorimachi T, Koike T, Takeuchi S, *et al.* Embolization of cerebral arteriovenous malformations achieved with polyvinyl alcohol particles: angiographic reappearance and complications. *Am J Neuroradiol* 1999;**20**:1323–8.

149. Mathis JA, Barr JD, Horton JA, *et al.* The efficacy of particulate embolization combined with stereotactic radiosurgery for treatment of large arteriovenous malformations of the brain. *Am J Neuroradiol* 1995;**16**:299–306.

150. Manninen PH, Gignac EM, Gelb AW, Lownie SP. Anesthesia for interventional neuroradiology. *J Clin Anesth* 1995;**7**:448–52.

151. Manninen PH, Chan AS, Papworth D. Conscious sedation for interventional neuroradiology: a comparison of midazolam and propofol infusion. *Can J Anaesth* 1997;**44**:26–30.

152. Pile-Spellman J, Young WL, Joshi S, *et al.* Adenosine-induced cardiac pause for endovascular embolization of cerebral arteriovenous malformations: technical case report. *Neurosurgery* 1999;**44**:881–6; discussion 886–7.

153. Han MH, Chang KH, Han DH, Yeon KM, Han MC. Preembolization functional evaluation in supratentorial cerebral arteriovenous malformations with superselective intraarterial injection of thiopental sodium solution. *Acta Radiol* 1994;**35**:212–16.

154. Moo LR, Murphy KJ, Gailloud P, Tesoro M, Hart J. Tailored cognitive testing with provocative amobarbital injection preceding AVM embolization. *Am J Neuroradiol* 2002;**23**:416–21.

155. Rauch RA, Vinuela F, Dion J, *et al.* Preembolization functional evaluation in brain arteriovenous malformations: the superselective Amytal test. *Am J Neuroradiol* 1992;**13**:303–8.

156. Young WL, Pile-Spellman J. Anesthetic considerations for interventional

neuroradiology. *Anesthesiology* 1994;**80**:427–56.

157. Jafar JJ, Tan WS, Crowell RM. Tissue plasminogen activator thrombolysis of a middle cerebral artery embolus in a patient with an arteriovenous malformation. Case report. *J Neurosurg* 1991;**74**:808–12.

158. Velat GJ, Reavey-Cantwell JF, Sistrom C, *et al.* Comparison of N-butyl cyanoacrylate and onyx for the embolization of intracranial arteriovenous malformations: analysis of fluoroscopy and procedure times. *Neurosurgery* 2008;**63**:ONS73–8; discussion ON78–80.

159. http://www.fda.gov/ohrms/dockets/ac/03/briefing/3975b1–02-clinical-review.htm. (Accessed at

160. Pierot LHD, Cognard C, Fransen H, *et al.* *Interventional Neuroradiology* 2009;**15**:121–4.

161. Jayaraman MV, Marcellus ML, Hamilton S, *et al.* Neurologic complications of arteriovenous malformation embolization using liquid embolic agents. *Am J Neuroradiol* 2008;**29**:242–6.

162. Aletich VADG. *Intracranial Arteriovenous Malformations: The Approach and Technique of*

Cyanoacrylate Embolization. Philadelphia: WB Saunders, 1999.

163. Houdart EME, Porcher R, Bresson D, Saint-Maurice JP, Bousser MG, Stapf C. *Interventional NeuroRadiology* 2009;**15**:121–4.

164. Piepgras DG, Sundt TM, Jr., Ragoowansi AT, Stevens L. Seizure outcome in patients with surgically treated cerebral arteriovenous malformations. *J Neurosurg* 1993;**78**:5–11.

165. Heikkinen ER, Konnov B, Melnikov L, *et al.* Relief of epilepsy by radiosurgery of cerebral arteriovenous malformations. *Stereotact Funct Neurosurg* 1989;**53**:157–66.

Intracranial dural arteriovenous fistulas

Thanh N. Nguyen, Jean Raymond, Alexander M. Norbash and Daniel Roy

Introduction

Dural arteriovenous fistulas (DAVF) are abnormal shunts between arteries and veins within the dura mater. They are acquired lesions[1-3] that occur most commonly without an obvious cause, but can also be found in association with trauma, surgery, tumors (most commonly meningiomas), or previous infections in the vicinity. They are often considered the result of a previous dural sinus inflammatory process, most often a thrombophlebitic episode. While DAVFs are extracerebral lesions, they may present with a wide range of neurologic symptoms, and their clinical presentation varies from an asymptomatic state to potentially cataclysmic events, such as life-threatening or fatal intracranial hemorrhage.[4] Much of the presentation depends on the venous drainage pattern, which is the most important determinant of prognosis. In benign fistulas, drainage does not involve the cerebral veins, and uncomplicated tinnitus or ocular symptoms are the most common forms of presentation. So-called "aggressive" or "dangerous" fistulas are characterized by retrograde cortical venous drainage,[5-7] and tend to present with intracranial hemorrhage, progressive neurological deficit, seizures, or intracranial hypertension.

By virtue of their rarity, variety, complexity, treatment failure rates and often multi-staged approach to treatment, DAVFs have puzzled and fascinated many since the early days of neurointerventional procedures. DAVFs have often been misunderstood, misdiagnosed, and poorly managed until a thorough knowledge of arterial and venous anatomy, and a mastering of principles and techniques of endovascular management have more recently offered cure for most patients. This chapter will review the epidemiology, pathophysiology, classification, natural history, clinical presentation, diagnosis, and management of DAVFs.

Epidemiology

Dural arteriovenous fistulas are uncommon lesions, comprising 6 to 15% of intracranial vascular malformations.[8-10] The apparent incidence of various types of fistulas is as much related to referral patterns to specialized institutions that report their case series as they are related to a true incidence to be found in a general population. In a prospective population-based study, the crude detection rate of DAVF was 0.16 per 100 000 adults per year (95% CI 0.08–0.27).[8] They can present from birth to old age (mean in the fifth decade).[6] There is no known correlation between age, cause of DAVF and presence of aggressive symptoms.[6]

The most common locations for DAVF are the transverse or sigmoid sinus,[5,6,11,12] (over 40% of reported locations), and the cavernous sinus region, which typically is affected to a greater degree in postmenopausal women.[13] Other locations include the superior sagittal sinus, petrosal sinuses, tentorium cerebelli, foramen magnum, sphenoparietal sinus, and anterior fossa. Aggressive DAVFs are more often seen in men. Dural AVFs can also be seen directly involving the ophthalmic or olfactory vein complexes, perhaps because these veins follow a trans-osseous course.[14] Reports have shown multiple DAVFs in approximately 7% of cases.[15] There are no clear associations between DAVF and the presence of other vascular malformations.

Pathophysiology

Pathophysiological perspectives may be separated into three overarching considerations:

(a) *Basis for thrombosis*. The etiopathogenesis of the disease and its relation to venous thrombosis, and individual risk factors for dural venous thrombosis.

(b) *Reactive inflammation*. The inflammatory cascade as it relates to recanalization, neovascularization, or mural pouch formation.

(c) *Architectural structure*. Potential explanations regarding the peculiar propensity for this location to develop A-V shunting in response to venous thrombosis.

Although much of the pathophysiology of DAVF remains unknown, the most convenient way of understanding the problem is as a secondary rather than primary disease of the wall of the dural venous sinuses. The sinus often shows signs of previous partial or complete thrombosis. The shunt consists of multiple reactive direct communications of various sizes between dural arteries of the vicinity and the sinus, collected to an anatomically defined segment of the dural venous sinus system. The dura seems to have this propensity for exuberant neovascularization, and direct arteriovenous shunts may result from angiogenesis in the proximity of arteries. Also, pre-existing arteriovenous communications can increase in size or grow in response to various angiogenic factors. Further description of the pathophysiology of DAVF merits first a review of the vascular anatomy of the dura.

Vascular anatomy of the dura

The normal dura mater is richly vascularized with an extensive shared supply. Most of its arterial supply arises from branches of the external carotid artery with some participation of the internal carotid, vertebral, and ophthalmic arteries. Detailed anatomical description of the arterial supply to the dura is beyond the scope of this chapter and the reader is referred to classical texts.[5,16] Extensive anastomoses exist between the meningeal arteries,[10,12] and this allows DAVFs to recruit feeders from distant arteries. The dominant supply to DAVFs are meningeal arteries, which were present in 95% of DAVFs in a series of 205 cases. Shared meningeal and cortical branch supply can be found in 5% of cases.[6] Pial supply to a DAVF typically originates from the development of trans-arachnoid anastomoses.

In contrast to vessels in the brain parenchyma, the arteries and veins within the dura are very close together. Therefore, following trauma, vascular rupture can more easily result in a fistulous communication. Postmortem studies have demonstrated AV shunts of 50 to 90 µ in diameter in normal dura, with a majority of shunts positioned lateral to the superior longitudinal sinus.[17] However, the function[18] and long-term potential for pathological transformation of these physiological dural AV shunts is unknown.

Role of sinus thrombosis and venous stenosis

The role of venous sinus thrombosis as a aute precedent or accompaniment to DAVF formation was demonstrated by Houser et al. by cerebral angiography.[3] In their series, two of 14 patients had angiographic evidence of sigmoid or transverse sinus occlusion before formation of DAVF in the pertinent sinus; ten patients with DAVF had compromised sinuses, of which eight demonstrated transverse or sigmoid sinus occlusion, and two demonstrated sinus stenosis.[3] In another study, cerebral sinus thrombosis was diagnosed in 27 (39%) of 69 patients with DAVF. Interestingly, 10 (37%) patients had cerebral sinus thrombosis (CST) in more than one location.[19] However, once CST is formed, most patients do not progress to DAVF.[18,20] In a series of 51 patients with lateral sinus

thrombosis with mean follow-up of 78 months, only one patient went on to develop a DAVF.[20]

Alternatively, sinus stenosis and thrombosis may less commonly occur as a consequence of a DAVF due to high flow angiopathy. The presence of venous thrombosis may affect the drainage of a dural fistula, impacting upon its clinical and hemodynamic behavior.[21] It may also explain the changes observed during the clinical evolution of fistulas from rerouting of venous drainage to other pathways (for example cavernous DAVF that can shift from ophthalmic drainage with ocular symptoms to petrous drainage with ophthalmological improvement but emergence of a bruit), to spontaneous closure of the fistula. In a study of 54 patients with untreated DAVF, patients without a venous sinus outflow occlusion at initial angiography were more likely to have symptom improvement or remain stable compared to patients with an occlusion who demonstrated infrequent improvement.[11] Cortical venous drainage can still develop without sinus occlusion,[3] when the flow exceeds the capacity of the sinus, although in many of these cases the question remains whether the sinus may have recanalized spontaneously following a prior occlusion with a reactive and remaining DAVF formation.

Because the disease can be associated by analogy to venous thrombosis, the pathogenesis can be analyzed using Virchow's triad (decreased flow, increased thrombogenicity, parietal injury). Thus local trauma or tumors may provoke venous outlet obstruction or parietal damage, while certain systemic risk factors may favor dural venous thrombosis.

Thrombophilic factors

Several hematologic abnormalities have been reported in patients with DAVF, though firm conclusions cannot be drawn due to the rarity of this disease and low incidence of mutations. Given the potential link between dural thrombophlebitis and DAVFs, associations with factors known to affect coagulation are unsurprising. In a pooled analysis, the factor V Leiden mutation was present in 9/121 (7.4%) patients compared to 3/178 (1.7%) volunteers (OR 4.7, 95% CI 1.2–17.7); the prothrombin gene mutation (G20210A) was present in seven of 121 patients, but only in one of 178 controls (OR 10.9, 95% CI 1.3–89.5).[22–25] Due to the low frequency of mutations in patients with DAVF, routine screening of prothrombotic mutations is not indicated.[22] Other hematologic parameters, such as basic coagulation profile, fibrinogen, and factor VIII were found normal in one study with 40 DAVF patients.[22]

Formation of the shunt

Venous sinus thrombosis may induce opening of normal or pre-existing intrinsic dural arteriovenous shunts during organization and recanalization of thrombus.[1,3,18] These microscopic shunts may be present from birth[10,26] or develop from abnormal growth of the vasa vasorum of the sinuses.[3] In rat

Table 14.1. Three classification schemes for dural arteriovenous fistulas: Djindjian, Cognard, and Borden

Djindjian	Cognard	Borden
Type I	Type I	Type I
– drainage into sinus or meningeal vein	– antegrade sinus drainage	– drainage into sinus or meningeal vein
Type II	Type II	Type II
– initial drainage into sinus with reflux into other sinuses or cortical veins	– antegrade and reflux sinus drainage	– drain into dural sinus or meningeal vein, but also retrograde into subarachnoid veins
	Type IIa	
	– retrograde venous drainage into sinus(es) only	
Type III	Type IIb	Type III
– initial drainage into cortical vein	– retrograde venous drainage into cortical vein(s) only	– drain into subarachnoid veins only
Type IV	Type IIa+b	
– initial drainage into cortical vein with giant venous pouch	– retrograde venous drainage into sinus(es) and cortical vein(s).	
	Type III	
	– drain directly into cortical vein without venous ectasia	
	Type IV	
	– drain into cortical vein with venous ectasia >5mm and 3x larger than diameter of draining vein	
	Type V	
	– drain into spinal perimedullary veins	

models, induced venous hypertension[27,28] and sinus thrombosis[27,29] were shown to elicit formation of DAVF.

There is some speculation that DAVFs arise from angiogenesis, or newly formed blood vessels, in response to an inflammatory cascade triggered by venous ischemia. A vicious cycle can occur: venous hypertension or thrombosis can lead to reduced perfusion, which leads to tissue hypoxia stimulating angiogenesis, perhaps due to higher levels of vascular endothelial growth factor (VEGF).[30] Angiogenesis by dural blood vessels could then promote shunting into dural sinuses.[27] Arterialization could further exacerbate venous hypertension and enlarge the dural fistula.

Risk factors for hemorrhage

DAVFs with cortical venous drainage typically present with intracranial hemorrhage, especially if no other drainage exists, or if ectasia of a draining vein is present. These patterns urge imperative treatment.[3,6,11] Location has been reported as another factor to consider, with DAVFs at the tentorium cerebelli, anterior cranial fossa, and superior sagittal sinus at higher risk for hemorrhage.[5,6,31,32] However, the tentorium cerebelli and anterior cranial fossa sites generally drain into cortical venous pathways, hence the risk of intracranial

hemorrhage is really due to cortical venous drainage rather than a peculiarity of the location.

Classification

At least three classifications have been proposed: those of Djindjian, Cognard, and Borden, but they are all variations of the same understanding (Table 14.1).[5–7] The classifications of DAVFs is determined by the direction of venous drainage, which separates benign from aggressive forms of the disease. In 1978, Djindjian and Merland used superselective angiography to classify DAVFs based on the pattern of venous drainage, with each subsequent type considered as a more aggressive form of the disease.[5] In this classification, type I fistulas drain into a sinus or meningeal vein; type II drain into a sinus with reflux into other sinuses(IIA) or cortical veins (IIB); type III drain directly into a cortical vein; type IV drain into a cortical vein with a giant associated venous pouch (dural or subdural) which can occasionally act as an intracranial space occupying lesion.

Cognard *et al.* further modified the original Djindjian classification by validating Djindjian's classification scheme with a series of over 200 patients.[6] They showed that no DAVF without cortical venous drainage bled, and expanded upon the patterns of venous drainage, particularly for Type II fistulas and fistula with spinal drainage. In this modified classification, type I fistulas exhibit antegrade drainage into a sinus; type II are located in the main sinus, with reflux of injected contrast into the sinus (IIa), cortical veins (IIb), or both (IIa + b); type III drain directly into a cortical vein without venous ectasia; type IV drain directly into a cortical vein with venous ectasia and type V have associated spinal perimedullary venous drainage. In general, tentorium cerebelli and anterior cranial fossa AVFs are type III and type IV dural fistulas because of their cortical venous drainage. The shunt lies in the wall of the intradural portion of a cortical vein proximal to its anastomosis with the corresponding sinus. When the anastomosis is stenosed or occluded (while the sinus may or may not be patent), the flow is directed in a retrograde manner into the cortical vein.[15] Patients with type IV dural fistulas can also develop progressive tumor-like symptoms due to mechanical compression of adjacent structures.[6]

Of note, the Cognard classification scheme only considered neurological brain parenchymal risk for cavernous sinus DAVFs and not the ophthalmologic risks. A cavernous sinus DAVF draining into the ophthalmic vein and without cortical venous reflux would be considered type IIa. The authors still highlight the ophthalmologic risk as a high priority.

Borden later simplified the classification scheme, unifying cranial and spinal fistula classification.[7] Type I DAVFs drain antegrade into dural venous sinuses or meningeal veins, and are considered benign. Type II DAVFs drain into dural sinuses or meningeal veins, although they can also drain in a retrograde manner to subarachnoid veins. Neurological deficits are seen with Type II DAVFs, due to secondary venous hypertension. Type III DAVFs drain into subarachnoid veins only, and typically present with intracranial hemorrhage.

Clinical presentation

DAVFs can present with a wide range of symptoms and signs, depending on their location and pattern of venous drainage. Most commonly patients present with tinnitus or ophthalmic manifestations in the more common transverse and cavernous locations. Although hemorrhagic presentations are less common, DAVFs should always be considered in the differential diagnosis of intracranial hemorrhages, particularly in the absence of more frequently seen conditions such as aneurysms or AVMs. Finally, the rarer lesions causing symptomatic venous hypertension can be associated with a wide variety of presentations. The high flow nature of a lesion can cause hemodynamic or high-output presentations, or the spinal drainage will be associated with a myelopathic presentation.

Symptoms may include pulsatile tinnitus, headache, diplopia, chemosis, proptosis, seizures, transient global amnesia, altered mental status including dementia or cognitive decline, and even progressive myelopathy. In children and infants,

there may be such high flow as to manifest signs and symptoms related to heart failure. Signs are also variable, and may manifest as an audible bruit, exophthalmos, chemosis, cranial nerve palsy, dysphasia, progressive dementia, or sensorimotor deficit. The onset of symptoms may be insidious, as with progressive neurological deficits, or fulminant, as with intracranial hemorrhage.[33]

Orbital symptoms related to cavernous DAVFs

Venous congestion is likely an important mechanism in the development of cranial nerve and orbital symptomatology in cavernous sinus DAVFs. Symptoms typical of dural cavernous carotid fistula include progressive conjunctival chemosis, proptosis, pulsating exophthalmos, and painful opthalmoparesis.[34] Later signs of cavernous sinus DAVF include visual acuity impairment and secondary or accelerating open angle glaucoma. Visual impairment may result from spontaneous choroidal detachment, strabismus, proptosis with corneal exposure, or retinal or optic nerve ischemia.[13] Decreased visual acuity mandates urgent treatment. Paradoxical symptoms in the contralateral orbit may occur if ipsilateral cavernous sinus thrombosis reroutes the venous drainage.[35] More subtle clinical manifestations of cavernous sinus fistulae can be found in middle-aged to elderly women; prominent congestion of episcleral and conjunctival veins are diagnostic clues.[36] The oculomotor nerves are the most common cranial nerves affected by a DAVF given the trajectory of these nerves through the cavernous sinus.

Tinnitus

Pulsatile tinnitus or bruit is the most common presenting symptom in DAVFs.[11] The sound becomes perceptible when there is venous drainage that involves a dural sinus in direct contact with the petrous pyramid.[35] Through bone conduction the sound is transmitted to the auditory apparatus.[37] This of course is most often the case in lesions of the transverse-sigmoid region, although due to bone conduction, auditory bruits are also not uncommon in cavernous sinus DAVFs, and those involving the petrosal sinus. The bruit is generally high pitched, worse with exercise, positional changes, stress and at night.[37] A softer bruit may be transmitted to the contralateral side.[5,37] A higher flow, or flow with little or no obstruction downstream, produces more intense tinnitus. Light pressure against the ipsilateral retro-auricular region or over the ipsilateral common carotid artery may improve the symptoms,[37,38] although typically such examinations need to be performed in extremely quiet rooms without background noise. An accompanying objective bruit is generally heard in cases with pulsatile tinnitus,[35] by placing a stethoscope over the ipsilateral mastoid bone.

Intracranial hemorrhage

Intracranial hemorrhage may be seen in aggressive fistulas with cortical venous drainage; many of these are fulminant.

The ictal event can consist of a severe headache and focal neurological deficit. Compartments affected by the intracranial hemorrhage can on occasion be localized to the subdural, or intraventricular spaces,[2,9,11] although they most commonly present with intraparenchymal and subarachnoid hemorrhage.[2,11]

Re-bleeding after initial hemorrhage can occur in up to 35% of patients. In a series of 20 patients who presented with intracranial hemorrhage, cortical venous drainage was demonstrated in all patients who underwent angiography. Of the 20 patients, seven suffered re-bleeding within 2 weeks after the first hemorrhage,[39] all with change in level of consciousness and worsened neurological status as a direct result of rebleeding. There was a predominance of type IV dural fistulae and posterior tentorial circulation location among those that rebled.

General neurological symptoms

Headache is a non-specific presentation of DAVF, but may be disabling. The headache can be due to underlying dural irritation, venous congestion, or intracranial hypertension. The headache may be ipsilateral to the fistula and may be aggravated by head position, exercise or Valsalva-like maneuver, and high blood pressure.[37] Hemorrhagic presentations can also be associated with headaches that have a "thunderclap" character and may be followed by coma.

High-flow large dural AVFs may overwhelm the pathways permitting normal cerebral venous drainage, thereby leading to increased intracranial pressure and communicating hydrocephalus.[2] Increased intracranial pressure has been attributed to an increase in the cerebral blood volume and pressure in the dural sinus, with a secondary decrease in CSF absorption (Monroe–Kellie doctrine). Intracranial hypertension can be seen in type IIa DAVFs.[6] Non-communicating hydrocephalus may also occur as a mechanical consequence, when a venous varix obstructs the outflow of cerebrospinal fluid in the posterior fossa,[2] leading to the classic triad of gait ataxia, urinary incontinence, and progressive cognitive decline. With increased intracranial pressure, patients may present with papilledema and secondary optic atrophy[40] and be erroneously diagnosed with benign intracranial hypertension.

Focal neurological symptoms

Focal neurological symptoms without hemorrhage are mainly seen in the presence of cortical venous drainage and venous congestion which interferes with normal venous drainage.[35] As a result, any territory may be affected, leading to seizures or deficits variable. Venous ischemia with edema, with or without infarction of the affected territory may occur.[37] Transient focal deficits have also been described.[3] Less commonly, local mass effect by a venous aneurysm or "venous lake" can result in a neurological deficit.[41] Symptoms such as dysphasia, motor weakness, transient ischemic attack, or focal seizure may surface, depending on the route of venous drainage. Visual changes can be seen in cases with altered venous flow from the occipital lobe or increased intracranial pressure. Cognitive or memory impairment may surface as a focal symptom in cases with impaired drainage of the temporal lobe, with secondary impaired regional blood flow, or as a generalized symptom, with or without increased intracranial pressure or hydrocephalus. In these cases, regional blood flow is diminished not only as a result of decreased venous outflow but also because of the elevation in intracranial pressure.

Myelopathy

Myelopathy is a rare clinical manifestation of intracranial DAVFs, occurring in approximately 3% of cases.[6,11] Drainage into perimedullary veins classifies the DAVF as type V, by the Cognard classification. Fistulas at the foramen magnum or at the tentorium have been described to drain via anastomotic connections towards the spinal perimedullary veins.[42,43] Drainage at this location may cause venous congestion leading to tissue edema of the spinal cord and progressive loss of cord function with urinary retention, numbness and paresthesias.[44–46] Patients present with progressive ascending myelopathy, manifest as lower extremity weakness followed by upper extremity weakness.[43,47] Rarely, if the edema progresses cephalad, the lower brainstem can be affected. Bulbar symptoms, such as dysphagia, can appear with lower brainstem involvement, as well as autonomic symptoms: orthostatic hypotension, tachycardia or bradycardia.[44–46]

Natural history
Benign DAVFs

DAVFs without cortical venous drainage are considered benign. In a series of 55 Borden type I DAVFs, 26 patients were followed for a mean of 32 months and showed symptom resolution or improvement in 21 (81%) patients. Five (19%) were unchanged.[48] Overall, 53/54 (98%) patients with Borden type I DAVFs were stable at follow-up (mean 33-month follow-up), whereas one patient deteriorated and died, likely secondary to raised intracranial pressure.[48]

The potential for transformation of a benign fistula to an aggressive type is low. A study of 117 patients with benign DAVFs showed that an aggressive clinical course occurred in 2% of patients over a median follow-up of 27.9 months (range 1 month to 17.5 years).[22] Another series showed absence of transformation in 84 type I DAVFs (47 followed 6 months to 23 years) other than one type I DAVF that progressed to type IIa due to increased flow.[6] Cognard et al. evoked several factors that may lead to worsening DAVF grade in a series of seven patients: stenosis or thrombosis of the draining veins in four cases, increased arterial flow in two, and appearance of a new fistula site or extension of the initial shunt in two.[49]

Table 14.2. Features considered in benign vs. aggressive dural arteriovenous fistulas

Benign	Aggressive
Clinical	Clinical
– asymptomatic	– hemorrhage
– headache	– focal neurological deficit
– tinnitus	– intracranial hypertension
– ocular symptoms without intracranial hypertension	– seizures
	– altered mental status
	– ascending myelopathy
Angiographic features	**Angiographic features**
– Drain into dural sinus	– leptomeningeal venous drainage
	– variceal or aneurysmal venous dilatation
	– Galenic drainage

There is some controversy in the follow-up of benign type I DAVFs. Clinical evaluation may not be reliable since positive changes in the symptoms such as a reduction of the bruit may be associated with development of cortical drainage which could remain asymptomatic until hemorrhage occurs. Due to the low probability of aggressive evolution, follow-up with catheter angiography appears ill-advised. Up until recently, non-invasive imaging could not distinguish reliably between benign and aggressive types but this is changing with the advent of time resolved MRA.

Aggressive DAVFs

The natural history of more aggressive lesions is very difficult to assess. Type III and IV intracranial DAVFs have been reported to have a hemorrhagic risk of approximately 1.8% per year.[39] The annual risk of mortality and morbidity with lesions with cortical venous reflux is 10 and 15%, respectively.[50] Presence of leptomeningeal venous drainage, variceal or aneurismal venous dilatations, and Galenic drainage are possible signs of a more aggressive fistula type (Table 14.2).[32]

Diagnosis

The gold standard test for diagnosis of DAVF is angiography. Benign types of dural fistulas are generally occult on CT or MR except for those located at the cavernous sinus where a dilatation of the superior ophthalmic vein with or without exophthalmia can be seen. In DAVFs with cortical drainage, CT and MR may show dilated veins or parenchymal reaction such as edema, infarction, hemorrhage or chronic white matter hyperintensities. Sensitivity and specificity of these techniques remain poor. Standard CTA and MRA lack the hemodynamic evaluation given by angiography as well as the spatial resolution necessary for small lesions. Time-resolved MRA is a promising technique that may become the imaging technique of choice for the diagnosis and follow-up of untreated DAVFs. In intracranial DAVFs with spinal venous drainage, MR may show spinal cord swelling as well as venous dilatations similar to what is seen in spinal dural fistulas.

Angiographic study of DAVFs

Angiographic evaluation for DAVFs should include selective injection of both internal and external carotid arteries as well as vertebral arteries. Vertebral artery injection may be omitted in case of cavernous or anterior fossa fistulas. Selective injection of both internal carotid and vertebral arteries is important for a complete evaluation of the pattern of cerebral venous drainage, and identification of pial or meningeal contributors to the DAVF. The location of the shunt should be identified, along with the arterial feeders (meningeal vs. pial). The topography of venous drainage should be identified with special attention directed towards identifying any cortical venous reflux or mural venous pouch. Risk factors for hemorrhage such as venous sinus stenosis, subtotal or total occlusion, and venous ectasia should be noted. One should also observe whether the sinus drainage carries any associated anomaly, stenosis, thrombosis or hypoplasia.[6]

In patients presenting with progressive cord myelopathy, findings of swollen cervical cord and dilated perimedullary veins, complete work-up must include external carotid artery injections and angiography of the vertebral area, if cervical or spinal artery catheterizations are negative.[43] Rapid recognition of an intracranial DAVF is important as early disconnection of the cranial DAVF drainage into spinal veins permits myelopathy recovery, before ischemic and gliotic changes become irreversible.[51]

Principles of management

The anatomy and behavior of dural fistulas being so variable, it is essential to tailor their management to each situation. Specific goals for each case should be first put forward, taking into account the natural history of the lesion (which mainly depends on its venous drainage pattern), its specific anatomical features and the patient's symptoms. As a rule of thumb, treatment should be conservative for benign lesions, while more aggressive approaches may be justified with hemorrhagic presentations. However, there is also no reason not to offer a low-risk procedure to a patient suffering from intolerable tinnitus. In aggressive lesions, that is fistulas associated with pial venous drainage, the aim should be angiographic obliteration. Most dural fistulas can be managed by endovascular means but some, mostly Borden type III or Cognard type III, IV and V, are sometimes more appropriately approached by surgery. Some difficult lesions need the judicious combination of endovascular techniques and surgery.

As with any arteriovenous shunt, the most effective and durable treatment consists of occlusion of the venous recipient of the fistula,[52] whether this is achieved by endovascular treatment or surgery. Two principles have to be respected. First, if venous occlusion is not at the fistulous point but downstream, persistent arterial input may lead to rupture of pial veins in case of type 3 fistulas or rerouting of flow in type 1 or 2 fistulas. The second point is that, when targeting the fistulous recipient, one should aim to avoid the occlusion of normal venous pathways, since this may lead to venous infarction or even life-threatening intracranial hematomas. With an endovascular approach, this goal may be achieved by a transarterial or transvenous approach and with several types of embolic agents. This is more a matter of personal technical comfort and may change from one anatomical situation to the other. In general, cavernous and transverse-sigmoid DAVFs are treated using a transvenous approach, most often using detachable coils, while type III–V fistulae are more commonly treated by an arterial approach, using a polymerizing agent or more recently ethylene-vinyl alcohol. Keeping these principles in mind, understanding the alternative venous outflow pathways when intentionally occluding veins and sinuses, and avoiding dogmatic attitudes should allow selection of the most appropriate technique for each specific situation.

Fistulas without pial venous drainage

The two most frequent sites of fistulas that are generally of the benign type are the transverse sinus and cavernous area. These two should be separated since their clinical behavior differs significantly. Even without pial drainage, cavernous fistulas are associated with disturbing functional symptoms such as diplopia as well as potentially loss of visual acuity due to increased ocular pressure. Thus, active treatment is more often indicated for cavernous fistulas than for type I fistulae of the transverse sinus.

Cavernous fistulas

These fistulas have been associated with the highest probability of spontaneous occlusion. Thus, in patients with mild symptoms and low ocular pressure, especially in the elderly, a conservative approach may be wise. Rapid decline of visual acuity on the other hand, is an indication for urgent intervention.

Manual compression of the neck vessels, although classically described as a first treatment, is probably not helpful and has fallen out of favor over time. The success reported by this simple procedure[53] may have been related to spontaneous occlusions. Because of the frequent bilateral supply and drainage of these lesions, the theoretical mechanism of this maneuvre seems disputable. There is also a theoretical risk of baroreceptor stimulation, particularly in elderly patients, as well as the risk of inadvertent permanent carotid occlusion.

Spontaneous occlusion of primary venous ophthalmic outflow may be associated with a dramatic increase in ocular symptomatology and urgent treatment should be considered, using either a trans-venous approach or trans-arterial approach. Trans-venous occlusion is currently the preferred approach because of higher efficacy and lower risk.[54] A retrograde inferior petrosal sinus approach is often achievable even when the inferior petrosal sinus is not visible at angiography.[55] Other approaches include contralateral inferior petrosal sinus through the intercavernous plexus, retrograde facial vein catheterization by jugular, femoral (Fig. 14.1) or direct facial or frontal vein puncture, or even direct puncture of the superior ophthalmic vein with or without surgical cut-down.[13,56–58] The first target should be the disconnection of the orbital veins from the fistula and then its complete occlusion. Caution must be exercised to avoid rerouting of venous drainage towards pial veins. Coils are most appropriate for this purpose. Because of the low thrombogenicity of standard platinum coils, some advocate the use of fibered coils or hydrogel or the adjunct of liquid embolic agents.[59–61] Poorly controlled liquid embolic agents run the risk of occluding the central retinal vein.

A transarterial approach with particles is rarely useful, except in palliation of acute presentations. The use of liquid embolic agents from an arterial approach is seldom advocated because of multiple arterial feeders involved in most instances and the numerous dangerous anastomoses with the carotid and vertebro-basilar systems.

Transverse-sigmoid sinus fistulas

Due to the benign natural history of Borden type I or Cognard type I and IIa dural fistulas, there are seldom indications for aggressive treatment of these lesions. However, patients may be significantly disturbed by their tinnitus and may demand treatment. Careful analysis of the angiogram may show that the affected sinus does not participate in the venous drainage of either the supratentorial or infratentorial circulations (Fig. 14.2). Also, compartments of a sinus may be involved by the fistula while others are free so that selective occlusion can be achieved while keeping the normal venous pathway patent.[62,63] In these situations, venous occlusion has been shown to be very effective and safe. When the targeted sinus is participating in normal cerebral drainage, arterial palliative embolization using particles may be used for symptom relief, but benefits are often transient. Embolization using diluted glue,[64] or more recently ethylene-vinyl alcohol, has been shown effective and durable for size and flow reduction with sometimes cure of the fistula while preserving sinus patency.

Fistulas with pial venous drainage

Due to their aggressive behavior, the intention when treating these fistulas is angiographic cure whenever possible. Anatomically and for technical reasons, these fistulas are divided into those involving a sinus with secondary pial reflux (Borden type II and Cognard type IIb and IIa+b) and others

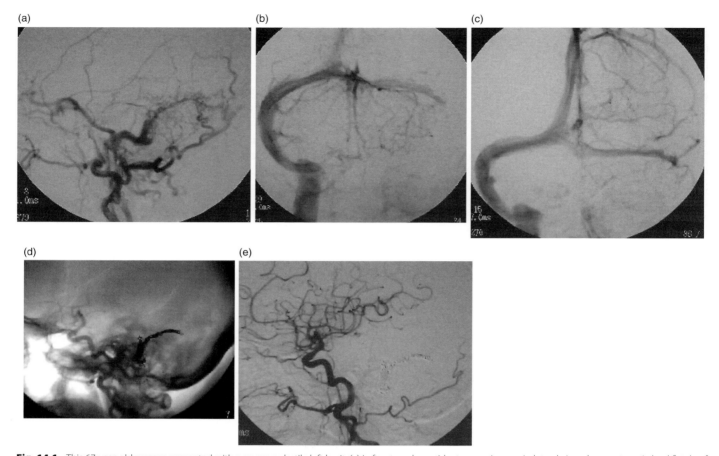

Fig. 14.1. This 67-year-old woman presented with a severe pulsatile left bruit. (a) Left external carotid artery angiogram in lateral view shows a type 1 dural fistula of the left transverse sinus with post-phlebitic changes. Venous phase of left vertebral injection (Towne's view) (b) and left internal carotid injection (AP view) (c) shows that the involved sinus no longer participates in the drainage of the brain. Lateral left external carotid artery, unsubtracted (d) and subtracted (e) images after transvenous embolization with coils showing closure of the fistula.

involving the intradural part of the pial vein without connection to the efferent sinus (Borden type III and Cognard type III, IV and V).

Fistulas with sinus involvement

The presence of pial reflux from a sinus indicates that this sinus is no longer participating in the normal venous drainage. The reduction of pressure in the venous system after closure of the fistula site then can only help. Thus, occlusion of the venous recipient of the fistula is not only efficient but also safe. Every effort should be made to occlude only the part of the sinus affected and leave the surrounding venous channels open to the extent possible. Most of these lesions are treated using a transvenous approach (Fig. 14.3). When the involved sinus is isolated from occlusions at both ends, access may still be possible by an arterial approach and this should be attempted. If not possible, a combined surgical–endovascular approach can be performed with a burr hole over the involved sinus followed by sinus packing under fluoroscopic guidance. This may be preceded by arterial embolization in high-flow lesions. Depending on the anatomy, reaching the

venous compartment with a liquid embolic agent from a trans-arterial approach may also be a valid option.

The use of sinus stenting has recently been advocated in a study[65] for the treatment of dural fistulas, with intended compression of the fistula pouch by the stent. This approach can only be used when the culprit sinus is patent. The efficiency and safety of this technique require confirmation.

Fistulas with direct cortical venous drainage

These fistulae, clearly the most aggressive, are also the most challenging to treat from an endovascular perspective. The multiplicity of arterial feeders, their tortuosity and the dangerous anastomoses often involved make the transarterial approach difficult. Diluted glue has been used most often in order to reach the vein.[64,66,67] Recently, ethylene-vinyl alcohol for trans-arterial embolization has been used with a high success rate.[68] This precipitate has the ability to reach arterial feeders retrogradely from one single injection with very little venous contamination and segmentation compared to glue (Fig. 14.4). When catheter positioning allows the safe pericatheter reflux necessary for controlled antegrade injections,

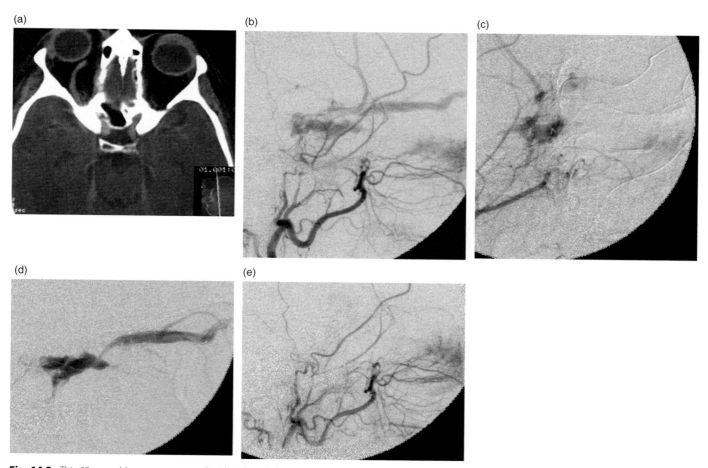

Fig. 14.2. This 62-year-old woman presented with right-sided exophthalmia, diplopia, chemosis and increased intra-ocular pressure. (a) Contrast-enhanced CT of the orbit showing right-sided exophthalmia and enlargement of the right superior ophthalmic vein (SOV). (b) Right external carotid artery (ECA) injection confirms the dural fistula of the cavernous sinus with retrograde filling of the SOV. (c) After failed attempt to catheterize the cavernous sinus from the inferior petrosal sinus, retrograde catheterization of the SOV via the facial vein from the femoral vein was achieved as shown on this oblique view of a right ECA injection. (d) Selective injection of the right cavernous sinus. (e) Right ECA injection after closure of the fistula with coils.

this technique has recently become the favored approach. Case reports of transvenous approach for direct type III fistulas have been published.[69] Unfortunately, a significant number of cases demonstrated complex venous drainage in which catheter navigation was difficult, if not impossible. The dural part of the vein should be reached for a safe embolization unless increased pressure in the system can occur with venous rupture.

Technique

After careful study of the DAVF including location of the shunt and venous drainage of normal brain, the intervention can be pursued. For transvenous coil embolization, percutaneous arterial and venous access are secured using modified Seldinger technique. A 6F or 7F guide catheter is introduced over a 0.035-inch guidewire into the common femoral and iliac veins, and subsequently advanced to the inferior vena cava, right atrium, and superior vena cava under fluoroscopic guidance. The guide catheter is advanced into the brachiocephalic vein and internal jugular vein. Simultaneous arterial injections with opacification of the internal jugular veins may be necessary to identify the origin and anatomical configuration of the vein for catheterization. On occasion, a tri-axial catheter system may be used, with a 7F guide catheter over a 0.038 catheter, over a microcatheter to increase the stability of microcatheter delivery to the shunt, especially if it involves crossing from one transverse sinus to another. With the guide catheter in the internal jugular vein, a microcatheter is advanced over a microguidewire under roadmap guidance from an arterial injection imaged in the venous phase. The microcatheter is approached as close as possible to the area of the shunt. After careful study of the venous drainage of the shunt compared to normal brain, consecutive coils are deployed to occlude the sinus of interest with caution not to occlude the outlets of normal venous drainage.

Embolization results

In the non-aggressive types of dural fistulas, results may be divided into complete angiographic cure and symptom relief

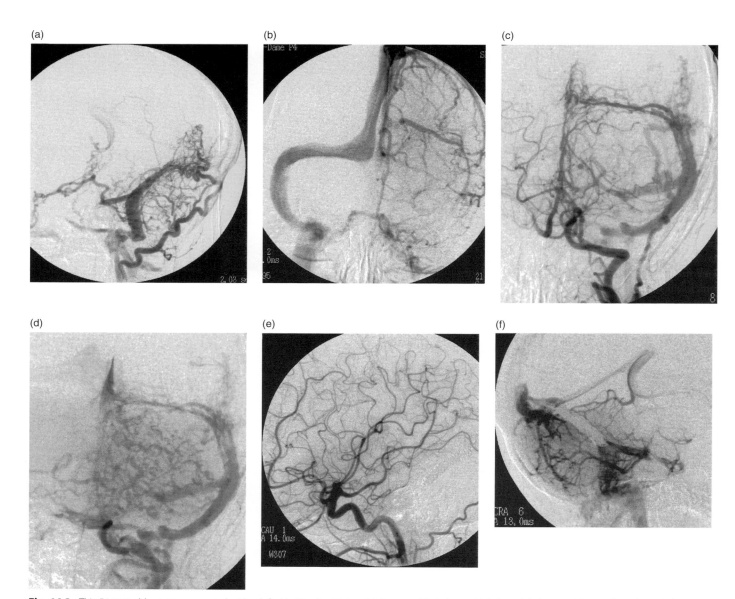

Fig. 14.3. This 54-year-old woman presented with a left-sided bruit with head fullness and imbalance. (a) Left occipital artery injection (lateral view) showing prominent opacification of the left transverse sinus with retrograde filling of pial veins of the posterior fossa as well as reflux into the Galen system via the superior petrosal sinus and lateral mesencephalic vein (Cognard type IIa+b). (b) Venous phase of the left internal carotid artery injection (AP view) showing no opacification of the left transverse sinus. Early (c) and late phase (d) of a left vertebral injection (Towne's view) showing the fistula and venous congestion in the posterior fossa. (e) Left common carotid injection (lateral view) 3 months after transvenous embolization of the fistula with coils. (f) Venous phase of a left vertebral injection (lateral view) 3 months after treatment showing normal appearance of the posterior fossa veins. The patient's symptoms completely disappeared.

even if a small shunt persists. Complete cure and clinical cure have been reported in over 90% of cases. For aggressive lesions, the goal is complete anatomical cure, and the results of embolization depend on the type and location of the fistula. Judicious use of different techniques including surgery should yield a high cure rate.[67]

Embolization complications

Most complications of embolization of dural fistulas are predictable, and perhaps avoidable with mastering of anatomical principles and meticulous technique. The overall risk of permanent neurological deficit ranges between 4% and 5% with a mortality between 0% to 4%.[25–27] Beside the intrinsic risks of angiography and vascular access, complications may arise from arterial or venous compromise. On the arterial side, complications may be related to cerebral embolization due to the passage of the embolic agent through anastomoses between external carotid artery branches and either the internal carotid or vertebro-basilar arteries. Therefore, knowledge of these ubiquitous anastomoses is particularly important Ischemia of cranial nerves may occur with the use of liquid embolic agents

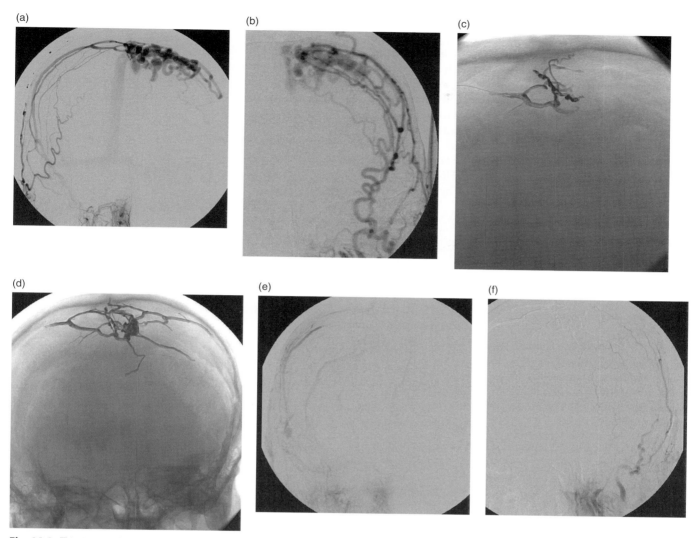

Fig. 14.4. This 65-year-old man presented with non-specific headaches. MRI (not shown) revealed vascular dilatation at the vertex consistent with the presence of an arteriovenous shunt. (a) Right ECA injection (AP view) and (b) left ECA injection (AP view) show a Cognard type IV dural fistula near the superior sagittal sinus fed by branches of both middle meningeal arteries. (c), (d) show progressive filling of the fistula feeders with Onyx during a single injection from the right side. The fistula was completely circumscribed by retrograde filling of the left-sided feeders with very little venous contamination with the embolic material. Right (e) and left (f) ECA injections (AP view) after embolization showing complete closure of the fistula.

in arteries at the base of the skull. Provocative testing is probably of no use and in any case cannot allow an injection that is known for anatomical reasons to be unsafe.

Transvenous embolization carries the risk of vessel perforation or of jeopardizing venous drainage of normal brain or rarely of retinal vein occlusions. A complete evaluation and understanding of both the supratentorial and infratentorial venous phase of the angiogram are very important. Inappropriate occlusion of a venous compartment may also lead to rerouting of the venous drainage of a fistula towards other paths and may transform a benign lesion into a dangerous one.

Transient nerve palsies may be seen following aggressive transvenous packing of cavernous sinus fistulas, especially VIth nerve palsies.[12,23] Transient XIIth nerve palsy following transvenous embolization of anterior condylar canal fistula is also possible. These transient nerve dysfunctions are believed to be related to the inflammatory reaction accompanying thrombosis, and steroids or other anti-inflammatory agents may be used for treatment. Finally, we have observed several cases of transient labyrinthine dysfunction after occlusion of the sigmoid sinus that we believe may be related to endolymphatic hydrops of the adjacent saccus endolymphaticus.[24]

Neurosurgical management

Surgery should be considered when complete cure of a fistula is indicated and cannot be obtained by endovascular approach.

The role of neurosurgery in the treatment of dural fistulas involving sinuses is limited nowadays, although in complex cases, especially when the sinus involved is isolated from segmental occlusions and endovascular approach is impossible from both the venous and arterial routes, surgery may be the sole method possible in accessing the lesion.[20] In a number of cases of fistulas, especially those involving the ethmoidal region, most frequently supplied by ophthalmic artery branches, and, less frequently the tentorial or foramen magnum fistulas, surgical disconnection of the vein[21] remains a safe and effective method of treatment. However, these recommendations may change in the future as new techniques evolve.

Radiosurgery

The efficacy of radiosurgery in the management of intracranial dural fistulas is not well documented. A recent paper from the Karolinska Institute[22] reported their experience over 25 years. The occlusion rate was 68%, with reduction of flow in additional 24% with few complications. However, flow reduction may not guarantee freedom from hemorrhagic risks. The delay between treatment and documented therapeutic occlusion remains a drawback when dealing with aggressive lesions. In some low risk but symptomatic fistulas where endovascular therapy has failed or surgery seems unreasonable, radio surgery could be contemplated.

Conclusion

DAVFs are uncommon but potentially aggressive lesions, particularly in the presence of cortical venous drainage. Comprehensive angiographic evaluation is important to determine appropriate therapy. Advances in endovascular therapy have recently allowed a high cure rate of these lesions.

References

1. Chaudhary MY, Sachdev VP, Cho SH, Weitzner I Jr, Puljic S, Huang YP. Dural arteriovenous malformation of the major venous sinuses: An acquired lesion. *Am J Neuroradiol* 1982;**3**:13–19.

2. Castaigne P, Bories J, Brunet P, Merland JJ, Meininger V. Les fistules arterioveineuses meningees pures a drainage veineux cortical. *Rev Neurol* 1976:169–181.

3. Houser OW, Campbell JK, Campbell RJ, Sundt TM Jr. Arteriovenous malformation affecting the transverse dural venous sinus – an acquired lesion. *Mayo Clin Proc* 1979;**54**:651–61.

4. Kosnik EJ, Hunt WE, Miller CA. Dural arteriovenous malformations. *J Neurosurg* 1974;**40**:322–9.

5. Djindjian R, Merland JJ. *Superselective Arteriography of the External Carotid Artery.* New York: Springer-Verlag, 1978:405–11.

6. Cognard C, Gobin GP, Pierot L, *et al.* Cerebral dural arteriovenous fistulas: clinical and angiographic correlation with a revised classification of venous drainage. *Radiology* 1995;**194**:671–80.

7. Borden JA, Wu JK, Shucart WA. A proposed classification for spinal and cranial dural arteriovenous malformations and implications for treatment. *J Neurosurg* 1995;**82**:166–79.

8. Al-Shahi R, Bhattacharya JJ, Currie DG, *et al.* Scottish Intracranial Vascular Malformation Study Collaborators. Prospective, population-based detection of intracranial vascular malformations in adults: the scottish intracranial vascular malformation study (sivms). *Stroke* 2003;**34**:1163–9.

9. Cordonnier C, Al-Shahiu R, Bhattacharaya JJ, *et al.* Differences between intracranial vascular malformation types in the characteristics of their presenting hemorrhages: Prospective-population-based study. *J Neurol Neurosurg Psych* 2007:May 8; [Epub ahead of print]

10. Newton TH, Cronqvist S. Involvement of dural arteries in intracranial arteriovenous malformations. *Radiology* 1969;**93**:1071–8.

11. Brown RD, Wiebers DO, Nichols DA. Intracranial dural arteriovenous fistulae: Angiographic predictors of intracranial hemorrhage and clinical outcome in nonsurgical patients. *J Neurosurg* 1994;**81**:531–8.

12. Aminoff M. Vascular anomalies in the intracranial dura mater. *Brain* 1973;**96**:601–12.

13. Goldberg RA, Goldey SH, Dukwiler G, Vinuela F. Management of cavernous sinus-dural fistulas. Indications and techniques for primary embolization via the superior ophthalmic vein. *Arch Opthalmol* 1996;**114**:707–14.

14. Piske RL, Lasjaunlas P. Extrasinusal dural arteriovenous malformations. *Neuroradiology* 1988:426–32.

15. Barnwell SL, Halbach VV, Dowd CF, Higashida RT, Hieshima GB, Wilson CB. Multiple dural arteriovenous fistulas of the cranium and spine. *Am J Neuroradiol* 1991;**12**:441–5.

16. Lasjaunias P, Berenstein A, Ter Brugge KG. Surgical neuroangiography. Vol. 2.1 In *Clinical Vascular Anatomy and Variations.* 2001;2nd edn. Heidelberg: Springer-Verlag Publications.

17. Rowbotham GF, Little E. Circulations of the cerebral hemispheres. *Br J Surg* 1965;**52**:8–21.

18. Graeb DA, Dolman CL. Radiological and pathological aspects of dural arteriovenous fistulas. Case report. *J Neurosurg* 1986;**64**:962–7.

19. Tsai LK, Jeng JS, Liu HM, Wang HJ, Yip PK. Intracranial dural arteriovenous fistulas with or without cerebral sinus thrombosis: Analysis of 69 patients. *J Neurol Neurosurg Psychiatry* 2004;**75**:1639–41.

20. Preter M, Tzourio C, Ameri A, Bousser MG. Long-term prognosis in cerebral venous thrombosis. *Stroke* 1996;**27**:243–6.

21. DeMarco JK, Dillon WP, Halbach VV, Tsuruda JS. Dural arteriovenous fistulas: evaluation with mr imaging. *Radiology* 1990;**175**:193–9.

22. Van Dijk JMC, Ter Brugge KG, Van der Meer FJ, Wallace C, Rosendaal FR. Thrombophilic factors and the formation of dural arteriovenous fistulas. *J Neurosurg* 2007;**107**:56–9.

23. Gerlach R, Yahya H, rohde S, Bohm M, Berkefeld J, Scharrer I, *et al.* Increased incidence of thrombophilic abnormalities in patients with cranial dural arteriovenous fistulae. *Neurol Res.* 2003;**25**:745–48

24. Jellema K, Tijssen CC, Fijnheer R, de Groot PG, Koudstaal PJ, van Gijn J. Spinal dural arteriovenous fistulas are not associated with prothrombotic factors. *Stroke* 2004;**35**:2069–71.

25. Kraus JA, Stuper BK, Berlit P. Association of resistance to activated protein c and dural arteriovenous fistulas. *J Neurol* 1998;**245**:731–3.

26. Kunc Z, Bret J. Congenital arterio-sinusal fistulae. *Acta Neurochir* 1969;**20**:85–103.

27. Lawton MT, JaCobowitz R, Spetzler RF. Redefined role of angiogenesis in the pathogenesis of dural arteriovenous malformations. *J Neurosurg* 1997;**87**:267–74.

28. Terada T, Higashida RT, Halbach VV, *et al.* Development of acquired arteriovenous fistulas in rats due to venous hypertension. *J Neurosurg* 1994;**80**:884–9.

29. Herman JM, Spetzler RF, Bederson JB, Kurbat JM, Zabramski JM. Genesis of a dural arteriovenous malformation in a rat model. *J Neurosurg* 1995;**83**:539–45.

30. Shin Y, Nakase H, Nakamura M, Shimada K, Konishi N, Sakaki T. Expression of angiogenic growth factor in the rat davf model. *Neurol Res* 2007;**14**:[Epub ahead of print]

31. Jamous Jamous MA, Satoh K, Satomi J, Matsubara S, Nakajima N, Uno M, Nagahiro S. Detection of enlarged cortical vein by magnetic resonance imaging contributes to early diagnosis and better outcome for patients with anterior cranial fossa dural arteriovenous fistula. *Neurol Med Chir (Tokyo); discussion 520–1.* 2004;**44**:516–20.

32. Awad IA, Little JR, Akarawi WP, Ahl J. Intracranial dural arteriovenous malformations: factors predisposing to an aggressive neurological course. *J Neurosurg* 1990;**72**:839–50.

33. Chen JC, Tsuruda JS, Halbach VV. Suspected dural arteriovenous fistula: Results with screening mr angiography in seven patients. *Radiology* 1992;**183**:265–71.

34. Vinuela F, Fox AJ, Debrun GM, Peerless SJ, Drake CG. Spontaneous carotid-cavernous fistulas: Clinical, radiological, and therapeutic considerations. *J Neurosurg* 1984;**60**:976–84.

35. Lasjaunias P, Chiv M, Ter Brugge K, Tolia A, Hurth M, Bernstein M. Neurological manifestations of intracranial dural arteriovenous malformations. *J Neurosurg* 1986;**64**:724–30.

36. Phelps CD, Thompson HS, Ossoinig KC. The diagnosis and prognosis of atypical carotid-cavernous fistula (red-eyed shunt syndrome). *Am J Ophthalmol* 1982;**93**:423–36.

37. Halbach VV, Higashida RT, Larsen DW, Dowd CF, McDougall CG, Hieshima GB, Wilson CB. Treatment of dural arteriovenous fistulas. In Maciunas RJ (ed). *Endovascular Neurological Intervention.* American Association of Neurological Surgeons, 1995:217–46.

38. Park IH, Kang HJ, Suh SI, Chae SW. Dural arteriovenous fistula presenting as subjective pulsatile tinnitus. *Arch Otolaryngol Head Neck Surg* 2006;**132**:1148–50.

39. Duffau H, Lopes M, Janosevic V, Early rebleeding from intracranial dural arteriovenous fistulas: Report of 20 cases and review of the literature. *J Neurosurg* 1999;**90**:78–84.

40. Kuhner A, Krastel A, Stoll W. Arteriovenous malformations of the transverse dural sinus. *J Neurosurg* 1976;**45**:12–19.

41. Mirabel S, Lindblom B, Halbach VV, Hoyt WF. Giant suprasellar varix: an unusual cause of chiasmal compression. *J Clin Neuroophthalmol* 1991;**11**:268–72.

42. Akkoc Y, Atamaz F, Oran I, Durmaz B. Intracranial dural arteriovenous fistula draining into spinal perimedullary veins: a rare cause of myelopathy. *J Korean Med Sci* 2006;**21**:958–62.

43. Van Rooij WJ, Shuzewski M, Beute GN. Intracranial dural fistulas with exclusive perimedullary drainage: the need for complete cerebral angiography for diagnosis and treatment planning. Case report. *Am J Neuroradiol* 2007;**28**:348–51.

44. Brunereau L, Gobin YP, Meder JF, Cognard C, Tubiana JM, Merland JJ. Intracranial dural arteriovenous fistulas with spinal venous drainage: Relation between clinical presentation and angiographic findings. *Am J Neuroradiol* 1996;**17**:1549–54.

45. Gobin YP, Royopoulos A, Aymard A, *et al.* Endovascular treatment of intracranial dural arteriovenous fistulas with spinal perimedullary venous drainage. *J Neurosurg* 1992;**77**:718–23.

46. Ricolfi F, Manelfe C, Meder JF, *et al.* Intracranial dural arteriovenous fistulae with perimedullary venous drainage. Anatomical, clinical and therapeutic considerations. *Neuroradiology* 1999;**41**:803–12.

47. Trop I, Roy D, Raymond J, Roux A, Bourgouin P, Leasge J. Craniocervical dural fistula associated with cervical myelopathy: Angiographic demonstration of normal venous drainage of the throacolumbar cord does not rule out diagnosis. *Am J Neuroradiol* 1998;**19**:583–6.

48. Davies MA, Saleh J, TerBrugge K, Willinski R, Wallace MC. The natural history and management of intracranial dural arteriovenous fistulae. *Interventional Neuroradiology* 1997;**3**:295–302.

49. Cognard C, Houdart E, Casasco A, Gabrillargues J, Chiras J, Merland JJ. Long-term changes in intracranial dural arteriovenous fistulae leading to worsening in the type of venous drainage. *Neuroradiology* 1997;**39**:59–66.

50. Van Dijik JMC, Ter Brugge KG, Willinsky RA, Wallace MC. Clinical course of cranial dural arteriovenous fistulas with long-term persistent cortical venous reflux. *Stroke* 2002;**3**:1233–6.

51. Wiesmann M, Padovan CS, Pfister HW, Yousry TA. Intracranial dural arteriovenous fistula with spinal medullary venous drainage. *Eur Radiol* 2000;**10**:1606–9.

52. Mullan S. Reflections upon the nature and management of intracranial and intraspinal vascular malformations and fistulae. *J Neurosurg* 1994;**80**:606–16.

53. Kay Y, Hamada JI, Morioka M, Yano S, Kuratsu JI. Treatment of cavernous sinus dural arteriovenous fistulae by external manual carotid compression. *Neurosurgery* 2007;**60**:253–8.

54. Kirsch M, Henkes H, Liebig T, Weber W, Esser J, Golik S, Kühne D. Endovascular management of dural carotid-cavernous sinus fistulas in 141 patients. *Neuroradiology* 2006;**48**:486–90.

55. Benndorf G, Bender A, Lehmann R, Lanksch W. Transvenous occlusion of dural cavernous sinus fistulas through the thrombosed inferior petrosal sinus: report of four cases and review of the literature. *Surg Neurol* 2000;**54**:42–54.

56. Biondi A, Milea D, Cognard C, Ricciardi GK, Bonneville F, van Effenterre R. Cavernous sinus dural fistulae treated by transvenous approach through the facial vein: Report of seven cases and review of the literature. *Am J Neuroradiol* 2003;**24**:1240–6.

57. Venturi C, Bracco S, Cerase A, Gennari P, Lorè F, Polito E, Casasco AE. Endovascular treatment of a cavernous sinous dural arteriovenous fistula by transvenous embolisation through the superior ophthalmic vein via cannulation of a frontal vein. *Neuroradiology.* 2003;**45**:574–78

58. Jahan R, Gobin YP, Glenn B, Duckwiler GR, Vinuela F. Transvenous embolisation of a dural arteriovenous fistula of the cavernous sinus through the contralateral ptrygoid plexus. *Neuroradiology* 1998;**40**:189–93.

59. Suzuki S, Lee DW, Jahan R, Duckwiler GR, Vinuela F. Transvenous treatment of sontaneous dural carotid-cavernous dural fistulas using a combination of detachable coils and onyx. *Am J Neuroradiol* 2006;**27**:1346–9.

60. Arat A, Cekirge S, Saatci I, Ozgen B. Transvenous injection of onyx for casting of the cavernous sinus for the treatment of a carotid-cavernous fistula. *Neuroradiology* 2004;**46**:1012–15.

61. Roy D, Raymond J. The role of transvenous embolization in the treatment of intracranial dural arteriovenous fistulas. *Neurosurgery* 1997;**40**:1133–41.

62. Mironov A. Selective transvenous embolization of dural fistulas without occlusion of the dural sinus. *Am J Neuroradiol* 1998;**19**:389–91.

63. Piske RL, Campos CM, Chaves JB, *et al.* Dural sinus compartment in dural arteriovenous shunts: A new angioarchitectural feature allowing superselective transvenous dural sinus occlusion treatment. *Am J Neuroradiol* 2005;**26**:1715–22.

64. Nelson PK, Russell SM, Woo HH, Alastra AJ, Vidovich DV. Use of a wedged microcatheter for curative transarterial embolization of complex intracranial dural arteriovenous fistulas: indications, endovascular technique, and outcome in 21 patients. *J Neurosurg* 2003;**98**:498–506.

65. Levrier O, Métullus P, Fuentes S, *et al.* Use of a self-expanding stent with balloon angioplasty in the treatment of dural arteriovenous fistulas involving the transverse and/or sigmoid sinus: Functional and neuroimaging-based outcome in 10 patients. *J Neurosurg* 2006;**104**:254–63.

66. Sarma D, ter Brugge K. Management of intracranial dural arteriovenous shunts in adults. *European Journal of Radiology* 2003;**46**:206–20.

67. Van Rooij WJ, Sluzewski M, Beute GN. Dural arteriovenous fistulas with cortical venous drainage: Incidence, clinical presentation, and treatment. *Am J Neuroradiol* 2007;**28**:651–5.

68. Arat A, Inci S. Treatment of a superior sagittal sinus dural arteriovenous fistula with onyx: technical case report. *Neurosurgery* 2006;**59**[ONS Suppl 1]:169–70.

69. Cloft HJ, Kallmes DF, Jensen JE, Dion JE. Percutaneous transvenous coil embolization of a type 4 sagittal sinus dural arteriovenous fistula: Case report. *Neurosurgery* 1997;**41**:1191–3.

Cerebral sinus thrombosis

Amit Singla and Randall C. Edgell

Incidence and risk factors for cerebral venous sinus thrombosis

Overview

Cerebral venous sinus thrombosis (CVST), i.e. thrombosis of the intracranial veins or sinuses, is the underlying cause of ca. 0.5% of all strokes, affecting approximately five people per million.[1] The incidence peaks in neonates and adults in their third decade of life with a female : male ratio of 5:1,5.[2]

CVST was first recognized about 150 years ago when Ribes provided the first detailed description of a patient with sagittal sinus thrombosis found on autopsy. CVST was originally considered a fatal disorder of infectious etiology, often diagnosed only at the time of autopsy.[3] Until recent times, because of the association between CVST and hemorrhage the use of anticoagulation was considered to be contraindicated.[4] As our understanding of this entity progressed, anticoagulation became the first line of treatment.[5–8] In spite of recent advances, however, CVST diagnosis and treatment remain challenging because of a remarkable diversity of clinical symptoms, modes of onset, and imaging features. Overall mortality remains high at 6–10%.[9,10]

In the present decade, progress has been made in our understanding of CVST from individual studies and from the International Study on Cerebral Vein and Dural Sinus Thrombosis (ISCVT). The ISCVT is the largest multinational observational study to date on CVST. The study included 624 adult patients with symptomatic CVST who were diagnosed at 89 participating centers in 21 countries, from May 1998 to May 2001.[11]

The distribution of the location of thrombosis based on data from the ISCVT is provided in Table 15.1. The sagittal (60%–75%) and lateral sinuses (70%–85%) were involved more frequently than the deep venous system. In about 75% of cases, multiple veins or sinuses were affected.[12] The location of venous thrombosis is important because deep cerebral and cerebellar vein thrombosis is associated with a higher mortality than thrombosis of superficial veins.[11]

Table 15.1. Frequency of occlusion sites in cerebral veins and sinus thrombosis as seen in the International Study on Cerebral Vein and Dural Sinus Thrombosis (ISCVT)

Sites of venous occlusion	% of cases
Superior sagittal sinus	62.0
Lateral sinus, left	44.7
Lateral sinus, right	41.2
Straight sinus	18.0
Deep venous system	10.9
Cortical veins	17.1
Jugular veins	11.9
Cerebellar veins	0.3

Anatomy

The cerebral venous system can be divided into a superficial and a deep system. The superficial system consists of the superior sagittal sinus and cortical veins that drain the surfaces of both cerebral hemispheres. The deep system is composed of the internal cerebral veins, the basal vein of Rosenthal, the vein of Galen, and the straight sinus. Both systems drain into the transverse sinuses, the sigmoid sinuses, and the jugular veins. The veins draining the brain do not follow the same course as the arteries that supply it. Generally, venous blood drains to the nearest venous sinus, except in the case of the deepest structures, that drain to deep veins. These drain, in turn, to the dural venous sinuses.[12,13]

The superficial venous system drains the entire neocortex together with a layer of subcortical white matter, separated from the periventricular white matter by a venous watershed. The superficial cerebral veins can be subdivided into three groups. These are interlinked with the anastomotic veins of Trolard and Labbe. However, the superficial cerebral veins are very variable and generally drain to the nearest dural sinus.

Thus the superolateral surface of the hemisphere drains to the superior sagittal sinus while the posteroinferior aspect drains to the transverse sinus.[14]

The deep venous system drains not only the choroid plexuses and the deep gray matter of the thalamus and striatum, but also the periventricular white matter and corpus callosum, hippocampus, and the cortical areas of the limbic lobe including the cingulate and parahippocampal gyri, the visual cortex, the diencephalon and rostral brainstem, and part of the cerebellum. In contrast to the superficial system, the deep system is rather constant with the exception of wide variations seen in the size of the basal vein. Hence thrombosis is more easily recognized here.[15]

Evidence from pathological anatomy indicates that the venous watershed exists not only in the white matter of the hemispheres, but also between the entire territories of the deep and superficial venous systems. Because of their anastomotic interconnections, only simultaneous obstruction of the veins of Galen and basal veins will effectively obstruct deep venous outflow.[16]

Etiology

The risk factors for venous thrombosis are generally linked to Virchow's triad that includes stasis of blood, changes in the vessel wall, and changes in the composition of blood.[10] The etiology of CVST is usually multifactorial. In ISCVT, 44% of the patients included had more than one cause or predisposing factor.[11] Local factors that may predispose to CVST include: infections of the ear, sinus, mouth, face, or neck; meningitis; brain tumors; vascular malformations; and head trauma. Other factors predisposing to CVST include various diagnostic and therapeutic procedures such as surgery, lumbar puncture, jugular catheters and some drugs – in particular oral contraceptives and anticancer drugs.[1] (Table 15.2)

Hereditary thrombophilia is found in 20 to 30% of patients with CVST.[13] Common inherited thrombophilic dispositions include factor V Leiden mutation, prothrombin-gene mutation 20210GA, antithrombin, protein C-, and protein S-deficiency. The factor V Leiden mutation (15%–17%) and prothrombin-gene-mutation (10%–12%) are the most frequently observed thrombophilias in patients with CVST whereas antithrombin, protein C, and protein S deficiencies are found in only 2%–6% of the patients. The presence of a thrombophilia amplifies the risk of CVST associated with other conditions such as anticardiolipin antibodies and puerperium.[17,18] Several studies have indicated that the combination of oral contraceptives and thrombophilia greatly increases the risk of CVST, particularly among women with hyperhomocysteinemia, factor V Leiden, or the prothrombin-gene mutation.[19–21] For classic congenital thrombophilia and hyperhomocysteinemia, the risk is increased when women receiving estrogen treatment have the protein C promoter CG haplotype.[17] Other studies are ongoing and it is very likely that new abnormalities in the coagulation and fibrinolysis systems will be identified in patients with CVST. Testing for congenital thrombophilia

Table 15.2. Causes of and risk factors associated with cerebral venous sinus thrombosis

Acquired prothrombotic states
Pregnancy
Puerperium
Homocysteinemia
Nephrotic syndrome
Antiphospholipid syndrome
Hematologic conditions
Polycythemia
Leukemia
Thrombocythemia
Infections
Otitis, mastoiditis
Meningitis
Systemic infectious disease antibodies
Mechanical causes
Head injury
Injury to sinuses, jugular vein or jugular vein catheterization
Neurosurgical procedures
Lumbar puncture
Drugs
Oral contraceptives
Asparaginase
Inflammatory disease
Systemic Lupus Erythematosus
Wegner's granulomatosis
Sarcoidosis
Inflammatory Bowel Disease
Behcet's syndrome
Genetic prothrombotic states
Antithrombin deficiency
Protein C and S deficiency
Factor V Leiden mutation
Prothrombin mutation
Miscellaneous
Dehydration
Cancer

should thus be standard in CVST even when there is a known cause because multiple etiologies are common. The presence of congenital thrombophilia potentiates the risk of venous thrombosis associated with other disorders. It is also important to look for the disorder in family members so that preventive measures in high-risk situations can be taken.[7,10]

Hyperhomocysteinemia is an independent and strong risk factor for CVST and is present in 27%–43% of patients and 8%–10% of controls, with an odds ratio denoting a strength of association ranging from four[22] to nearly seven.[23] Low folate concentrations may play a role in CVST, particularly during pregnancy and in those with a deficient nutritional status and low socioeconomic conditions. However, the mechanism through which low serum folate concentration predisposes individuals to CVST is still unknown.[24] Whether or not the correction of hyperhomocysteinemia, with folic acid alone or in combination with cobalamin and pyridoxine, helps reduce the risk of CVST, remains to be tested.

The association of CVST with pregnancy and puerperium is well known and may result in significant maternal mortality and morbidity especially in developing countries. CVST is seen more commonly in the puerperium because hypercoagulability worsens in the setting of volume depletion and trauma. The use of oral contraceptives is a frequent and important risk factor. An adjusted odds ratio ranging between 4 and 13 has been shown among women who use oral contraceptives.[19]

With increasing knowledge and interest, the list of causes of CVST continues to expand. Other causes mentioned in various cases reported in the literature include – tamoxifen,[25,26] anemia,[27,28] spontaneous intracranial hypotension,[10,29] erythropoietin[25,30] and high altitude sickness as reported in the Himalayas.[31] The search for a cause in CVST requires an extensive initial work-up and, when no cause is found, a long follow-up with repeated investigations is warranted.

Pathogenesis

To understand the symptoms and signs of sinus thrombosis, two different mechanisms should be distinguished: thrombosis of the cerebral veins, with local effects caused by venous obstruction, and thrombosis of the major sinuses, which causes intracranial hypertension. In the majority of patients, these two processes occur simultaneously.

The first mechanism, occlusion of the cerebral veins, can cause localized edema of the brain and venous infarction. Pathological examination shows enlarged, swollen veins, edema, ischemic neuronal damage, and petechial hemorrhages. The latter can merge and become large hematomas with a characteristic appearance on CT scans. Two different kinds of cerebral edema can develop. The first, cytotoxic edema, is caused by ischemia, which damages the energy-dependent cellular membrane pumps, leading to intracellular swelling. The second type, vasogenic edema, is caused by a disruption in the blood–brain barrier and leakage of blood plasma into the interstitial space. Vasogenic edema is reversible if the underlying condition is treated successfully. Both cytotoxic and vasogenic edema occur in CVST.[32]

The second mechanism is the development of intracranial hypertension as the result of occlusion of the major venous sinuses. Normally, the cerebrospinal fluid (CSF) is transported from the cerebral ventricles through the subarachnoid spaces at the base and surface of the brain to the arachnoid villi, where it is absorbed and drained into the superior sagittal sinus. Thrombosis of the sinuses leads to increased venous pressure, impaired absorption of CSF, and consequently, increased intracranial pressure. The obstruction to the drainage of CSF is located at the end of its transport pathway, and no pressure gradient develops between the subarachnoid spaces at the surface of the brain and the ventricles. Hence, the ventricles do not dilate, and hydrocephalus does not normally complicate sinus thrombosis.[32]

Clinical features

Cerebral venous sinus thrombosis is frequently a challenging diagnosis because patients can present with a multitude of signs and symptoms, including headache, focal neurological deficits, seizures, alterations of consciousness, and papilledema. The most frequent symptom of cerebral venous sinus thrombosis is severe headache, which is present in about 90% of all cases. It usually increases gradually over a couple of days but can also have an acute onset, mimicking a subarachnoid hemorrhage. Seizures occur in about 40 percent of patients, a far higher percentage than in patients with arterial stroke. Seizures are limited and focal in 50% of these patients but may generalize to a life-threatening status epilepticus.[8]

Focal neurologic signs, including sensory and motor deficits, aphasia, or hemianopsia develop in 40%–60% of patients with sinus thrombosis. Isolated intracranial hypertension with the triad of headache, vomiting, and blurred vision due to papilledema is the most homogenous pattern of clinical presentation accounting for 20%–40% of cerebral venous sinus thrombosis.[8] Characteristic, but rare, is the occurrence of unilateral hemispheric symptoms such as hemiparesis or aphasia, followed within days by symptoms from the other hemisphere; these are caused by the development of cortical lesions on both sides of the superior sagittal sinus. Thrombosis of the deep venous system – the straight sinus and its branches – causes centrally located, often bilateral thalamic lesions, with behavioral symptoms such as delirium, amnesia, and mutism, which can be the only manifestation of sinus thrombosis.[33] If large unilateral infarcts or hemorrhages compress the diencephalon and brainstem, patients may become comatose or die from cerebral herniation if untreated. Stupor or coma are found in 15%–19% of patients at hospital admission and are usually seen in patients with extensive thrombosis of the deep venous system with bilateral thalamic involvement or with generalized seizures. Coma at presentation is the most consistent and strongest predictor of poor outcome in patients with cerebral venous thrombosis.[2,8] The patients with infectious cavernous sinus thrombosis can present with headache, fever, and eye symptoms such as periorbital edema, proptosis, chemosis, and paralysis of eye movements due to involvement of the oculomotor, abducens, or trochlear nerves.[32]

Median delay between presenting symptoms and diagnosis was 7 days (interquartile range, 3 to 16) among the 624 patients in the ISCVT cohort.[34] Patients with disturbance of consciousness and of mental status, seizure, and with parenchymal lesions on admission CT/MR scans were diagnosed earlier, whereas men and those with isolated intracranial hypertension syndrome were diagnosed later. Persistent visual deficits were more frequent in patients diagnosed later. In patients with isolated intracranial hypertension syndrome, modified Rankin Scale score >2 at the end of follow-up was more frequent among patients diagnosed later.

Radiological features

A high index of suspicion is important for the diagnosis of CVST as routine neuroimaging studies such as CT or MRI may produce subtle findings that can be difficult to detect. The classic finding of sinus thrombosis on unenhanced CT images is a hyperattenuating thrombus in the occluded sinus. However, variability in the degree of thrombus attenuation makes this sign insensitive; hyperattenuation is present in only 25% of sinus thrombosis cases.[35] A well-described finding of sinus thrombosis with contrast-enhanced imaging is the empty delta sign, a central intra-luminal filling defect that represents a thrombus surrounded by contrast-enhanced dural collateral venous channels and cavernous spaces within the dural envelope. However, the empty delta sign on post-contrast CT is present in only up to 30% of cases.[36] The absence of a flow void and the presence of altered signal intensity in the sinus is a primary finding of sinus thrombosis on MR images. The finding of increased signal intensity on both T1-weighted images and T2-weighted images is almost always abnormal.[37]

Contrast angiography should be strongly considered if isolated cortical vein thrombosis is suspected.[38] MRI and magnetic resonance angiography (MRA) are regarded as the best tools for the diagnosis of CVST. Intra-arterial four vessel angiography which has long been the gold standard is less frequently relied upon today.[39] Diffusion-weighted imaging is extremely sensitive in detecting acute arterial strokes and can distinguish between cytotoxic and vasogenic edema. Cerebral venous infarctions are frequently hemorrhagic and are associated with considerable vasogenic edema. Both high and low apparent diffusion coefficient values can be present on diffusion-weighted imaging.[40]

Predictors of outcome

The ISCVT confirmed coma, cerebral hemorrhage, and malignancy as important prognostic factors for death or dependence in patients with cerebral venous thrombosis. In addition, male sex, age greater than 37 years, mental status changes, thrombosis of the deep cerebral venous system, and CNS infection were identified as variables that increase the risk of death or dependence. The most common cause of death was transtentorial herniation due to a unilateral hemorrhagic lesion or diffuse edema and bilateral lesions.[8] (see Tables 15.3 and Table 15.4.)

Table 15.3. Multivariate predictors of death and dependency: results of the International Study of Cerebral Vein and Dural Sinus Thrombosis (ISCVT)

Variables	Hazards ratio
Age >37 years	2.0
Male gender	1.6
Coma	2.7
Mental status changes	2.0
Central nervous system infection	3.3
Cancer thrombotic events	2.9
Intracerebral hemorrhage	1.9
Thrombosis of deep venous system	2.9

Table 15.4. Multivariate predictors of death and dependency in patients with intracerebral hemorrhage: results of the International Study of Cerebral Vein and Dural Sinus Thrombosis (ISCVT)

Variables	Odds ratio
Older age	2.0
Male gender	3.3
Motor deficits	2.9
Right lateral sinus thrombosis	2.6
Thrombosis of deep venous system	5.4

In a prospective randomized Dutch–European cerebral sinus thrombosis trial, the prognostic factors associated with poor outcome were papilledema, impaired consciousness, coma, age older than 33 years, diagnostic delay >10 days, intracerebral hemorrhage, and involvement of the straight sinus. Isolated intracranial hypertension and a delta sign on CT scan were associated with a good outcome.[2]

In the VENOPORT study the long-term prognosis of CVST patients was fairly good with 8% death and 1% dependency rates in the prospective series. Death, permanent disability, and recurrent CVST were infrequent in their study. Systemic deep venous thrombosis (Table 15.5) and seizures were the most common long-term complications. For the prospective cases, worsening after admission and encephalopathy as the presenting syndrome predicted death or dependency, while absence of aphasia and no worsening after admission predicted total recovery.[41]

A risk score was derived using a Cox proportional hazards regression model to predict modified Rankin Scale score >2 at 6 months in 624 patients in the ISCVT. The score was tested in two validation samples:[42] (1) the prospective Cerebral Venous Thrombosis Portuguese Collaborative Study Group (VENOPORT) sample with 91 patients; (2) a sample of 169 consecutive CVST patients admitted to five ISCVT centers after the end of the ISCVT recruitment period. The following variables were identified as predictors: malignancy 4.53; coma 4.19; thrombosis of the deep venous system 3.03; mental status

Table 15.5. Anatomic stratification of cerebral and dural vein thrombosis

Good prognosis	Prognosis variable	Poor prognosis
Cortical vein thrombosis	Posterior sagittal sinus	Confluence of sinuses with 2 or more adjacent sinuses involved
Anterior superior sagittal sinus	Transverse and sigmoid sinus	Deep venous sinuses involved
Isolated transverse sinus		Transverse sinus with contralateral aplasia or hypoplasia
Isolated sigmoid sinus		

Table 15.6. American Heart Association Recommendations

	Class/Level of evidence
For patients with cerebral venous sinus thrombosis, UFH or LMWH is reasonable even in the presence of hemorrhagic infarction.	Class IIa, Level B
Continuation of anticoagulation with an oral anticoagulant agent is reasonable for 3 to 6 mo, followed by antiplatelet therapy.	Class IIa, Level C

disturbance 2.18; male gender 1.60; intracranial hemorrhage 1.42. Using the risk score (range from 0 to 9) with a cut-off of $\geq = 3$ points, overall efficiency was 85.4, 84.4, and 90.1% in the derivation sample and validation samples 1 and 2, respectively. The CVST risk score may help identify high-risk CVST patients.

Medical treatment and outcome of cerebral venous thrombosis

Intravenous heparin and subcutaneous low-molecular-weight heparin are the primary treatments for patients with acute CVST with the intent to prevent thrombus propagation and pulmonary embolism and increase the chances of recanalization. Two randomized trials compared heparin with placebo. Both trials show a consistent and clinically meaningful trend in favour of anticoagulation (AC) and demonstrate the safety of AC therapy.[43,44]

The first trial, reported by Einhäupl et al.,[43] compared dose-adjusted unfractionated heparin (UFH) (partial thromboplastin time at least two times control) with placebo. The study was terminated early, after only 20 patents had been enrolled, because of the superiority of heparin therapy ($P<0.01$). Eight of the ten patients randomized to heparin recovered completely, and the other two had only mild neurological deficits. In the placebo group, only one patient had a complete recovery, and three died. The study group also reported a retrospective study of 43 patients with cerebral venous sinus thrombosis associated with intracranial bleeding; 27 of these patients were treated with dose-adjusted heparin. The mortality rate in the heparin group was considerably lower than in the non-anticoagulated group.

In the second randomized study of CVST ($n = 59$), reported by de Bruijn et al.,[44] nadroparin (90 anti-Xa units/kg twice daily) was compared with placebo. After 3 months of follow-up, 13% of the patients in the AC group and 21% in the placebo group had poor outcomes (RR reduction, 38%; $P = NS$). Two patients in the nadroparin group died versus 4 in the placebo group. Patients with intracranial bleeding were included, and no new symptomatic cerebral hemorrhages occurred in either group.

A meta-analysis of these two trials showed that the use of AC led to an absolute risk reduction in death or dependency of 13% with a relative risk reduction of 54%.[45] Thus, data from controlled trials favour the use of AC in patients with CVST because it may reduce the risk of fatal outcome and severe disability. From the results of these two small trials and observational data, it appears that both UFH and low-molecular-weight heparin (LMWH) are safe and probably effective in cerebral venous sinus thrombosis.

The American Heart Association /American Stroke Association provided comprehensive evidence-based recommendations on the management of CVST (see Table 15.6).[46] Simultaneously the European Federation of Neurological Societies task force searched MEDLINE, the Cochrane Central Register of Controlled Trials (CENTRAL), and the Cochrane library and provided their own guidelines for the management of CVST (see Table 15.7).[39]

It is not clear whether treatment with full-dose intravenous heparin is as effective as treatment with subcutaneous LMWH. A meta-analysis which compared the efficacy of fixed dose subcutaneous LMWH vs. adjusted dose unfractionated heparin for extracerebral venous thromboembolism found LMWH to be more effective with fewer major bleeding complications.[47] Other advantages of LMWH include the route of administration which increases the mobility of patients and the lack of laboratory monitoring and subsequent dose adjustments. The use of intravenous heparin is recommended in critically ill patients because the activated partial thromboplastin time (aPTT) will normalize within 1–2 h after discontinuation of the infusion if complications occur or surgical intervention is necessary.[7]

Heparin therapy should be continued until remission of the acute stage of the disease (normalizing level of consciousness or remission of mental confusion, improvement of headache and focal neurological deficits). The goal is to increase the aPTT to 1.5 to 2.0 times the baseline value. Subsequently, oral anticoagulation with warfarin is initiated with a target of achieving an international normalized ratio (INR) of 2.0 to 3.0. Therapeutic doses of intravenous heparin should be continued until the INR value achieves therapeutic values. In special circumstances such as pregnancy, oral AC should be avoided because of possible teratogenic effects.[48] Full dose heparin as a continuous IV infusion should be given for 5–10 days, followed by full dose heparin SC until term,

Table 15.7. European Federation of Neurological Societies Recommendations

1. **Heparin therapy**: Patients without contraindications for AC should be treated either with body weight-adjusted subcutaneous LMWH (180 anti-factor Xa U/kg/24 h administered by two subcutaneous injections daily) or dose-adjusted intravenous heparin with an at least doubled aPTT. LMWH should be preferred in uncomplicated CVST cases. Concomitant ICH related to CVST is not a contraindication for heparin therapy.

2. **Thrombolysis**: Among Patients showing deterioration despite adequate AC with other causes of deterioration ruled out, thrombolysis with urokinase or rtPA may be a therapeutic option in selected cases, possibly in those without ICH (insufficient current evidence).

3. **Duration of oral anticoagulation (AC)**: Oral AC may be given for 3 months if CVST was secondary to a transient risk factor, for 6–12 months in patients with idiopathic CVST and in those with mild hereditary thrombophilia. Indefinite AC should be considered in patients with two or more episodes of CVST and in those with one episode of CVST and severe hereditary thrombophilia (insufficient data).

4. **Anti-seizure prophylaxis**: Prophylactic antiepileptic therapy may be a therapeutic option in patients with focal neurological deficits and focal parenchymal lesions on admission CT/MRI. Optimal duration of anti-seizure prophylaxis is unclear.

5. **Elevated intracranial pressure**: In patients with IIH(isolated intracranial hypertension) and threatened vision possible therapeutic measures may include one or more lumbar punctures, acetazolamide, CSFshunting procedures and decompressive craniectomy (insufficient data).

Abbreviations used: AC, anticoagulation; LMWH, low molecular weight heparin; APTT, activated partial thromboplastin time; CVST, cerebral venous sinus thrombosis; ICH, intracranial hemorrhage; CT, computed tomography; MRI, magnetic resonance imaging; CSF, cerebrospinal fluid.

15 000–20 000 IU SC every 12 hours, adjusted to prolong the aPTT into the therapeutic range. Heparin treatment should be discontinued 24 hours before elective induction of labor.[48] Placental hemorrhages with subsequent placental insufficiency may appear during heparin therapy.

Controlled data about the benefit and optimal duration of oral anticoagulation in patients with CVST, does not exist. Oral anticoagulation may be given for 3 months if the CVST was secondary to a transient risk factor, for 6–12 months in patients with idiopathic CVST, and in those with "mild" hereditary thrombophilia such as protein S or C deficiency. Indefinite anticoagulation should be considered in patients with two or more episodes of CVST or in patients with a CVST and "severe" hereditary thrombophilia such as antithrombin III deficiency or a homozygous factor V Leiden mutation.[39]

Treatment of seizures

The prophylactic use of antiepileptic drugs (AED) in all patients with CVST is controversial. Whereas some authors recommend prophylactic treatment because of high incidence of seizures and their possible detrimental effects on the metabolic situation during the acute phase of the disease,[49] others restrict the use of anticonvulsants to those patients who clinically demonstrate seizure activity.[6] A recently published study identified the presence of focal sensory clinical deficits and the presence of focal edema or ischemic/hemorrhagic infarcts on admission computed tomographic (CT) scan or magnetic resonance imaging (MRI) as significant predictors of early symptomatic seizures.[50] These findings suggest that prophylactic treatment with AED may not be necessary in patients without any focal neurological deficits or focal parenchymal lesions on brain imaging (e. g., patients with isolated intracranial hypertension). Fosphenytoin is recommended for treatment of seizures in those patients who require a parenteral formulation. Alternatively, phenobarbital, levetiracetam, or valproate sodium injection may be utilized in the patient who is allergic to phenytoin. Delayed seizures usually occur within 12 months after the acute phase of CVST.[50,51] Late seizures are more common in patients with early symptomatic seizures compared with those patients who did not suffer seizures. Thus, prolonged treatment with AEDs for 1 year may be reasonable for patients with early seizures and hemorrhagic lesions on admission brain scan whereas in patients without these risk factors AED therapy may be discontinued after the first month.

Assessing recanalization and collateral formation

There has been substantial emphasis placed on categorizing recanalization and collateral formation in patients with acute arterial occlusion resulting in ischemic stroke. Such methods of semi-quantitatively classifying the severity of arterial occlusion for prognostic purposes and assessing the response to treatment have become an integral part of clinical studies. However, no such method exists for classifying either recanalization or collateral formation in patients with cerebral venous thrombosis. A method with two components was described that can be used to classify recanalization and collateral formation in patients with cerebral venous thrombosis[52] using serial magnetic resonance (MR) or computed tomographic (CT) venography or catheter based angiography with venous phase imaging. The recanalization is classified as follows (see Fig. 15.1): grade I, partial recanalization of one or more occluded dural sinuses with improved collateral flow; grade II, complete recanalization of one sinus but persistent occlusion of the other sinuses [A-no residual flow, B-non occlusive flow]; and grade III, complete recanalization. The collateral formation is classified as follows: grade I, collaterals bypass occluded segment of dural venous sinus and connect within the same sinus; grade II, collaterals bypass occluded segment and connect with a different sinus; and grade III, collaterals bypass the occluded segment and connect with different circulation. The classification recognizes the superficial and deep venous circulation as distinct pathways with different prognostic implications that can be linked through collateral pathways.

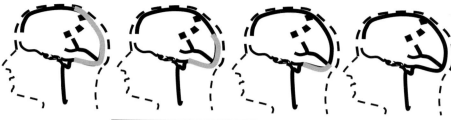

Fig. 15.1. Recanalization grades.

	Grade I	Grade II	Grade III
Recanalization grades	Partial recanalization (anterograde flow through part of the sinus) of one or more occluded dural venous sinuses with improved collateral flow or visualization of branches	Completed recanalization (anterograde flow through all the sinus) of one dural venous sinus but persistent occlusion in other venous sinuses A. No residual flow defect B. Non-occlusive flow defect	Complete recanalization of all occluded venous sinuses

Further studies are required to assess the inter-observer reliability of the proposed classification and assess the ease of use in clinical studies and practice.[53] In one study[53] six patients had both collaterals and recanalization, 11 patient had recanalization, and two patients had collateral formation only.

The proportion of patients with persistent headache was higher in those with none or partial recanalization compared to patients with complete recanalization. Identification of patterns of recanalization and/or collateral formation associated with minimal residual deficits may assist in selecting patients with cerebral venous thrombosis who can benefit from early transvenous thrombolysis.

Indications of endovascular treatment of cerebral venous sinus thrombosis

Due to the low incidence of CVST and high rate of favorable outcomes following medical treatment, it is difficult to prospectively compare the efficacy and safety of endovascular treatment to medical management alone. The role of endovascular treatment in CVST is limited to a selected group of patients.

Progression of neurological deficits despite therapeutic anticoagulation

The most widely used indication of endovascular therapy has been a "failure" of medical management. The failure of medical management in this setting has been defined using various criteria. A progression of neurological symptoms despite therapeutic AC is one criterion defining medical failure. Some authors feel that the neurological deterioration must be severe, or even life-threatening in nature to justify this approach. A second definition of failure is a patient who presents with

obtundation or coma who has failed to improve with therapeutic anti-coagulation over 24 to 48 hours.[54]

Intracranial hypertension refractory to first-line treatment

Intracranial hypertension occurs due to venous occlusion, engorgement, and limited cerebrospinal fluid clearance through the arachnoid villi and venous sinuses. If standard medical treatment is inadequate, reducing venous engorgement and pressure by rapid recanalization using endovascular techniques may be beneficial. Intracranial pressure (ICP) monitoring may be helpful in identifying the risk of neurological deterioration in patients with an impaired level of consciousness or neurological deterioration suspected due to elevated ICP.

Involvement of deep venous sinuses

Most authors have advocated waiting for progression of neurological deficits while on therapeutic doses of heparin before performing endovascular procedures. However, there have been concerns raised that intervening after neurological worsening has occurred might reduce the chances of favorable recovery. Another approach has been to use clinical and radiological criteria to identify a group of patients with low rates of favorable outcome and intervene at an early stage. Two studies have looked at predictors of poor outcome among patients with CVST.[2,8] Both studies identified involvement of deep venous sinuses as a predictor of poor outcome suggesting that such patients should be preferentially treated with endovascular treatment.

Poor candidates for anticoagulation

Some authors believe that the presence of subarachnoid hemorrhage adjacent to the thrombosed sinus places patients at

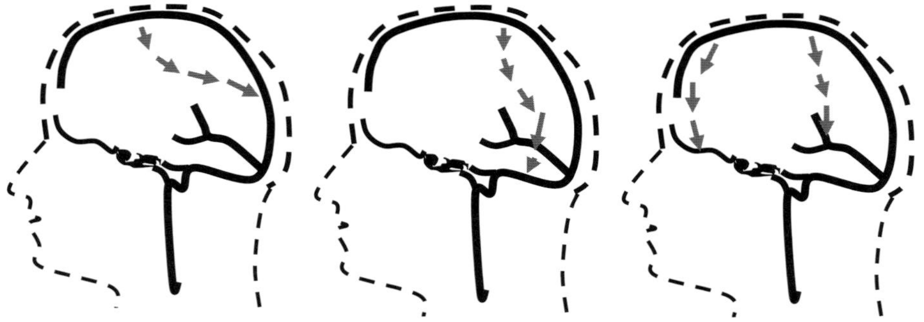

Fig. 15.2. Collateral grades.

Grade I	Grade II	Grade III
Collaterals bypass occluded segment of dural venous sinus but connect within the same sinus	Collaterals bypass occluded segment of dural venous sinus and connect with a different sinus	Collaterals bypass occluded segment of dural venous sinus and connect with a different circulation (through deep or cavernous venous sinus circulation)
If multiple patterns, than highest grade must be selected		

increased risk of life-threatening hemorrhage with anticoagulation and therefore justifies the used of endovascular mechanical thrombectomy.[55]

General principles of endovascular approach to CVST

Percutaneous arterial and venous access is obtained using modified Seldinger technique. A cerebral arterial angiogram is performed to identify the site of occlusion within the dural venous sinuses and alternate venous drainage channels that may have formed consequent to the occlusion. Examples of such alternate venous channels include cortical veins in the anterior part of the supratentorial compartment draining towards the deep venous channels (including the cavernous sinus) and cortical veins in the posterior part draining to the transverse sinuses consequent to superior sagittal sinus thrombosis. Figure 15.2 demonstrates various sites within the dural venous sinuses which can be bypassed through collaterals in the event of occlusion. Deep venous sinus drainage has limited ability to drain through alternate venous channels. Lack of opacification of a sinus such as the transverse sinus may be related to pre-existing hypo- or aplasia. Therefore, the MRV images should be reviewed prior to the angiogram to identify signal changes characteristic of thrombus within the sinuses. Another method for identifying hypoplasia includes using a Valsalva maneuver concomitant to the contrast injection which facilitates opacification of hypoplastic sinuses.

A 6F or 7F guide catheter is introduced over a 0.035-inch guidewire into the common femoral and iliac veins, and subsequently advanced to the inferior vena cava, right atrium, and superior vena cava under fluoroscopic guidance. The guide catheter is advanced into the brachiocephalic vein and internal jugular vein. Simultaneous arterial injections with opacification of the internal jugular veins may be necessary to identify the origin and anatomical configuration of the vein for catheterization. With the guide catheter in the internal jugular vein, a microcatheter is advanced over a microwire under guidance of a roadmap based on the venous phase of an arterial injection. The microcatheter is guided as close as possible to the area of occlusion. Traversing the occlusion may be difficult due to pre-existing trabeculae and organized thrombus. Venography using contrast injections from the microcatheter can be useful in delineating the morphology within the sinuses. After the microcatheter is placed within or past the thrombus, it may be used for infusion of thrombolytics. If indicated, an exchange length microwire may be used to retrieve the microcatheter and advance balloon angioplasty catheters or rheolytic catheters to the target position. It may be necessary to access the transverse sinus from the contralateral transverse sinus through the confluence of sinuses if occlusion is extensive and involves segments of the internal jugular vein.

Treatment techniques and results
Direct infusion of thrombolytic agents

The most commonly used endovascular technique for the treatment of cerebral sinus thrombosis is microcatheterization and direct infusion of thrombolytic agents. The first report describing this technique was published by Scott et al.[56] in 1988. There are presently a number of case reports and case series[57–62] describing a variety of thrombolytic drug regimens (see Table 15.8).

Generally, venous access is gained through the femoral vein with a 6 French or larger introducer sheath. A 5 or 6 French guide catheter is then navigated through the venous system and positioned in the jugular bulb or sigmoid sinus. A microcatheter is advanced over a microwire (0.014 inch) through the venous sinuses and a retrograde venogram is

Table 15.8. Regimens used for Cerebral Venous Sinus Thrombosis (CVST) thrombolysis

	Smith[63]1994	Spearman[64]1997	Rael[65] 1997	Kim[66]1997	Frey[67]1999	Yamini[68] 2001
Indication	Failed medical management	Rapid deterioration to coma	Coma that failed to improve with heparin	4/9 failed medical mangagement 5/9 first line	First line	Rapid progession to coma
Drug	urokinase	urokinase	urokinase	rt-PA	rt-PA	rt-PA
Bolus	80 000–250 000/ 15 min		250 000 U/2 hr	10 mg/10 min	1 mg/cm of clot	25 mg
Primary infusion rate	20 000–150 000 U/hr x 88 – 244hrs	5000–10 000 U/ min x 3 hrs	80 000 u/hr for 165 hrs	50 mg/3 hrs	1–2 mg/hr x 0.5 to 77 hrs	1mg/min x 19 hrs
Secondary infusion rate				5 mg/hr 100 mg max/day x 8 to 43 hrs		
Symptomatic intracranial hemorrhages	None	None	None	None	2/12	None
Clinical outcome	6/7 improved or normal	2/2 nearly complete recovery	1/1 complete recovery	9/9 improved to near normal	9/12 clinically improved	1/1 complete recovery

obtained. Once the microcatheter is within the thrombus, the microwire is removed and a bolus dose of thrombolytic is infused. This is followed by a prolonged infusion at a lower dose.

As illustrated in Table 15.8, most published reports of direct thrombolytic infusion for CVST describe the use of a bolus dose of the thrombolytic agent followed by a prolonged infusion. However, there is evidence from the treatment of pulmonary embolism that prolonged infusions may not be necessary. One randomized trial involving 53 patients found similar rates of recanalization when 50mg of rt-PA was infused over 15 minutes versus 100mg infused over 2 hours.[69] A second study involving 63 patients found similar rates of recanalization and hemorrhage among patients treated with a 10 mg bolus of rt-PA followed by 90 mg over 2 hours and those treated with a bolus of 4400 U/kg of urokinase and 4400 U/kg/hr over 12 hours.[70]

Mechanical disruption

A number of authors have described the use of microwires and microcatheters to mechanically disrupt clot in the cerebral sinuses. In so doing, they seek to enhance the effects of infused thrombolytics. This technique has not been described as effective when utilized in isolation.[59]

Chaloupka et al.[71] first described the use of angioplasty for mechanical clot disruption in 1999. The patient in this report presented with rapidly worsening neurological symptoms and complete occlusion of the superior sagittal sinus, confluence of the sinuses, and right transverse sinus. The patient received a bolus dose of urokinase. After failing to see improvement in flow, the authors entered the clot with a second 0.014-inch

microwire and microcatheter. A stiff, 300 cm, coronary wire was then used to exchange the microcatheter for a coronary angioplasty balloon. After primary angioplasty, a series of exchanges for progressively larger balloons ranging from 3.5 mm to 5 mm in diameter were introduced and inflated. The authors reported both excellent recanalization and clinical improvement with this technique. Soleau et al.[72] described the use of a Forgarty catheter inserted through a direct jugular puncture into the dural sinuses. The balloon tip was inflated and withdrawn in a retrograde manner in an attempt to disrupt clots within the cerebral sinus. They reported good results in six of eight patients.

Rheolytic thrombectomy

The only rheolytic thrombectomy catheter that has been used to treat dural sinus thrombosis to date and reported in the medical literature is the AngioJet catheter (Possis Medical, Minneapolis, MN). Since 1999, several groups have published case reports describing its use. Most reports describe femoral access using 7 French (some authors describe the use of a 90 cm sheath) or larger sheaths and guide catheters. Once a microcatheter has been positioned within the clot, it is exchanged for the AngioJet catheter (both the 4 and 5 French systems have been used). The catheter is then withdrawn through the clot at a rate of 0.2 to 1 cm/second. The device can only be used for 15 minutes or until 1000 ml of heparinized saline is utilized to prevent excessive hemolysis.[73]

The mechanism through which the AngioJet works is the following: saline exits the catheter tip at a rate of 50 mL/min via six small jets directed in a retrograde direction. A net negative pressure gradient is developed that creates a Venturi effect that breaks up thrombus and direct particulate debris with subsequent aspiration into an outflow lumen for collection in a disposable bag.[73] Recently a new device, the Penumbra System (Penumbra, Inc., Alameda, CA), capable of suction thrombolysis, has received Food and Drug Administration approval for use in ischemic arterial stroke. This device has the advantage of greater flexibility, but its use has not yet been described in the treatment of cerebral sinus thrombosis.

Prolonged microcatheter-based local thrombolytic infusion as salvage treatment for patients who fail transvenous endovascular treatment

A study determined the effectiveness of prolonged microcatheter-based local thrombolytic infusion in the treatment of patients with CVST who achieved none or suboptimal recanalization with endovascular treatment. Patients who underwent transvenous endovascular treatment at three hospitals were identified through local registries.[74] The final response to treatment was assessed and prolonged microcatheter-based local thrombolytic infusion was instituted in select patients as second line treatment. Serial angiograms were performed to assess treatment response and determine the duration of infusion. Eight patients underwent transvenous endovascular treatment. The treatment was considered suboptimal due to partial recanalization in one patient, no recanalization in two patients, and re-occlusion in two patients. All these patients were subsequently treated with a prolonged microcatheter-based local thrombolytic infusion. Follow up angiography demonstrated complete recanalization in two patients and improvement of partial recanalization in two additional patients. One patient died before follow-up imaging could be acquired. None of the patients developed intracranial hemorrhage associated with local thrombolytic infusion. Prolonged microcatheter-based local thrombolytic infusion resulted in additional recanalization in patients who had suboptimal response to acute transvenous endovascular treatment without any additional adverse events.

Long-term outcome of patients with CVST

A detailed account of rates of favorable outcome (Table 15.9) has been provided in the preceding sections. Some of the other sequelae that may follow treatment are described below:

Recurrence of CVST

Recurrence is seen in about 2%–12% of patients with CVST.[75] Most authors recommend using oral anticoagulation for 3 to 6 months and patients should be re-evaluated with MRI/MRV. Lifelong anticoagulation may be required for patients who experience two or more CVST events or a CVST event associated with an identified prothrombotic state.

Table 15.9. Studies that have evaluated the long-term outcome among patients with cerebral venous sinus thrombosis (CVST)

Study	Number of patients	Mean follow-up (months)	Death or dependency
Cerebral Venous Thrombosis Portuguese Collaborative Study Group	91	12	10%
International Study on Cerebral Vein and Dural Sinus Thrombosis	624	16	11%
Cerebral Venous Sinus Thrombosis Study Group (the Netherlands)	59	3	17%

Table 15.10. Location of Dural arterio-venous fistula (DAVF) associated with deep venous sinus thrombosis (DVST)[76]

Location of DAVF	% age of cases
cavernous sinus	30
skull base	19
transverse sinus	17
dural convexity	12
sigmoid sinus	10
torcular Herophili	7
superior sagittal sinus	4

Neuropsychological and neuropsychiatric sequelae

The neuropsychological deficits typically encountered are characterized by aphasia, abulia and depression.[51,75] Studies investigating professional status, cognitive performance, depressive symptoms and quality of life reported depression and anxiety in two-thirds of CVST patients despite an apparent good recovery in 87% of these patients. Thus, patients should be encouraged to return to previous occupations and hobbies and reassured about the very low risk of recurrence.

Development of dural arteriovenous fistula (DAVF)

Development of DAVF is another long-term complication of CVST (Table 15.10). There is evidence of an association between CVST and DAVF, although it may be difficult in some cases to ascertain if the thrombosis was a primary or secondary event. Two hypotheses have been proposed for the pathogenesis of DAVF formation in the setting of CVST.[76] Physiological arteriovenous shunts exist between the meningeal arterial networks and the dural venous sinuses. An increase in sinus and venous pressure by the obstruction of venous outflow by CVST may open these channels to create a DAVF. The second hypothesis suggests that venous hypertension induced by an obstruction to venous outflow may reduce cerebral perfusion and lead to ischemia, followed by angiogenesis. Arteriovenous shunting occurs as a result of aberrant angiogenic activity of the dural blood vessels. The occurrence of secondary thrombotic events is also a possibility probably because of the turbulent flow into the venous sinus due to DAVFs. Details about diagnosis and treatment are provided in another chapter in the book.

References

1. Bousser M-G, Ferro JM. Cerebral venous thrombosis: an update. *Lancet Neurol* 2007;**6**:162–70.

2. de Bruijn SF, de Haan RJ, Stam J. Clinical features and prognostic factors of cerebral venous sinus thrombosis in a prospective series of 59 patients. For The Cerebral Venous Sinus Thrombosis Study Group. *J Neurol Neurosurg Psychiatry* 2001;**70**:105–8.

3. RMF. Revue Médicale Française et Etrangère et Journal de Clinique de l'Hâtel-Dieu et de la Charité de Paris. 1825:5–41.

4. Bousser MG, Chiras J, Bories J, Castaigne P. Cerebral venous thrombosis–a review of 38 cases. *Stroke* 1985;**16**:199–213.

5. Ehtisham A'ad, Stern BJ. Cerebral venous thrombosis: a review. *Neurologist* 2006;**12**:32–8.

6. Ameri A, Bousser MG. Cerebral venous thrombosis. *Neurol Clin* 1992;**10**:87–111.

7. Masuhr F, Mehraein S, Einhaupl K. Cerebral venous and sinus thrombosis. *J Neurol* 2004;**251**:11–23.

8. Ferro JM, Canhao P, Stam J, Bousser M-G, Barinagarrementeria F. Prognosis of cerebral vein and dural sinus thrombosis: results of the International Study on Cerebral Vein and Dural Sinus Thrombosis (ISCVT). *Stroke* 2004;**35**:664–70.

9. Ferro JM, Correia M, Pontes C, Baptista MV, Pita F. Cerebral vein and dural sinus thrombosis in Portugal: 1980–1998. *Cerebrovasc Dis* 2001;**11**:177–82.

10. de Freitas GR, Bogousslavsky J. Risk factors of cerebral vein and sinus thrombosis. *Front Neurol Neurosci* 2008;**23**:23–54.

11. Bousser MG, Ross RR. *Cerebral Venous Thrombosis.***Vol 1**. London: WB Saunders 1997.

12. Sutton D, Stevens J. Vascular imaging in neuroradiology. In *Textbook of Radiology and Imaging*. **Vol 2**. New York, Churchill Livingstone 2003. 1682–1687.

13. Kido DK, Baker RA, Rumbaugh Calvin L. Normal cerebral vascular anatomy. In Abrams HL (ed.). *Angiograph, Vascular and Interventional Radiology* 1983;3rd edn. Boston, USA, Little, Brown and Company, 257–268.

14. Ono M, Rhoton ALJ, Peace D, Rodriguez RJ. Microsurgical anatomy of the deep venous system of the brain. *Neurosurgery* 1984;**15**:621–57.

15. Oka K, Rhoton ALJ, Barry M, Rodriguez R. Microsurgical anatomy of the superficial veins of the cerebrum. *Neurosurgery* 1985;**17**:711–48.

16. Andeweg J. Consequences of the anatomy of deep venous outflow from the brain. *Neuroradiology* 1999;**41**:233–41.

17. Weih M, Junge-Hulsing J, Mehraein S, Ziemer S, Einhaupl KM. [Hereditary thrombophilia with ischemic stroke and sinus thrombosis. Diagnosis, therapy and meta-analysis]. *Nervenarzt* 2000;**71**:936–45.

18. Bousser MG. Cerebral venous thrombosis: diagnosis and management. *J Neurol* 2000;**247**:252–8.

19. de Bruijn SF, Stam J, Koopman MM, Vandenbroucke JP. Case-control study of risk of cerebral sinus thrombosis in oral contraceptive users and in [correction of who are] carriers of hereditary prothrombotic conditions. The Cerebral Venous Sinus Thrombosis Study Group. *Br Med J* 1998;**316**:589–92.

20. Martinelli I, Sacchi E, Landi G, *et al.* High risk of cerebral-vein thrombosis in carriers of a prothrombin-gene mutation and in users of oral contraceptives. *N Engl J Med* 1998;**338**:1793–7.

21. Le Cam-Duchez V, Bagan-Triquenot A, Menard J-F, Mihout B, Borg J-Y. Association of the protein C promoter CG haplotype and the factor II G20210A mutation is a risk factor for cerebral venous thrombosis. *Blood Coagul Fibrinolysis* 2005;**16**:495–500.

22. Martinelli I, Battaglioli T, Pedotti P, Cattaneo M, Mannucci PM. Hyperhomocysteinemia in cerebral vein thrombosis. *Blood* 2003;**102**:1363–6.

23. Ventura P, Cobelli M, Marietta M, *et al.* Hyperhomocysteinemia and other newly recognized inherited coagulation disorders (factor V Leiden and prothrombin gene mutation) in patients with idiopathic cerebral vein thrombosis. *Cerebrovasc Dis* 2004;**17**:153–9.

24. Hotoleanu C, Porojan-Iuga M, Rusu ML, Andercou A. Hyperhomocysteinemia: clinical and therapeutical involvement in venous thrombosis. *Rom J Intern Med* 2007;**45**:159–64.

25. Finelli PF. Thrombosis of the cerebral veins and sinuses. *N Engl J Med* 2005;**353**:314–15.

26. Bushnell C. The cerebrovascular risks associated with tamoxifen use. *Expert Opin Drug Saf* 2005;**4**:501–7.

27. Balci K, Utku U, Asil T, Buyukkoyuncu N. Deep cerebral vein thrombosis associated with iron deficiency anaemia in adults. *J Clin Neurosci* 2007;**14**:181–4.

28. Stolz E, Valdueza JM, Grebe M, *et al.* Anemia as a risk factor for cerebral venous thrombosis? An old hypothesis revisited. Results of a prospective study. *J Neurol* 2007;**254**:729–34.

29. Tan K, Venketasubramanian N, Hwang CY, Lim CCT. My headache does not get better when I lie down: spontaneous intracranial hypotension complicated by venous thrombosis. *Headache* 2008;**48**:149–52.

30. Finelli PF, Carley MD. Cerebral venous thrombosis associated with epoetin alfa therapy. *Arch Neurol* 2000;**57**:260–2.

31. Basnyat B, Cumbo TA, Edelman R. Acute medical problems in the Himalayas outside the setting of altitude sickness. *High Alt Med Biol* 2000;**1**:167–74.

32. Stam J. Thrombosis of the cerebral veins and sinuses. *N Engl J Med* 2005;**352**:1791–8.

33. Kothare SV, Ebb DH, Rosenberger PB, *et al.* Acute confusion and mutism as a presentation of thalamic strokes secondary to deep cerebral venous thrombosis. *J Child Neurol* 1998;**13**:300–3.

34. Ferro JM, Canhao P, Stam J, *et al.* Delay in the diagnosis of cerebral vein and dural sinus thrombosis: influence on outcome. *Stroke* 2009;**40**:3133–8.

35. Virapongse C, Cazenave C, Quisling R, Sarwar M, Hunter S. The empty delta sign: frequency and significance in 76 cases of dural sinus thrombosis. *Radiology* 1987;**162**:779–85.

36. Vogl TJ, Bergman C, Villringer A, *et al.* Dural sinus thrombosis: value of venous MR angiography for diagnosis and follow-up. *AJR Am J Roentgenol* 1994;**162**:1191–8.

37. Leach JL, Fortuna RB, Jones BV, Gaskill-Shipley MF. Imaging of cerebral venous thrombosis: current techniques, spectrum of findings, and diagnostic pitfalls. *Radiographics* 2006;**26** Suppl 1: S19–41; discussion S42–41; discussion S42–3.

38. Wasay M, Azeemuddin M. Neuroimaging of cerebral venous thrombosis. *J Neuroimaging* 2005;**15**:118–128.

39. Einhaupl K, Bousser M-G, de Bruijn SFTM, *et al.* EFNS guideline on the treatment of cerebral venous and sinus thrombosis. *Eur J Neurol.* 2006;**13**: 553–559.

40. Bernstein R, Albers GW. Potential utility of diffusion-weighted imaging in venous infarction. *Arch Neurol* 2001;**58**:1538–9.

41. Ferro JM, Lopes MG, Rosas MJ, Ferro MA, Fontes J. Long-term prognosis of cerebral vein and dural sinus thrombosis. results of the VENOPORT study. *Cerebrovasc Dis* 2002;**13**:272–8.

42. Ferro JM, Bacelar-Nicolau H, Rodrigues T, *et al.* Risk score to predict the outcome of patients with cerebral vein and dural sinus thrombosis. *Cerebrovasc Dis* 2009;**28**:39–44.

43. Einhäupl KM, Villringer A, Meister W, *et al.* Heparin treatment in sinus venous thrombosis. *Lancet.* 1991;**338**:597–600.

44. de Bruijn SF, Stam J. Randomized, placebo-controlled trial of anticoagulant treatment with low-molecular-weight heparin for cerebral sinus thrombosis. *Stroke* 1999;**30**:484–8.

45. Stam J, De Bruijn SF, DeVeber G. Anticoagulation for cerebral sinus thrombosis. *Cochrane Database Syst Rev* 2002:CD002005.

46. Sacco RL, Adams R, Albers G, *et al.* Guidelines for prevention of stroke in patients with ischemic stroke or transient ischemic attack: a statement for healthcare professionals from the American Heart Association/American Stroke Association Council on Stroke: co-sponsored by the Council on Cardiovascular Radiology and Intervention: the American Academy of Neurology affirms the value of this guideline. *Circulation* 2006;**113**: e409–49.

47. van Dongen CJJ, van den Belt AGM, Prins MH, Lensing AWA. Fixed dose subcutaneous low molecular weight heparins versus adjusted dose unfractionated heparin for venous thromboembolism. *Cochrane Database Syst Rev* 2004:CD001100.

48. Ginsberg JS, Greer I, Hirsh J. Use of antithrombotic agents during pregnancy. *Chest* 2001;**119**: 122S–31S.

49. Eäupl KM, Masuhr F Cerebral venous and sinus thrombosis – an update, *Eur J Neurol* 1994;**1**:109–26.

50. Ferro JM, Correia M, Rosas MJ, Pinto AN, Neves G. Seizures in cerebral vein and dural sinus thrombosis. *Cerebrovasc Dis.* 2003;**15**:78–83.

51. Preter M, Tzourio C, Ameri A, Bousser MG. Long-term prognosis in cerebral venous thrombosis. Follow-up of 77 patients. *Stroke* 1996;**27**:243–6.

52. A Classification Scheme for Assessing Recanalization and Collateral Formation following Cerebral Venous Thrombosis. *J Vasc Interv Neurol* 2009;**2**:181–2.

53. Abeer Farrag MI, Gaurav K, Guliani *et al.* Occurrence of subacute recanalization and collateral formation in patients with cerebral venous thrombosis. *A Serial Venographic Study. Submitted Abstract.* 2010; American Academy of Neurology, Toronto.

54. Curtin KR, Shaibani A, Resnick SA, Russell EJ, Simuni T. Rheolytic catheter thrombectomy, balloon angioplasty, and direct recombinant tissue plasminogen activator thrombolysis of dural sinus thrombosis with preexisting hemorrhagic infarctions. *Am J Neuroradiol* 2004;**25**:1807–11.

55. Scarrow AM, Williams RL, Jungreis CA, Yonas H, Scarrow MR. Removal of a thrombus from the sigmoid and transverse sinuses with a rheolytic thrombectomy catheter. *Am J Neuroradiol* 1999;**20**:1467–9.

56. Scott JA, Pascuzzi RM, Hall PV, Becker GJ. Treatment of dural sinus thrombosis with local urokinase infusion. *Case report. J Neurosurg.* 1988;**68**:284–7.

57. Higashida RT, Helmer E, Halbach VV, Hieshima GB. Direct thrombolytic therapy for superior sagittal sinus thrombosis. *Am J Neuroradiol.* 1989;**10**: S4–6.

58. Barnwell SL, Higashida RT, Halbach VV, Dowd CF, Hieshima GB. Direct endovascular thrombolytic therapy for dural sinus thrombosis. *Neurosurgery.* 1991;**28**:135–42.

59. Eskridge JM, Wessbecher FW. Thrombolysis for superior sagittal sinus thrombosis. *J Vasc Interv Radiol* 1991;**2**:89–93; discussion 93–4.

60. Tsai FY, Higashida RT, Matovich V, Alfieri K. Acute thrombosis of the intracranial dural sinus: direct thrombolytic treatment. *Am J Neuroradiol* 1992;**13**:1137–41.

61. Canhao P, Falcao F, Ferro JM. Thrombolytics for cerebral sinus thrombosis: a systematic review. *Cerebrovasc Dis* 2003;**15**:159–66.

62. Horowitz M, Purdy P, Unwin H, *et al.* Treatment of dural sinus thrombosis using selective catheterization and urokinase. *Ann Neurol* 1995;**38**:58–67.

63. Smith TP, Higashida RT, Barnwell SL, *et al.* Treatment of dural sinus thrombosis by urokinase infusion. *Am J Neuroradiol* 1994;**15**:801–7.

64. Spearman MP, Jungreis CA, Wehner JJ, Gerszten PC, Welch WC. Endovascular thrombolysis in deep cerebral venous thrombosis. *Am J Neuroradiol* 1997;**18**:502–6.

65. Rael JR, Orrison WWJ, Baldwin N, Sell J. Direct thrombolysis of superior sagittal sinus thrombosis with coexisting intracranial hemorrhage. *Am J Neuroradiol* 1997;**18**:1238–42.

66. Kim SY, Suh JH. Direct endovascular thrombolytic therapy for dural sinus thrombosis: infusion of alteplase. *Am J Neuroradiol* 1997;**18**:639–45.

67. Frey JL, Muro GJ, McDougall CG, Dean BL, Jahnke HK. Cerebral venous thrombosis: combined intrathrombus rtPA and intravenous heparin. *Stroke* 1999;**30**:489–94.

68. Yamini B, Loch Macdonald R, Rosenblum J. Treatment of deep cerebral venous thrombosis by local

infusion of tissue plasminogen activator. *Surg Neurol* 2001;**55**:340–6.

69. Sors H, Pacouret G, Azarian R, *et al.* Hemodynamic effects of bolus vs 2-h infusion of alteplase in acute massive pulmonary embolism. A randomized controlled multicenter trial. *Chest* 1994;**106**:712–17.

70. Meyer G, Sors H, Charbonnier B, *et al.* Effects of intravenous urokinase versus alteplase on total pulmonary resistance in acute massive pulmonary embolism: a European multicenter double-blind trial. The European Cooperative Study Group for Pulmonary Embolism. *J Am Coll Cardiol* 1992;**19**:239–45.

71. Chaloupka JC, Mangla S, Huddle DC. Use of mechanical thrombolysis via microballoon percutaneous transluminal angioplasty for the treatment of acute dural sinus thrombosis: case presentation and technical report. *Neurosurgery* 1999;**45**:650–6; discussion 656–7.

72. Soleau SW, Schmidt R, Stevens S, Osborn A, MacDonald JD. Extensive experience with dural sinus thrombosis. *Neurosurgery* 2003;**52**:534–44; discussion 542–4.

73. Opatowsky MJ, Morris PP, Regan JD, Mewborne JD, Wilson JA. Rapid thrombectomy of superior sagittal sinus and transverse sinus thrombosis with a rheolytic catheter device. *Am J Neuroradiol.* 1999;**20**: 414–17.

74. Muna Irfan, Gaurav KGuliani *et al.* Prolonged microcatheter based local thrombolytic infusion as salvage treatment for patients who fail transvenous endovascular treatment for cerebral venous thrombosis. *Abstract submitted.* 2010; Annual Meeting of the American Academy of Neurology, Toronto.

75. Ferro JM, Canhao P. Complications of cerebral vein and sinus thrombosis. *Front Neurol Neurosci* 2008;**23**:161–71.

76. Tsai LK, Jeng JS, Liu HM, Wang HJ, Yip PK. Intracranial dural arteriovenous fistulas with or without cerebral sinus thrombosis: analysis of 69 patients. *J Neurol Neurosurg Psychiatry* 2004;**75**:1639–41.

Chapter 16

Intracranial and head and neck tumors: embolization and chemotherapy

Adnan I. Qureshi, Nauman Tariq, Rabia Qaiser, Herbert B. Newton and Stephen J. Haines

The extensive vascularity of neoplasms is vulnerable to super-selective intra-arterial injection of embolic particles and chemotherapeutic agents.[1] The highly vascular bed of neoplasms is easily identified on angiography, and can be amenable to selective microcatheterization. The purpose of this chapter is to review the use and techniques of these new endovascular modalities for treatment of intracranial and extracranial tumors.

Tumor vascularity

Angiogenesis is an essential process in the growth of tumors that also promotes its invasive and metastatic behavior. Angiogenesis is the sprouting of new microvessels that supply tumor tissues directly. It is supplemented by arteriogenesis (new arteries), caliber increase, and flow diversion in large arteries with the primary function of supplying blood to distal tumor capillary beds.

The extensive vascularity is categorized into primary and secondary arterial supply. The primary arterial supply is based on development of new small arteries and capillaries from the parent arteries and hypertrophy of parent arteries that supply the region of origin of tumor. As the tumor invades surrounding tissue and traverses various tissue planes, it recruits arterial supply from arteries supplying the invaded tissue (secondary arterial supply). The primary arterial supply is usually classified as Grade I or II based on angioarchitecture (see later section for description of classification). The secondary arterial supply is usually classified as Grade III. Some studies have described methodologies to examine the number and geometry of large arteries, the dynamics of contrast transport, and the amount of angiographic blush that is related to microvascular density.[2] The angiographic score is determined by the number of vessels that are identified in a pre-defined area within a selected region. Image histograms using grayscale intensity can be used to classify vessel diameters present in the region of interest. The contrast transit time is inversely proportional to the regional blood flow and can be measured.

Quantitation of tumor vascularity

Numerous techniques are used to quantify angiogenesis by measuring variables such as the angiographic score, capillary density, and regional blood flow.[2] The vascularization and hemodynamic characteristics of head and neck tumors have been characterized and quantified with a dynamic three-dimensional time-resolved echo-shared angiographic technique (TREAT) using regular contrast agent bolus[3]. In one study, 16 patients with head and neck tumors underwent three-dimensional-TREAT during contrast administration on a 1.5-T magnetic resonance imaging (MRI) scanner. Quantitative assessment included measurement of the contrast-to-noise ratio, determination of signal-intensity-over-time curves, time-to-peak enhancement within the carotid arteries and the tumor, and the delay between both. Data acquired by TREAT was compared with conventional digital subtraction angiography (DSA) in six patients. Tumor delineation with TREAT was very good or good in 11/16 patients, and better with TREAT than with DSA in 3/6 cases. Qualitative assessment of tumor vascularization on dynamic TREAT highly correlated with quantitative signal-intensity-over-time curves.

Mediators of tumor vascular changes

High expression of the vascular permeability factor/vascular endothelial growth factor (VEGF) in tumor tissue and normal brain plays a role in neovascularity and peritumoral edema. VEGF is a highly conserved 34–42-kD protein secreted by many tumor cells.[4] The most common forms of gene expressed are VEGF495, VEGF363, and VEGF567. Significant elevation of VEGF gene expression was observed in 81% of the highly vascular and edema-associated brain neoplasms in one study[5] (glioblastoma multiforme [GBM], capillary hemangioblastomas, meningiomas, and cerebral metastases). In contrast, only 13% of those brain tumors that are not commonly associated with significant neovascularity or cerebral edema (pituitary adenomas and nonastrocytic gliomas) had significantly increased levels of VEGF mRNA. Another study[4] revealed that

Textbook of Interventional Neurology, ed. Adnan I. Qureshi. Published by Cambridge University Press. © Cambridge University Press 2011.

eight VEGF-negative specimens exhibited no significant edema, whereas 26 VEGF-positive tumors exhibited significant peritumoral vasogenic brain edema. Dvorak and coworkers[6] found that VEGF is synthesized in tumor cells and accumulates in the endothelium of tumor vessels. VEGF expression was seen in adjacent pre-existing venules and small veins as early as 5 h after tumor transplant and plateaued at maximally intense levels in newly induced tumor vessels by approximately 5 days. VEGF increases the permeability of tumor vessels, plasma extravasation, angiogenesis, and tumor stroma formation.

Heparanase is an endoglycosidase,[7,8] which participates in degradation and remodeling of the extracellular matrix. The enzyme also releases angiogenic factors from the extracellular matrix and thereby induces an angiogenic response in vivo. Heparanase is preferentially expressed in human tumors and accelerates growth, angiogenesis, and invasiveness in experimental animals. A marked induction of tissue factor (TF) also occurs in response to heparanase over-expression in tumor and endothelial cells.[8] Tumor cells and the surrounding stroma are the principle source of growth factors and cytokines, which induce remodeling of the extracellular matrix. An increased production of matrix metalloproteinases (MMPs), MMP-2 and -9, has been also observed in advanced stages of tumor, favoring degradation of extracellular matrix and enhancing tumor dissemination.

MMPs are secreted by high-grade infiltrative gliomas like GBM and by macrophages,[9] and the production of macrophages is regulated by colony-stimulating factor (CSF)-1 expressed in several tumors. Suppression of CSF-1 or its receptors decreased tumor vascularity, reduced expression of angiogenic factors and MMPs, and decreased macrophage recruitment to the tumors. Monocyte chemoattractant protein-1 (MCP-1)[10] produced by tumor cells also plays a role in angiogenesis via macrophage recruitment and activation. AKT and focal adhesion kinase activation[11] play a role in blocking apoptosis, and thereby promote cell survival; AKT1 has been implicated as a major factor in many types of cancers. Copper is involved in multiple facets of angiogenesis[12] and tetrathiomolybdate, a potent copper chelator, suppresses angiogenesis.[13] Tumor angiogenesis may also be influenced by paracrine release of growth factors that bind to their corresponding endothelial cell surface receptors including receptors for fibroblast growth factors, VEGF-1 and VEGF-2, and the receptors Tie1 and Tie2.[14]

Vascular permeability

Increased cerebrovascular permeability to protein was demonstrated in all nineteen meningiomas and schwannomas studied by fluorescence microscopy and electron microscopy.[15] The increased permeability was attributed to open endothelial cell junctions, gaps between endothelial cells, and fenestrations in capillary endothelial membranes. The abnormal permeability to protein-bound tracers was found to be related to defective capillary endothelium. Endothelium cell abnormalities are not consistently found in surrounding edematous brain.

Coexistence of arteriovenous malformations

A review of the literature reveals 30 reported patients in whom an arteriovenous malformations (AVM) was found in association with intracranial tumors;[16] 14 were glial tumors (astrocytoma 7, GBM 1, oligodendroglioma 6), 7 meningiomas, 5 vestibular schwannomas, and a variety of other tumors. Of the seven patients who harbored both an AVM and a meningioma, only four had both lesions in the same cerebral hemisphere. However, Soria et al.[17] suggested a causal relationship because the lesions were in close spatial proximity in 18 of 30 reported cases. It remains unclear whether AVMs cause tumors due to chronic irritation or are a result of high flow in the tumor bed or secretion of vascular factors discussed above. However, the causal relationship between these entities in the event of co-existence is controversial.

Tumor embolization

Meningiomas

Prevalence and characteristics

Meningiomas account for 14%–26% of all primary intracranial tumors.[18] They tend to occur in persons aged between 40 and 70 years and more commonly in women.[19] Meningiomas are classified solely on the basis of histological anaplasia as benign (grade 1), atypical (grade II) displaying incipient signs of anaplasia, anaplastic (grade III), or sarcomatous (grade IV).[18] In grading anaplasia, six histological features are considered: loss of architecture, increased cellularity, nuclear pleomorphism, mitotic figures, focal necrosis, and brain infiltration.[20] Some authors consider "hemangiopericytic or hemangioblastic meningiomas" true hemangiopericytomas or hemangioblastomas, and exclude them from being classified as meninigiomas. From a clinical perspective, physicians also classify meningiomas as classic meningiomas, hemangiopericytomas or papillary meningiomas, atypical, and malignant meningiomas. Atypical and anaplastic tumors recur more frequently after complete resection and are found more frequently in falcine and lateral convexity regions (than are classic meningiomas). A study[19] correlated the MRI appearances with histopathological features in 35 meningioma patients and concluded that T1-weighted images predicted the presence of cysts and intratumoral blood vessels whereas T2-weighted images gave information about histological subtype, vascularity, and consistency. Meningiomas hyperintense to the cortex on T2-weighted images are usually soft, more vascular, and more frequently of syncytial or angioblastic subtype; tumors hypointense or hypoisointense on T2 tend to have a more hard consistency and are more often of fibroblastic or transitional subtype. It should be mentioned that, except for the angioblastic and

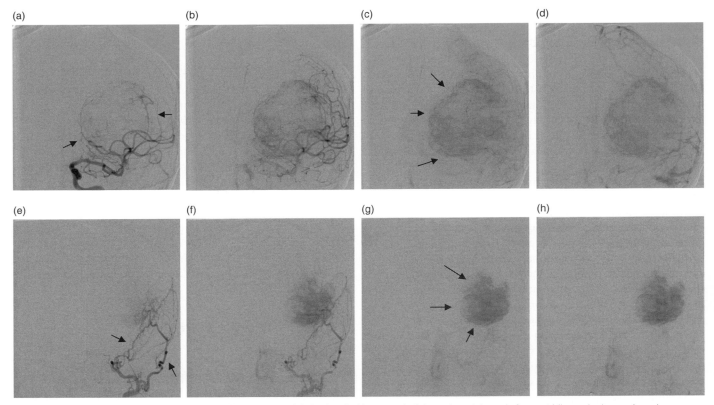

Fig. 16.1. (a)–(d) Various phases of contrast opacification (tumor blush identified by arrows) of the pial arterial supply from middle cerebral artery branches (see arrows) in a patient with frontal meningioma; (e)–(h) Various phases of contrast opacification (tumor blush identified by arrows in (g)) of the dural arterial supply from external carotid artery branches (see arrows in (e)) in a patient with frontal meningioma.

anaplastic/malignant varieties, other histologic patterns has not demonstrated a clear correlation with prognosis.

Tumor blood flow patterns

In one study,[21] blood flow was measured using the stable xenon-enhanced computed tomographic scan in intratumoral tissue, the cerebral hemispheres, and particularly in the peritumoral area of 12 patients with meningiomas. Tumor blood flow frequently showed a heterogeneous pattern of enhancement with high flow at the tumor periphery and a central area of hypoperfusion. Blood flow values were, on average, 28% lower in the peritumoral area than in the ipsilateral cerebral hemisphere. Blood flow values in the peritumoral edematous area were very low in certain cases.

Cerebral angiography in meningiomas

Angiography has been used to determine:[22] (1) the arterial supply and site of dural attachment of the tumor; (2) the location/displacement of key vascular structures in relation to the tumor, such as cortical draining veins and "arteries of passage," that is, major cerebral arteries supplying brain beyond the tumor; (3) the degree of invasion, encasement and/or occlusion of vascular structures, such as venous sinuses and arteries of passage; (4) the nature of the arterial blood

supply of the tumor: dural, pial or mixed; and (5) the precise degree of tumor vascularity.

Typically, the arterial pedicle enters the tumor at its meningeal attachment and supplies a radially arrayed tumor vascular pattern resulting in a "sunburst" or "spokeswheel" appearance (see Fig. 16.1). This is followed by the finding of a "delayed blush," that is, contrast persisting into the late venous phase. Meningiomas commonly have specific arterial feeders which are characteristic according to the location of the tumor.[20,22] Anterior fossa lesions receive their supply from internal and external systems; the latter include the artery of the falx and the ethmoidal arteries. Middle fossa tumors receive their supply from the internal carotid and external branches, including the artery of the foramen rotundum, the vidian arteries, the middle meningeal and accessory meningeal artery, and the ascending pharyngeal artery. Posterior fossa meningiomas obtain their blood supply from the posterior meningeal artery, the occipital artery, and the anterior meningeal branch of the vertebral artery.

Characteristics of arterial supply

The angiographic pattern of supply was studied in 173 of 230 meningiomas studied by CT scan in one study.[23] The vasculature of the tumors was classified into one of the following categories:

Table 16.1. Characteristics of angiographic supply based on study of meningiomas[23]

	Typical	Few vessels	No vessels	HPC like
Benign	66%	6%	26%	3%
Malignant	71%	10%	19%	0%
Overall	67%	6%	25%	3%

HPC, haemangiopericytoma

Table 16.2. Number of arterial feeders and magnitude of resection during surgery[26]

Arterial involvement	Total resection (%)	Near total resection (%)	Subtotal resection (%)	<0.0001
None	77.5	20	5.6	
Single	17.5	53.3	36.1	
Multiple	5	26.7	58.3	

(a) Typical vasculature of meningioma, feeding vessels from both meningeal arteries and the internal carotid artery, long-lasting tumor stain.

(b) Weak vascularization and tumor stain.

(c) No visible vasculature.

(d) Haemangiopericytoma-like vasculature: dual arterial supply, one to three main feeders giving rise to many irregular corkscrew-like vessels, dense, well-defined and long-lasting tumor stain, but early venous drainage. The summary of results is presented in Table 16.1.

Angiographic characteristics were unable to differentiate between the 152 benign and 21 malignant meningiomas. Malignant meningiomas expressed a variety of non-specific features including small feeding arteries with distal enlargement and ramification, marked vascularity and indistinct margins, and even minimum vascularity. Other investigators have also noted a poor correlation between the histological and angiographic findings in meningiomas. In a study of 147 patients who underwent radical surgery for intracranial meningioma, 25 (17%) had symptomatic recurrence.[24] Correlation between histological and angiographic findings of recurrent meningioma was against poor. Following extirpation of feeding meningeal vessels in convexity meningiomas in previous surgery, the principal blood supply was usually from the anterior, middle, and/or posterior cerebral arteries. The angiographic appearance was that of a "tree-root" or "sunburst" pattern, indicating neoplastic invasion of the pia mater and/or underlying brain tissue.

The correlation between angiographic neovascularization, peritumoral brain oedema and the expression of VEGF[25] was analyzed in 30 patients with meningiomas. All meningiomas with striking VEGF-expression were associated with vascular tumor supply from cerebral arteries, but VEGF-negative tumors were supplied in only 50% of the cases.

Number of arterial feeders and tumor resectability

The number of arteries supplying the tumor pre-operatively correlates with the chance of total, near-total, or partial resection during surgery. In one study,[26] the arterial involvement was assessed to design a scoring system. The number of feeding arteries was graded in three groups (0, 1, or ≥2 arteries) (see Table 16.2). In addition the following factors were assessed: (1)

tumor attachment size; (2) brainstem contact; (3) central cavity location; and (4) cranial nerve group involvement. Each factor was assigned a score of 0–2 points, and an additional point was added for previous surgical treatment or for radiation, giving a possible total score of 12 points. For cases scoring ≥8 points, the percentage showing neurological deterioration post-operatively exceeded the percentage showing improvement. The investigators found that with an increase in grade, fewer patients showed improvement in their pre-operative symptoms and more showed deterioration post-operatively. The table summarizes the association between arterial supply and resectability. Such a grading system requires independent validation before it can be recommended for general use.

Pial supply

The pial supply of meningiomas develops when there is close spatial relationship between the tumor surface and the adjacent brain parenchyma.[27–29] The arachnoid, which serves as a physiological barrier between the brain and the meningioma, is either penetrated by the cerebral vessels or infiltrated by the tumor. Three kinds of tumor–brain interfaces are described: smooth type, transitional type, and invasive type. These different microsurgical interfaces seem to correlate very precisely with computed tomographic images of halo-like and finger-like hypodense areas. In adjacent subarachnoid spaces, tumor secreted VEGF induces a proliferation of cerebral arteries, and development of capillaries across the arachnoid barrier into the tumor. Whether the development of pial blood supply is the primary or the secondary step to the disintegration of the arachnoid membrane is not yet clear. The relative frequency of various blood supply patterns is presented in Table 16.3.

Tumors fed mainly by the dural arterial supply usually leave the subarachnoid space preserved and are easily resectable.[27,28] The groups with prominent pial–cortical arterial supply are more likely to have pial membrane adherent to the tumor with crossing vessels visualized between the brain tissue and the tumor. The prominent pial–cortical arterial supply is also associated with peritumoral edema and intensity scores on T2-weighted MR images. In another study,[27] pre-operative angiograms were reviewed to identify angiographic characteristics of tumors that could be dissected by passing in the extrapial plane (i.e., "cleavable") and of those in which the dissection had to be subpial (i.e., "non-cleavable"). On

Table 16.3. Frequency of various combinations of blood supply to meningiomas[27,28]

Blood supply pattern	Frequency (Ildan *et al.*)	Frequency (Salpietro *et al.*)
Tumors stained with constrast had fed mainly by dural arterial supply and those not contrast enhanced had pial–cortical arterial supply	32 (42%)	40%
The pial–cortical arterial supply was found to participate in less than equal amounts as the meningeal – dural supply	26 (34%)	
The pial–cortical arterial supply was found to participate in at least equal amounts as the meningeal – dural supply	18 (24%)	59%

angiography, if the pial–cortical arterial supply participated in at least equal part with the meningeal–dural arterial supply, extrapial dissection was possible in only 35% of patients. If meningeal–dural arterial supply was predominant, extrapial dissection could be achieved in 84% of patients.

In a retrospective analysis,[30] the pial and dural blood supplies in 74 meningiomas was analyzed and classified as follows: 1, no pial supply; 2, pial supply smaller than dural supply; 3, pial supply equal to dural supply; 4, pial supply greater than dural supply; 5, no dural supply. The ratio of pial blush to tumor volume was approximated by evaluating the area of pial blush in anteroposterior and lateral angiograms. The three-dimensional localization of the pial blush in relation to the tumor surface was obtained from angiograms. The amount of edema and tumor size was calculated using computerized tomography. There were 49 meningiomas with peritumoral brain edema; of those tumors, 46 were supplied by pial vessels, and three were supplied exclusively by dural vessels. Tumors without peritumoral brain edema showed no pial blush. Meningiomas with a smaller pial supply than dural supply had significantly smaller mean peritumoral brain edema than tumors with a pial supply equal to or greater than the dural supply. In 70% of cases with pial blood supply, major portions of the edema were located adjacent to the tumor region supplied by pial vessels. Another study[31] suggested that histological subtype has no relationship to the production of cerebral edema, with one exception. Meningiomas with a hemangiopericytic component were the only histological subtype associated consistently with cerebral edema.

Encasement of adjacent arteries

A study reported on 15 operated cases of skull base meningioma encasing the main cerebral arteries.[32] Of 15 cases, four were sphenoid ridge meningiomas (all clinoidal types), three were planum sphenoidale, two were tuberculum sellae, olfactory groove and cerebellar tentorium, and one case was a cerebello-pontine angle and foramen magnum meningioma. Twelve tumors (80%) were large (diameter of 5 cm^2 or greater). Pre-operative tumor embolization was performed in two patients; external to internal carotid artery bypass was performed in one patient with severe stenosis of the internal carotid artery encased in the tumor. In five cases with the presence of inter-facing arachnoid membranes between the tumor and cerebral vessels, the tumor was totally removed. In the ten patients without interfacing arachnoid membranes, total removal was achieved in four of the ten patients by the sacrifice of the encased artery and in one patient injuring the arterial wall consequently. In the remaining five patients, the tumor could not be removed totally. In conclusion, greater difficulty with dissection was encountered in patients who did not have an arachnoid plane between the encased artery and the tumor.

Compression of adjacent arteries

A study of 12 patients with parasellar meningiomas[33] found that six patients demonstrated complete ICA involvement (encasement) and the other six showed partial ICA involvement (engulfment). The tumor was surgically excised and the ICA was successfully exposed in all cases in the engulfment group and in four of six cases in the encasement group. The ICA can be dissected even if it is involved at the center of the tumor if the tumor is soft and can be aspirated. Preservation of the perforating arteries was and more difficult. The angiographic finding of encasement of a long segment of the ICA is an unfavorable the predictor because of the high possibility that the perforating arteries are involved. Local stenosis of ICA is another unfavorable finding for surgical dissection because tumor may have invaded the arterial wall. Important findings predicting unsuccessful ICA dissection are involvement of a long segment of the ICA and local ICA stenosis on angiogram.

Dysplastic venous drainage and venous compression

In 30 patients[25] with intracranial meningiomas, dysplastic changes such as ectasia and distortion of veins with variance in diameter of tumor-draining cerebral veins were identified in the venous phase of angiography. Dysplastic changes of adjacent cortical, transmedullary, and deep cerebral veins (predominantly tumor draining) were found in 12 of 29 meningiomas. Dysplastic venous changes were associated with cerebral edema. Venous stasis[34] has been implicated in peritumoral edema in patients with meningioma due to: (1) compression of an adjacent cortical vein by the tumor with stasis at the site of compression and/or its distal portion; (2) compression of adjacent brain by the tumor with prolonged perfusion and delayed venous return; and (3) presence of an early draining vein linked to a nearby cortical vein with stasis at its periphery. Venous compression and stasis also seems to be related to the occurrence of hemorrhagic infarction after the resection of meningiomas.

Macroscopic tumor-vascularization

In 30 patients with intracranial meningiomas,[25] the presence of macroscopic tumor-neovascularization was differentiated from the existence of an exclusive tumor blush. An exclusive tumor blush was assumed, if the meningiomas were associated with a diffuse angiographic contrast-staining and additionally only the main feeding arterial vessels and their first junction could be visualized. In meningiomas with macroscopic tumor vascularization, additional distal branches of arterial tumor vessels had to be obvious like proximal arteries enlarged. Of the 30 patients, seven meningiomas demonstrated only a tumor blush and in 22 meningiomas, angiographic features of a macroscopic tumor vascularization were visualized. Macroscopic tumor-vascularization was associated with cerebral edema and was increased in meningiomas with strong VEGF staining.

Dural tail sign

The "dural tail" sign on gadolinium (Gd-DTPA)-enhanced MRI[35] has been described in association with meningiomas and represents a hypervascular, non-neoplastic reaction. While this sign was originally thought to be specific for meningiomas, subsequent case reports have described the presence of a dural tail in other intra- and extra-axial lesions. Giant aneurysm arising from the P2 segment of the right posterior cerebral artery,[35] adjacent to the tentorium, has been described with a prominent dural tail on Gd-DTPA-enhanced MRI.

Special site and etiology specific considerations for meningiomas

These are summarized in Table 16.4.

Embolization of meningiomas
Selection of patients

Pre-operative embolization of meningiomas is an option for use in selected cases prior to surgical resection of convexity and skull base lesions.[1,22,56]

Manelfe et al.[56] reviewed the results from 100 pre-operative embolizations and found that pre-operative embolization was useful in large tumors with pure or predominant external carotid artery supply (convexity meningiomas), in skull base meningiomas, and in middle fossa and paracavernous meningiomas. Embolization was also of value in falx and parasagittal meningiomas receiving blood supply from the opposite side and in posterior fossa meningiomas. However, since convexity meningiomas' blood supply is derived mainly from the external carotid artery system and is amenable to intraoperative cauterization before tumor resection, some investigators advocate the use of pre-operative embolization for convexity tumors only if they are of large size and highly vascular. One criterion proposed is for patients in whom tumors are ≥4 cm with at least 50% of their blood supply arising from the external carotid artery.[57]

Embolization is advocated for meningiomas located at the skull base. A retrospective analysis of pre-operative embolization of 280 feeding vessels in 167 cranial base meningiomas[58] defined as tumors originating from the olfactory groove, tuberculum sella, medial sphenoid wing, petro-clival region, or foramen magnum was performed. In 91% of patients embolized, good to excellent embolization was achieved without any permanent neurological complications. In 20 patients, embolization could not be performed due to the apparent risk of new neurologic deficits or lack of an appropriate vessel for embolization. Twenty-one patients (12.6%) had transient worsening of their neurologic deficit or a medical complication requiring hospitalization. Fifteen patients (9%) experienced permanent neurologic deficits or medical morbidity as a result of embolization. Another study[59] reviewed the results and complications of pre-operative embolization of hypervascular skull base tumors in 128 endovascular procedures in 66 patients including 41 skull base meningiomas, 18 paragangliomas of the temporal bone, and 7 juvenile nasopharyngeal angiofibromas. One death and two permanent disabilities were attributable to endovascular therapy. These complications occurred early in the investigators' experience and were related to thromboembolic events rather than complications of transcatheter embolization itself.

Recently, embolization has been recommended for tumors predicted to be very vascular or firm based on T_2 MRI imaging. Fifty patients diagnosed as having intracranial meningiomas were studied with 1.5 Tesla MRI.[60] The intensity of the tumors were categorized into three grades (low, iso, and high) compared to that of gray matter. Hyperintensity on protein density and T2-weighted images was a sign of a soft tumor. If the meningioma is believed to be firm (subjectively defined), pre-operative embolization will induce necrosis rendering it soft enough for easier surgical excision.

Effect of embolization on imaging parameters

Figure 16.2 demonstrates the changes in angiographic appearance and contrast enhancement after embolization. Gruber et al.[61] reported that total or near-total angiographic devascularization of the tumor parenchyma was accomplished in 38 (60%) of 63 consecutive patients who underwent pre-operative embolization of intracranial meningiomas with either an external carotid artery supply only ($n = 30$) or with contributions from the cavernous carotid artery, ophthalmic artery, vertebral artery, or pial feeders amenable to selective embolization ($n = 8$). Reasons for partial tumor embolization in the remaining 25 patients (40%) were: (1) the remnant feeders were considered easily accessible to surgical control; (2) the feeding branches were inaccessible via

Table 16.4. Special site- and etiology-specific considerations for meningiomas

Site/etiology	Considerations
Convexity, parasagittal, and lateral sphenoid wing meningiomas[20,36]	Arterial supply easily accessible. Patency of sagittal sinus, which may be left intact, reconstructed, or resected, depending on its pre-operative status and the tumor location
Olfactory groove meningiomas[20]	The sagittal sinus maybe ligated and removed with the tumor
Cribriform plate and planum sphenoidale meningiomas[37]	Removal may require bifrontal craniotomy and an interruption of the tumor's blood supply along the floor of the anterior cranial base. However, the presence of bulky tumor above makes it difficult to control bleeding from multiple bony foramina in the anterior cranial base and to expose these foramina. The blood supply to the dura in this region, and, therefore, to these tumors, is predominantly from the anterior and posterior ethmoid arteries. Pre-operative embolization of ethmoid arteries carries a risk of retinal ischemia. A frontoethmoidal approach to the arteries on both sides requires two separate skin incisions. Therefore, a subperiosteal, subperiorbital dissection and division of these arteries via a bicoronal skin incision is another alternative
Suprasellar meningiomas[38–40]	The magnitude of vascularity and tumor blush of intra- and suprasellar meningiomas is less prominent than in other locations. Left accessory middle meningeal artery originating from the dorsum sellae may be a source of supply in recurrent tumors
Optic sheath meningiomas[41–44]	Supplied by branches of the ophthalmic arteries, posterior ethmoidal arteries, anterior falx artery, and recurrent middle meningeal artery. Embolization of the ophthalmic and tumor feeding artery is possible with preservation of visual acuity and visual fields. In a report of 12 patients who underwent a total of 15 embolization attempts with preceding provocative testing on lesions involving the ophthalmic artery, 14 were successfully performed
Orbital meningiomas	An orbital meningioma may derive its blood supply from both the internal and external carotid systems. In cases in which the tumor's blood supply is derived from both systems, and only the external system is embolized, the benefit remains controversial
Cavernous sinus meningiomas[36,43,44]	The venous drainage of orbit and cavernous sinus requires study prior to operation
Clivus meningiomas[45–48]	Patients with blood supply from the basilar artery had a 4 times greater risk of permanent functional deterioration post-operatively. The enlarged tentorial marginal artery, dorsal meningeal artery, dural branches of the internal carotid artery, and inferior hypophyseal artery are amenable to embolization
Ventricular meningiomas[49]	Supplied by the lateral posterior choroidal artery amenable to embolization
Tentorial meningiomas[50–53]	Supplied by branches of the internal carotid artery, choroidal arteries, branches of the meningohypophyseal trunk, and branches of the posterior cerebral artery. Embolization only possible in 2 of 9 meningiomas in one study. Evidence of occlusion of the Galenic venous system and the development of collateral venous channels requires identification pre-operatively
Falcine meningioma[54]	Embolization via the terminal branch of the middle cerebral artery in the proximity of the tumor near or into the pre-falcine arterial anastomotic network around the superior sagittal sinus
Infratentorial (posterior fossa) meningiomas	No specific comments
Radiation-induced meningiomas[55]	Meningiomas induced by high-dose irradiation (greater than 2000 rad) require evaluation for large-vessel occlusive arteriopathy with transdural collateral vessels and invasion of the superior sagittal sinus

a microcatheter approach; or (3) microcatheter positions for embolization without reflux of embolic material into physiological branches was not achieved. Overall, 97 (77%) of 126 tumor feeders identified angiographically were selectively catheterized for embolization. In another study of 128 patients embolized with cellulose porous beads (200-microm diameter),[57] the percentage of blood supplied to the tumor by the internal and external carotid arteries was determined angiographically. Non-enhanced areas on postembolization MR imaging were calculated. In 72% of the patients with cellulose porous beads (CPB) embolization achieved reduction in the flow of the feeding artery by more than 50%. The non-enhanced area on MR imaging did not significantly correlate with the degree of external carotid artery supply or devascularization.

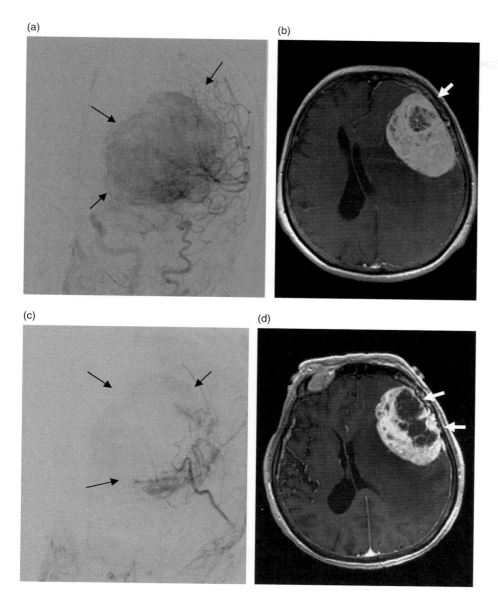

(a)

(b)

(c)

(d)

Fig. 16.2. Pre- and post-embolization angiographic and magnetic resonance images. (a) Pre-embolization arterial supply and tumor blush (see arrows) from both pial and dural sources. (b) Pre-embolization T1-weighted contrast enhanced image in transverse section. (c) Post-embolization obliteration of arterial supply and tumor blush (see arrows) from dural sources. (d) Post-embolization T1-weighted contrast enhanced image in transverse section demonstrating reduction in enhancement (see arrows).

Fifteen patients with meningiomas were prospectively studied[62] to determine the percentage of vascular supply to the tumor arising from the internal and external carotid arteries; the percentage of the tumor embolized was judged by angiography, by MRI, and by CT scanning. The data reveal an excellent correlation between the amount of tumor embolized as estimated by MRI and both the estimated blood loss at time of surgery and the presence of histological necrosis in the specimen. In another technique, selective intra-arterial injection of dilute MRI contrast identified the vascular distribution territories of meningeal tumors before and after embolization therapy.[63] Regions of the tumor that experienced loss of signal intensity after localized contrast injections into the external and common carotid as well as vertebral arteries were used to quantify the specific vessel's volume of distribution. MRI demonstrated the treated and untreated portions of the neoplasm

after therapy. In some instances, MRI revealed postembolization residual enhancement of the tumor not clearly identified on angiograms.

Bruening *et al.*[64] reported on 18 MRIs (nine patients) performed in a 1.5 T scanner before and following partial embolization using injection of particles (45–150 microns). During dynamic imaging a bolus of gadopentetate dimeglumine was injected. The tumor regional blood volume/gray matter regional blood volume ratio was 3 for untreated tumors and 0.1 for successfully embolized tumors. The regional blood volume in embolized meningiomas was significantly lower than that in untreated meningiomas. Vital tumor tissue showed positive enhancement in T1 and high regional blood volume; nonvital tissue lacked T1 enhancement and bolus effect in the first pass, thus leading to low or missing regional blood volume values. However, lack of bolus formation despite

T1 enhancement (6/9 postembolization regions), possibly due to slow collateral flow was also seen.

Pathological changes

Manelfe et al.[56] found embolic material on pathologic examination in 10%–30% of cases; fresh or recent ischemic and/or hemorrhagic necrosis consistent with technically successful embolization was demonstrated in 40%–60% of 100 embolized meningiomas. They did not find a good correlation between CT low density areas and necrosis on microscopic examination demonstrated after embolization. Morimura et al.[65] reported the following histopathological findings: (1) presence of emboli and thrombi within the tumor and/or dural vessels; (2) ischemic changes of the tumor cells; (3) pathologic evidence of infarction with or without inflammatory response; and (4) diffuse or nodular necrosis and surviving tumor cell clusters with an island-like appearance among 14 meningiomas treated with preoperative embolization. In another assessment of clinicopathologic features,[66] a good embolization result (>75% reduction in angiographic blush) was achieved in 52% of 64 meningiomas embolized. Histologically, embolized meningiomas showed higher frequencies of necrosis (89%), nuclear atypia (72%), macronucleoli (58%), sheeting (31%), high mitotic index (30%), and brain invasion (14%) when compared with non-embolized tissue. Median mitotic and MIB-1 indices were slightly elevated. A significant degree of necrosis (>10%) was found in 43% and correlated moderately with the extent of angiographic blush reduction and embolization particle size.

Metabolic changes

In a prospective study of 36 patients,[67] postembolization MRI (compared with pre-embolization MRI) revealed a variable pattern of secondary revascularization and devascularization. In all patients, peripheral secondary enhancement was present which histopathologically represented a thin layer of vital tumor tissue. Magnetic resonance spectroscopy revealed lactate in devascularized areas immediately after embolization. Lipids were not observed before the third day after embolization and were always associated with avascular and soft tissue at the time of surgery. In another study,[68] localized ^{31}P MR spectra of the brain were obtained by means of 2D-SI (voxel size: 36 cm^3) using 1.5-T whole-body MR tomography in 11 patients who underwent pre-operative embolization therapy; eight patients were examined before and after treatment. After embolization, alterations of pH and of the concentrations of high-energy phosphates (nucleoside-5′ triphosphate = NTP, phosphocreatine = PCr), inorganic phosphate (Pi), and membrane constituents were observed in the tumors. A [Pi] increase and decrease of [NTP], [PCr], and pH secondary to ischemic processes after tumor devascularization was observed. The most conspicuous findings using in vivo proton spectroscopy of meningiomas[69] were the observation of a transient lactate signal within 24 h

after embolization. Signals of tumor necrosis as shown by proton spectroscopy were complete within 4 days.

Molecular changes

In a molecular study of 35 benign intracranial meningiomas embolized 3 to 268 hours prior to surgical removal,[70] a perinecrotic increase in tumor cell proliferation was mainly due to macrophage-born mitogens. The proliferative indices peaked at the third to fourth day after embolization and started receding after the seventh day. The investigators concluded that perinecrotic proliferative activity in embolized meningiomas does not reflect true tumor proliferation and should not be used to identify the presence or degree of malignancy. In another study,[71] confluent necrosis and micronecrosis was the most common feature (48%). Other characteristic features included florid ischemic changes (16%), intravascular Ivalon particles (24%), and fibrinoid necrosis of vascular walls (12%). Immunostaining for the MIBI antigen and proliferating cell nuclear antigen (PCNA) demonstrated an increase in MIB1 and PCNA labeling indices in those tumors exhibiting necrotic foci, but this did not seem to have any prognostic significance. This study[72] indicates that cell death in embolized meningiomas is not only due to necrosis but also apoptosis and cell cycle arrest. The latter effects appear to be at least partly p53 dependent. The expression of p21 was not apparent 13 days after embolization, and apoptosis was observed until 6 days after embolization.[73] The expression of HIF-1alpha is increased by hypoxic stimulation during complete pre-operative embolization of meningiomas[74] and correlates with VEGF secretion. The VEGF121 and 165 isoforms were significantly upregulated in samples from patients who underwent partial or complete pre-operative embolization.[75]

Effect on intra-operative blood loss and transfusions

Endovascular devascularization of meningiomas decreases intra-operative blood loss and thus the need for intra-operative transfusions. A matched analysis[76] of patients undergoing surgery with and without embolization demonstrated that the mean value of estimated blood loss, 1403 ml vs. 1852 ml and number of transfusions, 1325 ml vs. 1747 ml were lower in embolized patients than in non-embolized patients. The length of post-surgical recovery, 30 days vs. 33 days, was non-significantly lower. There were no major complications caused by the embolization procedure. In another prospective study,[77] outcomes associated with meningioma resection were compared between two neurosurgical centers with differential use of pre-operative embolization. In Center A, embolization was performed for none of the 30 patients and in Center B, 30 consecutive patients underwent embolization. In Center B, the extent of tumor devascularization was evaluated using angiography and postembolization MRI. Intra-operatively, blood loss, the number of blood units transfused, and the observations of the neurosurgeon concerning hemostasis, tumor consistency, and intratumoral necrosis did not differ between the centers. There was some benefit for a subgroup of patients with subtotal devascularization (>90% of the tumor) on postembolization magnetic resonance imaging scans in Center B suggesting that only complete embolization had a noticeable effect on intra-operative blood loss. The rates of surgical morbidity, with permanent neurological worsening, were 20% ($n = 6$) in Center A and 16% ($n = 5$) in Center B. There was one permanent neurological deficit (3%) caused by embolization.

Another study evaluated the benefit of pre-operative superselective embolization for skull base meningiomas[78] in 20 patients who either underwent or did not undergo embolization. Intra-operative blood loss was lower in the embolized group in tumors smaller than 6 cm. In tumors larger than 6 cm, there was no difference in blood loss, perhaps because larger meningiomas tend to have tiny blood vessels that are unsuitable for pre-operative embolization. The embolized group tended to show a better clinical outcome than the non-embolized group.

A study compared the clinical efficacy, cost-effectiveness, and safety[79] between patients undergoing surgical resection for meningiomas with or without pre-operative embolization. The mean estimated blood loss (836 ml^3 vs. 533 ml^3), number of transfusions (1.56 units vs. 0.39 units), surgical resection time (338 minutes vs. 306 minutes), and length of hospitalization (15 days vs. 11 days) were greater in the patients who underwent surgical resection without embolization. However, only the estimated blood loss and number of transfusions variables were significantly different. The mean cost of hospitalization was not different ($29 605 for the embolized group and $38 449 for the non-embolized group). There were three major and nine minor complications in the non-embolized group and no major and six minor complications in the embolized group. There were four additional minor complications caused by the embolization procedure.

Appropriate interval between embolization and surgery

An intermediate interval between embolization and surgery (approximately 7 days) appears to provide the most optimal benefit in reducing intra-operative blood loss and achieving tumor softening. One study[80] compared whether immediate surgical resection (≤24 h) after embolization or delayed surgical resection (>24 h) was more effective in minimizing intra-operative blood loss in 50 patients with meningiomas. Intra-operative blood loss was greater for the immediate group than for the delayed group (29% with blood loss of >1000 ml vs. 0% with blood loss of >700 ml, median value of 475 ml vs. 338 ml). This difference was seen without any significant differences with respect to tumor volume, extent of embolization, degree of devascularization, necrosis,

duration of surgery, or length of the hospital stay. The interval between embolization and surgery and the tumor consistency at the time of surgery were recorded in 42 patients with intracranial meningiomas that received more than 50% of their blood supply from the external carotid artery.[81] On the polynomial regression curve, greatest tumor softening occurred 7–9 days after embolization. When the postembolization interval exceeded 10 days, no further softening occurred. There was no difference in intra-operative blood loss among strata of time intervals.

In a study of 128 patients[57] who underwent embolization with cellulose porous beads, 72% of the patients achieved reduction in the flow of the feeding artery by more than 50%. The non-enhanced area on MR imaging did not significantly correlate with the vascular obliteration. The interval between embolization and surgery was 8–26 days (mean 10 days). The tumor-softening effect and the rate of tumor removal were better among patients with a greater interval between embolization and surgical removal. The investigators recommended an interval of at least 7 days to maximize the benefit of embolization.

Although the embolic particles remain unabsorbed, recanalization starts occurring after the first weeks. Radiological findings in one patient who underwent embolization with polyvinyl alcohol (PVA) particles 694 days before surgery,[82] revealed contrast enhancement despite early obliteration 2 months after embolization. Moreover, angiography, demonstrated prominent tumor vascularity after 5 months despite angiographic confirmation of early obliteration. The histopathologic examination revealed the presence of extended necrotic lesions, a large number of macrophages that contained PVA particles, and destruction of the walls of the once-occluded vessels. In addition, there were many blood-filled vessels that had achieved recanalization.

Embolization without surgery

Embolization without subsequent surgery may cause substantial tumor shrinkage and may be used as a palliative measure. In an open, prospective study,[83] seven patients underwent embolization without subsequent surgery and were followed over a mean of 20 months. Marked tumor shrinkage occurred after embolization in six patients and was most pronounced during the first 6 months. There was improvement in clinical symptoms. In one patient, the tumor was unchanged despite complete angiographic obliteration.

Complications of embolization
Neurological complications

A review of the frequency of procedure-related neurologic complications associated with embolization of intracranial meningiomas in 185 patients[84] found that six patients (3.2%) had ischemic events with associated neurologic deficit.

Two had retinal ischemia and four patients presented with hemiparesis. Intracranial hemorrhage occurred in six patients (3.2%). In five of these patients, rapid microsurgical tumor removal resulted in a favorable outcome without persistent neurologic deficit. In one patient, a massive intratumoral, subarachnoid, and subdural hemorrhage was fatal.

Post-procedural intracranial hemorrhages

Post-procedural intracranial hemorrhages after embolization of meningiomas[85] occur due to distal occlusion of abnormal, friable microvasculature with continued pulsation within the proximal vessels. Previous workers have speculated that the risk of intratumoral hemorrhage increases with the use of small-diameter embolic agents, since each of the first three reported cases had been embolized with Gelfoam powder (40 ± 60 microns).[85,86] Some investigators recommend graduated increases in particle size during the embolization, such as beginning with 50 ± 150 micron particles and finishing with PVA 350 ± 500 microns for obliteration of proximal friable vessels.

Cerebral vasospasm

Nine (2%) of 470 consecutive patients who underwent cranial base tumor resection had evidence of cerebral vasospasm postoperatively; eight were symptomatic[87] with delayed neurological deterioration. There were seven meningiomas, one chordoma, and one trigeminal schwannoma. Vasospasm-related clinical symptoms were predominantly seen in the meningioma cases (range 1 to 30 days post-operatively). Factors that increased the occurrence of vasospasm were tumor size, total operative time, vessel encasement, vessel narrowing, and preoperative embolization. All eight patients with symptomatic vasospasm were treated with hypertensive and hypervolemic therapy; five patients also underwent intraluminal angioplasty and received intra-arterial papaverine alone. Angiographic improvement was seen in all and clinical improvement was seen in six of the eight symptomatic patients.

Glomus tumors

Characteristics

The glomus body is a tiny glandular structure comprising non-chromaffin staining cells clustered among thin-walled vascular channels. Glomus tumors arise from non-chromaffin paraganglionic cells derived from the primitive neural crest.[88–90] Glomus tumors are located around the jugular bulb and along the tympanic branch of the glossopharyngeal nerve, auricular branch of the vagus nerve, superior and inferior laryngeal nerve, aortic arch, nose, orbit, trachea, bladder, and mandible. The carotid body and glomus jugulare tumors are also called chemodectomas because they are assumed to originate from chemoreceptor tissue. Chemodectomas of the neck are more often seen in the carotid body and are considered histologically benign, although they might induce local or distant metastases.[91] Clinical presentation is often non-specific and may only consist of a slowly growing mass in the higher jugular-carotid region. Biopsy is avoided due to risk of massive bleeding and low diagnostic yield.

Therapeutic options

Surgery is the primary therapeutic option for young patients with small tumors less than 3 cm. A study of surgery results in 72 patients with glomus jugulare and nine with glomus vagale found a cure rate of 80% and 100%, respectively.[92] Radiotherapy with or without surgical resection are considered for elderly patients with malignant transformation, those with neurological deficit, or those in whom the tumor mass has already reached the skull base. Radiotherapy demonstrated a 65% tumor response rate and a 25% cure rate.

The primary goals of pre-operative embolization of glomus tumors is to reduce the blood loss in the surgical field, minimize the risk of operative complications, and prevent recurrence by contributing to complete resection. For patients with bilateral tumor involvement, pre-operative embolization is strongly considered because of the risk of swallowing and aspiration problems (caused by complete post-operative pharyngeal denervation), phonation, and breathing difficulty associated with surgical removal. In asymptomatic elderly patients with a slow tumor growth rate, embolization alone can be an option. In some tumors in which surgery is not indicated or is delayed, symptomatic relief and improvement in quality of life can be achieved by decreasing the vascularity and dimensions of the tumor using embolization.[92]

Blood supply

Selective angiography of internal and external carotid arteries, ascending pharyngeal branch of the thyrocervical trunk, and the occipital and vertebral arteries is recommended[93] (see Fig. 16.3). In one angiographic study of 17 non-surgical patients,[94] primary vascular supply was the ascending pharyngeal artery in five patients; the ascending pharyngeal artery and occipital artery in three patients; the ascending pharyngeal artery and superficial temporal artery in two patients; the occipital artery and superficial temporal artery in two patients; and the ascending pharyngeal artery, occipital artery, and superficial artery in one patient. In three patients with bilateral glomus jugulare tumors, the feeding vessels were the ascending pharyngeal artery and the occipital artery on both sides. In three patients with glomus caroticum tumors, the feeding vessels were from both internal and external carotid arteries. The other patients with a glomus caroticum tumor also had vessels from the ascending pharyngeal artery. The Arcellin projection is recommended for adequate visualization of the petrous carotid artery and distal sigmoid sinus in patients with suspected glomus tumor.[95]

(a)

(b)

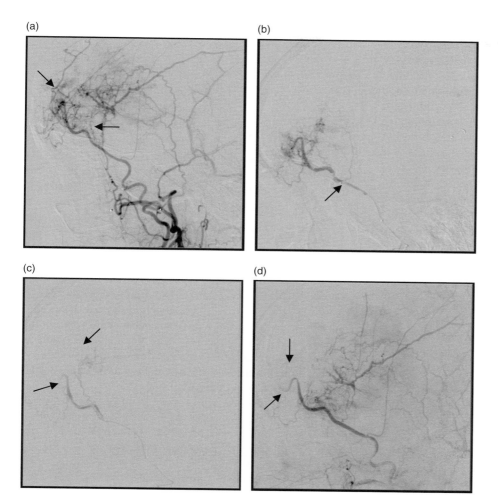

(c)

(d)

Fig. 16.3. Pre- and post-embolization angiographic images. (a) Pre-embolization dural arterial supply (see arrows) from branches of the external carotid artery. (b) Selective placement of the microcatheter in a branch of the external carotid artery (see arrow). (c) Post-embolization obliteration of arterial supply and tumor blush (see arrows) distal to microcatheter in an branch of external carotid artery after injection of particles. (d) Post-embolization obliteration of arterial supply and tumor blush (see arrows) from dural sources in an image acquired following contrast injection into the external carotid artery.

Technical success

Presurgical PVA embolization in 54 patients presenting with a total of 58 chemodectomas[96] (30 jugulare, 24 tympanicum, and 4 caroticum) resulted in complete and partial tumor embolization in 72% and 23% of patients, respectively; in 4% it was unsuccessful. A total of 16% of patients experienced minor events during the procedure including hypotension, bradycardia, and vertigo. Following embolization, tumors were completely excised in 98% of all patients. Although the majority experienced minor post-operative complications (69%), one patient developed meningitis. There were no reported deaths. In another study of 17 non-operable patients,[94] nine patients had complete embolization of the feeding vessels. Partial occlusion was obtained in one session in three patients with glomus jugulare tumors. In one patient with a glomus vagale tumor and in one patient with a glomus caroticum tumor, more than one trial was performed to achieve partial obliteration. Obliteration of the vessels was not successful in three patients (two glomus caroticum and one glomus jugulare tumor) due to tiny feeding vessels. Four patients (24%) with glomus jugulare tumors had temporary

pain and numbness at the site of catheter insertion for a few days after the procedure. Seven patients (41%) had either complete or partial regression of the symptoms during 4 to 15 months of follow-up.

Effectiveness of embolization

A comparison was made between 18 patients who underwent embolization and 17 who did not undergo embolization prior to surgical removal of a glomus jugular tumor.[97] The average operative time was 7 hours and 8 hours respectively among those who did and did not undergo pre-operative embolization. The average operative blood loss was 1122 ml^3 and 2769 ml^3 respectively. While the operative time and blood loss during surgery were lower among those who underwent pre-operative embolization, the risk of injury to cranial nerves IX, X, and XI was not affected. Another study compared six patients with carotid body tumors who underwent pre-operative embolization with 11 patients who underwent surgery without embolization.[98] The blood loss, surgical time, and number of neural injuries were lower in the patients who underwent pre-operative embolization. Only one of six patients had damage to the carotid bulb and required blood transfusion. La Muraglia *et al.*[99] analyzed the effect of pre-operative embolization on tumor dimensions during surgery in 17 patients with glomus caroticum tumors. Patients with embolization (65 cm[22]) and without embolization (63 cm^2) had similar tumor dimensions. The operation time and length of hospital stay was similar in the two groups. Intra-operative bleeding in the embolized group (372 ml) was less than that of the non-embolized group (609 ml). Embolization has also been used for partly embolizing glomus tumors prior to stereotactic radiosurgery.[100] Leber *et al.* reported on 13 patients treated with radiosurgery; six were treated because of recurrences after surgical removal. Two of them had partial embolization before radiosurgery. Within the follow-up period there was no tumor progression and no clinical deterioration in any of the patients.

Pre- and post-operative hemoglobin status was assessed in 27 patients with extracranial vascular tumors:[101] 13 patients had pre-operative embolization and the other patients directly underwent surgery. The percentage rate of change of pre-operative to post-operative hemoglobin was less in patients who underwent pre-operative embolization (9%) when compared with those who did not (18%). The ratio of pre-operative to post-operative hemoglobin in the two groups was also statistically significant (1 and 1.9).

Angiofibroma
Prevalence and characteristics

Juvenile nasopharyngeal angiofibroma is a rare tumour (0.05% of all of the head and neck tumors) that affects adolescent men.[102] The intensely vascular tumor originates from the posterolateral wall of the roof of the nose at the junction of the sphenoid and palatine bones, which also forms the superior margin of the sphenopalatine foramen. The tumors grow in the submucosa of the nasopharyngeal roof and invade the nasal cavity, sphenoid sinus, pterygomaxillary fossa, maxillary sinus, infratemporal fossa, orbit, and middle cranial fossa.[103,104] The tumor is classified based on the Fisch criteria[105,106] using computed tomography (CT) and MRI or both (see Table 16.5). Open or endoscopic surgery is the primary treatment modality

Table 16.5. Fisch's classification for grading angiofibromas[105]

Type I	Tumor is limited to the nasopharynx and nasal cavity with no bone destruction
Type II	Tumor is limited to the nasopharynx and nasal cavity with no bone destruction
Type III	Tumors invade the infratemporal fossa, orbit, and parasellar region but remain lateral to the cavernous sinus
Type IV	Tumors show massive invasion of the cavernous sinus, the optic chiasmal region, or the pituitary fossa

with radiotherapy reserved for patients with intracranial extension that prevents total excision.[107]

Blood supply

Analysis of tumor extension and blood supply is useful for controlling intra-operative bleeding, potential for pre-surgical embolization, and determining the appropriate surgical approach in patients with juvenile nasopharyngeal angiofibroma (see Fig. 16.4). The distinction between true and false internal carotid supply to these tumors, arterial supply to the cranial nerves, and identification of vascular anatomical variants that may represent potential hazards of embolization are important.[108] In one study of 21 patients,[109] the blood supply was exclusively ipsilateral in 18 patients, deriving mainly from the external carotid artery, and bilateral in three. There were no connections between the branches of the internal and external carotid arteries. Intratumoral embolization was achieved in all patients. The internal carotid artery and cavernous sinus are in proximity to the tumor. [110] Another study showed the arterial supply to be only ipsilateral in seven patients and predominantly ipsilateral in four patients.[111] The major arterial supply to these tumors is typically the ipsilateral internal maxillary artery, with occasional additional vessels from branches of the internal carotid or contralateral external carotid system.[106] The internal maxillary artery was the main supply in all 11 cases. In three cases, the ascending pharyngeal artery also contributed to the tumor supply. Further arterial supply was contributed by the internal carotid artery via dural perforating arteries originating from the carotid siphon, ethmoidal and via nasolacrimal branches of the ophthalmic artery. Post-embolization, a facial artery injection is required to identify the collaterals of the maxillary artery, and thus assess the completeness of maxillary artery embolization.[112]

Optimal time interval between embolization and surgery

Four days are the optimal time for operative intervention after embolization based on a case series including ten patients.[113] In another study of 12 patients with angiofibroma,[114] four were treated with a reabsorbable microparticulate substance (Gelfoam) while the remaining eight were treated with non-reabsorbable microparticulate substances (Ivalon, ITC contour, Terbal). The time interval between embolization and surgery ranged from a minimum of 1 day to a maximum of 4 days. The authors concluded that when using reabsorbable materials the interval should not exceed 48 hours because the supply vessels can quickly recanalize. For the materials which are not reabsorbed, the time interval can exceed 48 hours but must be less than 4 days because collateral circulation can arise.

Effectiveness of embolization

Several studies have suggested that pre-operative embolization may reduce intra-operative blood loss. In a national

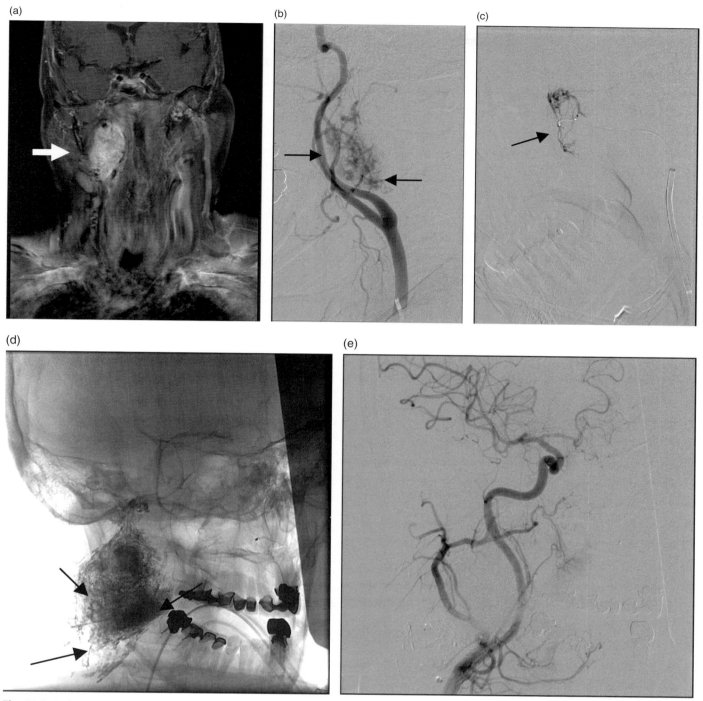

Fig. 16.4. A glomus tumor located at the carotid body. (a) A coronal image from a magnetic resonance imaging scan demonstrating enhancing tumor at the carotid bifurcation; (b) prominent tumor blush at the right carotid bifurcation measuring approximately 6 cm in diameter supplied by proximal branches of the right external carotid artery, specifically by the right ascending pharyngeal artery and right facial artery with minimal contribution from the right internal maxillary artery; (c) microcatheter placement in the main arterial feeder from external carotid artery branch (see arrow); (d) embolization of the glomus tumor with 20% n-BCA; 80% ethiodol and with two drops of glacial acetic acid. The radio-opaque cast is identified by arrows; (e) near complete obliteration of tumor vascularity after embolization.

retrospective cohort study of 443 patients with angiofibromas in Denmark over 22 years,[115] the intra-operative blood loss and need for peri-operative blood transfusion was reduced with pre-operative embolization (see Table 16.6).

Moulin et al.[116] found that a significant difference was noted between the embolized and the non-embolized patients with high-grade tumors but not between those with low-grade tumors, presumably because of less vascularity in low-grade tumors. Multiple embolization sessions may be required to achieve optimal results.[116,117]

With the availability of endoscopic surgery, the observed levels of intra-operative bleeding, occurrence of complications, and rates of recurrence in low-grade angiofibromas are close to those seen in embolized patients as reported in the literature.[118,119] However, the endoscopic approach is ineffective for stage IV angiofibromas and some stage III cases with major extension into the middle cranial fossa.[106] Pre-operative autologous donation and the cell saver system for immediate retransfusion of the collected blood after filtration have also minimized homologous blood transfusion.[120]

Complications associated with embolization

In one study of 20 patients with either extensive (Fisch class IIIa to IVb, $n = 17$) or less massive (Fisch class II, $n = 3$) nasopharyngeal angiofibromas, temporary visual disturbance or headache, or both, was seen in two of 20 patients after superselective tumor embolization, and further visual diminution was observed in one of six patients after balloon occlusion of the internal carotid artery.[123] Some studies have suggested that the recurrence rate of angiofibromas maybe higher with pre-operative embolization[124] presumably due to difficulty in discerning tumor margins in the absence of vascular margins. Other studies have suggested that the rate of recurrence is lower due to more complete removal of tumor due to lower intra-operative bleeding.[111,122]

Table 16.6. Summary of results evaluating the benefit of pre-operative embolization in terms of surgical blood loss

	Embolized patients		Non-embolized patients	
	Number	Blood loss	Number	Blood loss
Glad et al.[115]	10	650 ml	23	1200 ml
Li et al.[121]	11	677 ml	10	1136 ml
Siniluoto et al.[122]	5	510 ml	5	1510 ml
Moulin et al.[116]	13	538 ml	7	1038 ml

Technical aspects of the embolization procedure
Procedure objectives

The objectives are summarized below:

1. To control surgically inaccessible arterial feeders
2. To decrease surgical morbidity by reducing blood loss
3. To shorten the operative procedure time
4. To increase chances of complete surgical resection
5. To decrease the risk of damage to adjacent normal tissue
6. To relieve intractable pain
7. To decrease expected tumor recurrence, and
8. To allow better visualization of the surgical field with decreased overall surgical complications

Angiographic characteristics

The extensive vascularity of extra- and intracranial neoplasms is vulnerable to superselective intra-arterial injection of embolic particles. Angiographic images must be acquired to identify the main arteries supplying the vascular bed of the neoplasm. The tumor is identified by its characteristic aggregation of small diameter arteries, arterioles, and capillaries (blush). The current resolution of the angiographic images does not allow distinct visualization of arterioles and capillaries in peak opacification. Subsequently, selective catheterization into the parent artery such as the external carotid artery may be necessary to acquire images focusing on feeding arteries without concurrent opacification of surrounding unrelated arteries. The angiographic supply pattern determines the likelihood of success of the embolization procedure. A classification scheme[125] has been proposed that assigns a score from 1 to 3 (see Table 16.7) on the basis of the angiographic appearance of the vasculature. Increasing grade suggests a higher level of complexity for the embolization procedure. The classification is based on three factors: (1) End versus side origin; (2) Tree vs. plant configuration; and (3) Possibility of ischemic complications with reflux into proximal vasculature. The tree configuration is defined by presence of an angiographically identifiable trunk (see Fig. 16.5). The grade is assigned based on the predominant pattern of vasculature.

The venous outflow follows the usual venous drainage patterns with normal architecture.

Guidecatheter placement

Most embolization procedures can be performed using a 6F (or even a 5F) guidecatheter. The guidecatheter can be

Table 16.7. Proposed classification scheme for classifying the predominant pattern of arterial blood supply

Grade	Point of origin	Branching pattern	A	B
1	End arterial supply	Tree or plant configuration	Ischemic complications low risk with proximal reflux	Ischemic complications high risk with proximal reflux
2	Side arterial supply	Tree configuration		
3	Side arterial supply	Plant configuration		

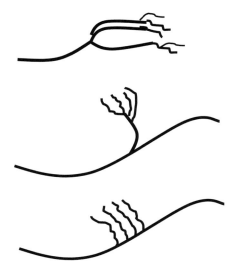

Fig. 16.5. Schematic representation of a proposed scheme for classifying the predominant pattern of arterial blood supply.

introduced into the external or internal carotid or vertebral artery using a 0.035-inch guidewire in most circumstances. The guidecatheter may be placed in the proximal vessel (such as the subclavian artery) if the parent artery is too small to accommodate the guidecatheter (thyrocervical trunk or small vertebral artery). The positioning of the guidecatheter may be an issue because its distal end may cause vasospasm or dissection in tortuous and small diameter arteries.

External carotid artery: embryonic development and anatomy

During development, the middle meningeal artery primarily arises from the supraorbital branch of the stapedial artery that stems from the dorsal part of the second branchial artery.[126] Later, by the formation of the external carotid artery connecting with the common trunk of the infraorbital and mandibular branches (maxillomandibular division) of the stapedial artery and by the atrophy of the proximal part of it, the middle meningeal artery is finally supplied by the external carotid artery. But in this example, it is supposed that the middle meningeal artery arose from a more distal position of the internal carotid artery owing to the persistence of the anastomosis between the dorsal part of the first branchial artery and the supraorbital branch and the interruption of the connection between the supraorbital branch and maxillomandibular division of the stapedial artery. Structural and morphometric investigations of the vessels of the neck region were carried out on 30 cadavers[127] to gain more knowledge of the anatomy for microvascular surgery. The non-common-truck type of the external carotid artery (in which each branch arises separately from the external carotid artery) was found in 77% of cases, the truncus linguofacialis type was found in 22%, and the truncus thyrolingualis type was found in 2%. The smallest internal diameter (the average was 1.2 mm) was found in the superficial cervical artery; the largest internal diameter (4.4 mm) was measured in the

external carotid artery; the longest arterial section (128 mm) was measured between the clavicle and mandibular margin; The vascular section or stem consisted of three parts: the supraclavicular part of the common carotid artery; the proximal section of the external carotid artery; and the first 3 cm of the facial artery; in 47% of cases, the facial, lingual, and superior thyroid veins joined together and formed a thyrolinguofacialis vein. The type with one external jugular vein accounted for 83% of cases, and the type with one anterior jugular vein for 67% of cases. The middle thyroid vein exhibited the smallest internal diameter (average of 2.0 mm). The largest internal diameter (7.9 mm) was measured in the internal jugular vein. The longest vessel to receive a vascular pedicle vein was the external jugular vein, the average length of which was 99.7 mm.

Selective microcatheter placement

Each of the supplying medium sized arteries (usually branches of the external carotid artery) is selectively catheterized with a microcatheter over a 0.010- or 0.014-inch microwire (see Fig. 16.6). Over the wire systems are preferable over flow-directed systems. The flow into the vascular bed of the tumor is not high enough to influence the course of a flow-directed microcatheter in most instances. Selective microcatheter contrast injections confirm the presence of hypervascularity in the tumor bed within the distribution of the catheterized artery. Any reflux of contrast into normal vasculature should be viewed with caution.

Super-selective vs. sub-selective positioning of catheter

The particles have to be injected slowly to avoid dangerous reflux. The most effective embolization occurs with the most distal loading of the vascular bed with super-selective microcatherization.[128] Wedging the catheter into the tumor vessels should be avoided because it can cause the tumor to rupture and/or hemorrhage. One study compared the efficacy of preoperative super-selective and sub-selective embolization for intracranial meningiomas.[129] Twenty-two patients underwent embolization with 45 to 150 mm PVA particles after super-selective catheterization of the feeding vessels with a microcatheter system and another 30 patients underwent subselective embolization with 150 to 300 mm Gelfoam particles after catheterization of the terminal external carotid artery just proximal to the orifice of the maxillary artery with a 4- or 5-F angiocatheter. The mean intra-operative blood loss (918 mL vs. 1450 mL), amount of blood transfused (4.9 units vs. 7.5 units), and surgical resection time (422 min vs. 529 min) were all lower in the super-selective group than in the sub-selective group. The occurrence of fresh ischemic necrosis (59% vs. 53%), hemorrhage (77% vs. 60%), and embolic material (55% vs. 13%) on pathologic examination were higher in the super-selective embolization group. No

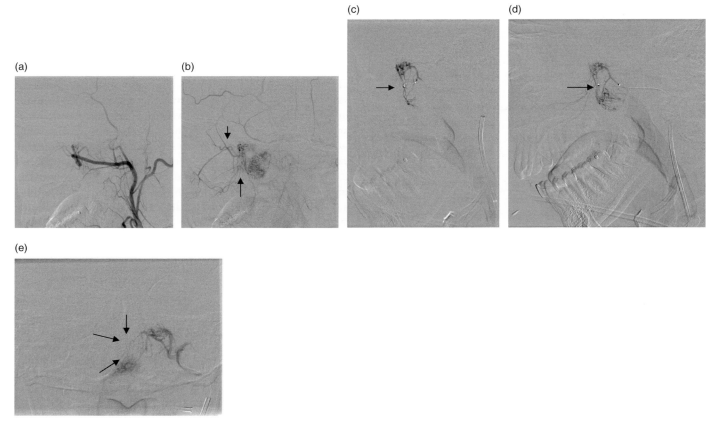

Fig. 16.6. Successful endovascular embolization of a left-sided nasopharyngeal juvenile angiofibroma with 100–300 micron PVA particles and tornado coils. (a) A lateral image demonstrating the branches of the external carotid artery; (b) opacification of the nasopharyngeal juvenile angiofibroma through branches of the internal maxillary artery (see arrows); (c), (d) microcatheter placement in the main arterial feeder from internal maxillary artery (see arrow); (e) at the end of the procedure there was no residual tumor blush visualized from images acquired in lateral plane from an external carotid artery injection (see arrows).

procedure-related complications occurred in the super-selective group, whereas two patients in the sub-selective group had post-operative scalp necrosis. The authors concluded that pre-operative embolization of meningiomas, if indicated, should be done with the super-selective technique whenever feasible.

Identifying the potential for new neurological deficits

The arterial supply to cranial nerves and the existence of anastomotic networks between external and internal carotid arteries should be recognized prior to embolization. The external carotid artery most importantly supplies the facial nerve and the lower cranial nerves from CN IX to XII. Thus, proximal embolization of any of the vessels supplying these nerves can result in cranial nerve palsies, which could be temporary and could recover after steroid injections and development of collaterals; however, distal embolization with either particles smaller than 80 μm or liquid materials can lead to permanent damage or even open channels with the intracranial contributions resulting in embolic strokes of the posterior fossa.

There are three major regions in these territories which form extracranial and intracranial anastomotic pathways.

1. The orbital region via the ophthalmic artery that is the interface between the internal maxillary and internal carotid territories.
2. The petrous-cavernous region via the inferolateral trunk, the petrous branches of the internal carotid artery, and the meningohypophyseal trunk to the carotid artery.
3. The upper cervical region via the ascending pharyngeal, the occipital, and the ascending and deep cervical arteries to the vertebral artery.

Injection into the middle maxillary artery (MMA) should be performed with caution because retinal blood supply can originate from the MMA[130] and there is the possibility of transdural anastomosis from the MMA to the superior cerebellar artery.[131] Anomalous meningeal branches of the ophthalmic artery can feed meningiomas of the brain convexity.[132] Similarly, spontaneous opening of a large occipital-vertebral artery anastomosis during embolization has been reported,[133,134] 27 histologic proven malignant gliomas judged by the surgeon as not to be operated upon.

Provocative tests

In addition to studying the angiographic anatomy, lidocaine and amytal provocation tests may identify the risk of complications associated with embolization. Provocative testing was performed[135] in 141 patients evaluated for embolization of meningioma. Eleven patients were not embolized because the test results were positive. The Patients with positive provocative tests had meningiomas in the cavernous sinus or petroclival region. The feeders were of middle meningeal artery origin and followed a posteromedial course toward the petrous apex or cavernous sinus. Three patients with negative provocative tests experienced complications which included intratumoral hemorrhage ($n = 2$) and post-embolization hearing disturbance ($n = 1$). In 21 patients with meningovascular tumors (meningiomas or angiofibromas),[136] 53 vessels underwent provocative testing using thiopental sodium, 15–20 mg (in 2 mL of sodium chloride solution), to detect anastomoses with cerebral vessels, then lidocaine, 10–20 mg (in 2 mL of sodium chloride solution), to identify vessels feeding cranial nerves. Injection of thiopental sodium into the occipital artery provided a positive result in one (2%) of the 53 cases. In arteries with negative provocative tests, the afferent was embolized with <300 micron particles without any complications.

Anatomical areas of arterial supply

CT scan acquired during angiography (angio-CT) may provide specific information about the tissue fed by the arterial branches selected for embolization such as ophthalmic branches by definite enhancement of the retina. In one study,[137] a total of 16 angio-CT, were performed for 11 tumors to study the regions of arterial supply of the middle meningeal artery ($n = 10$), internal carotid artery ($n = 4$), accessory meningeal artery ($n = 1$), and occipital artery ($n = 1$). A within subject comparison with DSA suggested that angio-CT had higher contrast and spatial resolution and allowed more definite visualization of tumor perfusion in nearly half of the cases. In one meningioma with multiple feeders, angio-CT provided more definite information on the vascular supply for each feeder than DSA. Arterial supply from the ICA territory was more clearly identified with angio-CT in three of four cases. All feeders of the external carotid arteries were embolized without complications. In one case, angio-CT identified vascular supply to the masticatory muscle and the microcatheter was re-positioned accordingly.

Injection of embolic material

The goal is to inject embolic material such as PVA particles, Gelfoam powder, fibrin glue, microfibrillar collagen, or gelatin microspheres (see Table 16.8) until the vascular blush is completely obliterated. The microcatheter is placed at a site where injection of embolic material can lead to maximal penetration and minimal reflux into normal vasculature. Vasodilator-assisted embolization may lead to higher penetration of embolic material. Intra-arterial nicardipine in doses of 0.5 to 1.0 mg (5 mg in 5 mL concentration) may be injected prior to embolization to induce temporary vasodilation within the arterioles. Particles are preferred over liquid embolic agents. The transient opacification during injection of embolic particles confirms the flow of embolic material in the correct vessels. Adequate obliteration is suggested by the accumulation and sluggish flow of contrast. Microcatheter- and guide catheter-injections are required to confirm the obliteration of the target vessels.

Size of embolic particles

Embolization is usually initiated with the smallest particles using high dilution to ensure adequate penetration into the tumor vascular bed except if there is a risk of flow through anastomotic channels into other distributions. Even if angiographic images suggest a single arterial supply, the vascular bed can form extensive collaterals leading to immediate or delayed supply from another medium-sized artery in the event of occlusion of the parent artery. Therefore, for sustained obliteration the occlusion must occur in the capillaries of the tumor bed. A gradual increase in the diameter of the particles injected may ensure smaller vessel obliteration prior to obliteration of larger proximal vessels. A study[138] found that the vessels located inside the tumors (mean 240 microns) are smaller than the extratumoral vessels (mean 400 microns). Therefore, larger particles may not adequately penetrate intratumoral vessels. One study[139] compared the efficacy of two embolization techniques: (1) administration of 150–300 micron PVA particles in the usual suspension; and (2) administration of 50–150 micron PVA particles in a highly diluted suspension for pre-operative meningioma embolization in 34 patients using CT, MR, 1H MR spectroscopy, MR volumetric measurements, intra-operative ultrasound, and histopathologic findings. Angiography after embolization demonstrated total elimination of tumor blush in all patients. Contrast-enhanced MR after the administration of 150 to 300 micron PVA particles revealed a reduction of tumor enhancement in only two out of 14 patients. In 12 of 20 patients embolized with small particles, 30% to 95% of the whole tumor was necrotic with 17% to 20% reduction of tumor volume in four cases, leading to recovery from the initial neurologic deficits. In three of 20 patients, post-embolization worsening of edema occurred with small particles. 1H MR spectroscopy of the tumors showed an increase of lactate and aliphatic lipid compounds after embolization, indicating tumor infarction. The appearance of the tumor at operation, ultrasound examination, and the histopathologic examination of different parts of the tumor confirmed the pre-operative MR findings suggesting superior obliteration with smaller particles.

Another study compared the efficacy of trisacryl gelatin microspheres[140] of various sizes including 150–300 micron ($n = 30$), PVA particles of 45 to 150 microns ($n = 15$), and PVA particles of 150 to 250 microns ($n = 15$). There was no

Table 16.8. Characteristics of embolic particles available

Company	Product name	Composition	Type	Sizes (µm)	Color coding	Indicated use
AngioDynamics	LC Bead	Polyvinyl alcohol hydrogel microsphere	Calibrated sphere	100–300, 300–500, 500–700	Labels are color coded and the beads are tinted blue	Embolization of HVTs and peripheral AVMs
BioSphere Medical	Embosphere Microspheres	Trisacryl crosslinked with gelatin	Spherical microsphere	40–120, 100–300, 300–500, 500–700, 700–900, 900–1200	Labels are color coded	Embolization of AVMs, HVTs, and symptomatic uterine fibroids
	EmboGold Microspheres					Embolization of HVTs and AVMs
	Quadrasphere	Super absorbent polymer	Expanding spherical microsphere	Dry sizes: 50–100, 100–150, 150–200		Embolization of HVTs and peripheral AVMs
Boston Scientific Corporation	Contour SE Microspheres	Spherical PVA	Sphere	100–300, 300–500, 500–700, 700–900, 900–1200	Packaging by size	Embolization of peripheral HVTs, including leiomyoma uteri and peripheral AVMs
CeloNova BioSciences, Inc.	Embozene Color-Advanced Microspheres	Hydrogel core with Polyzene-F coating	Sphere	40, 100, 250, 400, 500, 700, 900	Microspheres are dyed in size-specific colors, with color-coded syringes, labels, and boxes	Embolization of HVTs and AVMs
Terumo Interventional Systems	Bead Block	Acrylamido polyvinyl alcohol macromer	Sphere	100–300, 300–500, 500–700, 700–900, 900–1200	Spheres, syringe, and box by size	Embolization of HVTs and AVMs

Adapted from *Endovascular Today*, April 2009, p. 71, AVMs, arterio-venous mdl formations; HVTs, hypervascularized tumors.

significant difference in the extent of angiographic obliteration among the groups. The trisacryl gelatin microspheres were located more distally in tumor vessels than were the PVA particles of either size and resulted in lower intra-operative bleeding. There was no difference in intra-operative bleeding between the two sizes of PVA particles. The extent of intratumoral necrosis was not significantly different between the two embolic agents. In all groups, there was a mild inflammatory tissue reaction in the vicinity of the embolic agent.

Particles of small sizes can be used to occlude intratumoral arteries, whereas particles of large sizes can be chosen to occlude afferent pedicles. A study[141] determined the location of calibrated trisacryl gelatin microspheres in the arterial vasculature of 49 specimens of nasopharyngeal angiofibromas and paragangliomas treated operatively after embolization with particles of various sizes (100–300 µm to 900–1200 µm). Embolization was achieved with trisacryl gelatin microspheres of the following size ranges: 100–300 µm, 300–500 µm, 500–700 µm, 700–900 µm, and 900–1,200 µm. Sizes were increased step by step, according to size artery and the corresponding angiographic blush. Embolized vessels ($n = 1125$) were measured: 440 in paragangliomas and 685 in nasopharyngeal angiofibromas. Vessels were 89% intratumoral and 11% extratumoral. The diameter of the occluded vessels increased significantly with the size range of trisacryl gelatin microspheres used for embolization for each tumor type.[141]

In cases of dangerous anastomosis or collateral vessels, the particles must be large enough to avoid passage through the healthy branches with subsequent accidental occlusions. Embolization was started with 100–300-µm trisacryl gelatin microspheres except in arteries that were more likely to harbor an extracranial/intracranial anastomosis. In these arteries, embolization began with 300–500 µm trisacryl gelatin microspheres.[138] Embolization procedures differed slightly between the two pathologic conditions as a result of differences in the vasculature of the tumors. Paragangliomas are mostly fed by the ascending pharyngeal artery and the stylomastoid artery, which may show anastomosis to intracranial arteries, therefore embolization is initiated with particles of larger caliber. For AVMs or fistulas, the caliber of particles can be adjusted to the size of the shunt to be occluded. New pre-operative embolization strategies could also be developed by adapting the distal location and completion of devascularization to facilitate tumor resection.

Dilution of particles

Embolic particles mixed with diluted contrast are injected through the microcatheter. Adequate dilution of embolic material is essential to prevent excessive viscosity and plugging of the microcatheter. Dilution of particles is adapted to the size of particles and their concentration in the vial. Particles are suspended in a 50:50 mixture of saline solution and contrast medium. To get a homogeneous solution, injection into the microcatheter is achieved with a 3-mL Luer-lock syringe connected by means of a three-way stopcock to a 10-mL Luer-lock syringe filled with the solution containing the particles, and the suspension is smoothly agitated to maintain particles homogeneously suspended in the medium.[138] In case of insufficient dilution with a quick injection rate, small particles can form clusters in large vessels proximally to the site of occlusion[138] due to the high number of small particles present in each milliliter of suspension in commercial vials. Dry PVA preparations increase significantly in size when suspended in nonionic contrast or contrast-alcohol solutions. The saline-packaged PVA particles do not enlarge in contrast or contrast-alcohol solutions.[142]

Tissue reaction to embolic particles

Trisacryl gelatin microspheres appear in the tissues as round eosinophilic homogenous structures, generally surrounded by a vascular wall or an inflammatory reaction in histologic samples.[138] In the first few days after embolization, these microspheres are sometimes associated with fibrin thrombus and mild inflammation with macrophages and some polymorphonuclear cells. Later, during the first weeks, macrophages and giant cells predominate, with some associated fibrosis and lymphocytes. No trisacryl gelatin microspheres degradation has been observed, even in specimens obtained more than 6 months after embolization (as late as 7 years).

Embolization of internal carotid artery branches and pial vessels

Typically, embolization of feeders from the pial arterial system is not attempted unless: (1) there is pure or predominant pial supply; (2) no normal arteries are visualized in superselective angiography; (3) there are pre-existing irreversible neurological deficits related to tumor; (4) provocative test reveals no newly developed neurological symptoms and signs; and (5) it is technically feasible to advance a microcatheter proximal to the tumor.[143] In one study,[143] eight patients had lesions supplied by the ICA, or pial branches of the middle cerebral artery (MCA), anterior cerebral artery (ACA), or posterior cerebral artery (PCA). Seven tumors were extra-axial (six meningiomas, one solitary fibrous tumor) and one was intra-axial (metastatic hepatocellular carcinoma). All tumors were adjacent to the frontal or parietal lobe. Provocative testing by injection of sodium amytal (25 mg) or pentothal sodium (40 mg) was used to identify the blood supply to the motor or language cortex in four patients with tumors adjacent to the motor cortex. If no loss of speech or hemiparesis occurred within 5 min, feeding vessels were embolized. Pre-operative embolization was performed with PVA ranging from 150 to 250 mm in diameter, platinum microcoils, 25% mixture of histoacryl and lipiodol, or microfibril collagen. PVA particles were used to embolize small tumor vessels followed by a mixture of PVA particles and microfibril collagen to embolize proximal portions of feeding vessels in two patients. In three patients, a 25% mixture of histoacryl and lipiodol was used, and in one a coil was used. The angiographic obliteration was estimated to range from 40% to 80% based on serial MRIs. The choroidal blush was lost in one patient and retinal blush was lost in another patient although the patient had tumor related visual loss prior to embolization.

Al tumors were successfully removed with some operative difficulty in five in the non-embolized portion. In another report of two meningiomas,[144] the internal anterior-frontal (a branch of the anterior cerebral artery) artery and sulcal artery were embolized with gelfoam in one patient prior to surgical resection. No neurological deficit appeared after the embolization or the surgery in either case.

Direct tumor embolization

The percutaneous direct approach was initially used to treat tumors with difficult intravascular access[145,146] (see Fig. 16.7). DSA is recommended to identify all the collateral arterial supplies to the tumor and dangerous anastomotic feeders. After percutaneous puncture, reflux of blood was obtained followed by injection of contrast agent into the tumor to obtain local parenchymography, study local and regional venous drainage and anastomoses, and document absence of extravasation. Just before injecting the glue, one should inject a small amount of intratumoral contrast medium and analyze the images carefully for dangerous anastomoses. Temporary balloon occlusion of these internal carotid or vertebral arteries proximal to the feeders from these vessels during intratumoral embolization may be used in selected patients. Direct intratumoral embolization with histoacryl in 65 hypervascular lesions, including 29 juvenile nasopharyngeal angiofibromas, 22 glomus tumors, four metastases of the calvaria, four meningiomas, three hemangiopericytomas, one primary carcinoma of the sella, one hemangioblastoma, and one dural cavernoma of the sellar region[147] was reported. The report suggested that a feeder from the ophthalmic artery is a relative contraindication for direct puncture embolization with glue because of complications seen in a patient with juvenile nasopharyngeal angiofibroma, erosion the floor of the orbit, and recruitment of ophthalmic artery branches. The report also suggested that temporary balloon occlusion of the external carotid artery proximal to the feeders of a chemodectoma (located at the bifurcation of the common carotid artery) during intratumoral injection of the glue may prevent potential retrograde migration of the glue into the internal carotid artery.

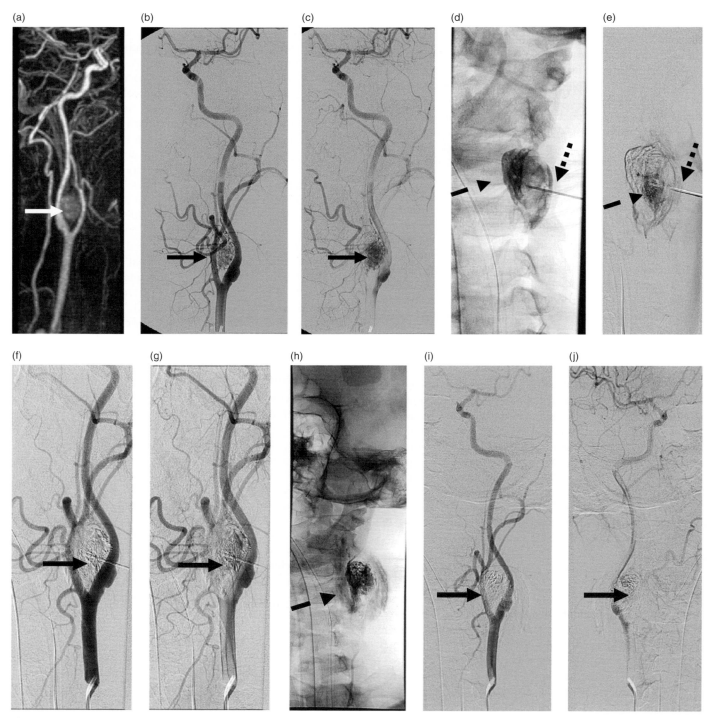

Fig. 16.7. Percutaneous embolization of glomus tumor located at the carotid body. (a) A magnetic resonance angiogram demonstrates a highly vascular mass located at the carotid bifurcation (arrow); (b), (c) an angiogram with common carotid artery injection demonstrating vascular opacification of the tumor in early and late arterial phases (see arrows); (d) and (e) percutaneous 20 gauge 3.5 inch needle insertion (see dotted arrow) and injection of radio-opaque n-BCA-ethiodol (see dashed arrows); (f), (g) a common carotid artery injection demonstrating obliteration of vascular opacification of the tumor in early and late arterial phases (see arrows); (h) additional injected radio-opaque n-BCA-ethiodol (see dashed arrows); (i), (j) a common carotid artery injection demonstrating near complete obliteration of vascular opacification of the tumor in early and late arterial phases (see arrows).

Casasco et al.[148] reported the results of direct tumor puncture performed percutaneously or via the nose and mouth to embolize ten nasopharyngeal fibromas, four tumors of the calvarium (three metastases and one hemangiopericytoma), one intrasellar hemangiopericytoma, and two glomus tumors. In one case, an intrasellar tumor was embolized via a transseptosphenoidal surgical approach. The embolization material used was n-BCA in 14 and alcohol in three patients. Angiographic obliteration was complete in 14 cases, and greater than 90% in three cases. Thirteen tumors were totally resected without requiring blood transfusion. Use of tungsten during embolization delineated tumor margins. During surgery, the limits of the exsanguinated tumor were very well defined. Of the four tumors embolized without surgery (three metastases and one glomus tumor), two metastases required retreatment after 6 and 8 months of remission, respectively. The volume of the glomus tumor decreased by 80% and remained unchanged after 8 months.

Gobin et al.[149] described successful percutaneous puncture of the external carotid artery or one of its branches distal to a surgical arterial ligation in 43 patients who underwent 64 embolization attempts. The punctured arteries were the trunk of the external carotid artery in 31 patients, the internal maxillary artery in nine, the facial artery in nine, the lingual artery in eight, the occipital artery in four, and the superficial temporal artery in three. Of 64 attempts, 57 were successful in one session, six were successful in two sessions, and one failed. Puncture-related complications were eight spontaneously resolving hematomas and six asymptomatic punctures of the internal carotid artery.

Inadvertent embolization

Infrequently, the embolic material may reflux proximally into a normal arterial branch or flow into a newly developed vascular channel secondary to high resistance into the primary hypervascular region. Recognizing the stage of obliteration where such risk increases is important. If advertent occlusion occurs, intra-arterial vasodilator injection into the affected distribution may facilitate the clearance of the particles. For cutaneous ischemia, transdermal vasodilator treatment may be helpful to recruit alternate collateral supply.

Microparticle-arteriovenous shunt occur during embolization[150] with pulmonary shunt index measured between 0% and 36% for branchial paragangliomas (glomus tumors) and between 82% and 95% for angiofibromas using Technetium[99m] Tc-labeled macroaggregated albumin particles with calibrated diameters between 25 and 50 microns. Paradoxical movement of embolic particle through a patent foramen ovale can occur during embolization leading to ischemic stroke.[151] Four cases of facial palsy following middle meningeal artery embolization, one case of aspiration pneumonia following glomus tumor embolization, and a case of pulmonary embolization following embolization of a spinal arteriovenous malformation were reported.[152] Gupta et al.[153] reported that one patient (carotid body tumor) developed mild unilateral seventh, ninth and tenth cranial nerve palsy, and one patient developed transient hemiparesis (nasopharyngeal angiofibroma) among 46 consecutive patients with 48 hypervascular head and neck tumors that had undergone preoperative embolization. The deficits resolved in both patients with steroids. One patient developed delayed glue migration into the middle cerebral artery territory 6 h after the procedure.

New embolic agents

Onyx liquid embolic agent (Micro Therapeutics, Inc, Irvine, CA) for delayed surgical resection,[154] hydroxyapatite ceramic microparticles, biocompatible embolic materials,[155] and phenytoin (250–500 mg) diluted with saline (25 mg/mL) injected slowly as a bolus[156] have been used for tumor embolization. In one study, 23 patients with meningioma were treated with high concentration mannitol[157] and 31 patients were treated with PVA particles alone. Satisfactory angiographic results were obtained in all 23 patients. Tumor necrosis was observed intra-operatively and confirmed pathologically. There was no significant difference in mean estimated blood loss between mannitol- and PVA-embolized patients (407 mL vs. 381 mL). In cell cultures, 1200 mOsm but not 300 mOsm of manitol led to death of endothelial and tumor cell lines.

Carotid blow out syndrome

Radiation carotid blowout syndrome in nasopharyngeal carcinoma may occur in various time intervals following exposure and can affect different arteries. A study of 14 patients with nasopharyngeal carcinomas and 15 carotid blowout syndromes secondary to radiation (average dose of 73 gray units) exposure after a mean period of 33 months were reported.[158] The blowout syndrome occured in the internal ($n = 10$), external ($n = 4$), or common carotid artery ($n = 1$). Endovascular treatment using detachable balloons in 11 and liquid adhesives or coils in four patients was successful in all 15 radiation carotid blowout syndromes with cessation of hemorrhage. One patient had hemiparesis after embolization.

Intra-arterial chemotherapy

Introduction

High-grade astrocytomas account for approximately 40% of all primary brain tumors. Despite the current standard treatments including surgical resection, radiation therapy, and chemotherapy, the median survival is approximately 8–10 months for patients with glioblastoma multiforme (GBM) and 36 months for patients with anaplastic astrocytoma.[159] For patients with disease recurrence/progression, available systemic chemotherapies offer modest clinical benefit with a 6-month progression-free survival of less than 15% for GBM and 31% for anaplastic astrocytoma and a median overall survival of 25 weeks and 47 weeks for recurrent GBM and anaplastic astrocytoma, respectively.[160] The Intra-arterial approach has been an attractive option to overcome some of the limitations of systemic chemotherapy.

Theoretical considerations

The intra-arterial administration of chemotherapeutic agents may result in a higher concentration of agent in the local blood supply and subsequently in the tumor.[161,162] When compared with intravenous administration, intra-arterial administration leads to a five-fold increase in the drugs local peak concentration.[163] The local peak concentration can be maximized by administering the drug in a smaller artery with slower flow to reduce the dilution and increase the extraction time. The extraction fraction within the target organ depends on capillary permeability (lipid solubility in brain). After the first pass, the drug circulates within the bloodstream and may be extracted minimally during the venous recirculation phase. The regional advantage equation expresses the combined effect of blood flow in the artery infused and total body clearance. The regional advantage equation is as follows in descending order: carmustine and other nitrosoureas, cisplatin, carboplatin, and etoposide.[163,164]

Regional concentration of chemotherapeutic agents

In a primate study,[165] intra-arterial carotid infusion of carbon-labeled BCNU resulted in five-fold greater delivery compared to intravenous administration. Intra-arterial administration of BCNU achieved 190% to 280% higher brain nucleic acid-bound drug levels in the infused hemisphere and 130% to 280% higher levels than in the non-infused hemisphere compared with the intravenous route. In addition, some brain regions directly subserved by the middle cerebral artery had bound drug levels four- to five-fold greater than those found in regions of non-infused brain. Namba et al.[166] introduced a superselective catheter into the anterior, middle, or posterior cerebral artery of patients with malignant glioma for intra-arterial chemotherapy. ^{99m}Tc-HMPAO was subsequently injected via a microcatheter introduced into the anterior, middle, or posterior cerebral artery of patients and regional concentration was measured using single photon emission computed tomography (SPECT). A higher dose of ^{99m}Tc-HMPAO was injected intravenously to obtain adequate background brain images. The concentration of ^{99m}Tc-HMPAO was about 50 times higher in tissue perfused by superselective injection into the anterior or middle cerebral artery that following intravenous injection.

Evolution of intra-arterial chemotherapy

Intra-arterial chemotherapy approaches have been used for low- and high-grade gliomas, and for cerebral lymphomas. Basso et al.[167] reviewed the results in terms of response and

toxicity from studies with intra-arterial administration of nitrosoureas (see Tables 16.9 and 16.10) and platinum derivatives (see Tables 16.11 and 16.12), and perspectives of the new strategy of blood–brain barrier disruption with osmotic agents or bradykinin analogs. Early intra-arterial regimens consisting of nitrosoureas were generally abandoned because the side effects outweighed the therapeutic advantage.[168–170] The theoretical efficacy of nitrosoureas is related to their high liposolubility and partial protein binding that contribute to their ability to cross the blood–brain barrier. Concerns regarding toxicity of nitrosourea administered intra-arterially[168–170] led to the consideration of other agents. Cisplatin demonstrated encouraging results for the treatment of glioblastomas and brain metastases when injected into the carotid artery,[171,172] but the drug's benefit was obscured by neurotoxicity, retinal damage, and ototoxicity.[173,174] Carboplatin has an antineoplastic spectrum similar to that of cisplatin[175,176] the side effects profile may be more favorable.[175–178] Recently, the intra-arterial administration of carboplatin has been evaluated for the treatment of intracranial neoplasms.[163,179–182] More recent studies suggest that toxicity can be reduced by the use of methotrexate-based regimens.[163] Manipulation of the blood–brain barrier has been described to increase the transport of chemotherapeutic agents into the tumor.[183,184] Initially, local infusion of hypertonic solutions was investigated to facilitate drug delivery.[183,184] Administration of RMP–7 (see Table 16.13), a bradykinin analog, increases the permeability of the brain tumor capillaries.[185,186] When administered with intra-arterial carboplatin, RMP-7 has been shown to increase the transport of carboplatin into the tumor bed by 2–12-fold.[185,186]

Indications for intra-arterial chemotherapy
Intra-arterial chemotherapy for newly diagnosed gliomas

Intra-arterial chemotherapy has been used prior to or concurrent with radiotherapy for newly diagnosed gliomas.[163] Table 16.14 summarizes the agents used either alone or in combination for newly diagnosed gliomas. A Phase III trial[169] compared the efficacy and safety of intra-arterial carmustine (BCNU) and intravenous BCNU (200 mg/m^2 every 8 weeks), each regimen without or with intravenous 5-fluorouracil (1 gm/m^2 three times daily given 2 weeks after BCNU) for the treatment of newly resected malignant gliomas. All patients also received radiation therapy. A total of 315 of the 505 patients were randomly assigned to receive intra-arterial (167 patients) or intravenous (148 patients) BCNU; 57 patients were excluded, primarily because of neuropathology error, and 190 patients could not receive intra-arterial BCNU. Log-rank analysis demonstrated reduced survival for the intra-arterial group patients predominantly in the anaplastic astrocytoma group compared to those receiving intravenous BCNU. Serious toxicity was observed in the intra-arterial

Table 16.9. Nitrosourea-based intra-arterial chemotherapy in high-grade gliomas recurrent after radiotherapy ± systemic chemotherapy

Author	Mechanism of action	Protocol	Complete/partial response(%)	SD	TTP	Overall survival (wks)	Toxicity (%)
Greenberg et al.[187]	BCNU-DNA and RNA alkylating agent and carbamoylation of amino acids in proteins	BCNU 200 mg/m2 [IC] every 6–8 weeks	54	16	20	54	Visual loss (12.5), leukoencephalopathy, (12.5), hydrocephalus (4)
Hochberg et al.[188]	See above	BCNU 240–600 mg/m2 [IC] or [SO] every 6 weeks	NR	NR	NR	50	Seizures (7)
Bradac et al.[189]	See above	BCNU 120–180mg/m2, [SS] every 6–8 weeks (dextrose as solvent)	29	35	NR	23 (in R/S patients)	Neurological impairment (24)
Vega et al.[190]	Nimustine – alkylates and crosslinks DNA, thereby causing DNA fragmentation, inhibition of protein synthesis, and cell death	ACNU 150 mg [IC] every 6–8 weeks	44		NR	26	25.7 (Gbm) 51.4 (Aa)	Visual loss (7.5) and fatal abdominal hemorrhage (2.5) (in the 40 total patients of the study)
Bobo et al.[191]	See above	BCNU 300 mg [SO], cisplatin 110–200 mg [SO] every 8 weeks	52	NR	NR	108	Neurological impairment (12)
Stewart et al.[192]	See above	BCNU 100 mg/m2 [IC] cisplatin 60 mg/m2 [IC] VM-26150 mg/m2 [IC] + Ara-C 1000 mg/m2 [IV] every 4 weeks	0	31	NR	14	Visual loss (12), neurological impairment, (38), seizures (19), fatal carotid thrombosis, (6), febrile neutropenia (25), fatal sepsis (6)
Hirano et al.[193]	See above	ACNU 50–100 mg [SS]	NR	NR	NR	91.7	Nausea (7.7), mild myelodepression (30,8), interstitial pneumonia (7.6)
Paccapelo et al.[194]	See above	ACNU 100 mg/m² [IC] every 6 weeks	28	51	38 (CR), 17(PR), 25 (SD)	82 (+Su + Rt) 70 (Su)	Visual loss (22), neurological toxicity (25), hematological toxicity (13)

Abbreviations used: Aa: Anaplastic astrocytoma; CR: Complete remission; IC: intracarotid infusion; iv.: Intravenous infusion; NR: Not reported; OS: Overall survival; PR: Partial remission; R/S: Responsive and stable patients (RC+RP+SO); Rt: Radiotherapy; Gbm: Glioblastoma multiforme; SD: Stabilization of disease; SO: Supraophthalmic infusion; SS: Superselective infusion; Su: Surgery; TTP: Time-to-progression; ACNU nimustine; BCNU, carmustine.
Adapted from Basso et al. Expert Rev Anticancer Ther. 2002;**2**:507–19 with permission.

group; 16 patients (10%) developed irreversible encephalopathy with cerebral edema on CT scan, and 26 patients (16%) developed visual loss ipsilateral to the infused carotid artery. Administration of 5-fluorouracil did not influence survival. Neuropathologically, intra-arterial BCNU produced white matter necrosis.

A prospective randomized trial compared the effectiveness of intra-arterial ACNU to intravenous ACNU in 82 newly diagnosed patients with supratentorial GBM who underwent surgery within 3 weeks.[198] The patients were randomly assigned to receive either intravenous or intra-arterial ACNU (80 mg/m2) once every 6 weeks concomitant with radiotherapy. Intraarterial ACNU was administered for the

first three courses followed by intravenous administration. Median survival and progression-free survival time was 59 and 24 weeks, respectively for the intra-arterial arm and 56 and 45 weeks, respectively, for the intravenous arm. There was no significant difference between the two treatment arms. Among the prognostic variables, age was the only significant factor for both survival and progression-free survival. With regard to toxicity, there was no significant difference between the two treatment arms. Leukoencephalopathy was not observed in the intra-arterial arm.

Another randomized study compared the effectiveness and side-effects of intra-arterial (17 patients) versus intravenous (16 patients) ACNU administration at the dose of

Table 16.10. Nitrosourea-based intra-arterial chemotherapy in newly diagnosed high-grade gliomas

Author	Mechanism of action	Protocol	Complete/ partial response (%)	SD (%)	TTP (wks)	Overall survival (wks)	Toxicity (%)
Greenberg et al.[187]	BCNU-DNA and RNA alkylating agent and carbamoylation of amino acids in proteins	BCNU 200 mg/m^2 [IC] every 6–8 weeks, before radiotherapy	75	8	25	54	Visual loss (50), leukoencephalopathy (33)
Hochberg et al.[188]	See above	BCNU 240 mg [IC] or SO every 6 weeks, before radiotherapy	NR	NR	NR	64 (IC) 50 (SO)	Seizures (8), neurological, impairment (17)
Bashir et al.[195]	See above	BCNU 400 mg [IC] every 4 weeks, before radiotherapy	44	NR	NR	37, (56 for patients receiving> 3 cycles)	Nausea/vomiting (24), visual loss (14), leukoencephalopathy (7), neurologic impairment (7)
Fauchon et al.[196]	See above	HECNU 120 mg/m^2 IC every 6–8 weeks, before radiotherapy	15	55	32	48	Visual loss (15), leukoencephalopathy (10)
Vega et al.[190]	Nimustine-alkylates and crosslinks DNA, thereby causing DNA fragmentation, inhibition of protein synthesis, and cell death	ACNU 150 mg, 55, every 6–8 weeks, before radiotherapy	26	NR	12.8	34.2 (Gbm) 34.2 (Aa)	Visual loss (7.5) and fatal abdominal hemorrhage (2.5) (in the 40 total patients of the study)
Shapiro et al.[169]	See above	BCNU 200 mg/m^2 [IC] ± 5-FU 1 g/m^2 for 3 days, iv., before radiotherapy vs. BCNU 200 mg/m2, iv ± 5-FU 1 g/m2 for 3 days, iv" before radiotherapy	NR	NR	NR	49.2 vs. 60	Ocular damage (15.5), fatal leukoencephalopathy (10)
Bobo et al.[191]	See above	BCNU 300 mg + cisplatin, 110–200 mg, SO, every 8 weeks, before radiotherapy	50	NR	NR	50	Neurological impairment (14)
Iwadate et al.[197]	See above	ACNU 100 mg cisplatin 100 mg [IC], ± mannitol concomitant with radiotherapy	54	23	33	52	Leukoencephalopathy, not fatal (8)
Hirano et al.[193]	See above	ACNU 50–100 mg SS, concomitant with radiotherapy	NR	NR	NR	66.9	Mild myelodepression (10), facial hemiparesis due to arterial embolism (5), interstitial pneumonia (5)
Kochii M[198]	See above	ACNU 80 mg/m^2, ia., every 6 weeks, versus ACNU 80 mg/m^2, iv., every 6 weeks, concomitant with radiotherapy	NR	NR	24 vs. 45	59 vs. 56	Two toxic deaths from neutropenic pneumonia (2.3%), renal failure (1.2%), liver dysfunction (1,2%) Grade 3–4 leukocytopenia (7.9% ia" 27% iv), and Grade 3–4 thrombocytopenia (10% ia" 8% iv)

Abbreviations used: Aa: Anaplastic astrocytoma; CR: Complete remission; Gbm: Glioblastoma multiforme; IC: Intracarotid infusion; iv; intravenous; NR: Not reported; Overall survival; PR: Partial remission; Rt Radiotherapy; SD: Stabilization of disease; SO: Supraophthalmic infusion; SS: Superselective infusion; TTP: Time-to-progression.
Adapted from Basso et al. Expert Rev Anticancer Ther. 2002;**2**:507–519 with permission.

Table 16.11. Platinum-based intra-arterial chemotherapy in high-grade gliomas recurrent after radiotherapy ± systemic chemotherapy

Author	Mechanism of action	Protocol	Complete/ partial response (%)	SO (%)	TTP (weeks)	Overall survival (weeks)	Toxicity (%)
Feun et al.[199]	Cisplatin-platinum complexes which bind to nucleophilic groups such as GC-rich sites in DNA, inducing intrastrand and interstrand DNA cross-links resulting in apoptosis and cell growth inhibition	Cisplatin 60–120 mg/m^2 [IC] every 4 weeks	30	25	33 (PR + CR) 16 (SO)	NR	Visual loss (20), hearing 1055 (15), neurological impairment (40), cerebral herniation (5)
Neuwelt et al.[200]	Methotrexate binds and inhibits the enzyme dihydrofolate reductase, resulting in inhibition of purine nucleotide and thymidylate synthesis, inhibition of DNA and RNA syntheses	MTX 1–4 g [IC] cyclophosphamide [IV] oral procarbazine every 4–6 weeks	23	11	NR	70	Visual loss (3), neurological impairment (66), seizures (55)
Newton et al.[171]	See above	Cisplatin 60–100 mg/m^2 [IC] every 4–6 weeks	8	NR	14	NR	Visual loss (17), seizures (25), neurological impairment (33)
Mahaley et al.[201]	See above	Cisplatin 60 mg/m^2 [IC] every 4 weeks	34	40	20 (PR + CR) 14 (SD) 4 (PD)	35 (PR + CR), 24 (SD), 14 (PD)	Visual loss (3), mild to toxicity, (22%), fatal endocranial hypertension (3), nephrotoxicity (37)
Follezou et al.[180]	Carboplatin- activated intracellularly to form reactive platinum complexes that bind to nucleophilic groups such as GC-rich sites in DNA, thereby inducing intrastrand and interstrand DNA cross-links resulting in apoptosis and cell growth inhibition	Carboplatin 400 mg/m^2 [IC] every 4 weeks	22	22	NR	NR	Visual loss (4), neurological, impairment (4)
Saris et al.[202]	See above	Cisplatin 70–100 mg/m^2 [IC] or [SO] pulsatile, every 6 weeks	10	30	NR	NR	Neurological impairment (10)
Stewart et al.[182]	See above	Carboplatin 200–400 mg/m^2 [IC] every 3 weeks	0	10	NR	8	Visual loss (50), neurological impairment (20)
Cloughesy et al.[179]	See above	Carboplatin 200–1400 mg [SS] pulsatile, up to 12 cycles	20	50	22	39	Seizures (20), partially reversible hemiparesis (5), nausea and vomiting (38)
Tamaki et al.[203]	See above	Cisplatin 45–100 mg ± ACNU, 100 mg [IC] or [SO] pulsatile	20	50	NR	NR	Neurotoxicity following SO, infusion (43)

Table 16.11. (cont.)

Author	Mechanism of action	Protocol	Complete/ partial response (%)	SO (%)	TTP (weeks)	Overall survival (weeks)	Toxicity (%)
Dropcho et al.[204]	See above	Cisplatin 75 mg/m2 [IC] or [SS] every 4 weeks, up to 8 cycles	10	22	7.3 (23.7 in R/5)	NR	Visual loss (5), seizures and/or permanent neurologic deterioration (37.5), hearing loss (2.5), neutropenia G3 (5), thrombocytopenia G3 (10)
Ashby et al.[205]	See above	Cisplatin 60 mg/m^2 iv.,. oral etoposide 50 mg/m^2 for 21 days, every 4 weeks, up to 9 cycles	10	30	18 weeks (R/S patients)	56.5 (R/S patients) 11 (PD)	1 toxic death due to sepsis and nephrotoxicity (4%), G3–4 neutropenia (33%), G3–4 thrombocytopenia (12%), G3 anemia (4%), seizures and reversible encephalopathy, (45%), 2 hearing loss (8%)

Abbreviations used: CR: Complete remission; IC: Intracarotid infusion: iv.: iV, Intravenous infusion; NR: Not reported; as: Overall survival; PO: Progression of disease during treatment. PR: Partial remission; RIS: Responsive and stable patients (RC+RP+SO); SO: Stabilization of disease; SD: Supraophthalmic infusion: SS: Superselective infusion; TIP: TIme-to-progression.
Adapted from Basso et al. Expert Rev Anticancer Ther. 2002;**2**:507–19 with permission.

80–100 mg/m^2 in newly diagnosed glioblastoma[214] after extensive surgical resection. Treatment was repeated every 5–8 weeks for a minimum of 2 and maximum of 14 cycles. No significant differences in systemic and hematological toxicity were observed between the two groups. Time to progression was 6 months for intra-arterial and 4 months for intravenous ACNU and total survival time was 17 months for intra-arterial and 20 months for intravenous ACNU.

Another analysis[215] used modeling technique to predict the survival among patients with malignant glioma who were eligible or ineligible for chemotherapy by three intra-arterial methods. Based on CT imaging and blind to outcome, an interventional neuroradiologist decided that: (1) for two-vessel treatment, 72.5% of the patients (74 of 102) were eligible; the eligible patients on average lived longer than the ineligible patients (15 vs. 4 months;) (2) for one-vessel treatment, 48% of the patients (49 of 102) were eligible; again, the eligible patients lived longer than the ineligible patients; and (3) for middle-cerebral artery treatment, 30% of the patients (31 of 102) were eligible. The eligible patients on average lived longer than the ineligible patients (15 vs. 4 months) for two vessel embolization. Trends were similar for patients with glioblastoma multiforme and anaplastic glioma. Patients who were eligible for intra-arterial chemotherapy lived significantly longer or somewhat longer (depending on the selection criteria used) than patients who were ineligible and

had better than expected outcomes. Therefore, non-randomized data should be interpreted with caution.

Intra-arterial chemotherapy for recurrent gliomas

Recurrent gliomas are defined by documented increase in tumor size radiologically after a progression-free interval of at least 3 months following radiotherapy in patients who have undergone surgery or biopsy and a radical course of radiotherapy.[212] There may be more encouraging results with intra-arterial ACNU particularly for recurrent gliomas and anaplastic astocytomas (see Table 16.14). The comparisons are based on historical controls. Thirty-three adult patients with anaplastic astrocytoma or GBM,[193] received post-operative intra-arterial ACNU chemotherapy and radiation. The outcomes in this group were compared to 37 intra-venous ACNU treated patients as the historical control. The median survival was 75 weeks for the former and 82 weeks for the latter. Although both groups were similar in terms of survival, toxicity was less frequent in the intra-arterial group.

The efficacy of intra-arterial cisplatin was compared with intravenous PCNU for treating primary brain tumors, in 311 adult patients with supratentorial tumors (confirmed histologically)[216] who had completed radiotherapy (4500–6020 cGy to the tumor bed) before randomization. Results were analyzed for the 311 patients in the randomized population (RP), and

Table 16.12. Platinum-based intra-arterial chemotherapy in newly diagnosed high-grade gliomas

Author	Mechanism of action	Patients	Protocol	Complete/ partial response (%)	SO (%)	TTP (weeks)	Overall survival (weeks)	Toxicity (%)
Recht et al.[206]	Cisplatin-platinum complexes which bind to nucleophilic groups such as GC-rich sites in DNA, inducing intrastrand and interstrand DNA cross-links resulting in apoptosis and cell growth inhibition	25	Cisplatin 90 mg/m² [IC] for two cycles, pior to radiotherapy followed by BCNU [IV]	16	52	53	60	Neurological impairment (8), hearing loss (8)
Madajewicz et al.[207]	See above	83	Cisplatin 60 mg/m², VP-16 40 mg/m² [IC] prior to or concomitantly with radiotherapy, every 3 weeks	48	NR	NR	30–85.7	Seizures (2,9%), headache (2.9%) transient confusion (4.7%), leukomalacia (0.6), nausea (25%), urinary retention (4.7%)
Larner JM[208]	FU- antimetabolite inhibits thymidylate synthetase, resulting in disruption of DNA synthesis and cytotoxicity	25	5-FU 200–600 mg [SO] every 4 weeks, concomitant with radiotherapy	NR	NR	NR	63 (Gbm) 34 (Aa)	Neurological impairment (16), cerebral hemorrhage (1)
Dropcho et al.[209]	See above	22	Cisplatin 75 mg/m² [IC] every 4 weeks	45	18	23	63	Visual loss (5), hearing loss (9), seizures (9), neurological impairment (4), endocranial hypertension with herniation (4)
Tfayli et al.[174]	See above	105 (+ 63 metastatic patients)	CDDP 40–60 mg/m², VP-16 2040 mg/m² [IC] during or after radiotherapy every 3 weeks, up to 6 cycles	NR	NR	NR	NR	Nausea/vomiting (25), seizures (3), headache (3), confusion with urinary retention/ incontinence (4.7), leukomalacia (0.6), blurred vision (3), groin hematoma (1.6%)

Abbreviations used: CR: Complete remission; IC: Intracarotid infusion; iv.: iv, Intravenous infusion; NR: Not reported; Overall survival; PR: Partial remission; Rt: Radiotherapy; SD: Stabilization of disease; SO: Supraophthalmic infusion Adapted from Basse et al. Expert Rev Anticancer Ther. 2002; **2**: 507–19, with permission.

for the 281 patients in the Valid Study Group (VSG) meeting protocol eligibility requirements (64% were stratified as progressive; 12% had received prior chemotherapy). The group randomized to PCNU had the longer survival in both RP and VSG. In the VSG, median survival was 10 months for the intra-arterial cisplatin group, and 13 months for the intravenous PCNU group. PCNU lead to greater hematotoxicity; cisplatin led to greater renal toxicity and some

Table 16.13. Blood–brain barrier disruption with RMP-7 in high-grade gliomas

Author	Mechanism of action	Protocol	Complete/ partial response (%)	SD (%)	TTP (%)	Overall survival (weeks)	Toxicity (%)
Doolittle et al.[210]	Cyclophosphamide - synthetic alkylating agent converted to the active metabolites aldophosphamide and phosphoramide mustard, which bind to DNA, inhibiting DNA replication and initiating cell death	25% mannitol [IA] before carboplatin 200 mg/m^2 [IA] cyclophosphamide 330 mg/m^2 [IV] VP-16 200 mg/m^2 [IV] for 2 days every 4 weeks 21	NR	NR	NR	NR	In the 221 patients: subintimal tear (5%), peripheral or pulmonary thromboembolism (17.6), stroke (1.3), confusion (5.4), nephrotoxicity (1.8), 2 early deaths within 48 h (9)
Black et al.[211]	See above	Carboplatin (AUC 5–7) [IV]+ 300 ng/kg RMP-7 [IV], every 4 weeks, up to 12 cycles	32 5	19 5	30.3 19.6	NR NR	Flushing (90%), thrombocytopenia and neutropenia G3–4, cerebral demyelination (1), headache, seizures (12.6), abdominal pain (22%)
Gregor et al.[212]	See above	Carboplatin 600 mg [IC] or [SS] + 300 ng/kg RMP-7, from 2–8 cycles	0	31	12.5	43.9 (after 46 weeks)	NR
LeMay et al.[213]	Carboplatin- activated intracellularly to form reactive platinum complexes that bind to nucleophilic groups such as GC-rich sites in DNA, thereby inducing intrastrand and interstrand DNA cross-links resulting in apoptosis and cell growth inhibition	Carboplatin 34–377 mg/m^2 [SS], from 1–13 cycles (+ RMP-7 in the same artery)	33	NR	NR	52 (at 1 year)	Neurological complications (33.3%), one ischemic stroke (4%), hematological toxicity Gl-2 (33.3%)

Abbreviations used: CR: Complete remission; IC: Intracarotid infusion; iv,: iv, Intravenous infusion; NR: Not reported; Overall survival; PR: Partial remission; SD: Stabilization of disease; SS: Superselective infusion: TTP: Time-to-progression.
Adapted from Basso et al. Expert Rev Anticancer Ther. 2002;**2**:507–19 with permission.

ototoxicity. Some cisplatin patients experienced complications associated with IA administration, including six cases of encephalopathy.

Combination alternating treatment has been proposed for recurrent gliomas to provide activity against tumor cells that may be resistant to one agent such as V79 spheroids, the non-cycling, hypoxic cell subpopulations resistant to cisplatin.[217] Cisplatin combination chemotherapy with a drug which preferentially kills hypoxic cells such as BCNU, etoposide, and mitomycin C[218] might prove useful. Combining the two agents produced the expected "complementary" activity, and in addition, synergism was observed between the drugs at exposure levels practical for clinical use. Some drug combination demonstrates synergistic activity of these drugs in preclinical models, such as the capacity of temozolomide to deplete intracellular levels of O-alkylguanine-DNA alkyltransferase (AGAT), the DNA repair enzyme involved in resistance to BCNU.[6] The strong relationship between AGAT expression and BCNU resistance suggests that modulation of nitrosourea resistance by depletion of AGAT is a reasonable therapeutic strategy.[219]

The combination of intracarotid BCNU and cisplatin appears to provide a modest increase in activity over intracarotid cisplatin alone;[199] however, neurologic and retinal toxicity may also be increased. In one study, 43 patients with recurrent malignant glioma were treated with alternating sequential intracarotid BCNU (two doses, 300 to 400 mg each) and cisplatin (two doses, 150 mg to 200 mg each) using alternating courses at 4-week to 6-week intervals.[220] Eight of 40 patients (20%) that could be evaluated after the first course of BCNU showed partial or minor response; median survival was 9 months. Cerebral or ocular toxicity and failure to show clinical improvement were the most common reasons for removal from the study. In a phase I dose finding study, 18 patients with progressive or recurrent intracerebral malignant neoplasms after radiation therapy were treated with 36 courses of intracarotid BCNU and cisplatin,[221] repeated every 4–6 weeks upon patients' recovery from toxicity. Intraarterial

Table 16.14. A summary of intra-arterial chemotherapeutic agents for treating neoplasms

Newly diagnosed gliomas

	Single agents	Combination
	Carmustine	Carmustine + PCV
	Nimustine	Carmustine+ 5-Fluorouracil
	He CNU	Cisplatin + Lomustine
	Cisplatin	Cisplatin + Carmustine
	5-Fluorouracil	
Median time to progression	12–32 weeks	33–50 weeks
Median survival time	1 year (32–73 weeks)	1 year (40–228) weeks

Recurrent gliomas

	Carmustine	Carmustine + PCV
	Nimustine	Carmustine+ PCV
	PCNU, He CNU	Carmustine + IA Cisplatin+ Teniposide
	Cisplatin	Carmustine + IA Cisplatin+ oral Lomustine
	Carboplatin	Carmustine + IA Cisplatin
	Diaziquone	Vincristine + Procarbazine
	Etoposide	Carmustine + Cisplatin + Teniposide + IV Cisplatin + IV Cystarabins + IV Teniposide
		Cisplatin + IA Etoposide
		Cisplatin + oral Etoposide
		Cisplatin + IA Etoposide + IV Cyclophosphamide
		Cisplatin + IV Etoposide
Median time to progression	13–33 weeks	14–36 weeks
Median survival time	8 to 82.5 weeks	13–108 weeks

Primary central nervous system lymphomas

	Methotrexate	
	Carboplatin	
Median survival time	42–48 months	

Metastatic tumors

	IA Carboplatin + IV Etoposide	
Median time to progression	16 weeks	
Median survival time	20 weeks	

cisplatin or BCNU alone was administered if the blood counts were still subnormal. Major toxic effects included ipsilateral retinal (amaurosis) in four patients and neurologic toxicity in two patients (minor focal seizure, reversible obtundation in one patient, and transient hemiparesis in one patient). Tumor regression was observed in patients previously treated with radiation and/or systemic chemotherapy, including four of nine who had recurrent malignant gliomas, and two of nine who had metastatic tumors. Recommended dose for phase II trials is BCNU 100 mg/m^2 and cisplatin 60 mg/m^2 every 4–6 weeks. Retinal and neurologic toxicity are possible side effects.

In the phase II study, 118 courses of intracarotid BCNU (100 mg/m^2) and cisplatin (60 mg/m^2) were administered to 36 patients with malignant brain tumors recurrent or progressive after radiation therapy[222] at 4–6 week intervals. Of 23 patients with recurrent glioma, who could be evaluated nine (39%) had tumor regression by CT scan and three had stable disease. The median time to tumor progression for responding patients was 37 weeks. For all patients with primary tumors it was 14 weeks. Four of 11 patients with brain metastases had a response and two had stable disease. Major neurologic toxicity of intracarotid BCNU and cisplatin appeared to be cumulative and consisted of reversible hemiparesis in 3%, TIA in 1%, expressive aphasia in 9%, lethargy in 3%, seizures in 12%, and reversible confusion in 1%. Retinal toxicity consisted of mild blurring of vision in 4 patients and ipsilateral blindness in five patients. Three of 22 patients who had received supra-ophthalmic infusion later developed evidence of leukoencephalopathy.

Intra-arterial chemotherapy for inoperable gliomas

Another study[223] compared the survival among patients with 27 histologically proven malignant non-operable gliomas (17 anaplastic astrocytomas and 10 glioblastomas) who were treated with three courses of intra-arterial ACNU, at intervals of 6 weeks, and a localized 60 Gy radiotherapy between the first and the second ACNU treatment. For the anaplastic astrocytomas, median survival was 21 months (higher than the expected survival of 15 months), with a survival rate of 37% at 24 months. For patients with GBM, median survival was 10 months (expected survival of 8 months). The results were compared with two previous trials, concerning inoperable patients, treated by combination of radiotherapy and systemic chemotherapy. Survival rates were at least equivalent.

Intra-arterial chemotherapy for primary brain lymphoma

Primary central nervous system lymphoma can respond to multidrug chemotherapy (including methotrexate-based or carboplatin-based regimens[163] with blood–brain barrier disruption) with durable tumor control and outcomes that are comparable or superior to other treatment regimens.

The treatment may be offered as first-line treatment prior to irradiation and frequently in conjunction with blood–brain barrier disruption. The median survival ranges from 42 to 48 months. A multicenter study reported an overall response rate of 82% (58% complete; 24% partial) in 149 newly diagnosed patients with central nervous system lymphoma treated with osmotic BBBD and intra-arterial methotrexate and BBBD.[224] Median overall survival was 3 years (25% estimated survival at 9 years); progression-free survival was 1.8 years, with 5-year and 7-year progression-free survival of 31% and 25%, respectively. In low-risk patients (age < 60 years and KPS ≥ 70), median survival was approximately 14 years. Focal seizures (9%) were the most frequent side effect.

A total of 37 relapsed central nervous system lymphoma patients, most of whom failed therapy with methotrexate-based chemotherapy, were treated with IA carboplatin-based chemotherapy with BBBD.[225] The median time for survival from first IA carboplatin treatment was 7 months with seven out of 37 patients surviving ≥27 months. Nine patients had complete radiographic response, four patients had partial radiographic response, 12 had stable disease, ten had progressive disease, and two could not be evaluated.

Intra-arterial chemotherapy for brain metastasis

Median survival following metastatic brain tumors is only 16–24 weeks after conventional radiation therapy. Newton et al.[254] reported that IA carboplatin (200 mg/m² per day) and intravenous (IV) etoposide (100 mg/m² per day) in 24 patients (18 with prior systemic therapy) for 2 days every 3–4 weeks resulted in six complete responses (25%), six partial responses (25%), one minor response (4.2%), seven cases of stable disease (32%), and five cases of progressive disease. Stewart et al. reported on 37 patients with intra-cranial primary or metastatic tumors treated with an IA combination of BCNU, cisplatin, and VM-26.[226] Thirteen of 19 (68%) primary brain tumors and nine of 16 (56%) brain metastases responded. The response rate was lower in patients previously treated with both radiotherapy and intravenous chemotherapy (54% vs. 82%) and also was dose related (100% at the highest doses tested versus 57% at the lower doses). Ipsilateral retinal and neurological toxicity were dose-limiting, with major toxicity (permanently decreased vision or hemiparesis) occurring in five of nine (56%) patients receiving doses of BCNU greater than or equal to 100 mg/m² plus cisplatin, 60 mg/m², plus VM-26, 175 mg/m². Only 9% of the patients treated with a lower VM-26 dose developed permanent severe toxicity. The investigators recommended BCNU, 100 mg/m²; cisplatin, 60 mg/m²; and VM-26, 150 mg/m² for future studies.

Combination of intra-arterial chemotherapy and radiation therapy

A systematic review and meta-analysis compared radiotherapy alone with radiotherapy plus chemotherapy for 3004 adults with high-grade glioma from 12 randomized controlled trials[227] and demonstrated significant prolongation of survival associated with chemotherapy, with a 15% relative decrease in the risk of death. This effect was equivalent to an absolute increase in 1-year survival of 6% from 40% to 46% and a 2-month increase in median survival time, and was seen in patient groups defined by age, sex, histology, performance status, or extent of resection.

Radiation therapy can be further divided into radiosurgery boost, external beam radiotherapy, and stereotactic fractionated radiation therapy.[228] For patients with malignant glioma, there is Level I–III evidence that the use of radiosurgery boost followed by external beam radiotherapy and BCNU does not confer benefit in terms of overall survival, or quality of life as compared with external beam radiotherapy and BCNU. The use of radiosurgery boost is associated with increased toxicity. For patients with malignant glioma, there is insufficient evidence regarding the benefits/harms of using radiosurgery at the time of progression or recurrence. There is also insufficient evidence regarding the benefits/harms in the use of stereotactic fractionated radiation therapy for patients with newly diagnosed or progressive/recurrent malignant glioma.[228]

Concomitant treatment

Concomitant chemotherapy with platinum increases the efficacy of radiotherapy by downregulating O^6methylguanine-DNA-methyltransferase (MGMT) responsible for repairing alkylating agent damage in DNA. Another agent, temozolomide, methylates and depletes O^6-alkylguanine DNA alkyltransferase (AGT) levels (a MGMT promoter) thus impairing DNA repair mechanism. A randomized phase III trial by the European Organization for Research and Treatment of Cancer (EORTC) and National Cancer Institute of Canada Clinical Trials Group (NCIC) reported improved median and 2-year survival for patients with glioblastoma treated with concomitant and adjuvant temozolomide and radiotherapy.[229]

Intra-arterial infusion of high-dose cisplatin (150 mg/m²) on days 2, 9, 16, and 23 concomitant with delivery of external beam radiotherapy (total dose, 70 Gy; 2 Gy, 35 fractions; 1 fraction/day for 7 weeks)[230] in 79 patients with inoperable stage IV head and neck cancer demonstrated complete local tumor response in 72 patients (91%) and a partial response in three patients. The complete response rate of neck node metastases was 90%. Sodium thiosulfate was administered intravenously to provide effective cisplatin neutralization. The median overall survival time was 2.2 years, with a 3-year overall survival probability of 43%. Acute toxicities included hematologic toxicity (22%), mucositis (43%), skin reactions (24%), toxicity of the upper gastrointestinal tract (57%), nausea (20%), and subjective deafness (10%). Treatment-related deaths wer observed in 3.8%. Six (18%) of 33 patients with complete remission needed tube feeding 2 years after treatment without intercurrent salvage surgery.

In 43 patients with inoperable stage III and IV head and neck cancer, super-selective intra-arterial infusions of cisplatin (100–120 mg/m^2 per week) with simultaneous intravenous infusion of thiosulfate to neutralize cisplatin toxicity and conventional extra-beam radiotherapy (65 Gy/26 f/6.5 weeks),[231] the 3-year progression-free rate was 70%, and 3-year overall survival was 54%. Thirty-five patients (81%) experienced non-hematologic toxicities including mucositis ($n = 16$), nausea/vomiting ($n = 8$), and neurologic signs ($n = 2$). There are 29 surviving patients without evidence of disease, all of whom are able to have oral intake without feeding-tube support.

Intra-arterial chemotherapy preceding radiotherapy

In the neo-adjuvant setting, the goal of chemotherapy is to reduce tumor burden, which may improve response to subsequent radiotherapy. Of the 27 patients[206] with malignant supratentorial gliomas treated with a pre-irradiation chemotherapy protocol consisting of two courses of intracarotid CDDP, 90 mg/m^2, followed by i.v. BCNU, 200 mg/m^2, tumor size on postchemotherapy computed CT scan was decreased by greater than 50% in 13%. In only 4% had tumors increased in size. In a phase II study, 26 patients with newly diagnosed anaplastic astrocytomas and GBM received four infusions of intra-carotid cisplatin (75 mg/m^2 every 4 weeks) before radiotherapy if the tumor was located within the vascular territory of one internal carotid artery.[209] Ten patients (45%) showed a >25% decrease in the enhancing tumor area before radiotherapy with stabilization or improvement of neurologic deficits, and three patients (14%) had a greater than 70% decrease in tumor area.

A comparison of survival between 79 patients with malignant gliomas who received pre-irradiation intra-arterial chemotherapy with BCNU combined with vincristine intravenously and 96 patients treated with only post-operative whole-brain irradiation[232] demonstrated that chemotherapy benefited patients with anaplastic astrocytoma, who were not corticosteroid-dependent, with pre-treatment performance status of 0–2 and with a frontal lobe location of the tumor. A comparison of 75 patients with grade I or II gliomas who received four cycles of combined intra-arterial chemotherapy followed by radiation with 57 patients who only received radiotherapy,[233] suggested that IA chemotherapy increased 5-year survival from 45% to 73%. The main benefit of combining chemotherapy and radiation in astrocytomas seems thus to come from a marked improvement of the overall survival in older patients (>40 years).

The data suggests that chemotherapy completed prior to radiotherapy yields better results than if given concomitantly. In an analysis of 63 and 20 patients with GBM and anaplastic astrocytoma, respectively, intra-arterial (intracarotid and/or intra-vertebral) cisplatin, 60 mg/m^2, and etoposide, 40 mg/m^2 and radiation therapy[207] were given either concomitantly or sequentially, starting with chemotherapy. The median survival for patients with GBM who received chemotherapy prior to radiation therapy was 20 months vs. 7 months for those patients who underwent concomitant chemotherapy/radiation. Patients with anaplastic astrocytoma who received chemotherapy prior to radiation had a median survival of 45 months compared with 12 months for patients who received treatment concomitantly.

Intra-arterial chemotherapy and blood–brain barrier disruption
Duration of blood–brain barrier disruption

Disruption of the blood–brain barrier was ascertained using ^{99m}Tc-glucoheptonate (TcGH) single-photon emission computerized tomography (SPECT) scanning, and demonstrated good-to-excellent disruption in 29 procedures and poor-to-moderate disruption in the other nine studies performed[232] in patients with primary central nervous system lymphoma and primitive neuroectodermal tumors treated with intra-arterial mannitol. For the patients with good-to-excellent disruption, 27, 2-fold increase in blood–brain barrier permeability was demonstrated at 1 minute and maintained up to 40 minutes. Then permeability declined at a quick pace between 40 and 120 minutes and then slower between 120 and 240 minutes. Permeability had returned to normal at 480 minutes after mannitol infusion. In some sessions, RMP-7 is infused concomitantly with chemotherapeutic agents.[212] The increase in permeability is seen immediately after the start of the injection. After about 30 minutes, the effect rapidly disappears due to receptor tachyphylaxis and internalization of B2 receptors. Therefore, IA emotherapeutic agent injection must start within 10 minutes of RMP-7 administration to maximize drug delivery.[235] The vascular permeability effect of RMP-7 is minimally impaired by dexamethasone. In a study of nine patients,[211] 10–300 ng/kg of intra-arterial RMP-7 infused in the supraopthalmic internal carotid artery at 1 ml/min over 15 minutes increased the gadolinium EDTA transport in to the tumor by 46% as measured by serial PET scan.

Clinical studies

Intra-arterial mannitol infusion for temporary blood–brain barrier disruption provided a survival benefit in patients receiving intra-arterial chemotherapy. Ninety-eight patients (34 with malignant gliomas and 64 with brain metastases) were randomly assigned to either an intra-arterial mannitol infusion (50 ml of 20% mannitol was injected at a rate of 50 ml/min) or a non-mannitol infusion immediately prior to ACNU and cisplatin administration (100 mg/body at a rate of 20 mg/min) through the common carotid artery.[197] Of the patients with malignant gliomas, the median survival time was 68 weeks and 47 weeks for patients with or without mannitol treatment, respectively. Of the patients with brain metastases, the median survival was 47 weeks and 24 weeks for patients with or without mannitol treatment, respectively, a significant difference. The aim of this study was to determine the safety and efficacy of IA chemotherapy with osmotic opening of the blood–brain barrier was assessed in 221 adult patients (2464 procedures) (BBB) for the treatment of primary central nervous system lymphoma, primitive neuroectodermal tumor (PNET), germ cell tumor, cancer metastasis to the brain, or low or high grade glioma tumors.[210] In patients with chemotherapy-sensitive tumors, such as primary central nervous system lymphoma, PNET, germ cell tumor, and cancer metastasis to the central nervous system, enhanced delivery results in a high degree of tumor response, with an efficacy profile that is reproducible across multiple centers. In one study,[181] blood–brain barrier disruption therapy with RMP-7 as an adjunct to administration of carboplatin was associated with a lower rate of local complications compared with intra-arterial carboplatin alone.

Technical aspects of intra-arterial chemotherapy

Timing of intra-arterial chemotherapy

The timing of intra-arterial treatment is variable and is usually performed after surgery to benefit from post-surgical transient blood–brain barrier disruption.[167] Intra-arterial chemotherapy is used either prior to or concomitantly to radiotherapy to ensure administration prior to post-radiation vascular damage.[167,188] A more detailed discussion has been provided in previous sections.

Ancillary steps

The guide catheter is placed in the proximal vessel (internal carotid artery and rarely in the vertebral artery). An intravenous heparin bolus (3000 U to 5000 U) is given to achieve an activated coagulation time between 250 and 300 seconds. In patients with large tumors or pronounced peritumoral brain edema, 1500 mL mannitol (150 mg/mL) infusion may be started intravenously immediately following the chemotherapeutic infusion. Dexamethasone (4 mg) × four doses maybe given the day before treatment and then titrated and discontinued over 10 days. All patients are routinely put on anticonvulsant medication prior to treatment.

Microcatheter placement

A microcatheter is selectively placed in the target artery. The location of the microcatheter may reduce the rate of some complications. For internal carotid artery infusion, the microcatheter is placed in the supraclinoid portion of the artery, distal to the origin of the ophthalmic artery to reduce the risk of retinal damage.[167] If a large posterior communicating artery is visualized, the microcatheter is placed distal to the origin of the posterior communicating artery. For vertebral artery infusions, the microcatheter is placed distal to the anterior inferior

cerebellar artery to reduce the chances of inner ear toxicity,[167] even as distal as the junction between the P2 and P3 segment of the posterior cerebral artery. Several pulsatile contrast injections are performed through the microcatheter[179] to define the territory perfused, identify any inhomogeneity in distribution, and the stability of the microcatheter.

Hochberg et al.[188] compared the results of 192 infra-ophthalmic and 66 supra-ophthalmic carotid artery infusions of high dose intra-arterial BCNU (400 mg every 4 weeks) in 79 patients with malignant glioma. The major ocular complications (pain and diminished visual acuity) associated with infra-ophthalmic carotid artery infusion were avoided by selective supra-ophthalmic carotid artery administration. However, both approaches were associated with white-matter changes, seen as diminished absorption on computerized tomography scans, in 20% of patients treated following irradiation therapy. In another study, the effects of intra-arterial chemotherapy on the visual system of 29 consecutive patients with gliomas were studied.[236] Infra-ophthalmic carotid infusion of cisplatin or BCNU was associated with clinically apparent anterior visual pathway lesions and electroretinography demonstrated retinal dysfunction in patients without clinical abnormalities. Supra-ophthalmic carotid infusion of cisplatin or BCNU caused no retinal or optic nerve lesions. Electroretinography was abnormal in only one of these patients. While visual toxicity may be reduced, cortical events may be more frequent in patients with super-selective chemotherapy. Dropcho et al.[204] studied patients with recurrent malignant gliomas located within the territory of one or two major cerebral arteries. Fifteen patients received infusions into the ICA and 26 patients into one or two major Cerebral axteries (most often into the M1 segment). The response rate did not significantly differ between patients receiving ICA versus selective intracerebral infusion, although the latter group contained a higher proportion of glioblastoma. Ipsilateral visual loss occurred in two patients after internal carotid artery infusion but in none of the selective infusion patients. Seizures and/or transient or permanent neurologic deterioration occurred in four patients (27%) after internal carotid artery infusion and in 11 patients (44%) after selective intracerebral infusion.

Vertebral artery infusions proved feasible,[237] although difficult and more toxic than carotid infusions in 26 patients predominantly with gliomas treated with intra-arterial BCNU, VM-26, and cisplatin combined with the systemic chemotherapy. Reversible neurological toxicity was common, but tolerable. One patient developed ipsilateral blindness, and two patients developed prolonged neurological toxicity. Pulmonary toxicity was also seen.

After the infusion has been completed, an angiogram is performed to ensure that no local complications such as dissection or vasospasm had occurred. Intracranial vessels are also imaged by angiography to avoid undetected compromise of the intracranial circulation due to secondary thromboembolic events. The patient is transferred to the regular floor for overnight observation and discharged the next day if no complications have occurred.

Distribution of chemotherapeutic agents

If the flow of blood is laminar in the segment of infusion, the distribution drug is not homogenous.[238] A streaming phenomenon may occur that leads to focal necrosis due to excessive distribution in downstream branches. The streaming is greater when the infusion is in the internal carotid artery compared to branches such as middle and anterior cerebral artery with more turbulent flow. Bobo et al.[191] found that the rate of neurological deficits was 6% if ≥ 3 branches were supplied by the infused artery compared to 42% for those with only two branches. The investigators recommended reducing the dose of cisplatin and BCNU when infusing into arteries with two or fewer branches. The authors also recommended intermittent bolus injections instead of infusion pumps to reduce streaming and the vector of outflow at 90 degrees from the axis of the catheter. Cloughesy et al.[179] calculated the dose-based local cerebral blood flow estimation. The calculations were made assuming that the middle cerebral artery, anterior cerebral artery, posterior cerebral artery, and perforating arteries supply 60%, 20%, 15%, and 5% of the hemispheric flow, respectively. The hemispheric dose was predetermined (200 mg/hemisphere of carboplatin and escalated to 1400 mg/hemisphere in this study). If the microcatheter was placed in the middle cerebral artery, 60% of the hemispheric dose was administered. In a study of 113 patients (462 procedures) treated, the hemispheric dose administered according to the algorithm was strongly predictive of seizure and neurologic deficit.[239] A diastole-phased pulsatile injection has been proposed in a pilot study[202] to ensure more homogenous drug distribution. Measurement of actual regional flow through the target artery to calculate drug dosage and injection rate has been proposed to reduce the streaming effect.

Rate of infusion

The solution is infused over 30–60 min. The rate of infusion and dilution may be important for the prevention of local complications. Blacklock et al.[238] studied the distribution of carbon-14 labeled iodoantipyrine in primates under various rates of intracarotid infusion. The distribution of iodoantipyrine was heterogeneous with 13-fold variability of drug concentration in adjacent cerebral sections with slow infusions (1%–2% of arterial blood flow). Increased infusion rate to 20% of internal carotid artery flow reduced the heterogeneity to a lesser extent comparable to intravenous administration. Nakagawa et al.[240] reviewed their experience of administering selective intra-arterial chemotherapy consisting of a combination of etoposide and cisplatin to 20 patients with malignant glioma to establish a safe technique for superselective intra-arterial chemotherapy. Initially, two cerebrovascular accidents in two patients (after etoposide in one and after etoposide plus cisplatin in the other) were observed with 100 mg/m^2 of etoposide and 100 mg/m^2 of cisplatin delivered via the horizontal segment of the middle cerebral artery (M1) or the tip of the basilar artery, with a 20-minute infusion time. Subsequently, the investigators diluted etoposide, and reduced the doses of both drugs to 80 mg or 50 mg/m^2, and finally to 60 mg/m^2, and infused both of them over 60 minutes. In addition, for prevention of local spasm, papaverine hydrochloride and nicardipine were given via the same catheter at 5-minute intervals during administration of etoposide and cisplatin. No complications developed in the latter cases. Infusions may be made in more than one artery in the same setting if required.

Value of initial angiographic findings

During intra-arterial chemotherapy of brain tumors, the initial vessels chosen for infusion are based on the vascular distribution of the tumor suggested by CT or MR imaging. However, angiography may identify information that requires an alteration of the vessel infusion plan in 6% of the patients.[255] A review of pre-infusion angiography in 78 patients with primary and metastatic brain tumors demonstrated substantial perfusion of the tumor from a different arterial supply in three patients and contralateral supply in two patients related to a hypoplastic or aplastic A1 segment. Eight patients (10.3%) were identified with incidental cerebral aneurysms.[256] The aneurysms were saccular and varied in size from 2–4 mm; seven of the eight patients underwent 35 intra-arterial chemotherapy procedures after detection of the aneurysm without any aneurysmal complications.

Hemoperfusion of the jugular blood

In a small study[241] of four patients with malignant cerebral gliomas, intra-arterial BCNU was injected into the internal carotid artery with ipsilateral jugular drainage pumped extracorporeally at 300 mL/min through a hemoperfusion cartridge containing a non-ionic adsorbant resin. Each patient received 220 mg/m^2 BCNU, infused over 45 minutes through a toposcopic catheter positioned with the tip in the ICA beyond the origin of the ophthalmic artery. Hemoperfusion of the jugular blood during intracarotid infusion reduced the systemic exposure by 56% to 87% and increased total body clearance of BCNU by two- to eight-fold.

Blood–brain barrier disruption protocols

In a multicenter protocol for BBBD,[210] patients are hydrated with D$_5$ 1/2NS at 100–150 mL/hour for a minimum of 6 hours. Because seizures (generally focal) occur during approximately 6% of blood–brain barrier disruption treatments, patients are pre-medicated with an anticonvulsant and procedures are performed under general anesthesia. To prevent bradycardia, atropine is administered intravenously immediately prior to blood–brain barrier disruption. An intra-arterial catheter is placed in an internal carotid artery

Table 16.15. Various definitions of response to treatment

Categories	Definitions
Complete response	The disappearance of all known disease, determined by two observations not less than four weeks apart; OR no tumor enhancement on CT brain scan and the patient was off steroids with stable or improved neurologic status
Partial response	50% or more decrease in total tumor load of the lesions that have been measured to determine the effect of therapy by two observations not less than four weeks apart. Bidimensional: single lesion, greater than or equal to 50% decrease in tumor area (multiplication of longest diameter by the greatest perpendicular diameter); multiple lesions, a 50% decrease in the sum of the products of the perpendicular diameters of the multiple lesions. Unidimensional: greater than or equal to 50% decrease in linear tumor measurement. In addition there can be no appearance of new lesions or progression of any lesion; OR, a reduction greater than or equal to 50% in tumor volume determined by CT scan with decreased or no use of steroids
Stable disease	An increase of less than 25% in tumor volume with stable steroid dose, or a reduction of less than 50%
Progressive disease	An increase of greater than or equal to 25% in tumor volume compared with baseline volume

Table 16.16. Performance status classification can be according to the Karnofsky scale

Grade	Definitions
Grade 0	Able to carry out all normal activity without restriction
Grade 1	Restricted in physically strenuous activity but ambulatory and able to do light work
Grade 2	Ambulatory and capable of all self-care but unable to carry out any work. Up and about more than 50% of waking hours
Grade 3	Capable of only limited self-care, confined to bed or chair more than 50% of waking hours
Grade 4	Completely disabled. Cannot carry on any self-care. Totally confined to bed or chair.

Table 16.17. Predictors of response to intra-arterial chemotherapy

Patient's age

Tumor histology[232]

Corticosteroid dependency[232]

Pre-treatment performance status[232]

Frontal lobe location[232]

Tumor regression seen on CT-scan after chemotherapy before irradiation

Pronounced decrease of tumor metabolism on PET after the first course of intra-arterial chemotherapy[244]

Time from diagnosis to intra-arterial chemotherapy[245]

Net tumor volume and vascularity.[245] In vitro sensitivity of tumor cells to different kinds of anticancer agents using flow cytometric (FCM) detection of apoptosis[246,247]

at C1–2 or in a vertebral artery at C4–5, depending on tumor location. Warmed mannitol (25%) is administered at 4–10 mL/second into the cannulated artery for 30 seconds. Depending on tumor histology, one of two chemotherapy regimens is used. Patients with high- and low-grade glioma, PNET, germ cell tumor, and cancer metastasis to the brain are treated with carboplatin (200 mg/m^2 each day, for a total dose of 400 mg/m^2) administered intra-arterially 5 minutes after the mannitol, cyclophosphamide (330 mg/m^2 each day, for a total dose of 660 mg/m^2) administered intravenously 10 minutes before the mannitol, followed by intravenous etoposide (200 mg/m^2 each day, for a total dose of 400 mg/m^2). A second chemotherapy regimen may be administered to patients with central nervous system lymphoma and brainstem glioma consisting of methotrexate (2500 mg each day, for a total dose of 5000 mg) administered intra-arterially, and cyclophosphamide (500 mg/m^2 each day, for a total dose of 1000 mg/m^2) and etoposide (150 mg/m^2 each day, for a total dose of 300 mg/m^2) given intravenously. In patients treated with methotrexate, NaHCO$_3$ was added to intravenous fluids and titrated to achieve a urine pH greater than 6.5.

In some sessions, RMP-7 is infused concomitantly with chemotherapeutic agents.[212] Intra-arterial chemotherapeutic agent injection must start within 10 minutes of administration to maximize drug delivery.[235] In a study of nine patients,[211] 10–300 ng/kg of intra-arterial RMP-7 was infused in the supra-opthalmic internal carotid artery at 1 mL/min over 15 minutes. The carboplatin infused 5 minutes after infusion of RMP-7. When carboplatin infused with RMP-7, each compound administered in an alternate manner every 30 seconds. Carboplatin was administered for another 3 minutes after infusion of RMP-7 was terminated.

Measures and predictors of response

The objective response in measurable disease[242] is used to define response to treatment as summarized in Table 16.15.

Performance status classification can be according to the Karnofsky scale (10 points)[243] or preferably using a 5-grade scale as shown in Table 16.16.

The predictors of response to intra-arterial chemotherapy are summarized in Table 16.17.

Complications

Overall rates of complications

A review of 100 super-selective intra-arterial infusion procedures of carboplatin performed in 24 patients[181] reported a total of 13 neurological complications (eight patients). Seizures, the most common complication, were observed in seven procedures, and were accompanied by transient focal deficits in three procedures. Five procedures were complicated by transient neurologic deficits (hemiparesis in two, confusion in one, and visual field deficits in one procedure). One patient developed ischemic stroke during the procedure. Asymptomatic angiographic dissection was seen in one patient. Procedures performed in women were associated with a higher frequency of neurological complications. In another study of 462 procedures in 113 patients,[239] six (1.3%) complications were asymptomatic; 12 (2.6%), transient neurologic; three (0.6%), permanent minor neurologic; three (0.6%), permanent major neurologic; and 32 (7.0%), seizures.[239] In a review of 392 consecutive IA chemotherapy procedures performed in 48 patients,[248] groin hematomas occurred in 10 (2.6%), and 2 asymptomatic carotid arterial dissections (0.5%) were reported. Only one patient required surgery for a delayed popliteal embolus. There were seven (1.8%) transient neurologic events, which consisted of paresis and visual disturbances. Six (1.5%) transient seizure events were recorded.

Stewart et al.[182] reported the results of intra-carotid infusion of carboplatin (200–400 mg/m^2) in 15 patients with either glioblastoma or metastatic tumors. Three of four patients who received 400 mg/m^2 of carboplatin developed retinal toxicity. Three of nine patients who received 300 mg/m^2 had decreased ipsilateral vision and one other developed worsening of a pre-existing hemiparesis. Focal seizures and transient aphasia occurred in one patient each. Follezou et al.[180] described 23 patients with malignant glioma who were treated with an intra-arterial infusion of 400 mg/m^2 of carboplatin every 4 weeks. One patient developed central neurotoxicity and another developed a reversible decrease in visual acuity. Cloughesy et al.[179] reported the use of escalating doses of carboplatin (up to 1400 mg/hemisphere) infused either in the supraclinoid internal carotid artery or basilar artery above the anterior inferior cerebellar artery in 21 patients with recurrent glioma. One patient had permanent neuromotor decline. The predominant complication was hematopoietic toxicity.

Among a total of 385 intra-arterial cisplatin and concomitant radiation therapy procedures for advanced head and neck cancer in 105 patients there were,[249] 22 (5.7%) groin hematomas, two asymptomatic common carotid artery dissections, two acute occlusions of the external iliac artery, three permanent, and three transient neurologic events. All patients were treated with selective intra-arterial tumor-directed cisplatin (150 mg/m^2 weekly × four), simultaneous intravenous thiosulfate (9 g/m^2) for systemic neutralization of cisplatin, and conventional external-beam radiation to the primary tumor and nodal disease (total dose of 66–74 Gy). Overall, there were 41 grade III/IV chemotoxic events related to treatment. Chemotoxic events included 29 mucosal events, nine hematologic events, two otologic events, and one gastrointestinal event. No renal events occurred.

Visual toxicity

Orbital pain is the most frequent symptom of intra-arterial BCNU-related ocular toxicity. The toxicity may be the combined result of arterial toxicity of the drug and unknown or uncontrolled promoting factors resulting in ischemic optic neuropathy or retinal vasculopathy. The ocular complications associated with intra-carotid arterial infusion of BCNU seem to be avoided with new nitrosourea compounds soluble in water and oil such Hydoxyethyl-CNU (HeCNU) (Asta-Werke, Heidelberg, Germany), A prospective study[168] of intra-arterial chemotherapy with a new nitrosourea HeCNU as a complementary treatment after surgery, after tumor recurrence, and prior to radiotherapy, reported the effects on the visual system of 68 patients with malignant gliomas. Eleven patients (16%) suffered a visual complication after two or more courses of chemotherapy that included mild to major decrease of visual acuity and in some cases ocular pain, palpebral edema, and conjunctival injection. The delay in onset of ocular symptoms varied from 1 week to 9 months. No relationship was found between the occurrence of visual toxicity and patient age, number of courses of HeCNU, the vascular axis treated, total systemic dose or dose by carotid artery, suggesting a possible specific sensitivity of some patients to chemotherapy. Antiplatelet therapy with or without sequential pulse corticotherapy before and following each course is proposed to prevent such vascular complications.

White matter changes

The Intra-arterial approach is associated with white-matter changes, non-specific gyral enhancement, and delayed calcification[236] indicative of neurotoxicity. The changes are seen as diminished absorption on computerized tomography scans, in 20% of patients treated following irradiation therapy.[188] This toxicity appears to preclude intra-arterial BCNU treatment in the immediate post-irradiation period. A study[250] on late (6–25 years) adverse effects of therapeutic brain radiotherapy using assessment of MRI, quality of life, and neuroendocrine function in 33 adult brain tumor patients demonstrated that all patients had white matter changes with increased signal intensity on T2 and FLAIR images. Discrete lesions (grade 1), beginning confluence of lesions (grade 2), and large confluent areas (grade 3) were present in 8, 8, and 17 patients, respectively. Patients treated with intra-arterial chemotherapy and patients at higher age at follow-up had significantly more grade 3 changes. Significantly worse clinical status and quality of life was found in patients with white matter changes grade 3 or atrophy. The rates of leukoencephalopathy are lower when relatively low doses of chemotherapeutic agents the low concentration of alcohol, and the relatively low perfusion rates are used.

Myelosuppresion

Thrombocytopenia (platelet count less than 100 000 cells/mm), leukopenia (leukocyte count less than 4000 cells/mm) or anemia (hemoglobin less than 11 g/dl) can be seen after IA chemotherapy. The severity of complications is graded according to the World Health Organization (WHO) toxicity scale.[242]

Ototoxicity

High-frequency hearing loss was noted in a large portion of patients[251] who received carboplatin and BBBD via the vertebral artery. Clinical trials using sodium thiosulfate administered intravenously 2 hours after carboplatin reduced the frequency of hearing loss.[252] Audiological assessment was conducted at baseline and within 24 h before each monthly treatment with sodium thiosulfate was administered as one (20 g/m^2) or two (20 g/m^2 and 16 g/m^2) 15-min doses, depending on baseline

hearing status. The initial group received the first dose 2 h (or 2 and 6 h) after carboplatin and a subsequent group received 4 h (or 4 and 8 h) after carboplatin. Audiological data were compared with a historical comparison group and demonstrated significantly lower rates of ototoxicity with increased delay in sodium thiosulfate. STS delayed to 4 h after carboplatin significantly decreased time to development of ototoxicity and rate of ototoxicity compared with historical controls.

New developments

Combined approach of IA chemotherapy and interstitial hyperthermia in rats with isotransplanted C(6) gliomas[253] resulted in increased uptake of adriamycin with hyperthermia. Hyperthermia of the tumors was achieved using radiofrequency antenna (RF-heating) and a heating device that maintained the tumor temperature above 40 °C. Combination treatment resulted in longer overall survival time in comparison to the other treatments. This method may be a new strategy for treating gliomas.

References

1. Qureshi AI. Endovascular treatment of cerebrovascular diseases and intracranial neoplasms. *Lancet* 2004;**363**:804–13.

2. Gounis MJ, Lieber BB, Webster KA, Wakhloo AK. A novel angiographic methodology for the quantification of angiogenesis. *IEEE Trans Biomed Eng* 2008;**55**:996–1003.

3. Michaely HJ, Herrmann KA, Dietrich O, Reiser MF, Schoenberg SO. Quantitative and qualitative characterization of vascularization and hemodynamics in head and neck tumors with a 3d magnetic resonance time-resolved echo-shared angiographic technique (treat)–initial results. *Eur Radiol* 2007;**17**:1101–10.

4. Strugar JG, Criscuolo GR, Rothbart D, Harrington WN. Vascular endothelial growth/permeability factor expression in human glioma specimens: Correlation with vasogenic brain edema and tumor-associated cysts. *J Neurosurg* 1995;**83**:682–9.

5. Berkman RA, Merrill MJ, Reinhold WC, *et al.* Expression of the vascular permeability factor/vascular endothelial growth factor gene in central nervous system neoplasms. *J Clin Invest* 1993;**91**:153–9.

6. Dvorak HF, Sioussat TM, Brown LF, *et al.* Distribution of vascular permeability factor (vascular endothelial growth factor) in tumors: Concentration in tumor blood vessels. *J Exp Med* 1991;**174**:1275–8.

7. Vlodavsky I, Elkin M, Abboud-Jarrous G, *et al.* Heparanase: one molecule with multiple functions in cancer progression. *Connect Tissue Res* 2008;**49**:207–10.

8. Vlodavsky I, Ilan N, Nadir Y, *et al.* Heparanase, heparin and the coagulation system in cancer progression. *Thromb Res* 2007;**120** Suppl 2:S112–20.

9. Aharinejad S, Sioud M, Lucas T, Abraham D. Target validation using rna interference in solid tumors. *Methods Mol Biol* 2007;**361**:227–38.

10. Ohta M, Kitadai Y, Tanaka S, *et al.* Monocyte chemoattractant protein-1 expression correlates with macrophage infiltration and tumor vascularity in human gastric carcinomas. *Int J Oncol* 2003;**22**:773–8.

11. McKenzie S, Sakamoto S, Kyprianou N. Maspin modulates prostate cancer cell apoptotic and angiogenic response to hypoxia via targeting akt. *Oncogene* 2008;**27**:7171–9.

12. Cox C, Teknos TN, Barrios M, Brewer GJ, Dick RD, Merajver SD. The role of copper suppression as an antiangiogenic strategy in head and neck squamous cell carcinoma. *Laryngoscope* 2001;**111**:696–701.

13. Hassouneh B, Islam M, Nagel T, Pan Q, Merajver SD, Teknos TN. Tetrathiomolybdate promotes tumor necrosis and prevents distant metastases by suppressing angiogenesis in head and neck cancer. *Mol Cancer Ther* 2007;**6**:1039–45.

14. Mowlavi A, Malafa MP. Angiogenesis in primary tumor cells of metastatic and nonmetastatic malignant melanoma. *Plast Reconstr Surg* 2000;**106**:514.

15. Long DM. Vascular ultrastructure in human meningiomas and schwannomas. *J Neurosurg* 1973;**38**:409–19.

16. Castillo M, Thompson JE, Mukherji SK. Association of an intracranial arteriovenous malformation and a meningioma. *Neuroradiology* 1998;**40**:574–6.

17. Soria E, Fine E, Hajdu I. Association of intracranial meningioma with arteriovenous malformation. *Surg Neurol* 1990;**34**:111–17.

18. Maier H, Ofner D, Hittmair A, Kitz K, Budka H. Classic, atypical, and anaplastic meningioma: Three histopathological subtypes of clinical relevance. *J Neurosurg* 1992;**77**:616–23.

19. Maiuri F, Iaconetta G, de Divitiis O, Cirillo S, Di Salle F, De Caro ML. Intracranial meningiomas: Correlations between mr imaging and histology. *Eur J Radiol* 1999;**31**:69–75.

20. Black PM. Meningiomas. *Neurosurgery* 1993;**32**:643–57.

21. Tatagiba M, Mirzai S, Samii M. Peritumoral blood flow in intracranial meningiomas. *Neurosurgery* 1991;**28**:400–4.

22. Engelhard HH. Progress in the diagnosis and treatment of patients with meningiomas. Part i: Diagnostic imaging, preoperative embolization. *Surg Neurol* 2001;**55**:89–101.

23. Servo A, Porras M, Jaaskelainen J, Paetau A, Haltia M. Computed tomography and angiography do not reliably discriminate malignant meningiomas from benign ones. *Neuroradiology* 1990;**32**:94–7.

24. Lee KF, Lin SR, Whiteley WH, Tsai FY, Thompson NL, Jr., Suh JH. Angiographic findings in recurrent meningioma. *Radiology* 1976;**119**:131–9.

25. Bitzer M, Opitz H, Popp J, *et al.* Angiogenesis and brain oedema in intracranial meningiomas: Influence of vascular endothelial growth factor. *Acta Neurochir (Wien)* 1998;**140**:333–40.

26. Adachi K, Kawase T, Yoshida K, Yazaki T, Onozuka S. Abc surgical risk scale for skull base meningioma: A new scoring system for predicting the extent of tumor removal and neurological outcome. *J Neurosurg* 2009; **111**: 1053–61.

27. Ildan F, Tuna M, Gocer AP, *et al.* Correlation of the relationships of brain-tumor interfaces, magnetic resonance imaging, and angiographic findings to predict cleavage of meningiomas. *J Neurosurg* 1999;**91**:384–90.

28. Salpietro FM, Alafaci C, Lucerna S, Iacopino DG, Todaro C, Tomasello F. Peritumoral edema in meningiomas: Microsurgical observations of different brain tumor interfaces related to computed tomography. *Neurosurgery* 1994;**35**:638–41; discussion 641–2.

29. Sindou MP, Alaywan M. Most intracranial meningiomas are not cleavable tumors: Anatomic-surgical evidence and angiographic predictibility. *Neurosurgery* 1998;**42**:476–80.

30. Bitzer M, Wockel L, Luft AR, *et al.* The importance of pial blood supply to the development of peritumoral brain edema in meningiomas. *J Neurosurg* 1997;**87**:368–73.

31. Smith HP, Challa VR, Moody DM, Kelly DL, Jr. Biological features of meningiomas that determine the production of cerebral edema. *Neurosurgery* 1981;**8**:428–33.

32. Sato M, Matsumoto M, Kodama N. [treatment of skull base meningioma encasing the main cerebral artery]. *No Shinkei Geka* 1997;**25**:239–45.

33. Ishikawa M, Nishi S, Aoki T, *et al.* Predictability of internal carotid artery (ica) dissectability in cases showing ica involvement in parasellar meningioma. *J Clin Neurosci* 2001;**8** Suppl 1:22–5.

34. Hiyama H, Kubo O, Tajika Y, Tohyama T, Takakura K. Meningiomas associated with peritumoural venous stasis: Three types on cerebral angiogram. *Acta Neurochir (Wien)* 1994;**129**:31–8.

35. Good CD, Kingsley DP, Taylor WJ, Harkness WF. "Dural tail" Adjacent to a giant posterior cerebral artery aneurysm: case report and review of the literature. *Neuroradiology* 1997;**39**:577–80.

36. Forbes G. Radiologic evaluation of orbital tumors. *Clin Neurosurg* 1985;**32**:474–513.

37. McDermott MW, Rootman J, Durity FA. Subperiosteal, subperiorbital dissection and division of the anterior and posterior ethmoid arteries for meningiomas of the cribriform plate and planum sphenoidale: technical note. *Neurosurgery* 1995;**36**:1215–18; discussion 1218–19.

38. Abe T, Matsumoto K, Homma H, Kawamura N, Iwata T, Nemoto S. Dorsum sellae meningioma mimicking pituitary macroadenoma: case report. *Surg Neurol* 1999;**51**:543–6; discussion 546–7.

39. Donovan JL, Nesbit GM. Distinction of masses involving the sella and suprasellar space: Specificity of imaging features. *Am J Roentgenol* 1996;**167**:597–603.

40. Nozaki K, Nagata I, Yoshida K, Kikuchi H. Intrasellar meningioma: Case report and review of the literature. *Surg Neurol* 1997;**47**:447–452; discussion 452–4.

41. Terada T, Kinoshita Y, Yokote H, *et al.* Preoperative embolization of meningiomas fed by ophthalmic branch arteries. *Surg Neurol* 1996;**45**:161–6.

42. Sorimachi T, Maruya J, Mizusawa Y, Ito Y, Takeuchi S. Glaucoma as a complication of superselective ophthalmic angiography. *Am J Neuroradiol* 2003;**24**:1552–3.

43. Boulos PT, Dumont AS, Mandell JW, Jane JA, Sr. Meningiomas of the orbit: Contemporary considerations. *Neurosurg Focus* 2001;**10**:E5.

44. Lefkowitz M, Giannotta SL, Hieshima G, *et al.* Embolization of neurosurgical lesions involving the ophthalmic artery. *Neurosurgery* 1998;**43**:1298–303.

45. Sekhar LN, Swamy NK, Jaiswal V, Rubinstein E, Hirsch WE, Jr., Wright DC. Surgical excision of meningiomas involving the clivus: Preoperative and intraoperative features as predictors of postoperative functional deterioration. *J Neurosurg* 1994;**81**:860–8.

46. Kusaka N, Tamiya T, Sugiu K, *et al.* Combined use of trufill dcs detachable coil system and guglielmi detachable coil for embolization of meningioma fed by branches of the cavernous internal carotid artery. *Neurol Med Chir (Tokyo)* 2007;**47**:29–31.

47. Hirohata M, Abe T, Morimitsu H, Fujimura N, Shigemori M, Norbash AM. Preoperative selective internal carotid artery dural branch embolisation for petroclival meningiomas. *Neuroradiology* 2003;**45**:656–60.

48. Tymianski M, Willinsky RA, Tator CH, Mikulis D, TerBrugge KG, Markson L. Embolization with temporary balloon occlusion of the internal carotid artery and in vivo proton spectroscopy improves radical removal of petrous-tentorial meningioma. *Neurosurgery* 1994;**35**:974–7; discussion 977.

49. Terada T, Yokote H, Tsuura M, *et al.* Presumed intraventricular meningioma treated by embolisation and the gamma knife. *Neuroradiology* 1999;**41**:334–7.

50. Asari S, Maeshiro T, Tomita S, *et al.* Meningiomas arising from the falcotentorial junction. Clinical features, neuroimaging studies, and surgical treatment. *J Neurosurg* 1995;**82**:726–38.

51. Odake G. Meningioma of the falcotentorial region: Report of two cases and literature review of occlusion of the galenic system. *Neurosurgery* 1992;**30**:788–93; discussion 793–4.

52. Rostomily RC, Eskridge JM, Winn HR. Tentorial meningiomas. *Neurosurg Clin N Am* 1994;**5**:331–48.

53. Quinones-Hinojosa A, Chang EF, Chaichana KL, McDermott MW. Surgical considerations in the management of falcotentorial meningiomas: advantages of the bilateral occipital transtentorial/transfalcine craniotomy for large tumors. *Neurosurgery* 2009;**64**:260–268; discussion 268.

54. Rossitti S. Preoperative embolization of lower-falx meningiomas with ethylene vinyl alcohol copolymer: technical and anatomical aspects. *Acta Radiol* 2007;**48**:321–6.

55. Harrison MJ, Wolfe DE, Lau TS, Mitnick RJ, Sachdev VP. Radiation-induced meningiomas: experience at the mount sinai hospital and review of the literature. *J Neurosurg* 1991;**75**: 564–74.

56. Manelfe C, Lasjaunias P, Ruscalleda J. Preoperative embolization of intracranial meningiomas. *Am J Neuroradiol* 1986;**7**:963–72.

57. Kai Y, Hamada JI, Morioka M, et al. Clinical evaluation of cellulose porous beads for the therapeutic embolization of meningiomas. *Am J Neuroradiol* 2006;**27**:1146–50.

58. Rosen CL, Ammerman JM, Sekhar LN, Bank WO. Outcome analysis of preoperative embolization in cranial base surgery. *Acta Neurochir (Wien)* 2002;**144**:1157–64.

59. Gruber A, Bavinzski G, Killer M, Richling B. Preoperative embolization of hypervascular skull base tumors. *Minim Invas Neurosurg* 2000;**43**:62–71.

60. Yamaguchi N, Kawase T, Sagoh M, Ohira T, Shiga H, Toya S. Prediction of consistency of meningiomas with preoperative magnetic resonance imaging. *Surg Neurol* 1997;**48**:579–83.

61. Gruber A, Killer M, Mazal P, Bavinzski G, Richling B. Preoperative embolization of intracranial meningiomas: A 17-years single center experience. *Minim Invas Neurosurg* 2000;**43**:18–29.

62. Grand C, Bank WO, Baleriaux D, et al. Gadolinium-enhanced mr in the evaluation of preoperative meningioma embolization. *Am J Neuroradiol* 1993;**14**:563–9.

63. Martin AJ, Cha S, Higashida RT, et al. Assessment of vasculature of meningiomas and the effects of embolization with intra-arterial mr perfusion imaging: a feasibility study. *Am J Neuroradiol* 2007;**28**:1771–7.

64. Bruening R, Wu RH, Yousry TA, et al. Regional relative blood volume mr maps of meningiomas before and after partial embolization. *J Comput Assist Tomogr* 1998;**22**:104–10.

65. Morimura T, Takeuchi J, Maeda Y, Tani E. Preoperative embolization of meningiomas: its efficacy and histopathological findings. *Noshuyo Byori* 1994;**11**:123–9.

66. Perry A, Chicoine MR, Filiput E, Miller JP, Cross DT. Clinicopathologic assessment and grading of embolized meningiomas: a correlative study of 64 patients. *Cancer* 2001;**92**: 701–11.

67. Bendszus M, Warmuth-Metz M, Klein R, et al. Sequential mri and mr spectroscopy in embolized meningiomas: correlation with surgical and histopathological findings. *Neuroradiology* 2002;**44**:77–82.

68. Blankenhorn M, Bachert P, Semmler W, et al. [phosphorus-31-mr spectroscopy imaging in preoperative embolization treatment of meningioma]. *Rofo* 1999;**170**:568–74.

69. Jungling FD, Wakhloo AK, Hennig J. In vivo proton spectroscopy of meningioma after preoperative embolization. *Magn Reson Med* 1993;**30**:155–60.

70. Patsouris E, Laas R, Hagel C, Stavrou D. Increased proliferative activity due to necroses induced by pre-operative embolization in benign meningiomas. *J Neurooncol* 1998;**40**:257–64.

71. Ng HK, Poon WS, Goh K, Chan MS. Histopathology of post-embolized meningiomas. *Am J Surg Pathol* 1996;**20**:1224–30.

72. Nakasu S, Nakajima M, Nakazawa T, Nakasu Y, Handa J. P53 accumulation and apoptosis in embolized meningiomas. *Acta Neuropathol* 1997;**93**:599–605.

73. Nakasu S, Nakajima M, Nakazawa T, Nakasu Y, Handa J. Alteration of bcl-2 and bax expression in embolized meningiomas. *Brain Tumor Pathol* 1998;**15**:13–17.

74. Jensen RL, Soleau S, Bhayani MK, Christiansen D. Expression of hypoxia inducible factor-1 alpha and correlation with preoperative embolization of meningiomas. *J Neurosurg* 2002;**97**:658–67.

75. Park K, Kim JH, Nam DH, et al. Vascular endothelial growth factor expression under ischemic stress in human meningiomas. *Neurosci Lett* 2000;**283**:45–8.

76. Zhang XB, Jin ZY. [clinical application of presurgical embolization of meningiomas]. *Zhongguo Yi Xue Ke Xue Yuan Xue Bao* 2003;**25**:168–71.

77. Bendszus M, Rao G, Burger R, et al. Is there a benefit of preoperative meningioma embolization? *Neurosurgery* 2000;**47**:1306–11; discussion 1311–12.

78. Oka H, Kurata A, Kawano N, et al. Preoperative superselective embolization of skull-base meningiomas: Indications and limitations. *J Neurooncol* 1998;**40**: 67–71.

79. Dean BL, Flom RA, Wallace RC, et al. Efficacy of endovascular treatment of meningiomas: evaluation with matched samples. *AJNR Am J Neuroradiol* 1994;**15**:1675–80.

80. Chun JY, McDermott MW, Lamborn KR, Wilson CB, Higashida R, Berger MS. Delayed surgical resection reduces intraoperative blood loss for embolized meningiomas. *Neurosurgery* 2002;**50**:1231–5; discussion 1235–7.

81. Kai Y, Hamada J, Morioka M, Yano S, Todaka T, Ushio Y. Appropriate interval between embolization and surgery in patients with meningioma. *Am J Neuroradiol* 2002;**23**:139–42.

82. Kuroiwa T, Tanaka H, Ohta T, Tsutsumi A. Preoperative embolization of highly vascular brain tumors: clinical and histopathological findings. *Noshuyo Byori* 1996;**13**:27–36.

83. Bendszus M, Martin-Schrader I, Schlake HP, Solymosi L. Embolisation of intracranial meningiomas without subsequent surgery. *Neuroradiology* 2003;**45**:451–5.

84. Bendszus M, Monoranu CM, Schutz A, Nolte I, Vince GH, Solymosi L. Neurologic complications after particle embolization of intracranial meningiomas. *Am J Neuroradiol* 2005;**26**:1413–19.

85. Kallmes DF, Evans AJ, Kaptain GJ, et al. Hemorrhagic complications in embolization of a meningioma: case report and review of the literature. *Neuroradiology* 1997;**39**:877–80.

86. Suyama T, Tamaki N, Fujiwara K, Hamano S, Kimura M, Matsumoto S. Peritumoral and intratumoral hemorrhage after gelatin sponge embolization of malignant meningioma: case report. *Neurosurgery* 1987;**21**:944–6.

87. Bejjani GK, Sekhar LN, Yost AM, Bank WO, Wright DC. Vasospasm after cranial base tumor resection: Pathogenesis, diagnosis, and therapy. *Surg Neurol* 1999;**52**:577–83; discussion 583–4.

88. Glasscock MF, Jackson CG. Neurologic skull base surgery for glomus tumors. *Laryngoscope* 1993;**103** (suppl 60):1–71.

89. Matishak MZ, Symon L, Cheeseman A, Pamphlett R. Catecholamine-secreting paragangliomas of the base of the skull. Report of two cases. *J Neurosurg* 1987;**66**:604–8.

90. Brackman D, Kinney S, Fu K. Glomus tumor: diagnosis and management. *Head Neck Surg* 1987;**9**:306–11.

91. Maurizi M, Almadori G, Ferri E, *et al.* [carotid body tumors: The clinical, diagnostic and therapeutic aspects]. *Acta Otorhinolaryngol Ital* 1992;**12**:527–45.

92. Ogura JH, Spector GJ, Gado M. Glomus jugulare and vagale. *Ann Otol Rhinol Laryngol* 1978;**87**:622–9.

93. Moret J, Picard L. *Semin Intervent Rad* 1987;**4**:291–308.

94. Tasar M, Yetiser S. Glomus tumors: therapeutic role of selective embolization. *J Craniofac Surg* 2004;**15**:497–505.

95. Carmody RF, Seeger JF, Horsley WW, Smith JR, Miller RW. Digital subtraction angiography of glomus tympanicum and jugulare tumors. *Am J Neuroradiol* 1983;**4**:263–5.

96. Girolami G, Heuser L, Hildmann H, Sudhoff H. [selective embolization and surgical resection for head and neck glomus tumours – clinical outcome analysis]. *Laryngorhinootologie* 2008;**87**:181–5.

97. Murphy TP, Brackmann DE. Effects of preoperative embolization on glomus jugulare tumors. *Laryngoscope* 1989;**99**:1244–7.

98. Ward PH, Liu C, Vinuela F, Bentson JR. Embolization: An adjunctive measure for removal of carotid body tumors. *Laryngoscope* 1988;**98**:1287–91.

99. LaMuraglia GM, Fabian RL, Brewster DC, *et al.* The current surgical management of carotid body paragangliomas. *J Vasc Surg* 1992;**15**:1038–44; discussion 1044–5.

100. Leber KA, Eustacchio S, Pendl G. Radiosurgery of glomus tumors: midterm results. *Stereotact Funct Neurosurg* 1999;**72** Suppl 1:53–9.

101. Bapuraj JR, Mani NB, Khandelwal NK, Thennarasu K, Sharma SC. New parameter of hemoglobin status as an indicator of efficacy of preoperative angioembolization in extracranial hypervascular tumours. *J Otolaryngol* 2002;**31**:313–16.

102. Gullane PJ, Davidson J, O'Dwyer T, Forte V. Juvenile angiofibroma: A review of the literature and a case series report. *Laryngoscope* 1992;**102**:928–33.

103. Jorissen M, Eloy P, Rombaux P, Bachert C, Daele J. Endoscopic sinus surgery for juvenile nasopharyngeal angiofibroma. *Acta Otorhinolaryngol Belg* 2000;**54**:201–19.

104. Harrison DF. The natural history, pathogenesis, and treatment of juvenile angiofibroma. Personal experience with 44 patients. *Arch Otolaryngol Head Neck Surg* 1987;**113**:936–42.

105. Fisch U. The infratemporal fossa approach for nasopharyngeal tumors. *Laryngoscope* 1983;**93**:36–44.

106. Mann WJ, Jecker P, Amedee RG. Juvenile angiofibromas: Changing surgical concept over the last 20 years. *Laryngoscope* 2004;**114**:291–3.

107. Waldman SR, Levine HL, Astor F, Wood BG, Weinstein M, Tucker HM. Surgical experience with nasopharyngeal angiofibroma. *Arch Otolaryngol* 1981;**107**:677–82.

108. Lasjaunias P. Nasopharyngeal angiofibromas: Hazards of embolization. *Radiology* 1980;**136**:119–23.

109. Giavroglou C, Constantinidis J, Triaridis S, Daniilidis J, Dimitriadis A. [angiographic evaluation and embolization of juvenile nasopharyngeal angiofibroma]. *HNO* 2007;**55**:36–41.

110. Yi Z, Li ZC, Lin C, Ye S. Huge lobulated juvenile angiofibroma: Sites of extension and selection of procedures for management. *J Otolaryngol* 2003;**32**:211–16.

111. Antonelli AR, Cappiello J, Di Lorenzo D, Donajo CA, Nicolai P, Orlandini A. Diagnosis, staging, and treatment of juvenile nasopharyngeal angiofibroma (jna). *Laryngoscope* 1987;**97**:1319–25.

112. Platzbecker H, Kohler K. Embolization in the head and neck region. *Acta Radiol Suppl* 1991;**377**:25–6.

113. Iablonskii SV, Shchenev SV, Nikanorov A, Myl'nikov AA. [use of x-ray endovascular occlusion in combined treatment of juvenile angiofibroma of the skull base in children]. *Vestn Otorinolaringol* 1998:37–40.

114. De Vincentiis M, Gallo A, Minni A, Torri E, Tomassi R, Della Rocca C. [preoperative embolization in the treatment protocol for rhinopharyngeal angiofibroma: Comparison of the effectiveness of various materials]. *Acta Otorhinolaryngol Ital* 1997;**17**:225–32.

115. Glad H, Vainer B, Buchwald C, *et al.* Juvenile nasopharyngeal angiofibromas in Denmark 1981–2003: diagnosis, incidence, and treatment. *Acta Otolaryngol* 2007;**127**:292–9.

116. Moulin G, Chagnaud C, Gras R, *et al.* Juvenile nasopharyngeal angiofibroma: comparison of blood loss during removal in embolized group versus nonembolized group. *Cardiovasc Intervent Radiol* 1995;**18**:158–61.

117. Oueslati S, Gamra OB, Kharrat S, *et al.* [nasopharyngeal angiofibroma: report of 15 cases treated by embolization]. *J Radiol* 2008;**89**:579–84.

118. Fonseca AS, Vinhaes E, Boaventura V, *et al.* Surgical treatment of non-embolized patients with nasoangiofibroma. *Braz J Otorhinolaryngol* 2008;**74**:583–7.

119. El-Banhawy OA, Ragab A, El-Sharnoby MM. Surgical resection of type iii juvenile angiofibroma without preoperative embolization. *Int J Pediatr Otorhinolaryngol* 2006;**70**:1715–23.

120. Schick B, Kahle G. Radiological findings in angiofibroma. *Acta Radiol* 2000;**41**:585–93.

121. Li JR, Qian J, Shan XZ, Wang L. Evaluation of the effectiveness of preoperative embolization in surgery for nasopharyngeal angiofibroma. *Eur Arch Otorhinolaryngol* 1998;**255**:430–2.

122. Siniluoto TM, Luotonen JP, Tikkakoski TA, Leinonen AS, Jokinen KE. Value of

pre-operative embolization in surgery for nasopharyngeal angiofibroma. *J Laryngol Otol* 1993;**107**:514–21.

123. Zhang M, Garvis W, Linder T, Fisch U. Update on the infratemporal fossa approaches to nasopharyngeal angiofibroma. *Laryngoscope* 1998;**108**:1717–23.

124. Petruson K, Rodriguez-Catarino M, Petruson B, Finizia C. Juvenile nasopharyngeal angiofibroma: long-term results in preoperative embolized and non-embolized patients. *Acta Otolaryngol* 2002;**122**:96–100.

125. Qureshi ai, a new classification scheme based on angiographic arterial supply to neoplasms. *J Vasc Interv Neurol* 2009;**2**:153–4.

126. Kawai K, Yoshinaga K, Koizumi M, Honma S, Tokiyoshi A, Kodama K. A middle meningeal artery which arises from the internal carotid artery in which the first branchial artery participates. *Ann Anat* 2006;**188**:33–8.

127. Shima H, von Luedinghausen M, Ohno K, Michi K. Anatomy of microvascular anastomosis in the neck. *Plast Reconstr Surg* 1998;**101**:33–41.

128. Probst EN, Grzyska U, Westphal M, Zeumer H. Preoperative embolization of intracranial meningiomas with a fibrin glue preparation. *Am J Neuroradiol* 1999;**20**:1695–702.

129. Ng SH, Wan YL, Wong HF, *et al.* Preoperative embolization of meningiomas: Comparison of superselective and subselective techniques. *J Formos Med Assoc.* 1998;**97**:153–158.

130. Hayashi N, Kubo M, Tsuboi Y, *et al.* Impact of anomalous origin of the ophthalmic artery from the middle meningeal artery on selection of surgical approach to skull base meningioma. *Surg Neurol* 2007;**68**: 568–571; discussion 571–2.

131. Ohata K, Nishio A, Takami T, Goto T. Sudden appearance of transdural anastomosis from middle meningeal artery to superior cerebellar artery during preoperative embolization of meningioma. *Neurol India* 2006;**54**:328.

132. Maiuri F, Donzelli R, de Divitiis O, Fusco M, Briganti F. Anomalous meningeal branches of the ophthalmic artery feeding meningiomas of the brain convexity. *Surg Radiol Anat* 1998;**20**:279–84.

133. Spetzler RF, Modic M, Bonstelle C. Spontaneous opening of large occipital-vertebral artery anastomosis during embolization. Case report. *J Neurosurg* 1980;**53**:849–50.

134. Kendall B, Moseley I. Therapeutic embolisation of the external carotid arterial tree. *J Neurol Neurosurg Psychiatry* 1977;**40**:937–50.

135. Kai Y, Hamada J, Morioka M, *et al.* Preoperative cellulose porous beads for therapeutic embolization of meningioma: provocation test and technical considerations. *Neuroradiology* 2007;**49**:437–43.

136. Serbinenko FA, Lysachev AG, Arustamian SR. [main anastomoses of external carotid artery branches with the beds of the internal carotid and the vertebral artery and a role of pharmacological tests in the determination of their functional value at tumor embolization]. *Zh Vopr Neirokhir Im N N Burdenko* 2002: 15–18.

137. Hirai T, Korogi Y, Ono K, Uemura S, Yamashita Y. Preoperative embolization for meningeal tumors: Evaluation of vascular supply with angio-ct. *Am J Neuroradiol* 2004;**25**: 74–6.

138. Laurent A, Wassef M, Chapot R, Houdart E, Merland JJ. Location of vessel occlusion of calibrated tris-acryl gelatin microspheres for tumor and arteriovenous malformation embolization. *J Vasc Interv Radiol* 2004;**15**:491–6.

139. Wakhloo AK, Juengling FD, Van Velthoven V, Schumacher M, Hennig J, Schwechheimer K. Extended preoperative polyvinyl alcohol microembolization of intracranial meningiomas: Assessment of two embolization techniques. *Am J Neuroradiol* 1993;**14**:571–82.

140. Bendszus M, Klein R, Burger R, Warmuth-Metz M, Hofmann E, Solymosi L. Efficacy of trisacryl gelatin microspheres versus polyvinyl alcohol particles in the preoperative embolization of meningiomas. *Am J Neuroradiol* 2000;**21**:255–61.

141. Laurent A, Wassef M, Chapot R, *et al.* Partition of calibrated tris-acryl gelatin microspheres in the arterial vasculature of embolized nasopharyngeal angiofibromas and paragangliomas. *J Vasc Interv Radiol* 2005;**16**: 507–13.

142. Derdeyn CP, Moran CJ, Cross DT, Dietrich HH, Dacey RG, Jr. Polyvinyl alcohol particle size and suspension characteristics. *Am J Neuroradiol* 1995;**16**:1335–43.

143. Yoon YS, Ahn JY, Chang JH, Cho JH, Suh SH, Lee BH, Lee KS. Pre-operative embolisation of internal carotid artery branches and pial vessels in hypervascular brain tumours. *Acta Neurochir (Wien)* 2008;**150**:447–52; discussion 452.

144. Kaji T, Hama Y, Iwasaki Y, Kyoto Y, Kusano S. Preoperative embolization of meningiomas with pial supply: successful treatment of two cases. *Surg Neurol* 1999;**52**:270–3.

145. Liang Y, Wang D, Huang W, Ling F, Liu Y, Lu F. Direct intratumoral embolization of hypervascular tumors of the head and neck. *Chin Med J (Engl)* 2003;**116**:616–19.

146. Pierot L, Boulin A, Castaings L, Chabolle F, Moret J. [embolization by direct puncture of hypervascularized orl tumors]. *Ann Otolaryngol Chir Cervicofac* 1994;**111**:403–9.

147. Casasco A, Houdart E, Biondi A, *et al.* Major complications of percutaneous embolization of skull-base tumors. *Am J Neuroradiol* 1999;**20**:179–81.

148. Casasco A, Herbreteau D, Houdart E, *et al.* Devascularization of craniofacial tumors by percutaneous tumor puncture. *Am J Neuroradiol* 1994;**15**:1233–9.

149. Gobin YP, Pasco A, Merland JJ, Aymard AA, Casasco A, Houdart E. Percutaneous puncture of the external carotid artery or its branches after surgical ligation. *Am J Neuroradiol* 1994;**15**:79–82.

150. Schroth G, Haldemann AR, Mariani L, Remonda L, Raveh J. Preoperative embolization of paragangliomas and angiofibromas. Measurement of intratumoral arteriovenous shunts. *Arch Otolaryngol Head Neck Surg* 1996;**122**:1320–5.

151. Horowitz MB, Carrau R, Crammond D, Kanal E. Risks of tumor embolization in the presence of an unrecognized patent foramen ovale: Case report. *Am J Neuroradiol* 2002;**23**:982–4.

152. Bentson J, Rand R, Calcaterra T, Lasjaunias P. Unexpected complications following therapeutic embolization. *Neuroradiology* 1978;**16**:420–3.

153. Gupta AK, Purkayastha S, Bodhey NK, Kapilamoorthy TR, Kesavadas C. Preoperative embolization of hypervascular head and neck tumours. *Australas Radiol* 2007;**51**:446–52.

154. Shi ZS, Feng L, Jiang XB, Huang Q, Yang Z, Huang ZS. Therapeutic embolization of meningiomas with onyx for delayed surgical resection. *Surg Neurol* 2008;**70**:478–81.

155. Kubo M, Kuwayama N, Hirashima Y, Takaku A, Ogawa T, Endo S. Hydroxyapatite ceramics as a particulate embolic material: Report of the clinical experience. *Am J Neuroradiol* 2003;**24**:1545–7.

156. Kasuya H, Shimizu T, Sasahara A, Takakura K. Phenytoin as a liquid material for embolisation of tumours. *Neuroradiology* 1999;**41**:320–3.

157. Feng L, Kienitz BA, Matsumoto C, et al. Feasibility of using hyperosmolar mannitol as a liquid tumor embolization agent. *Am J Neuroradiol* 2005;**26**:1405–12.

158. Luo CB, Teng MM, Chang FC, Chang CY, Guo WY. Radiation carotid blowout syndrome in nasopharyngeal carcinoma: Angiographic features and endovascular management. *Otolaryngol Head Neck Surg* 2008;**138**:86–91.

159. Scott CB, Scarantino C, Urtasun R, et al. Validation and predictive power of radiation therapy oncology group (rtog) recursive partitioning analysis classes for malignant glioma patients: a report using rtog 90–06. *Int J Radiat Oncol Biol Phys* 1998;**40**:51–5.

160. Desjardins A, Reardon DA, Vredenburgh JJ. Current available therapies and future directions in the treatment of malignant gliomas. *Biologics* 2009;**3**:15–25.

161. Nakashima M, Shibata S, Tokunaga Y, et al. In-vivo microdialysis study of the distribution of cisplatin into brain tumour tissue after intracarotid infusion in rats with 9l malignant glioma. *J Pharm Pharmacol* 1997;**49**:777–80.

162. Takeda N, Diksic M. Relationship between drug delivery and the intra-arterial infusion rate of sarcnu in c6 rat brain tumor model. *J Neurooncol* 1999;**41**:235–46.

163. Newton HB. Intra-arterial chemotherapy of primary brain tumors. *Curr Treat Options Oncol* 2005;**6**:519–30.

164. Ginos JZ, Cooper AJ, Dhawan V, et al. [13n]cisplatin pet to assess pharmacokinetics of intra-arterial versus intravenous chemotherapy for malignant brain tumors. *J Nucl Med* 1987;**28**:1844–52.

165. Levin VA, Kabra PM, Freeman-Dove MA. Pharmacokinetics of intracarotid artery 14c-bcnu in the squirrel monkey. *J Neurosurg* 1978;**48**:587–93.

166. Namba H, Kobayashi S, Iwadate Y, et al. Assessment of the brain areas perfused by superselective intra-arterial chemotherapy using single photon emission computed tomography with technetium-99m-hexamethyl-propyleneamine oxime–technical note. *Neurol Med Chir (Tokyo)* 1994;**34**:832–5.

167. Basso U, Lonardi S, Brandes AA. Is intra-arterial chemotherapy useful in high-grade gliomas? *Expert Rev Anticancer Ther* 2002;**2**:507–19.

168. Defer G, Fauchon F, Schaison M, Chiras J, Brunet P. Visual toxicity following intra-arterial chemotherapy with hydroxyethyl-cnu in patients with malignant gliomas. A prospective study with statistical analysis. *Neuroradiology* 1991;**33**:432–7.

169. Shapiro WR, Green SB, Burger PC, et al. A randomized comparison of intra-arterial versus intravenous bcnu, with or without intravenous 5-fluorouracil, for newly diagnosed patients with malignant glioma. *J Neurosurg* 1992;**76**:772–81.

170. Stewart DJ, Grahovac Z, Russel NA, et al. Phase i study of intracarotid pcnu. *J Neurooncol* 1987;**5**:245–50.

171. Newton HB, Page MA, Junck L, Greenberg HS. Intra-arterial cisplatin for the treatment of malignant gliomas. *J Neurooncol* 1989;**7**:39–45.

172. Stewart DJ, Wallace S, Feun L, et al. A phase i study of intracarotid artery infusion of cis-diamminedichloroplatinum(ii) in patients with recurrent malignant intracerebral tumors. *Cancer Res* 1982;**42**:2059–62.

173. Maiese K, Walker RW, Gargan R, Victor JD. Intra-arterial cisplatin-associated optic and otic toxicity. *Arch Neurol* 1992;**49**:83–6.

174. Tfayli A, Hentschel P, Madajewicz S, et al. Toxicities related to intraarterial infusion of cisplatin and etoposide in patients with brain tumors. *J Neurooncol* 1999;**42**:73–7.

175. Go RS, Adjei AA. Review of the comparative pharmacology and clinical activity of cisplatin and carboplatin. *J Clin Oncol* 1999;**17**:409–22.

176. Murry DJ. Comparative clinical pharmacology of cisplatin and carboplatin. *Pharmacotherapy* 1997;**17**:140S–5S.

177. Alberts DS. Carboplatin versus cisplatin in ovarian cancer. *Semin Oncol* 1995;**22**:88–90.

178. Ruckdeschel JC. The future role of carboplatin. *Semin Oncol* 1994;**21**:114–18.

179. Cloughesy TF, Gobin YP, Black KL, et al. Intra-arterial carboplatin chemotherapy for brain tumors: a dose escalation study based on cerebral blood flow. *J Neurooncol* 1997;**35**:121–31.

180. Follezou JY, Fauchon F, Chiras J. Intraarterial infusion of carboplatin in the treatment of malignant gliomas: a phase ii study. *Neoplasma.* 1989;**36**:349–52.

181. Qureshi AI, Suri MF, Khan J, et al. Superselective intra-arterial carboplatin for treatment of intracranial neoplasms: experience in 100 procedures. *J Neurooncol* 2001;**51**:151–8.

182. Stewart DJ, Belanger JM, Grahovac Z, et al. Phase i study of intracarotid administration of carboplatin. *Neurosurgery* 1992;**30**:512–16; discussion 516–17.

183. Bonstelle CT, Kori SH, Rekate H. Intracarotid chemotherapy of glioblastoma after induced blood–brain barrier disruption. *Am J Neuroradiol* 1983;**4**:810–12.

184. Fenstermacher J, Gazendam J. Intra-arterial infusions of drugs and hyperosmotic solutions as ways of enhancing cns chemotherapy. *Cancer Treat Rep* 1981;**65** Suppl 2:27–37.

185. Inamura T, Nomura T, Bartus RT, Black KL. Intracarotid infusion of rmp-7, a bradykinin analog: A method for selective drug delivery to brain tumors. *J Neurosurg* 1994;**81**:752–8.

186. Matsukado K, Inamura T, Nakano S, Fukui M, Bartus RT, Black KL. Enhanced tumor uptake of carboplatin and survival in glioma-bearing rats by intracarotid infusion of bradykinin analog, rmp-7. *Neurosurgery*

1996;**39**:125–133; discussion 133–4.

187. Greenberg HS, Ensminger WD, Chandler WF, *et al.* Intra-arterial bcnu chemotherapy for treatment of malignant gliomas of the central nervous system. *J Neurosurg* 1984;**61**:423–9.

188. Hochberg FH, Pruitt AA, Beck DO, DeBrun G, Davis K. The rationale and methodology for intra-arterial chemotherapy with bcnu as treatment for glioblastoma. *J Neurosurg* 1985;**63**:876–80.

189. Bradac GB, Soffietti R, Riva A, Stura G, Sales S, Schiffer D. Selective intra-arterial chemotherapy with bcnu in recurrent malignant gliomas. *Neuroradiology* 1992;**34**:73–6.

190. Vega F, Davila L, Chatellier G, *et al.* Treatment of malignant gliomas with surgery, intraarterial chemotherapy with acnu and radiation therapy. *J Neurooncol* 1992;**13**:131–5.

191. Bobo H, Kapp JP, Vance R. Effect of intra-arterial cisplatin and 1,3-bis (2chloroethyl)-1-nitrosourea (bcnu) dosage on radiographic response and regional toxicity in malignant glioma patients: proposal of a new method of intra-arterial dosage calculation. *J Neurooncol* 1992;**13**:291–9.

192. Stewart DJ, Grahovac Z, Hugenholtz H, *et al.* Feasibility study of intraarterial vs intravenous cisplatin, bcnu, and teniposide combined with systemic cisplatin, teniposide, cytosine arabinoside, glycerol and mannitol in the treatment of primary and metastatic brain tumors. *J Neurooncol* 1993;**17**: 71–9.

193. Hirano Y, Mineura K, Mizoi K, Tomura N. Therapeutic results of intra-arterial chemotherapy in patients with malignant glioma. *Int J Oncol* 1998;**13**:537–42.

194. Paccapelo A, Piana C, Rychlicki F, *et al.* Treatment of malignant gliomas: a new approach. *Tumori.* 1998;**84**:529–33.

195. Bashir R, Hochberg FH, Linggood RM, Hottleman K. Pre-irradiation internal carotid artery bcnu in treatment of glioblastoma multiforme. *J Neurosurg* 1988;**68**:917–19.

196. Fauchon F, Davila L, Chatellier G, *et al.* Treatment of malignant gliomas with surgery, intra-arterial infusions of 1-(2-hydroxyethyl)chloroethylnitrosourea,

and radiation therapy: A phase ii study. *Neurosurgery* 1990;**27**:231–4.

197. Iwadate Y, Namba H, Saegusa T, Sueyoshi K. Intra-arterial mannitol infusion in the chemotherapy for malignant brain tumors. *J Neurooncol* 1993;**15**:185–93.

198. Kochii M, Kitamura I, Goto T, *et al.* Randomized comparison of intra-arterial versus intravenous infusion of acnu for newly diagnosed patients with glioblastoma. *J Neurooncol* 2000;**49**: 63–70.

199. Feun LG, Wallace S, Stewart DJ, *et al.* Intracarotid infusion of cis-diamminedichloroplatinum in the treatment of recurrent malignant brain tumors. *Cancer* 1984;**54**:794–9.

200. Neuwelt EA, Howieson J, Frenkel EP, *et al.* Therapeutic efficacy of multiagent chemotherapy with drug delivery enhancement by blood–brain barrier modification in glioblastoma. *Neurosurgery.* 1986;**19**:573–82.

201. Mahaley MS, Jr., Hipp SW, Dropcho EJ, *et al.* Intracarotid cisplatin chemotherapy for recurrent gliomas. *J Neurosurg.* 1989;**70**:371–8.

202. Saris SC, Blasberg RG, Carson RE, *et al.* Intravascular streaming during carotid artery infusions. Demonstration in humans and reduction using diastole-phased pulsatile administration. *J Neurosurg* 1991;**74**:763–72.

203. Tamaki M, Ohno K, Niimi Y, *et al.* Parenchymal damage in the territory of the anterior choroidal artery following supraophthalmic intracarotid administration of cddp for treatment of malignant gliomas. *J Neurooncol* 1997;**35**:65–72.

204. Dropcho EJ, Rosenfeld SS, Vitek J, Guthrie BL, Morawetz RB. Phase ii study of intracarotid or selective intracerebral infusion of cisplatin for treatment of recurrent anaplastic gliomas. *J Neurooncol* 1998;**36**:191–8.

205. Ashby LS, Shapiro WR. Intra-arterial cisplatin plus oral etoposide for the treatment of recurrent malignant glioma: A phase ii study. *J Neurooncol* 2001;**51**:67–86.

206. Recht L, Fram RJ, Strauss G, *et al.* Preirradiation chemotherapy of supratentorial malignant primary brain tumors with intracarotid cis-platinum (cddp) and i.V. Bcnu. A phase ii trial. *Am J Clin Oncol* 1990;**13**:125–31.

207. Madajewicz S, Chowhan N, Tfayli A, *et al.* Therapy for patients with high grade astrocytoma using intraarterial chemotherapy and radiation therapy. *Cancer* 2000;**88**:2350–6.

208. Larner JM, Kersh CR, Constable WC, *et al.* Phase i/ii trial of superselective arterial 5-fu infusion with concomitant external beam radiation for patients with either anaplastic astrocytoma or glioblastoma multiforme. *Am J Clin Oncol* 1991;**14**:514–18.

209. Dropcho EJ, Rosenfeld SS, Morawetz RB, *et al.* Preradiation intracarotid cisplatin treatment of newly diagnosed anaplastic gliomas. The cns cancer consortium. *J Clin Oncol* 1992;**10**: 452–8.

210. Doolittle ND, Miner ME, Hall WA, *et al.* Safety and efficacy of a multicenter study using intraarterial chemotherapy in conjunction with osmotic opening of the blood-brain barrier for the treatment of patients with malignant brain tumors. *Cancer* 2000;**88**:637–47.

211. Black KL, Cloughesy T, Huang SC, *et al.* Intracarotid infusion of rmp-7, a bradykinin analog, and transport of gallium-68 ethylenediamine tetraacetic acid into human gliomas. *J Neurosurg* 1997;**86**:603–9.

212. Gregor A, Lind M, Newman H, *et al.* Phase ii studies of rmp-7 and carboplatin in the treatment of recurrent high grade glioma. Rmp-7 european study group. *J Neurooncol* 1999;**44**:137–45.

213. LeMay DR, Kittaka M, Gordon EM, *et al.* Intravenous rmp-7 increases delivery of ganciclovir into rat brain tumors and enhances the effects of herpes simplex virus thymidine kinase gene therapy. *Hum Gene Ther* 1998;**9**:989–95.

214. Imbesi F, Marchioni E, Benericetti E, *et al.* A randomized phase iii study: Comparison between intravenous and intraarterial acnu administration in newly diagnosed primary glioblastomas. *Anticancer Res* 2006;**26**:553–8.

215. Kirby S, Brothers M, Irish W, *et al.* Evaluating glioma therapies: Modeling treatments and predicting outcomes. *J Natl Cancer Inst* 1995;**87**:1884–8.

216. Hiesiger EM, Green SB, Shapiro WR, *et al.* Results of a randomized trial comparing intra-arterial cisplatin and intravenous pcnu for the treatment of

primary brain tumors in adults: Brain tumor cooperative group trial 8420a. *J Neurooncol* 1995;**25**:143–54.

217. Durand RE. Synergism of cisplatin and mitomycin c in sensitive and resistant cell subpopulations of a tumor model. *Int J Cancer* 1989;**44**:911–17.

218. Durand RE. Cisplatin and ccnu synergism in spheroid cell subpopulations. *Br J Cancer* 1990;**62**:947–53.

219. Plowman J, Waud WR, Koutsoukos AD, Rubinstein LV, Moore TD, Grever MR. Preclinical antitumor activity of temozolomide in mice: Efficacy against human brain tumor xenografts and synergism with 1,3-bis(2-chloroethyl)-1-nitrosourea. *Cancer Res* 1994;**54**:3793–9.

220. Rogers LR, Purvis JB, Lederman RJ, *et al.* Alternating sequential intracarotid bcnu and cisplatin in recurrent malignant glioma. *Cancer* 1991;**68**:15–21.

221. Feun LG, Wallace S, Yung WK, *et al.* Phase-i trial of intracarotid bcnu and cisplatin in patients with malignant intracerebral tumors. *Cancer Drug Deliv* 1984;**1**:239–45.

222. Feun LG, Lee YY, Yung WK, *et al.* Phase ii trial of intracarotid bcnu and cisplatin in primary malignant brain tumors. *Cancer Drug Deliv* 1986;**3**:147–56.

223. Chauveinc L, Sola-Martinez MT, Martin-Duverneuil M, *et al.* Intra arterial chemotherapy with acnu and radiotherapy in inoperable malignant gliomas. *J Neurooncol* 1996;**27**:141–7.

224. Angelov L, Doolittle ND, Kraemer DF, *et al.* Blood–brain barrier disruption and intra-arterial methotrexate-based therapy for newly diagnosed primary cns lymphoma: a multi-institutional experience. *J Clin Oncol* 2009;**27**:3503–9.

225. Tyson RM, Siegal T, Doolittle ND, Lacy C, Kraemer DF, Neutwelt EA. Current status and future of relapsed primary central nervous system lymphoma (pcnsl). *Leuk Lymphoma* 2003;**44**:627–33.

226. Stewart DJ, Grahovac Z, Benoit B, *et al.* Intracarotid chemotherapy with a combination of 1,3-bis(2-chloroethyl)-1-nitrosourea (bcnu), cis-diaminedichloroplatinum (cisplatin), and 4′-o-demethyl-1-o-(4,6-o-2-thenylidene-beta-d-glucopyranosyl) epipodophyllotoxin (vm-26) in the

treatment of primary and metastatic brain tumors. *Neurosurgery* 1984;**15**:828–33.

227. Stewart LA. Chemotherapy in adult high-grade glioma: a systematic review and meta-analysis of individual patient data from 12 randomised trials. *Lancet* 2002;**359**:1011–18.

228. Tsao MN, Mehta MP, Whelan TJ, *et al.* The american society for therapeutic radiology and oncology (astro) evidence-based review of the role of radiosurgery for malignant glioma. *Int J Radiat Oncol Biol Phys* 2005;**63**:47–55.

229. Stupp R, Hegi ME, Mason WP, *et al.* Effects of radiotherapy with concomitant and adjuvant temozolomide versus radiotherapy alone on survival in glioblastoma in a randomised phase iii study: 5-year analysis of the eortc-ncic trial. *Lancet Oncol* 2009;**10**:459–66.

230. Balm AJ, Rasch CR, Schornagel JH, *et al.* High-dose superselective intra-arterial cisplatin and concomitant radiation (radplat) for advanced head and neck cancer. *Head Neck* 2004;**26**:485–93.

231. Homma A, Furuta Y, Suzuki F, *et al.* Rapid superselective high-dose cisplatin infusion with concomitant radiotherapy for advanced head and neck cancer. *Head Neck* 2005;**27**:65–71.

232. Watne K, Hannisdal E, Nome O, Hager B, Hirschberg H. Prognostic factors in malignant gliomas with special reference to intra-arterial chemotherapy. *Acta Oncol* 1993;**32**:307–10.

233. Watne K, Hannisdal E, Nome O, *et al.* Combined intra-arterial chemotherapy followed by radiation in astrocytomas. *J Neurooncol* 1992;**14**:73–80.

234. Siegal T, Rubinstein R, Bokstein F, *et al.* In vivo assessment of the window of barrier opening after osmotic blood–brain barrier disruption in humans. *J Neurosurg* 2000;**92**:599–605.

235. Thomas HD, Lind MJ, Ford J, Bleehen N, Calvert AH, Boddy AV. Pharmacokinetics of carboplatin administered in combination with the bradykinin agonist cereport (rmp-7) for the treatment of brain tumours. *Cancer Chemother Pharmacol* 2000;**45**:284–90.

236. Kupersmith MJ, Frohman LP, Choi IS, *et al.* Visual system toxicity following intra-arterial chemotherapy. *Neurology* 1988;**38**:284–9.

237. Stewart DJ, Grahovac Z, Hugenholtz H, Russell N, Richard M, Benoit B. Combined intraarterial and systemic chemotherapy for intracerebral tumors. *Neurosurgery* 1987;**21**:207–14.

238. Blacklock JB, Wright DC, Dedrick RL, *et al.* Drug streaming during intra-arterial chemotherapy. *J Neurosurg* 1986;**64**:284–91.

239. Gobin YP, Cloughesy TF, Chow KL, *et al.* Intraarterial chemotherapy for brain tumors by using a spatial dose fractionation algorithm and pulsatile delivery. *Radiology* 2001;**218**:724–32.

240. Nakagawa H, Fujita T, Kubo S, *et al.* Selective intra-arterial chemotherapy with a combination of etoposide and cisplatin for malignant gliomas: preliminary report. *Surg Neurol* 1994;**41**:19–27.

241. Oldfield EH, Dedrick RL, *et al.* Reduced systemic drug exposure by combining intra-arterial chemotherapy with hemoperfusion of regional venous drainage. *J Neurosurg* 1985;**63**:726–32.

242. Miller AB, Hoogstraten B, Staquet M, Winkler A. Reporting results of cancer treatment. *Cancer* 1981;**47**:207–14.

243. Karnofsky DA, Burchenal JH. The clinical evaluation of chemotherapeutic agents in cancer. In Macleod CM, ed. *Evaluation of Chemotherapeutic Agents.* New York: Columbia Press, 1949, 191–205.

244. Langen KJ, Roosen N, Kuwert T, *et al.* Early effects of intra-arterial chemotherapy in patients with brain tumours studied with pet: Preliminary results. *Nucl Med Commun* 1989;**10**:779–90.

245. Chow KL, Gobin YP, Cloughesy T, Sayre JW, Villablanca JP, Vinuela F. Prognostic factors in recurrent glioblastoma multiforme and anaplastic astrocytoma treated with selective intra-arterial chemotherapy. *Am J Neuroradiol* 2000;**21**:471–8.

246. Cortazar P, Johnson BE. Review of the efficacy of individualized chemotherapy selected by in vitro drug sensitivity testing for patients with cancer. *J Clin Oncol* 1999;**17**:1625–31.

247. Iwadate Y, Fujimoto S, Namba H, Yamaura A. Promising survival for patients with glioblastoma multiforme

treated with individualised chemotherapy based on in vitro drug sensitivity testing. *Br J Cancer* 2003;**89**:1896–900.

248. Gelman M, Chakeres DW, Newton HB. Brain tumors: Complications of cerebral angiography accompanied by intraarterial chemotherapy. *Radiology* 1999;**213**:135–40.

249. Gemmete JJ. Complications associated with selective high-dose intraarterial cisplatin and concomitant radiation therapy for advanced head and neck cancer. *J Vasc Interv Radiol* 2003;**14**:743–8.

250. Johannesen TB, Lien HH, Hole KH, Lote K. Radiological and clinical assessment of long-term brain tumour survivors after radiotherapy. *Radiother Oncol* 2003;**69**:169–76.

251. Williams PC, Henner WD, Roman-Goldstein S, *et al.* Toxicity and efficacy of carboplatin and etoposide in conjunction with disruption of the blood-brain tumor barrier in the treatment of intracranial neoplasms. *Neurosurgery* 1995;**37**:17–27; discussion 27–8.

252. Neuwelt EA, Brummett RE, Doolittle ND, *et al.* First evidence of otoprotection against carboplatin-induced hearing loss with a two-compartment system in patients with central nervous system malignancy using sodium thiosulfate. *J Pharmacol Exp Ther* 1998;**286**:77–84.

253. Morita K, Tanaka R, Kakinuma K, Takahashi H, Motoyama H. Combination therapy of rat brain tumours using localized interstitial hyperthermia and intra-arterial chemotherapy. *Int J Hyperthermia* 2003;**19**:204–12.

254. Newton HB, Snyder MA, Stevens C, *et al.* Intra-arterial carboplatin and intravenous etoposide for the treatment of brain metastases. *J Neuro-Oncol* 2003;**61**: 35–44.

255. Newton HB, Figg GM, Slone W, Bourekas E. Incidence of infusion plan alterations after angiography in patients undergoing intra-arterial chemotherapy for brain tumors. *J Neuro-Oncol* 2006;**78**;157–60.

256. Bourekas EC, Figg GM, Slone W, Newton HB: Incidence and complication rate of incidental aneurysms discovered during intra-arterial chemotherapy of brain tumors. *Am J Neuroradiol* 2006;**27**;297–9.

Diagnostic and provocative testing

Haralabos Zacharatos, Ameer E. Hassan, M. Fareed K. Suri and Adnan I. Qureshi

Provocative testing

Provocative testing is based on the administration of an anesthetic agent selectively in the vascular distribution of interest, followed by neurological examination in an attempt to identify any new neurological deficits. The purpose of the test is to determine the neurological functions (if any) attributed to the target brain region prior to obliterating the vascular supply by embolization or surgical resection.

Introduction: selective WADA test

Patients suffering from chronic, intractable medial temporal lobe epilepsy who are candidates for temporal lobectomy traditionally have undergone the conventional intracarotid artery amobarbital (Wada) test prior to surgery. The conventional Wada test consists of an injection of a GABA$_A$-agonist, amobarbital, a short-acting barbiturate, into one or both internal carotid arteries, followed by neuropsychological tests that are designed to identify speech regions, the seizure focus, and predict post-operative memory function following temporal lobe surgical resection.[1–17] Non-selective intracarotid Wada procedures have been shown to have inconsistencies in their results and have led to difficulty in localization of memory,[18] language,[19] and neurobehavioral functional areas.[19] The reasons for these inconsistencies are: (1) non-selective Wada testing does not selectively inhibit the arterial territory supplying the lesion but inhibits the entire hemisphere making it hard to localize precisely the area of eloquence, memory and language; and (2) GABA$_A$-agonists (such as amobarbital) only inhibit gray matter and not white matter structures. Selective Wada techniques enable inhibition of the arterial territory of a selective branch supplying a specific functional and anatomic location in the brain, allowing for a reliable prediction of postoperative memory function.[20] Exclusive delivery of amobarbital to the mediobasal temporal lobe structures is of particular interest if selective amygdalohippocampectomy is the intended treatment.[5,21–26]

Anatomical considerations
Blood supply of the limbic system

The major components of the limbic system, the amygdala, hippocampal formation (the structure most widely accredited with memory encoding), and the parahippocampal gyrus, are located within the medial part of the temporal lobe.[27] Global memory processing is thought to require most of the structures within the medial temporal lobe. The middle cerebral, internal carotid, anterior choroidal and posterior cerebral arteries are the major vessels that either directly or through collaterals supply the medial part of the temporal lobe.[27] Huther et al. found that segments of the main arteries were responsible for supplying the cortical structures of the temporomesial region: (1) the proximal M1 segment of the middle cerebral artery (between the carotid bifurcation and the division of the middle cerebral artery); (2) the terminal segment of the internal carotid artery; (3) the cisternal segment of the anterior choroidal artery (before the anterior choroidal artery enters the choroidal fissure); and (4) the segments of the posterior cerebral artery (between the posterior communicating artery and the origin of parieto-occipital and calcarine arteries).[27]

A large number of anastomoses between different cerebral arteries have been documented in the temporomesial region, suggesting that there is potential for a selectively injected short acting anesthetic agent to diffuse to other regions.[27]

The hippocampus has an anterior and a posterior arterial supply. The posterior cerebral artery, not the internal carotid artery, is the main arterial supply of the medial temporal lobe with the exception of the amygdala, the uncus and a small portion of the anterior hippocampal formation.[28–33] The anterior choroidal artery supplies the amygdaloid body, the anterior hippocampus, and the fascia dentata (dentate gyrus).[28] The posterior cerebral artery exclusively supplies the posterior hippocampus. There is an overlapping arterial supply to the anterior hippocampus via the anterior choroidal artery and the posterior cerebral artery.[27,34–38] The entire hippocampus is anesthetized when amobarbital is injected

Textbook of Interventional Neurology, ed. Adnan I. Qureshi. Published by Cambridge University Press. © Cambridge University Press 2011.

into the ambient (P2) segment of the posterior cerebral artery.[39] Erdem *et al.* studied the microsurgical anatomy of the arterial supply to the hippocampus in 30 hemispheres. The majority of the blood supply perfusing the hippocampal formation was contributed by the posterior cerebral artery, directly and indirectly through its branches.[34] The hippocampal branches of the anterior choroidal artery and the hippocampal branches of the posterior cerebral artery anastomose at the uncal sulcus. The anterior choroidal artery, after passing through the choroid fissure, contributes branches to the lateral plexus and medial perforating branches within the choroid plexus.[34]

Anterior choroidal artery

The medial temporal lobe is supplied by branches of the cisternal segment of the anterior choroidal artery originating from the internal carotid artery.[29,32] There is considerable variability in the anatomy of the anterior choroidal artery. In some cases, branches of the posterior cerebral artery, not the anterior choroidal artery, supply the anterior third of the hippocampus and even the amygdala. The diameter of the first three centimeters of the anterior choroidal artery may indicate the number of branches that originate from it. If the diameter of the anterior choroidal artery decreases within the first three centimeters of its course, this indicates that the number of branches originating in this part of the artery will be high. There is also a high probability that the uncal branches will supply the anterior parts of the parahippocampal gyrus and the hippocampus. The caudal or dorsal uncal branches are reported to originate at a distance of 0.1–10 mm and 10.1–16 mm from the origin of the anterior choroidal artery from the internal carotid artery.[28]

Posterior cerebral artery

The ambient (P2) segment of the posterior cerebral artery gives off the hippocampal arteries. The hippocampal arteries form an arcade in the choroidal fissure, which ultimately supplies the hippocampal formation. A minor contribution from the anterior choroidal artery is seen at the anterior hippocampal formation. Extending from the basilar artery bifurcation to the ambient (P2) cistern is the peduncular (P1) segment of the posterior cerebral artery. Placing the catheter tip in the mid to distal peduncular segment would be optimal, when administering the amobarbital for provocative testing.[32,40] The posterior cerebral artery supplies the medial temporal lobe structures including the hippocampal formation, the parahippocampal gyrus and half of the inferior temporal gyrus and underlying white matter.[29–33,41] The medial temporal memory circuit at the level of the hippocampal formation will be interrupted with a selective amobarbital injection into the posterior cerebral artery, while leaving frontal, parietal and peri-Sylvian temporal functions intact. A direct "fetal" type origin of the posterior cerebral artery from the internal carotid artery occurs in approximately 10% of the adult population. In the absence of a fetal type origin, an amobarbital injection into

Table 17.1. Undesired side effects of conventional Wada procedure[42,46–61]

Phantom limb movements
Euphoria
Agitation/aggression
Crying
Behavioral disturbances: fear, verbal/physical disinhibition
Attentional disturbances
Aphasia

the internal carotid artery will not reach most of the medial temporal lobe – specifically, not the hippocampal formation – but will anesthetize most of the ipsilateral hemisphere.[29,32,40]

Conventional intracarotid amobarbital test limitations

Critics of the conventional intracarotid sodium amobarbital test question the reliability of the test for predicting postoperative memory function for two main reasons.[42] First, the internal carotid artery perfuses the uncus, amygdala and anterior hippocampus but not the posterior two-thirds of the hippocampus in the majority of patients.[27,34–40,42–45] Second, as a result of inactivating widespread hemispheric structures, memory testing is confounded by simultaneous inhibition of multiple areas. (see Table 17.1) The complication rate in the conventional intracarotid amobarbital procedure is approximately 0–5%.[42]

Selective WADA procedures

Selective Wada tests deliver amobarbital to specific regions of the brain, avoiding the confounding effects of inhibiting the entire brain's hemisphere. Sodium amobarbital can selectively be injected into the posterior cerebral artery, the anterior choroidal artery, or into the internal carotid artery during temporary balloon occlusion distal to the origin of the anterior choroidal artery [8,9,25,28,40,43,62,63]. Selective Wada testing has also been performed in the middle cerebral artery territory, suggesting that it can contribute to the risk assessment concerning post-surgical motor deficits before functional hemispherectomy; however, the indications are not well defined.[5,64,65] The medial temporal lobe regions are perfused in only approximately 30% of the patients with the conventional intracarotid amobarbital procedure.[28]

Indications for selective WADA testing

Selective anesthesia of the peduncular (P1) segment of the posterior cerebral artery is performed [7,40,66,67] when the assessment of memory function is the primary concern[5,64]; without contributing significantly to the euphoric and dysphoric responses seen with the non-selective intracarotid artery amobarbital test.[19]

Selective anesthesia of the middle cerebral artery vascular territory has been undertaken for evaluation of language function in patients who have a demonstrated persistent massive anterior cross-flow during an internal carotid artery angiogram; despite an optimally adjusted injection pressure.[28,46,67] The indication also may include bilateral structural and/or functional temporal lobe deficits according to neuroimaging methods (computed tomography, magnetic resonance imaging, Tc-hexamethylpropyleneamine oxime-single photon emission computed tomography and positron emission tomography with the glucose analog [18F] fluorodeoxyglucose).[28] Patients who have failed non-selective intracarotid amobarbital testing or had acute drug reactions which interfered with subsequent memory testing are candidates for either the selective posterior cerebral artery or anterior choroidal artery amobarbital test.[7,67,68] Selective anesthesia of the territory of the peduncular (P1) segment of the posterior cerebral artery is performed when the assessment of memory function is the primary concern without contributing significantly to the euphoric and dysphoric responses seen with the non-selective intracarotid artery amobarbital test.[68] Selective anesthesia of the territory of the middle cerebral artery has been undertaken for evaluation of language functions in patients when the internal carotid artery angiograms showed persistent massive anterior cross-flow, despite having an optimally adjusted injection pressure.[68] Standard internal carotid artery provocative testing is inaccurate when the anterior cross-flow of blood is present.[68]

Selective anterior choroidal artery amobarbital injections

Principles and indications

Selective perfusion of the anterior medial temporal lobe structures is attempted through the selective injection of amobarbital into the anterior choroidal artery or the internal carotid artery during temporary balloon occlusion distal to the origin of the anterior choroidal artery.[8] The test is performed in patients suffering from intractable temporal lobe epilepsy, who are at risk of severe post-operative verbal memory decline or global amnesia. The method leads to functional inactivation almost restricted to the hippocampal formation. Isolating the hippocampal formation enables a test of memory function without aphasia, attention deficits or behavioral disturbances.[46] Vulliemoz et al. concluded that the selective anterior choroidal injection can be used to screen for severe post-operative amnesia in inconclusive cases but cannot predict individual post-operative outcome, even when the perfusion pattern is taken into account using single photon emission computed tomography.[67] They performed selective anterior choroidal artery amobarbital testing on 17 patients with temporal lobe epilepsy and observed major variations in the selective anterior choroidal artery perfusion pattern that did not correlate with the verbal memory scores. Even though there were no patients who experienced a severe verbal memory

decline post-operatively, results during the selective anterior choroidal artery amobarbital test were found to give an insufficient estimate of the individual decline in post-operative verbal memory.

The study conducted by Wieser et al. showed a statistically significant correlation between the memory results of the anterior selective injections and the outcome following the selective amygdalohippocampectomy.[28] The postoperative verbal memory performance was well predicted by the selective amobarbital temporal lobe test, but prediction of nonverbal ("figural") memory was less accurate, i.e., the selective anterior temporal lobe amobarbital procedures underestimate the risk of post-operative figural memory performance.[28]

Anticipated clinical deficits

The observed clinical deficits associated with selective anterior choroidal arterial injections are caused by the functional interruption of pathways in the posterior limb of the internal capsule. Selective catheterization and injection of amobarbital into the anterior choroidal artery has been associated with a variety of clinical deficits: motor deficits, language disturbance, cranial nerve VII palsy, somatosensory disturbances, visual field defects and ptosis. Anesthesia of the optic tract leads to hemianopsia.[28] The ophthalmic nerve, which has sensory, motor, sympathetic, and parasympathetic fibers, is supplied by the ophthalmic artery. Miosis and eventually ptosis can be seen after the paralysis of sympathetic fibers. Anesthesia of the motor fibers can also lead to miosis and ptosis and the loss of the parasympathetic input will lead to mydriasis.[28]

Technical challenges

A variable perfusion pattern of amobarbital has been reported after it was selectively injected into the anterior choroidal artery and this may explain the lack of predictive value for certain memory functions.[67] Widespread involvement of structures involved in memory function, like the frontal, temporal and parieto-occipital lobes, as well as subcortical structures (thalamus), have been seen. Interpreting significant memory decline in patients with an extensive pattern of perfusion can lead to results that do not accurately predict the eventual memory deficits following selective surgical resection.[69] The variability can be attributed to a combination of anatomical variations and technical aspects like reflux and catheter displacement.[67]

Concurrent balloon occlusion distal to origin of anterior choroidal artery

Sodium amobarbital can be selectively injected into the internal carotid artery during temporary balloon occlusion distal to the origin of the anterior choroidal artery, with subsequent amobarbital inactivation of the territories of the anterior choroidal arteries, the posterior communicating artery and the ophthalmic artery. A variety of neurologic deficits are associated with this procedure: motor deficits, language disturbance, cranial nerve VII palsy, somatosensory disturbances, visual field defects and ophthalmic artery defects (ptosis, miosis, and mydriasis).[28] According to Wieser et al., the ophthalmic deficits were seen with balloon occlusion of the internal carotid artery technique only if the catheter tip was not accurately placed at the orificium of the anterior choroidal artery.[28] Theoretically, there is also a risk of involuntary disconnection of the balloon, potentially causing a hypoxic/anoxic environment for the anterior or middle cerebral artery territories.[28]

Selective posterior cerebral artery injection

Principles and indications

Selective posterior cerebral artery amobarbital injection inactivates the mesial temporal lobe more precisely compared with conventional intracarotid artery amobarbital testing, because it delivers the amobarbital more effectively to the ipsilateral hippocampal formation.[7,28,40,43,66,70–72] The posterior cerebral artery amobarbital injection tests only memory function, but not language function.[7,28,40,43,66,72] The selective posterior cerebral artery technique requires immediate memory testing following the injection to assess function during the time when the drug has its peak effect. Selective posterior cerebral artery injection in the dominant hemisphere avoids the occurrence of aphasia because amobarbital does not affect the temporal speech area.[32,40] The anterior and posterior temporal arteries that arise from the posterior cerebral artery supply only the inferior surface of the temporal lobe but not the temporal speech area.[40] The preliminary results of the report by Jack et al. suggest that selective left-sided injection into the posterior cerebral artery produces a greater impairment in verbal recall under antegrade amnesia testing conditions than right-sided injection.[40] This parallels the known response to surgical resection for temporal lobe seizure.[73] Patients perform more poorly on post-operative verbal memory testing after left lobectomy compared with right lobectomy. This observation supports the idea that amobarbital injection into the posterior cerebral artery may more accurately predict the effect of the operation.[40]

Technical considerations

The selective posterior cerebral artery injection is more time consuming than the non-selective intracarotid artery amobarbital procedure. The presence of increased tortuosity of the vertebral arteries at the C1 and C2 level will limit catheter control.[7,40] The patient must be cooperative enough to lie motionless in order to create an angiographic roadmap for selective catheterization. The tip of the microcatheter should be placed in the mid to distal peduncular (P1) segment of the posterior cerebral artery, which will enable amobarbital perfusion of the vascular bed distal to the peduncular (P1) segment, including the following structures: subiculum, dentate gyrus, hippocampus and associated white matter tracts.[40]

Anticipated deficits

The neurological deficits observed with the posterior cerebral artery amobarbital injection are explained by dysfunction of structures that are supplied by branches of the peduncular (P1) and ambient (P2) segment of the posterior cerebral artery. The proximal portion of the posterior cerebral artery originating at the bifurcation of the basilar artery and extending to the point where the posterior cerebral artery courses posteriorly and superiorly to enter the ambient cistern is identified as the peduncular (P1) segment of the posterior cerebral artery.[32,40] Marginal amobarbital perfusion of the vascular bed derived from the peduncular (P1) segment may be seen secondary to the placement of the microcatheter.[32,33,40] Amobarbital perfusion of small branches that supply the ipsilateral corticospinal tract in the cerebral peduncle and arise from the peduncular (P1) segment will lead to contralateral hand weakness.[28]

Contralateral hemisensory symptoms, such as dysesthesia with decreased sensation of touch, appear to be a result of amobarbital perfusion of the thalamus.[28] Excellent amobarbital perfusion of the ambient (P2) segment will lead to the development of these symptoms because of the significant blood supply the thalamus receives from branches of the ambient (P2) segment such as: (1) thalamo-geniculate-perforating branches; and (2) posterior lateral choroidal artery.[32,33]

Amobarbital perfusion of branches of the ambient (P2) segment that supply the visual cortex, such as the calcarine artery and accessory branches from the posterior temporal and parieto-occipital arteries as well as to the ipsilateral lateral geniculate body from the posterior lateral choroidal artery, lead to contralateral hemianopsia.[28,32] Contralateral hemianopsia and hemisensory impairment last for approximately 3–5 minutes and rarely interfere with the memory testing if the testing items are properly presented in the preserved visual field.[7,32,33,40]

Complications

The risks associated with catheter manipulation are greater in intracranial vessels compared with extracranial arteries. Transient signs of vasospasm, subarachnoid hemorrhage secondary to vessel perforation, cranial nerve VII palsy, aphasia (1–3 minutes), severe headache, diplopia, speech comprehension difficulties, and nausea have been reported with the selective posterior cerebral artery procedure.[7,25,66] One potential complication that also must be considered is the possibility of an accidental reflux of amobarbital into the basilar artery during the selective posterior cerebral artery test, leading to respiratory failure.[40] Wada and Rasmussen reported a case of inadvertent injection of 200 mg of amytal directly into a vertebral artery while attempting an intracarotid artery amobarbital test via direct puncture in the neck.[3] This patient required ventilatory support for 15 minutes, however his cardiovascular status remained stable throughout; no long term sequelae were observed.[40] Brain stem inactivation can also theoretically impair cardiovascular centers leading to hypotension.

Selective middle cerebral artery injection

Principles and indications

In the pre-surgical evaluation of patients with drug resistant epilepsy, the selective amobarbital middle cerebral artery injection with subsequent testing is performed infrequently.[5] The selective middle cerebral artery injection may be indicated in patients who will need functional hemispherectomy in order to treat a developmental or early acquired hemispheric lesion involving the motor cortex.[5] This technique is used to functionally inactivate the affected motor cortex prior to functional hemispherectomy, particularly in patients with incompletely maintained fine motor control (e.g., flexion of fingers, opposition of thumb) of the contralateral hand and fingers. By functionally inactivating the target motor cortex and disconnecting it from the healthy brain, it is possible to identify whether any contralateral hand plegia will develop post-operatively. Similarly, selective middle cerebral artery injection has been successfully used to identify the pre-operative vascular territory with the greatest risk of causing neurological deficit in a patient with a fusiform aneurysm of the anterosuperior division of the right middle cerebral artery.[74] Selective middle cerebral artery Wada injection using amobarbital, has also been successfully used to evaluate whether, and in which areas, ictal epileptic discharges could be suppressed in two children with electrographic status epilepticus in sleep.[5]

Adjunctive use of single photon emission computed tomography (SPECT)

Amobarbital injection may be simultaneously combined with ^{99m}Tc hexamethyl-propyleneamine oxime and the regions of inactivity assessed by single photon emission computed tomography reflecting the effect of the amobarbital. Both ^{99m}Tc hexamethyl-propyleneamine oxime (octanol partition coefficient of 80) and amobarbital (octanol partition coefficient 71) are lipophilic. The use of single photon emission computed tomography after simultaneous intra-arterial injection of amobarbital and ^{99m}Tc hexamethyl-propyleneamine oxime can be used to monitor the hypoactivity (low regional cerebral blood flow) induced by the amobarbital within the hippocampus.[2,25,28,64,75–78] Understanding the regions of hypoactivity induced by selectively administering amobarbital helps in the interpretation of the results obtained during neuropsychological testing.[2,27]

Adjunctive use of cerebral angiography

Cerebral angiographic images are used to identify anatomic variations that may affect the distribution of the anesthetic agent.[79] Differences in injection volume and pressure, greater viscosity of the contrast medium, position of the catheter, and variation of the cardiac cycle, may lead to an inaccurate assessment of arterial anatomy. The contralateral anterior circulation may fill, through the anterior communicating artery, in the event that a higher pressure or volume injection is used; therefore similar injection volume and pressure (preferably low to avoid cross filling) should be used during contrast and amobarbital injection.[28,79]

Cerebral angiography is also used to assess the size and anatomy of the posterior cerebral artery. The posterior cerebral artery can be of adult or fetal type. The fetal type fills from the internal carotid artery via the posterior communicating artery and needs to be identified prior to attempting internal carotid or posterior cerebral artery amobarbital injections.[25]

Adjunctive use of electro-encephalography (EEG)

Clinical neurological deficits may not be adequate in estimating the regional inactivation following amobarbital injection. A reliable interpretation of the effects of the selective tests can be performed using either intracranial EEG recorded from depth electrodes or foramen ovale electrodes in combination with scalp EEG.[28,80,81] Wieser et al. showed that foramen ovale electrodes reliably detected hippocampal EEG activity, whereas scalp recording alone may not detect hippocampal EEG changes.[80] Vulliemoz et al. utilized EEG to exclude the occurrence of subclinical seizures during selective anterior choroidal artery amobarbital injection.[67]

Selective pre-embolization provocative testing

The use of lidocaine and brevital in superselective provocative testing can increase the sensitivity and predictive value of pre-surgical or pre-embolization testing, potentially reducing the frequency of treatment-related morbidity.[19,40,64,66,82,83] A detailed account has been provided in the chapter on arteriovenous malformations. The co-administration of the local anesthetic, lidocaine, to inhibit white matter tracts, helps detect eloquent brain function not revealed by the individual administration of the gray matter specific brevital or amobarbital. The deficits detected by the addition of lidocaine are clinically relevant to treatment planning. All the studies using sequential administration of GABAA-agonists for gray matter and lidocaine for white matter tract inhibition have been with superselective injection and have been shown to be safe, feasible, and effective in treatment planning.[19]

Treatment implications

Selective amygdalohippocampectomy is the treatment of choice in patients who suffer from intractable medial temporal lobe epilepsy. The post-operative memory performance can be reliably predicted and most importantly the occurrence of post-operative unexpected severe amnesia can be avoided using the selective anterior and posterior circulation amobarbital injections with subsequent neurological assessment.[28,84–89] Approximately 70%–80% of patients who undergo unilateral anterior temporal lobectomy with selective amygdalohippocampectomy are seizure-free at follow-up.[28,40,90–95]

Venous sampling

Invasive central venous sampling diagnostic tests have been used to evaluate the hormonal composition of the venous environment in either the cavernous sinus, inferior petrosal sinus or the internal jugular vein. By sampling the blood in the venous environment surrounding the pituitary gland, the systemic dilution effect is minimized, allowing for a more accurate measurement of pituitary specific hormones. Bilateral cavernous sinus sampling, bilateral inferior petrosal sinus sampling and bilateral internal jugular venous sampling are the diagnostic tests that have been used to study the unilateral concentration of pituitary hormones. The venous sampling is used for detecting pituitary origin of Cushing's disease and for localizing the pituitary tumor to a particular side. The sensitivity and specificity of these diagnostic tests have improved over the course of three decades with better understanding of the technique and interpretation of testing.[96–98]

Anatomy of venous drainage of the pituitary gland

Clinically significant adenomas are located in the anterior lobe of the pituitary gland. Immediately lateral to the pituitary fossa are venous channels called the cavernous sinuses. The major portion within the cavernous sinus is occupied by the carotid artery. Cranial nerves run through the lateral wall of the cavernous sinus. Three sinuses that run transversely across the sella turcica interconnect the cavernous sinuses. Lying between the anterior surface of the anterior pituitary lobe and the anterior margin of the sella turcica is the anterior intercavernous sinus. Between the posterior surface of the posterior pituitary lobe and the posterior clinoid plate lies the posterior intercavernous sinus. Crossing the floor of the sella turcica just in front of the groove between the anterior and posterior lobes is the inferior intercavernous sinus.

On the surface of the pituitary gland there are two plexiform venous networks that drain laterally either into the intercavernous sinuses or directly into the cavernous sinuses. The small hypophyseal veins exiting directly from the anterior lobe enter the surface of the plexiform networks. Ipsilateral drainage of each half of the anterior lobe occurs into the corresponding cavernous sinus and ultimately into the inferior petrosal sinus.[98–100] The inferior petrosal sinus is a dural sinus that extends from the posterior aspect of the cavernous sinus approximately 23–28 mm laterally and posteriorly to the internal jugular vein (see Fig. 17.1))[101]. It is positioned just laterally to the clivus, along the posterior inferior edge of the petrous ridge. The inferior petrosal sinus usually exits the cranial cavity through the jugular foramen, through an opening separated from the rest of the foramen by the anterior petro-occipital ligament.[101] In the majority of individuals, the inferior petrosal sinus becomes a vein, approximately 2 cm in diameter, as it enters the jugular foramen, prior to draining into the internal jugular vein.[101,102] As the inferior petrosal sinus travels through the dura it receives venous blood from the dura, pons, medulla, internal auditory meatus and the

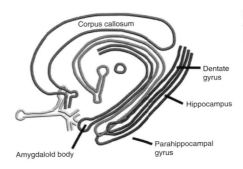

Fig. 17.1. Pituitary venous drainage. See plate section.

anterior condylar vein (a vein that communicates with a plexus surrounding the hypoglossal nerve in the condylar foramen, i.e., the hypoglossal canal).[103] Both inferior petrosal sinuses communicate with one another through the basilar venous plexus along the clivus and with the marginal sinus at the anterior margin of the foramen magnum.[101] The inferior petrosal sinus decreases in diameter from 7–10 mm at the cavernous sinus to 2–4 mm as it approaches the jugular foramen indicating that blood flow in the inferior petrosal sinus seems to be directed mainly to the vertebral venous plexus.[102]

Anatomic variants

There is substantial variability at the rostrocaudal level at which the inferior petrosal sinus enters the internal jugular vein. Shiu *et al.* documented variability in the junction between the inferior petrosal sinus and the internal jugular vein.[104] Based on studies looking at cavernous sinus venography, Shiu *et al.* described the appearance and relative frequency of four separate and distinct types of venous drainage of the inferior petrosal sinus (Type I–IV) (see Table 17.2).[104,105,106] (see Fig. 17.2[101,104])

Bilateral inferior petrosal sinus sampling is anatomically possible in 99% of people.[107] Miller *et al.* found that in four out of 692 patients (less than 0.6%), there was no connection between the inferior petrosal sinus and the internal jugular vein.[101] In another prospective study of 136 patients with Cushing's syndrome who underwent bilateral inferior petrosal sinus sampling, no anastomosis between the inferior petrosal sinus and the internal jugular vein was observed in approximately 1% of the patients.[107] In the same study the incomplete type IV venous drainage was found in 5% of patients.[107]

Miller *et al.* also described an incomplete type IV drainage configuration, where most of the venous drainage from the inferior petrosal sinus was via the anterior condylar vein and the vertebral venous plexus, but a small connection persisted between the inferior petrosal sinus and the internal jugular vein, which was amenable to catheterization.[101]

Symmetry of pituitary venous drainage

Venous flow through the cavernous and inferior petrosal sinuses, as determined through venography, can be

Table 17.2. Venous drainage patterns of the inferior petrosal sinus

Types	Prevalence	Characteristics
Type I	45%	Inferior petrosal sinus drains directly into the internal jugular bulb
Type II	24%	The sinus anastomosis, either directly or through a communicating vein, to the anterior condylar vein, which extends from the marginal sinus around the foramen magnum to the vertebral venous plexus
Type III	24%	Inferior petrosal sinus exists as a plexus of veins rather than as a single vessel. The inferior petrosal sinus drains into the internal jugular vein and (via the marginal sinus and the anterior condylar vein) into the vertebral venous plexus, which also forms an anastomosis extensively with the basilar venous plexus coursing along the surface of the clivus
Type IV	7%	Inferior petrosal sinus drains directly into the vertebral venous plexus. There is no connection between the inferior petrosal sinus and the internal jugular vein in a true type IV pattern; instead, the inferior petrosal sinus drains directly into the anterior condylar vein

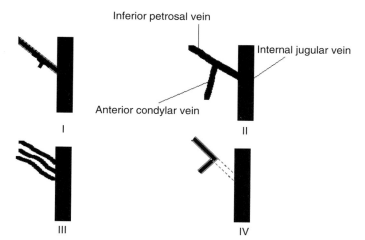

Fig. 17.2. Venous anatomy: Type I–IV. Type I: anastomosis between the inferior petrosal sinus and the internal jugular vein; the anterior condylar vein is small or absent. Type II: a prominent anastomosis between the large anterior condylar vein and the inferior petrosal sinus is present. Type III: the inferior petrosal sinus exists as several small channels, which may form a plexus. Type IV: the inferior petrosal sinus empties directly into the anterior condylar vein, never anastomosing with the internal jugular vein.

asymmetric or symmetric. Pituitary venous drainage is described as symmetric when the majority of the venous effluent from each side of the pituitary drains into the ipsilateral inferior petrosal sinus. Approximately 60% of individuals have symmetric pituitary venous drainage.[101,108,109] Symmetric venous flow increases the sensitivity of lateralization when bilateral inferior petrosal sinus sampling is performed. Mamelak *et al.* defined symmetric venous anatomy if both cavernous and inferior petrosal sinuses were patent, filled from a unilateral injection of contrast material and drained primarily into the inferior petrosal sinus ipsilateral to the site of injection. If cross-filling of the contralateral cavernous sinus and inferior petrosal sinus occurred bilaterally in approximately equal proportions, the venous drainage pattern was considered symmetric. Any other type of drainage pattern was considered asymmetric.[108]

In the case of asymmetric unilateral venous drainage patterns, cavernous sinus venous blood will mix significantly with the blood of the contralateral inferior petrosal sinus, with confounding of the lateralization data obtained from bilateral sampling.[108] The location of the adenoma in the pituitary gland may also influence the magnitude and laterality of the gradient. Artificial elevation of adrenocorticotropin hormone concentrations would be seen in the situation where hormone rich blood from the cavernous sinus on the side of the tumor is directed into the contralateral inferior petrosal sinus. Shunting of blood away from one inferior petrosal sinus to the other would reduce the adrenocorticotropin hormone concentration in that sinus, resulting in incorrect lateralization of the adenoma. The most common asymmetric venous drainage pattern is blood from both cavernous sinuses draining into the right inferior petrosal sinus, with no significant drainage into the left.[108]

Prior to bilateral inferior petrosal sinus sampling, a complete venogram of the basilar sinuses should be obtained to identify asymmetric drainage patterns that may affect interpretation of lateralization data.[108] Lateralization data obtained from patients who are found to have asymmetric venous drainage must be interpreted with great caution. In a study of 23 patents with Cushing's disease, conducted by Mamelak *et al.*, the cavernous sinus and inferior petrosal sinus were catheterized bilaterally and the flow of venous blood was observed using venous angiography.[108] Fourteen patients (61%) had bilaterally symmetric venous drainage and nine patients (39%) were asymmetric. Bilateral inferior petrosal sinus sampling correctly lateralized the tumor in 12 out of the 14 patients with symmetric drainage. In contrast, correct lateralization was observed in four out of the nine patients with asymmetric drainage. In a recent study by Lefournier *et al.*, the accuracy of lateralization of pituitary tumors increased to 86% when patients had symmetric venograms and the catheters were positioned in a low or middle location within the bilateral inferior petrosal sinuses.[109]

Inferior petrosal sinus sampling

Bilateral inferior petrosal sinus sampling is the preferred method of the venous sampling techniques used in the identification of the etiology of adrenocorticotropin hormone dependent Cushing's syndrome in children, adults and during pregnancy.[110,111] Bilateral inferior petrosal sinus sampling provides a higher sensitivity and better specificity than other available biochemical testing strategies in patients who do not have a pituitary lesion greater than 1 cm in size on magnetic resonance imaging (MRI).[112] Data collected during the procedure enable the pituitary micro-adenoma to be lateralized, providing the neurosurgeon information needed to appropriately select the treatment approach. The procedure has also been used in the evaluation of patients with pituitary micro-adenomas secreting growth hormone.[101,113–116]

As with any diagnostic procedure, false positive and false negative results can occur.[117–120] Technical difficulties and complications associated with the bilateral inferior petrosal sinus sampling procedure also must be considered.

The pretest probability of a pituitary source of adrenocorticotropin hormone (Cushing's disease) is estimated to be approximately 90% in unselected patients presenting with adrenocorticotropin hormone dependent Cushing's syndrome (See Table 17.3[112,121,122]). The challenge of differentiating between Cushing's disease and ectopic adrenocorticotropin hormone syndrome requires the measurement of plasma adrenocorticotropin hormone levels, non-invasive dynamic tests, and imaging studies, like MRI (see Table 17.4).[112] A combination of these tests is usually necessary as none of these tests have a 100% specificity[122] (see Table 17.5[112,117,122,123]).

Seventy to 80% of endogenous Cushing syndrome is a result of adrenocorticotropin hormone (ACTH) dependent Cushing's syndrome. Eighty to 90% of ACTH dependent Cushing's syndrome is caused by ACTH secreting pituitary adenomas. Ten–20% of adrenocorticotropin hormone (ACTH) dependent Cushing's syndrome is caused by adrenocorticotropin hormone (ACTH) producing ectopic tumors.

Indications for inferior petrosal sinus sampling

Relying solely on imaging and non-invasive biochemical tests may potentially result in inappropriate trans-sphenoidal surgery.[124] Incidental pituitary lesions have been reported to occur in 6.1% of the patients in an autopsy series of unselected patients.[125,126] An MRI study found that approximately 10% of the normal adult population had abnormalities compatible with asymptomatic pituitary microadenomas.[127] To make the diagnosis of Cushing's disease, it has been reported that bilateral inferior petrosal sinus sampling is more sensitive than pituitary MRI.[128] Bilateral inferior petrosal sinus sampling procedure is the gold standard for establishing the origin of adrenocorticotropin hormone secretion. Bilateral inferior petrosal sinus sampling is recommended for patients with an already established diagnosis of Cushing's syndrome whose biochemical (non-invasive testing) or radiological (pituitary MRI) studies are discordant or equivocal in identifying the pituitary or ectopic origin of the abnormal adrenocorticotropin hormone production (see Fig. 17.3).[110,122,129–136] Among

Table 17.3. Endogenous Cushing's syndrome summary

Endogenous Cushing's syndrome
• ACTH dependent Cushing's syndrome (70%–80%)
A. ACTH secreting pituitary adenomas: Cushing's disease (80%–90%)
B. ACTH producing ectopic tumors (10%–20%)
• Bronchial Carcinoids: most common

Table 17.4. Descending order of prevalence of neoplastic causes of excess adrenocorticotropin hormone secretion

Pituitary corticotroph adenomas
Ectopic adrenocorticotropin hormone secreting tumors
Ectopic corticotropin releasing hormone secreting tumors (very rare)

Table 17.5. Non-invasive biochemical tests used to distinguish between pituitary and ectopic adrenocorticotropin hormone dependent Cushing's syndrome

Dexamethasone suppressed CRH stimulation test
High dose dexamethasone suppression test
Low dose dexamethasone suppression test
Peripheral metyrapone stimulation test
Peripheral CRH test
Peripheral desmopressin stimulation test
Plasma ACTH concentration

ACTH: adrenocorticotropin hormone, CRH: corticotropin releasing hormone.

pituitary Cushing's patients, 18%–65% do not have concordant results between biochemical and imaging studies.[132]

A review of the literature does not establish a consensus among investigators regarding the precise indications for the bilateral inferior petrosal sinus sampling. Some investigators recommend the bilateral inferior petrosal sinus sampling procedure in patients with ACTH dependent Cushing's syndrome with a pituitary MRI without evidence of any abnormalities.[135] However, some investigators recommend performing the inferior petrosal sampling in all patients with a positive MRI study and discordant biochemical tests.[136]

Technical aspects of inferior petrosal sinus catheterization

The bilateral inferior sinus sampling procedure is performed with posteroanterior fluoroscopy and with the patient's head held in a neutral position. The origin of the inferior petrosal sinus is best identified in the lateral plane; concomitant anteroposterior images identify reflux into the opposite inferior petrosal sinus.[101]

Once the catheter is in the internal jugular vein, the catheter tip is rotated so that it is directed medially and anteriorly. The

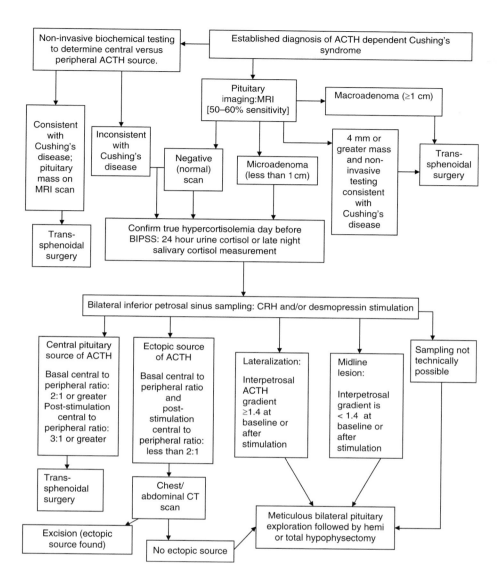

Fig. 17.3. Bilateral inferior petrosal sinus sampling algorithm. Abbreviations: BIPSS, bilateral inferior petrosal sinus sampling; ACTH, adrenocorticotropin hormone; MRI, magnetic resource imaging.

catheter tip is held several centimeters below the expected level of the inferior petrosal sinus. While the catheter is in this position, the guidewire (only a guidewire coated with hydrophilic material should be used) is advanced until it enters a medially directed vein. The trajectory of guide wire movement can indicate its position. Miller *et al.* suggested that guide wire movement, superiorly and medially or medially and then superiorly, is indicative of placement within the inferior petrosal sinus. Miller *et al.* caution against advancing the catheter more than 1 to 1.5 cm into the inferior petrosal sinus. If the guidewire continues to advance medially, almost to the midline, or starts to head inferiorly instead of superiorly, the wire may have entered the anterior condylar vein. In this situation, the catheter tip should be withdrawn slightly and the guide wire should be re-advanced with its tip directed superiorly to engage and enter the anterior portion of the inferior petrosal sinus.[101]

The side-to-side variability in the venous anatomy of the inferior petrosal sinuses will determine how difficult it is to catheterize them. It has been shown that a small inferior petrosal sinus on one side is associated with a larger sinus on the contralateral side. Similarly, a variable junction between the inferior petrosal sinus and the internal jugular vein according to its type of venous drainage pattern (type I–IV) will also contribute to the level of difficulty of the procedure. When faced with a situation where one inferior petrosal sinus is extremely difficult to catheterize, the operator is encouraged to catheterize the contralateral inferior petrosal sinus in order to visualize the anatomy of the other inferior petrosal sinus through contrast reflux.[101]

In the event of a rare, true type IV drainage pattern (no connection between the internal jugular vein and the inferior petrosal sinus) Miller *et al.* attempted, but failed to access the inferior petrosal sinus using the vertebral vein.[101] On the other hand, Landolt *et al.* were able to successfully navigate the catheter into the inferior petrosal sinus via the vertebral vein.[137]

Direct percutaneous internal jugular vein access may be necessary in the case of femoral vein occlusion, such as: (1) the presence of an inferior vena cava filter; or (2) aberrant anatomy of the great veins. Miller *et al.* cannulated the internal jugular vein using direct ultrasound guided puncture of the internal jugular veins as inferiorly as possible in the neck because most Cushing's syndrome patients have short, thick necks.[101]

The sensitivity of the bilateral inferior petrosal sinus sampling has been shown to be operator dependent. An increased sensitivity for the procedure was obtained when additional expertise and skills were obtained after a very large number of procedures.[97]

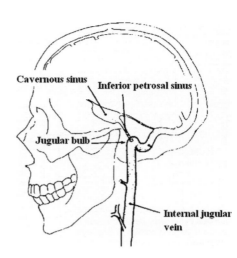

Fig. 17.4. Lateral view of the skull outlining the ipsilateral cavernous sinus, inferior petrosal sinus and internal jugular vein. The anteromedial aspect of the jugular bulb is where the inferior petrosal sinus enters the internal jugular vein.

Comparison of bilateral inferior petrosal sinus and internal jugular venous sampling

Bilateral inferior petrosal sinus sampling is more sensitive than bilateral internal jugular venous sampling with or without corticotropin releasing hormone stimulation.[132,138,139] Earlier studies of basal internal jugular venous sampling were disappointing, possibly because catheter placement in the jugular bulb may have been above the entry of inferior petrosal sinus effluent[140,141] or because corticotropin releasing hormone stimulation was not used (see Fig. 17.4). Although bilateral internal jugular vein sampling is technically a simpler procedure, bilateral inferior petrosal sinus sampling is recommended as the confirmatory test when there is a lack of a central to peripheral adrenocorticotropin hormone gradient (suggestive of an ectopic adrenocorticotropin hormone syndrome) and when there is only a gradient above the cut-off on basal (pre-corticotropin releasing hormone stimulation) sampling with bilateral internal jugular venous sampling.[138,139]

Comparison of bilateral inferior petrosal sinus and cavernous sinus sampling

Bilateral cavernous sinus sampling is an alternative venous sampling technique that is technically more difficult than inferior petrosal sinus sampling.[101,142,143] In comparison to bilateral internal jugular venous and bilateral inferior petrosal sinus sampling, bilateral cavernous sinus sampling is the most proximal measurement to the pituitary gland. When comparing the bilateral cavernous sinus to the bilateral inferior petrosal sinus sampling techniques, a consensus has not been reached regarding which technique is more sensitive in: (1) identifying whether the ACTH producing microadenoma is located within the pituitary or from an ectopic source; and (2) lateralizing the microadenoma to a particular side of the pituitary gland.[96,108,109,124,144–147] Cavernous sinus sampling has a similar morbidity when compared to inferior petrosal sinus sampling alone.[142,143,147] It can be associated with cranial nerve palsies and venous thrombosis.[148]

Central to peripheral adrenocorticotropin hormone ratio: basal and post-stimulation results

A central (inferior petrosal sinus) to peripheral ACTH concentration ratio is used to distinguish between pituitary Cushing's disease and the occult ectopic ACTH syndrome. Simultaneous measurements of ACTH levels are taken from each inferior petrosal sinus and from a peripheral vein. The central to peripheral ratios are calculated at baseline (pre-stimulation) and at various time points after intravenous peripheral corticotropin releasing hormone and/or desmopressin injection. The inferior petrosal sinus time point with the highest central to peripheral ACTH ratio is used for interpretation. A central pituitary source of ACTH overproduction is presumed if the inferior petrosal sinus to peripheral (central to peripheral) ratio is 2:1 or greater at baseline or if the ratio is 3:1 or greater at any time after the peripheral administration of corticotropin releasing hormone and/or desmopressin.[97,117,149–153] If the threshold criterion is not met, a peripheral (ectopic) source can be presumed.[154,155] In most patients who have occult ectopic adrenocorticotropin hormone syndrome, a central to peripheral ratio of less than 2 is found before and after corticotropin releasing hormone and/or desmopressin administration.[97,149,150,156] The central to peripheral ratio that has the highest diagnostic sensitivity for Cushing's disease was found to occur at 5 minutes post-stimulation.[97] Serial sampling is important due to the pituitary gland's transient secretion of ACTH pre- and post-stimulation.

Pituitary stimulation: principles and indications

The negative feedback suppression of the normal pituitary corticotrophs by long standing hypercortisolemia, associated with ACTH dependent Cushing's syndrome, suppresses the normal pituitary tissue. In that situation the normal pituitary corticotrophs do not secrete basal ACTH and do not release

ACTH with corticotropin releasing hormone stimulation. Any increase in ACTH concentration following stimulation is a result of the secreting actions of neoplastic tissue, since the normal pituitary corticotrophs are being suppressed. Using corticotropin releasing hormone and/or desmopressin stimulation, the sensitivity of detecting the pituitary origin of Cushing's disease and laterality of the tumor using the bilateral inferior petrosal sinus sampling procedure increases.[97,118,157,158] Investigators have used multiple stimulants, such as thyrotropin releasing hormone, corticotropin releasing hormone, desmopressin, metyrapone, and growth hormone secreting hormone in an attempt to increase the sensitivity of bilateral inferior petrosal sinus sampling.[114,159–161]

Corticotropin releasing hormone

Ovine and human corticotropin releasing hormone stimulation have been used with no clear superiority of one over the other. Peripheral adrenocorticotropin releasing hormone and cortisol responses to ovine corticotropin releasing hormone were significantly higher than with human corticotropin releasing hormone in a study conducted by Nieman et al.[162] In contrast, a separate study found that either human or ovine corticotropin releasing hormone may be used because human corticotropin releasing hormone was found to be as effective a secretagogue as ovine corticotropin releasing hormone.[97,163] The principal difference between the two peptide sequences is in their pharmacokinetic properties. The human-sequence peptide binds to an endogenous binding peptide (corticotropin releasing hormone binding peptide), which shortens its half-life.[97,164]

Desmopressin

A significant subgroup (4%–15%) of patients with Cushing's disease fail to demonstrate diagnostic gradients during bilateral inferior petrosal sinus sampling after corticotropin releasing hormone stimulation. In an effort to improve the diagnostic sensitivity of stimulation testing, corticotropin releasing hormone and desmopressin may be used alone or sequentially.[97,165,166] Desmopressin is a long-acting vasopressin analog with a high affinity for the V2 vasopressin receptor, but a relatively low affinity for the V3 receptor that predominates in the normal pituitary gland.[133] It increases ACTH secretion in 80%–90% of patients with Cushing's disease, but only rarely in normal individuals or patients with pseudo-Cushing's syndrome.[167] Some ectopic ACTH-secreting tumors (20%–50%) may respond to desmopressin, limiting its usefulness in distinguishing the source of adrenocorticotropin hormone.[133,168–172]

Value of corticotropin releasing hormone concentrations in the petrosal sinus

In some patients, the distinction between pituitary Cushing's disease and ectopic ACTH syndrome may be difficult. In an attempt to differentiate Cushing's syndrome from pseudo-Cushing states or normal physiology, human corticotropin releasing hormone levels in the inferior petrosal sinuses were measured in one study.[173] The human corticotropin releasing hormone levels were at, or below, the limits of detection of the assay in normal individuals, ectopic ACTH syndrome patients, pseudo-Cushing's patients, true Cushing's disease patients, and in patients with Cushing's syndrome of adrenal origin. It should be noted that in patients who do not have Cushing's disease or the ectopic ACTH syndrome, administration of any opioid or benzodiazepine may lead to an inhibition of corticotropin releasing hormone secreting neurons; leading to a falsely low corticotropin releasing hormone value.[173–177] The study concluded that measuring the human corticotropin releasing hormone levels in the inferior petrosal sinuses was not useful in determining whether individual patients may have hypersecretion of corticotropin releasing hormone causing their ACTH secretion.[173]

Accuracy of identifying pituitary origin of Cushing's disease using bilateral inferior petrosal sinus sampling

The sensitivity of the bilateral inferior petrosal sinus sampling technique has varied. Studies have consistently demonstrated that the use of corticotropin releasing hormone stimulation increases the sensitivity of this diagnostic test in comparison to performing it without stimulation. Two early major series reported a 100% sensitivity and specificity for the identification of pituitary origin for Cushing's disease by using a threshold of central to peripheral ACTH ratios of 3:1 after the administration of ovine corticotropin releasing hormone.[118,178] As the bilateral inferior petrosal sinus sampling, technique with peripheral corticotropin hormone stimulation has been used more frequently, the diagnostic accuracy has been found to fall within an approximate range of 88% to 100%, with occasional reports of false negative and false positive tests.[97,112,117,118,128,131,154,167,178–185] The sensitivity of the bilateral inferior petrosal sinus sampling technique for identifying a pituitary source without stimulation has been between 61.7% and 85%.[152,154]

Stimulation with the combination of corticotropin releasing hormone and desmopressin has been shown to increase the sensitivity of the bilateral inferior petrosal sinus sampling. A post-stimulation central to peripheral ACTH ratio of greater than 2, following human corticotropin releasing hormone and desmopressin injection, produced a sensitivity of 97.9% and specificity of 100% for identifying pituitary origin Cushing's disease.[152] A subsequent re-analysis of the data using a post-stimulation central to peripheral ACTH ratio of three or greater as the threshold value demonstrated a sensitivity of 91.5%.[152]

Accuracy of identifying laterality of pituitary production of adrenocorticotropin hormone using bilateral inferior petrosal sinus sampling

Lateralization of a pituitary corticotropin producing adenoma can be determined through bilateral venous sampling even when the lesion is not visualized on pituitary MRI or even during surgical exploration.[186] Within the sella, the location of a corticotropin producing tumor can selectively increase the levels of ACTH in the pituitary venous drainage ipsilaterally. Calculating an interpetrosal gradient between the left and right sides can identify the side of the tumor. In addition, the presence of a unilateral increase in ACTH concentration emphasizes the necessity of simultaneous sampling of both inferior petrosal sinuses to avoid false negative results or misclassification of an ectopic ACTH source.[98,108,112,141, 187,188] An interpetrosal ACTH gradient greater than or equal to 1.4 at baseline, or after ovine/human corticotropin releasing hormone, indicates evidence of lateralization.[189] A value less than 1.4 indicates a midline lesion with approximately 70% accuracy. In order to calculate this ratio, the greatest ACTH value obtained during simultaneous serial measurements of both respective inferior petrosal sinuses is chosen.[178] Interpetrosal ACTH gradient alone may not be sufficient to lateralize the pituitary adenoma reliably.[180] The accuracy of tumor localization is not improved despite corticotropin releasing hormone stimulation.[159,190] The sensitivity of lateralization ranges from 47% to 100% in various studies.[101,117,128,137,147,148,158,178,187,190–198] A combined analysis of several reports found that the mean diagnostic accuracy of using the interpetrosal ratio of greater than 1.4 to define laterality, was 78% (range 50%–100%), compared with the findings of pituitary surgery.[117]

Occasional reversal of the lateralizing gradient has been seen from the pre- to the post-ovine corticotropin releasing hormone stimulation values. Miller et al. reported this reversal in 5% of cases,[199] de Herder et al.[200] in 27% of cases, and Lefournier et al. in 10% of the patients.[109] If a reversal of the lateralization gradient is seen from the pre- to the post-corticotropin releasing hormone values, the test cannot accurately be relied on to lateralize the adenoma.[137]

The interpetrosal gradient may direct the surgeon to begin an initial examination of the pituitary gland on the side ipsilateral to the measured gradient: a full exploration is required to avoid missing tumors in approximately 22% of the patients.[117,122] Misleading results may be found in patients who have undergone prior pituitary surgery.[189] In a study that included patients with previous pituitary surgery, the sensitivities of lateralization of bilateral inferior petrosal sinus sampling were 53% without corticotropin releasing hormone stimulation and 59% after ovine corticotropin releasing hormone stimulation. None of the four patients who had previous trans-sphenoidal hypophysectomy were precisely localized by bilateral inferior petrosal sinus sampling.[189]

Multiple site sampling to increase diagnostic yield

Multiple-site, bilateral simultaneous venous sampling of adrenocorticotropin hormone may be valuable for lateralizing the adenoma in patients with Cushing's disease. There is data supporting higher accuracy with multiple site sampling compared with single site sampling.[201] Simultaneous, bilateral venous sampling for ACTH from the anterior, middle and posterior cavernous sinus and inferior petrosal sinus in patients with Cushing's disease was found to correctly identify the side of the microadenoma after corticotropin releasing hormone stimulation, in all 18 of the patients studied.[201]

False-positive results

Although the predictive value of a positive bilateral inferior petrosal sinus sampling is high, false positive results do occur.[154] A false positive test describes a situation where the inferior petrosal sinus to peripheral ratio is above the threshold criteria indicating a pituitary source; however, the tumor is not located in the pituitary.[154] Multiple causes exist for false positives with bilateral inferior petrosal sinus sampling: pseudo-Cushing's syndrome, pituitary corticotroph hyperplasia secondary to an ectopic neuroendocrine corticotropin releasing hormone, cyclic Cushing's syndrome (cyclic secretion of ACTH) during the eucortisolemic phase, treatment with cortisol blocking drugs (e.g., ketoconazole, metyrapone, mitotane, aminoglutethamide) which result in the desuppression of the normal pituitary corticotrophs which might then respond to corticotropin releasing hormone or desmopressin and adrenal Cushing's syndrome (adrenal tumors with intermittent cortisol production), (see Table 17.6).[112,113,117,154,183,202–205]

Bilateral inferior petrosal sinus sampling also produces falsely elevated results in patients who have had a bilateral adrenalectomy because these patients will not have elevated cortisol levels and their normal pituitary corticotrophs will not be suppressed.[113] Ectopic tumors with intermittent ACTH secretion will also contribute to the development of false positives.[183,206] False-positives can also be seen in normal individuals without hypercortisolemia who have high ACTH levels due to a normal pulsatile pituitary corticotroph ACTH release leading to an absolute increase in ACTH levels and central to peripheral ACTH ratios, obtained via bilateral inferior petrosal sinus sampling.[112,202] Extrasellar tumors, usually found on surgical exploration, can also lead to false positive results.[207,208]

False-negative results

A false-negative value is defined as a negative bilateral inferior petrosal sinus sampling study in a patient where the tumor is actually in the pituitary gland. A low pre-stimulation inferior petrosal sinus to peripheral ACTH ratio and a low post-stimulation ratio can suggest an occult ectopic ACTH syndrome or a false negative test. False-negatives have also been described in localizing the side of the pituitary tumor.[133,154,178,180,187]

Table 17.6. False-positive etiologies.

Asymmetric pituitary venous drainage
Pseudo Cushing's syndrome
Pituitary corticotroph hyperplasia secondary to ectopic neuroendocrine CRH secretion
Cyclic Cushing's syndrome (cyclic secretion of ACTH) during eucortisolemic phase
Cortisol blocking drugs: ketoconazole, metyrapone, mitotane and aminoglutethamide
Adrenal Cushing's syndrome (intermittent cortisol producing adrenal tumors)
Bilateral adrenalectomy
Intermittent ectopic ACTH secreting adenoma
Normal individuals with high pulsatile pituitary ACTH secretion
Extrasellar location of ACTH microadenoma

ACTH: adrenocorticotropin hormone; CRH: corticotropin releasing hormone.

Table 17.7. False-negative etiologies

Asymmetric/aberrant pituitary venous drainage
Inability to pass the catheter into position due to jugular occlusion
Anatomical abnormalities: inability to sample bilateral inferior petrosal sinuses
Anomalous venous drainage: hypoplastic inferior petrosal sinus
Lack of inferior petrosal sinus drainage of pituitary
Human error: lack of experience
Human error: wrong positioning of catheter tip, wrong venous sample obtained
Human error: inadequate CRH and/or desmopressin stimulation dosage administered
Minimally responsive pituitary adenoma to CRH and/or desmopressin stimulation
Unilateral central venous sampling
History of previous pituitary surgery leading to altered venous drainage pattern
Pituitary corticotroph adenoma originating ectopically in the sphenoid sinus
Cyclical ACTH producing pituitary adenomas (off phase)
Poor handling of the ACTH assay
Poor sample processing technique (failure to appropriately cool samples)

ACTH: adrenocorticotropin hormone; CRH: corticotropin releasing hormone.

In past studies, false-negative cases have been described, but many patients were presumed to have ectopic tumors.[179,180,184] A variety of reasons have been cited to account for false negative results: patients with aberrant pituitary venous drainage, inability to sample bilateral pituitary venous effluent adequately, anatomical abnormalities precluding satisfactory catheterization of at least one inferior petrosal sinus, unilateral or bilateral jugular venous occlusion, venous complex draining the pituitary without separate inferior petrosal sinus drainage, anomalous venous drainage from the pituitary gland caused by a hypoplastic inferior petrosal sinus, and altered venous drainage after previous trans-sphenoidal surgery (see Table 17.7).[154,178–180,182,184,187,209–211] Aberrant venous drainage not detected by bilateral inferior petrosal sinus sampling may be seen with an abnormally located pituitary corticotropin adenoma, if originating ectopically in the sphenoid sinus.[207,208]

Pituitary corticotropin producing adenomas demonstrate varying degrees of responsiveness to exogenous corticotropin releasing hormone. A false negative bilateral inferior petrosal sinus sample may be obtained in the case where the pituitary adenoma is minimally responsive to exogenous corticotropin releasing hormone and therefore the expected increase in ACTH secretion after stimulation is not observed. Some pituitary adenomas show a cyclical production pattern of ACTH; therefore, the sensitivity of bilateral inferior petrosal sinus sampling will depend upon whether the adenoma is in the on or off phase.[154]

Technical points to increase the accuracy of the technique

Pre-procedure assessment

On the day of the bilateral inferior petrosal sinus sampling procedure, the patient must be confirmed to be hypercortisolemic by measuring a 24-hour urine sample for urine free cortisol concluding on the morning of the sampling procedure or a late night salivary cortisol measurement the night before the procedure. The patient should not be taking any medication that may block cortisol production at the time of the procedure or have had an adrenalectomy.[101,112,154] Iatrogenic or exogenous hypercortisolism and pseudo Cushing's syndrome must be excluded in order for a true endogenous Cushing's syndrome to be diagnosed (see Table 17.8).[117,123,212–214] More frequent sampling may be required depending on the periodicity of the cyclic production because a single elevated urine free cortisol value on the day of the sampling may be insufficient to exclude inadequate suppression of pituitary corticotrophs.[154]

A summary of the bilateral inferior petrosal sinus sampling procedure is outlined in Table 17.9.[101,104,108,111,112,138,154,215]

Angiographic evaluation

Prior to sampling, venous angiography has been used to determine whether the venous drainage pattern is symmetric or asymmetric. Using fluoroscopic guidance and road mapping techniques, the catheters are guided into position within each of the inferior petrosal sinuses prior to sampling. The position of the catheter tip is confirmed by obtaining a venogram of

369

Table 17.8. Pseudo Cushing's syndrome etiologies

Adrenal disorders that autonomously secrete glucocorticoids
Alcoholism
Anorexia nervosa
Depression
Generalized resistance to glucocorticoids
Iatrogenic or exogenous hypercortisolism
Pregnancy

Hypercortisolism can be seen with these conditions. Iatrogenic or exogenous hypercortisolism must be excluded in order for a true endogenous Cushing's syndrome to be diagnosed.

Table 17.9. Summary of bilateral inferior petrosal sinus procedure

Conscious sedation
Sterile preparation of bilateral femoral veins at the groin with insertion of venous sheaths
Heparin infusion
Fluoroscopically-guided placement of catheters into the bilateral inferior petrosal sinuses
Venography to determine symmetrical or asymmetrical venous flow
Contrast enhanced fluoroscopy to confirm reflux into ipsilateral cavernous sinus
Baseline blood samples
CRH and/or desmopressin stimulation
Post-stimulation blood samples
Catheter removal and groin pressure until venous hemostasis

CRH: corticotropin releasing hormone.

each catheter after the catheters are placed in the inferior petrosal sinuses.[101] Antero-posterior images acquired during the venograms are used to interpret venous drainage patterns. Lateral projections help in defining: (1) anatomical junction between the cavernous sinus and inferior petrosal sinus;[108] (2) the anatomy of the inferior petrosal sinus; and (3) venous drainage pattern (type I–IV) particularly in the internal jugular vein. Mamelak *et al.* recommended a slow, manual injection of 1 mL of contrast material in order to avoid overwhelming or altering the venous flow patterns within the venous sinuses.[108] Lefournier *et al.* and Miller *et al.* administered 5 mL of iopamidol 300 contrast material through a soft, slow injection by hand.[101,109] The minimum requirement for a venogram is to observe reflux of the contrast material at least as far as the ipsilateral cavernous sinus.[98] Without reflux into the cavernous sinus, pituitary venous effluent will not be adequately reflected in the sample. Miller *et al.* recommended normal reflux of injected contrast material extending into the

ipsilateral cavernous sinus, through the intercavernous sinuses, into the contralateral cavernous sinus, and down the contralateral inferior petrosal sinus to the contralateral internal jugular vein for adequate assessment.[101]

Stimulation and sampling technique

Simultaneous blood samples can be obtained from each of the three ports: left inferior petrosal sinus, right inferior petrosal sinus, and from the peripheral vein via the femoral vein sheath. Typically, two sets of simultaneous baseline samples are drawn and then three sets of stimulated (corticotropin releasing hormone and/or desmopressin) samples are drawn. Subsequently, stimulation has been achieved with a peripheral, slow (over 1 minute) intravenous bolus of corticotropin releasing hormone at a dose of 1 µg/kg (maximum 100 µg) and/or desmopressin (10 µg/kg).[97,101,138,154,167] The general schedule of sampling following stimulation is usually as follows: −5 minutes (pre-stimulation), −1 minute (pre-stimulation), +3–5 minutes (post-stimulation), +8–10 minutes (post-stimulation) and +13–15 minutes (post-stimulation).[101,112,138,152]

Multiple sites within the inferior petrosal sinuses can be sampled to reduce the variability in ACTH levels attributable to slight variations in catheter placement and size of the venous sinus.[108] A sample collection takes approximately 20–40 seconds, therefore blood drawing should commence approximately 20 seconds prior to the nominal sample time.[101] A variety of sample volumes ranging from 3 ml to 10 ml have been recommended by investigators for measurement of ACTH.[101,138152]

Sample handling and hormone assay technique

Prior to sampling, an appropriate number of labeled lavender-top tubes, with ethylenediaminetetraacetic acid, should have been placed in an ice water bath. After successfully drawing each sample into a syringe, it is then transferred to the appropriately labeled and numbered lavender-top tube using a 16 gauge needle.[101] These samples can either be processed by the investigators or the hospital's laboratory. All samples should be centrifuged within one hour of collection in a refrigerated centrifuge for 10 minutes at 1500 g and 4–5°C.[112] The plasma is decanted into polypropylene tubes and placed on dry ice in an insulated container. These specimens are then sent for ACTH assay at 1:1, 1:10 and 1:100 dilutions.[101]

Catheters used for sampling

The inferior petrosal sinuses were originally sampled with catheters that were designed to have a specific bend at their tip.[104,215] An investigator who was a part of the Miller *et al.* group (D.L.M.) developed a design for left and right petrosal sinus catheters based on a straight 5-F catheter (Imager 35–103 [100 cm long, no side holes]; Medi-tech/Boston Scientific, Watertown, MA).[101] The catheter for the left side had a 75° bend, whereas the right sided catheter was set at an angle of 95°. Steam was used to shape these catheters. The distance from the tip to the shaft was 28 mm in each case. The catheters did not have any holes on their side. An angled-tip, hydrophilic-coated guide wire was used in conjunction with the catheters.[101]

Intra-procedural heparin

To prevent sinus thrombosis related to catheterization, heparin should be infused before catheters are advanced.[112] Miller *et al.* routinely administered 3000–4000 IU of heparin as an intravenous bolus through the femoral vein sheath before the catheters were advanced into the internal jugular veins. In addition, Miller *et al.* added heparin (5000 IU/L) to the flush solution and used this solution, via continuous drip, to irrigate both petrosal sinus catheters and the femoral vein sheath whenever they were not being manipulated.[101] Pre- and post-procedure assessment of the coagulation system, platelets, and hematocrit is recommended.

Complications associated with inferior petrosal sinus sampling

Bilateral inferior petrosal sinus sampling is generally a safe outpatient procedure with minimal morbidity and mortality. Miller *et al.* reported no deaths or serious complications in 335 procedures. Miller *et al.* also estimated with 95% confidence that the theoretical risk of serious complication or death was at most 0.9%.[101] Headache is a common manifestation that may be provoked secondary to the contrast injection or the insertion of the catheter into a small inferior petrosal sinus. Ipsilateral ear pain may also occur if the catheter is inserted into a small inferior petrosal sinus. The patient may also hear strange noises in the ear on the side of the catheter insertion. Intravenous narcotics can be used to help relieve the discomfort during the procedure. Reassurance about the transient nature of these symptoms is valuable for the patient.[101]

The most common complication has been a groin hematoma, estimated to have a frequency of around 3%–4%.[101] Cushing's syndrome patients are quite prone to developing ecchymoses, even with peripheral venipuncture. During the procedure there is an infusion of iodinated contrast material which increases the risk of acute renal insufficiency that may be exacerbated by pre-existing renal insufficiency or hypovolemia.[112] Some of the more rare complications seen with the procedure include deep venous thrombosis and pulmonary thromboembolism,[117,122,180,216–218] pontocerebellar junction stroke,[219] brainstem vascular damage (vessel perforation),[147,220] cranial nerve palsy,[221] venous subarachnoid hemorrhage,[222] obstructive hydrocephalus, and intracranial hematoma.[97,109,112,138,147,216,219,221–223] Variant venous anatomy or specific catheter use may lead to neurologic complications. The adverse sequelae may be reduced or averted if the bilateral inferior petrosal sinus sampling is aborted upon development of new neurologic signs or symptoms.[147] Cerebrovascular accidents have been attributed to placement of a catheter in small intracranial vessels, which occurs during bilateral inferior petrosal sinus sampling but not during jugular venous sampling.[132] Exposure to radiation during the fluoroscopic evaluation of catheter tip position is also another concern as well as catheter-related infections.[112]

Implications for treatment

The ideal therapy for ACTH-dependent Cushing's syndrome requires surgical removal of the ACTH-producing neoplasm.[154,180] The treatment of choice for children and adults with Cushing's disease is trans-sphenoidal adenomectomy. Mamelak *et al.* proceeded directly with trans-sphenoidal exploration in any patient with a visible adenoma more than 4 mm in size on MRI because the likelihood of it being an incidental finding was quite small.[110] Pituitary microsurgery can cure 50% and normalize cortisol levels in an additional 30%–40% of patients with Cushing's disease.[193] Trans-sphenoidal exploration should also be considered in all cases of unsuccessful bilateral inferior petrosal sinus sampling and in those cases in which no ectopic source can be identified after further body imaging, due to the high pre-test probability for Cushing's disease, even if the bilateral inferior petrosal sinus sampling is negative. This is true especially if peripheral ACTH levels rise significantly with corticotropin releasing hormone stimulation.[112,154,184] Patients with a bilateral inferior petrosal sinus sampling that suggest a central source will need trans-sphenoidal surgery. If no discrete pituitary tumor can be identified after meticulous bilateral exploration, then a hemi- or total hypophysectomy may be performed based on accurate lateralization data. Bilateral adrenalectomy is considered an option as an alternative to total hypophysectomy in patients with negative surgical pituitary explorations. Hemi- or total hypophysectomy is considered successful if pathological studies demonstrate a pituitary adenoma. Following the resection of the pituitary adenoma, the hormonal assays and the clinical course will be consistent with the remission of Cushing's disease.[108,154]

Intravascular ultrasound
Introduction

Intravascular ultrasound is an invasive technique used to assess the morphologic appearance and characteristics of the intraarterial vessel. The successful application of conventional (gray scale) intravascular ultrasound within the coronary arteries has led to its application within the extracranial and intracranial arteries. Intravascular ultrasound imaging has become the gold standard in randomized clinical trials for atherosclerosis imaging.[224] With excellent resolution, intravascular ultrasound provides cross sectional images of both the arterial wall and lumen, identifies intimal flaps and irregularities as well as the composition and extent of atherosclerotic plaque.[225–229] Intravascular ultrasound can also identify and characterize carotid artery aneurysm, dissection or thrombus.[230] The evolution of intravascular ultrasound technology has led to the development of more sophisticated diagnostic tools such as color flow and virtual histology intravascular ultrasound.[231]

Intravascular ultrasound has successfully been used to assist in making measurements during intracranial percutaneous transluminal carotid artery balloon angioplasty and stent placement.[232] It has been instrumental in the identification of factors leading to coronary stent under-expansion, poor apposition, subacute stent thrombosis and plaque protrusion.[233] Real time, dynamic intravascular ultrasound imaging of the cervical common carotid artery and internal carotid artery has the capability of detecting defects that are not always readily apparent by conventional contrast angiography, such as residual stenosis, suboptimal plaque coverage, arterial dissection, poor wall apposition of the stent, superficial calcification, atherosclerotic plaque progression or regression and plaque ulceration.[234-236] The sensitivity and specificity of intravenous ultrasound are higher than angiography and magnetic resonance imaging for studying the vessel lumen.[237,238] The growth of endovascular practice and intravascular ultrasound capabilities has set the stage for broader use of this technology in interventional neurology across the US.

Images produced by conventional intravascular ultrasound

The reflected signals that are collected by the transducer enable the creation of the images seen on the conventional, gray scale intravascular ultrasound.[231] The elastin and collagen organization within the arterial wall provides the substrate which leads to the ultrasound scattering differences between the individual layers. The intima (inner layer) reflects ultrasound brightly, presenting as white (hyperechoic). The media presents as dark (hypoechoic) and echolucent. The surrounding adventitia, the outermost layer, is white (hyperechoic). The arterial wall of the normal elastic arteries typically has a homogeneous appearance when imaged by intravascular ultrasound, secondary to the elastin in the media. A hypoechoic (dark) media is seen when muscular arteries are visualized, due to the presence of arterial smooth muscle cells.[239,240] The common carotid artery and the distal internal carotid artery both have a muscular and elastic component. Manninen et al. consistently found a three layered morphology in the distal internal carotid artery segment visualized by intravascular ultrasound, during life and after death. The common carotid artery typically had a characteristic homogeneous structure.[240] The arterial wall of the internal carotid artery bulb can have marked variation because it is typically a transitional zone. With regards to various parts of the carotid arterial wall imaged by intravascular ultrasound, there appears to be a continuum of findings.

Limitations of conventional intravascular ultrasound

Frequency of the transducer, gain settings, depth of penetration and focal depth are some of the factors that affect the sensitivity of the intravascular ultrasound imaging. The location and orientation of the imaging probe within the arterial lumen also influences the appearance of the vessel wall structure.[239] A lateral impulse response artifact can occur when the sonographic catheter is eccentrically placed, resulting in an image that suggests the presence of an intimal flap or ulceration.[229,241] The dark images obtained through conventional, gray scale intravascular ultrasound can make it difficult to distinguish between the lumen and the dark, echolucent plaque. Accurate delineation of the medial adventitial interface, leading to the appropriate sizing and imaging of lesions, has been achieved with intravascular ultrasound of the carotid arteries between 20–30 MHz.[229,231,240,242,243] Manninen et al. found that optimal resolution in arteries 3 to 6 mm in diameter was obtained by a 30 MHz transducer, giving a maximum radius of penetration of approximately 5 mm.[240] Miskolczi et al. observed that a 30 MHz sonographic system performed adequately at a distance of 2 to 3 mm (the distance between the intimal surface of the carotid artery and the transducer if the catheter was placed in a central position).[229] There are images that may not be visualized because they fall below the resolution limit of the intravascular ultrasound system being used.

Color flow intravascular ultrasound

Color flow intravascular ultrasound provides a greater understanding of intra-luminal blood flow, lumen size, success of treatment, and the interface between the vessel wall and the blood stream.[231] Real time images are produced from the transducer of the intravascular ultrasound apparatus at 30 frames per second. The difference between two sequential adjacent frames is detected by computer software, producing the color flow intravascular ultrasound images. Red demonstrates the movement of echogenic blood particles through the artery. Tight stenosis, resulting in an increase in the speed of blood through that segment, leads to a transition in the color representation from red to orange.

The main benefit of color flow intravascular ultrasound lies in its ability to distinguish luminal blood flow from the dark echolucent vessel wall.[244-246] Color flow intravascular ultrasound can also demonstrate soft echolucent plaques, plaque ulcerations, thrombus and arterial dissections.[244] In the case of arterial dissections, the probe should be placed in the true lumen where there is better blood flow visualization.[231] A reduction in contrast angiography and total radiation dosage was observed after the introduction of color flow intravascular ultrasound.[244] Diethrich et al. used color flow intravascular ultrasound with fluoroscopy alone to treat patients and deploy stents and endoluminal grafts, avoiding the use of contrast angiography in patients with renal failure or contrast allergy.[231] Following intervention, the demonstration of blood flow through color flow intravascular ultrasound allows the treating physician to evaluate the success of the treatment, without the use of angiography.[231]

Another clinical application of the color flow ultrasound is accurate stent deployment at the site of the origin of the common carotid artery, from the aortic arch.[247] Due to the curvature of the aortic arch, relying on angiography alone for accurate stent placement is difficult. Fluoroscopy can be used to visualize the radio-opaque color flow intravascular ultrasound transducer and guide it into position. Once the transducer is moved from the stenosis into the aorta, the color flow intravascular ultrasound will detect a sudden change in the size of color flow. This sudden change in color flow enables the precise identification of the origin ultimately leading to a more accurate stent deployment.[248]

Limitations of color flow intravascular ultrasound

The short diameter of the field of view is a limitation of color flow intravascular ultrasound. The entire vessel lumen may not be filled with color, especially if the probe is against the vessel wall in a large artery. Blood flow may not be detected in case large caliber sheaths are used secondary to the possibility that the catheter itself may impede the flow of blood through the vessel.[231] The image resolution is very high with this technique although flow velocities cannot be calculated. Color flow imaging cannot be performed when virtual histology intravascular ultrasound images are obtained because the software that is used to acquire and interpret the data is different for each modality. Also, color flow intravascular ultrasound images are not gated with the heart rate.[231]

Virtual histology map generated by intravascular ultrasound

The components of the vessel wall reflect the ultrasound signal at different frequencies and intensities, creating an opportunity for histological details to be appreciated through the generation of a virtual histology intravascular ultrasound map. This is the only available technique for real-time dynamic assessment of plaque morphology. This modality enables the creation of a virtual histology map of the atherosclerotic plaque, distinguishing between different components. The plaque may contain a varying amount of fibrous material, fibro-fatty content, calcium deposits as well as a lipid core.[231] A histological classification and a color coded map of the plaque can be produced by comparing virtual histology maps with true histological sections of diseased coronary arteries. A color-coded map currently provides detailed information about the contents of the plaque: dark green represents fibrous material, yellow/green represents fibro-fatty, white represents calcified, and red represents the necrotic lipid core.[249–251] Accurate information regarding the composition of the carotid atherosclerotic plaque can guide the neurointerventionalist to determine the resistance to balloon dilation or the potential for embolic phenomena.[231,252]

Limitations of virtual histology maps

Interpretation of the results of virtual histology maps requires experience. An increase in computing speed and improved software for interpretation is also needed. The modalities of color flow and virtual histology intravascular ultrasound cannot be used simultaneously. The process is time consuming, since adjustments to the borders that delineate the plaque are usually necessary requiring multiple retractions of the catheter with the intravascular ultrasound transducer. The metal stent struts are recognized as calcification, colored white, on virtual histology intravascular ultrasound, limiting its value after percutaneous carotid stent placement.[231]

Lipid microbubbles

Contrast enhanced intravascular ultrasonography with lipid microbubbles to allow imaging of inflammation and perfusion within atherosclerotic plaques is under investigation.[253] Studies suggest that proliferation of the vasa vasorum (blood vessels in the adventitial layer) in coronary atherosclerotic plaques is a preceding or concomitant factor associated with plaque inflammation and instability.[254–256] The carotid arteries are also perfused by vasa vasorum and therefore potentially subject to the same phenomenon.[257–259] Lipid microbubbles have been used extensively to help better understand inflamed plaques because lipid microbubbles have a tendency to be phagocytosed by macrophages within the inflamed plaque. Subsequently, these phagocytosed microbubbles generate characteristic echogenic features that can be used to identify their distribution within the plaque with real time intravascular ultrasonography.[253]

Lipid deposition within the plaque

Intravascular ultrasound studies of the coronary arteries and carotid arteries can delineate plaque lipid deposition. Echolucent (hypoechoic) zones within the atherosclerotic plaque, visualized through intravascular ultrasound, represent areas of lipid deposition.[260] Potkin et al. found that in vitro intravascular ultrasound correctly identified 78% (seven out of nine) lipid containing plaques, that were confirmed by histological analysis.[261] The sensitivity of the identification of these lipid depositions depends on the amount of lipid present within the atherosclerotic plaque. If the echolucent area is smaller than a quarter of the plaque the sensitivity will be lower.[262] The interpretation of echolucent areas is complex because similar signal can be generated by loose tissue and shadowing from calcium. The sensitivity to differentiate between fibrous and fatty tissue has been shown to vary depending on the intravascular ultrasound system used.[263]

The stage of plaque progression that the carotid lesion has reached may be used to identify an unstable atherosclerotic plaque that is more prone to embolize. Pathologic studies in coronary arteries have demonstrated that plaque rupture is more frequent in eccentric, lipid-rich, soft plaques with a thin, fibrous cap overlying it.[252,264–267,268,269] A large histopathological study found an association between stroke and carotid artery plaque rupture and mural thrombosis.[270] Following the initial rupture, the thrombotically active plaques may remain unstable. Further cerebral events may develop during this "vulnerable plaque" state, because of subsequent embolization.[270,271] Studies of the coronary arteries have shown an association between sudden death and rupture of a plaque with a necrotic lipid core (echolucent center). Intravascular ultrasound may be used to evaluate high risk asymptomatic patients suspected to have carotid lesions, even without a hemodynamically significant stenosis, in order to identify if their carotid atherosclerotic plaques contain a high proportion of a necrotic lipid core.[272,273] Intravascular ultrasound data may be able to identify patients at high risk for a massive shower of microemboli or large particulate embolism.[274–276] Further study of virtual histology intravascular ultrasound is required for better clarification of its full potential, especially with regards to validating the interpretation of plaque progression.[242,276–279]

Carotid plaque ulcerations

Intravascular ultrasound has been utilized to visualize small carotid plaque ulcerations. The risk of cerebral embolism may be increased in the presence of carotid plaque ulcerations which may act as thromboembolic substrates or release plaque material into the arterial lumen.[229] An apparent hole (small cavity) in the plaque is the hallmark sign of an ulceration on intracarotid ultrasound. Fisher and Ojemann applied the phrase "cul de sac" to explain the shape of the ulceration.[280] The prevalence of carotid ulceration varies. Streifler et al. and Fürst et al. found that there was a high prevalence of ulceration in a selected group of patients that underwent endarterectomy.[281,282] An in vitro study of human carotid arteries conducted by Miskolczi et al. found that 29% of the arteries had at least one ulceration and accurately identified all ulcerated arteries and individual ulcerations with intravascular ultrasonography (90% to 100% sensitivity).[229] According to Miskolczi et al. the minimum pre-defined depth of the ulceration (a minimum 0.5 mm or greater) was within the resolution limits of the intravascular ultrasound system (30 MHz, 3.5F sonographic probe). When compared to gross histologic measurements of the ulcerations, the intravascular ultrasound measurements underestimated the carotid plaque ulcerations' depth of penetration (1.05 ± 0.44 mm vs. 1 ± 0.36 mm) and orifice diameter (1.95 ± 0.72 mm vs. 1.76 ± 0.59 mm).[229] They concluded that intravascular ultrasound was a more sensitive technique for the identification of small ulcerations in comparison to digital subtraction angiography, B-mode sonography, duplex sonography, and color flow sonography.[229]

Detection of plaque calcification

Intravascular ultrasound can effectively identify calcium deposits within the atherosclerotic plaque.[236] Atherosclerotic plaques that contain calcifications are characterized by a bright echo signal (hyperechoic) with distal shadowing, which may hide other plaque components and deeper vessel structures.[262] Determination of the actual dimensions of the carotid atherosclerotic plaque and the percentage stenosis may be difficult in situations where intravascular ultrasound identifies superficial, plate-like calcifications.[240] Kostama et al found that intravascular ultrasound underestimated the total calcified plaque

cross sectional area by 39% because the ultrasound beam could not penetrate the intralesional calcium deposits.[283] The identification of arterial calcification is very important because calcification can lead to a non-compliant lesion resistant to balloon angioplasty. The presence of heavy intra-arterial calcification, especially in combination with arterial tortuosity, also causes difficulties in tracking devices, lesion dilation, stent positioning and adequate stent expansion.

Coronary plaque calcification has been detected with a sensitivity between 86% and 97%, in comparative studies done using both histology and intravascular ultrasound.[284,285] Friedrich et al. also studied 50 fresh coronary vessel segments with intravascular ultrasound and compared their results with the corresponding histologic sections. Intravascular ultrasound correctly identified 89% (16 of 18) of cases with dense calcified plaques, 17% (2 of 12) of cases with microcalcification (small calcium flecks less than or equal to 0.5 mm), and 100% (three of three) of the cases with a combination of calcified plaque surrounded by small calcium flecks.[286] In an intravascular ultrasound study of the carotid arteries, Manninen et al. similarly found that the macroscopic calcifications were consistently detected, but disseminated microcalcifications were usually missed.[240]

Atherosclerotic plaque characterization

The atherosclerotic plaque and its components can be delineated from the hypoechoic (dark) media layer in the internal carotid artery and can be visualized secondary to the high spatial resolution provided by intravascular ultrasound.[240,287,288,289,290] The area of the arterial lumen and the area of the vessel's external elastic membrane can be measured allowing for the calculation of the atherosclerotic plaque area.[289] Coronary artery vessels have demonstrated an ability to remodel themselves at the location of the coronary atherosclerotic plaque. Positive remodeling represents the compensatory increase in the local vessel size in response to an increase in plaque burden. Negative remodeling represents the local shrinkage of vessel size in response to an increase in plaque burden.[289] Intravascular ultrasound can also be used to evaluate carotid artery vessel wall remodeling secondary to the presence of an atherosclerotic plaque.

Approximately 20%–25% of all strokes are caused by carotid artery stenosis in their extracranial course.[291] Intravascular ultrasound has also been used to follow the successful progressive reduction of atherosclerotic plaques in patients who have been actively treated with a variety of pharmacological agents such as a statin or recombinant ApoA-1 Milanophospholipid complexes.[224,225,243,292–295]

Classification of plaque types

The detection of vulnerable (unstable) plaques, i.e., intra-arterial plaques that have a high probability of rupture, can be achieved using intravascular ultrasound.[273,296] Vulnerable (soft) plaques contain a large lipid core typically making up 40% of the entire plaque.[262] Atherosclerotic plaques containing an increased amount of calcification are interpreted as more stable and mature. Intravascular ultrasound enables the following characteristics of the coronary/carotid atherosclerotic plaque to be viewed: (1) size of the lipid (echolucent) core; (2) thickness of the fibrous cap; (3) presence of inflammatory cells (macrophages); (4) amount of remodeling and extent of plaque-free vessel wall; and (5) three-dimensional morphology.[297] The differentiation of "soft" (unstable) from "fibrotic" (stable) plaque is highly dependent on the gain settings used during intravascular ultrasound.[298] Structures sized over 160 microns can be estimated accurately by intravascular ultrasound.[262]

Comparison of intravascular ultrasound and angiography

Intravascular ultrasound has an advantage over angiography because it provides images from within the vessel, has greater resolution, does not have to penetrate through extravascular soft tissues and provides three-dimensional assessment.[299] When looking for intimal thickening, concentric plaques, plaque surface ulceration, and the presence of calcifications within the carotid arteries, intravascular ultrasound has proven to be more sensitive than digital subtraction angiography.[300] Manninen et al. showed that contrast-enhanced angiography of a variety of carotid arteries did not detect ten cases of calcification that were all visualized with intravascular ultrasound.[240] Digital subtraction angiography visualized 5 of 17 (29%) intimal thickenings that were all successfully imaged with intravascular ultrasound.[240] Angiographic contrast agents injected within the coronary arteries can provide no information regarding perivascular blood flow within the vasa vasorum.[253] Intravascular ultrasound can detect blood flow in perivascular vessels as a result of contrast-generated signal from flowing microbubbles after proper image analysis.[253]

Case reports and observational studies support the advantages of visualizing the common carotid artery using intravascular ultrasound over the common carotid angiogram, when evaluating the degree of stenosis within the arterial lumen. A 50% stenosis of the left common carotid artery was revealed through an angiogram, whereas an 87% stenosis with complex superficial calcification was observed through the intravascular ultrasound in the same patient. Intravascular ultrasound was also able to demonstrate protrusion of the superficial calcification within the lumen of the common carotid artery.[299] The results of digital subtraction angiography can be obscured by heavy calcification of the vessel border.[299] Digital subtraction angiography of the carotid arteries also missed two concentric stenoses greater than 20%, that were detected by intravascular ultrasound.[240] Similarly, intravascular ultrasound revealed some degree of stenosis in 80% of angiographically normal left main coronary arteries after percutaneous transluminal coronary angioplasty.[301] Intravascular ultrasound has also been used to assess a stenotic lesion within the distal left posterior cerebral artery.[232]

A more accurate assessment of carotid artery stent dimensions can be obtained through intravascular ultrasound, when compared to quantitative carotid angiography. Intravascular ultrasound allows for a more accurate evaluation of stent dimensions, expansion, and apposition. When compared to quantitative carotid angiography, Clark et al. found that intravascular ultrasound measured the internal carotid artery stent minimum lumen diameter significantly smaller (3.65 ± 0.68 vs. 4.31 ± 0.76 mm; $P < 0.001$).[236] Intravascular ultrasound measurements of the minimum lumen diameter of the distal internal carotid artery reference segment (non-stented) were similar to quantitative carotid angiography (4.60 ± 0.74 vs. 4.74 ± 0.71 mm; $P = 0.21$).[236] In 11% of cases, intravascular ultrasound also found stent malapposition.[236] After an optimal angiographic result, intravascular ultrasound findings led to additional treatment in 9% of cases (ten patients): four patients required stent expansion, three patients required additional stents to achieve better plaque coverage and three patients were found to have stent malapposition.[236]

At the lesion site, intravascular ultrasound has been found to be more sensitive than angiography in the detection of calcium within the arteries (61% vs. 46%; $P < 0.05$).[236] When three or four quadrants of the carotid arteries were found to have superficial lesion calcification by intravascular ultrasound, there was a 31% incidence of ischemic stroke; however, there was a 1% incidence of ischemic stroke in patients without severe superficial calcification intra-arterially.[236] Reduced stent expansion and less stent symmetry were seen in patients who had severe superficial calcium identified intra-arterially by intravascular ultrasound.[236] An increased risk of stroke after carotid stent placement is observed in patients with heavy atherosclerotic plaque calcification.[302]

Intravascular ultrasound and percutaneous carotid artery stent placement

Intravascular ultrasound has become an integral component of carotid stent placement by helping decide the correct stent diameter and the amount of balloon inflation pressure required during angioplasty.[234,235,237,303–305] In preparing for balloon angioplasty, identification of arterial calcification is important because the calcification can produce a non-compliant lesion that necessitates the use of high balloon inflation pressures.[306] In addition, the images provide an accurate method to understand if the stent deployed post-angioplasty has expanded the lumen to the desired size or if there is a need for any post-stent balloon angioplasty.[235,242,307] The length of the stent necessary to completely cover coronary lesions has been determined through the measurements made by intravascular ultrasound.[308] When evaluating carotid artery atherosclerotic plaques, intravascular ultrasound has been used in a similar fashion.

Post-stent miminum lumen diameter and minimum lumen area

Intravascular ultrasound can provide measurements of the minimum lumen diameter and minimum lumen area during

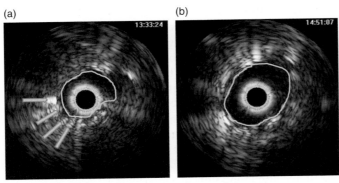

(a) 13:33:24   (b) 14:51:07

Fig. 17.5. (a) Intravascular ultrasound images demonstrating severe stenosis with plaque outside the struts of the carotid stent (arrows). No plaque inside the stent is identified. (b) There was improvement in vessel lumen diameter at post-stent angioplasty.

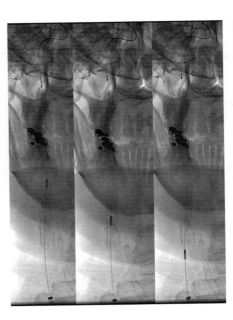

Fig. 17.6. Angiographic images demonstrating retraction of intravascular ultrasound probe using motorized device (not shown) after carotid stent placement to visualize any residual stenosis and apposition of stent to the surrounding vessel wall.

pre- and post-percutaneous carotid artery balloon angioplasty and stent placement. Gray scale intravascular ultrasound accurately determines the post stent lumen diameter[309] (see Fig. 17.5). Irshad *et al.* recommend using the gray scale or color flow intravascular ultrasound, instead of virtual histology maps, when confirming proper stent deployment.[242] Good judgment is needed in situations where further treatment is needed because overzealous treatment may risk neurological complications, despite the information provided through the intravascular ultrasound procedure.[247,248,309]

Intravascular ultrasound and restenosis

Vascular remodeling, after angioplasty and stenting, can be evaluated through intravascular ultrasound. Post-angioplasty lumen diameter, area and plaque percentage are factors quantifiable by intravascular ultrasound that predispose to restenosis.[310] A higher risk of restenosis has been found when a small post-procedural carotid stent diameter and reduced stent expansion were recognized by intravascular ultrasound.[236,311–313] Stent under-expansion and deformity was not reliably detected prior to the development of intravascular ultrasound imaging.[314,315] Intravascular ultrasound imaging has suggested that balloon expandable endovascular stents within carotid arteries may be subject to two types of compressive forces, that will lead to stent deformation and restenosis: (1) two point compressive force causing eccentric deformation; and (2) multidirectional compressive force causing complete circumferential encroachment of the stent struts around the catheter.[314,316,317] Rosenfield *et al.* found that intravascular ultrasound was more sensitive than angiography when detecting restenosis of endovascular stents secondary to stent compression.[314] Restenosis may occur in the absence of any obvious neo-intimal hyperplasia.[314] The quantitative assessment of arterial luminal volume through intravascular ultrasound also determines the extent of restenosis (see Fig. 17.6).

Intravascular ultrasound: aneurysm and dissection

Intravascular ultrasound can act in a complementary manner to other neuroradiological studies such as magnetic resonance imaging and 3D-computed tomography angiography in the treatment of cervical aneurysms. Intravascular ultrasound has been utilized to measure the extent of arterial dissections after balloon angioplasty in the carotid and coronary circulation.[318–320] It has been applied to measure the most distal and proximal extents of an intracranial dissection and to gauge whether the entire length of the dissection has been covered by the stents after treatment.[232] The true extent of an intracranial dissection of the left internal carotid artery, that angiographically extended from the level of the carotid canal to the cavernous-carotid segment and was occlusive, was assessed by advancing the intravascular ultrasound catheter past the area of the lesion to the normal artery. Color flow intravascular ultrasound imaging can demonstrate trace flow of blood into the true lumen of an arterial dissection. It is very important to confirm that the entire dissection is covered by stents because recanalization can occur from a distal damaged section, in the event that only the proximal entry point of the dissection is treated.[232]

Aneurysm wall composition, intra-aneurysmal contents (e.g., thrombus or calcification) and the aneurysm neck can be better defined using intravascular ultrasound imaging.[234,321,322] A dissecting or pseudo-aneurysm is indicated by intravascular ultrasound when a defect of both the hypoechoic (dark) signal of the normal media and hyperechoic (white) signal of the adventitia is found.

Safety of intravascular ultrasound

Intravascular ultrasound has been a relatively safe procedure. Manninen *et al.* did not encounter any adverse effects in 22 patients who underwent intravascular ultrasound imaging of their carotid arteries.[240] Similarly, Weissman *et al.* did not encounter an adverse event in the 102 patients that had their distal internal carotid artery and common carotid artery imaged by intravascular ultrasound.[323] An observational study was conducted by Clark *et al.* to assess the safety and utility of intravascular ultrasound during percutaneous carotid artery stent placement and the procedural success was found to be 97%.[236] At 30 days post-procedure, the stroke rate and combined stroke or death rate was 5% and 6%, respectively.[236] One patient had a common carotid artery perforation, but ultimately had a successful procedure.[236] The ultrasound catheter itself may disrupt an atherosclerotic plaque, releasing plaque material into the intra-arterial environment, which may lead to embolic stroke. Some investigators recommend using intravenous heparin while performing the intravascular ultrasound study to avoid the development of thrombosis.

Future utility of intravascular ultrasound

A reduction in the rate of ischemic strokes during and after the percutaneous carotid artery stenting procedure may be achieved through use of intravascular ultrasound. Intravascular ultrasound can be used to identify intraluminal embolic material or carotid plaque histology patterns that are more likely to cause embolic events.[309] In conjunction with intravascular ultrasound, the usage of distal embolic protection devices may reduce the incidence of procedure-related stroke in high risk patients.[236,324–330] Intraluminal lesions, which can represent a ruptured plaque or thrombus, have been identified with intravascular ultrasound post-stent evaluation before the removal of the distal embolic protection device leading to their treatment, ultimately reducing post stent embolic events.[309] Intravascular ultrasound can also potentially be used during the treatment of an acute ischemic stroke, in order to help identify the exact location of the causative occlusion and its composition (calcific versus fibrous vs. soft clot). The treatment modality subsequently used can ultimately be based on the information provided. Similarly, intravascular ultrasound may be used to identify carotid artery atherosclerotic plaques in high risk, asymptomatic patients so that treatment can be rendered prior to the development of stroke, transient ischemic attack, or retinal ischemic events.

References

1. Wada J. An experimental study on the neural mechanism of the spread of epileptic impulse. *Folia Psychiatr Neurol Jpn* 1951;**4**:289–301.

2. Castillo M, Mukherji SK, McCartney WH. Cerebral amobarbital sodium distribution during Wada testing: utility of digital subtraction angiography and single-photon emission tomography. *Neuroradiology* 2000;**42**:814–17.

3. Wada J, Rasmussen T. Intracarotid injection of sodium amytal for the lateralization of cerebral speech dominance. 1960. *J Neurosurg* 2007;**106**:1117–33.

4. Milner BBC, Rasmussen T. Study of short term memory after intracarotid injection of sodium amytal. *Trans Am Neurol Assoc* 1962;**87** 224–6.

5. Urbach H, Von Oertzen J, Klemm E, *et al.* Selective middle cerebral artery Wada tests as a part of presurgical evaluation in patients with drug-resistant epilepsies. *Epilepsia* 2002;**43**:1217–23.

6. Jones-Gotman M. *Commentary: Psychological Evaluation-testing Hippocampal Function.* New York: Raven Press, 1987.

7. Yen DJ, Lirng JF, Shih YH, *et al.* Selective posterior cerebral artery amobarbital test in patients with temporal lobe epilepsy for surgical treatment. *Seizure* 2006;**15**: 117–24.

8. Wieser HGLT, Valavanis A. Selective amytal memory tests: correlation with postoperative results (Abstract). *Epilepsia* 1989;**30**:724.

9. Wieser H. *Anterior Cerebral Artery Amobarbital Test.* New York: Raven Press, 1991.

10. Landis TRM, Wieser HG, Schiess R. Dissociated memory function during a new "selective" amytal procedure. *J Clin Exp Neuropsychol* 1988;**10**:83.

11. Groth-Marnat G, Gallagher, R, Hale, JB, Kaplan, E. *The Wechsler Intelligence Scales.* New York: John Wiley & Sons, Inc, 2000.

12. Delis DC, Kramer, J.H., Kaplan, E., *et al. California Verbal LearningTest Manual* (Research Edition). San Antonio,TX: Psychological Corporation/Harcourt Brace, 1987.

13. Wechsler D. *Wechsler Memory Scale–Revised (WMS-R) Manual. The Psychological Corporation.* San Antonio, TX: Harcourt Brace Jovanovich, Inc, 1987.

14. Kaplan E, Goodglass, H., Weintraub, S. *The Boston Naming Test.* 2nd edn. Philadelphia: Lea & Febiger, 1983.

15. Hermann BP, Seidenberg M, Schoenfeld J, Peterson J, Leveroni C, Wyler AR. Empirical techniques for determining the reliability, magnitude, and pattern of neuropsychological change after epilepsy surgery. *Epilepsia* 1996;**37**:942–50.

16. Sawrie SM, Chelune GJ, Naugle RI, Luders HO. Empirical methods for assessing meaningful neuropsychological change following epilepsy surgery. *J Int Neuropsychol Soc* 1996;**2**:556–64.

17. Wechsler D. *Wechsler Memory Scale.* 3rd edn. San Antonio, TX: The Psychological Corporation; 1997a.

18. Kubu CS, Girvin JP, McLachlan RS, Pavol M, Harnadek MC. Does the intracarotid amobarbital procedure predict global amnesia after temporal lobectomy? *Epilepsia* 2000;**41**:1321–9.

19. Fitzsimmons BF, Marshall RS, Pile-Spellman J, Lazar RM. Neurobehavioral differences in superselective Wada testing with amobarbital versus lidocaine. *Am J Neuroradiol* 2003;**24**:1456–60.

20. von Oertzen J, Klemm E, Urbach H, *et al.* SATSCOM–Selective amobarbital test intraarterial SPECT coregistered to MRI: description of a method assessing selective perfusion. *Neuroimage* 2000;**12**:617–22.

21. Rausch R, Babb TL. Hippocampal neuron loss and memory scores before and after temporal lobe surgery for epilepsy. *Arch Neurol* 1993;**50**:812–17.

22. Saling MM, Berkovic SF, O'Shea MF, Kalnins RM, Darby DG, Bladin PF. Lateralization of verbal memory and unilateral hippocampal sclerosis: evidence of task-specific effects. *J Clin Exp Neuropsychol* 1993;**15**:608–18.

23. Loring DW, Meador KJ, Lee GP, *et al.* Wada memory performance predicts

seizure outcome following anterior temporal lobectomy. *Neurology* 1994;**44**:2322–4.

24. Sperling MR, Saykin AJ, Glosser G, *et al.* Predictors of outcome after anterior temporal lobectomy: the intracarotid amobarbital test. *Neurology* 1994;**44**:2325–30.

25. Urbach H, Klemm E, Linke DB, *et al.* Posterior cerebral artery Wada test: sodium amytal distribution and functional deficits. *Neuroradiology* 2001;**43**:290–4.

26. Wieser HG, Yasargil MG. Selective amygdalohippocampectomy as a surgical treatment of mesiobasal limbic epilepsy. *Surg Neurol* 1982;**17**:445–57.

27. Huther G, Dorfl J, Van der Loos H, Jeanmonod D. Microanatomic and vascular aspects of the temporomesial region. *Neurosurgery* 1998;**43**: 1118–36.

28. Wieser HG, Muller S, Schiess R, *et al.* The anterior and posterior selective temporal lobe amobarbital tests: angiographic, clinical, electroencephalographic, PET, SPECT findings, and memory performance. *Brain Cogn* 1997;**33**:71–97.

29. Carpenter MB, Noback CR, Moss ML. The anterior choroidal artery; its origins course, distribution, and variations. *AMA Arch Neurol Psychiatry* 1954;**71**:714–22.

30. Muller J, Shaw L. Arterial vascularization of the human hippocampus. 1. Extracerebral relationships. *Arch Neurol* 1965;**13**:45–7.

31. Yasargil MG, Teddy PJ, Roth P. Selective amygdalo-hippocampectomy. Operative anatomy and surgical technique. *Adv Tech Stand Neurosurg* 1985;**12**:93–123.

32. Margolis MINT, Hoyt WF. The posterior cerebral artery. II. Gross and Roentgenographic Anatomy. St. Louis: Mosby, 1974.

33. Stephens RB.SD. *Arteries and Veins of the Human Brain.* Springfield, IL: Charles C Thomas, 1969.

34. Erdem A, Yasargil G, Roth P. Microsurgical anatomy of the hippocampal arteries. *J Neurosurg* 1993;**79**:256–65.

35. Saeki N, Rhoton AL, Jr. Microsurgical anatomy of the upper basilar artery and the posterior circle of Willis. *J Neurosurg* 1977;**46**:563–78.

36. Marinkovic S, Milisavljevic M, Puskas L. Microvascular anatomy of the hippocampal formation. *Surg Neurol* 1992;**37**:339–49.

37. Rhoton AL, Jr., Fujii K, Fradd B. Microsurgical anatomy of the anterior choroidal artery. *Surg Neurol* 1979;**12**:171–87.

38. Hussein S, Renella RR, Dietz H. Microsurgical anatomy of the anterior choroidal artery. *Acta Neurochir (Wien)* 1988;**92**:19–28.

39. Klemm E, Urbach, H., Reul, J., *et al.* Functional inactivation of the hippocampus identified by high resolution intraarterial 99m Tc-HMPAO SPECT and angiography: comparison of the intracarotidal and the selective posterior cerebral artery amobarbital test. (Abstract). *Eur J Nucl Med* 1998;**25** (PS-305):1060.

40. Jack CR, Jr., Nichols DA, Sharbrough FW, Marsh WR, Petersen RC. Selective posterior cerebral artery Amytal test for evaluating memory function before surgery for temporal lobe seizure. *Radiology* 1988;**168**:787–93.

41. Horel JA. The neuroanatomy of amnesia. A critique of the hippocampal memory hypothesis. *Brain* 1978;**101**:403–45.

42. Rausch R, Silfvenius, H, Wieser, HG, Dodrill, CB, Meador, KJ, Jones-Gotman, M. *Intraarterial Amobarbital Procedures.* 2nd edn. New York: Raven Press, 1993.

43. Jack CR, Jr., Nichols DA, Sharbrough FW, et al. Selective posterior cerebral artery injection of amytal: new method of preoperative memory testing. *Mayo Clin Proc* 1989;**64**:965–75.

44. Brechtelsbauer D.KE, Urbach H., *et al.* Functional inactivation of the hippocampus in the intracarotid Wada-test. Correlation of angiography and high resolution SPECT. *Klin Neuroradiol* 1998;**8**:182–5.

45. Urbach H, Kurthen M, Klemm E, *et al.* Amobarbital effects on the posterior hippocampus during the intracarotid amobarbital test. *Neurology* 1999;**52**:1596–602.

46. Quiske AS-BA, Juengling F, Zentner J, Klisch J. Selective or Superselective Wada Test for Postoperative Memory Prediction? (Case report). *Klin Neuroradiology* 2003;**13**: 45–8.

47. Terzian H. Behavioural and EEG effects of intracarotid sodium amytal injection. *Acta Neurochir (Wien)* 1964;**12**:230–9.

48. Lee GP, Loring DW, Meador KJ, Flanigin HF, Brooks BS. Severe behavioral complications following intracarotid sodium amobarbital injection: implications for hemispheric asymmetry of emotion. *Neurology* 1988;**38**:1233–6.

49. de Paola L, Mader MJ, Germiniani FM, *et al.* Bizarre behavior during intracarotid sodium amytal testing (Wada test): are they predictable? *Arq Neuropsiquiatr* 2004;**62**:444–8.

50. Lu LH, Barrett AM, Cibula JE, Gilmore RL, Fennell EB, Heilman KM. Dissociation of anosognosia and phantom movement during the Wada test. *J Neurol Neurosurg Psychiatry* 2000;**69**:820–3.

51. Masia SL, Perrine K, Westbrook L, Alper K, Devinsky O. Emotional outbursts and post-traumatic stress disorder during intracarotid amobarbital procedure. *Neurology* 2000;**54**:1691–3.

52. O'Shea MF, Saling MM, Berkovic SF. Behavioural status during the intracarotid amobarbital procedure (Wada test): relevance for surgical management. *J Neurol Neurosurg Psychiatry* 1999;**67**:549.

53. Ahern GL, Herring AM, Labiner DM, Weinand ME, Hutzler R. Affective self-report during the intracarotid sodium amobarbital test: group differences. *J Int Neuropsychol Soc* 2000;**6**: 659–67.

54. Rossi GF, Rosadini, G. *Experimental Analysis of Cerebral Dominance in Man.* New York: Grune & Stratton, 1967.

55. Milner B.BC. Discussion in: Rossi GF, Rosadini G. *Experimental Analysis of Cerebral Dominance in Man.* New York: Grune & Stratton, 1967.

56. Lee GP, Loring DW, Meader KJ, Brooks BB. Hemispheric specialization for emotional expression: a reexamination of results from intracarotid administration of sodium amobarbital. *Brain Cogn* 1990;**12**:267–80.

57. Risse GLFM, Mercer DK, Hempel AM, Gates JR, Moriarty GL. The incidence and severity of affective responses following intracarotid injections of amobarbital. *Epilepsia* 1994;**35** (Suppl. 8):77.

58. Tengesdal M. Experiences with intracarotid injections of sodium amytal. A preliminary report. *Acta Neurol Scand Suppl* 1963;**39**:Suppl 4:329–43.

59. Fedio P, Weinberg LK. Dysnomia and impairment of verbal memory following intracarotid injection of sodium amytal. *Brain Res* 1971;**31**:159–68.

60. Kurthen M, Linke DB, Reuter BM, Hufnagel A, Elger CE. Severe negative emotional reactions in intracarotid sodium amytal procedures: further evidence for hemispheric asymmetries? *Cortex* 1991;**27**:333–7.

61. Claverie BRA. Positive emotional reactions in intracarotid sodium amytal (Wada) procedures. *J Epilepsy* 1994;**7**:137–43.

62. Petersen RSF. *Posterior Cerebral Artery Amobarbital Test*. New York: Raven Press, 1991.

63. Brassel F, Weissenborn K, Ruckert N, Hussein S, Becker H. Superselective intra-arterial amytal (Wada test) in temporal lobe epilepsy: basics for neuroradiological investigations. *Neuroradiology* 1996;**38**:417–21.

64. Hajek M, Valavanis A, Yonekawa Y, Schiess R, Buck A, Wieser HG. Selective amobarbital test for the determination of language function in patients with epilepsy with frontal and posterior temporal brain lesions. *Epilepsia* 1998;**39**:389–98.

65. Brundert S, Elger CE, Solymosi L, Kurthen M, Linke D. [The selective amobarbital test in epileptology]. *Radiologe* 1993;**33**:213–18.

66. Stabell KE, Bakke SJ, Andresen S, *et al.* Selective posterior cerebral artery amobarbital test: its role in presurgical memory assessment in temporal lobe epilepsy. *Epilepsia* 2004;**45**:817–25.

67. Vulliemoz S, Pegna AJ, Annoni JM, *et al.* The selective amobarbital test in the anterior choroidal artery: perfusion pattern assessed by intraarterial SPECT and prediction of postoperative verbal memory. *Epilepsy Behav* 2008;**12**:445–55.

68. Stabell KE, Andresen S, Bakke SJ, *et al.* Emotional responses during unilateral amobarbital anesthesia: differential hemispheric contributions? *Acta Neurol Scand* 2004;**110**:313–21.

69. Kopelman M. Disorders of memory. *Brain* 2002;**125**:2152–90.

70. Jone-Gotman M, Smith, ML, Wieser, HG *Intra-arterial Amobarbital Procedure*. 1st edn. Philadelphia: Lippincott-Raven Publisher, 1998.

71. Weissenborn K, Ruckert N, Brassel F, Becker H, Dietz H. A proposed modification of the Wada test for presurgical assessment in temporal lobe epilepsy. *Neuroradiology* 1996;**38**:422–9.

72. Ivnik RJ, Sharbrough FW, Laws ER, Jr. Anterior temporal lobectomy for the control of partial complex seizures: information for counseling patients. *Mayo Clin Proc* 1988;**63**:783–93.

73. Ivnik RJ, Sharbrough FW, Laws ER, Jr. Effects of anterior temporal lobectomy on cognitive function. *J Clin Psychol* 1987;**43**:128–37.

74. Escosa-Bage M, Sola RG, Liberal-Gonzalez R, Caniego JL, Castrillo-Cazon C. Fusiform aneurysm of the middle cerebral artery. *Rev Neurol* 2002;**34**:655–8.

75. Wieser H.G.MS. Improved multipolar foramen ovale electrode monitoring. *J Epilepsy* 1988;**1**:13–22.

76. Perret E. The left frontal lobe of man and the suppression of habitual responses in verbal categorical behaviour. *Neuropsychologia* 1974;**12**:323–30.

77. Regard M, Strauss E, Knapp P. Children's production on verbal and non-verbal fluency tasks. *Percept Mot Skills* 1982;**55**:839–44.

78. Bouwer MS, Jones-Gotman M, Gotman J. Duration of sodium amytal effect: behavioral and EEG measures. *Epilepsia* 1993;**34**:61–8.

79. Jeffery PJ, Monsein LH, Szabo Z, *et al.* Mapping the distribution of amobarbital sodium in the intracarotid Wada test by use of Tc-99m HMPAO with SPECT. *Radiology* 1991;**178**:847–50.

80. Wieser HG, Elger CE, Stodieck SR. The 'foramen ovale electrode': a new recording method for the preoperative evaluation of patients suffering from mesio-basal temporal lobe epilepsy. *Electroencephalogr Clin Neurophysiol* 1985;**61**:314–22.

81. Hufnagel A, Elger CE, Boker DK, Linke DB, Kurthen M, Solymosi L. Activation of the epileptic focus during intracarotid amobarbital test. Electrocorticographic registration via subdural electrodes. *Electroencephalogr Clin Neurophysiol* 1990;**75**:453–63.

82. Rauch RA, Vinuela F, Dion J, *et al.* Preembolization functional evaluation in brain arteriovenous malformations: the ability of superselective Amytal test to predict neurologic dysfunction before embolization. *Am J Neuroradiol* 1992;**13**:309–14.

83. Rauch RA, Vinuela F, Dion J, et al. Preembolization functional evaluation in brain arteriovenous malformations: the superselective Amytal test. *Am J Neuroradiol* 1992;**13**:303–8.

84. Penfield W, Milner B. Memory deficit produced by bilateral lesions in the hippocampal zone. *AMA Arch Neurol Psychiatry* 1958;**79**:475–97.

85. Milner B, Penfield W. The effect of hippocampal lesions on recent memory. *Trans Am Neurol Assoc* 1955:42–8.

86. Scoville WB, Milner B. Loss of recent memory after bilateral hippocampal lesions. *J Neurol Neurosurg Psychiatry* 1957;**20**:11–21.

87. Markowitsch HJ. Can amnesia be caused by damage of a single brain structure? *Cortex* 1984;**20**:27–45.

88. Mishkin M, Appenzeller T. The anatomy of memory. *Sci Am* 1987;**256**:80–9.

89. von Cramon DY, Hebel N, Schuri U. Verbal memory and learning in unilateral posterior cerebral infarction. A report on 30 cases. *Brain* 1988;**111** (Pt 5):1061–77.

90. Penfield W, Flanigin H. Surgical therapy of temporal lobe seizures. *AMA Arch Neurol Psychiatry* 1950;**64**:491–500.

91. Penfield W, Baldwin M. Temporal lobe seizures and the technic of subtotal temporal lobectomy. *Ann Surg* 1952;**136**:625–34.

92. Feindel W. Factors contributing to the success or failure of surgical intervention for epilepsy. *Adv Neurol* 1975;**8**:281–98.

93. Schomer DL. Current concepts in neurology. Partial epilepsy. *N Engl J Med* 1983;**309**:536–9.

94. Bengzon AR, Rasmussen T, Gloor P, Dussault J, Stephens M. Prognostic factors in the surgical treatment of temporal lobe epileptics. *Neurology* 1968;**18**:717–31.

95. Meyer FB, Marsh WR, Laws ER, Jr., Sharbrough FW. Temporal lobectomy

in children with epilepsy. *J Neurosurg* 1986;**64**:371–6.

96. Teramoto A, Yoshida Y, Sanno N, Nemoto S. Cavernous sinus sampling in patients with adrenocorticotrophic hormone-dependent Cushing's syndrome with emphasis on inter- and intracavernous adrenocorticotrophic hormone gradients. *J Neurosurg* 1998;**89**:762–8.

97. Kaltsas GA, Giannulis MG, Newell-Price JD, et al. A critical analysis of the value of simultaneous inferior petrosal sinus sampling in Cushing's disease and the occult ectopic adrenocorticotrophin syndrome. *J Clin Endocrinol Metab* 1999;**84**:487–92.

98. Doppman JL, Oldfield E, Krudy AG, et al. Petrosal sinus sampling for Cushing syndrome: anatomical and technical considerations. Work in progress. *Radiology* 1984;**150**:99–103.

99. Xuereb GP, Prichard MM, Daniel PM. The arterial supply and venous drainage of the human hypophysis cerebri. *Q J Exp Physiol Cogn Med Sci* 1954;**39**:199–217.

100. Green HT. The venous drainage of the human hypophysis cerebri. *Am J Anat* 1957;**100**:435–69.

101. Miller DL, Doppman JL. Petrosal sinus sampling: technique and rationale. *Radiology* 1991;**178**:37–47.

102. Boskovic MSV, Josifov J. Uber die Sinus petrosi und ihre Zulusse. *Gegenbaurs Morphol Verb* 1963:420–9.

103. Peardon Donaghy R. *Surgery of the Dural Sinuses.* New York: Springer-Verlag, 1985.

104. Shiu PC, Hanafee WN, Wilson GH, Rand RW. Cavernous sinus venography. *Am J Roentgenol Radium Ther Nucl Med* 1968;**104**:57–62.

105. Wackenheim ABJ. *The Veins of the Posterior Fossa: Normal and Pathologic Findings.* Berlin: Springer-Verlag; 1978.

106. Stolic E, Mrvaljevic D. [Origins of the vertebral veins]. *C R Assoc Anat* 1970;**149**:1027–36.

107. Miller DL, Doppman JL, Chang R. Anatomy of the junction of the inferior petrosal sinus and the internal jugular vein. *Am J Neuroradiol* 1993;**14**: 1075–83.

108. Mamelak AN, Dowd CF, Tyrrell JB, McDonald JF, Wilson CB. Venous angiography is needed to interpret inferior petrosal sinus and cavernous sinus sampling data for lateralizing adrenocorticotropin-secreting adenomas. *J Clin Endocrinol Metab* 1996;**81**:475–81.

109. Lefournier V, Martinie M, Vasdev A, et al. Accuracy of bilateral inferior petrosal or cavernous sinuses sampling in predicting the lateralization of Cushing's disease pituitary microadenoma: influence of catheter position and anatomy of venous drainage. *J Clin Endocrinol Metab* 2003;**88**:196–203.

110. Magiakou MA, Mastorakos G, Oldfield EH, et al. Cushing's syndrome in children and adolescents. Presentation, diagnosis, and therapy. *N Engl J Med* 1994;**331**:629–36.

111. Pinette MG, Pan YQ, Oppenheim D, Pinette SG, Blackstone J. Bilateral inferior petrosal sinus corticotropin sampling with corticotropin-releasing hormone stimulation in a pregnant patient with Cushing's syndrome. *Am J Obstet Gynecol* 1994;**171**:563–4.

112. Utz A, Biller BM. The role of bilateral inferior petrosal sinus sampling in the diagnosis of Cushing's syndrome. *Arq Bras Endocrinol Metabol* 2007;**51**: 1329–38.

113. Frank SJ, Gesundheit N, Doppman JL, et al. Preoperative lateralization of pituitary microadenomas by petrosal sinus sampling: utility in two patients with non-ACTH-secreting tumors. *Am J Med* 1989;**87**:679–82.

114. Frey H, Torjesen PA, Enge IP, Stiris MG, Reinlie S. [Analysis of blood from the inferior sinus petrosus in patients with Cushing syndrome and acromegaly]. *Tidsskr Nor Laegeforen* 1994;**114**:2257–61.

115. Crock PA, Gilford EJ, Henderson JK, et al. Inferior petrosal sinus sampling in acromegaly. *Aust N Z J Med* 1989;**19**:244–7.

116. Doppman JL, Miller DL, Patronas NJ, et al. The diagnosis of acromegaly: value of inferior petrosal sinus sampling. *Am J Roentgenol* 1990;**154**:1075–7.

117. Newell-Price J, Trainer P, Besser M, Grossman A. The diagnosis and differential diagnosis of Cushing's syndrome and pseudo-Cushing's states. *Endocr Rev* 1998;**19**:647–72.

118. Findling JW, Kehoe ME, Shaker JL, Raff H. Routine inferior petrosal sinus sampling in the differential diagnosis of adrenocorticotropin (ACTH)-dependent Cushing's syndrome: early recognition of the occult ectopic ACTH syndrome. *J Clin Endocrinol Metab* 1991;**73**:408–13.

119. Lindsay JR, Nieman LK. Differential diagnosis and imaging in Cushing's syndrome. *Endocrinol Metab Clin North Am* 2005;**34**:403–21, x.

120. Raff HKM, Findling JW. *DDAVP increases inferior petrosal sinus ACTH concentration in patients with pituitary and ectopic ACTH-dependent Cushing's syndrome* (Abstract). 1997.

121. Findling J. Differential diagnosis of Cushing's syndrome. *Endocrinologist* 1996;**7**:17S–23S.

122. Vilar L, Freitas Mda C, Faria M, et al. Pitfalls in the diagnosis of Cushing's syndrome. *Arq Bras Endocrinol Metabol* 2007;**51**:1207–16.

123. Kaye TB, Crapo L. The Cushing syndrome: an update on diagnostic tests. *Ann Intern Med* 1990;**112**: 434–44.

124. Graham KE, Samuels MH, Nesbit GM, et al. Cavernous sinus sampling is highly accurate in distinguishing Cushing's disease from the ectopic adrenocorticotropin syndrome and in predicting intrapituitary tumor location. *J Clin Endocrinol Metab* 1999;**84**:1602–10.

125. Teramoto A, Hirakawa K, Sanno N, Osamura Y. Incidental pituitary lesions in 1,000 unselected autopsy specimens. *Radiology* 1994;**193**:161–4.

126. Ezzat S, Asa SL, Couldwell WT, et al. The prevalence of pituitary adenomas: a systematic review. *Cancer* 2004;**101**:613–9.

127. Hall WA, Luciano MG, Doppman JL, Patronas NJ, Oldfield EH. Pituitary magnetic resonance imaging in normal human volunteers: occult adenomas in the general population. *Ann Intern Med* 1994;**120**:817–20.

128. Booth GL, Redelmeier DA, Grosman H, Kovacs K, Smyth HS, Ezzat S. Improved diagnostic accuracy of inferior petrosal sinus sampling over imaging for localizing pituitary pathology in patients with Cushing's disease. *J Clin Endocrinol Metab* 1998;**83**:2291–5.

129. Reimondo G, Paccotti P, Minetto M, et al. The corticotrophin-releasing hormone test is the most reliable noninvasive method to differentiate pituitary from ectopic ACTH secretion

in Cushing's syndrome. *Clin Endocrinol (Oxf)* 2003;**58**:718–24.

130. Midgette AS, Aron DC. High-dose dexamethasone suppression testing versus inferior petrosal sinus sampling in the differential diagnosis of adrenocorticotropin-dependent Cushing's syndrome: a decision analysis. *Am J Med Sci* 1995;**309**:162–70.

131. Wiggam MI, Heaney AP, McIlrath EM, et al. Bilateral inferior petrosal sinus sampling in the differential diagnosis of adrenocorticotropin-dependent Cushing's syndrome: a comparison with other diagnostic tests. *J Clin Endocrinol Metab* 2000;**85**:1525–32.

132. Ilias I, Chang R, Pacak K, et al. Jugular venous sampling: an alternative to petrosal sinus sampling for the diagnostic evaluation of adrenocorticotropic hormone-dependent Cushing's syndrome. *J Clin Endocrinol Metab* 2004;**89**:3795–800.

133. Testa RM, Albiger N, Occhi G, et al. The usefulness of combined biochemical tests in the diagnosis of Cushing's disease with negative pituitary magnetic resonance imaging. *Eur J Endocrinol* 2007;**156**:241–8.

134. Arnaldi G, Angeli A, Atkinson AB, et al. Diagnosis and complications of Cushing's syndrome: a consensus statement. *J Clin Endocrinol Metab* 2003;**88**:5593–602.

135. Bochicchio D, Losa M, Buchfelder M. Factors influencing the immediate and late outcome of Cushing's disease treated by transsphenoidal surgery: a retrospective study by the European Cushing's Disease Survey Group. *J Clin Endocrinol Metab* 1995;**80**:3114–20.

136. Newell-Price J, Bertagna X, Grossman AB, Nieman LK. Cushing's syndrome. *Lancet* 2006;**367**:1605–17.

137. Landolt AM, Valavanis A, Girard J, Eberle AN. Corticotrophin-releasing factor-test used with bilateral, simultaneous inferior petrosal sinus blood-sampling for the diagnosis of pituitary-dependent Cushing's disease. *Clin Endocrinol (Oxf)* 1986;**25**:687–96.

138. Erickson D, Huston J, 3rd, Young WF, Jr., et al. Internal jugular vein sampling in adrenocorticotropic hormone-dependent Cushing's syndrome: a comparison with inferior petrosal sinus sampling. *Clin Endocrinol (Oxf)* 2004;**60**:413–9.

139. Doppman JL, Oldfield EH, Nieman LK. Bilateral sampling of the internal jugular vein to distinguish between mechanisms of adrenocorticotropic hormone-dependent Cushing syndrome. *Ann Intern Med* 1998;**128**:33–6.

140. Drury PL, Ratter S, Tomlin S, et al. Experience with selective venous sampling in diagnosis of ACTH-dependent Cushing's syndrome. *Br Med J (Clin Res Ed)* 1982;**284**:9–12.

141. Corrigan DF, Schaaf M, Whaley RA, Czerwinski CL, Earll JM. Selective venous sampling to differentiate ectopic ACTH secretion from pituitary Cushing's syndrome. *N Engl J Med* 1977;**296**:861–2.

142. Teramoto A, Nemoto S, Takakura K, Sasaki Y, Machida T. Selective venous sampling directly from cavernous sinus in Cushing's syndrome. *J Clin Endocrinol Metab* 1993;**76**:637–41.

143. Vandorpe RA, Fox AJ, Pelz DM, Lee DH. Direct sampling of the cavernous sinus in Cushing's disease. *Can Assoc Radiol J* 1994;**45**:234–7.

144. Yoshida Y, Sanno N, Teramoto A. Multiple pituitary hormone gradients from cavernous sinus sampling in patients with Cushing's disease. *Acta Neurochir (Wien)* 2000;**142**:1339–44.

145. Flitsch J, Ludecke DK, Knappe UJ, Grzyska U. Cavernous sinus sampling in selected cases of Cushing's disease. *Exp Clin Endocrinol Diabetes* 2002;**110**:329–35.

146. Doppman JL, Nieman LK, Chang R, et al. Selective venous sampling from the cavernous sinuses is not a more reliable technique than sampling from the inferior petrosal sinuses in Cushing's syndrome. *J Clin Endocrinol Metab* 1995;**80**:2485–9.

147. Miller DL, Doppman JL, Peterman SB, Nieman LK, Oldfield EH, Chang R. Neurologic complications of petrosal sinus sampling. *Radiology* 1992;**185**:143–7.

148. Doppman JL, Krudy AG, Girton ME, Oldfield EH. Basilar venous plexus of the posterior fossa: a potential source of error in petrosal sinus sampling. *Radiology* 1985;**155**:375–8.

149. Vilar L, Naves LA, Freitas Mda C, et al. [Endogenous Cushing's syndrome: clinical and laboratory features in 73 cases]. *Arq Bras Endocrinol Metabol* 2007;**51**:566–74.

150. Castinetti F, Morange I, Dufour H, et al. Desmopressin test during petrosal sinus sampling: a valuable tool to discriminate pituitary or ectopic ACTH-dependent Cushing's syndrome. *Eur J Endocrinol* 2007;**157**:271–7.

151. Belli S, Oneto A, Mendaro E. [Bilateral inferior petrosal sinus sampling in the differential diagnosis of ACTH-dependent Cushing's syndrome]. *Rev Med Chil* 2007;**135**:1095–102.

152. Tsagarakis S, Vassiliadi D, Kaskarelis IS, Komninos J, Souvatzoglou E, Thalassinos N. The application of the combined corticotropin-releasing hormone plus desmopressin stimulation during petrosal sinus sampling is both sensitive and specific in differentiating patients with Cushing's disease from patients with the occult ectopic adrenocorticotropin syndrome. *J Clin Endocrinol Metab* 2007;**92**:2080–6.

153. Machado MC, de Sa SV, Domenice S, et al. The role of desmopressin in bilateral and simultaneous inferior petrosal sinus sampling for differential diagnosis of ACTH-dependent Cushing's syndrome. *Clin Endocrinol (Oxf)* 2007;**66**:136–42.

154. Swearingen B, Katznelson L, Miller K, et al. Diagnostic errors after inferior petrosal sinus sampling. *J Clin Endocrinol Metab* 2004;**89**:3752–63.

155. Martines V, Mansueto G, Tosi F, Caruso B, Castello R, Procacci C. Selective venous sampling in diagnosing ACTH-dependent hypercortisolism. *Radiol Med (Torino)* 2003;**105**:356–61.

156. Vilar LCC. *Diagnosis and Differential Diagnosis of Cushing's Syndrome*. 3rd edn. Rio de Janeiro: Guanabara Koogan, 2006.

157. Zarrilli L, Colao A, Merola B, et al. Corticotropin-releasing hormone test: improvement of the diagnostic accuracy of simultaneous and bilateral inferior petrosal sinus sampling in patients with Cushing syndrome. *World J Surg* 1995;**19**:150–3.

158. Tabarin A, Greselle JF, San-Galli F, et al. Usefulness of the corticotropin-releasing hormone test during bilateral inferior petrosal sinus sampling for the diagnosis of Cushing's disease. *J Clin Endocrinol Metab* 1991;**73**:53–9.

159. McNally PG, Bolia A, Absalom SR, Falconer-Smith J, Howlett TA. Preliminary observations using endocrine markers of pituitary venous

dilution during bilateral simultaneous inferior petrosal sinus catheterization in Cushing's syndrome: is combined CRF and TRH stimulation of value? *Clin Endocrinol (Oxf)* 1993;**39**:681–6.

160. Strack TR, Schild HH, Bohl J, Beyer J, Schrezemeir J, Kahaly G. Selective bilateral blood sampling from the inferior petrosal sinus in Cushing's disease: effects of corticotropin-releasing factor and thyrotropin-releasing hormone on pituitary secretion. *Cardiovasc Intervent Radiol* 1993;**16**:287–92.

161. Cuneo RC, Lee W, Harper J, *et al.* Metyrapone pre-treated inferior petrosal sinus sampling in the differential diagnosis of ACTH-dependent Cushing's syndrome. *Clin Endocrinol (Oxf)* 1997;**46**:607–18.

162. Nieman LK, Cutler GB, Jr., Oldfield EH, Loriaux DL, Chrousos GP. The ovine corticotropin-releasing hormone (CRH) stimulation test is superior to the human CRH stimulation test for the diagnosis of Cushing's disease. *J Clin Endocrinol Metab* 1989;**69**:165–9.

163. Trainer PJ, Faria M, Newell-Price J, *et al.* A comparison of the effects of human and ovine corticotropin-releasing hormone on the pituitary-adrenal axis. *J Clin Endocrinol Metab* 1995;**80**:412–17.

164. Woods RJ, Grossman A, Saphier P, *et al.* Association of human corticotropin-releasing hormone to its binding protein in blood may trigger clearance of the complex. *J Clin Endocrinol Metab* 1994;**78**:73–6.

165. Dahia PL, Ahmed-Shuaib A, Jacobs RA, *et al.* Vasopressin receptor expression and mutation analysis in corticotropin-secreting tumors. *J Clin Endocrinol Metab* 1996;**81**:1768–71.

166. Newell-Price J, Perry L, Medbak S, *et al.* A combined test using desmopressin and corticotropin-releasing hormone in the differential diagnosis of Cushing's syndrome. *J Clin Endocrinol Metab* 1997;**82**:176–81.

167. Tsagarakis S, Kaskarelis IS, Kokkoris P, Malagari C, Thalassinos N. The application of a combined stimulation with CRH and desmopressin during bilateral inferior petrosal sinus sampling in patients with Cushing's syndrome. *Clin Endocrinol (Oxf)* 2000;**52**:355–61.

168. Tsagarakis S, Tsigos C, Vasiliou V, *et al.* The desmopressin and combined CRH-desmopressin tests in the differential diagnosis of ACTH-dependent Cushing's syndrome: constraints imposed by the expression of V2 vasopressin receptors in tumors with ectopic ACTH secretion. *J Clin Endocrinol Metab* 2002;**87**:1646–53.

169. Tsagarakis S, Vasiliou V, Kokkoris P, Stavropoulos G, Thalassinos N. Assessment of cortisol and ACTH responses to the desmopressin test in patients with Cushing's syndrome and simple obesity. *Clin Endocrinol (Oxf)* 1999;**51**:473–7.

170. Moro M, Putignano P, Losa M, Invitti C, Maraschini C, Cavagnini F. The desmopressin test in the differential diagnosis between Cushing's disease and pseudo-Cushing states. *J Clin Endocrinol Metab* 2000;**85**:3569–74.

171. Scott LV, Medbak S, Dinan TG. ACTH and cortisol release following intravenous desmopressin: a dose-response study. *Clin Endocrinol (Oxf)* 1999;**51**:653–8.

172. Arlt W, Dahia PL, Callies F, *et al.* Ectopic ACTH production by a bronchial carcinoid tumour responsive to desmopressin in vivo and in vitro. *Clin Endocrinol (Oxf)* 1997;**47**:623–7.

173. Yanovski JA, Nieman LK, Doppman JL, *et al.* Plasma levels of corticotropin-releasing hormone in the inferior petrosal sinuses of healthy volunteers, patients with Cushing's syndrome, and patients with pseudo-Cushing states. *J Clin Endocrinol Metab* 1998;**83**:1485–8.

174. Calogero AE, Bagdy G, Szemeredi K, Tartaglia ME, Gold PW, Chrousos GP. Mechanisms of serotonin receptor agonist-induced activation of the hypothalamic-pituitary-adrenal axis in the rat. *Endocrinology* 1990;**126**:1888–94.

175. Calogero AE, Gallucci WT, Chrousos GP, Gold PW. Interaction between GABAergic neurotransmission and rat hypothalamic corticotropin-releasing hormone secretion in vitro. *Brain Res* 1988;**463**:28–36.

176. Kalogeras KT, Calogero AE, Kuribayiashi T, *et al.* In vitro and in vivo effects of the triazolobenzodiazepine alprazolam on hypothalamic–pituitary–adrenal function: pharmacological and clinical implications. *J Clin Endocrinol Metab* 1990;**70**:1462–71.

177. Rittmaster RS, Cutler GB, Jr., Sobel DO, *et al.* Morphine inhibits the pituitary-adrenal response to ovine corticotropin-releasing hormone in normal subjects. *J Clin Endocrinol Metab* 1985;**60**:891–5.

178. Oldfield EH, Doppman JL, Nieman LK, *et al.* Petrosal sinus sampling with and without corticotropin-releasing hormone for the differential diagnosis of Cushing's syndrome. *N Engl J Med* 1991;**325**:897–905.

179. Colao A, Faggiano A, Pivonello R, Pecori Giraldi F, Cavagnini F, Lombardi G. Inferior petrosal sinus sampling in the differential diagnosis of Cushing's syndrome: results of an Italian multicenter study. *Eur J Endocrinol* 2001;**144**:499–507.

180. Bonelli FS, Huston J, 3rd, Carpenter PC, Erickson D, Young WF, Jr., Meyer FB. Adrenocorticotropic hormone-dependent Cushing's syndrome: sensitivity and specificity of inferior petrosal sinus sampling. *Am J Neuroradiol* 2000;**21**:690–6.

181. Invitti C, Pecori Giraldi F, de Martin M, Cavagnini F. Diagnosis and management of Cushing's syndrome: results of an Italian multicentre study. Study Group of the Italian Society of Endocrinology on the Pathophysiology of the Hypothalamic-Pituitary-Adrenal Axis. *J Clin Endocrinol Metab* 1999;**84**:440–8.

182. Doppman JL, Chang R, Oldfield EH, Chrousos G, Stratakis CA, Nieman LK. The hypoplastic inferior petrosal sinus: a potential source of false-negative results in petrosal sampling for Cushing's disease. *J Clin Endocrinol Metab* 1999;**84**:533–40.

183. Yamamoto Y, Davis DH, Nippoldt TB, Young WF, Jr., Huston J, 3rd, Parisi JE. False-positive inferior petrosal sinus sampling in the diagnosis of Cushing's disease. Report of two cases. *J Neurosurg* 1995;**83**:1087–91.

184. Lopez J, Barcelo B, Lucas T, *et al.* Petrosal sinus sampling for diagnosis of Cushing's disease: evidence of false negative results. *Clin Endocrinol (Oxf)* 1996;**45**:147–56.

185. Findling JW, Raff H. Diagnosis and differential diagnosis of Cushing's syndrome. *Endocrinol Metab Clin North Am* 2001;**30**:729–47.

186. Dwyer AJ, Frank JA, Doppman JL, *et al.* Pituitary adenomas in patients with Cushing disease: initial experience with Gd-DTPA-enhanced MR imaging. *Radiology* 1987;**163**:421–6.

187. Manni A, Latshaw RF, Page R, Santen RJ. Simultaneous bilateral venous sampling for adrenocorticotropin in pituitary-dependent cushing's disease: evidence for lateralization of pituitary venous drainage. *J Clin Endocrinol Metab* 1983;**57**:1070–3.

188. Findling JW, Aron DC, Tyrrell JB, *et al.* Selective venous sampling for ACTH in Cushing's syndrome: differentiation between Cushing disease and the ectopic ACTH syndrome. *Ann Intern Med* 1981;**94**:647–52.

189. Lin LY, Teng MM, Huang CI, *et al.* Assessment of bilateral inferior petrosal sinus sampling (BIPSS) in the diagnosis of Cushing's disease. *J Chin Med Assoc* 2007;**70**:4–10.

190. Yamada S, Shishiba Y, Sawano S, Aiba T. ACTH determination in a petrosal sinus venous specimen after corticotrophin releasing factor provides the best clue on the laterality of microadenoma in Cushing's disease. *Endocrinol Jpn* 1989;**36**:269–74.

191. Boolell M, Gilford E, Arnott R, McNeill P, Cummins J, Alford F. An overview of bilateral synchronous inferior petrosal sinus sampling (BSIPSS) in the pre-operative assessment of Cushing's disease. *Aust N Z J Med* 1990;**20**:765–70.

192. Landolt AM, Schubiger O, Maurer R, Girard J. The value of inferior petrosal sinus sampling in diagnosis and treatment of Cushing's disease. *Clin Endocrinol (Oxf)* 1994;**40**:485–92.

193. Mampalam TJ, Tyrrell JB, Wilson CB. Transsphenoidal microsurgery for Cushing disease. A report of 216 cases. *Ann Intern Med* 1988;**109**:487–93.

194. Merola B, Colao A, Rossi R, *et al.* Bilateral and simultaneous inferior petrosal sinus sampling in the early diagnosis of an ACTH-producing pituitary microadenoma and its detection by magnetic resonance one year later. *Horm Res* 1992;**37**:64–7.

195. Snow RB, Patterson RH, Jr., Horwith M, Saint Louis L, Fraser RA. Usefulness of preoperative inferior petrosal vein sampling in Cushing's disease. *Surg Neurol* 1988;**29**:17–21.

196. Vignati F, Berselli ME, Scialfa G, Boccardi E, Loli P. Bilateral and simultaneous venous sampling of inferior petrosal sinuses for ACTH and PRL determination: preoperative localization of ACTH-secreting microadenomas. *J Endocrinol Invest* 1989;**12**:235–8.

197. Zovickian J, Oldfield EH, Doppman JL, Cutler GB, Jr., Loriaux DL. Usefulness of inferior petrosal sinus venous endocrine markers in Cushing's disease. *J Neurosurg* 1988;**68**:205–10.

198. Oldfield EH, Chrousos GP, Schulte HM, *et al.* Preoperative lateralization of ACTH-secreting pituitary microadenomas by bilateral and simultaneous inferior petrosal venous sinus sampling. *N Engl J Med* 1985;**312**:100–3.

199. Miller DL, Doppman JL, Nieman LK, *et al.* Petrosal sinus sampling: discordant lateralization of ACTH-secreting pituitary microadenomas before and after stimulation with corticotropin-releasing hormone. *Radiology* 1990;**176**:429–31.

200. de Herder WW, Uitterlinden P, Pieterman H, *et al.* Pituitary tumour localization in patients with Cushing's disease by magnetic resonance imaging. Is there a place for petrosal sinus sampling? *Clin Endocrinol (Oxf)* 1994;**40**:87–92.

201. Kai Y, Hamada J, Nishi T, Morioka M, Mizuno T, Ushio Y. Usefulness of multiple-site venous sampling in the treatment of adrenocorticotropic hormone-producing pituitary adenomas. *Surg Neurol* 2003;**59**:292–8; discussion 8–9.

202. Yanovski JA, Cutler GB, Jr., Doppman JL, *et al.* The limited ability of inferior petrosal sinus sampling with corticotropin-releasing hormone to distinguish Cushing's disease from pseudo-Cushing states or normal physiology. *J Clin Endocrinol Metab* 1993;**77**:503–9.

203. Freda PU, Wardlaw SL, Bruce JN, Post KD, Goland RS. Differential diagnosis in cushing syndrome. Use of corticotropin-releasing hormone. *Medicine (Baltimore)* 1995;**74**:74–82.

204. O'Brien T, Young WF, Jr., Davila DG, *et al.* Cushing's syndrome associated with ectopic production of corticotrophin-releasing hormone, corticotrophin and vasopressin by a phaeochromocytoma. *Clin Endocrinol (Oxf)* 1992;**37**:460–7.

205. Case records of the Massachusetts General Hospital. Weekly clinicopathological exercises. Case 52–1987. A 20-year-old woman with Cushing's disease and a pulmonary nodule. *N Engl J Med* 1987;**317**:1648–58.

206. Young J, Deneux C, Grino M, Oliver C, Chanson P, Schaison G. Pitfall of petrosal sinus sampling in a Cushing's syndrome secondary to ectopic adrenocorticotropin-corticotropin releasing hormone (ACTH-CRH) secretion. *J Clin Endocrinol Metab* 1998;**83**:305–8.

207. Bethge H, Arlt W, Zimmermann U, *et al.* Cushing's syndrome due to an ectopic ACTH-secreting pituitary tumour mimicking occult paraneoplastic ectopic ACTH production. *Clin Endocrinol (Oxf)* 1999;**51**:809–14.

208. Al-Gahtany M, Bilbao J, Kovacs K, Horvath E, Smyth HS. Juxtaposition of an ectopic corticotroph adenoma of the sphenoid sinus with orthotopic intrasellar corticotroph hyperplasia in a patient with Cushing disease. Case report. *J Neurosurg* 2003;**98**:891–6.

209. Findling JW, Kehoe ME, Raff H. Identification of patients with Cushing's disease with negative pituitary adrenocorticotropin gradients during inferior petrosal sinus sampling: prolactin as an index of pituitary venous effluent. *J Clin Endocrinol Metab* 2004;**89**:6005–9.

210. Aniszewski JP, Young WF, Jr., Thompson GB, Grant CS, van Heerden JA. Cushing syndrome due to ectopic adrenocorticotropic hormone secretion. *World J Surg* 2001;**25**:934–40.

211. Doppman JL, Nieman L, Miller DL, *et al.* Ectopic adrenocorticotropic hormone syndrome: localization studies in 28 patients. *Radiology* 1989;**172**:115–24.

212. Findling JW, Raff H. Screening and diagnosis of Cushing's syndrome. *Endocrinol Metab Clin North Am* 2005;**34**:385–402, ix–x.

213. Findling JW, Raff H. Cushing's Syndrome: important issues in diagnosis and management. *J Clin Endocrinol Metab* 2006;**91**:3746–53.

214. Meier CA, Biller BM. Clinical and biochemical evaluation of Cushing's syndrome. *Endocrinol Metab Clin North Am* 1997;**26**:741–62.

215. Hanafee W, Rosen LM, Weidner W, Wilson GH. Venography of the cavernous sinus, orbital veins, and basal venous plexus. *Radiology* 1965;**84**:751–3.

216. Obuobie K, Davies JS, Ogunko A, Scanlon MF. Venous thrombo-embolism following inferior petrosal sinus sampling in Cushing's disease. *J Endocrinol Invest* 2000;**23**:542–4.

217. Blevins LS, Jr., Clark RV, Owens DS. Thromboembolic complications after inferior petrosal sinus sampling in patients with cushing's syndrome. *Endocr Pract* 1998;**4**:365–7.

218. Diez JJ, Iglesias P. Pulmonary thromboembolism after inferior petrosal sinus sampling in Cushing's syndrome. *Clin Endocrinol (Oxf)* 1997;**46**:777.

219. Sturrock ND, Jeffcoate WJ. A neurological complication of inferior petrosal sinus sampling during investigation for Cushing's disease: a case report. *J Neurol Neurosurg Psychiatry* 1997;**62**:527–8.

220. Gandhi CD, Meyer SA, Patel AB, Johnson DM, Post KD. Neurologic complications of inferior petrosal sinus sampling. *AJNR Am J Neuroradiol* 2008;**29**:760–5.

221. Lefournier V, Gatta B, Martinie M, et al. One transient neurological complication (sixth nerve palsy) in 166 consecutive inferior petrosal sinus samplings for the etiological diagnosis of Cushing's syndrome. *J Clin Endocrinol Metab* 1999;**84**:3401–2.

222. Bonelli FS, Huston J, 3rd, Meyer FB, Carpenter PC. Venous subarachnoid hemorrhage after inferior petrosal sinus sampling for adrenocorticotropic hormone. *AJNR Am J Neuroradiol* 1999;**20**:306–7.

223. Seyer H, Honegger J, Schott W, et al. Raymond's syndrome following petrosal sinus sampling. *Acta Neurochir (Wien)* 1994;**131**:157–9.

224. Nissen SE, Tuzcu EM, Schoenhagen P, et al. Effect of intensive compared with moderate lipid-lowering therapy on progression of coronary atherosclerosis: a randomized controlled trial. *JAMA* 2004;**291**:1071–80.

225. Guedes A, Tardif JC. Intravascular ultrasound assessment of atherosclerosis. *Curr Atheroscler Rep* 2004;**6**:219–24.

226. Waller BF, Pinkerton CA, Slack JD. Intravascular ultrasound: a histological study of vessels during life. The new 'gold standard' for vascular imaging. *Circulation* 1992;**85**:2305–10.

227. Lockwood GR, Ryan LK, Gotlieb AI, et al. In vitro high resolution intravascular imaging in muscular and elastic arteries. *J Am Coll Cardiol* 1992;**20**:153–60.

228. Gatzoulis L, Watson RJ, Jordan LB, et al. Three-dimensional forward-viewing intravascular ultrasound imaging of human arteries in vitro. *Ultrasound Med Biol* 2001;**27**:969–82.

229. Miskolczi L, Guterman LR, Flaherty JD, Hopkins LN. Depiction of carotid plaque ulceration and other plaque-related disorders by intravascular sonography: a flow chamber study. *AJNR Am J Neuroradiol* 1996;**17**:1881–90.

230. Tozzi P, Mueller X, Mallabiabarrena I, von Segesser LK. Intravascular ultrasound underestimates vessel dimensions. *Eur J Vasc Endovasc Surg* 2000;**19**:501–3.

231. Diethrich EB, Irshad K, Reid DB. Virtual histology and color flow intravascular ultrasound in peripheral interventions. *Semin Vasc Surg* 2006;**19**:155–62.

232. Wehman JC, Holmes DR, Jr., Hanel RA, Levy EI, Hopkins LN. Intravascular ultrasound for intracranial angioplasty and stent placement: technical case report. *Neurosurgery* 2006;**59**:ONSE481–3; discussion ONSE3.

233. Uren NG, Schwarzacher SP, Metz JA, et al. Predictors and outcomes of stent thrombosis: an intravascular ultrasound registry. *Eur Heart J* 2002;**23**:124–32.

234. Satler LF, Hoffmann R, Lansky A, et al. Carotid stent-assisted angioplasty: preliminary technique, angiography, and intravascular ultrasound observations. *J Invas Cardiol* 1996;**8**:23–30.

235. Reid DB, Diethrich EB, Marx P, Wrasper R. Intravascular ultrasound assessment in carotid interventions. *J Endovasc Surg* 1996;**3**:203–10.

236. Clark DJ, Lessio S, O'Donoghue M, Schainfeld R, Rosenfield K. Safety and utility of intravascular ultrasound-guided carotid artery stenting. *Catheter Cardiovasc Interv* 2004;**63**:355–62.

237. Blessing E, Hausmann D, Sturm M, Wolpers HG, Amende I, Mugge A. Intravascular ultrasound and stent implantation: intraobserver and interobserver variability. *Am Heart J* 1999;**137**:368–71.

238. Tobis JM, Mallery JA, Mahon D, et al. Intravascular ultrasound imaging: a new method for guiding interventional vascular procedures. *Echocardiography* 1990;**7**:415–24.

239. Nishimura RA, Edwards WD, Warnes CA, et al. Intravascular ultrasound imaging: in vitro validation and pathologic correlation. *J Am Coll Cardiol* 1990;**16**:145–54.

240. Manninen HI, Rasanen H, Vanninen RL, et al. Human carotid arteries: correlation of intravascular US with angiographic and histopathologic findings. *Radiology* 1998;**206**:65–74.

241. Finet G, Maurincomme E, Tabib A, et al. Artifacts in intravascular ultrasound imaging: analyses and implications. *Ultrasound Med Biol* 1993;**19**:533–47.

242. Irshad K, Millar S, Velu R, Reid AW, Diethrich EB, Reid DB. Virtual histology intravascular ultrasound in carotid interventions. *J Endovasc Ther* 2007;**14**:198–207.

243. Jensen LO, Thayssen P, Pedersen KE, Stender S, Haghfelt T. Regression of coronary atherosclerosis by simvastatin: a serial intravascular ultrasound study. *Circulation* 2004;**110**:265–70.

244. Irshad K, Reid DB, Miller PH, Velu R, Kopchok GE, White RA. Early clinical experience with color three-dimensional intravascular ultrasound in peripheral interventions. *J Endovasc Ther* 2001;**8**:329–38.

245. Reid DB, Douglas M, Diethrich EB. The clinical value of three-dimensional intravascular ultrasound imaging. *J Endovasc Surg* 1995;**2**:356–64.

246. White RA, Scoccianti M, Back M, Kopchok G, Donayre C. Innovations in vascular imaging: arteriography, three-dimensional CT scans, and two- and three-dimensional intravascular ultrasound evaluation of an abdominal aortic aneurysm. *Ann Vasc Surg* 1994;**8**:285–9.

247. Irshad K, Bain D, Miller PH, *et al.* *Angioplasty and Stenting of the Carotid and Supra-Aortic Trunks.* London: Martin Dunitz, 2004.

248. Irshad K, Rahman N, Bain D, *et al.* *Textbook of Peripheral Vascular Interventions.* London: Martin Dunitz, 2004.

249. Vince DG, Davies SC. Peripheral application of intravascular ultrasound virtual histology. *Semin Vasc Surg* 2004;**17**:119–25.

250. Nair A, Kuban BD, Obuchowski N, Vince DG. Assessing spectral algorithms to predict atherosclerotic plaque composition with normalized and raw intravascular ultrasound data. *Ultrasound Med Biol* 2001;**27**: 1319–31.

251. Nair A, Kuban BD, Tuzcu EM, Schoenhagen P, Nissen SE, Vince DG. Coronary plaque classification with intravascular ultrasound radiofrequency data analysis. *Circulation* 2002;**106**:2200–6.

252. Stary HC, Chandler AB, Dinsmore RE, *et al.* A definition of advanced types of atherosclerotic lesions and a histological classification of atherosclerosis. A report from the Committee on Vascular Lesions of the Council on Arteriosclerosis, American Heart Association. *Arterioscler Thromb Vasc Biol* 1995;**15**:1512–31.

253. Vavuranakis M, Papaioannou TG, Kakadiaris IA, *et al.* Detection of perivascular blood flow in vivo by contrast-enhanced intracoronary ultrasonography and image analysis: an animal study. *Clin Exp Pharmacol Physiol* 2007;**34**:1319–23.

254. Moulton KS, Vakili K, Zurakowski D, *et al.* Inhibition of plaque neovascularization reduces macrophage accumulation and progression of advanced atherosclerosis. *Proc Natl Acad Sci U S A* 2003;**100**:4736–41.

255. Moreno PR, Purushothaman KR, Fuster V, *et al.* Plaque neovascularization is increased in ruptured atherosclerotic lesions of human aorta: implications for plaque vulnerability. *Circulation* 2004;**110**:2032–8.

256. Moreno PR, Purushothaman KR, Fuster V, O'Connor WN. Intimomedial interface damage and adventitial inflammation is increased beneath disrupted atherosclerosis in the aorta: implications for plaque vulnerability. *Circulation* 2002;**105**:2504–11.

257. Galili O, Herrmann J, Woodrum J, Sattler KJ, Lerman LO, Lerman A. Adventitial vasa vasorum heterogeneity among different vascular beds. *J Vasc Surg* 2004;**40**:529–35.

258. Heistad DD, Marcus ML, Larsen GE, Armstrong ML. Role of vasa vasorum in nourishment of the aortic wall. *Am J Physiol* 1981;**240**:H781–7.

259. Williams JK, Armstrong ML, Heistad DD. Vasa vasorum in atherosclerotic coronary arteries: responses to vasoactive stimuli and regression of atherosclerosis. *Circ Res* 1988;**62**: 515–23.

260. Rasheed Q, Dhawale PJ, Anderson J, Hodgson JM. Intracoronary ultrasound-defined plaque composition: computer-aided plaque characterization and correlation with histologic samples obtained during directional coronary atherectomy. *Am Heart J* 1995;**129**:631–7.

261. Potkin BN, Bartorelli AL, Gessert JM, *et al.* Coronary artery imaging with intravascular high-frequency ultrasound. *Circulation* 1990;**81**: 1575–85.

262. Schaar JA, Mastik F, Regar E, *et al.* Current diagnostic modalities for vulnerable plaque detection. *Curr Pharm Des* 2007;**13**:995–1001.

263. Hiro T, Leung CY, Russo RJ, Karimi H, Farvid AR, Tobis JM. Variability of a three-layered appearance in intravascular ultrasound coronary images: a comparison of morphometric measurements with four intravascular ultrasound systems. *Am J Card Imaging* 1996;**10**:219–27.

264. Davies MJ, Thomas A. Thrombosis and acute coronary-artery lesions in sudden cardiac ischemic death. *N Engl J Med* 1984;**310**:1137–40.

265. Levin DC, Fallon JT. Significance of the angiographic morphology of localized coronary stenoses: histopathologic correlations. *Circulation* 1982;**66**: 316–20.

266. Beach KW, Hatsukami T, Detmer PR, *et al.* Carotid artery intraplaque hemorrhage and stenotic velocity. *Stroke* 1993;**24**:314–9.

267. Fryer JA, Myers PC, Appleberg M. Carotid intraplaque hemorrhage: the significance of neovascularity. *J Vasc Surg* 1987;**6**:341–9.

268. von Maravic C, Kessler C, von Maravic M, Hohlbach G, Kompf D. Clinical relevance of intraplaque hemorrhage in the internal carotid artery. *Eur J Surg* 1991;**157**:185–8.

269. Yamagishi M, Terashima M, Awano K, *et al.* Morphology of vulnerable coronary plaque: insights from follow-up of patients examined by intravascular ultrasound before an acute coronary syndrome. *J Am Coll Cardiol* 2000;**35**:106–11.

270. Spagnoli LG, Mauriello A, Sangiorgi G, *et al.* Extracranial thrombotically active carotid plaque as a risk factor for ischemic stroke. *J Am Med Assoc* 2004;**292**:1845–52.

271. Virmani R, Kolodgie FD, Burke AP, *et al.* Atherosclerotic plaque progression and vulnerability to rupture: angiogenesis as a source of intraplaque hemorrhage. *Arterioscler Thromb Vasc Biol* 2005;**25**:2054–61.

272. Kuchulakanti P, Rha SW, Cheneau E, *et al.* Identification of "vulnerable plaque" using virtual histology in angiographically benign looking lesion of proximal left anterior descending artery. *Cardiovasc Radiat Med* 2003;**4**:225–7.

273. Virmani R, Kolodgie FD, Burke AP, Farb A, Schwartz SM. Lessons from sudden coronary death: a comprehensive morphological classification scheme for atherosclerotic lesions. *Arterioscler Thromb Vasc Biol* 2000;**20**:1262–75.

274. Sabetai MM, Tegos TJ, Nicolaides AN, *et al.* Hemispheric symptoms and carotid plaque echomorphology. *J Vasc Surg* 2000;**31**:39–49.

275. Tegos TJ, Sohail M, Sabetai MM, *et al.* Echomorphologic and histopathologic characteristics of unstable carotid plaques. *AJNR Am J Neuroradiol* 2000;**21**:1937–44.

276. Verheye S, De Meyer GR, Van Langenhove G, Knaapen MW, Kockx MM. In vivo temperature heterogeneity of atherosclerotic plaques is determined by plaque composition. *Circulation* 2002;**105**:1596–601.

277. Naghavi M, Libby P, Falk E, *et al.* From vulnerable plaque to vulnerable patient: a call for new definitions and risk assessment strategies: Part I. *Circulation* 2003;**108**:1664–72.

278. Virmani R, Burke AP, Kolodgie FD, Farb A. Pathology of the thin-cap

fibroatheroma: a type of vulnerable plaque. *J Interv Cardiol* 2003;**16**:267–72.

279. Fujii K, Kobayashi Y, Mintz GS, et al. Intravascular ultrasound assessment of ulcerated ruptured plaques: a comparison of culprit and nonculprit lesions of patients with acute coronary syndromes and lesions in patients without acute coronary syndromes. *Circulation* 2003;**108**:2473–8.

280. Fisher CM, Ojemann RG. A clinico-pathologic study of carotid endarterectomy plaques. *Rev Neurol (Paris)* 1986;**142**:573–89.

281. Streifler JY, Eliasziw M, Fox AJ, et al. Angiographic detection of carotid plaque ulceration. Comparison with surgical observations in a multicenter study. North American Symptomatic Carotid Endarterectomy Trial. *Stroke* 1994;**25**:1130–2.

282. Fürst H, Hartl WH, Jansen I, Liepsch D, Lauterjung L, Schildberg FW. Color-flow Doppler sonography in the identification of ulcerative plaques in patients with high-grade carotid artery stenosis. *AJNR Am J Neuroradiol* 1992;**13**:1581–7.

283. Kostama H, Donovan J, Kasaoka S, Tobis J, Fitzpatrick L. Calcified plaque cross-sectional area in human arteries: correlation between intravascular ultrasound and undecalcified histology. *Am Heart J* 1999;**137**:482–8.

284. Di Mario C, The SH, Madretsma S, et al. Detection and characterization of vascular lesions by intravascular ultrasound: an in vitro study correlated with histology. *J Am Soc Echocardiogr* 1992;**5**:135–46.

285. Sechtem U, Arnold G, Keweloh T, Casper C, Curtius JM. [In vitro diagnosis of coronary plaque morphology with intravascular ultrasound: comparison with histopathologic findings]. *Z Kardiol* 1993;**82**:618–27.

286. Friedrich GJ, Moes NY, Muhlberger VA, et al. Detection of intralesional calcium by intracoronary ultrasound depends on the histologic pattern. *Am Heart J* 1994;**128**:435–41.

287. Glagov S, Weisenberg E, Zarins CK, Stankunavicius R, Kolettis GJ. Compensatory enlargement of human atherosclerotic coronary arteries. *N Engl J Med* 1987;**316**:1371–5.

288. Nissen SE, Yock P. Intravascular ultrasound: novel pathophysiological insights and current clinical applications. *Circulation* 2001;**103**:604–16.

289. Schoenhagen P, Ziada KM, Kapadia SR, Crowe TD, Nissen SE, Tuzcu EM. Extent and direction of arterial remodeling in stable versus unstable coronary syndromes: an intravascular ultrasound study. *Circulation* 2000;**101**:598–603.

290. Varnava AM, Mills PG, Davies MJ. Relationship between coronary artery remodeling and plaque vulnerability. *Circulation* 2002;**105**:939–43.

291. Kazmierski MK. [Stenosis of the carotid arteries]. *Wiad Lek* 2003;**56**:260–5.

292. Nissen SE, Tsunoda T, Tuzcu EM, et al. Effect of recombinant ApoA-I Milano on coronary atherosclerosis in patients with acute coronary syndromes: a randomized controlled trial. *JAMA* 2003;**290**:2292–300.

293. Matsuzaki M, Hiramori K, Imaizumi T, et al. Intravascular ultrasound evaluation of coronary plaque regression by low density lipoprotein-apheresis in familial hypercholesterolemia: the Low Density Lipoprotein-Apheresis Coronary Morphology and Reserve Trial (LACMART). *J Am Coll Cardiol* 2002;**40**:220–7.

294. Petronio AS, Amoroso G, Limbruno U, et al. Simvastatin does not inhibit intimal hyperplasia and restenosis but promotes plaque regression in normocholesterolemic patients undergoing coronary stenting: a randomized study with intravascular ultrasound. *Am Heart J* 2005;**149**:520–6.

295. Okazaki S, Yokoyama T, Miyauchi K, et al. Early statin treatment in patients with acute coronary syndrome: demonstration of the beneficial effect on atherosclerotic lesions by serial volumetric intravascular ultrasound analysis during half a year after coronary event: the ESTABLISH Study. *Circulation* 2004;**110**:1061–8.

296. Falk E. Stable versus unstable atherosclerosis: clinical aspects. *Am Heart J* 1999;**138**:S421–5.

297. Lendon CL, Davies MJ, Born GV, Richardson PD. Atherosclerotic plaque caps are locally weakened when macrophages density is increased. *Atherosclerosis* 1991;**87**:87–90.

298. Kimura BJ, Bhargava V, DeMaria AN. Value and limitations of intravascular ultrasound imaging in characterizing coronary atherosclerotic plaque. *Am Heart J* 1995;**130**:386–96.

299. Tresukosol D, Wongpraparut N, Lirdvilai T. The value of intravascular ultrasound-facilitated internal carotid artery stenting in a patient with heavily calcified and ambiguous common carotid artery stenosis. *J Invasive Cardiol* 2007;**19**:E203–6.

300. Eikelboom BC, Riles TR, Mintzer R, et al. Inaccuracy of angiography in the diagnosis of carotid ulceration. *Stroke* 1983;**14**:882–5.

301. Hermiller JB, Buller CE, Tenaglia AN, et al. Unrecognized left main coronary artery disease in patients undergoing interventional procedures. *Am J Cardiol* 1993;**71**:173–6.

302. Burstein JM, Hong T, Cheema AN. Side-strut stenting technique for the treatment of aorto-ostial in-stent restenosis and deformed stent struts. *J Invasive Cardiol* 2006;**18**:E234–7.

303. Diethrich EB, Ndiaye M, Reid DB. Stenting in the carotid artery: initial experience in 110 patients. *J Endovasc Surg* 1996;**3**:42–62.

304. Aviram G, Shmilovich H, Finkelstein A, et al. Coronary ostium-straight tube or funnel-shaped? A computerized tomographic coronary angiography study. *Acute Card Care* 2006;**8**:224–8.

305. Chetcuti SJ, Moscucci M. Double-wire technique for access into a protruding aorto-ostial stent for treatment of in-stent restenosis. *Catheter Cardiovasc Interv* 2004;**62**:214–7.

306. Demer LL. Effect of calcification on in vivo mechanical response of rabbit arteries to balloon dilation. *Circulation* 1991;**83**:2083–93.

307. Reid DB, Irshad K, Miller S, Reid AW, Reid W, Diethrich EB. Endovascular significance of the external carotid artery in the treatment of cerebrovascular insufficiency. *J Endovasc Ther* 2004;**11**:727–33.

308. Oemrawsingh PV, Mintz GS, Schalij MJ, Zwinderman AH, Jukema JW, van der Wall EE. Intravascular ultrasound guidance improves angiographic and clinical outcome of stent implantation

for long coronary artery stenoses: final results of a randomized comparison with angiographic guidance (TULIP Study). *Circulation* 2003; **107**:62–7.

309. Wehman JC, Holmes DR, Jr., Ecker RD, *et al.* Intravascular ultrasound identification of intraluminal embolic plaque material during carotid angioplasty with stenting. *Catheter Cardiovasc Interv* 2006;**68**: 853–7.

310. Investigators TGT. Guidance by Ultrasound Imaging for Decision Endpoints (GUIDE) Trial Investigators: IVUS-determined predictors of restenosis in PTCA and DCA: Final report from the GUIDE Trial, Phase II. *J Am Coll Cardiol* 1996;**27**.

311. Clark DJ, Lessio S, O'Donoghue M, Tsalamandris C, Schainfeld R, Rosenfield K. Mechanisms and predictors of carotid artery stent restenosis: a serial intravascular ultrasound study. *J Am Coll Cardiol* 2006;**47**:2390–6.

312. Kasaoka S, Tobis JM, Akiyama T, *et al.* Angiographic and intravascular ultrasound predictors of in-stent restenosis. *J Am Coll Cardiol* 1998;**32**:1630–5.

313. Schiele F, Meneveau N, Vuillemenot A, *et al.* Impact of intravascular ultrasound guidance in stent deployment on 6-month restenosis rate: a multicenter, randomized study comparing two strategies–with and without intravascular ultrasound guidance. RESIST Study Group. REStenosis after Ivus guided STenting. *J Am Coll Cardiol* 1998;**32**:320–8.

314. Rosenfield K, Schainfeld R, Pieczek A, Haley L, Isner JM. Restenosis of endovascular stents from stent compression. *J Am Coll Cardiol* 1997;**29**:328–38.

315. Painter JA, Mintz GS, Wong SC, *et al.* Serial intravascular ultrasound studies fail to show evidence of chronic Palmaz–Schatz stent recoil. *Am J Cardiol* 1995;**75**:398–400.

316. Elson JD, Becker GJ, Wholey MH, Ehrman KO. Vena caval and central venous stenoses: management with Palmaz balloon-expandable intraluminal stents. *J Vasc Interv Radiol* 1991;**2**:215–23.

317. Bjarnason H, Hunter DW, Crain MR, Ferral H, Miltz-Miller SE, Wegryn SA. Collapse of a Palmaz stent in the subclavian vein. *AJR Am J Roentgenol* 1993;**160**:1123–4.

318. Schwarzacher SP, Metz JA, Yock PG, Fitzgerald PJ. Vessel tearing at the edge of intracoronary stents detected with intravascular ultrasound imaging. *Cathet Cardiovasc Diagn* 1997;**40**: 152–5.

319. Stone GW, Hodgson JM, St Goar FG, *et al.* Improved procedural results of coronary angioplasty with intravascular ultrasound-guided balloon sizing: the CLOUT Pilot Trial. Clinical Outcomes With Ultrasound Trial (CLOUT) Investigators. *Circulation* 1997;**95**:2044–52.

320. Metz JA, Mooney MR, Walter PD, *et al.* Significance of edge tears in coronary stenting: Initial observations from the STRUT (Stent Treatment Region assessed by Ultrasound Tomography) registry (abstr 2606). *Circulation* 1995;92.

321. Tsuura M, Terada T, Nakai K, Itakura T. Endovascular stent placement for cervical internal carotid artery aneurysm causing cerebral embolism: usefulness of neuroradiological evaluation. *Acta Neurochir* (*Wien*) 1999;**141**:503–7.

322. Manninen HI, Koivisto T, Saari T, *et al.* Dissecting aneurysms of all four cervicocranial arteries in fibromuscular dysplasia: treatment with self-expanding endovascular stents, coil embolization, and surgical ligation. *Am J Neuroradiol* 1997;**18**:1216–20.

323. Weissman NJ, Mintz GS, Laird JR Jr, Satler LF, Canos D, Leon MB. Carotid artery intravascular ultrasound: safety and morphologic observations during carotid stenting in 102 patients (Abstract). *J Am Coll Cardiol* 2000;**35**.

324. Reimers B, Corvaja N, Moshiri S, *et al.* Cerebral protection with filter devices during carotid artery stenting. *Circulation* 2001;**104**:12–15.

325. Macdonald S, McKevitt F, Venables GS, Cleveland TJ, Gaines PA. Neurological outcomes after carotid stenting protected with the NeuroShield filter compared to unprotected stenting. *J Endovasc Ther* 2002;**9**:777–85.

326. Henry M, Polydorou A, Henry I, Hugel M. Carotid angioplasty under cerebral protection with the PercuSurge GuardWire System. *Catheter Cardiovasc Interv* 2004;**61**:293–305.

327. Bosiers M, Peeters P, Verbist J, *et al.* Belgian experience with FilterWire EX in the prevention of embolic events during carotid stenting. *J Endovasc Ther* 2003;**10**:695–701.

328. Al-Mubarak N, Colombo A, Gaines PA, *et al.* Multicenter evaluation of carotid artery stenting with a filter protection system. *J Am Coll Cardiol* 2002;**39**: 841–6.

329. Castriota F, Cremonesi A, Manetti R, *et al.* Impact of cerebral protection devices on early outcome of carotid stenting. *J Endovasc Ther* 2002;**9**: 786–92.

330. Parodi JC, La Mura R, Ferreira LM, *et al.* Initial evaluation of carotid angioplasty and stenting with three different cerebral protection devices. *J Vasc Surg* 2000;**32**:1127–36.

Chapter 18

Spinal vascular and neoplastic lesions

Osman S. Kozak, Edgard Pereira and Adnan I. Qureshi

Vascular supply of the spinal cord: arterial system

Basic properties of the arterial supply

The arterial supply of the spinal cord can be roughly divided into two almost independent systems, or longitudinal anastomotic chains: the anterior spinal artery and the paired posterior spinal arteries. Sulcal penetrating arteries from the anterior spinal artery supply the central portion and the anterior two thirds of the spinal cord, while the posterior one third receives its supply from the pial network provided by the posterior spinal arteries. The periphery of the cord is supplied mainly by a pial plexus from the posterior spinal arteries with some contribution from the anterior spinal artery. The anterior and posterior spinal arteries are formed by the segmental arteries originating from the thoraco-abdominal aorta and, at its cephalad and caudal ends, from the tributaries of the subclavian and iliac arteries.

The segmental spinal arteries originate from the vertebral and deep cervical arteries in the neck and intercostal and lumbar arteries in the thorax and abdomen, respectively. Each segmental artery enters the intervertebral foramen at every level and divides into an anterior and a posterior branch to supply the spine and its content. The posterior branch is further divided into a muscular branch and a radicular branch. The radicular branch is classified as radicular, radiculopial, and radiculomedullary artery according to their contribution to the spinal cord. The radicular artery is a branch restricted to the supply of the spinal nerve root, and is present in every vertebral level. The radiculopial artery supplies the superficial pial plexus in addition to the nerve root. The radiculomedullary artery supplies the nerve root, pial plexus, and spinal cord. The radiculomedullary arteries contribute to the supply of the anterior spinal artery, while the radiculopial arteries contribute to the posterior spinal arteries. Upon reaching the midline fissure on the spinal cord ventral surface, the radiculomedullary artery divides into a distinct anatomic pattern. One branch ascends while the other curves down giving a characteristic hairpin appearance on angiograms (Fig. 18.1). In the embryo,

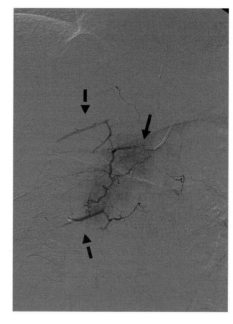

Fig. 18.1. An injection from the pedicle of the right lumbar artery (see bold arrow) demonstrates the multiple anastomoses between the segmental arteries. The injection opacifies also adjacent levels above and below (see dashed arrows) and one on the left side. The retrocorporeal anastomosis (diamond shape) is well depicted. The presence of multiple anastomoses increases the risk of inadvertent embolization of normal arteries.

segmental arteries at each vertebral level originate 31 pairs of radicular arteries that reach the ventral aspect of the spinal cord to form a longitudinal vascular channel on each side of the midline. Progressive fusion of these channels along the midline and regression of these arteries will give rise to 3–15 radiculomedullary arteries (averaging 7), throughout the length of the cord that participate in the supply of the anterior spinal axis. In contrast, 10–20 radiculopial arteries continue to supply the paired posterior spinal arteries. Segmental arteries are connected across the midline and between levels above and below, through highly effective extradural and extraspinal anastomotic systems. These anastomoses provide an excellent collateral circulation that can be visualized by the injection of one segmental artery (Fig. 18.1). These anastomoses protect the spinal cord against ischemia. In the sacral and lower lumbar regions, sacral arteries and the iliolumbar artery derived from the internal iliac arteries are the most important supply to the caudal spine.[1–3]

Textbook of Interventional Neurology, ed. Adnan I. Qureshi. Published by Cambridge University Press. © Cambridge University Press 2011.

Anterior spinal artery

The anterior spinal artery is a single anastomotic vessel that lies in anterior central sulcus and supplies blood to the anterior two-thirds of the spinal cord via the central branches and penetrating branches of the pial plexus. In reality, it is the archaic continuation of the basilar artery, derived from fusion of the embryonic paired longitudinal arterial axis. Although originally described as discontinuous, the anterior spinal artery has been portrayed in more recent studies as continuous, but with an ongoing heavy dependence on segmental supply.[4] It originates in the upper cervical region from the anterior spinal branches of the intradural vertebral arteries, just below the basilar artery. It is fed by anterior spinal branches of vertebral arteries, deep (C6–T1) and ascending (C4–C6) cervical arteries, and by the thoracic (intercostal) and lumbar segmental arteries. At the conus, it continues with the posterior spinal arteries forming an anastomotic basket, comparable to that of the circle of Willis. The anterior spinal artery progresses down to the conus medullaris ending as a fine artery at the filum terminale.

There are usually 8–10 unpaired radiculomedullary arteries arising from the aorta, vertebrals, and internal iliac arteries to supply the anterior spinal cord. The cervical and first two or three thoracic segments of cord are supplied by the radiculomedullary arteries that arise from subclavian or vertebral arteries. The mid-thoracic region of the cord (T3–T7) is supplied from the arteries accompanying T4 or T5 root. A single large radiculomedullary artery, known as the artery of Adamkiewicz, commonly supplies the rest of the cord, from T8 to the conus. This artery originates commonly between T9 and T12, but more frequently from the T12 segmental artery on the left side. It is a slender vessel measuring 0.5 to 1 mm in diameter. It arises from a left-sided lumbar segmental artery in 80% of the individuals. It reaches the cord in 85% of the cases between the T9–L2 in or between T3–T8 in 15%. It is often the only ventral feeder to the lower thoracic and lumbosacral cord. The artery of Adamkiewicz has a large anterior branch and a small posterior branch. The anterior branch ascends and gives off a small ascending branch and a larger descending branch. The descending branch goes inferior and makes an anastomotic loop with the posterior spinal arteries.

Posterior spinal artery

Posterior spinal arteries are not true arteries, but a pair of dominant vascular channels formed at the expense of the pial network running along the dorsal aspect of the cord. They supply the posterior one-third of the cord.[5] The developmental regression is less pronounced dorsally, and 10–20 radiculopial arteries will persist. Rostrally, the posterior spinal arteries originate from the preatlantal part of the vertebral artery or occasionally from the posterior inferior cerebellar arteries. Throughout the length of the spine, many anastomoses exist between the radiculopial arteries of segments above and below along the midline. At the lower end of the cord, they anastomose with the anterior spinal artery via the rami cruciantes forming the arterial basket described above.

Collaterals and variants

Despite its inherent weakness to a sudden decrease in blood supply, the spinal cord vasculature is capable of adapting to a gradual arterial blockage. Virtually any intercostal artery has the potential to provide collateral support for the cord. This resembles a pathological equivalent of the delay phenomenon, with permanent and irreversible dilation of the choke vessels within 48 to 72 hours. A rich collateral circulation supporting the spinal cord was demonstrated in patients with chronic aortic disease and intercostal artery occlusions.[6]

Spinal cord vasculature follows the angiosome concept. There are four angiosome territories: vertebral, subclavian, intercostal thoracic, and lumbar. They are joined by longitudinal anastomotic channels along the anterior and posterior spinal cord. These anastomoses are poorly developed in the thoracolumbar region, rendering this area vulnerable to ischemia. The anterior cord relies on fewer feeder arteries than the posterior cord, and the anterior thoracolumbar cord depends almost solely on the artery of Adamkiewicz for its supply.

Although the segmental anatomy of the spinal cord is relatively simple, with a pair of arterial trunks originating from the aorta at most of the thoracic and lumbar vertebral levels, knowledge of certain variations is important. The direct origin of the radiculomedullary artery from the aorta is a rare but a significant variant. If it is missed, the spinal angiography would be incomplete.[7] It is almost always located at low thoracic levels and associated with presence of a common intercostal trunk. When it is located on the left side, there is high tendency to carry a major spinal cord feeder (radiculomedullary branch).[8,9]

Vascular supply of the spinal cord: venous system

The venous drainage of the spinal cord can be divided into three systems: the intrinsic, the extrinsic, and the extradural (epidural) venous plexus. Different from the arterial system, the venous system does not present an axial territory dominance, and the blood drainage from the dorsal and ventral aspect of the cord is equally distributed.

Intrinsic venous system

The intrinsic venous system is composed of an extensive network of venous capillaries anastomosing in the axial plane (radial veins) and sagittal plane (sulcal veins), and by larger transmedullary anastomotic veins. The intrinsic veins of the spinal cord parenchyma drain radially in to most parts of the spinal cord except in the lower thoracic cord to the conus, where the sulcal veins are more prominent than the radial veins. Transmedullary anastomotic veins provide the anastomoses between the intrinsic (radial and sulcal) veins, and between the median veins on both sides of cord. Presumably, these channels maintain pressure and flow between the anterior and posterior vein reservoirs.

Extrinsic venous system

The extrinsic venous system is formed by the pial network, longitudinal collectors, and radicular veins. The pial network collects the intrinsic venous perforators. It is a large anastomotic system around the surface of the spinal cord. At the level of the spinal pia mater, blood is accumulated in two longitudinal anastomoses (collectors): the anterior and posterior median spinal veins. At multiple levels, radicular veins drain the anterior and posterior spinal veins into the epidural venous plexus. Radicular veins almost never accompany the radicular arteries. A large vein is usually seen at the thoracolumbar segment. Absence of valves in these veins may permit metastases of abdominal infectious processes and tumors to the spinal cord.

Spinal cord ischemia

Incidence

Compared with brain ischemia, spinal cord infarction is exceedingly rare, accounting for only 1% of all strokes. Its diagnosis can be very challenging.[10–14] and recognition of typical patterns of spinal cord involvement needs a thorough understanding of its vascular anatomy (see Fig. 18.2).

Etiology

Various causes of spinal cord infarction have been reported: vertebral artery dissection, atherosclerosis of the vertebral arteries with severe stenosis, hypotension, dissecting aortic aneurysm, thoracic/aortic surgery, aortic cross-clamping above the renal artery (below that level anastomotic flow via the artery of Adamkiewicz usually provides protection), fibrocartilaginous embolism, epidural anesthesia, vasculitis, and trauma.[14,15] There is clear identifiable etiology in up to 60% of the patients.[13,16] Hypertension is the most common vascular risk factor.[17]

Clinical presentation

Usually, the onset of symptoms occurs over minutes, and unlike cerebral infarcts, more than 80% of the cases are associated with pain, which is almost always localized to the level of the spinal cord lesion. Transverse cord symptoms and radicular pain are common initial complaints. Neurological deficits are often confined to the anterior spinal artery territory with involvement of the anterior and lateral spinothalamic and corticospinal tracts. The symptoms consist of flaccid para- or tetraparesis, bladder dysfunction, bilateral dissociated sensory deficit with loss of temperature, and pain below the level of infarction. Posterior columns are typically spared with preservation of proprioception, light touch, and vibration sense.[18]

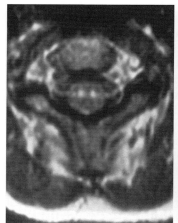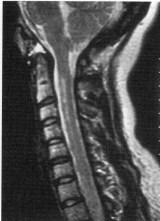

Fig. 18.2. Left, T2-weighted magnetic resonance axial scan at C3 level showing bilateral cervical spinal cord hyperintensities ("snake-eye" conformation). Right, Sagittal MR scan visualizes expansion of this lesion from C2 to C5 vertebral levels.

Within the spinal cord, the central portion of the cord is a watershed zone, and a central cord syndrome may result after prolonged hypotension. This gray matter disorder involves crossing spinothalamic tracts near the central canal. The expected pattern is one of segmental findings: loss of pain and temperature sensation; loss of tendon reflexes; segmental atrophy and weakness; and may include long tract signs (spastic weakness, brisk reflexes, extensor plantar response, and/or urinary urgency) below the lesion.[4]

Pathophysiology

The blood from the dominant arteries provides important segmental supply to maintain a perfusion anterior spinal artery distribution. Normally, two small radicular branches supply the cord between C8 and T9, this being the remainder of the spinal cord supplied largely by the arteria radicularis magna (artery of Adamkiewicz) with minor contribution from the infrarenal radicular arteries. This pattern of supply leaves the cord at T1–T5, and T8–T9 prone to ischemic damage.[4] Several clinical studies, however, have not supported the existence of a single predominant midthoracic watershed zone.[11] The usual anatomic distribution of the cervical radicular arteries also prompted the hypothesis of a minor watershed zone at C4 (see Table 18.1).

Sulcal penetrating arteries from the anterior spinal artery are end-arteries with few anastomoses. The few feeding vessels to the anterior spinal artery make this system appear quite vulnerable and explain the typical anterior location of spinal cord infarcts. The pial network has many feeders and extensive anastomoses, which explains the rarity of posterior spinal artery infarcts. Radicular arteries also supply the vertebral bodies and vascular occlusion may result in bone infarcts adjacent to the cord segment with infarction, which helps in the identification of the spinal infarct.

Table 18.1. Clinical features associated with the spinal cord syndromes

Stroke syndrome	Clinical features
Anterior spinal artery infarct	Bilateral motor deficit with spinothalamic sensory deficit
Anterior unilateral infarct	Hemiparesis with contralateral spinothalamic sensory deficit
Posterior unilateral infarct	Hemiparesis with homolateral lemniscal sensory deficit
Central infarct	Bilateral spinothalamic sensory deficit without motor deficit
Posterior spinal artery infarct	Bilateral motor deficit with lemniscal sensory deficit
Transverse infarct	Bilateral motor deficit with complete sensory deficit

Table 18.2. Spinal vascular lesions

1. Neoplastic vascular lesions

a. Hemangioblastoma

b. Cavernous malformation

2. Spinal aneurysms

3. Arteriovenous lesions

a. Arteriovenous fistulas

I–Extradural

II–Intradural (dorsal or ventral)

b. Arteriovenous malformations

I–Extradural–intradural

II–Intradural

–Intramedullary

Compact

Diffuse

– Extramedullary

III–Conus medullaris

Diagnostic studies

Magnetic resonance imaging (MRI) with diffusion-weighted images is the diagnostic modality of choice.[19,20] Moderate cord swelling and "pencil-like" T2-weighted hyperintensities are often present in the acute phase, followed by contrast enhancement in the subacute phase.[21] The high vulnerability of the gray matter of the anterior horns may lead also to a typical "snake" eye configuration of cord infarction with bilateral T2-weighted hyperintensities.[21,22] (Fig. 18.3) Within the cervical cord, the ischemic lesions often cause medial and centrally located hyperintensities, as opposed to lateral abnormalities seen in demyelinating lesions.[21] While endovascular treatment has not been described for patients with acute spinal cord ischemia, a rapid diagnosis can open the possibility of super-selective administration of thrombolytics or differentiate it from lesions appropriate for endovascular therapy.

Outcome

The natural history of patients with spinal cord ischemia is not well described because most reported cases are secondary to complication of surgical procedures or to prolonged arterial hypotension.[13] The percentage of the patients with significant functional improvement ranges from 23 to 60%.[13,16,17,23] The chance of ambulation increases significantly if the patient regains any movement within one month of the event.[17]

Spinal cord vascular malformations
History and incidence

Spinal vascular malformations are rare and insufficiently studied conditions characterized by considerable variation. Although they represent 3% to 16% of all spinal compressive lesions, they can be responsible for up to 30% of the myelopathies of "unknown cause".[24–26] They were first described in the nineteenth century as tumors.[26] Virchow provided the earliest classification of spinal vascular lesions based on pathological

finding, and also described them as neoplasms. He divided them in two large groups: angioma cavernosum, in which there was parenchyma between the blood vessels; and angioma recemosum (hamartoma), in which the vessels were separated by parenchyma. Later it was recognized that vascular neoplasms and vascular malformations were distinct entities. Heboldt in 1885 and Gaupp in 1888, referred to these lesions as "hemorrhoids of the pia mater", hence recognizing their ability to cause subarachnoid hemorrhage. Berenbruch in 1890 gave the first clinical description of a spinal vascular malformation and recognized the lesion as a vascular entity at autopsy.

Classification

Because many spinal vascular lesions are complex or lack a clear distinguishing feature, there is considerable overlap in their classification. With the advent of digital subtraction angiography for evaluation of spinal vascular pathology new classifications have been proposed, based on patterns of blood flow and the anatomy of circulation and adjacent structures. As a result, our understanding of the spinal vascular malformations and our ability to treat these lesions, both surgically and endovascularly, has improved significantly.[27] Despite these advances, there remain widespread disagreement and confusion on the nomenclature. The most used classification was proposed by Spetzler et al., which divided the spinal vascular malformations in three broad categories[28] (Table 18.2). This classification offers a more logical and practical framework. For the purpose of this chapter, however, spinal vascular malformations will be divided into arteriovenous malformations (AVMs) and arteriovenous fistula (AVFs).

(a) 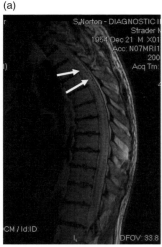 (b) 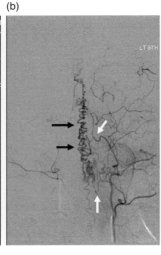 (c)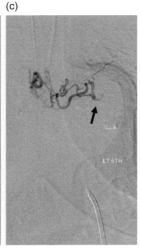

Fig. 18.3. An extradural arteriovenous fistula located in high thoracic region. (a) Multiple flow void signals (see arrows) extending in the dorsal aspect of the spinal cord on sagittal view; (b) selective catheterization of left fifth thoracic pedicle demonstrates the arterial feeders (see arrows) into dorsal venous channels (see black arrows); (c) selective microcatheter placement in left fifth thoracic pedicle branches (see arrows) that supply the fistula for selective injection of embolic material.

Pathophysiology

The underlying pathophysiology of the vascular malformations of the spinal cord has not been clearly identified. Intradural (parenchymal) lesions are believed to be congenital and they predominate in a younger age population. These lesions recruit arterials and thin-walled venous vessels, and often present with acute parenchymal hemorrhage. Dural AVF tend to occur in the elderly population, are believed to be acquired lesions, and typically develop over months to years. The high-pressure arterial flow is transmitted to the venous system resulting in venous stasis that causes spinal cord edema and ischemia.

Clinical symptoms

The majority of the patients with spinal vascular malformation present a progressive or step-wise deteriorating myelopathy. This is followed by conus medullaris syndrome with back and lower extremity pain.[29] Abrupt axial or radicular back pain can also be secondary to spinal epidural hematomas.[30] Most of the clinical features of myelopathy secondary to spinal vascular malformations, such as progressive lower extremity weakness, paresthesias, and sensory loss, are also seen in patients with and without AVMs. Urinary incontinence and perineal paresthesias, on the other hand, predominate in patients with AVM (64% for AVM and 23% for non-AVM patients), though these symptoms are absent in one third of the AVM patients.[25] AVM patients are generally older than non-AVM patients, but the age distribution overlaps.

MRI is not sensitive for early detection of AVMs. While increased T2 signal in the cord with flow voids are associated with AVMs, flow voids were visualized in only 50–57% of the AVM patients.[25,29] Spinal angiography is warranted in all patients with unexplained myelopathy and MRI demonstrating increased T2 signal and flow voids. Clinical factors favoring the presence of spinal AVMs include: age older than 35, urinary incontinence, and perineal sensory changes.[25]

Neurophysiological characteristics and localization

Neurophysiologic tests can be helpful in the diagnosis of spinal vascular malformations. Widespread lower motor neuron signs are present in about 95% of patients with spinal dural AVF and may include several myotomes. Electromyography shows increased rate of polyphasic and pathological spontaneous activity affecting several myotomes.[31] Frequently, there is discrepancy between the localization of the fistula and the symptomatic spinal level, suggesting that the symptoms are due to inadequate venous drainage rather than the arteriovenous shunting itself. Somotosensory evoked potentials (SEPs) may show absent or prolonged latencies and pathological wave forms in the presence of normal sensory conduction velocities. Examination of the lumbar and cortical SEPs can help to differentiate radicular lesions from cord lesions. In earlier stages of the disease, prolonged cortical latencies with normal lumbar latencies suggest a cord lesion instead of a radicular lesion.[32]

Arteriovenous fistulas

Spinal dural AVFs are the most common vascular malformations of the spinal cord accounting for 70% of all vascular cord lesions. They are classified according to their anatomical location into intradural or extradural.

Extradural spinal AVFs

These are rare lesions also known as epidural AVFs (see Fig. 18.3 and 18.4). An extradural arterial branch, often arising from the radicular artery, communicates directly with the epidural venous plexus, causing prominent engorgement of the venous plexus due to the high flow and pressure. The typical clinical presentation is a progressive neurological deficit and radicular pain from direct compression of the adjacent nerve roots or spinal cord by the enlarged venous plexus or due to ischemia from arterial steal or venous hypertension.

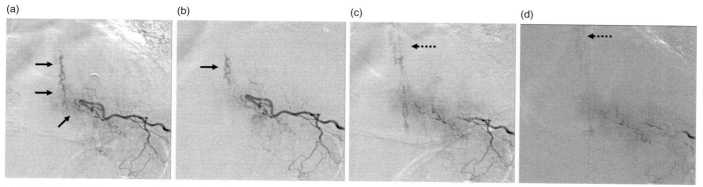

Fig. 18.4. Sequential contrast opacification through a extradural arteriovenous venous fistula deriving arterial supply from lumbar artery. The arterial supply is depicted by solid arrows and venous drainage is depicted by dashed arrows.

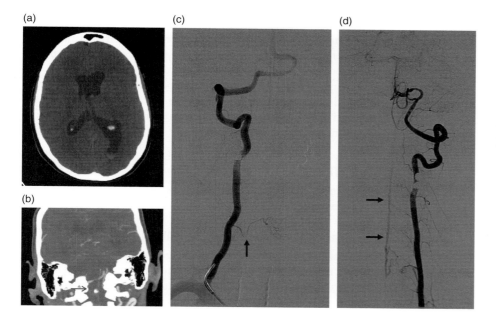

Fig. 18.5. An intradural arteriovenous fistula located in the high cervical region. (a) a transverse section of computed tomographic (CT) scan demonstrated subarachnoid and intraventricular hemorrhage; (b) the CT scan with contrast in coronal plain shows enhancement of the midline vein that drains the fistula; (c) right vertebral artery injection demonstrates medial branch (see arrow) contributing to arteriovenous fistula; (d) left vertebral artery injection demonstrates medial branch (see arrow) contributing to arteriovenous fistula with early filling of venous outflow channel (see arrows).

The treatment of choice is embolization via endovascular approach. The goal of the embolization is to eliminate the three parts of the lesion: the feeding artery, the fistula itself, and the proximal part of the draining vein. As these lesions often have high flow rates, flow-directed or detachable coils or the combination of coils with liquid embolic agents is used.

Intradural spinal AVFs

Intradural AVFs are divided into dorsal and ventral types.

Dorsal spinal AVFs (Type I spinal AVFs)

These are the most common spinal vascular malformation accounting for 80%–85% of all cases. They are also known as "dural spinal AVFs" or historically "angioma recemosum." A dural branch from a radicular artery (usually single) forms an abnormal communication with a dural vein establishing a fistula without a nidus at the nerve root entry or dural sleeve.

As a result, the perimedullary venous plexus is exposed to the high arterial blood pressure with subsequent hypertrophy and dilatation. Spinal dural AVF is a preventable cause of paralysis, but unfortunately its diagnosis is often delayed and many patients present late in the course. Patients present with progressive radiculomyelopathy secondary to decreased spinal cord perfusion caused by venous hypertension.[33] Subarachnoid hemorrhage can rarely occur. MRI often demonstrates T2-weighted hyperintensity in the central areal of the cord and flow voids secondary to increased venous flow in the perimedullary plexus in the surrounding subarachnoid space (see Fig. 18.5). Involvement of conus medullaris is typical on MRI. The tortuous vascular structures may be better visualized on fast imaging employing steady state acquisition (FIESTA) and also differentiate pulsation artifact from flow voids. The treatment can be accomplished either by direct surgical exposure or, more commonly, by endovascular embolization. Complete obliteration of the fistula and proximal draining vein, sparing the perimedullary venous plexus, is the goal of the treatment. Incomplete elimination of the fistula or occlusion of the arterial feeding vessel alone will result in later recruitment of new arterial supply, and progressive neurological deterioration.[29] As the anterior spinal artery is not involved in the malformation, embolization can be performed with relative safety. The success depends upon identification of the precise site of arteriovenous connection. The preferred agents include n-butyl cyanoacrylate and Onyx. Obliteration of the dural AVFs can lead to significant neurological recovery.[34]

Ventral intradural spinal AVFs (Type IV AVMs)

These lesions are also referred to as perimedullary AVFs. They are typically located ventral to the cord near the conus medullaris with the fistulous connection located intradural but in extramedullary. Feeding arteries arise primarily from the anterior spinal artery and rarely from the posterior spinal arteries. Flow-related aneurysms and venous ectasias are common. These lesions can be further classified according to the size and number of feeding arteries. Type I perimedullary AVFs are small, low-flow lesions causing only moderate venous hypertension. They are often located at the conus or terminal filum and the arterial supply is from the anterior spinal artery. Type II perimedullary AVFs represent larger fistulous connections in the pia composed for several distinct shunts that are fed by an engorged anterior spinal or posterior spinal artery. Type III perimedullary AVFs, the most common form, are giant lesions with multiple dilated feeding arteries converging into a single fistula with a significantly dilated and complex venous drainage that includes perimedullary veins lying over the anterior and posterior surface of the cord.[35] Patients present usually between their third and sixth decade of life with myelopathy related to parenchymal hemorrhage, compression from enlarged venous varices, or ischemia secondary to vascular steal phenomenon. In the absence of an intramedullary component, the chance of complete cure with treatment is high. Endovascular approach with embolization or surgical resection has been reported with promising outcomes.[36] Presence of intra- or extra-medullary shunting is important in determining the treatment. The goal of the treatment is elimination of the shunt.[33] Superselective microcatheterization is critical to prevent any inadvertent embolization of the normal tissue.

Arteriovenous malformation

Spinal cord AVMs are rare lesions representing approximately 10% of the AVMs diagnosed in the central nervous system. In these lesions a tangle of malformed vessels or nidus substituting the normal capillary network is interposed between an artery and a vein. The clinical presentation varies from mild neurological symptoms to severe motor deficits secondary to myelopathy. Non-specific early symptoms can delay proper diagnosis and treatment leading to irreversible neurological deficits. Most spinal AVMs are associated with venous

hypertension or steal phenomenon (shunting of blood away from normal capillaries into low resistance circuits of AVMs) resulting in ischemia or hemorrhage. In many cases, an irregular vascular pattern may be seen on myelography and represent arterialized draining veins, rather than the AVM itself. Several classifications have been proposed based on the anatomic location and arterial supply (see below).

Extradural–intradural spinal AVMs

These lesions are also classified as Type III (juvenile) AVMs. They are mostly encountered in young adults and adolescents. These lesions commonly involve tissues from all embryological origins. They have intramedullary, extramedullary, at times, extraspinal, components. Typically, they are rather large and complex lesions with multiple arterial feeders over several vertebral segments. Patients often present with myelopathy from the compression resulting from the large fistulas and the high flow. They can rarely be treated without significant associated morbidity. Therefore, the treatment options are mainly palliative. MRI plays an important role in the diagnosis of these lesions demonstrating the malformations within the cord and associated edema, ischemia, and hemorrhage in surrounding tissue.

Intradural spinal AVMs

These lesions are divided into two groups as intramedullary or extramedullary (see Table 18.3).

Intramedullary spinal AVMs (Type II AVMs)

These lesions are also known as "glomus AVMs" or historically referred to as "angioma venosum racemossum". They are equally distributed among men and women, and present at a younger age compared to the type I AVMs/dorsal spinal AVFs. The nidus of the AVM is compact and located within the intramedullary compartment. Arterial feeding branches originate from the anterior and/or posterior spinal arteries. Venous drainage is through the arterialized coronal venous plexus. These lesions have high pressure with rapid flow and early venous drainage. Patients often present with acute myelopathy from intramedullary hemorrhage (60%) leading to significant neurological deficits (47%). The risk of recurrent bleeding is 10% within the first month and 40% within the first year.[33,35] Presence of large arterial feeders originating directly from the anterior spinal artery and predominantly anterior location are predictors of higher rates of recurrent hemorrhages.[37] Mortality rates as high as 18% have been reported. Treatment options include endovascular and/or surgical approaches. Patients may need repeated embolization procedures. A high rate of upto 80% for long-term cure is reported, and good functional outcome is seen in 86% of the patients treated by endovascular techniques. Despite successful occlusion of the malformation, chronic dysthetic pain can persist.[37]

Table 18.3. Classification of spinal arteriovenous malformation

Types	Angio-architecture	Arterial feeder(s)	Nidus	Venous drainage	Treatment
I	Dural AVF	Single (radicular artery)	None	Dural veins and perimedullary venous plexus	Elimination of shunt (curative)
II	Intramedullary AVM	Multiple (anterior or posterior spinal artery)	Intramedullary	Perimedullary venous plexus	Embolization of arterial feeders (palliative without surgery)
III	Extra- and intra-dural AVM	Multiple spinal arteries	Intra-medullary	Variable	Reduce venous hypertension (palliative)
IV	Intradural AVF (three subtypes)	Single (can be multiple-anterior or posterior spinal artery)	None	Perimedullary venous plexus	Elimination of shunt (curative)

Abbreviations used: AVF, arteriovenous fistula; AVM, arteriovenous malformation.

Extramedullary spinal AVMs

These lesions are known as "type 4 spinal AVMs" or "ventral intradural spinal AVFs" or "perimedullary AVFs". As the underlying lesion is truly fistulous, they were reviewed in the AVFs section.

Conus medullaris AVMs

These lesions may present with combinations of cauda equina symptoms and myelopathy. Due to the widespread involvement of vessels, endovascular treatment is rarely curative but can assist in the surgical resection by reducing the vascularity.

Spinal angiography

Digital subtraction angiography remains as the gold standard for diagnosis and evaluation of spinal cord vascular malformations. Common indications for spinal angiography are evaluation of vascular malformations, vascular tumors of the spine, preoperative vascular assessment in patients undergoing surgery involving the descending aorta, or prior to ventrolateral surgical approaches to the spine.

Spinal cord assessment commonly starts with an aortogram, which is often helpful to localize a lesion, especially in children. A pigtail catheter is positioned at the thoracic and then at the abdominal aorta in order to cover the totality of the spinal cord. A low pressure injection of 24 mL to 30 mL of contrast during 2 seconds will allow opacification of the segmental arteries which are located in the dorsal aspect of the aorta. Subsequently, individual intercostal and lumbar arteries are catheterized. The authors' preference is to use 4 F Simmons I, Headhunter, or Cobra catheters for selective catheterization. For lumbar arteries, renal catheters may be another option. Subclavian arteries and their branches including vertebral, thyrocervical, and costocervical arteries are imaged if the lesion is located in the cervical and/or higher thoracic region along with external carotid arteries. There should be high emphasis on the venous phase as it is essential for a complete study, especially for the examination of dural AVFs. The venous phase from the artery of Adamkiewicz using high quality angiography with adequate magnification can support or exclude the presence of a dural AVF. The presence of venous stasis in the spinal circulation of patients with dural AVF has been well documented. Thus, when a diagnosis of dural AVF is entertained, the demonstration of a normal venous phase practically excludes presence of dural AVF and eliminates selective intercostal injections, unless the abnormality is only confined to cervical level, in which case the venous phase from the artery of Ademkiewicz can be normal.[38] By contrast, demonstration of stasis is consistent with dural AVF, and complete angiography should be performed.[39]

Considering the length of the procedure and large contrast volumes, certain measures should be considered to reduce the risk and improve the quality of the examination. Pre-procedural magnetic resonance angiography may identify the affected segments and delineate target vessels for selective catheterization during spinal angiography. Digital subtraction capability is essential and general anesthesia is usually employed. Low osmolality contrast agents cause less discomfort and nephrotoxicity.[40,41] For this purpose, iohexol is suggested as the preferential agent.[42] A good bowel preparation or use of glucagon can decrease artifacts from intestinal gas or motility.

Three-dimensional spinal angiography

Rotation angiography with reconstruction is commonly used for evaluation of intracranial aneurysm and other vascular anomalies, but its use in spinal angiography was investigated in few studies. Three-dimensional angiography is helpful in determining the presence of aneurysms within the malformation, its complex, vascular architecture, and its relationship with the surrounding structures to facilitate the treatment plan.[43,44] It is important to recognize that there is temporal resolution with three dimensional angiography. Therefore, it cannot be used to determine the transit time within the anterior spinal artery circulation. Three-dimensional angiography does not replace conventional angiography, but complements it, and reduces the total radiation dose by eliminating various oblique projections. Intra-procedural Dyna-CT with axial tomography reconstructions may be helpful in identifying the entry point of arterial feeders into dural AVF and differentiating epidural from dural AVFs. Images are acquired during contrast injection into target artery.

Limitations of spinal angiography

Infrequently, spinal angiography may fail to identify or adequately visualize spinal dural AVF.[45] If the clinical and radiological examinations suggest a spinal dural AVF, surgical exploration may be indicated, despite negative angiographic results, in the absence of definite diagnosis.[46]

Determining the exact relationship of the vascular malformation with the anatomical surrounding is not possible with angiography, therefore adjunct evaluation with MRI or Dyna-CT is recommended before making final treatment planning.[47]

Intra-operative spinal angiography

The utility of intra-operative spinal angiography has not been well established. Several case reports, however, have demonstrated the safety and feasibility of intra-operative angiography for the treatment of spinal AVMs.[48] There was a high correlation between the intra-operative and post-operative angiography to detect unexpected residual AVMs in one-third of the cases.[48]

Additional indications for spinal angiography

Neurogical complications remain one of the major concerns in descending thoracic and abdominal aorta surgeries. Paraplegia after repair of the thoracic aorta is a recognized event, with an incidence of about 5%.[4] The purpose of the pre-operative angiogram would be to avoid spinal cord ischemia by identifying the segmental arteries that contribute to the spinal cord vasculature, especially the artery of Adamkiewicz. However, radiographic evidence of this artery with highly variable level of origin remains of questionable advantage for such purpose. Spinal angiography is helpful when a lateral extracavitary surgical approach for spinal cord decompression and fusion is planned or in patients with thoracic and thoracoabdominal aortic aneurysm repairs.[49–52] Conversely, several studies did not find any significant impact of pre-operative angiography on the neurological outcome of thoracic and abdominal aortic replacement.[4,53]

Its use also was investigated in chronic inflammatory conditions of the spine. It is frequently used to evaluate aneurysmal bone cyst and tumors of the vertebral bodies and surrounding tissues.

Endovascular treatment of AVMs

The eloquence of the spinal cord and the complexity of the vascular lesions limit surgery excision to superficial-lateral or dorsal malformations. The new generation of embolic agents and devices have improved the safety and efficacy of the endovascular approach and made this therapy the modality of choice for most spinal AVMs. The goal of the endovascular treatment is to achieve a hemodynamic equilibrium between the spinal cord and the vascular malformation in order to minimize the risk of hemorrhage, to relieve the compression of surrounding tissue, and to prevent the progression of cord ischemia.[33] Significant clinical recovery and functional improvement can result even with partial AVM occlusion.[54,55]

Surgical excision versus endovascular treatment

The treatment of spinal cord vascular malformations varies according to the complexity and type of lesion. With the rapid evolution of the endovascular tools, the scope of the endovascular therapy has broadened significantly. Specific locations, size, and number of feeding arteries, degree of the arteriovenous shunting, and clinical presentation determine the best treatment and associated outcomes. Endovascular therapy has been increasingly used as first-line therapy in spinal AVMs largely due to its proved efficacy and inherent minimally invasive nature.[56]

Surgical treatment of perimedullary AVFs, historically safe and efficient,[57] is being replaced by endovascular techniques.[58] Initial surgical approach can be considered for type I and II perimedullary AVFs (or type IV spinal AVMs), when the fistula is located on the dorsal surface of the spinal cord and at the level of the conus medullaris. However, endovascular treatment should be considered when the fistula is located on the ventral side of the spinal cord and above the conus medullaris or when the feeding artery is relatively large. For type III perimedullary AVFs, endovascular approach is the preferred modality.[36,59]

Technical aspects

Various embolic agents are used in the treatment of spinal vascular malformations. Detachable latex balloons were reported to be safe and effective in selective types of malformations, when a single arteriovenous shunt is present. However, its limited availability and the popularity of liquid agents has long replaced their use.[59] Superselective microcatheterization is important to ensure embolic material delivery to the target lesion without compromising normal arterial branches. The goal is distal occlusion of the feeding artery or nidus without blocking the venous outflow. Proximal occlusions often result in collateral reconstitution and recanalization of the lesion. Inadvertent occlusion of the venous drainage without elimination of the fistula may cause hemorrhage. Embolic agents can be classified as liquid or particulate material. Liquid agents include N-butyryl cyanoacrylate (nBCA), ethylene vinyl alcohol copolymer dissolved in dimethyl sulfoxid (Onyx liquid embolic system), and sclerosing agents such as ethanol. Particulate agents primarily consist of polyvinyl alcohol (PVA) particles.

Embolization with PVA

PVA was the agent of choice in the past. The size of the particles is determined according to the size of the lesion and its collaterals. Due to the high recanalization rate (up to 50%), many patients require retreatment.[60,61,62] With the newer embolic agents, the use of PVA is limited to pre-operative embolizations and lesions of small size or when superselective catheterization is not technically possible. The most concerning complication is the embolization of the anterior spinal artery with subsequent ischemia.

Embolization with nBCA

nBCA is the most frequently used agent for the embolization of spinal vascular malformations. It offers high stability with low recanalization rates and satisfactory filling of the nidus.[60] Successful endovascular embolization can be achieved in 90% of the cases with a recurrence rate of 10%–15%.[63,64] Favorable clinical outcomes were reported even for very long follow-up times.[64] However, its use is technically demanding and requires considerable skill to prevent inadvertent proximal reflux, excessive venous penetration, or gluing of the catheter at the site of injection.[54] Superselective microcatheterization is critical. Manipulation of the nBCA viscosity and polymerization time aids in a more precise deposition. In high-flow lesions, pharmacologically induced hypotension or cardiac arrest can also be considered prior to the nBCA injection.[33] Corticosteroids can be used pre- and post-procedure to minimize any local inflammatory reaction secondary to the nBCA.

Embolization with Onyx

Onyx is a new liquid embolic agent, with limited but promising results in the treatment of spinal vascular malformations.[54,65,66] It is a biocompatible non-adhesive polymer that is dissolved in DMSO for endovascular delivery. The agent is mixed with tantalum to render the solution radio-opaque. During injection, the DMSO solvent rapidly diffuses, causing precipitation of the polymer. Several advantages of Onyx over the nBCA were reported including the ability to inject it slowly over several minutes, the lower risk of premature occlusion of the venous drainage, and the reduced possibility of adhering the microcatheter to surrounding vessels.[54] It also remains more cohesive and it does not appear to initiate a thrombotic cascade. Complete occlusion rates up to 36% were reported, with a clinical improvement in 82% of treated patients.

Anesthesia and monitoring

Provocative functional tests are often used to test the physiologic importance of pedicles prior to embolization. The provocative test may overestimate the deficits anticipated with embolization.[67] However, neurophysiologic monitoring may increase the yield of such provocative tests particularly when patient is under general anesthesia.[68] A retrospective analysis of 60 provocative tests performed during 84 angiographic procedures (in 52 patients) reported a high negative predictive value.[69] Tests included 47 sodium amytal (50 mg) and 56 lidocaine (40 mg) microcatheter injections at the position of intended embolization under general anesthesia with monitoring of cortical SEPs and transcranial motor evoked potentials (MEPs). If SEPs and MEPs did not change, embolization was performed with nBCA. If SEPs or MEPs changed, nBCA embolization was not performed from that catheter position. One false-negative result occurred, with an increase in spasticity after embolization despite no abnormalities during provocative testing. Nineteen injections (four after amytal injection and 15 after lidocaine injections) resulted in abnormalities on neurophysiologic monitoring. Seven injections in a posterior spinal artery feeder resulted in loss of SEPs or MEPs. Eleven injections in the anterior spinal artery feeder and one in the posterior inferior cerebellar artery feeder resulted in loss of MEPs.

Outcome of embolization

Obliteration of pre-procedure flow voids on immediate post-embolization MRI is used as a marker for technical success. The clinical success of the endovascular therapy is between 36% and 83%.[54,60,66] There is a limited number of studies addressing the long-term outcome of this therapy, but successful prevention of any hemorrhage is seen in 98% of the patients in whom the endovascular treatment was complete. Morbidity rates associated with embolization is between 11% and 19%, and it is usually evident within 24 hours of the procedure. Complications are usually related to inadvertent embolization of the normal spinal cord tissue. In almost all of these cases, the embolization was performed through the anterior spinal artery. Thrombus formation within the medullary veins is also reported as a delayed complication.[33,70]

The main predictor of the outcome is the duration of the symptoms, so early diagnosis and intervention are critical for a favorable outcome.

Radiotherapy

Stereotactic radiosurgery has emerged as an alternative to microsurgical resection and endovascular embolization, especially in cases where these therapies are limited by the angioarhitecture or AVM size and location. Although it has affected the treatment of cerebral AVMs profoundly, its application in the treatment of spinal malformations is still limited. In a small number of case series its safety and effectiveness was demonstrated.[71] Its use is often reserved for the treatment of type II and III AVMs as type I and IV AVMs can be easily treated with surgery or endovascular embolization. Complete cure is achieved only in a minority of patients, but some protective effect is suggested even after partial treatment.[71] The disadvantage of radiosurgery is the long time needed for complete obliteration of the AVM (the latency period), where the patients still remain at risk for hemorrhage.

Cavernous malformations

Once believed to be extremely rare, cavernous malformations are being diagnosed more frequently due to wide spread availability of MRI scans. Spinal cavernous malformations represent only 3%–5% of all central nervous system cavernous malformations. They can be familial or acquired. The familial form is associated with a dominant trait located on chromosome 7q. They also may be induced following radiation exposure of the spinal cord. From a histological perspective, spinal cavernous malformations are identical to those that occur in the brain. These lesions are characterized by thin, endothelial and subendothelial stroma-lined vascular channels, devoid of smooth muscle layers. They can be located either in the epidural or intradural-intramedullary region.

Cavernous malformations are often diagnosed after a new hemorrhagic event or progressively neurological deterioration related to spinal cord compression. Symptoms depend on the location of the lesion within the spinal cord. MRI often shows evidence of blood breakdown products at different stages. The lesions are well demarcated, with mixed signal intensity. The core is surrounded by a rim of low intensity that corresponds to hemosiderin. The clinical history of patients with spinal cord cavernous malformation is acute neurological decline that improves but without returning to baseline status. After repeated hemorrhages, significant and permanent impairment can occur.

There is no endovascular treatment for patients with cavernous malformations, but rapid diagnosis can differentiate them from lesions with endovascular treatment options. Surgical resection is the primary treatment. Intramedullary cavernous angiomas are avascular and resectable lesions. Although the natural history of spinal intramedullary cavernous angiomas are not well known, an operation should be performed in symptomatic cases with repeated hemorrhages to prevent regrowth and further neurological deterioration. Whether asymptomatic lesions should be excised is controversial. The duration of symptoms less than 3 years correlated significantly with a better surgical outcome.[33,72]

Spinal vascular aneurysms

Isolated spinal aneurysms are rare.[73] They are generally associated with spinal AVFs and AVMs. They often manifest with bleeding related to rupture but also can present as compressive lesions. Ruptured spinal aneurysms often present with sudden onset of back pain. Intracranial subarachnoid hemorrhage can also be seen as initial presentation for the spinal aneurysms in cervical location.[74] Their pathophysiology differs from that of intracranial aneurysms. They occur along the course of an artery and seldom appear at branching points. The majority of them are fusiform in shape. Hemodynamic factors related to high flow appear to be the most significant underlying factor for their growth and rupture.

Surgery has been the classic treatment modality for spinal vascular aneurysms. As these aneurysms are often fusiform, surgical wrapping or parent vessel sacrifice may be required.[73] Recent reports mention the use of endovascular treatment for such lesions and include occlusion of the aneurysm or the parent vessel, if there is flow distal to the lesion.[73]

Spinal cord neoplasms
Introduction

Primary spinal cord tumors can be classified by the cellular elements of origin, including neurons, supporting glial cells, and meninges. Alternatively, they can also be classified according to the compartment of origin as intramedullary or extramedullary. Most primary spinal cord tumors are astrocytomas or ependymomas. Metastatic lesions involving the spinal cord affect about 5%–10% of the patients with cancer.[2] Only the neoplastic lesions with similar behavior to vascular malformations with respect to high vascularity and propensity to hemorrhage are included in this section. Unlike intramedullary lesions, it is not necessary to perform a full spinal angiogram for evaluation of spinal tumors. In general, catheterization of one or two levels above and below the tumor is sufficient.

Principles of embolization

Endovascular treatment for spinal tumors can be either presurgical embolization or palliative (see Fig. 18.6). Especially in hypervascular intradural tumors, embolization can facilitate the successful excision by reducing intra-operative bleeding and ensuring an unimpeded view of the surgical field.[75] In unresectable tumors, embolization can improve the symptoms and alleviate pain by decreasing the mass effect. Superselective catheterization of the arterial feeders is crucial to obliterate the tumor bed. The occurrence of numerous anastomotic channels around the spinal column mandate a thorough analysis of all possible arterial feeders in the levels adjacent to the tumor. The microcatheter should be advanced as close as possible to the tumor vascular bed to limit embolization to the lesion and prevent inadvertent occlusion of normal vessels. As the flow is usually slow, over-the-wire microcatheters should be preferred. Occlusion of a proximal branch of the feeder vessel may be required not only to prevent accidental embolization of normal tissue but also to redirect the embolic agent to the tumor vascular bed. Proximal occlusion usually does not cause ischemia of the normal tissue, because there are sufficient anastomoses in the adjacent structures. Special attention should be paid to identify the anterior spinal artery as its

(b)

(d)

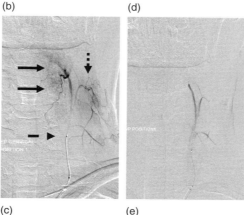

(a)

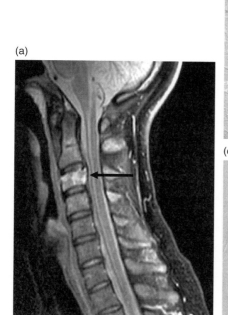

(c)

(e)

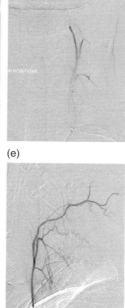

Fig. 18.6. A tumor of the third cervical vertebral body. (a) a sagittal view of the tumor on MRI (see arrow); (b) a microcatheter injection into the anteroposterior projection (dashed arrow) in the deep cervical artery demonstrating vascular supply to the vertebral tumor (see solid arrows) and soft tissue (see dotted arrow); (c) a microcatheter injection into the anteroposterior projection (dashed arrow) in the deep cervical artery demonstrating vascular supply to the vertebral tumor (see solid arrows) and soft tissue (see dotted arrow); (d), (e) anteroposterior and lateral views demonstrating complete obliteration of arterial supply to the tumor in vertebral body and soft tissue after embolization.

presence in the same pedicle is a contraindication for embolization. Posterior spinal arteries often can be sacrificed without ischemic complications.[75] Spinal tumors that can be treated by embolization are shown in Table 18.4.

Embolic agents

Various embolic agents are used for the embolization of the spinal tumors.[76] The embolic agent can be chosen according to the vasculature and tumoral blush. Gelfoam, frequently used in the past, was largely abandoned because of early recanalization and ineffective embolization. Currently PVA, nBCA, and Onyx are the preferable agents.[75] PVA particles of 150- to 250-mm diameter can penetrate into the capillary bed as the capillaries within the tumor average 200 mm in diameter. Larger particles such as 250 mm–350 mm or 350 mm–500 mm are indicated if dangerous anastomoses are seen during the superselective catheterization. nBCA is often considered as a first-line agent, with PVA particles being reserved for cases where distal catheterization is not possible. Because of its liquid nature, nBCA penetrates deeply into the tumor, and renders a high degree of permanent devascularization. nBCA injection is usually performed under general anesthesia and apnea. Despite its polymerization into solid state, its use does not hinder the surgery, but facilitates its manipulation and excision.[76] SEPs and provocative amytal testing to identify vulnerable areas within the distribution of selected arterial

Table 18.4. Spinal tumors that can be treated with pre-operative embolization

Benign tumors:
Hemangioma and hemangioblastoma
Paragangioma
Osteoblastoma
Aneursymal bone cyst
Meningioma
Schwannoma
Hemangiopericytoma
Malignant tumors:
Chondrosarcoma
Chordoma
Giant cell tumor
Osteogenic sarcoma
Plasmocytoma
Myeloma
Metastatic tumors:
Renal cell carcinoma
Thyroid carcinoma

(a)

(c)

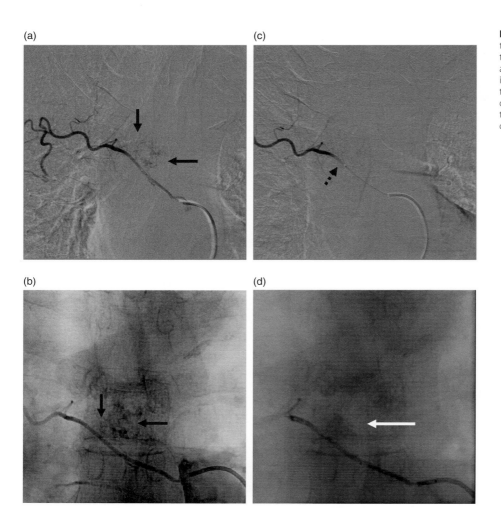

Fig. 18.7. A hemangioblastoma of the fifth thoracic vertebra deriving supply from the right thoracic artery (selective injection). (a), (b) The arterial supply of the hemangioblastoma is identified by bold arrows. (c) The distal part of the microcatheter position is identified by a dotted arrow. (d) A selective injection of the right thoracic artery after alcohol embolization reveals complete obliteration of vascularity (arrow).

(b)

(d)

feeders can be performed to prevent any inadvertent embolization of the spinal arteries supplying normal tissue during the procedure.

Hemangioblastoma

Hemangioblastomas (HBs) are rare lesions accounting for 1%–5% of all spinal cord tumors.[77] They are true intradural tumors with prominent hypervascularity (see Fig. 18.7). A total of 75% of HBs are intramedullary and usually located in the posterior half of the spinal cord. The majority is located in the cervical and thoracic region. Lesions of the conus medullaris and the cauda equina are uncommon. They occur either as sporadic lesions or as an expression of von Hippel–Lindau disease, and 80% of the cases are solitary. Angiographically, HBs can be recognized by non-dilated feeders, heterogeneous opacification of involved vertebral bodies with contrast pooling.[78] Adjacent blood vessels can be seen as serpentine-enhancing structures above and below the mass. In gadolinium-enhanced MRI images, the tumor typically appears as a bright enhanced lesion. Although MRI can safely identify

the lesions, angiography is often needed for detailed analysis of the vascular condition, and for planning the treatment strategy.

With current microneurosurgical techniques, removal of these lesions can be performed with low morbidity and it can be considered even in asymptomatic cases. However, periprocedural complications are not rare as these tumors are frequently located within the eloquent spinal cord tissue. In the lower spinal region, the anterior spinal artery often supplies the HBs increasing the risk of bleeding during surgical removal. Presurgical embolization can greatly facilitate surgical excision by reducing tumor vascular supply, thereby intraoperative blood loss.

Metastases

Metastatic spread to the spinal column constitutes a common problem in patients with cancer. Surgical removal of these tumors can be complicated by excessive blood loss. Metastases of renal cell carcinoma, in particular, are very vascular lesions. Their appearance on spinal angiograms reveal large, irregular arterial feeders and a rich vascular blush with prominent arteriovenous shunts and dilated draining veins.[79] Presurgical spinal angiography and embolization of spinal metastasis from renal cell carcinoma reduce the surgical complications and improve outcomes.[80,81] In addition to transarterial embolization, direct percutaneous embolization can also improve the extent and completeness of the surgical excision.[82] It may also be used in cases where transarterial embolization is not possible. Embolization may also be used as a palliative treatment for spinal cord compression and obviate the need for open surgical decompression.[79] PVA particles and nBCA both have been used with high success rates and safety.

References

1. Thron A. *Vascular Anatomy of the Spine*. Oxford: Oxford University Press, 2002.

2. Herst RW. Spinal angiography. In Baum S, ed. *Abrams' Angiography*. Little, Brown and Company, 1997.

3. Uflacker R. *Atlas of Vascular Anatomy: an Angiographic Approach*. Williams & Wilkins; 1997.

4. Shamji MF, Maziak DE, Shamji FM, Ginsberg RJ, Pon R. Circulation of the spinal cord: An important consideration for thoracic surgeons. *Ann Thorac Surg* 2003;**76**:315–21.

5. Lasjaunias P, Vallee B, Person H, Ter Brugge K, Chiu M. The lateral spinal artery of the upper cervical spinal cord. Anatomy, normal variations, and angiographic aspects. *J Neurosurg* 1985;**63**:235–41.

6. Hong MK, Pan WR, Wallace D, Ashton MW, Taylor GI. The angiosome territories of the spinal cord: exploring the issue of preoperative spinal angiography. Laboratory investigation. *J Neurosurg Spine* 2008;**8**:352–64.

7. Chiras J, Merland JJ. The dorsospinal artery. A little known anatomical variant. Its importance in spinal angiography. *J Neuroradiol* 1979;**6**:93–100.

8. Siclari F, Fasel JH, Gailloud P. Direct emergence of the dorsospinal artery from the aorta and spinal cord blood supply. Case reports and literature review. *Neuroradiology* 2006;**48**:412–14.

9. Lefournier V, Bessou P, Gailloud P, Vasdev A, Rufenacht D, Boubagra K. Direct emergence of the dorsospinal artery from the aorta supplying the anterior spinal artery: report of two cases. *Am J Neuroradiol* 1998;**19**:1961–2.

10. Sandson TA, Friedman JH. Spinal cord infarction. Report of 8 cases and review of the literature. *Medicine (Baltimore)* 1989;**68**:282–92.

11. Cheshire WP, Santos CC, Massey EW, Howard JF, Jr. Spinal cord infarction: Etiology and outcome. *Neurology* 1996;**47**:321–30.

12. Pau Serradell A. [acute ischemic spinal cord disease. Spinal cord infarction. A clinical study and mri in 8 cases]. *Rev Neurol (Paris)* 1994;**150**:22–32.

13. Novy J, Carruzzo A, Maeder P, Bogousslavsky J. Spinal cord ischemia: Clinical and imaging patterns, pathogenesis, and outcomes in 27 patients. *Arch Neurol* 2006;**63**:1113–20.

14. Yousef OM Appenzeller P, Kornfeld M. Fibrocartilagenous embolism: An unusual cause of spinal cord infarction. *Am J Forens Med Pathol* 1998;**19**:395–9.

15. Mikulis DJ, Ogilvy CS, McKee A, Davis KR, Ojeman RG. Spinal cord infarction and fibrocartilagenous emboli. *Am J Neuroradiol* 1992;**13**:155–60.

16. Cheng MY, Lyu RK, Chang YJ, *et al.* Spinal cord infarction in chinese patients. Clinical features, risk factors, imaging and prognosis. *Cerebrovasc Dis* 2008;**26**:502–8.

17. Salvador de la Barrera S, Barca-Buyo A, Montoto-Marques A, *et al.* Spinal cord infarction: Prognosis and recovery in a series of 36 patients. *Spinal Cord* 2001;**39**:520–5.

18. S. Lamin JJB. Vascular anatmomy of the spinal cord and cord ischemia. *Practi Neurol* 2003:92–5.

19. Kuker W, Weller M, Klose U, Krapf H, Dichgans J, Nagele T. Diffusion-weighted mri of spinal cord infarction–high resolution imaging and time course of diffusion abnormality. *J Neurol* 2004;**251**:818–24.

20. Masson C, Leys D, Meder JF, Dousset V, Pruvo JP. [spinal cord ischemia]. *J Neuroradiol* 2004;**31**:35–46.

21. Weidauer S, Nichtweiss M, Lanfermann H, Zanella FE. Spinal cord infarction: Mr imaging and clinical features in 16 cases. *Neuroradiology* 2002;**44**:851–7.

22. Pullicino P. Bilateral distal upper limb amyotrophy and watershed infarcts from vertebral dissection. *Stroke* 1994;**25**:1870–2.

23. Waters RL, Sie I, Yakura J, Adkins R. Recovery following ischemic myelopathy. *J Trauma* 1993;**35**:837–9.

24. da Costa L, Dehdashti AR, terBrugge KG. Spinal cord vascular shunts: Spinal cord vascular malformations and dural arteriovenous fistulas. *Neurosurg Focus* 2009;**26**:E6.

25. Strom RG, Derdeyn CP, Moran CJ, *et al.* Frequency of spinal arteriovenous malformations in patients with unexplained myelopathy. *Neurology* 2006;**66**:928–31.

26. Black P. Spinal vascular malformations: an historical perspective. *Neurosurg Focus* 2006;**21**:E11.

27. Kim LJ, Spetzler RF. Classification and surgical management of spinal arteriovenous lesions: Arteriovenous fistulae and arteriovenous malformations. *Neurosurgery* 2006;**59**:S195–201; discussion S193–13.

28. Spetzler RF, Detwiler PW, Riina HA, Porter RW. Modified classification of spinal cord vascular lesions. *J Neurosurg* 2002;**96**:145–56.

29. Hemphill JC, 3rd, Smith WS, Halbach VV. Neurologic manifestations of spinal epidural arteriovenous malformations. *Neurology* 1998;**50**:817–19.

30. Brunori A, Scarano P, Simonetti G, Delitala A, Chiappetta F. Spontaneous spinal epidural hematomas: Is the role of dural arteriovenous malformations underestimated? *Eur Spine J* 1996;**5**:264–7.

31. Schrader V, Koenig E, Thron A, Dichgans J. Neurophysiological characteristics of spinal arteriovenous malformations. *Electromyogr Clin Neurophysiol* 1989;**29**:169–77.

32. Koenig E, Thron A, Schrader V, Dichgans J. Spinal arteriovenous malformations and fistulae: clinical, neuroradiological and neurophysiological findings. *J Neurol* 1989;**236**:260–6.

33. Veznedaroglu E, Nelson PK, Jabbour PM, Rosenwasser RH. Endovascular treatment of spinal cord arteriovenous

malformations. *Neurosurgery* 2006;
59:S202–209; discussion S203–13.

34. Song JK, Vinuela F, Gobin YP, *et al.*
Surgical and endovascular treatment of
spinal dural arteriovenous fistulas:
long-term disability assessment and
prognostic factors. *J Neurosurg*
2001;**94**:199–204.

35. Gueguen B, Merland JJ, Riche MC, Rey
A. Vascular malformations of the spinal
cord: Intrathecal perimedullary
arteriovenous fistulas fed by medullary
arteries. *Neurology* 1987;**37**:969–79.

36. Cho KT, Lee DY, Chung CK, Han MH,
Kim HJ. Treatment of spinal cord
perimedullary arteriovenous fistula:
Embolization versus surgery.
Neurosurgery 2005;**56**:232–41;
discussion 232–41.

37. Connolly ES, Jr., Zubay GP,
McCormick PC, Stein BM. The
posterior approach to a series of glomus
(type ii) intramedullary spinal cord
arteriovenous malformations.
Neurosurgery 1998;**42**:774–85;
discussion 785–6.

38. Trop I, Roy D, Raymond J, Roux A,
Bourgouin P, Lesage J. Craniocervical
dural fistula associated with cervical
myelopathy: angiographic
demonstration of normal venous
drainage of the thoracolumbar cord
does not rule out diagnosis. *Am
J Neuroradiol.* 1998;**19**:583–6.

39. Willinsky R, Lasjaunias P, Terbrugge K,
Hurth M. Angiography in the
investigation of spinal dural
arteriovenous fistula. A protocol
with application of the venous phase.
Neuroradiology 1990;**32**:114–16.

40. Nelson PK, Setton A, Berenstein A.
Vertebrospinal angiography in the
evaluation of vertebral and spinal cord
disease. *Neuroimaging Clin N Am*
1996;**6**:589–605.

41. Lamb JT. Angiography with amipaque.
Neuroradiology 1978;**16**:612–13.

42. Kendall B. Spinal angiography with
iohexol. *Neuroradiology* 1986,**28**:72–3.

43. Prestigiacomo CJ, Niimi Y, Setton A,
Berenstein A. Three-dimensional
rotational spinal angiography in the
evaluation and treatment of vascular
malformations. *Am J Neuroradiol*
2003;**24**:1429–35.

44. Matsubara N, Miyachi S, Izumi T, *et al.*
Usefulness of three-dimensional digital
subtraction angiography in endovascular
treatment of a spinal dural arteriovenous

fistula. *J Neurosurg Spine* 2008;
8:462–7.

45. Alleyne CH, Jr., Barrow DL, Joseph G.
Surgical management of angiographically
occult spinal dural arteriovenous
fistulae (type i spinal arteriovenous
malformations): Three technical case
reports. *Neurosurgery* 1999;**44**:891–4;
discussion 894–5.

46. Byrne E, Anderson RM, Henderson K,
Cummins J, McNeill P, Gilford E.
Spinal arteriovenous malformations:
Some diagnostic difficulties with
illustrative cases. *Clin Exp Neurol*
1987;**24**:55–61.

47. Kasdon DL, Wolpert SM, Stein BM.
Surgical and angiographic localization
of spinal arteriovenous malformations.
Surg Neurol 1976;**5**:279–83.

48. Schievink WI, Vishteh AG, McDougall
CG, Spetzler RF. Intraoperative spinal
angiography. *J Neurosurg* 1999;
90:48–51.

49. Tartaro A, Simonson TM, Maeda M,
Yuh WT. Preoperative spinal
angiography for lateral extracavitary
approach to thoracic and lumbar
spine. *Am J Neuroradiol* 1995;
16:1947–48.

50. Yamada N, Okita Y, Minatoya K, *et al.*
Preoperative demonstration of the
adamkiewicz artery by magnetic
resonance angiography in patients with
descending or thoracoabdominal aortic
aneurysms. *Eur J Cardiothorac Surg*
2000;**18**:104–11.

51. Ogino H, Sasaki H, Minatoya K,
Matsuda H, Yamada N, Kitamura S.
Combined use of adamkiewicz artery
demonstration and motor-evoked
potentials in descending and
thoracoabdominal repair. *Ann Thorac
Surg* 2006;**82**:592–6.

52. Heinemann MK, Brassel F, Herzog T,
Dresler C, Becker H, Borst HG.
The role of spinal angiography in
operations on the thoracic aorta: myth
or reality?*Ann Thorac Surg*
1998;**65**:346–51.

53. Minatoya K, Karck M, Hagl C, *et al.*
The impact of spinal angiography on
the neurological outcome after surgery
on the descending thoracic and
thoracoabdominal aorta. *Ann Thorac
Surg* 2002;**74**:S1870–2; discussion
S1872–8.

54. Corkill RA, Mitsos AP, Molyneux AJ.
Embolization of spinal intramedullary
arteriovenous malformations using the

liquid embolic agent, onyx: a single-center
experience in a series of 17 patients.
J Neurosurg Spine 2007;7:478–85.

55. Rodesch G, Lasjaunias P. Spinal cord
arteriovenous shunts: from imaging
to management. *Eur J Radiol*
2003;**46**:221–32.

56. Medel R, Crowley RW, Dumont AS.
Endovascular management of spinal
vascular malformations: history and
literature review. *Neurosurg Focus*
2009;**26**:E7.

57. Huffmann BC, Gilsbach JM, Thron A.
Spinal dural arteriovenous fistulas:
a plea for neurosurgical treatment.
Acta Neurochir (Wien). 1995;
135:44–51.

58. Hodes JE, Merland JJ, Casasco A,
Houdart E, Reizine D. Spinal vascular
malformations: Endovascular
therapy. *Neurosurg Clin N Am*
1999;**10**:139–52.

59. Ricolfi F, Gobin PY, Aymard A,
Brunelle F, Gaston A, Merland JJ. Giant
perimedullary arteriovenous fistulas of
the spine: Clinical and radiologic
features and endovascular treatment.
Am J Neuroradiol 1997;**18**:677–87.

60. Rodesch G, Hurth M, Alvarez H, David
P, Tadie M, Lasjaunias P. Embolization
of spinal cord arteriovenous shunts:
Morphological and clinical follow-up
and results–review of 69 consecutive
cases. *Neurosurgery* 2003;**53**:40–49;
discussion 49–50.

61. Nichols DA, Rufenacht DA, Jack CR,
Jr., Forbes GS. Embolization of spinal
dural arteriovenous fistula with
polyvinyl alcohol particles: Experience
in 14 patients. *Am J Neuroradiol* 1992;
13:933–40.

62. Touho H, Karasawa J, Ohnishi H,
Yamada K, Shibamoto K. Superselective
embolization of spinal arteriovenous
malformations using the tracker
catheter. *Surg Neurol* 1992;
38:85–94.

63. Song JK, Gobin YP, Duckwiler GR,
Murayama Y, Frazee JG, Martin NA,
Vinuela F. N-butyl 2-cyanoacrylate
embolization of spinal dural
arteriovenous fistulae. *Am J Neuroradiol*
2001;**22**:40–7.

64. Sherif C, Gruber A, Bavinzski G,
et al. Long-term outcome of a
multidisciplinary concept of spinal
dural arteriovenous fistulae treatment.
Neuroradiology 2008;**50**:67–74.

65. Warakaulle DR, Aviv RI, Niemann D, Molyneux AJ, Byrne JV, Teddy P. Embolisation of spinal dural arteriovenous fistulae with onyx. *Neuroradiology* 2003;**45**:110–12.

66. Molyneux AJ, Coley SC. Embolization of spinal cord arteriovenous malformations with an ethylene vinyl alcohol copolymer dissolved in dimethyl sulfoxide (onyx liquid embolic system). Report of two cases. *J Neurosurg* 2000;**93**:304–8.

67. Katsuta T, Morioka T, Hasuo K, Miyahara S, Fukui M, Masuda K. Discrepancy between provocative test and clinical results following endovascular obliteration of spinal arteriovenous malformation. *Surg Neurol* 1993;**40**:142–5.

68. Berenstein A, Young W, Ransohoff J, Benjamin V, Merkin H. Somatosensory evoked potentials during spinal angiography and therapeutic transvascular embolization. *J Neurosurg* 1984;**60**:777–85.

69. Niimi Y, Sala F, Deletis V, Setton A, de Camargo AB, Berenstein A. Neurophysiologic monitoring and pharmacologic provocative testing for embolization of spinal cord arteriovenous malformations. *Am J Neuroradiol* 2004;**25**:1131–8.

70. Morgan MK, Marsh WR. Management of spinal dural arteriovenous malformations. *J Neurosurg* 1989;**70**:832–6.

71. Sinclair J, Chang SD, Gibbs IC, Adler JR, Jr. Multisession cyberknife radiosurgery for intramedullary spinal cord arteriovenous malformations. *Neurosurgery* 2006;**58**:1081–9; discussion 1081–9.

72. Zevgaridis D, Medele RJ, Hamburger C, Steiger HJ, Reulen HJ. Cavernous haemangiomas of the spinal cord. A review of 117 cases. *Acta Neurochir (Wien)* 1999;**141**:237–45.

73. Gonzalez LF, Zabramski JM, Tabrizi P, Wallace RC, Massand MG, Spetzler RF. Spontaneous spinal subarachnoid hemorrhage secondary to spinal aneurysms: diagnosis and treatment paradigm. *Neurosurgery* 2005;**57**: 1127–131; discussion 1127–31.

74. Rengachary SS, Duke DA, Tsai FY, Kragel PJ. Spinal arterial aneurysm: case report. *Neurosurgery* 1993;**33**: 125–9; discussion 129–30.

75. Shi HB, Suh DC, Lee HK, Lim SM, *et al.* Preoperative transarterial embolization of spinal tumor: embolization techniques and results. *Am J Neuroradiol* 1999;**20**:2009–15.

76. Rodesch G, Gaillard S, Loiseau H, Brotchi J. Embolization of intradural vascular spinal cord tumors: report of five cases and review of the literature. *Neuroradiology* 2008; **50**:145–51.

77. Biondi A, Ricciardi GK, Faillot T, Capelle L, Van Effenterre R, Chiras J. Hemangioblastomas of the lower spinal region: report of four cases with preoperative embolization and review of the literature. *Am J Neuroradiol* 2005;**26**:936–45.

78. Smith TP, Gray L, Weinstein JN, Richardson WJ, Payne CS. Preoperative transarterial embolization of spinal column neoplasms. *J Vasc Interv Radiol* 1995;**6**:863–9.

79. Kuether TA, Nesbit GM, Barnwell SL. Embolization as treatment for spinal cord compression from renal cell carcinoma: case report. *Neurosurgery* 1996;**39**:1260–2; discussion 1262–3.

80. Sundaresan N, Choi IS, Hughes JE, Sachdev VP, Berenstein A. Treatment of spinal metastases from kidney cancer by presurgical embolization and resection. *J Neurosurg* 1990; **73**:548–54.

81. Sundaresan N, Scher H, DiGiacinto GV, Yagoda A, Whitmore W, Choi IS. Surgical treatment of spinal cord compression in kidney cancer. *J Clin Oncol* 1986;**4**:1851–186.

82. Schirmer CM, Malek AM, Kwan ES, Hoit DA, Weller SJ. Preoperative embolization of hypervascular spinal metastases using percutaneous direct injection with n-butyl cyanoacrylate: technical case report. *Neurosurgery*. 2006;**59**:E431–2; author reply E431–2.

Chapter 19

Central retinal artery occlusion

Alberto Maud, Muhammad Zeeshan Memon, M. Fareed K. Suri and Adnan I. Qureshi

Introduction

Central retinal artery occlusion (CRAO) is an acute condition that can lead to severe and permanent loss of vision in the affected eye due to ischemia. Delay in treatment after symptom onset is common because there is no standardized approach for this disease. The traditional conservative treatment is able to achieve a good outcome in approximately 15% of the cases. In the last decade there was increasing enthusiasm about the use of acute local thrombolysis in the ophthalmic artery in the first few hours after onset of CRAO. It appears that there is potential benefit from intra-arterial thrombolysis in patients with acute CRAO, but this alternative is only offered in certain urban teaching hospitals and clinical trials are needed to confirm this beneficial effect.[1] This chapter will review the main anatomical aspects of the vascular anatomy of the orbit and retina, pathophysiology, clinical presentation, and treatment approach of patients with acute CRAO, focusing on the intra-arterial thrombolytic treatment.

Vascular anatomy of the eye

The central retinal artery is the major source of blood supply to the retina. Several investigators have described the anatomy of the central retinal artery.[2–11] A thorough review of published work reveals lack of unanimity regarding the anatomical description of this artery. This controversy stems from the fact that there is wide natural variation in the origin, course, branches, and anastomoses of this artery. Singh *et al.*[2] in their investigation of 106 specimens showed that no two specimens, even from the two eyes of the same person, demonstrated consistency in their pattern of origin, course, branches, distribution, and anastomoses. The number of specimens examined in each series by the various investigators has been rather small. Furthermore, the reported results depended upon the technique used by the investigators to identify the course, the small branches, and the anastomoses. As different workers employed different techniques to delineate these details, there is wide variation in the findings reported.

The following is a brief description of the most common pattern of origin, course, branches, and anastomoses of the central retinal artery. Minor variations were omitted.

Ophthalmic artery

The main vessel supplying the orbital structures is the ophthalmic artery. It arises from the anterior wall of the internal carotid artery as it leaves the cavernous sinus medial to the anterior clinoid process. The origin of the ophthalmic artery is intradural in about 90% of cases, but in about 10% of cases, the artery originates extradurally from the cavernous segment of the internal carotid artery.[12] Rarely, it can arise as two trunks from the internal carotid artery and middle meningeal artery. The ophthalmic artery then enters the orbit through the optical canal inferolateral to the optic nerve and gives off various branches that supply the orbital structures. Once it pierces the dura of the optic nerve, it has a short trajectory through a dural sheath until it becomes intra-orbital. The intra-orbital portion has three segments. The first part extends from the site of entry into the orbit to the portion where the artery crosses under the optic nerve. The second part is the segment of the artery that crosses the optic nerve, and the third part is the portion of the artery that lies medial to the nerve and extends to the origin of the optic nerve.[13] Terminal branches of the ophthalmic artery include: the first major branch which is the central artery of the retina, the lateral posterior ciliary artery, the lacrimal artery, various muscular arteries, the medial posterior ciliary artery, the posterior ethmoid artery, the supraorbital artery, the anterior ethmoid artery, and the medial palpebral artery (Fig. 19.1.)

Visual acuity is a function of the fovea only. The peripheral retina is important for the visualization of moving targets and it is crucial for visual navigation.

The posterior ciliary arteries divide into many small, tortuous branches that pierce the sclera around the optic nerve and form an anastomotic ring known as the circle of Zinn and Haller.[14,15] These branches are called short posterior ciliary arteries and they supply the region around the macula and around the optic nerve. They also give rise to the cilioretinal

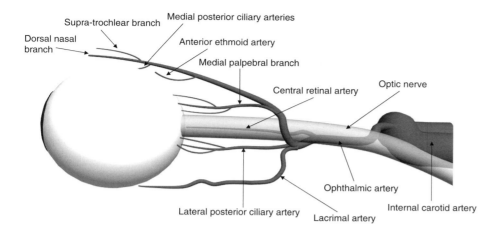

Fig. 19.1. The course and main branches of the ophthalmic artery. See plate section.

arteries that supply the retina between the region of the optic nerve and the macula, including the papillomacular bundle, which are the fibers carrying signals from the foveal region to the optic nerve. The foveal region is at the center of the macula and is avascular. It is surrounded by a perimacular choriocapillaris ring.[16] Between two and four posterior ciliary arteries pierce the sclera medially and laterally from the optic nerve and supply the internal structures of the anterior portion of the eye. These vessels are called long posterior ciliary arteries.

Retinal blood vessels

The retina is supplied by two sets of arteries and veins, the ciliary vessels of the choroid (posterior cilliary arteries) and branches of the central retinal artery and veins. The central retinal vessels enter and leave the retina at the optic disk. The retina is dependent on both circulations as neither is sufficient alone to keep its full viability and functionality.[17] Even in cases with clear cherry red spot and marked retinal infarction, fluorescein angiography done immediately will show a variable amount of slow retinal flow coming from the collateral circulation, mainly from cilliary vessels. However, this residual retinal circulation is not enough to prevent retinal infarction.

Central artery of the retina

The small central artery of the retina arises as the first branch of the ophthalmic artery and then enters the dural sheath of the optic nerve 1.2 cm behind the eye ball. It is responsible for the blood supply to the entire retina except the perimacular and perioptic nerve regions which are irrigated by ciliary arteries.

Course of the central artery of the retina

For descriptive purposes, the whole course of the central retinal artery may be divided into three distinct parts.[11]

1. *Intra-orbital* This extends from the origin of the artery to its entry into the space between the optic nerve and the

dural sheath. The central retinal artery usually has a tortuous intra-orbital course. The tortuosity is marked near the point of entrance into the dural sheath. The arterial segments are usually fixed to each other by thin fibrous tissue near its entrance into the dural sheath. The intra-orbital part usually lies free in fatty areolar tissue around the optic nerve, lightly adherent to the sheath of the nerve.[9]

2. *Intravaginal* This lies in the space between the optic nerve and the dural sheath. In its intravaginal course the artery usually runs forward for a short distance in the subdural space and for a much greater distance in the subarachnoid space. The artery carries a prolongation from the dura, and it also carries from the arachnoid a tube-like prolongation which surrounds it in the subarachnoid space. The intravaginal part of the artery is usually 0–9 mm to 2–5 mm. long. The artery may be accompanied by the central retinal vein.

3. *Intraneural* This part lies within the substance of the optic nerve. The artery enters the nerve by invaginating into the pial membrane. The intraneural part of the central retinal artery has two distinct sections: vertical and horizontal. The vertical section runs upwards and slightly forwards to reach the center of the nerve, whereas the horizontal section runs forwards in the center of the optic nerve and passes through the center of the lamina cribrosa to reach the optic disc, where it divides into its terminal branches.

Branches of the central retinal artery

The central retinal artery during its entire course gives off several branches of various sizes without any constant pattern of origin. No branches arise near the lamina cribrosa region. These branches supply the dural sheath of the optic nerve and the optic nerve itself. After traveling in the optic nerve substance and reaching the level of the optic nerve head, it divides into two equally sized superior and inferior branches. These branches further divide into superior and inferior nasal and superior and inferior temporal, each supplying the corresponding retinal quadrant.

Anastomoses

The extra-ocular branches of the central retinal artery establish numerous anastomoses with other branches of the ophthalmic artery. The anastomoses are mostly between the pial branches of the central retinal artery and the ophthalmic artery.[2] The following types of anastomoses can be established by the central retinal artery:

1. The most commonly seen anastomosis is between the central retinal artery and pial branches from other sources.
2. The second most common anastomosis is between the central retinal artery and the pial branches from the collateral branches of the orbital arteries.
3. Pial branches arising from different parts of the central retinal artery form anastomoses with each other.

In summary, the central retinal artery participates in many anastomoses and these channels allow collateral circulations to be formed. These collateral channels may be of great physiological importance, but their exact role is not known, especially in cases of CRAO.

Pathophysiology of retinal artery occlusion

Anatomic considerations

Occlusion of the central retinal artery deprives the entire inner retina of its blood supply unless a cilioretinal artery is present (15%–30% of individuals). The central retinal artery needs to penetrate the lamina cribrosa to reach and feed the retinal fundus. The lamina cribrosa is an inelastic meshwork of glial-lined collagen fibers near the sclera. At the point of penetration, the central retinal artery is narrowest in diameter, and the fibrous tissue around the artery presents a mechanical barrier to the expansion of the artery, thus making it vulnerable to occlusion by sclerotic, inflammatory or embolic phenomena.

Pathogenesis

Retinal stroke is the term used to describe a variety of retinal arterial occlusive diseases that clinically present as central retinal artery occlusion or single or multiple retinal branch occlusions. The majority of the occlusions of the central retinal artery occur in the region of the lamina cribrosa, regardless of the cause. The most common mechanism of retinal stroke is embolism from proximal sources. The embolic material varies from fibrin-platelet thrombi to cholesterol plaques and small calcium fragments. Embolism is a dynamic process and disappearance or distal migration of the originally visualized embolus is not uncommon. When a patient with retinal stroke has an ophthalmoscopically visible embolus in the retinal arterioles with the typical appearance of cholesterol plaque, carotid disease is almost always responsible, although aortic arch atheroma is another potential embolic source.

The etiology of retinal occlusive disease can be classified into six main causes:

1. *Embolism* Emboli arising from atherosclerotic plaques of the common carotid artery bifurcation, the proximal cervical internal carotid artery, and from the aortic arch are the most common embolic source. Cardioembolism is the second most common cause and atrial fibrillation is a major source. However, any major cardiac source of cerebral embolism can result in retinal stroke. Using prospectively collected data from two stroke prevention projects, the Stroke Prevention in Atrial Fibrillation (SPAF) I through III and the North American Symptomatic Carotid Endarterectomy Trial (NASCET), Anderson et al.[18] were able to demonstrate that retinal ischemia was more typical of carotid stenosis than atrial fibrillation. Odds of hemispheric: retinal ischemic events were 25:1 for atrial fibrillation compared to 2:1 in a patient population with symptomatic severe internal carotid stenosis. However, transient retinal ischemia has a better prognosis regarding subsequent stroke compared to transient cerebral ischemia in patients with severe internal carotid stenosis.[19]

2. *Vasculitis* The central retinal artery can be affected in many systemic vasculitic disorders. The most common systemic vasculitis associated with retinal ischemia is giant cell arteritis (GCA). Visual symptoms and signs are extremely common in patients with GCA and they can be the first manifestation of the disease. CRAO may occur in patients with GCA, although only 5%–10% of patients with CRAO have GCA. CRAO due to giant cell arteritis has some particular features when compared to proximal embolism from a carotid stenosis: permanent visual loss is less frequently preceded by transient monocular visual loss; occlusion of the contralateral retinal artery is more common; and branch retinal occlusion is less common. More widespread ischemia involving other ocular structures is the rule (ischemic orbitopathy) in patients with GCA and it includes anterior ischemic optic neuritis (the most common cause of visual loss in patients with GCA), posterior ischemic optic neuropathy, choroidal ischemia (responsible for retinal detachment and pigmentary changes), and even ocular muscles, ocular nerves, the optic chiasm, the ciliary ganglion, and posterior ciliary nerves can be affected. The typical fundoscopic appearance of the retinal and optic nerve lesions associated with GCA are helpful in determining the diagnosis.

3. *Local atherosclerotic thrombosis* Although less frequent than embolic occlusion, local atherosclerosis may lead to CRAO and it is commonly associated with hypertension and diabetes mellitus. The ophthalmic artery and the central retinal artery are not a common location for intracranial stenosis due to atherosclerosis. Moreover,

atherosclerosis is a chronic process in which the recruitment of collaterals tends to compensate the stenotic vessel. The eye is well known for its abundance of collaterals from other territories, mainly external carotid artery branches.

4. *Vasospasm* Central retinal artery vasospasm is a rare cause of occlusion but may be underreported. It has been implicated as the mechanism underlying migraine and Raynaud's phenomenon but is also a common associated phenomenon in inflammatory syndromes such as systemic vasculitis or GCA. Vasospasm may not only be a primary cause of amaurosis fugax, but can also occur as a result of platelet aggregation, leading to the release of serotonin in damaged vessels.[20] Retinal- or ophthalmic-artery vasospasm should be considered as the cause of amaurosis fugax when thromboembolic disease and carotid artery hypoperfusion have been carefully excluded as causes.

5. *Systemic hypotension* Blood flow in the central retinal artery can be compromised by high intraocular pressure (as is the case in glaucoma) or by systemic hypotension and severe carotid stenosis. It is well known that tight stenosis in patients with carotid disease favors retinal as opposed to brain ischemia. However, a hemodynamic effect does not appear to be more important in the pathogenesis of retinal events than hemispheric ones in patients with severe proximal internal carotid stenosis.[18]

6. *Hypercoagulable state* Hypercoagulable disorders are most often the etiology of retinal vein occlusion. However, in the absence of a clear proximal embolic source or in the absence of an arterial inflammatory process (vasculitis), a hypercoagulable state can also be the cause of CRAO. A recent prospective observational study of patients with CRAO looked for genetic and serologic markers of thrombophilia and hypofibrinolysis. Patients with CRAO were found to have a higher incidence of familial and acquired thrombophilia (low protein C, homocysteinemia, and lupus anticoagulant) compared with controls.[21] In certain cases of CRAO, associated with thrombophilia and hypofibrinolysis anticoagulation is indicated for prevention of further thromboembolic events.

Clinical features
Clinical signs and symptoms

Sudden painless visual loss is the typical presentation, although visual loss sometimes may be accompanied by sudden ipsilateral ocular pain and an amorphous flash of light.[22] Unilateral acute loss of visual acuity is the most common presentation of acute CRAO. Patients with CRAO have almost always extremely poor visual acuity in the affected eye. Blindness is confirmed by the failure of the pupil to react to light with an initial Snellen acuity of counting fingers or worse.[23] However, some patients can present with isolated visual field deficit with

relatively preserved visual acuity. The presence of a patent cilioretinal artery accounts for these cases in which the macula is not entirely affected by ischemia. However, when the thrombus extends more proximally to the ophthalmic artery, a cilioretinal artery will not be able to preserve the viability of the retina. Visual acuity is a function of the fovea only; for this reason, Goldmann's kinetic perimetry should always accompany the evaluation of patients with CRAO. Central scotoma is invariably present in CRAO. Improvement in the visual acuity without improvement in the central scotoma means that the patient has learned to fixate eccentrically rather than having a genuine improvement in visual acuity.[24,25]

In the case of branch retinal occlusion, a partial or incomplete visual field defect can be present usually as a partial altitudinal or quadrantic defect. Some patients experience transient monocular blindness before persistent visual loss occurs, whereas others have no warning symptoms before they lose vision.[26] It is not uncommon to find asymptomatic small distal branch retinal artery occlusion during an ophthalmoscopic examination that includes computerized visual field and direct ophthalmoscopic testing.

Differential diagnosis of central retinal artery occlusion

Several ocular diseases can produce acute transient or permanent loss of vision besides CRAO. Initial ophthalmologic evaluation is crucial in order to rule out other conditions such as temporal arteritis, retinal vasculitis, central serous choroidopathy, vitreous hemorrhage, retinal detachment, optic neuritis, traumatic optic neuropathy, and retinal vein occlusion. From the neuroendovascular point of view, it is important to separate CRAO from non-arteritic acute ischemic optic neuropathy (ION) because the pathophysiology, treatment, and prognosis are different (Table 19.1). While CRAO is considered a retinal stroke, ION is a stroke of the optic nerve. ION can be further classified as anterior optic ischemic neuropathy (AION), the most common type in which the head of the optic nerve (optic disk) is affected, and posterior ischemic optic neuropathy (PION), in which the retrobulbar portion of the optic nerve is infarcted. AION is rarely an embolic event; on the contrary, it is commonly associated with cerebral small vessel disease, type II diabetes mellitus and systemic hypertension. PION is far less common than AION, but may occur in the setting of severe perioperative hypotension and other causes of hemodynamic shock.

Fundoscopic examination

Ophthalmoscopic findings in a patient with CRAO depend on the extension of the occlusion and the duration between the event and the examination. Acute CRAO is characterized by diffuse pale swelling of the retina, macular "cherry red" spot and attenuation of the retinal vessels plus sheathed arteries, and presence of "box-carring" ("cattle trucking") of the blood

Table 19.1. Differences between central retinal arterial occlusion and non-arteritic anterior ischemic optic neuropathy

	CRAO[†]	Non-arteritic AION[‡]
Arterial territory involved	Central retinal artery or branches	Posterior ciliary arteries
Clinical presentation	Sudden painless severe loss of visual acuity. Transient monocular blindness can precede the permanent visual loss	Acute loss of visual acuity. Stuttering presentation is not uncommon
Visual acuity	Severely affected most of the time. Sometimes relatively preserved in cases of patent cilioretinal artery	Decreased visual acuity in various degrees depending on the damage of the papillomacular nerve fibers
Visual field	Central scotoma	Altitudinal visual field defect
Most likely mechanism	Embolism from proximal sources	Atherothrombotic: microatheroma and lipohyalinosis of small perforating vessel
Association with atherosclerotic carotid disease	Relevant	Irrelevant
Association with small vessel cerebral disease, systemic hypertension and diabetes	Irrelevant	Relevant
Prognosis	Unless there is rapid acute recovery, the prognosis of visual recovery is very poor	Visual acuity and visual field defect may improve in up to 40% of patients in the first 3–6 months, but subsequent involvement of the contralateral eye is common

[†]CRAO: central retinal artery occlusion.
[‡]AION: anterior ischemic optic neuritis.

column in the retinal vessels.[22,23] Normal vessel appearance is not infrequent and direct observation of the emboli is rare.[27] The optic disk usually appears pale because of attenuation of the surface vessels. Within 3 weeks, the retinal arteries remain thin, but they tend to recanalize and the optic disk usually remains pale.

Findings on fluorescein angiography

Fluorescein angiography is a technique for examining the circulation of the retina using the dye tracing method. It involves injection of sodium fluorescein into the systemic circulation, and then obtaining an angiogram by photographing the fluorescence emitted after illumination of the retina with blue light. It allows the visualization of the posterior ciliary arteries, choroidal flush (or "pre-arterial phase"), retinal arterial stage, capillary transition stage, early venous stage, venous stage, and late venous stage in approximately 20 seconds after the intravenous injection of the dye.[28] In the case of CRAO there is evidence of absence or marked stasis of the retinal arterial circulation, except in eyes with transient CRAO. A fluorescein angiogram allows study of the presence of cilioretinal optic disk collaterals. These vessels are enlarged in the case of CRAO as a compensatory mechanism in order to ensure blood supply to the ischemic retina. These collaterals come from the posterior ciliary arteries and they usually develop in the late phase of the CRAO. Sometimes in patients with cilioretinal artery sparing, they can be prominent around

the optic disk and they may be misdiagnosed as disk neovascularization.[27]

Prognosis of retinal artery occlusion

CRAO typically causes severe and permanent visual loss in the affected eye. In general, the prognosis is dismal, and meaningful recovery of visual acuity is only achieved in less than 10% of the cases.[24,29,30] It is estimated that up to 22% of patients with acute CRAO can experience spontaneous improvement in visual acuity.[31] Approximately one-third of human eyes with CRAO have a patent cilioretinal artery that may allow for preserved central visual acuity if it supplies the foveal region.

Branch retinal artery occlusion is a less ominous condition with less widespread ischemia of the retina compared with CRAO.[32] In the case of branch retinal artery occlusion the visual field defect tends to be partial and the decrease in visual acuity is less profound with rates of spontaneous recovery of up to 80%.

Treatments for central retinal artery or branch occlusion

Since the first description of CRAO was published in 1859 by Albrecht von Graefe, several treatment modalities were attempted in order to improve outcome. They can be divided into two major categories: (1) conservative treatment, including mechanical (ocular massage and paracentesis), and pharmacologic; and (2) invasive treatment including acute surgical embolus removal and selective intra-arterial thrombolysis in the ophthalmic artery.

In general, there are no controlled trials that address the efficacy of conservative and invasive treatment for patients with acute CRAO. The outcome measures vary greatly from one study to another. Assessment of visual outcome does not always include formal visual field testing and definition is solely based on visual acuity improvement after treatment. On the other hand, there is no uniformity on how visual field improvement is defined. Full recovery of vision on the affected eye should be the mainstay of any treatment, but this happens only in a few cases, and marginal and meaningless recovery of vision is sometimes included as a significant visual outcome.

Medical treatment of CRAO

The medical treatments involve therapies directed towards decreasing intraocular pressure and increasing retinal blood flow, vasodilators, antithrombotics, intravenous or systemic fibrinolysis, and rheologic modification of the blood. These treatments have limited ability to prevent ischemic damage in the retina.[33] Most of the recommendations are based on very small series or on personal communications, and none of them has been evaluated in a controlled clinical trial.

Mechanical dislodgement of the embolus

Globe massage is a relatively safe maneuver that has been used since the early description of CRAO. Most ophthalmologists agree that attempting to dislodge a visible retinal embolus by ocular massage may be useful in some patients.

Intraocular pressure reduction by medical treatment

A reduction in intraocular pressure favors the inflow of a higher amount of blood volume, which is expected to dislodge a non-attached embolus from the central retinal artery to a distal branch. Reduction of intraocular pressure can be achieved by pharmacological and mechanical measures.[34] The use of oral glycerol or intravenous diuretics like mannitol and acetazolamide or the use of topical glaucoma medications (beta blockers, topical timolol maleate) can reduce intraocular pressure and increase retinal blood flow.

Anterior chamber paracentesis

Anterior chamber paracentesis suddenly lowers the intraocular pressure, causing dilatation of the retinal vessels and theoretically allowing an embolus to pass further down the arterial tree into an arteriole less crucial to central vision. There are several case series and personal communications about the effectiveness of anterior chamber paracentesis in CRAO.[29,35,36] The efficacy of paracentesis ranges from as high as 26% to a marginal benefit of 5.6%; however all these communications are based on small numbers of patients, retrospectively collected and with important selection bias.

Vasodilators and rheologic modification of the blood

Vasodilatation of the ocular vessels is achieved by systemic vasodilating medication, including calcium channel blockers (oral or intravenous). Prostaglandin E1 (intravenous) is a potent vasodilator of the microcirculation used in peripheral vascular disease. Sublingual nitroglycerin and isosorbide dinitrate are other vasodilating medications commonly used. Manipulation of the blood content and rheologic modification in the dynamics of the red blood cells have been attempted in order to improve vision in cases of CRAO. These methods range from hemodilution and hyperbaric oxygen to medications that modify the arterial blood content.

Hemodilution has been used based on the fact that reduced hematocrit levels lower plasma viscosity, which may lead to improved retinal circulation and perfusion. Hyperbaric oxygen has the ability to increase the arterial oxygen content and it is thought that this can delay retinal damage after CRAO. Beiran *et al.* found a better visual outcome in 80% of the patients (35 patients) with CRAO treated with hyperbaric oxygenation and conservative measures compared with only 30% of improvement in a control group of 37 patients treated with only conservative treatment.[37] However, this is a comparative retrospective study based on chart review and marginal improvement in the visual outcome was also labeled as a good outcome.

Pentoxifylline is an oral agent used in peripheral vascular disease to improve perfusion of stenotic vessels by increasing red blood cell deformability, reducing blood cell viscosity, and potentially decreasing platelet aggregation and thrombus formation. It was suggested that pentoxifylline might improve retinal blood flow following CRAO. A small, non-randomized, prospective study of ten patients with thrombosis of the retinal artery showed improvement in the peak and end diastolic flow velocities in patients treated with pentoxifyllin (1800 g daily) for 4 weeks compared with placebo. The peak systolic and end diastolic flow velocities increased by 500% and 400%, respectively, in five patients treated with pentoxifyllin vs. 288% and 200%, respectively, in a placebo group of five patients.[38] The interpretation of this small non-controlled trial is difficult considering that the authors did not mention visual outcome, and duration from onset of the symptoms, which may clearly influence the rate of spontaneous recanalization.

Antithrombotic medications

Antithrombotic medications including antiplatelets and anticoagulants are currently reserved for secondary prevention of cerebral and ocular infarction.[39] There is no evidence that supports the use of acute anticoagulation in patients with acute CRAO and data is extrapolated from evidence accumulated in cerebral ischemia.[40] Although there is no direct evidence, aspirin is the most common antiplatelet drug used in patients with CRAO. The vast majority of small series and clinical trials in patients with CRAO include aspirin in their conservative arm. However, the precise effect of aspirin in these cases is difficult to evaluate because of combined use with other medications with different therapeutic effects. Anticoagulation should be reserved for the secondary prevention of ocular or cerebral ischemia in patients with an underlying disease that justifies its use such as atrial fibrillation or hypercoagulable disorders.[39]

Thrombolysis in the treatment of acute CRAO

Thrombolytic treatment is the most specific treatment attempted for retinal arterial occlusion because it can directly lyse the thrombus responsible for the acute visual loss. The goal of thrombolytic treatment is rapid restoration of the retinal blood flow, which is essential for preserving retinal tissue.

In CRAO, as in cerebral infarction, thrombolytic agents can be administered intravenously or intra-arterially through selective catheterization of the ophthalmic artery. The tolerance of retinal tissue to acute ischemia appears to be higher than that of brain tissue.[41] In experiments in monkeys, the retina could tolerate up to 240 minutes of ischemia without developing permanent damage.[41] Although the experience in retinal ischemia in rhesus monkeys may not exactly reflect what happens in humans with acute CRAO, it clearly supports the concept of a longer treatment window for retinal ischemia (compared with brain ischemia). In several retrospective studies of thrombolysis in acute retinal ischemia, thrombolytic medication was administered up to 20 hours after symptom onset.[42]

Most of the occluding thrombi in the retinal circulation are made up of a combination of fibrin and platelets.[43] This matrix of embolic material provides the ideal substrate for fibrinolytic drugs to exert their pharmacologic properties. It is thought that, in cases of visible calcific embolus obstructing the central retinal artery, the effect of fibrinolytic medication would be less pronounced.

Intravenous administration of thrombolytics

Since the approval by the US Food and Drug Administration (FDA) in 1996[44] of intravenous recombinant tissue plasminogen activator (rt-PA) for acute ischemic stroke within 3 hours of onset, there have been several small retrospective case series about the use of rt-PA in cases of acute ocular ischemia.[42,45–47] Extrapolation from the experience with intravenous rt-PA to the treatment of acute ischemic stroke has been used in these small retrospective series and personal communications for selecting patients with acute CRAO to receive intravenous thrombolytic treatment. These include a negative head computerized tomography that rules out intracranial hemorrhage

and classic contraindications for administering systemic fibrinolysis. The main point of discrepancy is the delay of the treatment onset in patients with acute CRAO with some studies reporting treatment windows of even up to days.

In one small prospective pilot study of intravenous thrombolysis by Kattah et al., 12 patients with acute CRAO were treated with 0.9 mg kg^{-1} of intravenous rt-PA.[48] Inclusion criteria were acute CRAO within the preceding 24 hours and no contraindications for use of systemic t-PA. In all patients who were found to have an intraocular pressure 12 mmHg or higher, an anterior-chamber paracentesis was performed. All enrolled patients were anticoagulated for months after acute treatment with intravenous rt-PA. The mean time from symptom onset to treatment was 5.5 hours. Ten patients had improved visual acuity and in four patients, the visual acuity improvement was significant with up to eight Snellen chart lines. Two patients did not improve and, in six patients, recovery was only partial. There were no hemorrhagic complications. Based on this pilot study, rt-PA appears to have a role in the treatment of acute CRAO within 24 hours of onset.

Intra-arterial thrombolysis for central retinal artery occlusion
Technique

Intra-arterial thrombolytic treatment is an invasive treatment option for patients with acute CRAO. This treatment consists of catheterization of the femoral artery and endovascular navigation through the aortic arch and further catheterization of the cervical internal carotid artery using a 5F or 6F guidecatheter. We recommend using a 0.010-inch microwire and a 0.010-inch microcatheter to catheterize the ophthalmic artery. The origin of the ophthalmic artery from the internal carotid artery can be tortuous. Once the microwire engages the origin, the microwire is navigated to a distance of 5 mm and the microcatheter advanced over the microwire. In most instances, the microcatheter can only be advanced 2 mm –3 mm into the ophthalmic artery (Fig. 19.2). In the event that the cervical internal carotid artery cannot be traversed due to occlusion or high grade stenosis, alternate filling of the ophthalmic artery via anastomoses from branches of the internal maxillary artery (external carotid artery) may be occurring. The guide catheter is placed in the external carotid artery and the microcatheter is placed in the internal maxillary artery proximal to the anastomosis for infusion. If a clear anastomotic filling of the ophthalmic artery is not visualized, revascularization of the occluded or stenotic internal carotid artery must be considered using angioplasty and stent placement to access the ophthalmic artery. Once the microcatheter is in place, we use intra-arterial reteplase (prepared as 1 unit in 5 ml of normal saline) and infuse a maximum of 4 units (1 unit over 5 minutes). Other thrombolytics can be used, but should be prepared in high concentrations to avoid administering high volumes within the ophthalmic artery.

(a)

(b)

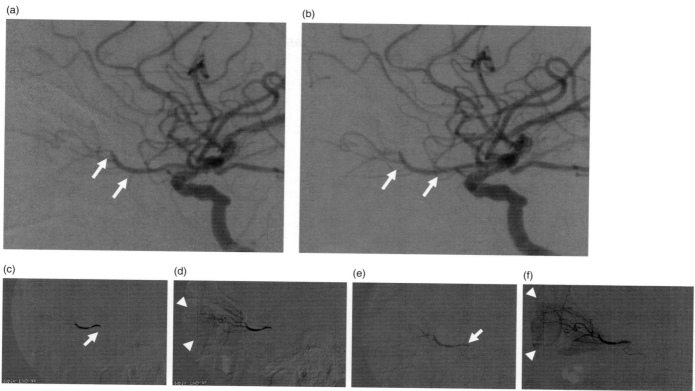

(c)   (d)   (e)   (f)

Fig. 19.2. (a) Lateral view of the ophthalmic artery (see arrows) in a patient with central retinal artery occlusion; (b) post-procedure lateral view of the ophthalmic artery (see arrows). Note that it is difficult to identify any changes in retinal artery flow from images acquired from internal carotid artery injections; (c) super-selective injection from a microcatheter (see arrow) placed in the ophthalmic artery (early arterial phase); (d) super-selective injection from a microcatheter placed in the ophthalmic artery (late arterial phase) – note the poor opacification of distal ophthalmic branches (see arrow heads); (e) super-selective injection from a microcatheter placed in the ophthalmic artery after intra-arterial thrombolysis (early arterial phase); (f) super-selective injection from a microcatheter placed in the ophthalmic artery (late arterial phase) – note the robust opacification of ophthalmic and retinal arteries and capillaries suggestive of improved flow after thrombolysis (see arrow heads).

Issues related to interpretation of clinical studies

The evidence for intra-arterial thrombolytic use in patients with CRAO is limited by several shortcomings. First, there is not a single controlled clinical trial evaluating the efficacy of intra-arterial thrombolysis in patients with acute CRAO. The literature is limited to class 4 level of evidence, which also makes difficult the interpretation of meta-analyses of published data. Second, the improvement in visual outcome in patients treated with intra-arterial thrombolysis varies depending on the definition. Third, there are many publication biases. Case reports and small cases series are usually only published in the case of good outcome leading to publication bias. Fourth, the treatment protocol and onset of treatment varies greatly. There is no uniformity in the studies regarding treatment window, with a wide range of treatment onset from 4 hours to 3 days after symptom onset.

Results of clinical studies

Mames et al.[49] found that 4 out of 17 patients (24%) with CRAO treated with local fibrinolysis in the ophthalmic artery using urokinase or rt-PA had improvement of two or more lines in the Snellen test compared with 16 of 46 patients (35%)

treated with ocular massage, intravenous acetazolamide and paracentesis. In contrast, one of the largest retrospective series published by Schmidt et al.[50] compared 62 patients with CRAO treated with selective local thrombolysis in the ophthalmic artery with 116 patients treated with conservative treatment including ocular massage, acetazolamide, anterior-chamber paracentesis, hemodilution, pentoxifyllin, and aspirin. The mean time of treatment onset was 10 hours. A significantly higher number of patients had visual improvement in the intra-arterial group (10 out of 62 patients). Interestingly, in this group thrombolysis was started within 6 hours after symptom onset.

Fernandez et al.[51] reported their experience in five patients with CRAO who underwent selective intra-arterial treatment with urokinase. The rate of improvement in visual outcome was superior in the treated group compared with the group treated conservatively. In this series, intra-arterial thrombolytic treatment was not only safe, but also beneficial. Arnold et al.[52] reported a retrospective analysis of 37 patients with acute CRAO treated with intra-arterial thrombolysis using urokinase. This arm included also some patients who received both intra-arterial and intravenous thrombolysis. They were compared with 19 patients receiving conservative treatment. All patients

Table 19.2. Published studies investigating outcome of intra-arterial thrombolysis for central retinal artery occlusion (CRAO)

Authors, year	No. of patients	Study type	Fibrinolytic agent	Time to treatment	Pretreatment VA	Post-treatment VA	Angiographically confirmed?	Comments
Annonier et al. 1984,[56] 1988[57]	2, 5	Case series	Urokinase	NA	NA	NA	NA	1988 study is the continuation of the 1984 study
Mach et al. 1992[58]	1	Case report	Urokinase	NA	NA	NA	NA	Czech
Schumacher et al. 1991,[59] 1993[60]	6, 23	Cohort	Urokinase (n = 18)	4 h to 2.5 days	20/200 or worse in 100% (23/23)	Marked or total improvement in 26% (6/23) Partial improvement in 48% (11/23)	NA	1993 paper is the continuation of the 1991 and 1992 study
Schmidt et al. 1992[61]	14		rt-PA (n = 5)			Poor results in 26% (6/23)		
Brassel, 1993[62]	NA	Review	NA	NA	NA	NA	NA	
Turner et al. 1993[63]	NA	Animal study	NA	NA	NA	NA	NA	German
Van Cauwenberge, 1993[64]	NA	Review	NA	NA	NA	NA	NA	French
Vulpius et al. 1996[65]	9	Case series	rt-PA	10–37 h	HM in 33% (3/9)	12/20 in 33% (3/9) Improvement in visual acuity in 63% (5/8)	NA	German
Ma et al. 1996[66]	4	NA	Urokinase	NA	NA	NA	NA	Chinese
Weber et al. 1998[67]	17	Cohort	Urokinase	4.2 h (range: 1–6 h)	20/250 or worse	20/30 or better in 29% (5/17) vs. 0% (10/15) in control group, P = 0.01 Some improvement in 35% (6/17) No change in 35% (6/17) vs 67% (10/15), P = 0.01	No	
Weill et al. 1998[68]	7	Case series	Urokinase	12.5 h (range: 9–20)	LP in 57% (4/7) HM in 29% (2/7) 4/10 P2 in 14% (1/7)	20/20 in 43% (3/7) >20/40 in 28% (2/7) No change in 29% (2/7)	NA	French
Wirostko et al. 1998[69]	1	Case report	Urokinase	4 h	CF	20/20	No	
Hattenbach, 1998[70]	NA	Review	NA	NA	NA	NA	NA	German

Study	n	Study type	Agent	Time to treatment	Initial VA	Outcome	RCT	Comments
Richard et al. 1999[71]	53 (46 CRAO, 7 BRAO)	Case series	rt-PA	14 h (range: 3–50 h)	HM, FC, some LP or no LP in 70% (37/53)	Overall improvement in 66% (35/53), P<0.0001 Improvement of more than two lines in 47% (25/53) Improvement of one to two lines in 19% (10/53) 9% (4/46) achieved 20/20 or better 20% (9/43) achieved 20/40 or better 41% (19/43) achieved 20/400 or better	Yes	
Padolecchia et al. 1999[72]	3	Case series	rt-PA	Unknown	Unknown	All patients showed a visual improvement	Unknown	
Framme et al. 2001[73]	17	Comparative study	Urokinase (n = 7), rt-PA (n = 10)	<8 h	Unknown	Improvement of more than two lines in 24% (4/17) vs. 36% (16/45) in the control group No change in 71% (12/17) vs. 64% (29/45) Decline of more than two lines in 6% (1/17) vs. 0% (0/45)	Unknown	German
Korner-Stiefbold, 2001[74]	NA	Review	NA	NA	NA	NA	NA	German
Kattah et al. 2002[75]	12	Case series	rt-PA	5.75 h	HM in 67% (8/12) LP in 25% (3/12) FC in 8% (1/12)	20/25 to 20/800 in 83% (10/12) No change in 8% (1/12) Decline in 8% (1/12)	No	Did not use intra-arterial thrombolysis but intravenous rt-PA
Schmidt et al. 2002[76]	62	Cohort	Urokinase or rt-PA	9 h	Diminished, highly reduced, or no LP	Overall improvement in 58% (36/62) vs 29% (34/116) in the control group (P = 0.0022) Distinct or partial improvement in 80% (8/10) with incomplete CRAO vs. 66% (19/29) in the control group, 51% (24/47) with subtotal CRAO vs. 18% (15/83) in the control group, 80% (4/5) with total CRAO vs. 0% (0/4) in the control group No change or deterioration in 20% (2/10) with incomplete CRAO vs. 34% (10/29) in the control group, 49% (23/47) with subtotal CRAO vs. 82% (68/83) in the control group,	Yes	Continuation of data from Schumacher et al, 1991,[16] 1993[18] and Schmidt et al, 1992[17]

Table 19.2. (cont.)

Authors, year	No. of patients	Study type	Fibrinolytic agent	Time to treatment	Pretreatment VA	Post-treatment VA	Angiographically confirmed?	Comments
						20% (1/5) with total CRAO vs 100% (4/4) in the control group		
Fernandez et al. 2002[77]	5	Case series	Urokinase	11 h	NA	5/5 (100%) showed improvement in perfusion of retinal arteries 4/5 (80%) showed improvement in VA	NA	Spanish
Butz et al. 2003[78]	22	Case series	Urokinase (n = 7), rt-PA (n = 15)	7.6 h (1.8) h	HM or worse in 77% (17/22)	20/20 in 5% (1/22) HM to 20/32 in 36% (8/22) No change in 59% (13/22)	No	
Diaconu et al. 2004[79]	1	Case report	NA	NA	NA	NA	NA	Romanian
Arnold et al. 2005[80]	37	Case-control study	Urokinase	4 h	<0.01 in 57% (21/37) 0.01 to 0.05 in 43% (16/37) >0.05 in 0% (0/37)	>0.6 logMAR in 22% (8/37) vs. 0% (0/19) in the control group, P = 0.04	No	
Plant and Landau, 2005[81]	NA	Editorial commentary	NA	NA	NA	NA	NA	
Pettersen et al. 2005[82]	6	Case series	rt-PA			Improvement by two or more lines in 50% (3/6) Improvement by one line in 50% (3/6) 20/300 or better achieved in 0% (0/6)		

CRAO, central retinal artery occlusion; FC, finger counting; HM, hand movements; LP, light perception; rt-PA, recombinant tissue plasminogen activator; VA, visual acuity. Reproduced with permission from BMJ Publishing Group Ltd, publishers of *British Journal of Ophthalmology*.

were treated within 6 hours after symptom onset; 8 of 37 patients had improvement of visual acuity to more than 20/30 and the best response was observed in patients treated within four hours after onset. None of the 19 patients in the conservative treatment showed improvement in visual function.

Systematic review of clinical studies

A recent review of thrombolysis for CRAO was published by Biousse et al.[53] All reports of thrombolysis in CRAO were included. Cases of branch retinal artery occlusion were excluded. The primary outcome was complete or full recovery of visual acuity, improvement of visual acuity by at least eight Snellen lines or four Snellen lines. A total of 35 articles (including a prior meta-analysis published in 2000) were included in this review: 249 patients with acute CRAO were included, and the delay between onset and treatment ranged between 3 hours and 14 days (mean: 10.3 ± 8 hours, median: 8 hours). Full recovery of vision occurred in 15% of patients; visual acuity improved by four Snellen lines in 35% of patients, and by at least eight Snellen lines in 20% of patients. These results suggested that intra-arterial thrombolysis is better than conservative (non-thrombolytic) treatment in patients with CRAO. A correlation between improvement and treatment delay was not found and the linear regression analysis of the relationship between improvement and treatment delay showed no significant relationship. Complications were

reported in 10% of the patients. Twelve patients had a transient ischemic attack, six had minor ischemic stroke and two patients had a major stroke. There were two cases of intracerebral hemorrhage and three cases of groin hematoma. The incidence of systemic and intracerebral hemorrhage was low.

A more specific systematic review focusing only on intra-arterial thrombolysis was published by Noble et al. It included eight studies with a total of 158 patients (Table 19.2). Onset to treatment time was, on average, 8 hours. The majority of patients showed some degree of improvement in visual acuity after treatment. Visual improvement occurred in 93% of the patients, with 13% achieving 20/20 or better, 25% achieving 20/40 or better, and 41% achieving 20/200 or better. This data suggests that intra-arterial thrombolysis may produce superior visual outcomes compared with conventional treatment.[54]

National utilization of intra-arterial thrombolysis

A study determined the rates, hospital outcomes, and hospital charges incurred for patients with CRAO treated with thrombolysis using a Nationwide Inpatient Survey (NIS), and compared them with patients treated without thrombolysis.[1] NIS is the largest all-payer in-patient care database in the US. There were 1379 admissions with the primary diagnosis of CRAO in 2001–2003. Intra-arterial thrombolysis was used in 27(1.9%) of the patients with CRAO, exclusively in urban teaching

Table 19.3. Exclusion criteria for the European Assessment Group for Lysis in the Eye (EAGLE) study

Eye disease	Therapy with Marcumar/warfarin
Branch retinal artery occlusion (BRAO)	Allergic reaction to contrast agent
Cilioretinal arteries supplying the macula	Hemorrhagic diathesis
Combined arterial-venous occlusion	Aneurysms
Proliferative diabetic retinopathy	Inflammatory vascular diseases (e.g., giant cell arteritis, Wegener's granulomatosis)
Elevated intraocular pressure (>30 mmHg)	Endocarditis
Systemic diseases	Gastric ulcer
Severe general diseases	Patient participation in other studies during the prior 4 weeks
Systemic arterial hypertension (systolic pressure >200 mmHg), despite medical therapy	**Other exclusion criteria**
Acute systemic inflammation (erythrocyte sedimentation rate >30 mm within the first hour/C-reactive protein >1.0 mg/dl)	No willingness or ability of the patient to participate in all follow-ups
Antithrombin-III deficiency	Pregnancy
Thrombocytopenia (<100 000/ml): pathologic clotting time	Written consent not given
Acute pancreatitis with elevated pancreatic enzymes	Patient is not mobile (bedridden)
Medical history	Other conditions/circumstances likely to lead to poor treatment adherence (e.g., history of poor compliance, alcohol or drug dependency)
Heart attack within the last 6 weeks	
Intracerebral bleeding or neurosurgical operation within the last 4 weeks	

hospitals. There was no in-hospital mortality or intracranial hemorrhage reported among the patients treated with thrombolysis. All patients treated with intra-arterial thrombolysis were discharged home. The study concluded that there is potential benefit from intra-arterial thrombolysis in CRAO, which is only offered in certain centers.

Ongoing prospective randomized trial

The European Assessment Group for Lysis in the Eye (EAGLE) is a multicenter study of the treatment of central retinal occlusion study which is ongoing.[55] This is the first prospective randomized clinical trial evaluating the effect of intra-arterial rt-PA compared with conservative treatment, which includes ocular massage, therapies to lower intra-ocular pressure, aspirin, heparin, and isovolemic dilution. The inclusion criteria are as follows:

1. Age between 18 and 75 years
2. CRAO no older than 20 hours
3. Visual acuity worse than 0.5 (logMAR), corresponding to a decimal of visual acuity of 0.32
4. No exclusion criteria (Table 19.3.).

The primary outcome is improvement in visual acuity (logMAR scale) from the initial examination to the 1 month follow-up after CRAO using letter-by-letter scoring on ETDRS charts. The secondary outcomes are: change in visual field using Goldmann's kinetic perimetry, improvement in retinal circulation using fluorescein angiography, safety and number of procedures including complications, prognosis in relation to delay of treatment after onset of symptoms, severity of CRAO, and pre-existing systemic disease.

The study was started in three European countries (Germany, Austria, and Switzerland) in 2002. The recruitment goal is 200 patients, 100 in each arm. So far, 47 patients have been enrolled.

Conclusions

Based on the available evidence, there is a suggestion that intra-arterial thrombolysis may result in recovery of vision compared with conservative treatment in patients with acute CRAO. However, the magnitude of the benefit is still unknown and the subgroup of patients who will benefit the most from intra-arterial thrombolysis is not clearly defined. There is currently not enough evidence to offer intra-arterial thrombolysis to all patients with acute CRAO as a standard of care. It seems reasonable to consider intra-arterial thrombolytic treatment in patients with CRAO within a few hours of symptom onset using well-defined protocols with uniform endpoint ascertainment and periodic review. In order to offer timely intra-arterial treatment to patients with CRAO, 24-hour access to fluorescein angiography, and interventional neurology is required. Emergent ophthalmologic assessment must be streamlined. When more data regarding efficacy of intra-arterial thrombolysis for CRAO become available, a cost-effectiveness analysis is warranted to determine the feasibility of this treatment.

References

1. Suri MF, Nasar A, Hussein HM, Divani AA, Qureshi AI. Intra-arterial thrombolysis for central retinal artery occlusion in United States: Nationwide In-patient Survey 2001–2003. *J Neuroimaging* 2007;**17**:339–43.

2. Singh S, Dass R. The central artery of the retina. I. Origin and course. *Br J Ophthalmol* 1960;**44**:193–212.

3. Wolff E. Some aspects of blood supply to the optic nerve. *Trans Ophthal Soc UK* 1939;**59**:157.

4. Wolff E *The Anatomy of the Eye and Orbit*. 4th edn. London: Lewis, 1954:121–351.

5. Kershner CM. *Blood Supply of the Visual Pathway*. Boston.: Meadow, 1943.

6. Sudakevitch T. The variations in the system of the trunks of the posterior ciliary arteries. *Br J Ophthal* 1947;**31**:738–60.

7. Traquair HM. *An Introduction to Clinical Perimetry*. 6th edn. London: Kimpton, 1949:299.

8. François J. Aleetens A. Vascularization of the optic pathway: I, Lamina cribosa and optic nerve. *Br J Ophthal* 1954.

9. Wybar KC. Anastomas between the retinal and ciliary arterial circulations. *Br J Ophthal* 1956;**40**(2):65–81.

10. Steele EJ, Blunt, M.J. http://www.ncbi.nim.nih.gov/pmc/articles/PMC505867/pdf/brjoptha100407-0025.pdf. *J Anat (Lond)* 1956:486.

11. Singh S, Dass R. The central artery of the retina. II. A study of its distribution and anastomoses. *Br J Ophthalmol* 1960;**44**:280–99.

12. Punt J. Some observations on aneurysms of the proximal internal carotid artery. *J Neurosurg* 1979;**51**:151–4.

13. Hayreh SS, Dass R. The ophthalmic artery: Ii. Intra-orbital course. *Br J Ophthalmol* 1962;**46**:165–85.

14. Zhao Y, Li FM. Microangioarchitecture of optic papilla. *Jpn J Ophthalmol* 1987;**31**:147–59.

15. Risco JM, Grimson BS, Johnson PT. Angioarchitecture of the ciliary artery circulation of the posterior pole. *Arch Ophthalmol* 1981;**99**:864–8.

16. Amalric P. The choriocapillaris in the macular area. Clinical and angiographic study. *Int Ophthalmol* 1983;**6**:149–53.

17. Olver JM, Spalton DJ, McCartney AC. Microvascular study of the retrolaminar optic nerve in man: the possible significance in anterior ischaemic optic neuropathy. *Eye* 1990;**4** (Pt 1):7–24.

18. Anderson DC, Kappelle LJ, Eliasziw M, Babikian VL, Pearce LA, Barnett HJ. Occurrence of hemispheric and retinal ischemia in atrial fibrillation compared with carotid stenosis. *Stroke* 2002;**33**:1963–7.

19. Benavente O, Eliasziw M, Streifler JY, Fox AJ, Barnett HJ, Meldrum H. Prognosis after transient monocular blindness associated with carotid-artery stenosis. *N Engl J Med* 2001;**345**:1084–90.

20. Flammer J, Pache M, Resink T. Vasospasm, its role in the pathogenesis of diseases with particular reference to

the eye. *Prog Retin Eye Res* 2001;**20**:319–49.

21. Glueck CJ, Wang P, Hutchins R, Petersen MR, Golnik K. Ocular Vascular Thrombotic Events: Central Retinal Vein and Central Retinal Artery Occlusions. *Clin Appl Thromb Hemost* 2007.

22. Ros MA, Magargal LE, Uram M. Branch retinal-artery obstruction: a review of 201 eyes. *Ann Ophthalmol* 1989;**21**:103–7.

23. Connolly BP, Krishnan A, Shah GK, et al. Characteristics of patients presenting with central retinal artery occlusion with and without giant cell arteritis. *Can J Ophthalmol* 2000;**35**:379–84.

24. Hayreh SS, Zimmerman MB. Central retinal artery occlusion: visual outcome. *Am J Ophthalmol* 2005;**140**:376–91.

25. Hayreh SS. Intra-arterial thrombolysis for central retinal artery occlusion. *Br J Ophthalmol* 2008;**92**:585–7.

26. Kline L. The natural history of patients with amaurosis fugax. *Ophthalmol Clin North Am* 1996:351–7.

27. Hayreh SS, Zimmerman MB. Fundus changes in central retinal artery occlusion. *Retina* 2007;**27**:276–89.

28. David NJ, Norton EW, Gass JD, Beauchamp J. Fluorescein angiography in central retinal artery occlusion. *Arch Ophthalmol* 1967;**77**:619–29.

29. Atebara NH, Brown GC, Cater J. Efficacy of anterior chamber paracentesis and Carbogen in treating acute nonarteritic central retinal artery occlusion. *Ophthalmology* 1995;**102**:2029–34; discussion 34–5.

30. Fraser S, Siriwardena D. Interventions for acute non-arteritic central retinal artery occlusion. *Cochrane Database Syst Rev* 2002:CD001989.

31. Augsburger JJ, Magargal LE. Visual prognosis following treatment of acute central retinal artery obstruction. *Br J Ophthalmol* 1980;**64**:913–17.

32. Yuzurihara D, Iijima H. Visual outcome in central retinal and branch retinal artery occlusion. *Jpn J Ophthalmol* 2004;**48**:490–2.

33. Mueller AJ, Neubauer AS, Schaller U, Kampik A. Evaluation of minimally invasive therapies and rationale for a prospective randomized trial to evaluate selective intra-arterial lysis for clinically complete central retinal artery occlusion. *Arch Ophthalmol* 2003;**121**:1377–81.

34. Ffytche TJ, Bulpitt CJ, Kohner EM, Archer D, Dollery CT. Effect of changes in intraocular pressure on the retinal microcirculation. *Br J Ophthalmol* 1974;**58**:514–22.

35. Ffytche TJ. A rationalization of treatment of central retinal artery occlusion. *Trans Ophthalmol Soc UK* 1974;**94**:468–79.

36. Blair NP, Baker DS, Rhode JP, Solomon M. Vitreoperfusion. A new approach to ocular ischemia. *Arch Ophthalmol* 1989;**107**:417–23.

37. Beiran I, Goldenberg I, Adir Y, Tamir A, Shupak A, Miller B. Early hyperbaric oxygen therapy for retinal artery occlusion. *Eur J Ophthalmol* 2001;**11**:345–50.

38. Incandela L, Cesarone MR, Belcaro G, et al. Treatment of vascular retinal disease with pentoxifylline: a controlled, randomized trial. *Angiology* 2002;**53** Suppl 1:S31–4.

39. Adams RJ, Albers G, Alberts MJ, et al. Update to the AHA/ASA recommendations for the prevention of stroke in patients with stroke and transient ischemic attack. *Stroke* 2008;**39**:1647–52.

40. Adams HP, Jr., del Zoppo G, Alberts MJ, et al. Guidelines for the early management of adults with ischemic stroke: a guideline from the American Heart Association/American Stroke Association Stroke Council, Clinical Cardiology Council, Cardiovascular Radiology and Intervention Council, and the Atherosclerotic Peripheral Vascular Disease and Quality of Care Outcomes in Research Interdisciplinary Working Groups: The American Academy of Neurology affirms the value of this guideline as an educational tool for neurologists. *Circulation* 2007;**115**:e478–534.

41. Hayreh SS, Kolder HE, Weingeist TA. Central retinal artery occlusion and retinal tolerance time. *Ophthalmology* 1980;**87**:75–8.

42. Beatty S, Au Eong KG. Local intra-arterial fibrinolysis for acute occlusion of the central retinal artery: a meta-analysis of the published data. *Br J Ophthalmol* 2000;**84**:914–16.

43. Jorgensen L, Torvik A. Ischaemic cerebrovascular diseases in an autopsy series. 2. Prevalence, location, pathogenesis, and clinical course of cerebral infarcts. *J Neurol Sci* 1969;**9**:285–320.

44. The National Institute of Neurological Disorders and Stroke rt-PA Stroke Study Group. Tissue plasminogen activator for acute ischemic stroke. *N Engl J Med* 1995;**333**:1581–7.

45. Rumelt S, Dorenboim Y, Rehany U. Aggressive systematic treatment for central retinal artery occlusion. *Am J Ophthalmol* 1999;**128**:733–8.

46. Mames RN, Shugar JK, Levy N, Brasington A, Margo CE. Peripheral thrombolytic therapy for central retinal artery occlusion. CRAO Study Group. *Arch Ophthalmol* 1995;**113**:1094.

47. Cilveti Puche A, Lapeira Andraca M, Garcia Campos J. [Fibrinolysis with rTPA in acute retinal arterial occlusion]. *Arch Soc Esp Oftalmol* 2000;**75**:287–90.

48. Kattah JC, Wang DZ, Reddy C. Intravenous recombinant tissue-type plasminogen activator thrombolysis in treatment of central retinal artery occlusion. *Arch Ophthalmol* 2002;**120**:1234–6.

49. Framme C, Spiegel D, Roider J, et al. [Central retinal artery occlusion. Importance of selective intra-arterial fibrinolysis]. *Ophthalmologe* 2001;**98**:725–30.

50. Schmidt DP, Schulte-Monting J, Schumacher M. Prognosis of central retinal artery occlusion: local intraarterial fibrinolysis versus conservative treatment. *Am J Neuroradiol* 2002;**23**:1301–7.

51. Fernandez FJ, Guelbenzu S, Barrena C, et al. [Selective ophthalmic artery fibrinolysis in acute central retinal artery occlusion]. *Arch Soc Esp Oftalmol* 2002;**77**:81–6.

52. Arnold M, Koerner U, Remonda L, et al. Comparison of intra-arterial thrombolysis with conventional treatment in patients with acute central retinal artery occlusion. *J Neurol Neurosurg Psychiatry* 2005;**76**:196–9.

53. Biousse V, Calvetti O, Bruce BB, Newman NJ. Thrombolysis for central retinal artery occlusion. *J Neuroophthalmol* 2007;**27**:215–30.

54. Noble J, Weizblit N, Baerlocher MO, Eng KT. Intra-arterial thrombolysis for central retinal artery occlusion: a

systematic review. *Br J Ophthalmol* 2008;**92**:588–93.

55. Feltgen N, Neubauer A, Jurklies B, *et al.* Multicenter study of the European Assessment Group for Lysis in the Eye (EAGLE) for the treatment of central retinal artery occlusion: design issues and implications. EAGLE Study report no. 1: EAGLE Study report no. 1. *Graefes Arch Clin Exp Ophthalmol* 2006;**244**:950–6.

56. Annonier P, Sahel J, Wenger JJ, *et al.* Local fibrinolytic treatment in occlusions of the central retinal artery. *J Fr Ophtalmol* 1984;**7**:711–16.

57. Annonier P, Benichou C, Flament J, *et al.* A Role of fibrinolysis in the treatment of retinal arterial occlusion. Discussion of 5 cases. *Bull Soc Ophtalmol Fr* 1988;**88**:1167–71.

58. Mach R, Kessler P, Susicky P, *et al.* Thrombolysis of arterial retinal occlusion using urokinase. *Cesk Oftalmol* 1992;**48**:42–7.

59. Schumacher M, Schmidt D, Wakhloo A K. Intra-arterial fibrinolysis in central artery occlusion. *Radiologe* 1991;**31**:240–3.

60. Schumacher M, Schmidt D, Wakhloo A K. Intra-arterial fibrinolytic therapy in central retinal artery occlusion. *Neuroradiology* 1993;**35**:600–5.

61. Schmidt D, Schumacher M, Wakhloo A K. Microcatheter urokinase infusion in central retinal artery occlusion. *Am J Ophthalmol* 1992;**113**:429–34.

62. Brassel F. Possibilities and limits of local intra-arterial fibrinolysis in thromboembolic vascular occlusions of the central nervous system. *Z Gesamte Inn Med* 1993;**48**:351–5.

63. Turner K, Guhl A, Hettesheimer H. Technik der selektiven kontrollierten retinalen Fibrinolyse im Modell. *Ophtalmologe* 1993;**90**:472–5.

64. Van Cauwenberge F. Fibrinolyse: indications en ophtalmologie. *Bull Soc Belge Ophtalmol* 1993;**247**:71–3.

65. Vulpius K, Hoh H, Lange H, *et al.* Selective percutaneous transluminal thrombolytic therapy with rt-PA in central retinal artery occlusion. *Ophthalmologe* 1996;**93**:149–53.

66. Ma Z, Li B, Dou H. Treatment of central retinal artery occlusion with thrombolysis via superselective ophthalmic artery catheterization. *Zhonghua Yan Ke Za Zhi* 1996;**32**:445–7.

67. Weber J, Remonda L, Mattle HP, *et al.* Selective intra-arterial fibrinolysis of acute central retinal artery occlusion. *Stroke* 1998;**29**:2076–9.

68. Weill A, Cognard C, Piotin M, *et al.* Persistent value of intra-arterial fibrinolysis 8 hours or more following central retinal artery occlusion or of its branches. *J Fr Ophtalmol* 1998;**21**: 466–70.

69. Wirostko WJ, Pulido JS, Hendrix LE. Selective thrombolysis of central retinal artery occlusion without long-term systemic heparinization. *Surg Neurol* 1998;**50**:408–10.

70. Hattenbach LO. Systemic lysis therapy in retinal vascular occlusions. *Ophthalmologe* 1998;**95**:568–75.

71. Richard G, Lerche RC, Knospe V, *et al.* Treatment of retinal arterial occlusion with local fibrinolysis using recombinant tissue plasminogen activator. *Ophthalmology* 1999;**106**:768–73.

72. Padolecchia R, Puglioli M, Ragone MC, *et al.* Superselective intra-arterial fibrinolysis in central retinal artery occlusion. *AJNR Am J Neuroradiol* 1999;**20**:565–7.

73. Framme C, Spiegel D, Roider J, *et al.* Central retinal artery occlusion. Importance of selective intra-arterial fibrinolysis. *Ophthalmologe* 2001;**98**:725–30.

74. Korner-Stiefbold U. Central retinal artery occlusion—etiology, clinical picture, therapeutic possibilities. *Ther Umsch* 2001;**58**:36–40.

75. Kattah JC, Wang DZ, Reddy C. Intravenous recombinant tissue-type plasminogen activator thrombolysis in treatment of central retinal artery occlusion. *Arch Ophthalmol* 2002;**120**:1234–6.

76. Schmidt DP, Schulte-Monting J, Schumacher M. Prognosis of central retinal artery occlusion: local intra-arterial fibrinolysis versus conservative treatment. *AJNR Am J Neuroradiol* 2002;**23**:1301–7.

77. Fernandez FJ, Guelbenzu S, Barrena C, *et al.* Selective ophthalmic artery fibrinolysis in acute central retinal artery occlusion. *Arch Soc Esp Oftalmol* 2002;**77**:81–6.

78. Butz B, Strotzer M. Manke C, *et al.* Selective intraarterial fibrinolysis of acute central retinal artery occlusion. *Acta Radiol* 2003;**44**:680–4.

79. Diaconu E, Stanciu V, Ciuca A. Systemic thrombosis in central retinal artery occlusion—case report. *Oftalmologia* 2004;**48**:25–7.

80. Arnold M, Koerner U, Remonda L, *et al.* Comparison of intra-arterial thrombolysis with conventional treatment in patients with acute central retinal artery occlusion. *J Neurol Neurosurg Psychiatry* 2005;**76**:196–9.

81. Plant GT, Landau K. Thrombolysis for central retinal artery occlusion. *J Neurol Neurosurg Psychiatry* 2005;**76**:160–1.

82. Pettersen JA, Hill MD, Dechuck AM, *et al.* Intra-arterial thrombolysis for retinal artery occlusion: the Calgary experience. *Can J Neurol Sci* 2005;**32**:507–11.

Chapter 20

Epistaxis

Alexandros L. Georgiadis, Steve M. Cordina, Haralabos Zacharatos and Adnan I. Qureshi

Introduction

Epistaxis is a common condition with a lifetime incidence estimated at 60% among the general population.[1] Most episodes are, however, self-limited. Only in 6% of cases do patients seek medical attention and hospitalization is rarely required (less than 2 of 10 000 cases).[2] The age distribution is bi-modal with the highest incidence seen in the elderly, followed by children under the age of ten.[3] Epistaxis is more common in the winter months, presumably due to dehumidification of the nasal mucosa.[4,5] Most cases are non-traumatic, especially among older patients,[3] and idiopathic.[6–8] Alcohol abuse, hypertension, and use of antiplatelet medications are encountered frequently among refractory cases.[9] Table 20.1 lists the most common conditions that can be associated with epistaxis. In rare cases, epistaxis can result from rupture of internal carotid artery (ICA) aneurysms,[10–12] intracranial arterio-venous malformations,[13] or anterior fossa dural arterio-venous fistulas.[14]

Nasal vascular supply

The internal and external carotid arteries both contribute to the blood supply of the nose. The septum receives blood from the anterior and posterior ethmoidal arteries (branches of the ophthalmic artery), from the posterior septal branch of the sphenopalatine artery, and from septal branches of the facial artery (see Fig. 20.1). In the anterior septum, vessels form a plexus (Kiesselbach plexus or Little's area) which is the most common site of hemorrhage (up to 90% of cases).[4] Blood supply to the lateral wall is from the ophthalmic artery (via the ethmoidal arteries and the angular artery) and from the sphenopalatine and descending palatine arteries (see Fig. 20.2). Only 10% of bleeds originate posteriorly, typically from the sphenopalatine artery.[15] These are more common among older patients and are more likely to be refractory.

Treatment options

Surgery and endovascular intervention are reserved for intractable epistaxis, most commonly defined as refractory to posterior nasal packing. Posterior packing can only be used for

Table 20.1. Overview of the most common causes of epistaxis

Causes of epistaxis	
Local	**Systemic**
Traumatic	*Coagulation disorders/ deficits*
Fracture, surgical procedures	Thrombocytopenia
Nasal intubation	Acquired and congenital coagulopathies
Digital trauma	Vitamin A, C, D, E, K deficiency
Antihistamine, steroid nasal sprays	Hepatic disease
Cocaine, snuff, heroine sniffing	Renal failure
Nasal oxygen, continuous positive airway pressure (CPAP)	Chronic alcohol abuse
Foreign bodies	Malnutrition
Structural	Polycythemia vera
Septal deformity, perforation	Multiple myeloma
Inflammatory disease	Leukemia
Viral upper respiratory infections	Antiplatelet drugs
Bacterial sinusitis	Anticoagulants
Allergic rhinitis	*Vascular disease*
Pyogenic granuloma	Atherosclerosis
Granulomatous disease	Collagen abnormalities
Environmental irritants	Hereditary hemorrhagic telangiectasia
Tumors, vascular malformations	*Cardiovascular conditions*
Aneurysms	Congestive heart failure
Angiofibroma	Mitral valve stenosis
Epidermoid carcinoma	*Hypertension – unproven*
Nasal papilloma	
Hemangioma	
Adenocarcinoma	

Textbook of Interventional Neurology, ed. Adnan I. Qureshi. Published by Cambridge University Press. © Cambridge University Press 2011.

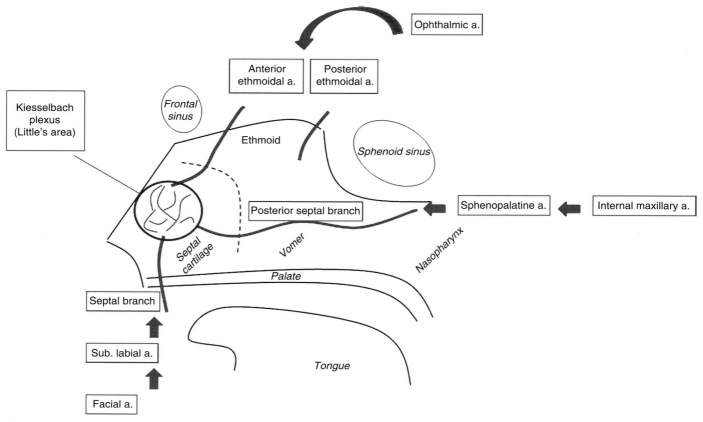

Fig. 20.1. The blood supply to the nasal septum. See plate section.

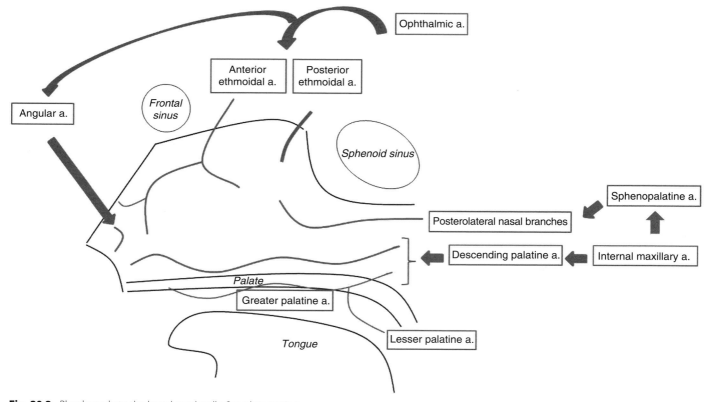

Fig. 20.2. Blood supply to the lateral nasal walls. See plate section.

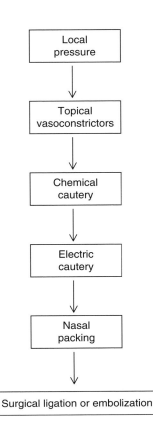

Fig. 20.3. Proposed treatment algorithm for epistaxis.

limited duration as it is often not tolerated well by patients and can have a number of side effects including infections and respiratory compromise.[16] Fig. 20.3 illustrates a suggested management algorithm.[4] Depending on the site of hemorrhage (anterior or posterior), the surgical option consists of ligation of the ethmoidal arteries or of the sphenopalatine artery.

Endovascular embolization for epistaxis was first described in 1974.[17] Advantages of this technique are: (1) the responsible vessel can potentially be directly identified; (2) general anesthesia can usually be avoided; (3) superselective catheterization with microcatheters enables the operator to target more distal vessels than is the case with surgical ligation. Diagnostic angiography can reveal the site of bleeding by showing active extravasation, and areas of increased vascularity of the mucosa, vascular malformations, tumors, or telangiectatic vessels.

Some authors recommend embolization as the primary treatment for refractory epistaxis,[16,18–20] while others consider it as an adjunct to surgery.[21]

Comparison of surgical and endovascular treatments

Surgical ligation and endovascular treatment are roughly comparable in terms of efficacy and complication rates.

In one study of 21 patients with intractable epistaxis,[22] 12 patients were treated with embolization, five with transantral ligation, and four required both. The success rates for embolization and surgery were 94% and 89%, respectively. No mortality or serious morbidity occurred with either technique. Endovascular treatment was slightly more expensive ($6783 vs. $5941).

In a series of 39 patients,[23] the failure rate of embolization (21%) was similar to that of internal maxillary artery (IMAX) ligation, with or without ethmoid artery ligation (27%). The complication rate was 16% for embolization and 18% for ligation. The cost of embolization was lower ($4545 vs. $6185) in this study.

Della Faille and colleagues[24] found that, in cases when ethmoidal artery bleeding was not suspected, embolization led to fewer complications and recurrences, shorter hospital stay, and improved post-operative comfort.

A review of 20 studies published between 1973 and 1995[23] suggested that surgery is associated with less treatment failures and less major complications. The rates of minor complications, however, were higher with surgery. It should be noted that, since the 1970s, technical advances have increased the efficacy and decreased the complications of endovascular procedures. Endoscopic sphenopalatine artery ligation, introduced in 1992, seems to be the most promising surgical method for the future.[25]

Endovascular treatment

The procedure is performed with nasal packing in place. Before starting, necessary measures should be taken, as needed, to establish hemodynamic stability. The decision to intubate and provide general anesthesia should be made on a case-by-case basis, depending on the patient's ability to lay still, the perceived risk of aspiration and hemodynamic fluctuations, and the likelihood of anesthesia-related sequelae.

Diagnostic angiography begins with catheterization of the ICA on the symptomatic side, if this is known. Typically, a 6-French guide-catheter, such as the Envoy™ (Cordis Corp) is used. If there is excessive aortic arch and/or proximal cerebral vessel tortuosity, a Simmons II™ (Cordis Corp) catheter can be employed. Following a proximal injection, the extent of blood supply to the nose from the ethmoidal arteries and the presence of a choroidal blush should be assessed. Extensive vascularization of the nose through the ethmoidal arteries indicates that embolization is unlikely to be successful, since ICA branches cannot be safely embolized. If no choroidal blush is present, the ophthalmic artery should be expected to arise from the external carotid artery (ECA) circulation, specifically from the middle meningeal artery (MMA). In this case, embolization is contra-indicated since material reflux into the ophthalmic artery can lead to retinal ischemia. The catheter is then positioned in the proximal ECA for an initial injection to provide an overview of the ECA circulation. Subsequently, a micro-catheter is introduced through the guide into the IMAX for a selective injection. A commonly used combination is the Prowler™ 10 or 14 micro-catheter (Cordis Corp) over a Transend™ (Boston Scientific/Target Therapeutics) 0.010″ or 0.014″ micro-wire. Choroidal blush should not be visualized from IMAX injection. The ophthalmic artery should not arise from the MMA. One should look for sites of possible contrast extravasation and for the presence of tumors and vessel anomalies, such as malformations or telangiectasias. Variations of the common patterns of the ECA branches are quite common. Note should be made of variations that could potentially lead to complications. For example, in 5% of cases, the ascending pharyngeal artery can arise from a common lingual-facial artery trunk.[26] This is important to know because the ascending pharyngeal artery supplies the lower cranial nerves. Collaterals to the ICA circulation are always present to some extent, even if angiographically not visible. Depending on the extent of collateralization, embolization can be possible only with special caution and in some cases it should be avoided altogether. Figure 20.4 offers an overview of potential collateral pathways between the ECA, ICA and vertebral arteries. Figure 20.5 illustrates some of the anatomy of the IMAX and facial artery branches.

A selective micro-catheter injection into the facial artery is the best way to assess this vessel's contribution to nasal blood supply. Depending on the findings, embolization of facial artery branches might be indicated.

The IMAX is the principal target vessel. The micro-catheter is advanced past the MMA and accessory meningeal arteries. Placement of the micro-catheter past the middle deep temporal artery can help reduce post-embolization pain and trismus.[27]

Embolization can be performed with coils, polyvinyl alcohol (PVA), trisacryl gelatin microspheres (Embosphere®,

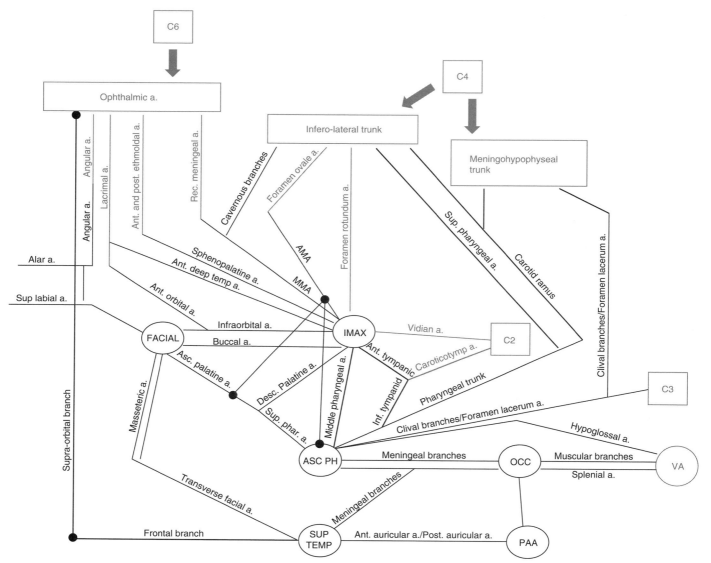

Fig. 20.4. Overview of the most important collateral pathways between the internal carotid, external carotid, and vertebral arteries. First-order branches of the external carotid artery are encircled. First-order branches of the internal carotid artery are highlighted in boxes. Black lines represent external carotid artery branches; Gray lines represent internal carotid artery branches. The names of internal carotid artery branches are shown in red. Abbreviations used: a, artery; AMA, accessory meningeal artery; MMA, middle meningeal artery; Ant, anterior; Post, posterior; Asc, ascending; Desc, descending; Sup, superior; Occ, occipital artery; IMAX, internal maxillary artery; ASC PH, ascending pharyngeal artery; SUP TEMP, superior temporal artery; PAA, C2-C6, internal carotid artery divisions; VA, vertebral artery. See plate section.

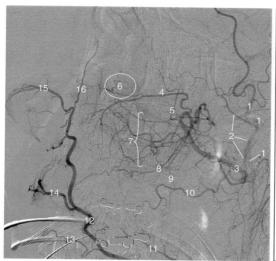

External carotid artery injection, lateral projection:
 1: Superficial temporal artery
 2: Middle meningeal artery
 3: Internal maxillary artery
 4: Inferior orbital artery
 5: Deep temporal artery
 6: Anterior orbital branches (from 4)
 7: Sphenopalatine artery branches (medial to septum and lateral to conchae)
 8: Descending palatine artery
 9: Buccal artery
10: Transverse facial artery
11: Lingual artery
12: Facial artery
13: Inferior labial artery
14: Superior labial artery
15: Septal arteries (from 12)
16: Angular artery

Fig. 20.5. Anatomy of facial and internal maxillary artery branches.

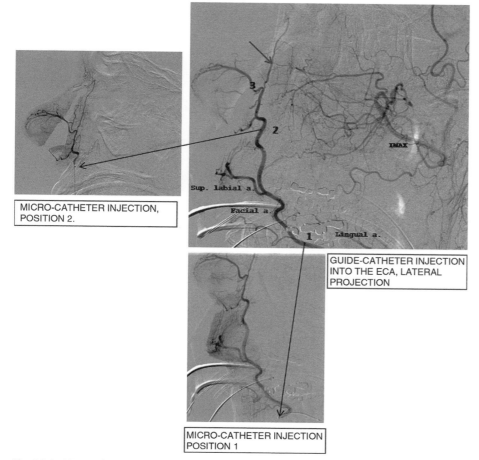

MICRO-CATHETER INJECTION, POSITION 2.

GUIDE-CATHETER INJECTION INTO THE ECA, LATERAL PROJECTION

MICRO-CATHETER INJECTION POSITION 1

Fig. 20.6. Micro-catheter exploration of the facial artery in preparation for embolization. The micro-catheter is advanced in a stepwise fashion. First it is brought to position 1. The gray arrows point at the position of the micro-catheter tip. A contrast injection reveals that it is still proximal to the superior labial artery. It is then advanced further over the micro-wire under fluoroscopy and brought into position 2. A contrast injection shows that it is now past the superior labial artery. However, a large branch (gray arrow) is identified as the angular artery which is known to anastomose with the angular branch of the ophthalmic artery. In order to avoid inadvertent embolization of the ophthalmic artery circulation, the micro-catheter is further advanced into position 3. Embolization proceeded after micro-catheter injection (not shown) confirmed placement past the origin of the angular artery. Abbreviations used: a, artery; Sup, superior; IMAX, internal maxillary artery; ECA, external carotid artery.

Table 20.2. Overview of studies published since 1990 that included at least 30 patients treated with embolization

Study	Number of patients	Vessels embolized (Rate in %)					Embolization material			Success rate in %		Rate of complications in %	
		IMAX		FACIAL		OTHER	PVA	Coils	GS	Immediate	Short-term[a]	Major	Minor
		IL	CL	IL	CL								
Vitek et al. 1991[19]	30	100		13					☐	87	97[b]	3	N/A
Siniluoto et al. 1993[38]	31	100					•		☐	71	71	0	10
Elden et al. 1994[37]	97	100	100	33	N/A		☐			88	88	3	23
Elahi et al. 1995[18]	54	100	20				☐			91	96[b]	6	7
Tseng et al. 1998[6]	112	100	21	24	2		☐		•	93	86	2	15
Moreau et al. 1998[21]	45	100	71	4			☐			95	97[b]	4	4
Leppanen et al. 1999[36]	37	100					☐	•		89	89	3	8
Oguni et al. 2000[35]	37	100	57	51	5			•	•	100	95	0	45
Christensen et al. 2005[7]	70	94	70	43		10	•	•	•	88	75	1	N/A

☐ Primarily employed method (when known), • adjunct method,
[a]Until discharge from the hospital.
[b]Following additional embolization.
Abbreviations used: PVA, Polyvinyl alcohol; GS, gelatin sponge; IMAX, internal maxillary artery; IL, ipsilateral; CL, contralateral; N/A, information is not available.

BioSphere Medical Inc, Rockland, MA), and gelatin sponge pledgets (Gelfoam®, Pfizer). PVA particles are the most widely used. They range in size from 50 to 700 μm. Because of their hydrophobic property and shape irregularity, PVA particles tend to form aggregates that block relatively proximal vessels. There are data that support that tris-acryl gelatin microspheres, which are spherical and hydrophilic, cause more reliable results owing to deeper penetration.[28,29] However, there are no randomized comparisons between various embolic agents in the neuro-intervention literature. No difference was found between the two types of particles in a large randomized study of uterine artery embolization for treatment of leiomyomas.[30]

Smaller particles lodge more distally and cause more permanent occlusion.[31] At the same time, the risk of tissue necrosis is higher, as is the risk of material reflux and penetration into small collateral vessels with inadvertent embolization of other circulations. Occlusion of capillaries and immediate precapillary level arteries (diameter of 10–150 μm) leads to tissue necrosis because of the lack of collateral pathways at that level.[32] Therefore, particles sized 50–150 μm are used sparsely, if at all. PVA particles are diluted in a solution containing iodinated contrast agent so that the injected material is radioopaque and angiographically visible. The particles are injected under continuous fluoroscopy in small gentle pushes, waiting for the contrast to clear. Slower injections can help avoid reflux and may lead to deeper penetration.[33] Pure-contrast injections are performed intermittently to assess distal runoff and to look for dangerous collateral pathways that could have developed

Table 20.3. Overview of reported complications following embolization for epistaxis

Reported complications of embolization for epistaxis
Facial pain[6,16]
Facial numbness[51]
Facial edema
Facial paresis[51]
Ophthalmoparesis
Fever[16]
Trismus[16]
Sinusitis
Ischemic sialadenitis[47]
Otitis
Septal perforation
Necrosis of skin or mucosa[50]
Palate ulceration[48,50]
Retinal artery occlusion/Visual deficits[49,52]
Seizures[18]
Mental status changes[6]
Transient neurological deficits[36]
Stroke[6,7]

Reprinted with permission from: Geibprasert S, et al., 2009.

Table 20.4. Summary of the cranial nerve blood supply

Cranial nerve	Location	Arterial supply	
III, IV	Cisternal	Mesencephalic perforators (common trunk for CN III)	Vertebrobasilar system
	Cavernous sinus	CN III: ILT only; CN IV: marginal artery of the tentorium cerebelli (meningohypophyseal trunk) + ILT	
	Superior orbital fissure	Anteromedial branch of ILT	
VI	Cisternal		Vertebrobasilar system
	Dorsum sella	Jugular branch of AscPhA, medial branch of lateral clival artery, meningohypophyseal trunk	
	Cavernous sinus	ILT	
	Superior orbital fissure	Anteromedial branch of ILT	
V	Cisternal	Basilar vestige of trigeminal artery (between SCA and AICA)	
	Meckel cave	Lateral artery of trigeminal ganglion, cavernous branch of MMA, carotid branch of AscPhA, ILT	
V2	Foramen rotundum	Artery of foramen rotundum	ILT, distal IMA
V3	Foramen ovale	Posteromedial branch	ILT, AMA
VII, VIII	Cisternal + IAC	Internal auditory artery	AICA
	Geniculate ganglion	Petrosal branch of MMA, stylomastoid branch of posterior auricular/occipital artery	
IX, X	Cisternal, jugular foramen	Jugular branch of neuromeningeal trunk	VA, AscPhA
XI	Spinal root	C3 segmental branch	Cervical arteries, musculospinal branch of AscPhA
	Cranial root	Jugular branch of neuromeningeal trunk	AscPhA
XII	Cisternal hypoglossal canal	Hypoglossal branch of neuromeningeal trunk	VA, AscPhA

AscPhA indicates ascending pharyngeal artery; SCA, superior cerebellar artery; IAC, internal auditory canal; AICA, anterior inferior cerebellar artery; VA, vertebral artery; AICA, anterior inferior cerebellar artery; ILT, inferior lateral trunk; IMA, internal maxillary artery; MMA, middle meningeal artery; AMA, accessory meningeal artery.

during the procedure.[34] Embolization is discontinued when there is stasis or marked slowing of flow, or when there is reflux of material into other arteries that cannot be avoided by technique modification.

Following PVA embolization, gelatin sponge pledgets are often injected into the distal IMAX. Coils can also be employed. However, the use of coils is usually deferred (except for cases of traumatic epistaxis) owing to the small size of the target vessels and the fact that re-treatment is rendered impossible through the coil within the vessel. Prior to retrieving the micro-catheter, a guide-catheter injection is performed to assess the degree of devascularization. If it is felt that treatment of the facial artery is warranted, then the micro-catheter should be introduced into the vessel and advanced as far distally as is necessary and feasible so that the embolization is as selective as possible. It is good practice to retrieve the first microcatheter and replace it with a new microcatheter prior to catheterizing the new artery. Figure 20.6 illustrates that principle.

As can be seen in Table 20.2,[6,7,18,19,21,35–38] there is considerable variation in practice among endovascvular surgeons regarding the vessels that are targeted for embolization. The IMAX ipsilateral to the bleeding is treated virtually consistently. The facial artery will also be treated by most practitioners if its contribution is regarded significant. However, some authors advocate routinely embolizing multiple vessels: both IMAX,[37] the ipsilateral IMAX and facial arteries, or even both IMAX and the ipsilateral facial artery.[39] The rationale is that sufficient collateral flow can develop from these vessels to cause recurrence of bleeding. Moreover, the symptomatic side cannot always be accurately identified clinically or angiographically, the latter especially when packing is in place. Still, treatment of the ipsilateral IMAX alone[19,36] if the side of bleeding is correctly identified can result in success rates in the vicinity of 90%, not significantly different from the rates achieved with multi-vessel embolization regimens (see Table 20.2).

Our protocol is as follows. If we know with certainty which side is the source of bleeding, we embolize the ipsilateral IMAX alone. If there is any doubt, we proceed with bilateral IMAX embolization. Smaller particles are used on the symptomatic side. The ipsilateral facial artery is treated only if its contribution is felt to be extensive. Following the procedure, we prefer to have the nasal packings removed in the angiographic suite in the presence of ear-nose-throat team that can re-pack the nose if needed. Should bleeding recur, further embolization is performed. If not, the patients are monitored for 24 hours and are then discharged if they are stable and not in need of further acute work up.

Hereditary hemorrhagic telangiectasia (HHT)

HHT, also known as Osler–Weber–Rendu syndrome, is an autosomal-dominant disorder associated with telangiectasias and skin, mucosal, visceral, pulmonary, and cerebral arterio-venous malformations.[40,41] On the skin, telangiectasias (small arterio-venous shunts) are seen as 1–2 mm red spots that disappear with pressure. Epistaxis is the most common symptom (93% of patients)[42] and often the presenting symptom among affected individuals and is one of the criteria used for establishing the diagnosis.[43] Among the large number of available treatment options, endonasal laser coagulation or argon plasma coagulation and septodermoplasty are considered to have the best results.[44] Embolization is usually recommended for emergency treatment and for cases refractory to other therapeutic modalities. It offers good results in terms of immediate and short-term cessation of bleeding,[15,45] but recurrence and treatment failure are more common than in idiopathic epistaxis.[15,37,46]

Complications

In the larger published series, complication rates have been between 0% and 6% (minor) and 4% and 45% (major) (see Table 20.2). The more serious complications occur secondary to reflux of embolic material into the ICA circulation. This is a complication that tends to occur towards the end of the procedure[19] and with overly forceful injections. As mentioned above, use of very small particles increases the risk of tissue necrosis. Table 20.3[6,7,16,18,36,47–52] lists the complications that have been reported in the literature. Treatment of these complications is mostly symptomatic. Skin slough will rarely require plastic surgery.[53] An empiric trial of high-dose intravenous steroids might be beneficial in cases of cranial nerve palsy under the presumption that ischemia and edema of the nerve sheath are contributing to the symptoms.[54] Table 20.4[55] offers an overview of the blood supply of the cranial nerves that are at risk during embolization.

References

1. Gifford TO, Orlandi RR. Epistaxis. *Otolaryngol Clin North Am* 2008;**41**: 525–36, viii.

2. Viehweg TL, Roberson JB, Hudson JW. Epistaxis: diagnosis and treatment. *J Oral Maxillofac Surg* 2006;**64**:511–18.

3. Pallin DJ, Chng Y-M, McKay MP, *et al.* Epidemiology of epistaxis in US emergency departments, 1992 to 2001. *Ann Emerg Med* 2005;**46**:77–81.

4. Schlosser RJ. Clinical practice. Epistaxis. *N Engl J Med* 2009;**360**:784–9.

5. Walker TWM, Macfarlane TV, McGarry GW. The epidemiology and chronobiology of epistaxis: an investigation of Scottish hospital admissions 1995–2004. *Clin Otolaryngol* 2007;**32**:361–5.

6. Tseng EY, Narducci CA, Willing SJ, Sillers MJ. Angiographic embolization for epistaxis: a review of 114 cases. *Laryngoscope* 1998;**108**:615–19.

7. Christensen NP, Smith DS, Barnwell SL, Wax MK. Arterial embolization in the management of posterior epistaxis. *Otolaryngol Head Neck Surg* 2005;**133**:748–53.

8. Awan MS, Iqbal M, Imam SZ. Epistaxis: when are coagulation studies justified?. *Emerg Med J* 2008;**25**:156–7.

9. Jackson KR, Jackson RT. Factors associated with active, refractory epistaxis. *Arch Otolaryngol Head Neck Surg* 1988;**114**:862–5.

10. Lehmann P, Saliou G, Page C, *et al.* Epistaxis revealing the rupture of a carotid aneurysm of the cavernous sinus extending into the sphenoid: treatment using an uncovered stent and coils. Review of literature. *Eur Arch Otorhinolaryngol* 2009;**266**:767–72.

11. Roebuck JC, Pereira KD. Idiopathic internal carotid artery aneurysm rupture in an infant: a case report. *Ear Nose Throat J* 2009;**88**:835–7.

12. Singh H, Thomas J, Hoe WLE, Sethi DS. Giant petrous carotid aneurysm: persistent epistaxis despite internal carotid artery ligation. *J Laryngol Otol* 2008;**122**:e18.

13. de Tilly LN, Willinsky R, TerBrugge K, *et al.* Cerebral arteriovenous malformation causing epistaxis. *AJNR Am J Neuroradiol* 1992;**13**:333–4.

14. Baskaya MK, Suzuki Y, Seki Y, *et al.* Dural arteriovenous malformations in the anterior cranial fossa. *Acta Neurochir (Wien)* 1994;**129**:146–51.

15. Andersen PJ, Kjeldsen AD, Nepper-Rasmussen J. Selective embolization in the treatment of intractable epistaxis. *Acta Otolaryngol* 2005;**125**:293–7.

16. Strutz J, Schumacher M. Uncontrollable epistaxis. Angiographic localization and embolization. *Arch Otolaryngol Head Neck Surg* 1990;**116**:697–9.

17. Sokoloff J, Wickbom I, McDonald D, *et al.* Therapeutic percutaneous embolization in intractable epistaxis. *Radiology* 1974;**111**:285–7.

18. Elahi MM, Parnes LS, Fox AJ, Pelz DM, Lee DH. Therapeutic embolization in the treatment of intractable epistaxis. *Arch Otolaryngol Head Neck Surg* 1995;**121**:65–9.

19. Vitek J. Idiopathic intractable epistaxis: endovascular therapy. *Radiology* 1991;**181**:113–16.

20. Merland JJ, Melki JP, Chiras J, Riche MC, Hadjean E. Place of embolization in the treatment of severe epistaxis. *Laryngoscope* 1980;**90**:1694–704.

21. Moreau S, De Rugy MG, Babin E, Courtheoux P, Valdazo A. Supraselective embolization in intractable epistaxis: review of 45 cases. *Laryngoscope* 1998;**108**:887–8.

22. Strong EB, Bell DA, Johnson LP, Jacobs JM. Intractable epistaxis: transantral ligation vs. embolization: efficacy review and cost analysis. *Otolaryngol Head Neck Surg* 1995;**113**: 674–8.

23. Cullen MM, Tami TA. Comparison of internal maxillary artery ligation versus embolization for refractory posterior epistaxis. *Otolaryngol Head Neck Surg* 1998;**118**:636–42.

24. della Faille D, Schmelzer B, Vidts G, *et al.* Posterior epistaxis: our experience with transantral ligation and embolisation. *Acta Otorhinolaryngol Belg* 1997;**51**:167–71.

25. Kumar S, Shetty A, Rockey J, Nilssen E. Contemporary surgical treatment of epistaxis. What is the evidence for sphenopalatine artery ligation?. *Clin Otolaryngol Allied Sci* 2003; **28**:360–3.

26. Cavalcanti DD, Reis CVC, Hanel R, *et al.* The ascending pharyngeal artery and its relevance for neurosurgical and endovascular procedures. *Neurosurgery.* 2009;**65**:114–20; discussion 120.

27. Willems PWA, Farb RI, Agid R. Endovascular treatment of epistaxis. *Am J Neuroradiol* 2009;**30**: 1637–45.

28. Bendszus M, Klein R, Burger R, *et al.* Efficacy of trisacryl gelatin microspheres versus polyvinyl alcohol particles in the preoperative embolization of meningiomas. *Am J Neuroradiol.* 2000;**21**:255–61.

29. Andrews RT, Binkert CA. Relative rates of blood flow reduction during transcatheter arterial embolization with tris-acryl gelatin microspheres or polyvinyl alcohol: quantitative comparison in a swine model. *J Vasc Interv Radiol* 2003;**14**:1311–16.

30. Spies JB, Allison S, Flick P, *et al.* Polyvinyl alcohol particles and tris-acryl gelatin microspheres for uterine artery embolization for leiomyomas: results of a randomized comparative study. *J Vasc Interv Radiol* 2004;**15**:793–800.

31. Weaver EM, Chaloupka JC, Putman CM, *et al.* Effect of internal maxillary arterial occlusion on nasal blood flow in swine. *Laryngoscope* 1999;**109**:8–14.

32. Turowski B, Zanella FE. Interventional neuroradiology of the head and neck. *Neuroimaging Clin N Am* 2003;**13**:619–45.

33. Choe DH, Han MH, Kang GH, Yeon KM, Han MC. An experimental study of embolic effect according to infusion rate and concentration of suspension in transarterial particulate embolization. *Invest Radiol* 1997;**32**:260–7.

34. Nguyen T, Roy D, Cuilbert F. Meningioma embolization with particles. *In* Qureshi AI, Georgiadis AL, eds. *Atlas of Interventional Neurology.* Demos Medical, 2008;196–7.

35. Oguni T, Korogi Y, Yasunaga T, *et al.* Superselective embolisation for intractable idiopathic epistaxis. *Br J Radiol* 2000;**73**:1148–53.

36. Leppanen M, Seppanen S, Laranne J, Kuoppala K. Microcatheter embolization of intractable idiopathic epistaxis. *Cardiovasc Intervent Radiol* 1999;**22**:499–503.

37. Elden L, Montanera W, Terbrugge K, *et al.* Angiographic embolization for the treatment of epistaxis: a review of 108 cases. *Otolaryngol Head Neck Surg* 1994;**111**:44–50.

38. Siniluoto TM, Leinonen AS, Karttunen AI, Karjalainen HK, Jokinen KE. Embolization for the treatment of posterior epistaxis. An analysis of 31 cases. *Arch Otolaryngol Head Neck Surg* 1993;**119**:837–41.

39. Shah QA. Bilateral tri-arterial embolization for the treatment of epistaxis. *J Vasc Interventional Neurol.* 2008;**1**(4):102–5.

40. Sharathkumar AA, Shapiro A. Hereditary haemorrhagic telangiectasia. *Haemophilia* 2008;**14**:1269–80.

41. Easey AJ, Wallace GMF, Hughes JMB, *et al.* Should asymptomatic patients with hereditary haemorrhagic telangiectasia (HHT) be screened for cerebral vascular malformations? Data from 22,061 years of HHT patient life. *J Neurol Neurosurg Psychiatry* 2003;**74**:743–8.

42. Pau H, Carney AS, Murty GE. Hereditary haemorrhagic telangiectasia (Osler–Weber–Rendu syndrome): otorhinolaryngological manifestations. *Clin Otolaryngol Allied Sci* 2001;**26**:93–8.

43. Shovlin CL, Guttmacher AE, Buscarini E, *et al.* Diagnostic criteria for hereditary hemorrhagic telangiectasia (Rendu–Osler–Weber syndrome). *Am J Med Genet* 2000;**91**:66–7.

44. Geisthoff UW, Fiorella ML, Fiorella R. Treatment of recurrent epistaxis in HHT. *Curr Pharm Des* 2006;**12**:1237–42.

45. Braak SJ, de Witt CA, Disch FJM, Overtoom TTC, Westermann JJ. Percutaneous embolization on hereditary hemorrhagic telangiectasia patients with severe epistaxis. *Rhinology* 2009;**47**:166–71.

46. Layton KF, Kallmes DF, Gray LA, Cloft HJ. Endovascular treatment of epistaxis in patients with hereditary hemorrhagic telangiectasia. *Am J Neuroradiol.* 2007;**28**:885–8.

47. Duncan IC, Spiro FI, van Staden D. Acute ischemic sialadenitis following facial artery embolization. *Cardiovasc Intervent Radiol* 2004;**27**:300–2.

48. Guss J, Cohen MA, Mirza N. Hard palate necrosis after bilateral internal maxillary artery embolization for epistaxis. *Laryngoscope* 2007;**117**:1683–4.

49. Mames RN, Snady-McCoy L, Guy J. Central retinal and posterior ciliary artery occlusion after particle embolization of the external carotid artery system. *Ophthalmology* 1991;**98**:527–31.

50. Sadri M, Midwinter K, Ahmed A, Parker A. Assessment of safety and efficacy of arterial embolisation in the management of intractable epistaxis. *Eur Arch Otorhinolaryngol* 2006;**263**:560–6.

51. de Vries N, Versluis RJ, Valk J, Snow GB. Facial nerve paralysis following embolization for severe epistaxis (case report and review of the literature). *J Laryngol Otol* 1986;**100**:207–10.

52. Ashwin PT, Mirza S, Ajithkumar N, Tsaloumas MD. Iatrogenic central retinal artery occlusion during treatment for epistaxis. *Br J Ophthalmol* 2007;**91**:122–3.

53. Hassan Z, Law EJ, Still JM. Repair of extensive tissue slough of the face which followed insertion of coils to control epistaxis. *Plast Reconstr Surg* 2004;**113**:769–71.

54. Connors III JJWJC. Chapter 13. Epistaxis. In *Interventional Neuroradiology.* Connors III JJ, Wojak JC, eds. Saunders, 1999;147–56.

55. Geibprasert S, Pongpech S, Armstrong D, Krings T. Dangerous extracranial–intracranial anastomoses and supply to the cranial nerves: vessels the neurointerventionalist needs to know. *Am J Neuroradiol* 2009;**30**: 1459–68.

Stanley H. Kim, Anant I. Patel, Nancy Gruell, Kirk Conrad and Young J. Yu

Introduction

Vertebroplasty and kyphoplasty are minimally invasive procedures to relieve back pain in patients with vertebral compression fractures (VCF) from various causes such as osteoporosis, malignancy, and hemangioma. These two procedures are based on similar principles which consist of injecting acrylic cement called polymethylmethacrylate (PMMA) into a fractured vertebral body via a percutaneously placed cannula to strengthen the vertebral body. Kyphoplasty, developed in 1997, evolved from vertebroplasty which was first performed in 1984. However, many of the primary care physicians who frequently encounter patients with osteoporotic or pathological VCFs are often not aware of the differences between these procedures. The procedures differ in the methodology of cement delivery into the vertebral body and the effect on reduction of compression deformity. Different types of vertebral compression fractures may be better treated by one procedure than the other. There are also differences in cost and reimbursement. To this date, no randomized studies have compared the two procedures in terms of efficacy or safety.

This chapter will briefly summarize the history, diagnosis, indications, technique, complications, and outcome of vertebroplasty and kyphoplasty. A few difficult and challenging cases will be illustrated. The authors acknowledge that this review is based on individual opinions and variations on many issues, such as indications and optimal timing of the procedures and the number of vertebral body levels to be treated may be controversial in the absence of randomized clinical trials. As products and techniques used undergo evolution in the future and more data become available, some of these recommendations may be modified.

History of vertebroplasty and kyphoplasty

Galibert and Deramond of the Department of Radiology of the University Hospital of Amiens, France, were the first to perform percutaneous vertebroplasty in a 54-year-old woman with neck pain from a C2 hemangioma.[1] They injected PMMA percutaneously using a 15-gauge needle into the C2 cervical vertebral body. The excellent pain relief achieved by the procedure led to application of the technique in cases of VCF and vertebral metastasis.[2] In 1997, Jensen and colleagues (radiologists) reported the first case series of percutaneous PMMA vertebroplasty for the treatment of osteoporotic VCFs in the US.[3] Subsequently, the vertebroplasty procedure has become very popular especially among the interventional radiologists in the US. Medicare and private insurance companies have endorsed the use of vertebroplasty by providing dedicated reimbursement codes. Both vertebroplasty and kyphoplasty now use FDA approved bone cement called Simplex P (Stryker-Howmedica-Osteonics, Rutherford, NJ).

Kyphoplasty evolved from vertebroplasty. In 1997, Mark Reily, an orthopedic surgeon, percutaneously inserted an inflatable balloon tamp into a compressed vertebral body before injecting the PMMA cement to restore the vertebral height and reduce kyphotic deformity (Fig. 21.1). In 1998, Reily performed the first kyphoplasty for osteoporotic VCF and later that year, the FDA approved kyphoplasty (Kyphon Inc. Sunnyvale, USA). Since then, many surgeons in the orthopedic and neurosurgical community and interventional radiologists or neurointerventional surgeons have acquired training in performing this procedure. It is estimated that over 460 000 VCFs have been treated in the USA with kyphoplasty since the year 2000.

In the absence of a randomized trials comparing the efficacy and safety of these two procedures, it is not clear which one is superior. Both procedures are reported to be safe and effective in reducing or relieving pain from VCFs, especially for painful osteoporotic VCFs.[4,5] Between 90% and 95% of patients who undergo either procedure report pain relief from osteoporotic VCF.[6–9] Currently, there is continued effort among clinicians and manufacturers to improve upon the cement composition and the tools and techniques used to deliver the cement.

Although the exact mechanism of pain relief is not well known for either vertebroplasty or kyphoplasty, theories of pain relief include improved load bearing ability of the treated

Textbook of Interventional Neurology, ed. Adnan I. Qureshi. Published by Cambridge University Press. © Cambridge University Press 2011.

(a)

(b)

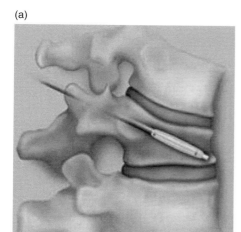

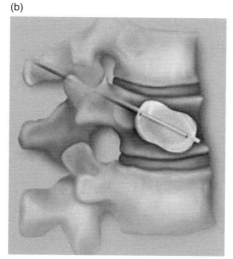

Fig. 21.1. (a), (b) Diagram of balloon tamp restoring the vertebral height.

Balloon tamp in place

The balloon tamp is inflated, and the collapsed vertebral bone is restored back to its normal height and shape.

vertebral body, direct tissue toxicity and thermal injury to pain fibers, and fracture reduction with potential restoration of normal spinal alignment.

Indications for vertebroplasty and kyphoplasty
Vertebroplasty

The indications are very similar for these two procedures (Tables 21.1 and 21.2). Vertebroplasty and kyphoplasty may be performed in symptomatic patients with osteoporotic VCF or VCF related to malignancy such as multiple myeloma or metastasis or hemangioma. The authors agree with the general concept that, ideally, patients who have failed conservative medical therapy including pain medications, bed rest, physical therapy, or brace, may be candidates for either procedure. However, over the last 20 years, there has been significant change of opinion among the treating physicians on the duration of symptoms of pain from the VCF before these procedures should be performed. In the early period, the consensus among physicians was to wait at least three months before recommending surgical intervention. But now, many physicians recommend surgical intervention within days or weeks of the symptomatic VCF if hospitalization is required and the pain is unresponsive to intravenous narcotics. Also, there have been reports of good outcome even for chronic symptomatic VCF lasting for 2 years.[10] The argument for early intervention is faster relief of pain, expedition of mobility or rehabilitation, discharge from the hospital, and reduction of complications related to prolonged bed rest and narcotic dependence.

It is important to establish that the pain localizes to the fracture level identified on the imaging study. If there is a discrepancy, the physician needs to investigate further the source of back pain and/or abnormal imaging finding. An asymptomatic chronic VCF is not an indication for these procedures. At present, there is no strong data to support prophylactic treatment of asymptomatic osteoporotic vertebral bodies or VCF. Although there are reports of pain relief with these procedures in the setting of acute traumatic non-osteoporotic VCF, the authors believe that, in general, conservative treatment or alternative surgical treatment should be considered in this group of patients at this time. In general, vertebroplasty is not considered an option for burst fractures. Extreme care should be taken in cases of disruption of posterior cortex of the vertebral body to avoid mild retropulsion of bone into the spinal canal when attempting vertebroplasty.

Kyphoplasty

The indications for kyphoplasty are similar to those mentioned earlier for vertebroplasty. Kyphoplasty may be preferable over vertebroplasty in patients presenting with disruption of the posterior cortex of the vertebral body or burst fracture. Since a balloon tamp is used to create a void in the fractured vertebral body, careful placement of the cement limited to the void area may reduce the chance of cement leakage into the spinal canal or outside the vertebral body. Kyphoplasty may be able to reduce end-plate depression and correct or reduce the kyphotic deformity, which may reduce the risk of potential long-term pulmonary complications and subsequent fractures.

Diagnosis
History and physical examination

Complete history and physical examination is essential prior to performing vertebroplasty and kyphoplasty. Often, there is a

Table 21.1. Indications and contraindications for vertebroplasty

Indications
1. Symptomatic osteoporotic VCF (acute or chronic)
2. Symptomatic tumor involvement or VCF secondary to multiple myeloma or metastasis
3. Symptomatic or destructive hemangioma

Contraindications
1. Vertebral wedge deformity >90% (vertebral plana) or severe enough to prevent safe percutaneous access into the vertebral body
2. Comminuted burst fracture in which bone is broken in multiple pieces
3. Inability to localize the pain level or discrepancy between the pain level and imaging findings
4. Inability to lie in prone position
5. Morbid obesity that prevents adequate radiological visualization of the vertebral body or skin and adipose tissue prevent the use of tools.
6. Uncorrectable coagulopathy or bleeding diathesis
7. Infection (systemic as well as spinal discitis, osteomyelitis, epidural abscess)
8. Acute traumatic non-osteoporotic VCF
9. Asymptomatic osteoporotic vertebral body
10. Significant neurologic symptoms
11. Allergy to any product used during the procedure
12. Vertebral bodies higher than thoracic spine T5 require treatment

Relative contraindications
1. Disruption of posterior cortex of vertebral body
2. Retropulsion of bone with significant canal compromise exceeding 20%
3. Radicular pain exceeding vertebral pain unrelated to vertebral collapse
4. Epidural tumor extension
5. Treatment of more than three levels at one time
6. Pedicle fracture may warrant extra-pedicular approach if feasible

Table 21.2. Indications and contraindications for kyphoplasty

Indications
1. Symptomatic osteoporotic VCF (acute or chronic)
2. Symptomatic tumor involvement or VCF secondary to multiple myeloma or metastasis
3. Symptomatic or destructive hemangioma

Contraindications
1. Vertebral wedge deformity > 90% (vertebral plana) or severe enough to prevent safe percutaneous access into the vertebral body
2. Inability to localize the pain level or discrepancy between the pain level and imaging findings
3. Inability to lie in prone position
4. Morbid obesity that prevents adequate radiological visualization of the vertebral body or skin and adipose tissue prevent the use of tools.
5. Uncorrectable coagulopathy or bleeding diathesis
6. Infection (systemic as well as spinal discitis, osteomyelitis, epidural abscess)
7. Acute traumatic non-osteoporotic VCF
8. Asymptomatic osteoporotic vertebral body
9. Significant neurologic symptoms
10. Allergy to any product used during the procedure
11. Vertebral bodies higher than thoracic spine T5 require treatment

Relative contraindications
1. Retropulsion of bone with significant canal compromise exceeding 20%
2. Radicular pain exceeding vertebral pain unrelated to vertebral collapse
3. Epidural tumor extension
4. Treatment of more than three levels at one time
5. Pedicle fracture may warrant extra-pedicular approach if feasible

Abbreviations used: VCF, vertebral compression fracture.

history of fall or trauma to the spine in cases of osteoporotic VCF. However, a clear history of antecedent trauma may be lacking and the diagnosis of osteoporotic VCF may be easily missed especially without any imaging studies. Any woman of post-menopausal age and potential risk of osteoporosis with complaint of back pain should undergo plain X-rays of the spine at the minimum to screen for possible VCF. Patients with a history of multiple myeloma or primary or metastatic tumor complaining of back pain should be evaluated for possible VCF or spinal metastasis.

Pre-operative imaging

All patients who are being considered for possible vertebroplasty or kyphoplasty should undergo magnetic resonance imaging (MRI) of the spine to identify acute or chronic vertebral body fracture. Additional features such as the presence of bone marrow edema on MRI study are very helpful in predicting which patients are most likely to respond favorably to these procedures. Alvarez demonstrated moderate to complete relief of pain in 96% of patients who had T1-hypotense and T2-hypertense changes on MRI prior to vertebroplasty (Fig. 21.2 (a),(b)).[11] In patients where MRI is contraindicated,

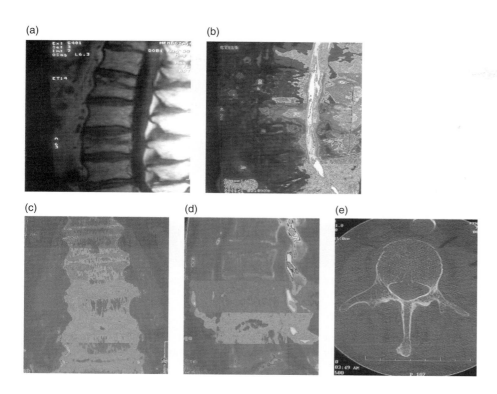

Fig. 21.2. (a)–(e) MRI of lumbar spine showing L1 (a) and L3 VCF (V). CT scan of lumbar spine showing the L3 VCF (c),(d),(e).

as in patients with a pacemaker, bone scintigraphy may be helpful in differentiating acute from chronic VCF. The authors recommend reviewing a computed tomography (CT) scan of the spine to acquire information about the quality and details of the vertebral body fracture and the size of the vertebral components such as the pedicle (Fig 21.2 (c),(d),(e)). CT scan also identifies the type of vertebral body fracture and the integrity of the posterior cortex of the body.

Technique of vertebroplasty

The goals of vertebroplasty are to strengthen the spine, improve mobility, decrease pain from symptomatic VCF, and to prevent neurological compromise. The procedure can be performed under local anesthesia with conscious moderate sedation or under general anesthesia depending on the comfort level of the patient, a operating physician preference, and the number of vertebral levels being treated. The authors prefer to perform complicated procedures under general anesthesia. The procedure can be performed in the operating room preferably with bi-plane fluoroscopic unit. Although a single C-arm fluoroscopy machine can be used, it will significantly prolong the procedure time and make the procedure extremely difficult and laborious due to constant need for reviewing AP and lateral views concurrently.

The patient is placed in a prone position on a pillow or chest roll with the arms placed above the shoulder. Extremity joints are adequately padded. The operative area is prepped in a sterile condition. The authors prefer to use the Parallax EZflow™ Cement Delivery System (Arthrocare Corp.; Austin, TX) because the kit includes all the tools and the cement needed

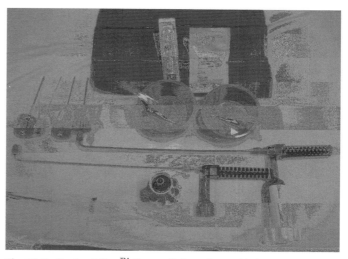

Fig. 21.3. Parallax EZflow™ Cement Delivery System (Arthrocare Corp.; Austin, TX) comes with Jamshidi needle, colored injector barrel, patented 17″ extension tubing to minimize radiation exposure, and Codman Cranioplasty Kit (CMW Laboratories, Blackpool, UK).

to perform vertebroplasty (Fig. 21.3). The procedure can be performed using a separate kit from the Cook Murphy bone biopsy kit (Cook Incorporated, Bloomington, IN). In any case, the vertebral body of interest is visualized on AP and lateral views and the physician must take time to confirm the correct level being treated as relying only on the report of MRI or CT scan can sometimes be misleading. The operator must be absolutely certain of the correct fractured body especially in cases of multiple VCFs. Subsequently, 10

(a)

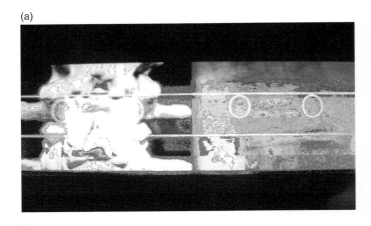

(b)

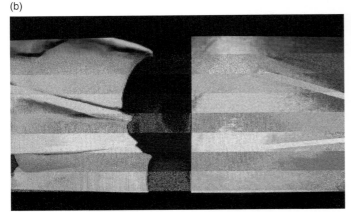

Fig. 21.4. (a), (b) Diagram showing AP (a) and lateral (b) views of the spine to visualize the pedicle and superior and inferior endplates of the fractured vertebral body.

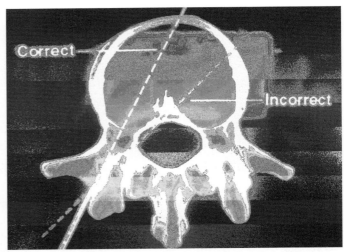

Fig. 21.5. Diagram demonstrating the risk of disruption of the medial wall of the pedicle if the needle is angled too medially.

mL^3 of 1% lidocaine without epinephrine (Abbot Laboratories: Chicago, IL) are injected subcutaneously over the pedicle region of interest.

Transpedicular approach

Transpedicular approach is usually performed for the lumbar and lower thoracic spine due to the presence of pedicles of adequate size. In the middle to upper thoracic spine, extrapedicular approach is usually used due to the presence of narrow pedicles. A 21-gauge spinal needle may be used to localize the center of the pedicle in AP and lateral views of the spine. It is important to visualize the pedicles and the superior and inferior endplates of the fractured vertebral body at the beginning of the procedure (Fig 21.4. (a),(b)). A small stab incision is made with an 11 blade knife just lateral to the lateral aspect of the pedicle identified from the AP view of the spine. Following the trajectory of the spinal needle, an 11-gauge bone biopsy needle is inserted percutaneously through the stab incision and advanced until the tip of the needle is at approximately the 10 o' clock position for the left side of the pedicle and at the 2 o'clock position for the right side of the pedicle. The rest of the procedure is performed under AP and

lateral X-ray fluoroscopic views. The bone biopsy needle is slowly advanced under continuous AP and lateral X-ray fluoroscopic views. The tip of the needle courses from the lateral aspect of the pedicle to the medial aspect of the pedicle on AP view, and is subsequently positioned at the junction of the pedicle and the posterior aspect of the vertebral body on the lateral X-ray. The medial wall of the pedicle may be violated and the bone biopsy needle may enter the spinal canal if the tip of the needle on AP X-ray has reached the medial wall of the pedicle well before it reached the junction of the pedicle and the posterior vertebral body cortex (Fig. 21.5). At this point, the bone biopsy needle can be advanced further, slowly to reach the anterior one-third of the vertebral body. Bone specimen can be taken at this time if indicated. Cement deposition in the anterior aspect of the body is important because the anterior half of the vertebral body sustains the majority of the load. Also, the main venous drainage of the body starts at the mid point of the body in the AP dimension. The AP view should demonstrate that the needle tip is near the midline of the vertebral body. A contrast dye is injected through the bone biopsy needle either with a 10 mL^3 syringe or through a short piece of extension pressure tubing to visualize venous drainage under live fluoroscopy. Digital subtraction angiography is performed to ensure that contrast from the vertebra is not shunting into the inferior vena cava. If such shunting is identified, the needle is withdrawn slightly to see if the shunting disappears. If shunting persists, vertebroplasty at this point can lead to pulmonary embolism. To avoid this complication, the surgeon can either reposition the needle or occlude the fistulous tract with a gelfoam or thickened PMMA cement. If the occlusion of the fistula is successful, the surgeon can proceed with vertebroplasty using the contralateral pedicle access and inject PMMA from the contralateral side. After venography has demonstrated absence of venous outflow into potential embolic tracts, the PMMA can be injected.

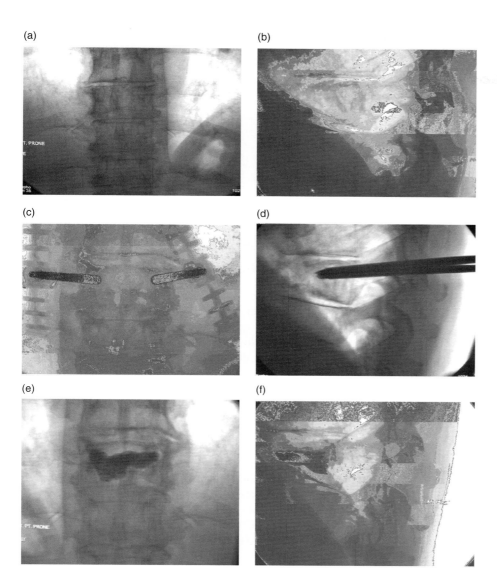

(a)

(b)

(c)

(d)

(e)

(f)

Fig. 21.6. A 53-year-old patient with a history of multiple myeloma presented with symptomatic T9 VCF (a),(b). Vertebroplasty was performed via bilateral pedicular approach with excellent pain relief (c),(d),(e),(f).

The PMMA is prepared by mixing the methylmethacrylate polymer powder and the methylmethacrylate as a monomer. The powder is placed in a $60 \, \text{mL}^3$ syringe and $17 \, \text{mL}^3$ of the powder is placed in two plastic bowls. Three grams of the barium sulfate powder are added to each bowl to opacify the polymer and mixed thoroughly. Subsequently, $7–8 \, \text{mL}^3$ of the liquid monomer are added to the opacified polymer and mixed thoroughly to a consistency of thick paste (e.g., toothpaste). The cement is then poured into a $10 \, \text{mL}^3$ syringe or in the case of Parallax kit, an injector barrel syringe, and injected slowly using continuous AP and lateral fluoroscopic images to ensure that the cement does not leak into the spinal canal or outside of the vertebral body or travel into the inferior vena cava. The injection will be met with resistance when the cement fills the vertebral body. Often, with placement of the needle tip in the midline of the body, the cement will diffuse across the midline into the contralateral side of the vertebral body. The volume of the cement injected depends upon the degree of vertebral compression, the size of the vertebral body, and any unwanted cement leakage. If the initial injection results in deposition of cement unilaterally within the body, a contralateral pedicular access and injection can be performed. Otherwise, unilateral pedicular vertebroplasty may be adequate in providing pain relief. The bilateral pedicular approach for vertebroplasty is illustrated in Fig. 21.6 (a)–(f). Although some patients may receive significant relief of pain with a small volume of cement injection, typically the volume of cement injected may be determined by the size and volume of the fractured vertebral body and the degree of compression and the presence of cement leakage. After satisfactory deposition of the cement, the needle is removed and sterile dressing is applied over the stab wound. The patient is observed in the recovery room for several hours and then allowed to sit and ambulate with assistance if needed. The authors usually observe patients overnight before discharging on oral pain medications as needed. Ambulation, out-patient physical therapy, or rehabilitation is recommended depending on the needs and condition of the patient. Continuation of the daily calcium and Vitamin D supplements and anti-osteoporotic medications is recommended to the patient prior to discharge. No bracing is needed.

Extra-pedicular or posterolateral approach

Thoracic vertebral bodies at about T9 or above or in patients with very small pedicles may preclude the transpedicular approach required for vertebroplasty. For such patients, extra-pedicular or posterolateral approach may be used. The transcutaneous insertion point is about 2 cm lateral to the lateral aspect of the pedicle. The entry point of the bone biopsy needle is superior and lateral to the pedicle just medial to the rib head or through the rib head. As a result, pedicle entry with the needle is just lateral to the site where the pedicle connects to the body.

Complications of vertebroplasty

In general, vertebroplasty is associated with a clinical complication rate of about 1% for patients treated for osteoporotic VCF or vertebral hemangioma and about 5% to 10% for those treated for malignant tumors[8,12–14] (see Table 21.3) Some reports identify a high rate of cement leakage, but most of the leakage reported is not clinically significant. However, cement leakage near a nerve root may result in acute radiculopathy which has been reported with an incidence as high as 5% in some case series.[15,16] A short course of steroids is recommended in these patients. Cement leakage may be more common in cases of malignant tumors because of higher frequency of underlying vertebral cortex destruction.

Outcome of vertebroplasty

A review of the literature suggests that vertebroplasty is a highly effective procedure for osteoporotic VCF and malignant VCF. The majority of patients (90%–95%) report pain relief following vertebroplasty. However, there are very few large series published to date. In addition, many of these studies lack reliable outcome instruments such as visual analog scales, disease-specific outcomes questionnaires, or quality of life global outcomes scales. Many studies used verbal response to pain scale with a follow-up period no longer than 24 hours. Layton *et al.* reported the short-term (2 hour) and long-term (2 years) outcome of vertebroplasty performed on 1000 patients with osteoporotic and malignancy-related VCFs.[17] Evaluation at each follow-up time point included pain response (subjective and visual analog pain score), change in mobility, change in pain medication utilization, and modified Roland–Morris Disability Questionnaire. Statistical analysis was performed on the pain response and change in the Roland–Morris score at each follow-up time point. They reported an immediate improvement in the degree of pain after vertebroplasty even at the 2-hour post-procedure

Table 21.3. Complications associated with vertebroplasty

1. Radiculopathy (5%)
2. Cement leakage (as high as 30% to 70%)
3. Fracture of the rib
4. Fracture of the pedicle
5. Pneumothorax
6. Spinal cord compression
7. Transient cerebrospinal fluid leak
8. Infection
9. Pulmonary emboli
10. Cerebral infarction from right-to-left shunt
11. Death (1/50,000 cases) secondary to allergic reaction

follow-up evaluation. This improvement in pain continued for all follow-up time points up to 2 years and was accompanied by a similar improvement in spine-related disability, mobility, and pain medication usage. They reported a complication rate of 1.8%; the majority of complications consisted of rib fracture from lying in the prone position. Although a 25% rate of cement leakage was observed during the procedure, only a 0.45% rate of clinically significant cement leakage was encountered (one patient developed pulmonary embolus and two patients developed radiculopathy).

The New England Journal of Medicine recently published two separate randomized prospective studies that failed to demonstrate any significant benefit of vertebroplasty over simulated or sham procedure in patients with painful osteoporotic vertebral compression fractures. However, these studies have significant potential pitfalls in the inclusion criteria that could have affected their outcome. The authors believe that each patient with osteoporotic compression fractures needs to be evaluated in detail in terms of the age of the fracture, concomitant spinal disease or fracture, timing of intervention, and technique of intervention. The results of these two studies are in direct contrast to the experience of the authors who have a combined experience of performing over 1000 cases of vertebroplasty and kyphoplasty. A brief overview of these two studies will be mentioned here.

The first study is a multicenter, randomized, double-blind, placebo-controlled trial from Australia that evaluated the short-term efficacy and safety of vertebroplasty over a sham procedure in reducing pain and improving physical function in patients with one or two painful osteoporotic vertebral compression fractures.[18] In this study, Buchbinder *et al.* evaluated 71 patients (35 of 38 in the vertebroplasty group and 36 of 40 in the sham procedure group) with one or two painful osteoporotic vertebral compression fractures of less than 12 months duration in symptoms. The median period of back pain due to the osteoporotic vertebral compression fractures was 9 weeks in the vertebroplasty group and 9.5 weeks in the sham procedure group. The investigators evaluated the patients with the use of mailed questionnaires at 1 week and 1, 3, and 6 months after the procedure. The primary outcome of the study was the overall pain as measured on a scale of 0 to 10 (with 0 being no pain and 10 being maximum imaginable pain, and 1.5 being the minimal clinically important difference). Secondary outcomes included quality of life, as measured with the use of the Quality of Life Questionnaire of the European Foundation for Osteoporosis (QUALEFFO), the Assessment of Quality of Life (AQoL) questionnaire, and the European Quality of Life-5 Dimensions (EQ-5D) scale, and Roland-Morris Disability Questionnaire (RDQ). Of 468 potential participants, 78 met the inclusion criteria and 71 completed the study at 6 months. The study found no significant differences between the vertebroplasty treated group and the sham procedure group in the primary outcome of overall pain at 3 months. Also, the study found no significant difference between the two groups in any other outcome, except for the total QUALEFFO score at 1 week, which favored the placebo group. The investigators admit that selection bias cannot be ruled out due to the fact that 30% of potentially eligible patients declined to participate in the study. The mean volume of cement injected into the vertebral body was 2.8 ± 1.2 mL. It is not clear whether there was any relationship between the volume of the cement injected and outcome. The volume of cement injected may be relevant as many of the physicians performing vertebroplasty or kyphoplasty report injection of cement in the range of 4 to 9 mL per level especially in the lumbar vertebral bodies that are larger in volume than the middle to upper thoracic vertebral bodies. There is no mention of how well the cement deposition had penetrated the fractured vertebral body on post-operative X-rays. It is not clear if there were any other factors such as degenerative disc herniation, spondylolisthesis, or concomitant facet fracture that could have accounted for back pain in addition to the vertebral compression fracture. There is no mention of the length of hospital stay or duration of bed dependency after the procedures. There is no mention of any medical complications such as systemic infections or deep vein thrombosis in patients that did not receive vertebroplasty and may have remained bed ridden for a prolonged period of time. We believe that these issues need to be evaluated in future randomized studies.

In the second randomized, controlled prospective trial, called the Investigational Vertebroplasty Efficacy and Safety Trial (INVEST), performed at five centers in the USA, five centers in the UK, and 1 center in Australia, Kallmes et al. evaluated the efficacy of vertebroplasty over a sham procedure in patients with painful osteoporotic vertebral compression fractures, ranging from one to three levels.[19] Of 131 patients evaluated in the study, 68 patients underwent vertebroplasty and 63 patients underwent a sham procedure. The main goal of this study was to test the hypothesis that patients with painful osteoporotic vertebral compression fractures who undergo vertebroplasty have a lower rate of disability and pain at 1 month. The control group underwent placement of local anesthesia near the fracture, without placement of cement. The study used modified Roland-Morris Disability (RDQ) and patient's ratings of average pain intensity during the preceding 24 hours at one month. Patients were allowed to cross over to the other study group after 1 month. The study reported that both groups had immediate improvement in disability and pain scores after the intervention. The two groups did not differ significantly on any secondary outcome measure at one month, but there was a trend toward a higher rate of clinically meaningful improvement in pain in the vertebroplasty group. The study concluded that there was no significant difference in the improvement in pain and in pain-related disability associated with osteoporotic compression fractures treated with vertebroplasty. However, the investigators acknowledge that the study had several limitations. First, the patients were allowed to cross over at 1 month because both physicians and patients did not wish to accept a longer period. The control group may have had other medical treatment that may have affected their outcome. There may have been other causes of back pain in addition to vertebral compression fracture. Over 36% of patients who had vertebroplasty had symptoms of back pain for longer than 6 months. The authors emphasize that some vertebral compression fractures may not respond to vertebroplasty at this very late stage of healing. The amount of cement injected into the fractured verterbrae is not mentioned in the study. Results of post-operative X-rays are not well mentioned in the study. Again, the length of hospital stay after either procedure and any medical complications of prolonged bed rest or bed dependency in the control group are not mentioned.

These two randomized studies have raised several important issues that may need to be addressed in future studies. There must be some information as to what is the cause of back pain in patients who did not receive significant relief of pain after the vertebroplasty procedure. This understanding of cause and effect or lack thereof may shed light on which specific population of patients with osteoporotic compression fractures may benefit from the vertebroplasty versus conservative medical management. Specifically, the age of the compression fracture, number of vertebral fractures treated per session, the amount of cement injected, and review of post-operative imaging to assess the result of the cement deposition and adjacent spinal anatomy may be important in understanding which of these osteoporotic vertebral compression fractures may benefit the most from vertebroplasty or kyphoplasty. Also of importance in a future study would be to compare the length of hospital stay and the medical complications between the vertebroplasty- or kyphoplasty- treated group versus the medically managed or control group as those factors have an impact on the cost of health care.

Technique of kyphoplasty

The main goals of kyphoplasty are to restore the vertebral height, reduce the kyphotic deformity and improve the safety of PMMA injection. Whether these goals actually result in better clinical outcome compared with vertebroplasty in terms of safety and efficacy may not be conclusively demonstrated without a randomized trial. The proponents of kyphoplasty emphasize that vertebroplasty makes no attempt to restore the vertebral height or correct kyphotic deformity and is associated with higher incidence of cement leakage. However, some series report that vertebroplasty in some cases can augment the vertebral body height. It remains unclear whether the location of the cement leakage is more relevant for the occurrence of clinically significant complications rather than the overall incidence of the cement leakage. More studies are needed to assess the long-term clinical consequences of reduction of kyphotic deformity and restoration of vertebral height.

Transpedicular approach

Pre-operative preparation is very similar to that needed for vertebroplasty. The authors usually perform bilateral pedicular access. However, in cases where a unilateral pedicle fracture exists, a unilateral pedicular approach for kyphoplasty contralateral to the fractured pedicle can be performed with good radiographic and clinical results. The authors prefer to perform the procedure in a bi-plane angiography suite under general anesthesia. A pillow or gel rolls are placed along the chest and across the pelvis. The back is prepped and draped in sterile fashion. The KyphX system or kit (Kyphon Inc.; Sunnyvale, CA) provides all of the tools necessary for the procedure (Fig. 21.7 (a)-(o)). Local anesthetic (1% lidocaine without epinephrine) is injected subcutaneously over the pedicle area of interest. On AP view, the pedicles must be well visualized and cranial or caudal angulations may be needed for optimal imaging. On lateral view, the superior and inferior endplates must be linear and not be seen in oblique alignment. A 21-gauge spinal needle may be used to localize the center of the pedicle in AP and lateral views of the spine. When performing a transpedicular approach (typically in the lumbar spine), a small stab incision is made with an 11 blade knife about 1 cm lateral to the lateral aspect of the pedicle seen from the AP view of the spine. Following the trajectory of the spinal needle, an 11-gauge Jamshidi needle is inserted percutaneously through the stab incision and advanced until the tip of the needle is at approximately the 10 o'clock position for the left side of the pedicle and at 2 o'clock position for the right side of the pedicle (Fig. 21.8 (a), (b)). The rest of the procedure is performed using continuous AP and lateral fluorscopic images. The Jamshidi needle is slowly advanced under AP and lateral X-ray fluoroscopy to ensure that the tip of the needle coursing from the lateral aspect of the pedicle to the medial aspect of the pedicle on AP view is concurrently placed at the junction of the pedicle and the posterior aspect of the vertebral body on the lateral views.

The medial wall of the pedicle and the spinal canal may be inadvertently entered by the Jamshidi needle if the tip of the needle on AP view has reached the medial wall of the pedicle well before it has reached the junction of the pedicle and the posterior vertebral body cortex. At this point, the Jamishidi needle can be advanced further until it reaches the posterior two-thirds of the vertebral body. The stylet is removed and a blunt guide pin is inserted through the Jamshidi needle to the anterior one-third of the vertebral body with subsequent removal of the Jamshidi needle (Fig. 21.8 (c), (d)). An osteointroducer is inserted over the guide pin until it reaches about one-third of the posterior vertebral body and the guide pin is subsequently removed (Fig. 21.8 (e), (f)). A biopsy needle can be inserted into the osteointroducer at this time and advanced until it reaches about 1 cm from the anterior wall of the vertebral body if a biopsy specimen is needed. Sometimes, no bone specimen is collected from the biopsy needle as it is aspirated with a $10\,mL^3$ syringe. Subsequently, a manual drill can be used to obtain a bone specimen. The drill is advanced through the osteointroducer to create a channel near the anterior wall of the vertebral body (Fig. 21.8 (g), (h)). The drill is removed and the bone fragments from the tip of the drill sent for pathological examination.

After removing the drill, an appropriate length of balloon tamp (10 mm to 20 mm length) is inserted into the introducer and advanced until it reaches the anterior wall of the vertebral body or the endplate depression area but remains about 1cm or greater away from the posterior cortex of the body (Fig. 21.8 (i), (j)). The radiopaque markers of the balloon must be outside the osteointroducer and be visible on AP and lateral images before the balloon is inflated. When both pedicles are accessed, the same procedure is performed via the contralateral pedicle (Fig. 21.8 (k)-(r)). Once both balloons are satisfactorily placed into the vertebral body, they are simultaneously inflated under fluoroscopy (to a pressure of usually no more than 220 psi) until the vertebral body height is restored or improved.

The PMMA cement is prepared while the balloons remain inflated in the body. The volume of the balloon is a good estimate of the amount of cement that will be needed to fill the void created by the balloon. The cement is loaded into a syringe and subsequently injected into multiple $1.5\,mL^3$ cannulas. When the cement has reached a thick paste consistency (e.g., toothpaste), the balloons are deflated and removed from the osteointroducer. The cement-filled cannula is inserted into the osteointroducer and observed under live fluoroscopy until the tip of the cannula reaches the anterior third of the vertebral body. Subsequently, a stylet is used to push the cement out of the cannula into the vertebral body usually alternating from one side of the pedicle to the other until the cement has filled approximately two-thirds of the posterior cortex of the body. The stylet and the cannula are used together to push anteriorly any cement coming back towards the pedicle followed by removal of the osteointroducer from both pedicles (Fig. 21.8 (s), (t)).

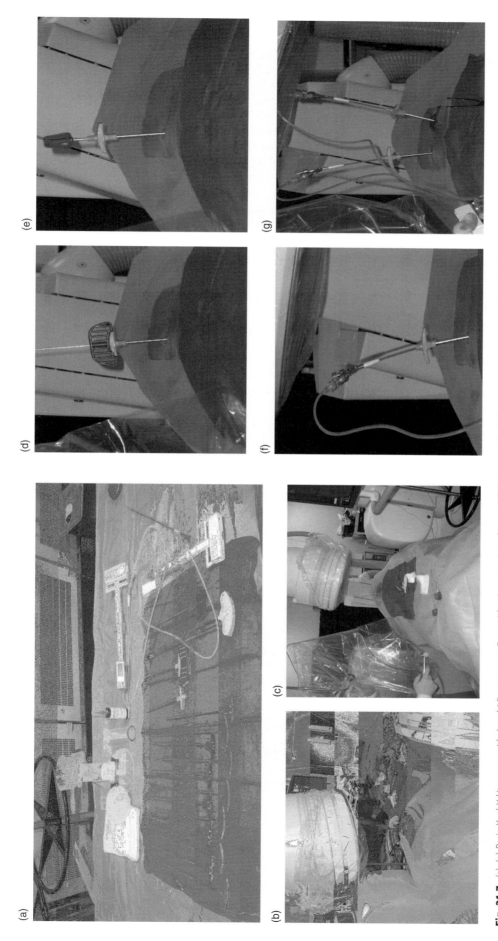

Fig. 21.7. (a)–(o) Basic KyphX kit comes with Jamshidi access needles, guide pins, osteointroducers, drill, biopsy needle, balloon tamps, cement cannulas and stylets, and PMMA bone cement (a). Basic steps of kyphoplasty include insertion of a Jamshidi needle (b) followed by placement of a guide pin through the Jamshidi needle (c), followed by removal of Jamshidi needle and placement of osteointroducer over the guide pin (d) followed by removal of guide pin and placement of either biopsy needle if indicated or manual drill (e) followed by insertion of a balloon tamp (f). The procedure can be repeated on the contra-lateral side of the pedicle if bilateral pedicle access is performed (g). While the balloons are inflated, the cement is prepared (h) and then inserted into cannulas (i) which are then inserted into the osteointroducers and into the anterior portion of the vertebral body (j),(k). The stylet is used to push the cement out of the cannula into the vertebral body (l),(m). New directional balloon tamps (n) and osteointroducers are also available if needed (o).

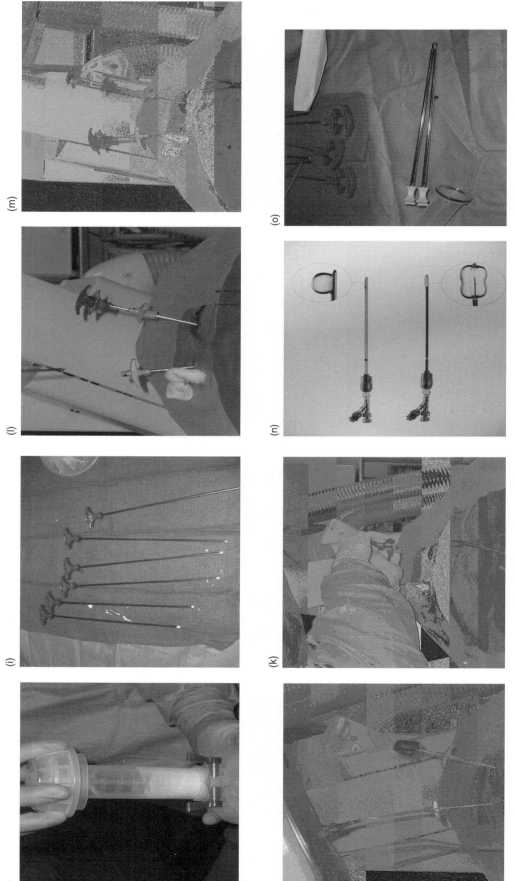

Fig. 21.7. (cont.)

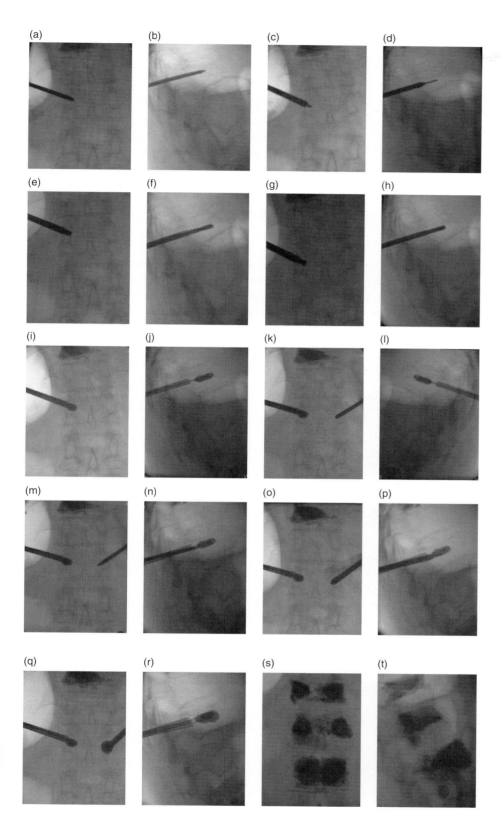

Fig. 21.8. (a)–(t) Thoracic T12 and Lumbar L1 and L2 kyphoplasty in a 53-year-old woman with a history of multiple myeloma. Step-by-step use of the instruments is illustrated.

When treating multiple levels, the balloons can be left in the osteointroducers until the cement is ready. Subsequently, the balloons are deflated and removed stepwise from each level and the cement can be deposited one level at a time to conserve time (Fig. 21.9 (a)–(j)). The stab incision on the back may be closed with 3-o nylon sutures. The patient is extubated and taken to the recovery room for a few hours and then observed overnight prior to discharge. No bracing is needed.

Extra-pedicular approach

Thoracic vertebra bodies from T9 and above have narrow and laterally directed pedicles, which make transpedicular approach difficult and often lead to suboptimal placement of the osteointroducer and balloon tamp. Therefore, an extra-pedicular approach is recommended. A small stab incision is made with an 11 blade knife about 2 cm lateral to the lateral aspect of the pedicle. The transcutaneous entry point of the Jamshidi needle is superior and lateral to the pedicle just medial to the rib head or even through the rib head. The pedicle is traversed just lateral to where the pedicle connects to the body. Care is required because an excessively lateral entry point can lead to pneumothorax and an excessively inferior entry point can result in segmental artery laceration.

New direction in fracture reduction

The KyphX Elevate inflatable balloon tamp (IBT) is an advanced balloon designed to provide single-plane preferential inflation resulting in a 50% greater superior/inferior profile comparison with the medial/lateral profile. These balloons are modifications of the original balloon tamp (Fig. 21.10).

Complications of kyphoplasty

In general, the rate of cement leakage is lower than that reported in case series of vertebroplasty. Prospective multi-center series reported 1.1% major complications with kyphoplasty.[20] Lieberman et al. reported a cement leak rate of 8.6% during kyphoplasty.[21] Similar to cases with vertebroplasty, the vast majority of cement leakages during kyphoplasty were asymptomatic. Other rare complications are listed in Table 21.4.

(a)

(b)

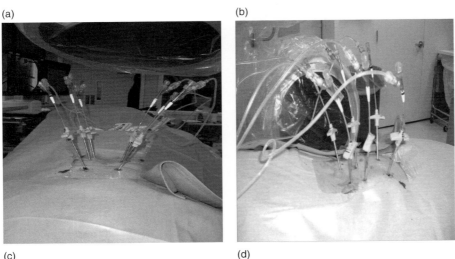

Fig. 21.9. A three-level kyphoplasty is performed where the balloon tamps are inflated sequentially (a),(b),(c),(d) while the cement is being prepared. Then, the balloons are removed and the cement containing cannulas are inserted into the osteointroducers sequentially (e)–(j).

(c)

(d)

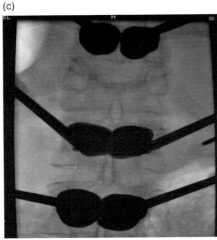
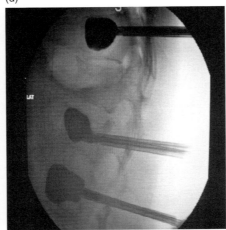

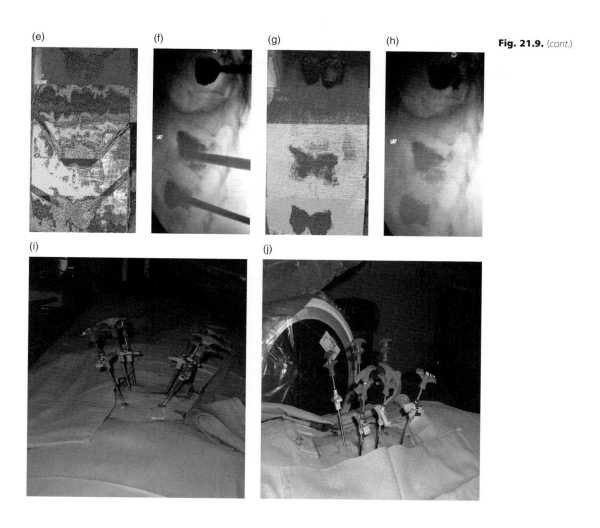

Fig. 21.9. (*cont.*)

Fig. 21.10. KyphX Elevate IBT.

Table 21.4. Complications associated with vertebroplasty

1. Cement leakage (8.6%)
2. Fracture of the rib
3. Pneumothorax
4. Spinal cord compression
5. Transient cerebrospinal fluid leak
6. Infection
7. Pulmonary emboli
8. Death (1/50 000 cases) secondary to allergic reaction

Outcome of kyphoplasty

Review of reports assessing the clinical outcome of kyphoplasty suggests that similar limitations exist as with vertebroplasty. The small number of patients and the mean length of follow-up of less than 2 years limits most studies. No randomized study has been performed to compare the results of kyphoplasty with those observed with conservative medical treatment. There are several recent studies demonstrating promising short-term clinical results. The high success rate of pain relief associated with this procedure makes randomization challenging. Grafe et al. reported greater improvement in pain and reduction of occurrence of new VCF at 12-month follow-up in the kyphoplasty treated group with chronic VCF (1 year or greater) compared with an unmatched medically treated patients.[22] Ledlie et al. reported the results of a retrospective study involving 65 patients treated with kyphoplasty for VCF related to osteoporosis or multiple myeloma or other malignancy at a single center with a 2-year follow-up.[23] This study showed that kyphoplasty significantly improved pain and function and resulted in significant vertebral height restoration that remained stable for at least 2 years following treatment. In this study, 9% of patients had a new fracture during 2 year follow-up. Garfin et al. reported the results of a prospective, multicenter, practice-based study of kyphoplasty in 100 patients with VCF resulting from osteoporosis, multiple myeloma, or malignancy. Kyphoplasty resulted in significant improvement in pain, and functional and mental health outcomes at one month after kyphoplasty and sustained at 24 months.[24] In this study, at least 10% of the vertebral height was restored in 82% of the fractures and the average mid-vertebral body height loss restored by 32%. Long-term follow-up studies using appropriate outcome measures will further strengthen the conclusions about the durability and efficacy of kyphoplasty.

Case 1: Kyphoplasty for lumbar L3 osteoporotic burst fracture

Clinical information

This patient was a 43-year-old volleyball coach who presented to the emergency department after falling backwards and landing on her buttocks, while playing volleyball. She experienced low back pain without neurological deficits and underwent a CT of the lumbar spine, which revealed a lumbar L3 burst fracture (Fig. 21.11 (a), (b)). MRI of the lumbar spine showed 30–50% loss of height centrally with an epidural hemorrhage extending anteriorly from L1 to L5-S1, most pronounced at the L3 vertebral body (Fig. 21.11 (c), (d)). The combination of the retropulsion of the posterior superior aspect and the ventral epidural hemorrhage resulted in canal stenosis with the canal measuring approximately 6–7 mm in maximal AP dimension. The canal measured 15–18 mm in the L1–2 level. Slight edema extended into the pedicles without a fracture line. She had a history of breast cancer, osteoporosis, and recent administration of chemotherapy for breast cancer. She was not a good candidate for a major procedure such as spinal vertebrectomy and fusion. Therefore L3 kyphoplasty was performed (Fig. 21.11 (e)–(n)). One day after kyphoplasty, MRI of the lumbar spine showed improved

appearance of the L3 compression fracture and resolving epidural hemorrhage and spinal canal stenosis (Fig. 21.11 (o)–(r)). She was subsequently seen by physical and occupational therapy and was able to ambulate without difficulty. She was discharged 3 days after her kyphoplasty and resumed working as a teacher 6 weeks after the fracture with complete relief of her back pain. This case illustrates that with good placement of the osteointroducer and careful slow injection of the cement, excellent clinical and radiographic result can be achieved.

Case 2: Kyphoplasty for complex thoracic T9-L1 osteoporotic VCF

Clinical information

An 86-year-old man with a history of osteoporosis and pacemaker placement presented with a 3-month history of gradual decline in activity due to severe thoracic back pain. At initial evaluation, he was wheelchair dependent, requiring regular narcotic pain medication without any urinary or bowel incontinence. He had developed depression due to decreased mobility and pain. He underwent a bone scan and a CT scan of the thoracic and lumbar spine that revealed acute vertebral fractures involving the vertebral bodies from T9 to L1. The superior endplate of the T10 vertebral body had displaced into the inferior endplate of T9 (Fig. 21.12 (a), (b)). The posterior cortex of T10 and T9 were intact. There was retropulsion of the T10 vertebral body into the spinal canal. The patient was considered at high risk for complications associated with major thoracotomy and anterior thoracic multi-level reconstruction. Due to severe osteoporosis, he was felt to be a poor candidate for posterior instrumentation and fusion. Kyphoplasty was performed at the T9 and T10 levels followed by T11, T12, and L1 using a 15 mm balloon tamp (Fig. 21.12 (c), (d)). The balloons were placed near the anterior portion of the bodies to prevent leakage into the spinal canal. The patient tolerated the procedure well and post-operative CT scan of the thoracic spine demonstrated penetration of the cement through the superior endplate of T10 into the inferior endplate of T9 connecting the two vertebral bodies (Fig. 21.12 (e), (f), (g), (h)). The patient had significant relief of back pain and was transferred to rehabilitation with the ability to walk with assistance on post-operative day 2.

Conclusion

Vertebroplasty and kyphoplasty are minimally invasive procedures with low complication rates and a very high success rate for relieving pain associated with VCF, particularly in patients with osteoporotic VCF. The potential advantage of kyphoplasty over vertebroplasty is that kyphoplasty can restore some or a significant amount of vertebral height and reduce kyphotic deformity of the spine to a greater extent. Whether these differences result in significantly better long-term clinical or radiological outcomes requires further follow-up studies.

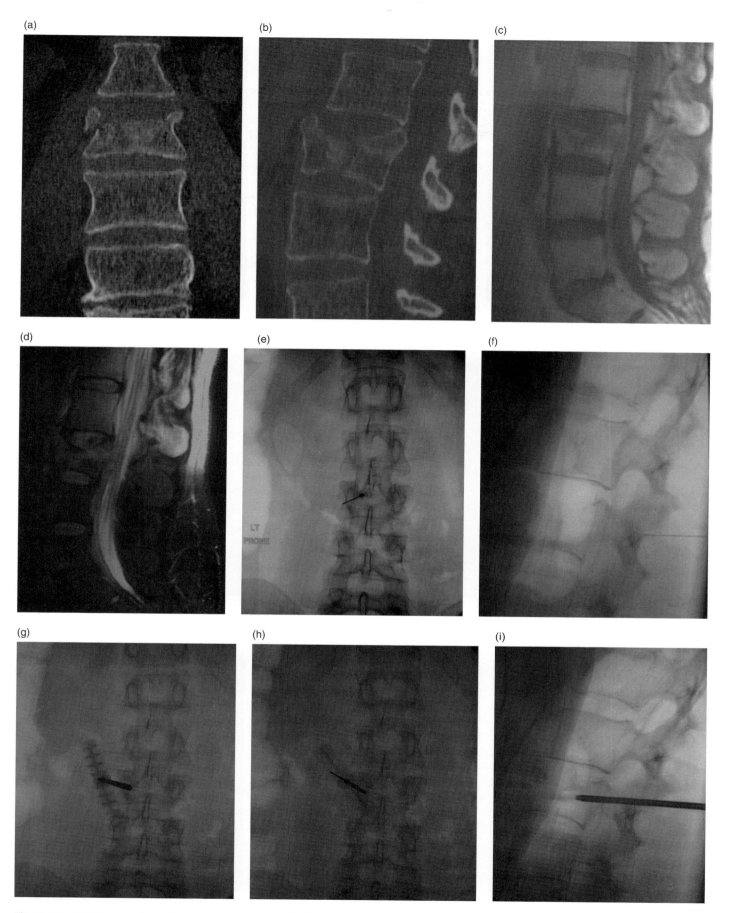

Fig. 21.11. (a)–(r) Pre-operative and post-operative imaging of lumbar L3 burst fracture with retropulsion.

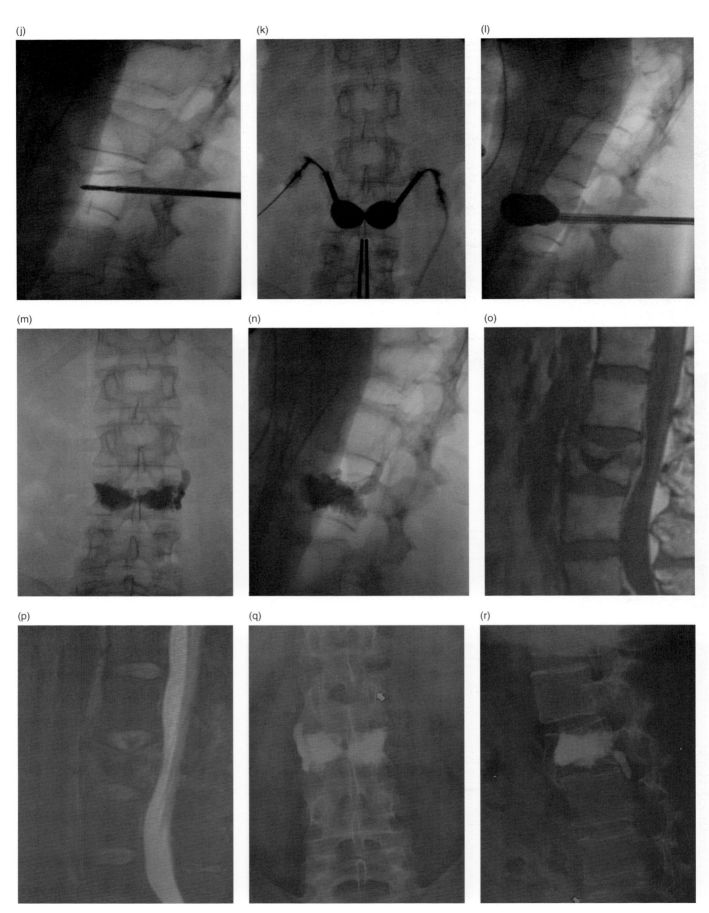

Fig. 21.11. (cont.)

(a)

(b)

(c)

(d)

(e)

(f)

(g)

(h)

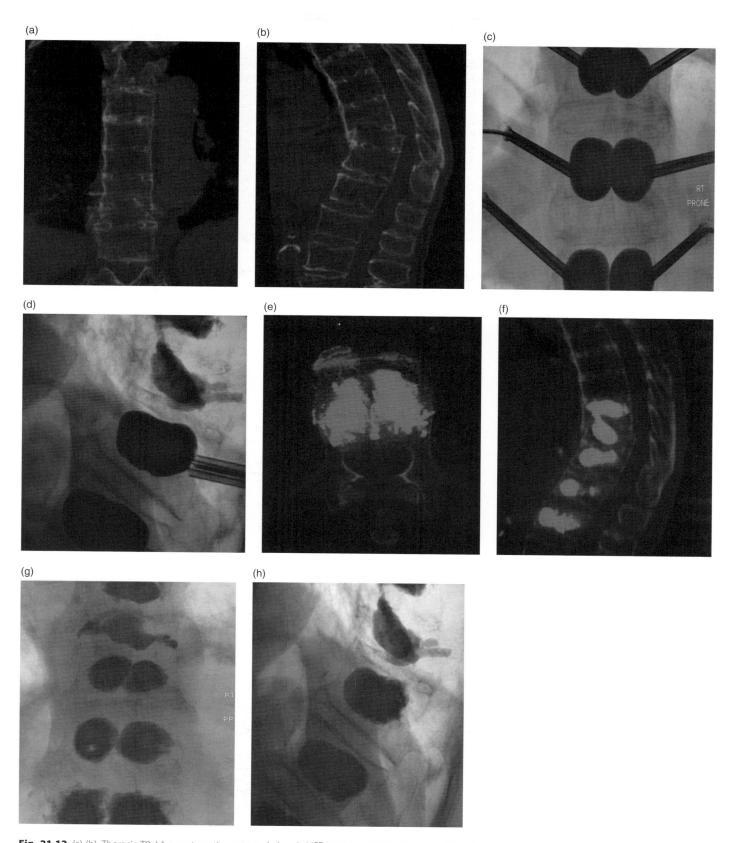

Fig. 21.12 (a)-(h). Thoracic T9–L1 symptomatic acute and chronic VCF in an osteoporotic 86-year-old-male.

From an economical standpoint, kyphoplasty costs about $3400 without bone cement compared with vertebroplasty that costs about $400 with the bone cement. Patients with complex VCFs such as burst fractures warrant extreme caution and experience on the part of the performing physician regardless of the procedure selected. Further modifications in the bone cement material and the cement delivery system may allow these procedures to be more effective in the future.

References

1. Galibert P, Deramond H, Rosat P, Le Gars D. [Preliminary note on the treatment of vertebral angioma by percutaneous acrylic vertebroplasty]. *Neurochirurgie* 1987;**33**:166–8.

2. Bascoulergue YDJ, Leclercq R, *et al.* (abstract). Percutaneous injection of methyl methacrylate for the treatment of various diseases: percutaneous vertebroplasty. *Radiology* 1988; **169P**:372.

3. Jensen ME, Evans AJ, Mathis JM, Kallmes DF, Cloft HJ, Dion JE. Percutaneous polymethylmethacrylate vertebroplasty in the treatment of osteoporotic vertebral body compression fractures: technical aspects. *Am J Neuroradiol* 1997; **18**:1897–904.

4. Taylor RS, Fritzell P, Taylor RJ. Balloon kyphoplasty in the management of vertebral compression fractures: an updated systematic review and meta-analysis. *Eur Spine J* 2007;**16**:1085–100.

5. Taylor RS, Taylor RJ, Fritzell P. Balloon kyphoplasty and vertebroplasty for vertebral compression fractures: a comparative systematic review of efficacy and safety. *Spine* 2006;**31**:2747–55.

6. Barr JD, Barr MS, Lemley TJ, McCann RM. Percutaneous vertebroplasty for pain relief and spinal stabilization. *Spine* 2000;**25**:923–8.

7. Cortet B, Cotten A, Boutry N, *et al.* Percutaneous vertebroplasty in the treatment of osteoporotic vertebral compression fractures: an open prospective study. *J Rheumatol* 1999;**26**:2222–8.

8. Deramond H, Depriester C, Galibert P, Le Gars D. Percutaneous vertebroplasty with polymethylmethacrylate. Technique, indications, and results. *Radiol Clin North Am* 1998;**36**: 533–46.

9. Garfin SRYH, Lieberman IH, *et al.* Early results of 300 kyphoplasties for the treatment of painful vertebral body compression fractures. In: *Proceedings AAOS annual meeting; 2001*; San Francisco; 2001.

10. Kaufmann TJ, Jensen ME, Schweickert PA, Marx WF, Kallmes DF. Age of fracture and clinical outcomes of percutaneous vertebroplasty. *Am J Neuroradiol* 2001;**22**:1860–3.

11. Alvarez L, Perez-Higueras A, Granizo JJ, de Miguel I, Quinones D, Rossi RE. Predictors of outcomes of percutaneous vertebroplasty for osteoporotic vertebral fractures. *Spine* 2005;**30**:87–92.

12. Cortet B, Houvenagel E, Puisieux F, Roches E, Garnier P, Delcambre B. Spinal curvatures and quality of life in women with vertebral fractures secondary to osteoporosis. *Spine* 1999;**24**:1921–5.

13. Cyteval C, Sarrabere MP, Roux JO, *et al.* Acute osteoporotic vertebral collapse: open study on percutaneous injection of acrylic surgical cement in 20 patients. *Am J Roentgenol* 1999;**173**:1685–90.

14. Deramond H. DC, Galibert P, Le Gars D. Percutaneous vertebroplasty with polymethylmethacrylate: Techniques, indications, and results. *Radiol Clin North Am* 1998;**117** (supplement) 352.

15. Chiras J, Depriester C, Weill A, Sola-Martinez MT, Deramond H [Percutaneous vertebral surgery. Technics and indications]. *J Neuroradiol* 1997;**24**:45–59.

16. Lee BJ, Lee SR, Yoo TY. Paraplegia as a complication of percutaneous vertebroplasty with polymethylmethacrylate: a case report. *Spine* 2002;**27**:E419–22.

17. Layton KF, Thielen KR, Koch CA, *et al.* Vertebroplasty, first 1000 levels of a single center: evaluation of the outcomes and complications. *AJNR Am J Neuroradiol* 2007;**28**:683–9.

18. Buchbinder R, Osborne RH, Ebeling PR, *et al.* A Randomized trial of vertebroplasty for painful osteoporotic vertebral fractures. *N Engl J Med.* 2009;**6**:557–68.

19. Kallmes DF, Cornstock BA, Heagerty PJ, *et al.* A randomized trial of vertebroplasty for osteoporotic spnal fractures. *N Engl J Med* 2009; **361**(6):569–79.

20. Lane JM, Girard F, Parvaianen H, *et al.* Preliminary outcomes of the first 226 consecutive kyphoplasties for the fixation of painful osteoporotic vertebral compression fractures (abstract). *Osteoporotsis Int (Suppl)* 2000; **11**:S206.

21. Lieberman IH, Dudeney S, Reinhardt MK, Bell G. Initial outcome and efficacy of "kyphoplasty" in the treatment of painful osteoporotic vertebral compression fractures. *Spine* 2001;**26**:1631–8.

22. Grafe IA, Da Fonseca K, Hillmeier J, *et al.* Reduction of pain and fracture incidence after kyphoplasty: 1-year outcomes of a prospective controlled trial of patients with primary osteoporosis. *Osteoporos Int* 2005;**16**:2005–12.

23. Ledlie JT, Renfro MB. Kyphoplasty treatment of vertebral fractures: 2-year outcomes show sustained benefits. *Spine* 2006;**31**: 57–64.

24. Garfin SR, Buckley RA, Ledlie J. Balloon kyphoplasty for symptomatic vertebral body compression fractures results in rapid, significant, and sustained improvements in back pain, function, and quality of life for elderly patients. *Spine* 2006;**31**: 2213–20.

Chapter 22

Clinical endovascular trials in stroke

Haitham M. Hussein and Adnan I. Qureshi

Introduction

Clinical trials evaluating endovascular interventions for the treatment of cerebrovascular diseases require the active involvement of a multidisciplinary team of physicians (vascular neurologists, interventionalists, and neuro intensivists) as well as statisticians. The involvement includes planning of the trial, recruitment of study patients, performance of the intervention, and assessment of clinical outcomes. It is essential that all groups understand each component of the clinical trial and its effect on the results of the trial. This chapter aims to describe and to highlight the importance of each component, through a summary of the design and methodological components of clinical trials that have influenced the practice of endovascular management of ischemic stroke in the past decade.

Endovascualr intervention in ischemic stroke can be categorized into two major groups: (a) acute management which deals with intra-arterial (IA) mechanical and/or pharmacological thrombolysis, and (b) primary or secondary prevention through revascularization of cervical or intracranial vessels. From the former group, we will present the Prolyse in Acute Cerebral Thromboembolism (PROACT) II study,[1] The Interventional Management of Stroke II (IMS II) study,[2,3] and the The Interventional Management of Stroke III (IMS III) study.[4,5] From the latter group, we will present the Carotid Revascularization Endarterectomy vs. Stenting Trial (CREST),[6-12] the Endarterectomy vs. Angioplasty in Patients with Symptomatic Severe Carotid Stenosis (EVA-3S) study,[13] the Stenting and Angioplasty with Protection in Patients at High Risk for Endarterectomy (SAPPHIRE) study,[14] and the Stent-Protected Angioplasty vs. Carotid Endarterectomy in Symptomatic Patients (SPACE) study.[15]

Definition of a clinical trial

Friedman et al.[16] defined a clinical trial as a prospective study comparing the effect and value of an intervention vs. a control treatment among human subjects. In this definition, the term intervention is used in the broadest sense, to include prophylactic, diagnostic, and therapeutic agents, device regimens, and procedures. Hobson[16] defined a clinical trial as a carefully and ethically designed experiment with the aim of answering some precisely framed question.

Table 22.1. Clinical trial criteria

Criterion	Question
Feasibility	Can the proposed intervention be performed?
Efficacy	Can it work?
Safety	Are the risks acceptable?

When is a clinical trial justified?

Certain criteria must be fulfilled before study of an intervention in a large clinical study, to avoid costly evaluations of interventions with little potential for development into meaningful therapy. The criteria provided in Table 22.1 were adapted from those proposed by Schwartz.[17] A Phase III clinical trial is conducted to provide information regarding safety and efficacy, i.e., a net benefit under ideal circumstances (Level 1 evidence).[17] In addition, Schwartz states, "The market is now requiring that in addition to being safe and efficacious, interventions also must be demonstrated to be both effective, i.e., to provide benefit under routine circumstances, and efficient, i.e., the benefit obtained is worth the cost."[17] Clinical health economics examine the efficiency and value of a therapy. Are the health benefits derived worth the monetary costs?

Not all procedures should be evaluated in randomized trials;[18] other criteria that must be considered are equipoise and timing. Clinical equipoise is defined by Freedman[19] as a state of genuine uncertainty within the expert medical community, not necessarily on the part of the individual investigator, about the preferred treatment. For example, a state of equipoise does not exist for treatment with intravenous (IV) recombinant tissue plasminogen activator (rt-PA) vs. no treatment for patients presenting with acute ischemic stroke within 3 hours of symptom onset (if they fulfill inclusion/exclusion

Textbook of Interventional Neurology, ed. Adnan I. Qureshi. Published by Cambridge University Press. © Cambridge University Press 2011.

criteria). This is based on the National Institute of Neurological Disorders and Stroke (NINDS) study, which showed that favorable outcomes (defined as a global odds ratio of complete or nearly complete neurological recovery at 3 months) were achieved in 31% to 50% of patients treated with rt-PA, as compared with 20% to 38% of patients given placebo. The benefit was similar 1 year after stroke.[20] Therefore, it is unethical to deprive such patients of a beneficial treatment, even in the context of a clinical trial. On the other hand, a state of equipoise dose exist when IV thrombolysis is compared to IV plus IA thrombolysis. This equipoise was the basis for initiation of the IMS trials.

When new technology is introduced, an effort must be made not to compare it with a standard form of therapy too soon after the development of the new technology. Inappropriate timing was demonstrated in a 1996 randomized trial comparing carotid artery angioplasty and stent placement (CAS) with carotid endarterectomy (CEA);[21] the trial was prematurely stopped because of the unacceptable risk associated with the endovascular procedure. The safety and feasibility of the procedure involving the new technology, as well as some evidence of effectiveness, should first be demonstrated in case series with large numbers of patients. In addition, expertise in performing the procedure must exist at multiple institutions. In time, interventionalists gained more experience in the procedure, and more specific subsets of patients who might benefit from CAS were identified. Several case series and registries were published indicating the potential benefits of CAS, as well as its comparable risks to CEA. By the early 2000s, several randomized trials were initiated comparing CAS to CEA, each with its specific qualification requirements for interventionalists to ensure their familiarity with the procedure.

Phases of a clinical trial

Pharmaceutical clinical trials are conducted in phases.[22,23,24] Surgical intervention and medical device trials often adopt the drug trial lexicon. Each clinical trial phase has a different purpose and helps scientists answer different questions. In Phase I studies, the goal is to determine the safety, dose range, and adverse side effects of a new drug or treatment among a small group of subjects ($n = 15$–30). No control group is required, but randomization may be used for different dose ranges. Healthy individuals are often the subjects in these trials. In Phase II studies, the goals are to determine effectiveness and to perform a more detailed evaluation of the safety of a new drug or treatment with a larger group ($n = 50$–300). A control group and randomization may be used, but such studies are not adequate for statistical testing of efficacy measures. In Phase III studies, the goal is to compare the effectiveness and safety of a study drug or treatment with those of a standard treatment, with large groups ($n = 100$–20 000). A control group and randomization are mandatory. In Phase IV studies, the goal is to provide post-marketing surveillance of the risks, benefits, and optimal use of the drug or therapy.

Phase IV trials demonstrate that the rates of specific outcomes for general patient populations ($n = 100$–50 000) are similar to those observed for trial populations. No control group or randomization is required. Phase IV randomized studies have occasionally been performed to compare competing therapies. Phase III studies are designed to provide definitive evidence for the effectiveness and safety of the procedure. For drug assessments, the Food and Drug Administration generally requires two Phase III studies. Therefore, it is not unusual for the testing process from Phase I to Phase III to require 10 years or more. Some Phase III trials are based on the results of Phase I and Phase II trials. For other Phase III trials, evidence from case series and extensive clinical experience is considered strong enough. This report concentrates on the design and performance of Phase III studies.

The trial objective (the research question)

The clinical trial must have a clear objective, with the intent to address a specific research question or hypothesis.[24] Table 22.2 indicates the primary research question in each of the five representative trials. Important considerations in the formulation of the research question are the target condition, the target population, the measures to determine the effectiveness of the intervention, the time until effectiveness occurs, and the magnitude of the difference indicating the superiority of the new treatment, compared with the existing treatment.

For a study intended to compare endovascular and surgical approaches for the treatment of carotid stenosis, the question, "Is either endovascular or surgical treatment of patients with carotid stenosis, more effective than the other?" is too general to be meaningful. The investigators must define the question to properly evaluate effectiveness for the target condition and population. The research question must define the measure to be used to determine the effectiveness of the new procedure and the time frame during which this change is expected to occur. The question, "Is either endovascular or surgical treatment of carotid stenosis more effective than the other in reducing the rate of any stroke, myocardial infarction (MI), or death during the 30-day periprocedural period, or ipsilateral stroke after 30 days?" defines the measure and the time frame but is still not specific enough. To establish the superiority of one treatment over another, the investigators must define the magnitude of the difference between the new treatment or intervention and the existing treatment that is to be detected in the study. However, the question, "Can either endovascular or surgical treatment of patients with carotid stenosis reduce the rate of any stroke, MI, or death during the 30-day periprocedural period, or ipsilateral stroke after 30 days by 25% or more compared with the other treatment?" is still not acceptable, because it lacks a definition of the population to which the new procedure is to be targeted. The specific question, "Can either endovascular or surgical treatment of patients with symptomatic extracranial carotid stenosis $\geq$50%, for whom both endovascular and surgical treatments are acceptable

Table 22.2. Research questions and assumptions of different clinical trials

Prolyse in Acute Cerebral Thromboembolism II Study

Do 9 mg of prourokinase administered intra-arterially within 6 h after symptom onset increase or decrease the rate of slight or no neurological disability (mRS scores of 0–2 at 90 d) among patients with angiographically proven occlusion of the middle cerebral artery and without hemorrhage or major early infarction signs on computed tomographic scans? It was assumed that 21% of patients treated without intra-arterially administered prourokinase would have slight or no neurological disability at 90 d (mRS scores of 0 or 1 at 90 d).

Interventional Management of Stroke II Study

Null Hypothesis: Does using a combination of low dose IV rt-PA (0.6 mg/kg) followed by delivery of additional IA rt-PA (up to 22 mg) in the setting of low-energy ultrasound via the EKOS microinfusion catheter at the site of IA occlusion for treatment of patients with acute ischemic stroke (NIHSSS ≥10) within 3 hours of symptom onset lead to rate of favorable outcome (defined as mRS of 0 to 1) of 29% or more at 3 months? Alternative Hypothesis: Rate of patients with favorable outcome is less than 29%. To be compared to historic control group is the NINDS trial placebo group whose rate of mRS 0 to 1 was 17% at 1 month. If the null hypothesis was rejected, then it would be concluded that it is futile to proceed to phase III trial.

Interventional Management of Stroke III Study

Does using a combined IV/IA approach (0.6 mg/kg IV rt-PA followed by IA therapy) to recanalization, lead to an absolute difference of 10% in favorable outcome (mild or no disability as measured by mRS of 0–2) at 3 months when compared to standard IV rt-PA alone, in patients presenting within 3 hours of symptom onset with moderate to severe strokes (NIHSSS ≥10)? There is also a non-inferiority margin set at 5% absolute difference.

Stenting and Angioplasty with Protection in Patients at High Risk for Endarterectomy (SAPPHIRE) trial

Compared to CEA, does the use of CAS for treatment of high risk patients with extracranial carotid stenosis (≥50% symptomatic or ≥80% asymptomatic) lead to similar or slightly higher rate (<3%) of death, stroke, or myocardial infarction within 30 days after the procedure or death or ipsilateral stroke between 31 days and 1 year?

Stent-Supported Percutaneous Angioplasty of the Carotid Artery versus Endarterectomy (SPACE) trial

Compared to CEA, does the use of CAS for treatment of patients with symptomatic extracranial carotid stenosis ≥50% lead to similar or slightly higher (<2.5%) rate of ipsilateral stroke (ischzemic stroke or intracerebral bleeding or both, with symptoms lasting more than 24 h) or death of any cause between randomization and 30 days after treatment?

Endarterectomy vs. Angioplasty in Patients with Symptomatic Severe Carotid Stenosis (EVA-3S) trial

Compared to CEA does the use of CAS for treatment of patients with symptomatic extracranial carotid stenosis ≥50% lead to similar or slightly higher (2%) rate of any stroke or death occurring within 30 days after treatment?

Carotid Revascularization Endarterectomy versus Stenting Trial (CREST)

Compared to CEA, does the use of CAS for treatment of patients with symptomatic extracranial carotid stenosis ≥50% lead to similar or insignificantly higher or lower (≤1.2%) rate of any stroke, myocardial infarction, or death during the 30-day peri-operative or peri-procedural period, or ipsilateral stroke after 30 days?

Abbreviations caused: MRS, modified Rankin scale; d, days; IV, intravenous; IA, intra-arterial; rt-PA, recombinant tissue plasminogen activator; NIHSSS, National Institutes of Health Stroke Scale Score; NINDS, National Institute of Neurologic Disorders and Stroke; CEA, Carotid Endarterectomy; CAS, Carotid artery stunt placement; H, hours.

options, reduce the rate of any stroke, MI, or death during the 30-day peri-procedural period, or ipsilateral stroke after 30 days by 25% or more compared to the other treatment?" was the research question posed by CREST.[6] This research question takes into consideration the important elements for a trial comparing these therapies.

Study population

The study sample should be a representative subset of the eligible population targeted for application of the new procedure, as defined by rigorous and unambiguous inclusion and exclusion criteria. The criteria must define a population that is at risk for the expected primary end point and is relatively homogeneous in composition, within the group as a whole or within well-defined strata (e.g., younger versus older subjects).

The variability in response is smaller for homogeneous or stratified groups than for more heterogeneous groups. Reduced variability allows smaller sample sizes for observation of a specified significant difference between two groups, at a fixed level of statistical power. Narrow inclusion and exclusion criteria confine enrollment in the study to a smaller subset of patients with the disease, but may impose limitations on the generalization of the results to the entire affected population. In addition, it is important to note that the inclusion and exclusion criteria may exclude a subset of patients who are of interest, but for whom the risk/benefit ratio is deemed unacceptable, by either the principal investigator or internal review board at the participating center or the data and safety monitoring committee for the trial.

Various inclusion and exclusion criteria were established to identify eligible subjects for different trials. In the IMS III trial [5], patients with moderate-to-large (National Institutes of Health Stroke Scale score (NIHSSS) $\geq$10) ischemic stroke between ages 18 and 80 are target for enrollment. In order to be eligible for the trial, subjects must have had moderate to large strokes (baseline NIHSSS $\geq$10) before initiation of IV rt-PA. In addition, IV rt-PA must be initiated within 3 hours of symptom onset. The protocol adheres to current medical practice regarding inclusion and exclusion criteria for revascularization therapies with only a few exceptions. Specifically, subjects older than 80 years, undergoing hemodialysis or peritoneal dialysis, or with blood glucose levels greater than 400 mg/dl have been excluded at this time due to possibly increased ICH rates based on the IMS II trial and prior IV and IA studies. [25] Imaging criteria for exclusion are consistent with the NINDS rt-PA stroke trial. Specifically, patients with large regions of clear hypodensity on CT scan, such as greater than one-third of the middle cerebral artery vascular territory, are excluded. An Alberta Stroke Program Early CT Score (ASPECTS) of $\leq$4 can be used as a guideline when evaluating >1/3 region of territory involvement. However, sulcal effacement and/or loss of gray–white matter differentiation alone are not contraindications for treatment.

In the EVA-3S trial, patients were eligible if they were 18 years of age or older, had had a hemispheric or retinal transient ischemic attack or a non-disabling stroke (or retinal infarct) within 120 days before enrollment, and had a stenosis of 60% to 99% in the symptomatic carotid artery, as determined by the North American Symptomatic Carotid Endarterectomy Trial (NASCET) method. [26] The degree of stenosis warranting treatment, set at 70% or more at the start of the trial, was modified, 3 years after the study initiation to 60% or more because endarterectomy was shown to benefit patients with symptomatic stenosis of 50% to 69%. [27] The presence of an ipsilateral carotid stenosis of 60% or more had to be confirmed by means of catheter angiography or both duplex scanning and magnetic resonance angiography of the carotid artery. Patients were excluded if one of the following was present: a modified Rankin Scale (mRS) score of 3 or more (disabling stroke); non-atherosclerotic carotid disease; severe tandem lesions (stenosis of proximal common carotid artery or intracranial artery that was more severe than the cervical lesion); previous revascularization of the symptomatic stenosis; history of bleeding disorder; uncontrolled hypertension or diabetes; unstable angina; contraindication to heparin, ticlopidine, or clopidogrel; life expectancy of less than 2 years; or percutaneous or surgical intervention within 30 days before or after the study procedure. The appearance of the stenotic lesion on angiography was not a factor in the selection of patients.

As can be observed in Figs. 22.1 to 22.5, the study populations in the trials highlighted in this chapter represented small proportions of the patients with a particular disease evaluated at the participating centers. Patients presenting to study centers can be divided into four groups, i.e., eligible and randomized, eligible and not randomized, not eligible and randomized, and not eligible and not randomized. A major

concern is that patients who are included in the clinical trial (eligible and randomized) represent those for whom a better clinical outcome could be expected because of the presence or absence of known prognostic factors or the investigators' experience, in comparison with patients who are eligible and not randomized. This form of bias, called the "cherry-picking phenomenon," was a major concern in the interpretation of the results of the ISAT Study. [28] In the International Subarachnoid Aneurysm Trial (ISAT), endovascular treatment (EVT) of ruptured intracranial aneurysm was compared to surgical treatment; 23.7% allocated to EVT were dependent or dead at 1 year compared to 30.6% allocated to surgery ($P = 0.0019$). Of the 9559 patients that were eligible for inclusion, 78% were excluded. 9% of the exclusions were for refusal to participate, and the remaining 69% were excluded from the study because of lack of equipoise, i.e., the aneurysm could not be treated by both procedures. Since almost all intracranial aneurysms can be treated by surgery, 69% of the aneurysms were excluded because of clinical concerns (e.g., large intracranial hematoma with increased bleeding risk with long-lasting deep anticoagulation) or because of morphological concerns (e.g., aneurysm with a configuration not suitable or ideal for coiling), this proportion could be interpreted as representing a selection or sample bias ("cherry picking"). [28]

In studies in which a new procedure is being compared to medical treatment, the cherry-picking phenomenon may reduce the ability to detect meaningful differences in effectiveness, because of the low risk of recurrent events in the medical treatment group. Moreover, cherry-picking leads to bias in the determination of the primary endpoint for the intended study population, with the results reflecting the morbidity and mortality rates associated with the procedure more than the natural history of the disease. [29]

It is reasonable to think that a more rigorous approach to patient recruitment is necessary to ensure randomization of the maximal number of eligible patients. Strategies such as external monitoring, involvement of centers and physicians committed to the trial, and effective methods for approaching patients for enrollment may limit the loss of eligible patients because of physician- and patient-related factors.

Another consideration regarding the study population of a trial is the possibility of randomization of non-eligible patients. In the SPACE trial, [15] 18 patients allocated to the CAS group were not treated (4 patients because of a diminished stenosis and 14 patients because of contraindications that arose between randomization and treatment), while in the CEA group, 1 patient died before treatment and 12 were not treated (1 because of a diminished stenosis, 2 because of occlusion of the carotid artery, and 9 because of contraindications found after randomization). The intention to treat analysis included all these patients in their allocated group. Similarly, in the SAPPHIRE study, [14] of the 167 patients randomly assigned to CAS, 8 patients were not treated (3 because of deterioration of their condition, 2 because of inability to meet the enrollment criteria, and 3 withdrew their consent). Of the 167 patients assigned to CEA, 16 patients were

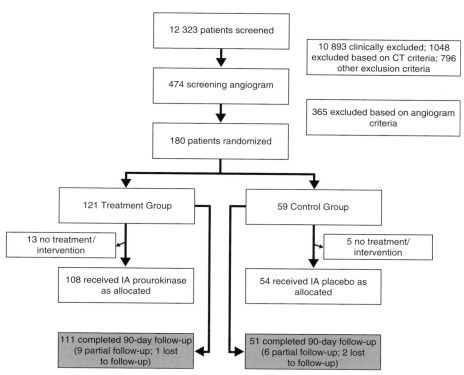

Fig. 22.1. Flow of patients in the PROACT II study (modified from Furlan *et al.* 1999).[1]

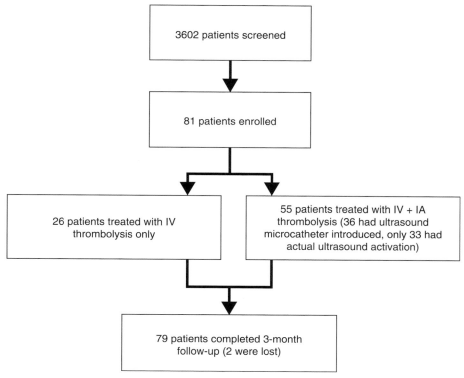

Fig. 22.2. Flow of patients in the IMS II trial (modified from the original publication *Stroke* 2007).[2]

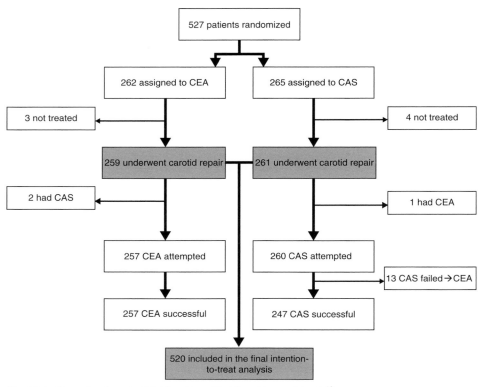

Fig. 22.3. Flow of patients in EVA-3S trial (modified from Mas *et al.* 2006).[13]
Abbreviations used: CEA, Carotid endarterectomy; CAS, Carotid artery stunt placement.

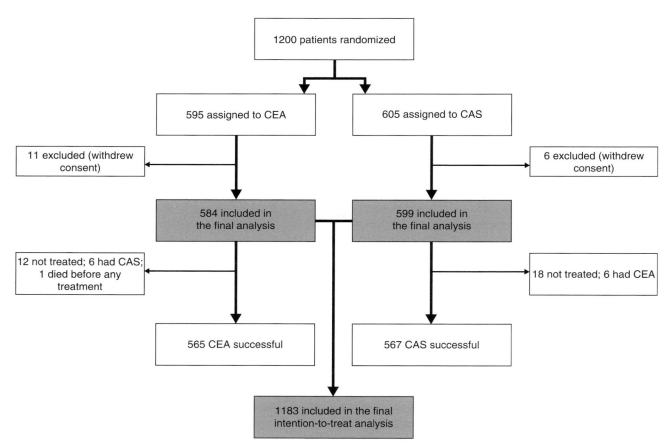

Fig. 22.4. Flow of patients in the SPACE trial (modified from original publication *Lancet* 2006).[15]
Abbreviations used: CEA, Carotid endarterectomy; CAS, Carotid artery stunt placement.

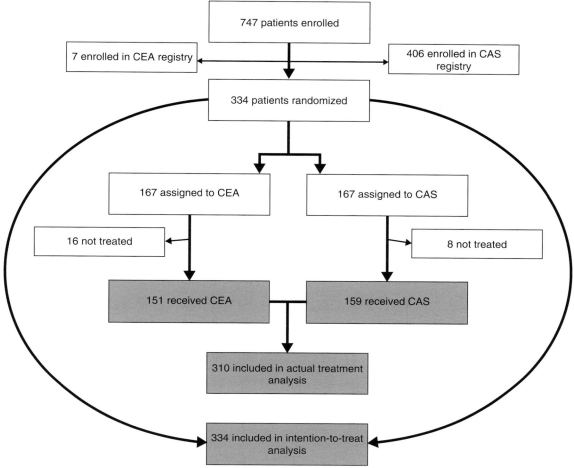

Fig. 22.5. Flow chart of patients in SAPPHIRE trial.[14]
Abbreviations used: CEA, Carotid endarterectomy; CAS, Carotid artery stunt placement.

not treated (4 because of deterioration of their condition, 4 because of inability to meet the enrollment criteria, and 8 withdrew their consent). Again, these patients' data was included in the final analysis.

Identification and selection of variables

Three categories of variables are assessed in a clinical study, i.e., safety variables, outcome variables, and baseline and/or screening variables. Safety variables are monitored continuously during the course of the study. The primary safety variables consist of adverse events, which are often categorized according to intensity (mild, moderate, severe, life-threatening, or resulting in death) and relationship to the study treatment (not, possibly, probably, or definitely related). Data on adverse events are reviewed in detail at regular intervals by the trial steering committee, the internal review board, and the data and safety monitoring committee and possibly by the Food and Drug Administration, depending on the type of trial. It is the responsibility of the data and safety monitoring committee

to ensure that patients' relative risks are not increased as a result of participation in the clinical trial.[29]

Outcome variables define and answer the research question and are also known as efficacy, response, endpoint, or dependent variables.[23,24] The primary outcome or endpoint variable must be objectively defined with respect to a time frame (e.g., short-term vs. long-term outcome). The primary endpoint can be a single event, such as slight or no neurological disability (e.g., mRS scores of 0 to 2 at 90 days), as in the PROACT II study,[1] or a composite of multiple outcomes (e.g., any stroke, MI, or death during the 30-day peri-procedural period, or ipsilateral stroke after 30 days), as in the CREST.[6] Secondary and tertiary end point events are documented throughout the study, as part of the data collection process, and are analyzed at the conclusion of the study. Endpoint events are determined or confirmed by an adjudicating committee, to ensure an objective definition. A more detailed discussion is provided below.

Baseline data typically consist of demographic, clinical, and laboratory characteristics of the subjects, e.g., blood chemistry testing results, data on the severity of the illness (target condition), and history and physical examination findings. Baseline data are obtained to describe the study patients and to determine whether the patients are representative of the target population. A subset of baseline data includes influencing variables, which are also known as covariates, prognostic factors, confounding factors, independent variables, or predictor variables.[23,24] These variables are generally assumed to be correlated with the outcome variables (e.g., correlation of age and initial stroke severity with outcome). Selected influencing variables that are highly correlated with the outcome variables are often used as stratification variables. Stratification ensures that only subjects with similar influencing variable findings are compared, with segregation of the subjects into strata (subgroups). The relationship between the influencing variables and outcomes can be examined separately in each stratum. The pitfall of not accounting for influencing variables, as in a non-randomized study, is that differences in the observed effects with different interventions may be merely the result of imbalances of influencing variables. For example, an excess number of elderly patients or patients with severe strokes may worsen outcomes for a treatment group without having true implications for the effects of the treatment being evaluated. The advantage of a randomized study is that influencing variables are balanced in the arms of the study, whether they are measured or not; therefore, a cause-and-effect conclusion can be drawn with statistical hypothesis testing. Baseline variables in the treatment and control groups are compared and periodically monitored by the data and safety monitoring committee, for identification of potential problems that might affect the progress of the trial. Such monitoring includes an examination of differences in baseline variables that might arise because of different dropout rates for the groups. Baseline information is routinely summarized at the time of study completion, to ensure that the randomization procedure was properly performed and the statistical test results are thus valid at the appropriate level of significance.

Sample size and statistical error rates

A trial investigating the scientific merit of a new treatment is based on a research question or objective proposing that one treatment is superior to another treatment. The evidence for treatment differences is defined in terms of a null hypothesis (there are no differences) and an alternative hypothesis (there are differences). The primary purpose of these hypotheses is to establish the basis for tests of statistical significance. Both hypotheses are framed within the context of a parameter that corresponds to the primary end point. The population sample data are used to estimate this parameter, a statistical test is performed, a P value is calculated, and the hypothesis testing is performed. In a standard comparison of two treatments, the null hypothesis states that, on average (rates and proportions are specific types of averages), the treatments are equivalent with respect to the primary end point (e.g., the 2-year survival rates are, on average, equivalent for Treatments A and B). The alternative hypothesis may be one- or two-sided and states

that, on average, the treatments are different with respect to the primary outcome. A one-sided (or one-tailed) test suggests a directional difference (e.g., Treatment A improves the survival rate, compared with Treatment B). A two-sided test does not specify the direction (e.g., the survival rate is different, either superior or inferior, for Treatment A, compared with Treatment B) and therefore is the preferred method. In trials consisting of three or more treatment comparisons, the alternative hypothesis states that at least one treatment is different from the others. Conclusions in statistical hypothesis testing either reject the null hypothesis (in favor of the alternative hypothesis) or fail to reject the null hypothesis.[29]

For example, in the IMS III trial,[5] the aim is to find a difference in outcome between the IV thrombolysis protocol versus a combined IV and IA protocol. The null hypothesis is that the proportion of patients with mRS 0–2 at 3 months is equal between the two protocols (absolute difference of ≤10%). If the null hypothesis is rejected (absolute difference >10%), then the conclusion would be that one protocol is superior. This is a superiority study two-sided hypothesis. Compare this to the EVA-3S trial,[13] which is a non-inferiority study with a one-sided hypothesis. The aim is to prove that CAS has similar (not worse) outcome than CEA. The null hypothesis is that the absolute difference in outcome (any stroke or death at 30 days) is > 2% (this is called non-inferiority margin). If the null hypothesis is rejected (absolute difference ≤ 2%), the investigators would conclude that there is no significant difference in outcome between the two interventions (i.e., CAS is not inferior to CEA). If the null hypothesis cannot be rejected, then the investigators would not be able to conclude non-inferiority.

All statistical tests have an inherent element of random error. Estimates of a population from a sample always include some degree of error. The error associated with this discrepancy is accounted for by the statistical analysis. A reduction in the hypothesis testing error rate represents a compromise regarding sample size, clinically meaningful average treatment differences, and costs of the treatments being compared. There are two types of errors in hypothesis testing, i.e., rejecting the null hypothesis when it is actually true and failing to reject the null hypothesis when it is actually false. These error rates are conditional probabilities and are defined as Type I (false-positive) and Type II (false-negative) errors, typically denoted by the Greek letters α and β, respectively. The α level (probability of rejecting the null hypothesis when it is true) is the threshold value for statistical significance. The β level (probability of not rejecting the null hypothesis when it is false) is usually expressed as statistical power, which is computed as $1-\beta$.[29]

The α level is typically set at either 0.05 or 0.01 before the trial is implemented. Most clinical trials set α at a level of 0.05, which suggests that the chance of concluding there is a treatment difference when one truly does not exist is 1 in 20. An α levels of 0.01 was used for testing the secondary outcomes and exploratory analyses in the IMS III study,[5] whereas an α level of 0.05 will be used to test the primary hypothesis. The

SPACE,[15] EVA-3S,[13] and PROACT II study[1] (13) all used α levels of 0.05. If the *P* value is less than α, then the conclusion is to reject the null hypothesis. A small *P* value indicates a result that is far from the null hypothesis, i.e., a high likelihood of a treatment difference.

Statistical power (1–β) is typically set at levels of 0.80 or 0.90 (sometimes written as 80% or 90%). A statistical power of 0.80 indicates a one in five chance of concluding there is no treatment difference when one actually exists. A statistical power of 0.90 indicates a one in ten chance of concluding there is no treatment difference when one exists. A power of 0.90 was used to calculate the sample size for CREST,[6] while a power of 0.80 was used for sample size calculations for the PROACT II study.[1] Therefore, if no therapeutic benefit was demonstrated with intra-arterially administered prourokinase, there was a one in five chance that there actually would be a therapeutic benefit in the general population that was not demonstrated in the study population (i.e., the association was missed in error because the sample size was small). In general, a trial with a power of less than 0.80 is not considered a definitive trial of treatment efficacy and is more likely to represent a pilot study. An underpowered study is usually the result of inadequate sample size.

To determine the sample size for a given trial, the statistical testing procedure must be specified in advance (e.g., *t* test or test of proportions). Then, α and β levels must be specified, as well as the clinically meaningful difference between treatment groups, which is defined in terms of the population parameter. Some degree of variability in the outcome measure must also be ascertained from pilot data, or a literature review, or by other means.

In calculating the sample size, it is also critical to take into consideration the numbers of dropouts and other study patients who will not be available for follow-up evaluations. If the trial planning committee determines that a substantial proportion of subjects will not be available, then the sample size should be increased accordingly. In the IMS III study,[5] a total sample size of 900 was determined, based on an anticipated effect size of 10% (the absolute difference between the IV and IV/IA subjects with favorable outcomes). Type I and Type II errors are probabilities of 0.05 and 0.20, respectively. The sample size of 900 includes inflation by 1.03 to safeguard against dilution of the effect size by patients lost to follow-up and/or treatment cross-over in approximately 1%–3% of the cases. The rates of morbidity and outcome events expected in the representative clinical trials are presented in Table 22.3.

Clinically meaningful differences between treatment arms must often be determined from the collective knowledge and experience of a group of experts in the medical community or by the investigators themselves. The differences may be dictated by a number of factors, such as cost reduction, lower morbidity rates, improved quality of life, or reduction in mortality rates. In CREST,[7] the sample size for the study is approximately 2500 symptomatic patients, which will be sufficient to detect a relative difference of 25% to 30% between CAS

and CEA groups with the previously mentioned statistical power of 0.90. Lesser differences would be considered sufficiently small to declare the treatments equivalent. In general, for detection of smaller differences, larger numbers of study patients must be recruited.

Interim or sequential analysis methods extend the concept of hypothesis testing at a single time point to multiple time points. In contrast to the performance of the primary statistical analysis at the completion of the trial, interim tests of efficacy are designed to test for treatment differences at one or more time points during the trial, defined on the basis of calendar time or patient accrual. The intent of interim or sequential testing is to stop the trial early if one treatment is vastly superior to the other, to promote that treatment to the medical community as soon as possible. As an example, the most basic interim analysis would be to test for treatment differences after one-half of the predetermined number of subjects has completed the trial, rather than the standard approach of analyzing the data at the conclusion of the trial. In a study protocol that incorporates interim or sequential testing, a conservative test of the null hypothesis is performed at the interim analysis point and one of the following conclusions is reached: stop the trial early because of the efficacy of one treatment over the other or continue the trial to the next interim point or to the final analysis. The three classic methods for performing interim analyses are the Pocock method, the O'Brien and Fleming method, and the Haybittle and Peto method.[30] Exact descriptions of each method are beyond the scope of this discussion. In contrast to interim analyses of efficacy, futility analyses are often requested by data and safety monitoring committees. Futility analysis estimates, with various statistical methods, the probability of finding a treatment-based difference at the completion of the trial, given the information that has been accrued at a prespecified point during the trial. The basic concept is to stop the trial early if there is only a very small probability of finding a treatment difference at the completion of the trial. The goal of a futility analysis is to conserve resources (i.e., why continue the trial to completion if the available information indicates a low probability of obtaining a statistically and clinically significant result?). Interim and futility analyses are described below in the context of data and safety monitoring committees.[29]

In the SPACE study,[15] an interim analysis was planned for once half the patients were accrued or 3 years after the start of the study, whichever came first. To ensure the specified type-1 error probability, a group sequential analysis was done with the Lan-DeMets α-spending function method. The output also contains the conditional power since the probability of rejecting the null hypothesis at the next and final look in view of the data obtained thus far and if the following and final look was to be done at the recommended ideal next look position. On the basis of the results of the interim analysis, a second interim analysis after 1200 randomized patients was recommended. After 1200 patients, a second interim analysis was done. Re-adjustment of the power to

Table 22.3. Rate of adverse events within 1 year in the SAPPHIRE trial analyzed by both intention to treat and actual treatment analyses[14]

Event	Intention to treat			Actual treatment		
	CAS (*N* = 167)	CEA (*N* = 167)	*P* value	CAS (*N* = 159)	CEA (*N* = 151)	*P* value
Primary end point*	20 (12.2%)	32 (20.1%)	0.05	19 (12.0%)	30 (20.1%)	0.05
Any Stroke	10 (6.2%)	12 (7.9%)	0.60	9 (5.8%)	11 (7.7%)	0.52
Major ipsilateral	**1 (0.6%)**	**5 (3.3%)**	**0.09**	**0**	**5 (3.5%)**	**0.02**
Major non-ipsilateral	1 (0.6%)	2 (1.4%)	0.53	1 (0.6%)	1 (0.7%)	0.97
Minor ipsilateral	6 (3.7%)	3 (2.0%)	0.34	6 (3.8%)	3 (2.2)	0.37
Minor non-ipsilateral	3 (1.9%)	4 (2.7%)	0.64	3 (2.0%)	3 (2.1%)	0.89
Myocardial infarction	**5 (3.0%)**	**12 (7.5%)**	**0.07**	**4 (2.5%)**	**12 (8.1%)**	**0.03**

*Death, stroke, or myocardial infarction at 30 days plus ipsilateral stroke or death from neurologic causes within 31 days to 1 yr.
Modified from Yadav *et al.* 2004.[14]
Abbreviations used: CEA, Carotid endarterectomy; CAS, Carotid artery stunt placement.

prove equivalence of both treatment modalities, with an absolute difference of 0.51% in the rate of primary-endpoint events with the initial planned sample size of 950 patients per group, led to a conditional power of only 52%. To reach an 80% power, more than 2500 patients would be needed. Therefore, the steering committee, also considering the absence of further funding, decided to stop recruitment after the second interim analysis.

In the IMS III study, three interim analyses will be performed after approximately 225 (25% of 900), 450 (50%), and 675 (75%) subjects complete the 3-month mRS assessment and tested at appropriate nominal levels that ensure an overall level of 0.05.

Methods of assignment of the intervention: allocation concealment and randomization

The method of treatment assignment in the trial must minimize the potential for the introduction of selection bias. Selection bias occurs when patients with one or more influencing factors appear more frequently in one comparison group than in others. For example, in trials involving patients with ischemic stroke, patients with greater stroke severity, as defined on the basis of NIHSS, are more likely to experience poor outcomes after any intervention.[31] If patients with higher NIHSS were enrolled in the new procedure group of a clinical trial, then the potential beneficial effect of the treatment would likely be obscured. Appropriate steps must be taken to ensure that imbalances among known or suspected prognostic factors are minimized. Imbalances can occur because of investigator or patient bias toward a particular treatment or by chance. Two strategies are used to reduce selection bias: allocation concealment and randomization. Allocation concealment seeks to prevent selection bias, protects the allocation sequence until assignment, and can always be successfully implemented, regardless of the intervention. Trials with inadequate allocation concealment have been demonstrated to yield larger estimates of treatment effects, compared with trials with adequate

concealment (after adjustment for other aspects of quality, odds ratios were exaggerated by 41% for inadequately concealed trials).[32,33] Allocation concealment also protects the trial from conscious or subconscious actions on the part of the study investigators that could lead to non-comparability, e.g., assigning (or selecting) the most seriously ill patients to the therapy considered by the physicians to be the more aggressive treatment. Determination of eligibility and procurement of the patient's agreement to participate must occur before randomization and treatment assignment.[24] In trials of medical treatment alone, double blinding (an approach in which the patients and treating physicians and possibly a distinct set of evaluators are unaware of the treatments allocated) ensures that patient preference does not influence study conduct. In surgical or endovascular treatment trials, the nature of the treatment cannot be hidden from either the investigator or the patient, and compliance with the treatment allocated can become an issue. In the SAPPHIRE study,[14] 167 patients were assigned to CAS, and 167 were assigned to CEA. Only 159 and 167 patients were actually treated by CAS and CEA, respectively. The data was analyzed in two ways: an intention to treat analysis and actual treatment analysis. Despite yielding generally similar results, there were a few differences between both analyses (Table 22.3).

The preferred method for protecting a trial against selection bias attributable to chance is randomization. During the process of randomization, patients are assigned to the intervention or control group, with each patient having equal chances of being selected for either group. Random-number tables and computer-generated programs are commonly used randomization methods.[25,34] The method of randomization used in a trial should be specified in the protocol. Systematic or patterned intervention assignments are best avoided. Assigning patients to interventions in a systematic manner (e.g., every other or every second patient) seems random; however, imbalances can occur, and selection bias is possible, because the intervention assignment is predictable. On occasion, randomization schemes may not provide an adequate balance of the prognostic factors among the comparison groups.[23,24] Stratification and other randomization strategies are then used to ensure that the groups are balanced in terms of influencing factors. As previously mentioned, stratification is performed to guard against imbalances with respect to these variables. Subgroups, called strata, are formed by grouping subsets of selected influencing variables. For this approach, patients are initially stratified according to their baseline characteristics (such as older age, categorized on the basis of some cutoff point) and then randomized. Therefore, approximately equal numbers of patients in one stratum (e.g., patients with high NIHSSS) are allocated to the new procedure and to the control treatment.

In the IMS III trial,[5] subjects are randomized in a 2 : 1 ratio, with more subjects assigned to the combined IV/IA group. This randomization regimen was chosen based on pilot data, suggesting a higher rate of favorable clinical outcome in the combined IV/IA group in the IMS I and II trials as compared with comparable historical controls from the NINDS rt-PA stroke trial. The design and implementation of the randomization scheme is conducted by the Data Coordination Unit (DCU). The randomization scheme was designed to ensure a 2 : 1 treatment group distribution within each baseline NIHSSS stratum (10–20 or >20), each performance site, and throughout the overall study. Randomization is implemented using a combination of a web-based minimization + biased coin scheme and sealed randomization envelopes placed at each clinical site. A patient is randomized by opening a prespecified sealed envelope that contains the treatment assignment. The prespecification of the envelope is performed through the web within 8 h after the previous patient is randomized and his/her enrollment data are entered into the database via the study website. This system was designed to allow for rapid randomization because it does not require a phone call, fax back system, or access to a website before treatment. To minimize any delay in the administration of a proven effective therapy (i.e., IV rt-PA), the standard dose of open-label IV rt-PA (0.9 mg/kg; 90 mg maximum) can be initiated before enrollment and randomization in the trial if standard eligibility criteria are met. In addition, the IV rt-PA can be initiated in a patient who cannot provide informed consent for the study and for whom an authorized legal representative is not yet available (standard of care). Randomization can be accomplished at any time before completion of 40 minutes of the IV rt-PA infusion (approximately two-thirds of the 0.9 mg/kg dose). This allows for time to complete the determination of trial eligibility, confirm interventional staff availability, obtain consent/HIPAA authorization from the patient and/or legal representative, and identify the randomization assignment. If the patient and/or authorized legal representative cannot provide informed consent for participation or the subject cannot be successfully randomized into the trial before completion of 40 minutes of IV rt-PA infusion, the remainder of the 0.9 mg/kg standard dose of rt-PA can be administered. The patient would then not be included as a participant in the IMS III study. A subject is considered to be included in the IMS III trial only when the sealed randomization envelope is opened. If the patient is entered in the trial and randomized to the IV rt-PA alone group, he/she will receive the full dose (0.9 mg/kg, 90 mg maximum) of rt-PA intravenously over an hour, as Food and Drug Administration (FDA) approved standard of care. The combined IV/IA group will undergo open-label rt-PA over 40 min only instead of 1 h (~0.6 mg/kg, 60 mg maximum) and then undergo immediate angiography.

In the PROACT II study,[1] patients were randomized into three strata on the basis of their NIHSS (scores of 4 through 10, 11 through 20, or 21 through 30).

In the EVA-3S study (H12)[13], patients who were suitable candidates for both techniques were randomly assigned to undergo endarterectomy or stenting. Randomization was carried out centrally by means of a computer-generated sequence, involving randomized blocks of two, four, or six patients that were stratified according to study center and degree of stenosis (stenosis of ≥90% or <90%).

In the SPACE trial,[15] the random allocation schedule was generated using a computer program. This was done by members of the data and statistic centre, who also obtained and analyzed the data. This centre was not involved in the clinical work and was separate from all clinical centers; therefore, no clinical centre was able to obtain information about the randomization sequence. Patient entry was by fax to the data center, which provided an eight-patient block randomization design per center. No stratification process was in place.

In the SAPPHIRE study,[14] patients were randomly assigned to a procedure only if all members of the team were in agreement that the patient was a suitable candidate for either CEA or CAS. If the surgeon assessing the patient concluded that CEA could not be safely performed, but the interventional physician judged that CAS was feasible, the patient was not randomly assigned to a procedure but instead was entered into a stent registry. Likewise, if the surgeon deemed the patient suitable for surgery but the interventional physician did not think that CAS was feasible, the patient was entered into a surgical registry. Patients were randomly assigned in a 1 : 1 ratio, with stratification according to the clinical center and according to whether the patient had symptomatic or asymptomatic disease. Randomization was performed with the use of a pseudo-random number generator, and the numbers were distributed by an automated, centralized telephone response system.

Masking (or blinding)

Three of the more serious types of bids that may occur in a clinical trial are investigator bias, evaluator bias, and sham or placebo effect bias. Investigator or evaluator bias occurs when an investigator or evaluator either consciously or subconsciously favors one group over another. For example, if investigators know which group received the intervention, then they may monitor that group more closely and thus treat them differently from the control group, in a way that could seriously affect the outcome of the trial. Sham or placebo effect bias occurs when patients are exposed to an inactive mode of therapy, but think they are being treated with an intervention and subsequently over-report disease improvement. The key to obtaining an unbiased estimate of effect for the active arm is to partition out or subtract the sham or placebo effect (e.g., the true effect of the active treatment is the measured effect of the active treatment minus the measured effect of the placebo or sham treatment). Blinded (or masked) trials may be single-blinded, doubled-blinded, or even triple-blinded. In a single-blinded trial, the subject is unaware of the treatment assignment. In a double-blinded trial, treating physicians (and possibly a distinct set of evaluators) and patients are unaware of the treatment. Double-blinding prevents most of the types of bids described above and tends to foster compliance in inactive treatment arms.[29] In certain situations, such as comparisons of endovascular and surgical treatments or surgical and medical treatments, double-blinding is not possible. Lack of double-blinding exaggerates estimates of treatment benefits by approximately 19%.[17,35,26,36] Strategies must be developed during planning to minimize the bias introduced by a lack of blinding. In the PROACT II study,[1] participating centers were required to designate a neurologist who was to remain blinded to the treatment assignments and angiographic results for the duration of the trial. The neurologist conducted clinical assessments of treatment efficacy, in a blinded manner, at 7 to 10 days, 30 days, and 90 days after the initial treatment. In triple-blinded studies, a third party (e.g., a sponsor such as a pharmaceutical company or the National Institutes of Health) is unaware of the treatment assignments.

Study centers and investigators

Because pooling of data across study sites and among investigators is usually necessary to attain the required sample size, the selection of study sites and investigators is critical for the planning of a clinical trial. The selected sites must have sufficient numbers of eligible patients who are representative of the target population for whom the investigational treatment is intended. It should be noted that, despite a common protocol and the best efforts of the study monitor, site-specific effects are possible and might invalidate pooling of the data. A careful analysis to exclude potential bias as a result of site-specific effects is an important part of the investigational protocol.

For trials involving the performance of a procedure, it is important that practitioners have adequate experience and expertise in performing the procedure before the beginning of the trial. In the EVA-3S trial,[13] the vascular surgeon had to have performed at least 25 CEA in the year before enrollment. The interventional physician had to have performed at least 12 CAS procedures or at least 35 stenting procedures in the supra-aortic trunks, of which at least five were in the carotid artery. Centers fulfilling all requirements except those with regard to the interventional physician could join the EVA-3S study and

randomly assign patients, but all stenting procedures had to be performed under the supervision of an experienced tutor (a clinician who qualified to perform stenting in this study) until the local interventional physician became self-sufficient (according to the tutor) and performed a sufficient number of procedures according to the predefined criteria. This clearly biased experience against CAS manifested in failure of stent placement in 13 (5%) out of 260 patients on whom CAS was attempted and who ended up getting CEA instead. Two of these patients had a stroke before CEA. The expected 30-day stroke or death rates on which the study was designed were 5.6% for CEA and 4% for CAS. This trial was stopped early for reasons of both safety and futility. The 30-day risk of any stroke or death was significantly higher after CAS (9.6%) than after CEA (3.9%). This difference was statistically significant (P = 0.01), resulting in a relative risk of 2.5 (95% CI, 1.2 to 5.1). The EVA-3S investigators reported that the 30-day incidence of stroke or death was similar among patients treated by interventional physicians who were experienced (11 of 105, or 10.5%), tutored during training (7 of 98, or 7.1%), and tutored after training (7 of 57, or 12.3%) (P = 0.54; chi-square statistic, 1.25). Based on that, they argued that the difference in training and experience did not affect the outcomes, although they did not exclude the possibility of an overall "learning curve" considering the novelty of CAS and the changes in technique recommended during the trial. In fact, the 30-day rate of stroke and death in the CAS group was 50% to 100% higher than reported in recent clinical studies involving stenting of the extracranial carotid artery[12,14,15,37,38,39] (H25,13,9,14,23,24). A major critique was of course the poor qualifications of the trial interventionalists.

On the other hand, CREST[12] (H9) recognized this challenge. A lead-in phase is built into the CREST study design to provide clinical centers with start-up and credentialing periods, during which each eligible interventionalist will perform as many as 20 CAS procedures. Results from each interventionalist are reviewed by the Interventional Management Committee (IMC), and committee approval is required before the interventionalist is certified to perform CAS in randomized patients. Each interventionalist who applied for CREST certification is required to submit data on standardized forms about their last 10 to 30 CAS procedures performed with any device. These data are reviewed by the CREST IMC. As a guideline, 30-day stroke and death is to be below 6% to 8%, and technical features are to include use of 0.014 wire systems rather than 0.035 wires, 6F guide sheaths, and initial application of anti-embolic devices. After approval to join CREST and before enrolling patients in the lead-in phase, study interventionalists without previous experience with the ACCULINK or ACCUNET systems are required to participate in a specially designed Carotid Stent Operator Certification Program. This program consists of intensive didactic and hands-on training that focused on the prerequisites for use of carotid stenting and embolic protection devices, and observation of live case demonstrations. The CAS procedures in the lead-in phase are then performed only by

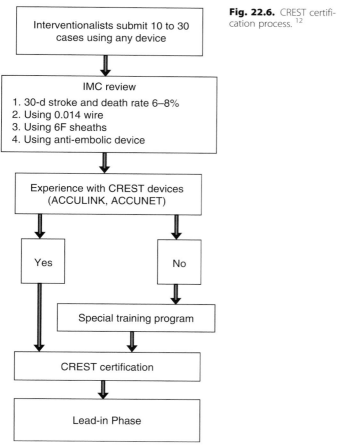

Fig. 22.6. CREST certification process. [12]

CREST-certified study interventionalists (Fig. 22.6 and 22.7). Patients with asymptomatic disease with stenosis of 70% or greater, and patients with symptomatic disease with stenosis 50% or greater are eligible for this lead-in phase. CREST investigators published part of the lead-in phase data in 2004. For events monitored through March 31, 2004, 789 patients had undergone CAS procedures performed by these 134 specialists. Thirty-day stroke and death rate was 4.6%, and MI was observed in 1.1% of patients. Serious adverse events have not been clustered at individual institutions, and no significant differences have been observed between vascular surgeons or neurosurgeons and other credentialed specialists (Cardiologists, Interventional Neuroradiologists, Interventional Radiologists and Neurologists).

Additional requirements for study site investigators include the ability to recruit eligible patients and a willingness to abide by the procedures established by the protocol. Potential investigators may overestimate their abilities to recruit and process study patients; therefore, a review of the demographic characteristics and records of patients treated during a recent calendar period is advisable. Monitoring techniques to ensure compliance with the protocol, with appropriate measures to avoid protocol violations, must be in place.

Clinical protocol: manual of operations

The clinical protocols for baseline evaluations, interventional or surgical procedures, and follow-up monitoring should be specifically defined in the manual of operations. This manual

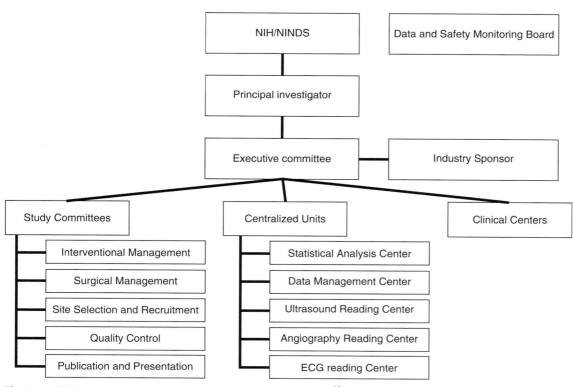

Fig. 22.7. CREST structural organization (modified from Hobson *et al.* 2001).[10]

should be made available to each participating site. The inclusion of standardized data collection forms ensures that all required data are collected for each participant.

Baseline evaluation

The accurate determination of baseline information allows evaluation of subjects' eligibility, stratification (if necessary), descriptive characterization of the target population or determination that the trial sample represents the target population, and measurement of baseline physical and laboratory parameters before the intervention is performed. The assessment of baseline data is important for the identification of prognostic factors that must be approximately balanced among intervention groups. These may include the patient's current disease status, concomitant medication and/or therapy regimens, age, sex, socioeconomic status, disease history, and other factors. The assessment of baseline data allows the selection and implementation of methods that minimize the effects of any potential bias on comparisons of outcome measures. If a prognostic factor is discovered during the course of the trial (not adjusted for with stratification) and if adequate baseline measurements exist, then adjustment or standardization methods can be applied during data analysis to minimize the effects of imbalances on comparisons between treatment groups.

Intervention

A prespecified regimen for the performance of the procedure should be used for every subject. In the SPACE trial,[15] patients allocated to CAS had to be given 100 mg aspirin plus 75 mg clopidogrel daily for at least 3 days before, and 30 days after, the intervention. The use of protection devices, predilation, and balloon size were left to the discretion of the interventional physician. All stent systems, dilation catheters, and protection devices had to have Communite Europeene certification and were approved for use in the study by the trial endovascular standards committee. For patients allocated to CEA, surgeons used their usual operative technique. All patients had to be given at least 100 mg aspirin before, during, and after surgery. Shunting during surgery was optional. Both general and local anesthesia could be used. All patients were examined clinically by the neurologist before and 1 day after surgery or intervention. Follow-up clinical and ultrasound examinations were scheduled after 7 and 30 days, and after 6, 12, and 24 months. In the PROACT II study,[1] placement of a microcatheter proximal to the middle cerebral artery occlusion was mandated for all patients, whether they received intra-arterially administered prourokinase or placebo. Both groups underwent intra-arterial infusion of the study drug and IV administration of heparin.

Follow-up evaluation

Two characteristics of follow-up monitoring are critical, i.e., completeness and duration. Completeness is defined as the proportion of patients entering the trial who return for every follow-up appointment. It is extremely important that this proportion be as close to 100% as possible, because statistical power decreases as patients are lost to follow-up monitoring. Follow-up compliance of less than 80% is generally considered poor and results in an incomplete trial. It is also important for compliance rates to be similar among comparison groups and study sites. Patients lost to follow-up monitoring may be more likely to have experienced poor outcomes or died, which may bias the study if the percentages are not similar for all comparison groups. Therefore, it is essential to determine the health status of all patients entered into the trial, even those who do not return to the clinic for all follow-up appointments, with telephone calls or questionnaires. The duration of follow-up monitoring is the period of time after the intervention during which the study subjects are scheduled to be observed and evaluated. The duration must be long enough for accurate estimation of the rates of known or suspected adverse events. Strategies may be required to adjust for patients lost to follow-up monitoring. In the PROACT II study,[1] the last available assessment was used for patients who missed the 90-day evaluation. For survivors for whom no follow-up data were available, mRS scores corresponding to failure (i.e., scores of 3–6) were imputed. Of the 121 patients randomized to receive intra-arterially administered prourokinase, 111 patients either died or completed follow-up evaluations. Among the ten patients for whom no follow-up data were available, the previous evaluation findings were used to determine the 90-day outcomes for nine patients and treatment was considered a failure for one patient.

Ascertainment of outcomes

Because the results of any study are determined by the accuracy of outcome assessments, it is important for a study to have an outcome that is objectively defined and can be reproducibly assessed. Definitions for events such as stroke, transient ischemic attack, and recurrent hemorrhage were provided in the protocols of the trials discussed in this chapter (Table 22.2). The method by which events are adjudicated varies between trials. In the SPACE trial,[14] outcome events were reviewed by the members of the data center. Additionally, all primary outcome, fatal outcome events and doubtful events were reported to, and adjudicated by, the external safety committee. Any disagreements were resolved by discussion. In the SAPPHIRE trial,[14] major adverse clinical events were adjudicated by an independent, blinded clinical-events committee appointed by the data-coordinating center and composed of neurologists, surgeons, and cardiologists. An independent data and safety monitoring board, not affiliated to the study sponsor or the study investigators, reviewed the data periodically to identify safety concerns. In the IMS III trial, an independent data safety and monitoring board, consisting of clinicians familiar with the treatment of stroke, biostatisticians, a neuro-interventionalist, and other experts has been established by NINDS to monitor the progress of the trial. Additionally, two stroke neurologists have been appointed as internal and external safety monitors. The internal safety monitor will review safety data on an ongoing basis, including monitoring the trend in serious adverse outcome events and submitting FDA Medwatch reports. The external safety monitor, an independent and experienced neurologist, will review all serious life-threatening bleeding events during this study and will be the final adjudicator of intracranial hemorrhage endpoints (symptomatic or asymptomatic and the relationship with study intervention) when there is disagreement between the local site and the internal medical monitor.

Definitions in the mRS [40] were used for ascertainment of primary outcomes in almost all the stroke trials, including the ones presented in this chapter. This is because of high inter-observer agreement. The agreement for differences of one grade on the mRS is 0.56 and that for two grades is 0.91.[40]

Other tools used include the NIHSSS (which reflects neurologic deficit severity rather than functional state), the Glasgow Outcome Scale (GOS),[41] and the Barthel Index (BI)[42] (both assess functional state). In the IMS II trial,[2] the primary measure of outcome was mRS of 0 or 1 at 3 months. Predefined secondary clinical efficacy endpoints included: (1) mRS of 0 to 2 at 3 months; (2) NIHSSS ≤ 2 at 24 hours; (3) other 3-month favorable subject outcomes as measured by a BI score of 95 to 100, GOS score of 0 to 1, and NIHSSS of 0 or 1; (4) quality of life at 3 months as defined by the EuroQol Questionnaire; and (5) a 3-month global outcome that included the mRS, NIHSSS, BI, and GOS. In CREST, performance of neurological status questionnaires will be handed to patients at baseline, 30 days and 6 months post-procedure. All patients with a positive neurological status questionnaire will be evaluated by a neurologist.

Data and safety monitoring and interim analyses

Any clinical trial is based on several initial assumptions, and it is not unusual that one or more of those assumptions are discovered to be incorrect after the trial has begun. An external data and safety monitoring committee is responsible for monitoring all aspects of the study, including aspects requiring access to blinded data. The committee includes experts not otherwise involved in the study, i.e., an independent group of clinical trialists, statisticians, stroke specialists, and patient advocates. The committee reviews the data from interim analyses at prespecified intervals, to assess the progress of the study. The committee may recommend the discontinuation of any treatment arm at any time for any of the following reasons.[29]

1. Compelling evidence from this or any other study of an adverse effect of the study treatment that is sufficient to override any potential benefit of the intervention for the target population.
2. Compelling evidence from this or any other study of a significant beneficial effect of the study treatment such that

continued denial to the other study group(s) would be unethical.
3. A very low probability of answering the study question within a reasonable time frame. If the new therapy is not widely used, then a negative trend with little chance of demonstrating a benefit might be reason to terminate the trial or even dismiss the therapy as not being of further interest. As previously mentioned, a futility analysis may be planned earlier in the study, to stop the clinical trial before the scheduled time if the treatment in question is found to be highly ineffective, thus exposing as few patient as possible to an ineffective therapy.

In the EVA-3S trail,[13] the trial was stopped early for reasons of both safety and futility. The 30-day risk of any stroke or death was significantly higher after CAS (9.6%) than after CEA (3.9%), resulting in a relative risk of 2.5 (95% CI, 1.2 to 5.1). The excess of primary outcome events after CAS was considered large enough (one additional stroke or death among each 17 patients treated by CAS) for the safety committee to recommend stopping the trial. In addition, the observed rates of the primary outcome made it very unlikely that the trial would show the non-inferiority of CAS (futility).

In the IMS II study,[2] the primary analysis of futility was conducted by 1-sample test for binomial proportions using normal approximation. Given the statistical parameters, the null hypothesis would be rejected if <22% subjects had a favorable outcome at 3 months. Because 33% of IMS II subjects had favorable outcome (mRS of 0 to 1), the futility criterion was not met.

Analysis and interpretation of results

The data in most clinical trials are analyzed on the basis of an intention to treat. This is an analytic approach that compares outcomes with every subject being analyzed according to the randomized group assignment. It is important to realize that patients randomized to a new procedure might not have actually received that treatment or might have, in effect, changed study groups (i.e., crossed over to the other treatment group). Figures 22.1 to 22.5 provide a detailed account of the numbers of patients who did not receive the treatment allocated or crossed over in the studies highlighted in this article. In addition, patients lost to follow-up monitoring must be counted as though they actually completed the study in their assigned group. Because no outcome can be observed after the patient is lost to follow-up monitoring, the therapy cannot be counted as a success and is considered a failure for such patients in an intention-to-treat analysis. Although an intention-to-treat analysis is the only type of analysis that preserves the integrity of randomization, other types of analyses may be considered in certain circumstances. In the SAPPHIRE trial,[14] 747 patients were enrolled in the study, and 334 patients underwent randomization. Of the 413 patients who were not randomly

Table 22.4. Characteristics of an optimal Phase III clinical trial of a new procedure

Background

- *Sufficient evidence (observational studies, previous relevant research, Phase I and II trials) exists to justify the need for evaluation of a new procedure (equipoise).*
- *Adequate experience has accrued (technical maturation), and the timing of the trial is appropriate.*

Objective

- *A primary objective measure of efficacy has been defined.*
- *A quantitative difference has been specified to define the superiority of one procedure over another.*
- *The patient population to be studied has been specified.*

Study population

- *Representative of the target population, relatively homogeneous, accessible, and readily identifiable with explicit inclusion and exclusion criteria.*
- *Feasible to study, with the lowest possible ratio of eligible non-randomized patients to eligible randomized patients.*

Sample size and statistical power

- *α level and statistical power ($1-\beta$).*
- *Planned interim analyses as a component of the study plan.*
- *Anticipated rate of events in the control group (on the basis of available data).*
- *Magnitude of difference necessary to define clinically meaningful superiority.*
- *Variability of the efficacy variable under consideration.*

Methods of assignment

- *Allocation concealment.*
- *Randomization, with or without stratification.*

Masking (or blinding)

- *Methods of blinding undertaken to avoid investigator and patient bias in post-procedural care and ascertainment of outcomes.*

Identification and selection of variables

- *Objective criteria for defining outcomes and influencing variables.*
- *Rationale for selection of outcomes and influencing variables.*

Study centers and investigators

- *Participating centers have investigators with adequate expertise (objective criteria).*
- *Participating centers possess the necessary organizational resources.*

Trial monitoring

- *External body performs independent auditing to verify conformity with eligibility criteria, recruitment and outcome data, and reporting of adverse events.*
- *External body reports to the principal investigators and the data and safety monitoring committee.*

Clinical protocol: manual of operations

- *Protocol for baseline evaluation. Any baseline data that might influence the results of the intervention or the overall prognosis are collected.*
- *Protocol for intervention. Trials may vary in defining the extent of specific steps for intervention. Standardization is important for components of the intervention or treatment that can affect the success or failure of the procedure.*
- *Protocol for follow-up evaluations, based on objective evidence suggesting that enough patients would reach the primary end points for a meaningful comparison.*

Ascertainment of outcomes

- *Outcomes must be objectively defined and reproducibly ascertained.*
- *An independent body of investigators must adjudicate the outcomes.*

Table 22.4. *(cont.)*

- *Adjudication preferably occurs at multiple levels.*

- *A structured system exists for determining, managing, monitoring, and reporting the occurrence of adverse events.*

- *Protocols for referring and/or treating subjects experiencing adverse events are available.*

Data and safety monitoring and interim analyses

- *Discontinue trial if there is compelling evidence from this or any other study of an adverse effect of the study treatment that is sufficient to override any potential benefit of the new procedure.*

- *Discontinue trial if there is compelling evidence from this or any other study of a significant beneficial effect of the new procedure, such that not offering it to other study group(s) would be unethical.*

- *Discontinue trial if there is a very low probability of addressing the study hypothesis within a feasible time frame.*

Analysis and interpretation of results

- *Outcome analysis, intention-to-treat, or target population analysis, with parametric or non-parametric methods.*

- *Method for analyzing the data for patients who did not receive the allocated intervention or treatment, crossed over to the other treatment arm, withdrew from the study, or were lost to follow-up monitoring.*

- *Rates of outcomes for each group, actual rate versus a rate predicted using survival analysis.*

- *Post hoc analysis to confirm uniformity among different clinical subgroups and participating centers.*

assigned to treatment, 406 were entered into the stent registry and seven were entered into the surgical registry. Of the 167 patients randomly assigned to stenting, 159 received the assigned treatment, while eight patients did not. Of the 167 patients assigned to surgery, 151 received the assigned treatment, while 16 patients did not. All 334 patients were followed. Data was analyzed using the intention to treat analysis with 167 patients in both the CAS and the CEA groups, and using the actual treatment analysis with only 159 patients in the CAS group and 151 patients in the CEA group (Table 22.3).

An understanding of comparisons of actual and estimated rates of outcome events is important. Trials may have a short follow-up period, as in the PROACT II study,[1] in which final outcomes were determined at 90 days after treatment. With such study designs, the investigators can wait until all patients have completed the 90-day follow-up period and then determine the rates of the primary endpoint for each group. At the time of the 90-day follow-up evaluation for the PROACT II study,[1] the primary endpoint (mRS scores of 0–2) was achieved by 40% of 121 patients randomized to receive pro-urokinase and 25% of 59 patients randomized to receive placebo.

In trials involving longer follow-up periods, randomized patients are in various stages of follow-up monitoring at a given time. Interim analyses can be complex, because the proportion of patients who have reached the 2- or 5-year endpoint may not be sufficient for statistically valid analyses for years. Investigators have used other methods to predict the rates of primary endpoint events on the basis of available data, to avoid unnecessarily continuing a trial and exposing patients to excess risk. Rates can be predicted with Kaplan–Meier survival curve estimates at 2 or 5 years or at any time point specified by the investigators. In survival analyses, the time

between the date of randomization and the last follow-up observation before analysis is recorded for each patient who is alive and has not experienced a primary endpoint event.[43] The percentage of survivors who have not experienced a primary event at the end of a specified interval (such as each month or at 1 yr) is used to estimate the probability that a typical patient will be alive without experiencing a primary endpoint event at the end of a given period.[43] The endpoint variable in survival analyses is actually the time to the event, not the event itself.

Parametric tests such as Student's *t* test and analysis of variance are used to compare the outcomes between the treatment and control groups. Parametric tests require that the outcome measure is normally distributed and sample sizes are close to equal between the two groups. If outcomes are not normally distributed, or if sample sizes are not equal, then non-parametric tests such as the Wilcoxon and Mann–Whitney tests are used.

Study subjects at different investigational sites are typically pooled, to obtain an adequate sample size for a clinical trial. Pooling must be justified by testing the balance of prognostic factors and verifying that all clinical procedures were performed in the manner prescribed in the protocol. On occasion, data acquired at one study site exhibit characteristics that distinguish them from data obtained at other sites. The trial coordinating center must investigate all relevant effects associated with that particular site and report on those instances, to determine the cause of the discrepancy. In the SPACE trail,[15] 50% of patients were recruited from seven centers. Three centers recruited more than 100 patients, six centers between 50 and 99, and 26 centers less than 50 patients. In the EVA-3S trial,[13] the homogeneity of the relative risks of stroke or death among centers was assessed using the Breslow–Day test. For this purpose, centers were categorized into three groups, based on the number of patients included in the study (<21, 21 to 40, and >40 patients). The relative risk of stroke or death did not differ significantly among the centers that enrolled fewer than 21 patients (relative risk, 1.9; 95% CI, 0.6 to 6.2), those that enrolled 21 to 40 patients (relative risk, 3.3; 95% CI, 0.7 to 15.2), and those that enrolled more than 40 patients (relative risk, 2.7; 95% CI, 0.9 to 8.1) (P = 0.83).

The participation of small centers increased the intercenter variance and diminished the quality of the data. Intercenter differences can be unavoidable because of variations in demographic characteristics and disease severity among study patients (e.g., older patients or patients with complex diseases referred for tertiary care). Variations in the management protocol among centers may also be responsible for differences.

Conclusions

Ongoing and future clinical trials will shape the practice of surgery and endovascular therapy for cerebrovascular diseases. A summary of the characteristics of an optimal Phase III randomized trial is presented in Table 22.4. A basic understanding of the designs and methods of clinical trials is essential for practitioners who are involved in the planning and execution of such trials and who will ultimately be responsible for implementation of the results in clinical practice.

References

1. Furlan A, Higashida R, Wechsler L, *et al.* Intra-arterial prourokinase for acute ischemic stroke. The proact ii study: a randomized controlled trial. Prolyse in acute cerebral thromboembolism. *J Am Med Assoc* 1999;**282**:2003–11.

2. The interventional management of stroke (ims) ii study. *Stroke* 2007;**38**:2127–35.

3. Tomsick T, Broderick J, Carrozella J, *et al.* Revascularization results in the interventional management of stroke ii trial. *Am J Neuroradiol* 2008;**29**:582–7.

4. Mauldin PS, Palesch, YY, Spilker, JS, Hill, MD, Khatri, P; Broderick, JP. Design of the economic evaluation for the interventional management of stroke (iii) trial. *Int J Stroke* 2008;**3**:138–44.

5. Khatri PH, Palesch, YY, Spilker, J, *et al.* Methodology of the interventional management of stroke iii trial. *Int J Stroke* 2008;**3**:130–7.

6. Hobson RW, 2nd. Crest (carotid revascularization endarterectomy versus stent trial): background, design, and current status. *Semin Vasc Surg* 2000;**13**:139–43.

7. Hobson RW, 2nd. Update on the carotid revascularization endarterectomy versus stent trial (crest) protocol. *J Am Coll Surg* 2002;**194**:S9–14.

8. Hobson RW, 2nd. Rationale and status of randomized controlled clinical trials in carotid artery stenting. *Semin Vasc Surg* 2003;**16**:311–16

9. Hobson RW, 2nd, Brott TG, Roubin GS, Silver FL, Barnett HJ. Carotid artery stenting: Meeting the recruitment challenge of a clinical trial. *Stroke* 2005;**36**:1314–15.

10. Hobson RW, 2nd, Howard VJ, Brott TG, Howard G, Roubin GS, Ferguson RD. Organizing the carotid revascularization endarterectomy versus stenting trial (crest): national institutes of health, health care financing administration, and industry funding. *Curr Control Trials Cardiovasc Med* 2001;**2**:160–4.

11. Hobson RW, 2nd, Howard VJ, Roubin GS, *et al.* Carotid artery stenting is associated with increased complications in octogenarians: 30-day stroke and death rates in the crest lead-in phase. *J Vasc Surg* 2004;**40**:1106–11.

12. Hobson RW, 2nd, Howard VJ, Roubin GS, *et al.* Credentialing of surgeons as interventionalists for carotid artery stenting: experience from the lead-in phase of crest. *J Vasc Surg* 2004;**40**:952–7.

13. Mas JL, Chatellier G, Beyssen B, *et al.* Endarterectomy versus stenting in patients with symptomatic severe carotid stenosis. *N Engl J Med* 2006;**355**:1660–71.

14. Yadav JS, Wholey MH, Kuntz RE, *et al.* Protected carotid-artery stenting versus endarterectomy in high-risk patients. *N Engl J Med* 2004;**351**:1493–501.

15. Ringleb PA, Allenberg J, Bruckmann H, *et al.* 30 day results from the space trial of stent-protected angioplasty versus carotid endarterectomy in symptomatic patients: a randomised non-inferiority trial. *Lancet* 2006;**368**:1239–47.

16. Friedman LMFC, DeMets DL. *Fundamentals of Clinical Trials.* St. Louis: Mosby Year Book, 1985.

17. Schwartz JS. Clinical economics and noncoronary vascular disease. *J Vasc Interv Radiol* 1995;**6**:116S–4S.

18. Meakins JL. Innovation in surgery: the rules of evidence. *Am J Surg* 2002;**183**:399–405.

19. Freedman B. Equipoise and the ethics of clinical research. *N Engl J Med.* 1987;**317**:141–5.

20. Kwiatkowski TG, Libman RB, Frankel M, *et al.* Effects of tissue plasminogen activator for acute ischemic stroke at one year. National institute of neurological disorders and stroke recombinant tissue plasminogen activator stroke study group. *N Engl J Med* 1999;**340**:1781–1787.

21. Naylor AR, Bolia A, Abbott RJ, *et al.* Randomized study of carotid angioplasty and stenting versus carotid endarterectomy: A stopped trial. *J Vasc Surg* 1998;**28**:326–334.

22. Begg C, Cho M, Eastwood S, *et al.* Improving the quality of reporting of randomized controlled trials. The consort statement. *J Am Med Assoc* 1996;**276**:637–639.

23. Institute NIoHaC. Cancer clinical trials: The in-depth program.

24. Administration USFaD. *Statistical Guidance for Clinical Trials of Non-Diagnostic Medical Devices.* Washington, DC: United States Food and Drug Administration, 1996.

25. Flaherty ML, Woo D, Kissela B, *et al.* Combined iv and intra-arterial thrombolysis for acute ischemic stroke. *Neurology* 2005;**64**:386–8.

26. North American symptomatic carotid endarterectomy trial. Methods, patient

characteristics, and progress. *Stroke* 1991;**22**:711–720.

27. Rothwell PM, Eliasziw M, Gutnikov SA, *et al.* Analysis of pooled data from the randomised controlled trials of endarterectomy for symptomatic carotid stenosis. *Lancet* 2003;**361**:107–16.

28. Molyneux A KR, Stratton I, Sandercock P, Clarke M, Shrimpton J, Holman. International subarachnoid aneurysm trial (isat) of neurosurgical clipping versus endovascular coiling in 2143 patients with ruptured intracranial aneurysms: A randomised trial. *Lancet* 2002;**360**:1267–74.

29. Qureshi AI, Hutson AD, Harbaugh RE, Stieg PE, Hopkins LN. Methods and design considerations for randomized clinical trials evaluating surgical or endovascular treatments for cerebrovascular diseases. *Neurosurgery* 2004;**54**:248–264; discussion 264–7.

30. Lewis RJ. An introduction to the use of interim data analyses in clinical trials. *Ann Emerg Med* 1993;**22**:1463–9.

31. Thijs VN, Lansberg MG, Beaulieu C, Marks MP, Moseley ME, Albers GW. Is early ischemic lesion volume on diffusion-weighted imaging an independent predictor of stroke outcome? A multivariable analysis. *Stroke* 2000;**31**:2597–602.

32. Schulz KF, Chalmers I, Altman DG. The landscape and lexicon of blinding in randomized trials. *Ann Intern Med* 2002;**136**:254–259.

33. Schulz KF, Chalmers I, Hayes RJ, Altman DG. Empirical evidence of bias. Dimensions of methodological quality associated with estimates of treatment effects in controlled trials. *J Am Med Assoc* 1995;**273**:408–12.

34. Hill B. *Principles of Medical Statistics.* New York: Oxford University Press, 1967.

35. Matchar DB DP. Cost of stroke. *Stroke Clin Updates.* 1994;**5**:9–12.

36. Beneficial effect of carotid endarterectomy in symptomatic patients with high-grade carotid stenosis. North american symptomatic carotid endarterectomy trial collaborators. *N Engl J Med* 1991;**325**:445–53.

37. Qureshi AI. Carotid angioplasty and stent placement after eva-3s trial. *Stroke* 2007;**38**:1993–6.

38. Schreiber TL CS, Massop D, Kumar V, Davis T, Ramee S. Report of the cases-pms study: patient demographics and 30-day major adverse events for the cordis precise nitinol stent and angioguardtm emboli capture guidewire condition of approval surveillance study. *The American College of Cardiology 55th Annual Scientific Session*, 2006.

39. Gray WA, Yadav JS, Verta P, *et al.* The capture registry: Results of carotid stenting with embolic protection in the post approval setting. *Catheter Cardiovasc Interv* 2007;**69**:341–8.

40. van Swieten JC, Koudstaal PJ, Visser MC, Schouten HJ, van Gijn J. Interobserver agreement for the assessment of handicap in stroke patients. *Stroke* 1988;**19**:604–7.

41. Teasdale G, Knill-Jones R, van der Sande J. Observer variability in assessing impaired consciousness and coma. *J Neurol Neurosurg Psychiatry* 1978;**41**:603–10.

42. Mahoney FI, Barthel DW. Functional evaluation: The barthel index. *Md State Med J.* 1965;**14**:61–65.

43. Lang TA, Secic M. How to Report Statistics in Medicine. *Annotated guidelines for authors, editors and reviewers.* Philadelphia: American College of Physicians, 1997.

Chapter 23

Qualification requirements for performing neuro-interventional procedures

Adnan I. Qureshi, Alex Abou-Chebl and Tudor G. Jovin

The chapter summarizes the existing data derived from regulatory bodies, professional organizations, and clinical trials with direct pertinence to indications and qualifications required for performing neurointerventional procedures and provide recommendations regarding qualifications required for performing individual neurointerventional procedures. Most of the text is reproduced from a previous publication from *Journal of Neuroimaging*[1] with permission. Endovascular procedures that have been introduced and improved upon over the last decade include carotid, vertebral and intracranial angioplasty and stent placement, intra-arterial thrombolysis, endovascular treatment of intracranial aneurysms using detachable coils and liquid embolic agents, embolization for arteriovenous malformations and neoplasms, endovascular treatment of vasospasm following subarachnoid hemorrhage, and intra-arterial chemotherapy for neoplasms.[2] The advent of interventional neurology as a subspecialty has created an opportunity for vascular neurologists to play an active role in the procedural aspects of diagnosis and management of cerebrovascular diseases. The need for training of vascular neurologists to perform diagnostic and interventional neuroimaging procedures has been recognized by the Accreditation Council for Graduate Medical Education (ACGME) by including vascular neurology among the three specialties in which physicians may pursue training in the newly recognized discipline of Endovascular Surgical Neuroradiology.[3]

The common ground shared by all professional societal statements is that there are three components of credentialing: cognitive, procedural, and clinical knowledge.[4] Almost all interventional neurologists with vascular neurology training will have all of the requisite cognitive and clinical skills. Vascular neurologists receive extensive training in clinical aspects of cerebrovascular disease using a well defined curriculum specified by the Accreditation Council for Graduate Medical Education (ACGME). The real question, therefore, is what is needed in terms of procedural (i.e., technical) training to obtain appropriate credentials and subsequently be granted privileges for performing individual procedures for

interventional neurologists. Specifically, "credentialing" (assuring professional competency) demonstrates that the qualification to perform the requested procedures exists and "privileges" (permission to perform procedures) are specific patient care responsibilities afforded to an individual practitioner by the hospital. Although used interchangeably, credentialing is a pre-requisite for obtaining privileges.

Specific aims of the present document

1. To develop a comprehensive document that summarizes the existing data derived from regulatory bodies, professional organizations, and clinical trials with direct pertinence to indications and qualifications required for performing endovascular procedures for cerebrovascular, other head and neck diseases, and spine interventions.
2. To provide recommendations based on review of existing data regarding qualifications required for performing individual neurointerventional procedures.

Need for the present document
Interventional neurology as a new sub-specialty of neurology

The advent of endovascular treatments for cerebrovascular diseases inspired many neurologists to take an interest in performing these procedures. This was a natural bridge between their involvements in patient selection and post-procedural management. With more training opportunities available, it is now expected that, in the next 5 years, there will be more than 50 interventional neurologists in the US.[5] Currently, the majority of neurology departments are not oriented towards invasive procedures and therefore lack experience in credentialing and auditing for interventional procedures. To circumvent this shortcoming, one option for graduating interventional neurology fellows is to be employed and credentialed under departments of radiology or neurosurgery. Although practical in the short term, this strategy will eventually limit

Textbook of Interventional Neurology, ed. Adnan I. Qureshi. Published by Cambridge University Press. © Cambridge University Press 2011.
Reproduced from Qureshi AI, Abou-Chebl A, Jovin TG. *J Neuroimaging* 2008;**18**:433–67, with permission.

involvement of neurology departments in the subspecialty. The present document is expected to serve as a template to assist neurology departments in developing credentialing criteria in conjunction with their respective hospital administrations.

Procedure-specific credentialing in hospitals

Because of the multidisciplinary nature of neuro-interventional procedures, physicians from different backgrounds are requesting privileges.[6] Credentialing committees in hospitals are sensitive to the problems of providing credentials under a broad category of "neuro-interventional procedures." The variety of procedures that are included under that category are diverse and competency in one procedure does not necessarily mean equivalent competency in others. Based on these considerations, hospitals are moving towards "procedure-specific credentialing." This change in paradigm has necessitated development of new documentation to provide more details for requiring training experience in each procedure. The concept of procedure-specific credentialing is consistent with the recommendations of accrediting organizations and professional associations that support well-defined criteria that judge experience and competency rather than evidence of certification, fellowship, or membership in a specialty body or society. There is also an increasing need to define privileging criteria for neurointerventional procedures that are new to the hospital and for which no privileging criteria currently exist. Establishing procedure-specific credentialing ensures that the eligibility to exercise a new procedure is determined by ascertaining competence, rather than promoting or limiting access to any particular specialty.

Lack of ACGME accredited programs

The ACGME, in June 2000, officially approved the Guidelines for Training in Endovascular Surgical Neuroradiology (as outlined later).[3] Since the inception of the guidelines, only four programs have achieved ACGME accreditation. The three programs represent only a fraction of the 42 existing Endovascular Surgical Neuroradiology programs in the US according to the list of all active programs provided by the American Society of Interventional and Therapeutic Neuroradiology (ASITN)[7] and 10 programs provided by the Interventional Section of the American Academy of Neurology. Therefore, most graduates and practicing endovascular physicians will not graduate from ACGME approved programs. Standardization of training for each procedure is limited by the lack of ACGME accreditation. The ACGME document also lacks details about the adequacy of training for each procedure and only provides a total number of endovascular procedures as a measure of adequate training.

Variations in guidelines from different professional organizations

Although originally this document targeted all physicians performing endovascular procedures, including interventional neurologists, the members of the Society of Vascular and

Interventional Neurology perceived the need to have a document that is specific for interventional neurologists. This is because the American College of Cardiology Foundation (ACCF), the Society for Cardiovascular Angiography and Interventions (SCAI), the Society for Clinical Vascular Surgery (SCVS), the Society for Vascular Medicine and Biology (SVMB), and the Society for Vascular Surgery (SVS) have published a separate document that has different credentialing criteria.[8,9] This lack of agreement amongst the professional societies has only added to the confusion despite the requirement by the Joint Commission on Accreditation of Healthcare Organizations (JCAHO) that criteria used to grant procedural privileges be uniformly and individually applied.[10] It is critical that each of the representative societies establish its own set of responsible guidelines for credentialing requirements for multidisciplinary procedures with the understanding that the final decision will be made locally.[11] The differences in backgrounds can be important. For instance, practitioners experienced in coronary, renal, lower extremity, and subclavian interventions may require fewer procedures to become proficient in carotid stent placement compared with those without such experience. However, practitioners who manage patients with cerebrovascular diseases as part of clinical practice may not need formal education in the cognitive and clinical skills component of the required training.

Published position statements on hospital privileges for procedures

The American Medical Association

The American Medical Association provides broad recommendations about hospital privileges (http://www.ama-assn.org/ama/pub/category/8345.html) as follows:

> The mutual objective of both the governing board and the medical staff is to improve the quality and efficiency of patient care in the hospital. Decisions regarding hospital privileges should be based upon the training, experience, and demonstrated competence of candidates, taking into consideration the availability of facilities and the overall medical needs of the community, the hospital, and especially patients. Privileges should not be based on numbers of patients admitted to the facility or the economic or insurance status of the patient. Personal friendships, antagonisms, jurisdictional disputes, or fear of competition should not play a role in making these decisions.

The American Medical Association also provides recommendations for accreditation (http://www.ama-assn.org/ama/pub/category/8516.html) as follows:

> Physicians who engage in activities that involve the accreditation, approval, or certification of institutions, facilities, and programs that provide patient care or medical education or certify the attainment of specialized professional competence have the ethical responsibility to apply standards that are relevant, fair, reasonable, and non-discriminatory. The accreditation of institutions and facilities that provide patient care should be based upon standards

that focus upon the quality of patient care achieved. Standards used in the accreditation of patient care and medical education, or the certification of specialized professional attainment should not be adopted or used as a means of economic regulation.

Pertinent to the performance of neurointerventional procedures is the recommendations on new medical procedures (http://www.ama-assn.org/ama/pub/category/8540.html) which state:

> Physicians have an obligation to share their knowledge and skills and to report the results of clinical and laboratory research. Both positive and negative studies should be included even though they may not support the author's hypothesis. This tradition enhances patient care, leads to the early evaluation of new technologies, and permits the rapid dissemination of improved techniques. The intentional withholding of new medical knowledge, skills, and techniques from colleagues for reasons of personal gain is detrimental to the medical profession and to society and is to be condemned.

The Joint Commission on Accreditation of Healthcare Organizations and the Centers for Medicare & Medicaid Services

The JCAHO, in its Accreditation Manual for Hospitals,[10] states that the criteria used to determine grants of privileges or medical staff membership must be designed to help establish an applicant's background, current competence, and physical and mental ability to discharge patient care responsibilities. Decisions on membership and granting of privileges must consider criteria that are directly related to the quality of health care, treatment, and services. If privileging criteria are used that are unrelated to quality of care, treatment, and services or professional competence, evidence exists that the impact of resulting decisions on the quality of care, treatment, and services is evaluated. The organized medical staff must have a credentialing process that is defined in the medical staff bylaws. The credentialing process must examine documentation of current licensure, relevant training or experience, and current competence. The documentation of current competence should address the types of operative procedures performed as the surgeon of record, or the skill demonstrated in performing invasive procedures, including information on appropriateness and outcomes for applicants in fields performing operative and other procedure(s).

The Centers for Medicare & Medicaid Services requires that the hospital's privileging process must be in compliance with the hospital Conditions of Participation and the process must be approved by the hospital's Governing Body (http://www.healthynh.com/nhha/nh_hospitals/ruralhealth/cah%20downloads/SC%2005–04%20Medical%20Staff%20Privileging.pdf). The hospital's Medical Staff bylaws must describe the privileging process to be used in the hospital. The process must include criteria for determining the privileges that may be granted to individual practitioners and a procedure for applying the criteria to individual practitioners. Any procedure privilege requested by and recommended for a practitioner beyond the specified list of privileges for their particular category of practitioner would require evidence of additional qualifications and competencies, and be a procedure that the hospital can support and is conducted within the hospital. The hospital's Governing Body and Medical staff must assure that every individual practitioner who provides a medical level of care and/or who conducts surgical procedures in the hospital is competent to perform all granted privileges. The bodies should also ensure the criteria for selection are individual character, competence, training, experience, and judgment; and not dependent solely upon certification, fellowship, or membership in a specialty body or society.

Published position statements on neuro-interventional procedures

The Accreditation Council for Graduate Medical Education

Endovascular surgical neuroradiology is a subspecialty that uses catheter technology, radiological imaging, and clinical expertise to diagnose and treat diseases of the central nervous system. The ACGME, in June 2000, officially approved the Guidelines for Training in endovascular surgical neuroradiology.[3] The radiology residency review committee (RRC), neurosurgery RRC, and neurology RRC agreed to submit program requirements in endovascular surgical neuroradiology for applicants from neurology in a timely fashion in a correspondence dated May 23, 2000. Subsequently, the program requirements for neurology were approved by the ACGME in May 2003.

The unique clinical and invasive nature of this subspecialty requires special training and skills. The objective of the training is to give residents an organized, comprehensive, supervised, one-year full-time educational experience in endovascular surgical neuroradiology. This experience includes the management of patients with neurological disease, the performance of neurointerventional procedures, and the integration of neurointerventional treatments into the clinical management of patients. The program must perform at least 100 therapeutic neurointerventional procedures per year, including treatment of aneurysms, brain and spine arteriovenous malformation, arteriovenous fistulas, tumors of the central nervous system, occlusive vascular diseases, revascularization, traumatic injury, maxillofacial vascular malformations, tumors and pathologic compression fracture of the spine. In addition, the program must provide adequate training and experience in invasive functional testing.

Residents entering from a neurology background must have fulfilled the following preparatory requirements:

1. Completed an ACGME-accredited residency in neurology.
2. Completed an ACGME-accredited 1-year vascular neurology program.[12]

3. Completed a 3-month course in basic radiology skills acceptable to the program director where the neuroradiology training will occur. The basic radiology skills and neuroradiology training may be acquired during elective time in the neurology residency.

4. Completed 3 months of clinical experience in an ACGME-accredited neurological surgery program, which may be acquired during elective time in neurology and/or vascular neurology training.

5. Completed at least 12 months of training, preferably consecutive, in neuroradiology. Candidates who do not come from a radiology training program shall have access to a 1–year period of training in neuroradiology in the institution sponsoring the endovascular surgical neuroradiology program. The purpose of this preparatory year is to gain experience in performance and interpretation of diagnostic cerebral angiography.

The Neurovascular Coalition: AAN, AANS, ASITN, ASNR, CNS, SIR

The American Academy of Neurology (AAN) has previously endorsed a carotid angioplasty and stent placement credentialing document prepared by the Neurovascular Coalition Writing Group.[9] This group includes the AAN, the American Association of Neurological Surgeons (AANS), ASITN, the American Society of Neuroradiology (ASNR), the Congress of Neurological Surgeons (CNS), the AANS/CNS Cerebrovascular Section, and the Society of Interventional Radiology (SIR). All collaborating neuroscience societies are of the unanimous opinion that the safety of the patient is paramount and to that end they have agreed on the following.

1. Defined formal training and experience in both the cognitive and technical aspects of the neurosciences are essential for the performance and interpretation of diagnostic and therapeutic cervical and cerebrovascular procedures. Therefore, in addition to procedural technical experience requirements, a minimum of 6 months of formal cognitive neuroscience training is required in an approved program in radiology, neuroradiology, neurosurgery, neurology, and/or vascular neurology for any practitioner performing cervical carotid interventional therapy.

2. All collaborating neuroscience societies endorse the principles of the several published standards from various societies for training and quality concerning cervicocerebral angiography and intervention. Credentialing to perform (and in some cases interpret) cervicocerebral angiograms for one single purpose (e.g., evaluation of carotid occlusive disease) theoretically approves performance and interpretation for all purposes or neurovascular conditions without distinction, some of which are: cerebrovascular trauma, vasculitis, congenital vascular malformations, venous anomalies, tumors, mass

effects, identification of embolic complications, differentiation of acute/subacute/chronic dissection from atherosclerotic disease, diagnosis of arteritides, identification of intracerebral aneurysms, and normal anatomical variation. Interpretative skills cannot be adequately conferred by casual training and experience. Therefore, limited credentialing for limited procedures with limited training is unacceptable.

3. All collaborating neuroscience societies recommend appropriately supervised cervicocerebral angiography training and resultant credentialing with an accumulated total of 100 diagnostic cervicocerebral angiograms before post-graduate training in cervicocerebral interventional procedures, including carotid stent placement.

4. All collaborating neuroscience societies specifically endorse the principles outlined by the ACGME for developing specialized training programs in endovascular surgical neuroradiology, vascular neurology and neurosurgery.

The Brain Attack Coalition

The Brain Attack Coalition[13] identified the following requirements for a comprehensive stroke center.

1. Health care personnel with specific expertise in a number of disciplines, including neurosurgery and vascular neurology.

2. Advanced neuroimaging capabilities such as magnetic resonance imaging (MRI) and various types of cerebral angiography.

3. Surgical and endovascular techniques, including clipping and coiling of intracranial aneurysms, carotid endarterectomy, and intra-arterial thrombolytic therapy.

4. Other specific infrastructure and programmatic elements such as an intensive care unit and a stroke registry.

A neurointerventional specialist was recommended as a necessary component of a comprehensive stroke center. An individual with such expertise is capable of performing extracranial and intracranial angioplasty and stenting for atherosclerosis or vasospasm and emergency catheter-directed intra-arterial stroke therapy. The endovascular treatment of patients with cerebral aneurysms, arteriovenous malformations, and arteriovenous fistulas requires these specialized skills. These neurointerventional procedures are technically and cognitively demanding and should only be performed by physicians with formal and specific training (or equivalent experience) in neurointerventional therapy, working in coordination with a multidisciplinary team. The Brain Attack Coalition recommends that the neurointerventional specialists accrue significant experience in a procedure because past studies have shown that more experience and an increasing number of procedures reduce complication rates.

It was recommended that a multidisciplinary team evaluate patients before and after some of the endovascular procedures outlined above to discuss treatment options and assess for complications during and after the intervention. A registry should be established to track treatments, outcomes, and complications. A quality assurance process should confirm that procedures and therapies are performed for appropriate indications, with rates of success and complications that meet acceptable standards. The committee should define a list of appropriate indicators that would trigger automatic chart review. When case reviews find significant deviations in the standards of care, the committee should recommend corrective action through appropriate methods.

Reviews of specific procedures
Cerebral digital subtraction angiography

Fundamental to the procedure-based practice of cerebrovascular disorders is acquiring proficiency in performance and interpretation of diagnostic cerebral angiography. This procedure is not only the gold standard for diagnosis of many vascular conditions affecting the brain,[14] but competence in performance and interpretation of diagnostic cerebral angiography is also a prerequisite for those who wish to pursue training in neurointerventional procedures. An estimated 133 883 cerebral angiograms are performed in the US every year by physicians from multiple disciplines.[15]

Training guidelines for digital subtraction angiography are officially stated by numerous medical societies, including the American Heart Association (AHA), the Society of Vascular Surgery (SVS), and Society of Interventional Radiology (SIR).[8,9,16–20] Physicians with expertise in diagnostic cerebral angiography must possess many of the cognitive skills required of the vascular specialist. Expertise in diagnostic cerebral angiography also requires knowledge of the indications, limitations, and complications of these procedures and an understanding of alternative diagnostic methods. Individuals performing diagnostic cerebral angiography must be aware of the risks and benefits for each procedure. Catheter-based procedures require knowledge of radiation physics and skills in operating radiographic imaging equipment. Knowledge and expertise regarding methods to achieve hemostasis and alternatives to manual compression such as compression devices and vascular closure devices are required, as is knowledge about the effect of local anesthesia and about conscious sedation. The ability to recognize and to manage procedure-related complications such as access site bleeding, arteriovenous fistula, pseudoaneurysm, infection, distal embolization, vessel rupture or occlusion, acute renal failure, and cholesterol embolization, is required.

A prerequisite for interventional training is the ability to perform and interpret cerebral angiograms. The ACGME Training Guidelines for neuroradiology stipulate that fellows be involved in 50 catheter angiograms during their training[21]. However, the Neuroimaging Section of the AAN and a joint statement of ASITN, Joint Section for Cerebrovascular Neurosurgery, CNS, ASNR, and the Ad Hoc Writing Group[4,16,17]

have suggested that trainees participate in a minimum of 100 diagnostic angiograms prior to being credentialed or prior to beginning neurointerventional training. The Neurovascular Coalition[9] stated that operator experience as measured by decreased complications and decreased fluoroscopy time necessary for the exam improves in a linear fashion up to 100 procedures. The statement further suggested that analysis of the trainee learning curve suggests that 200 procedures are necessary for a physician to become a competent and secure examiner of the carotid and intracranial vasculature. The statement further stated that effect of training and experience, and/or lack thereof, has been shown in previous analysis that demonstrated that fellowship-trained specialists have fewer neurological complications than even experienced angiographers, and both have far fewer complications than trainees under supervision. In contrast, the SCAI/SCVS/SVMB/SVS statement, which assumes the physician has prior catheter experience, only requires 50 cerebral angiograms[8] for proficiency in performing carotid artery stent placement.

The adequacy of a cerebral angiogram depends upon the procedural success and associated complications. Therefore, a crucial aspect of training in diagnostic angiography is the ability to adequately answer the diagnostic question by catheterizing the appropriate vessels, obtaining the appropriate views, and performing the correct interpretation of the images obtained. Improperly performed or interpreted angiograms can impose additional risks to patients if erroneous treatments are instituted as a consequence of diagnostic errors. The quality improvement guidelines for cerebral angiography by the ASNR, ASITN, and the SCVIR[16] defined a successful examination as a sufficient selective neuroangiographic technical evaluation and image interpretation to establish or exclude pathology of the extracranial and intracranial circulation. The acceptable rate for a practitioner was defined as 98%.

Overall, acceptable rate of major procedural complications was defined as 2% or less in the quality improvement guidelines for cerebral angiography by the ASNR, ASITN, and the SCVIR.[16] The risk of permanent neurological deficit as a result of stroke attributed to diagnostic cerebral angiography in previous studies ranges from 0.3%–5.7%.[22–29] In addition to the level of training and experience of the person performing the procedure, patient-related risk factors including older age, presence of atherosclerotic disease (especially involving the aortic arch and carotid arteries) and recent cerebral ischemic symptoms increase the risk of complications associated with cerebral angiography.[22–29] Given that elderly persons with symptomatic atherosclerotic disease are likely to constitute the bulk of patients typically encountered in the practice of vascular neurologists, the highest standards of training should be required of vascular neurologists interested in pursuing training in diagnostic angiography.

Summary and recommendations

A prerequisite for safely performing diagnostic cerebral angiography is adequate specialty education, which in the case of neurologists must include completion of an ACGME-approved neurology residency program and also formal training in vascular neurology or neurocritical care. Training in digital subtraction angiography must follow a clear curriculum and must be provided by individuals with documented adequate training in diagnostic angiography. Training should include hands-on experience, under supervision, as secondary and primary operator. There should be documentation of the number of procedures, success and failure rates, complication rates, and outcomes. In concordance with previous recommendations made by several medical societies and accreditation bodies, a minimum of 100 cases are required to meet accreditation standards for safe and competent performance of diagnostic cerebral angiography.[4] Those cases may be performed during the diagnostic portion of the interventional procedures. Maintenance of competence in diagnostic cerebral angiography is an ongoing process that ensures continuity and growth of the cognitive, clinical, and technologic skills acquired during training. Technical skills should be maintained via performance of at least 50 diagnostic cerebral angiograms annually with documentation of outcomes and complications.

Intra-arterial thrombolysis and mechanical thrombectomy

The intra-arterial approach has been promoted because a high concentration of thrombolytic agents can be delivered into the thrombus complimented by mechanical disruption to facilitate thrombolysis.[2] Despite the uncontrolled observation that recanalization rates may be higher with intra-arterial thrombolysis compared with intravenous,[2] clinical benefit may be counterbalanced by a delay in treatment with the intra-arterial approach. However, both intravenous and intra-arterial thrombolytic treatments appear to be underutilized in the acute stroke setting in the USA. In data derived from National Hospital Discharge Survey, there were 1 796 513 admissions for ischemic stroke between 1999 and 2001.[30] Of these admitted patients, 1314 (0.07%) underwent intra-arterial thrombolysis and 11 283 (0.6%) underwent intravenous thrombolysis. Lack of qualified physicians and resources within the hospitals is an important contributor to this underutilization.

The 2003 guidelines by the stroke council of the American Stroke Association (ASA)[31] recommended that intra-arterial thrombolysis is an option for treatment of selected patients with major stroke of <6 hours' duration due to large vessel occlusions of the middle cerebral artery. The guidelines acknowledged that case series data suggest this approach may also be of benefit in patients with basilar artery occlusion treated at longer intervals. The Brain Attack Coalition [13] considers intra-arterial lytics are considered to be a recommended component of a comprehensive stroke center. The recommendations mandate close monitoring of complication rates. The 2007 guideline from the American Heart Association/American Stroke Association Stroke Council [32] recommended that treatment requires the patient to be at an experienced stroke center with immediate access to cerebral angiography and qualified interventionalists. Facilities are encouraged to define criteria to credential individuals who can perform intra-arterial thrombolysis. Intra-arterial thrombolysis is reasonable in patients who have contraindications to use of intravenous thrombolysis, such as recent surgery. Although the MERCI device is a reasonable intervention for extraction of intra-arterial thrombi in carefully selected patients, the panel also recognizes that the utility of the device in improving outcomes after stroke is unclear.

Although no reports have studied the association between operator experience and peri-procedural complications of intra-arterial thrombolysis, there is some data pertaining to intravenous thrombolysis that suggests that inadequate patient selection and poor compliance with recommended protocols can increase the rate of intracranial hemorrhages following treatment.[33,34] There are also data that suggests that increased compliance with patient selection and peri-procedural care protocols reduces the rate of intracranial hemorrhages following intravenous treatment within the same settings.[35] The low rates of intracranial hemorrhages following intra-arterial thrombolytic treatment in selected single center studies also support some role of operator experience although it may be related to patient selection and peri-procedural care rather than just procedural skills.[36–38] The credentialing guidelines adopted by the Interventional Management of Stroke (IMS) study set a framework for individuals performing intra-arterial thrombolysis.[39] The recommendations suggest that the physician performing the procedure must be board eligible or certified in diagnostic radiology, neurosurgery, or vascular neurology. The physician must have experience in performance and interpretation of 100 cerebral angiographic procedures as primary operator and a minimum of a 1-year fellowship in endovascular surgical neuroradiology that meets or reflects the training requirements for performance and interpretation set forth by a national multidisciplinary council and ACGME. The experience should include at least ten intra-arterial thrombolysis procedures. In absence of formal training, qualifying training and experience would include successful completion of an accredited residency and completion of a 1-year post-graduate fellowship in an accredited program, or equivalent. In addition, training is required in cerebral angiography within an approved program, including performance and interpretation of a minimum of 200 cerebral angiograms. The criteria also require participation in 50 endovascular surgical neuroradiology procedures under the supervision of a director who qualifies as program director under the program requirements for residency education in endovascular surgical neuroradiology; and performance of 50 endovascular surgical neuroradiology procedures as primary operator with at least 10 intra-arterial thrombolytic procedures.

Summary and recommendations

New criteria need to be established to determine the qualifications of physicians who can perform intra-arterial thrombolysis based on recent statements from professional organizations and clinical trials. Treatment requires the patient to be treated at an experienced stroke center with immediate access to cerebral angiography and qualified interventionalists. In addition to meeting the training period and overall case volume requirements set by ACGME for endovascular surgical neuroradiology residency education, the physician requesting credentialing must have performed at least ten intra-arterial thrombolytic procedures. The committee recognizes that most practicing and graduating interventionalists will not be trained in an ACGME accredited program in surgical endovascular neuroradiology due to the recent institution of the accreditation process and current lack of accredited programs. Therefore, compliance with the ACGME requirements for overall case volume and training period in the absence of a formal accreditation (by relevant ACGME residency review committee) are considered adequate. The committee recognizes the important contribution of patient selection and peri-procedural care on the complication rates of the intra-arterial thrombolysis. It is recommended that either the interventionalist must possess the required training for patient selection and administration of intravenous thrombolysis and peri-procedural care in acute stroke patients or seek simultaneous consultation by a qualified individual.

Carotid angioplasty and stent placement

An accurate national estimate of symptomatic and asymptomatic carotid stenosis requiring treatment is not available. An estimated 151 000 carotid endarterectomies are performed every year,[15] which provides some data regarding the prevalence of carotid stenosis in the USA. Carotid angioplasty and stent placement is a new option for the treatment of selected patients with symptomatic or asymptomatic carotid artery stenosis. Over the past 10 years, the technical success rate for CAS has exceeded 97% and the complication rates have improved.[2] Carotid stent placement is a procedure that is performed by physicians from several disciplines and therefore is subject to overview by several professional organizations as described in the following sections.

A summary of recommendations from all professional organizations is presented in Table 23.1.[4,8,40,41] The ACCF/SCAI/SVMB/SIR/ASITN 2007 Clinical Expert Consensus Document on Carotid Stenting[41] reviews the first carotid angioplasty and stent placement training document from the ASITN/ASNR/SIR [40] and the subsequent AAN/AANS/ASITN/ASNR/CNS/SIR document[4] (see Table 23.1)[8,40,41] included preparatory requirements for both the performance of cerebral angiography and stent placement before performing carotid angioplasty and stent placement independently. The documents required a minimum of 100 supervised cerebral angiograms and either 25 non-carotid stent procedures with four supervised carotid stent procedures and 16 h of continuing medical education (CME), or ten supervised carotid angioplasty and stent placement procedures with

acceptable results. The 16 h of CME must include a didactic program of formal instruction in the cognitive and clinical elements, combined with hands-on technical instruction on the procedure and devices utilized during carotid angioplasty and stent placement. The SCAI/SVMB/SVS document[8] specifies that new operators in these specialties perform a minimum of 30 supervised diagnostic cervicocerebral angiograms (at least 15 as a primary operator) and a minimum of 25 supervised carotid interventions (at least 13 as primary operator) prior to performing carotid angioplasty and stent placement independently.

Fewer procedures required by the cardiology and vascular surgery organizations is based on the belief that previous experience with coronary (minimum of 300 diagnostic coronary angiograms and 250 coronary interventions)[42] and peripheral interventional procedures (minimum of 100 diagnostic peripheral angiograms and 50 peripheral interventions)[43] are transferable to neurovascular intervention. While the SCAI/SVMB/SVS clinical competence statement stipulates a minimum of 25 carotid angioplasty and stent placement procedures [8] (half as primary operator), a published statement by the ASITN, ASNR, SIR focusing on quality improvement guidelines for carotid angioplasty and stent placement recommended the following two alternative pathways for credentialing[40] (see also Table 23.1).

1. Twenty-five non–carotid stent complete procedures, plus attendance at and completion of a "hands-on" course in performance of carotid angioplasty and stent placement (16 hours of AMA category 1 CME), plus performance and completion of at least four successful and uncomplicated carotid angioplasty and stent placement procedures as principal operator under the supervision of an on-site qualified physician.

2. Ten consecutive carotid angioplasty and stent placement procedures as principal operator under the supervision of an on-site qualified physician on patients treated for appropriate indications documented by a log of cases performed and with acceptable success and complication rates according to the thresholds contained in this guideline and the ACR guideline for cervicocerebral angiography.

Some authors have reported, based on retrospective studies, that there is a learning curve for carotid angioplasty and stent placement and outcomes have improved with increasing physician and center experience.[44] The credentialing process for several clinical studies and associated results are presented in Table 23.2.[45] The SAPPHIRE trial,[46] Carotid Revascularization Endarterectomy vs. Stenting Trial (CREST) trial,[44] Endarterectomy vs. Angioplasty in Patients with Symptomatic Severe Carotid Stenosis (EVA-3S) trial,[47] and Stent-Supported Percutaneous Angioplasty of the Carotid Artery vs Endarterectomy (SPACE) trial[48] are all randomized trials with different credentialing criteria. The results are derived from the randomized group treated with carotid stent placement in all except that the CREST trial reports events monitored through March

Table 23.1. Various credentialing requirements from different professional organizations regarding carotid stent placement.

Organization	Background	Previous experience	Procedural experience
Society of Interventional Radiology (SIR), American Society of Interventional and Therapeutic Neuroradiology (ASITN), and American Society of Neuroradiology (ASNR)[40]	Substantial knowledge of cerebrovascular anatomy, knowledge of the clinical and imaging evaluation of patients with cerebrovascular disorders, including knowledge of the clinical manifestations and the natural history of cerebrovascular ischemic disease.	Performance (under the supervision of a qualified physician and with at least 50% performed as the primary operator) of at least 200 diagnostic cervicocerebral angiograms with documented acceptable indications and outcomes for physicians with no prior catheter experience, or at least 100 diagnostic cervicocerebral angiograms with documented acceptable indications and outcomes for physicians with experience sufficient to meet the American Heart Association requirements for peripheral vascular interventions.	25 non-carotid stent complete procedures, plus attendance at and completion of a "hands-on" course in performance of CAS (16 hours of AMA category 1 CME), plus performance and completion of at least four successful and uncomplicated CAS procedures as principal operator under the supervision of an on-site qualified physician; OR Ten consecutive CAS procedures as principal operator under the supervision of an on-site qualified physician on patients treated for appropriate indications documented by a log of cases performed and with acceptable success and complication rates according to the thresholds contained in this guideline and the American College of Radiolgy guidelines for cervicocerebral angiography.
The Society of Vascular Surgeons (SVS)[8]	Must have knowledge of all treatment options for extracranial cerebrovascular disease, and must demonstrate clinical competency as described in a SVS, ACC, ACP, SCAI, SVMB joint clinical competence statement on Vascular Medicine and Catheter-based Peripheral Vascular Interventions.	Demonstrate primary clinical responsibility for the management of carotid occlusive disease in 50 patients; performance of a minimum of 30 diagnostic cerebrovascular angiograms with 15 as a supervised primary operator	A minimum of 25 supervised CAS, at least half as primary operator
Society for Vascular Medicine and Biology (SVMB) and The Society for Cardiovascular Angiography and Interventions (SCAI) and SVS and The American College of Cardiology (ACC)[8]	Favor less stringent guidelines and acknowledge the transferable nature of basic and advanced catheter skills acquired in other vascular beds. The trainee should have acquired extensive knowledge of neurovascular anatomy and pathology through study of appropriate textbooks and review of others' angiograms.	An accredited post-graduate residency or fellowship training program (i.e. interventional cardiology, interventional radiology or endovascular surgery) in conjunction with peripheral angioplasty training that will include carotid training; OR, the practice pathway will occur with physicians who have completed their training and will be trained to perform carotid stenting in a clinical practice setting. Demonstrated expertise in non-cerebrovascular vessels can achieve the required level of technical skill by performing (30) supervised angiograms, half as primary operator, in a supervised setting.	A minimum of 25 CAS procedures (half as primary operator)

Table 23.1. (cont.)

Organization	Background	Previous experience	Procedural experience
Neurovascular coalition including AAN, AANS, ASITN, ASNR, CNS, the AANS/CNS Cerebrovascular Section, and the SIR.[4]	Formal training and experience in both the cognitive and technical aspects of the neurosciences. A minimum of 6 months of formal cognitive neuroscience training is required in an approved program in radiology, neuroradiology, neurosurgery, neurology, and/or vascular neurology.	Recommend appropriately supervised cervicocerebral angiography training and resultant credentialing with an accumulated total of 100 diagnostic cervicocerebral angiograms	The principles of training and quality assurance stated in the multisociety *Quality Improvement Guidelines for the Performance of Carotid Angioplasty and Stent Placement*, defined training pathway for any qualified practitioner for carotid stent training; specifically, endorsement of the principles of the ACGME and the training programs in Endovascular Surgical Neuroradiology, Vascular Neurology and Neuroradiology.

Abbreviations used: CAS, carotid artery stent placement; ACGME, Accreditation Council for Graduate Medical Education; AAN, American Academy of Neurology; AANS, American Association of Neurological Surgeons; and CNS, Congress of Neurological Surgeons.

31, 2004 in the non-randomized lead-in phase. As can be observed in Table 23.2, the one-month stroke and death rate were prominently higher in the EVA-3S trial compared with the other trials. The number of procedures required to qualify for participation in the trial as an interventionalist was lower than in other studies. The study also allowed a novice interventional physician to perform stent placement under the supervision of an experienced tutor (a clinician who qualified to perform stent placement in this study) until the novice became self-sufficient (according to the tutor) and performed a sufficient number of procedures according to the predefined criteria. This prompted concerns that the qualifications required in the EVA-3S trial (12 carotid stent placement procedures) are not adequate. Recently, however, results have been reported from a large registry of carotid angioplasty and stent placement performed in the The Carotid Acculink/Accunet Post Approval Trial to Uncover Rare Events (CAPTURE) with outcome data stratified according to prior physician experience.[49] In that study, there was no significant difference in outcome between those physicians with no or little previous carotid angioplasty and stent placement experience (<ten cases) and more experienced operators. The physicians with no previous carotid angioplasty and stent placement experience completed a didactic training course on carotid disease and had extensive peripheral interventional experience and experience in cerebral angiography. This apparent discrepancy may be attributable to the fact that the patients treated in the registry were predominantly asymptomatic. Presumably, the operator experience may be more important in patients at higher risk of peri-procedural events such as patients with recent retinal or cerebral ischemic symptoms.[47]

In addition to the training standards delineated above, successful completion of an industry-sponsored certification course may be required, to ensure proper use of specific FDA-approved stent and embolic protection systems. These programs are variable and include online (web-based) graded didactic training, metric-based simulator training to proficiency at regional training centers, and on-site proctoring. Cordis Endovascular

Systems has proposed a training program including an online didactic session, observation of actual cases, simulation using a simulator, a proctoring system, and training of adjunctive staff. The didactic training is done via the Internet, observation and simulation experiences are delivered at regional education centers, and the proctoring network and staff training are performed on-site at the physician's facility. The only evidence for efficacy of such programs is derived from results of a project where investigators were trained using an earlier version of the Cordis Endovascular Systems training system intended to support the SAPPHIRE study.[50] The training occurred at 36 centers. The 30-day site-reported adverse events included a death rate of 0.6%, stroke 2.6%, and myocardial infarction 1.4%, yielding a major adverse event rate of 4.3% in 491 patients. A subsequent larger study evaluated the results of the comprehensive training program in Carotid Artery Stenting with Emboli Protection Surveillance-Post-Marketing Study (CASES-PMS).[51] The data were derived from 1279 patients with inclusion and exclusion criteria matching those of the SAPPHIRE study. The rate of stroke, death, and MI at 1 month was 4.8%, similar to the rate observed in the SAPPHIRE study. Similar results were observed in the CAPTURE trial[49] (see Table 23.2).

Summary and recommendations

After review of correlation between qualification requirements and results of clinical trials and prospective registries, the ASITN/ASNR/SIR carotid angioplasty and stent placement quality improvement guidelines, the SCAI/SVMB/SVS clinical competence statement, and the training standards of vascular neurology residency programs, the committee recommends a minimum of 25 carotid angioplasty and stent placement cases be performed under supervision in fellowship training before an interventional neurologist should be granted credentials for carotid angioplasty and stent placement. There is some evidence that a smaller number of procedures may provide adequate experience to achieve low rates of peri-procedural stroke and death in asymptomatic patients who are at low risk for such events. However, since most practitioners will treat

Table 23.2. Credentialing requirements required and peri-operative complications observed in clinical studies involving carotid stent placement with distal protection

Clinical study	Design	Patients included	Credentialing requirements	1-month stroke and death rate
Stenting and angioplasty with protection in patients at high risk for endartectomy trial (SAPPHIRE)[46]	Randomized clinical trial at 29 centers (N = 167)	High surgical risk patients with symptomatic stenosis ≥50% or asymptomatic stenosis ≥80%	Required to submit experience and results. The median total number of carotid stent procedures performed per operator was 64 (range, 20 to 700) and the mean stroke, death, or myocardial infarction rate was 4%	4.8% (includes myocardial infarction)
Carotid Revascularization Endartectomy vs. stent trial (CREST)[44]	Lead-inphase for randomized clinical trial at 60 centers (N = 789)	Patients with symptomatic stenosis ≥50% or asymptomatic stenosis ≥70%	Required to submit data on 10–30 cases previously performed and depending on this data had to perform up to 20 lead-in cases	4.6% (no variation between various credentialed specialists)
Stent supported percutaneous angioplasty of the carotid artery vs. endarterectomy trial (SPACE)[48]	Randomized clinical trial at 35 centers (N = 605)	Patients with symptomatic stenosis ≥70%	Perform at least 25 successful consecutive percutaneous carotid angioplasty or stent procedures	7.8%
Endarterectomie versus angioplastie chez les patients ayant une stenose carotide symptomatique serree (EVA-3S)[47]	Randomized clinical trial in 20 academic and 10 nonacademic centers (N = 247)	Patients with symptomatic stenosis ≥60%	Perform at least 12 carotid stent procedures or at least 35 stent procedures in the supra-aortic trunks, of which at least 5 were in the carotid artery	9.6% (no significant differences in outcome related to the experience of the interventional physicians, although these analyses were only able to detect large differences)
Carotid artery stenting with emboli protection surveillance post-marketing study (CASES-PMS)[51]	Post-marketing surveillance study at 70 centers (N = 1279)	High surgical risk patients with symptomatic stenosis ≥50% or asymptomatic stenosis ≥80%	Training included didactic review, case observations and simulation training, and hands-on experience at the Regional Education Centers	4.8% (includes myocardial infarction)
The Carotid Acculink/Accunet Post Approval Trial to Uncover Rare Events (CAPTURE)[49]	Post-marketing surveillance study at 144 centers (N = 3500)	Predominantly asymptomatic patients (90%)	Guidant's physician training program tailored to the experience level of each physician; majority of physicians (71%) performing the procedures had a medium level of experience (performed 10 carotid stent procedures as the primary operator); only one third or less of patients enrolled at hospitals with a high level of experience	6.3% (includes myocardial infarction); no difference according to operator experience levels or physician specialties

patients with carotid stenosis associated with recent retinal or cerebral ischemic symptoms, a higher level of experience is recommended. The evidence is insufficient that industry sponsored courses can substitute for the existing training standards. This specific requirement is in addition to meeting the training period and overall case volume requirements set by ACGME for endovascular surgical neuroradiology residency education. The committee recognizes that most practicing and graduating interventionalists will not be trained in an ACGME accredited program in surgical endovascular neuroradiology due to the recent institution of the accreditation process and current lack of accredited programs. Therefore, compliance with the ACGME requirements for overall case volume and training period in the absence of a formal accreditation (by relevant ACGME residency review committee) are considered adequate. This credentialing document is only one aspect of granting physicians privileges. There are institutional, state, as well as federal guidelines, and for carotid angioplasty and stent placement in particular, physicians and hospitals must enroll patients in databases for quality and outcome measures. Interventional neurologists will also need to maintain their skills via continuing medical education and adequate case volume.

Endovascular treatment of intracranial aneurysms

Endovascular detachable coil treatment is being increasingly used as an alternative to craniotomy and clipping for ruptured and unruptured intracranial aneurysms.[52] There were 133 269 admissions for subarachnoid hemorrhage and 51 904 admissions for unruptured intracranial aneurysms during the period of 1996–2001 in the USA.[53] Although endovascular treatment was less frequently used than surgical treatment,[53,54] endovascular treatment for intracranial aneurysms is expected to increase[52] over the next few years. This increase will require a concomitant increase in the number of qualified physicians to meet the demand.

The best evidence for credentialing interventionalists is derived from the design of the International Subarachnoid Aneurysm Trial (ISAT).[55] The ISAT was a randomized, multicenter trial to compare the safety and efficacy of endovascular coiling with standard neurosurgical clipping for ruptured aneurysms judged to be suitable for both treatments. The study enrolled 2143 patients with ruptured intracranial aneurysms and randomly assigned them to neurosurgical clipping ($n = 1070$) or endovascular treatment by detachable platinum coils ($n = 1073$). The primary outcome was the proportion of patients with a modified Rankin scale score of 3–6 (dependency or death) at 1 year, which was observed in 190 of 801 (23.7%) patients allocated endovascular treatment compared with 243 of 793 (30.6%) allocated neurosurgical treatment ($P = 0.0019$). The early survival advantage was maintained for up to 7 years and was statistically significant (log rank $P = 0.03$).[56]

The study was conducted at neurosurgical centers treating a significant number of patients with acute subarachnoid hemorrhage with a referral base of at least 1.5 million. There was at least one experienced endovascular operator at each center. The endovascular operator was required to have wide interventional neuroimaging experience and must have treated at least 30 cases with the Gugliemi detachable coil device before randomizing patients in the trial. Because of the heterogeneity in subarachnoid hemorrhage management and wide outcome variation depending on the patient's clinical grade, age, aneurysm location, and the relatively small numbers of procedures each year for individual surgeons or endovascular operators, it was deemed inappropriate to demand, as a prerequisite to being a participating center, outcome figures from individual operators for managing patients in ISAT. After completion of the study, ISAT investigators compared the effect of treatment in the six largest recruiting centers and the sum of all the smaller centers, and found no evidence of heterogeneity of treatment effect. The technical success rates (successful completion of embolization) were 92.6% in the ISAT. However, it should be noted that the patients included in ISAT are not a random sample of all patients in the community with subarachnoid hemorrhage due to rupture of an aneurysm, but were selected in accordance with the eligibility criteria.

Another study identified all unruptured aneurysms treated with coil embolization at one institution from 1990 through 1997.[57] The influence of experience of the treating-physician on complications was evaluated. Complications occurred in 53% of the first five cases that each of three physicians treated, and in 10% of later cases. After an adjustment for all other predictors, including physician assessment of the risk of the procedure, the odds of a complication decreased with increasing physician experience (odds ratio, 0.69 for every five cases treated; 95% confidence interval: 0.50–0.96; $P = 0.03$). A retrospective cohort study used the Nationwide Inpatient Sample, 1996–2000 to evaluate the probability of in-hospital mortality and discharge other than to home in relation to treating physician volume of endovascular treatment of unruptured intracranial aneurysms, by quartile.[58] The best outcome was observed for endovascular physicians treating more than five patients with unruptured intracranial aneurysms a year. No single cutoff point was statistically significant for physician volume (annual volume of endovascular treatment of unruptured aneurysms). The studies confirm that the risk of complications with coil embolization of unruptured aneurysms appears to decrease dramatically with physician experience. In the absence of adjustments for previous experience with other endovascular techniques at study onset, the rate of learning may not be generalizable to other centers.

Summary and recommendations

Physicians who receive credentials for endovascular treatment of intracranial aneurysms must have performed at least 30 endovascular procedures for intracranial aneurysms. There is some evidence that a smaller number of procedures may provide adequate experience to achieve low rates of peri-procedural stroke and death in patients with unruptured aneurysms who are at low risk for such events. However, since most practitioners will treat patients with ruptured intracranial aneurysms, a higher level of experience is recommended. This specific requirement is in addition to meeting the training period and overall case volume requirements set by ACGME for endovascular surgical neuroradiology residency education as specified earlier. The committee recognizes that most practicing and graduating interventionalists will not be trained in an ACGME accredited program in surgical endovascular neuroradiology due to the recent institution of the accreditation process and current lack of accredited programs. Therefore, compliance with the ACGME requirements for overall case volume and training period in the absence of a formal accreditation (by relevant ACGME residency review committee) are considered adequate. Prior to using specific devices, the recommended training required by manufacturers must be completed including the Neuroform® Microdelivery Stent System and Enterprise™ Vascular Reconstruction Device and Delivery System.

Intracranial stent placement

Intracranial stenosis is responsible for 8% to 10% of all ischemic strokes and approximately 100 000 patients with symptomatic intracranial stenosis are seen in the USA every year.[59]

Results from clinical studies demonstrate the feasibility and intermediate-term effectiveness (for secondary stroke prevention) of angioplasty or stent placement for treatment of intracranial atherosclerotic disease.[2] The procedure can be performed with an acceptable risk of peri-procedural stroke and death. The procedure is offered at specialized centers for patients with symptomatic intracranial stenosis that are considered at high risk for recurrent ischemic events. Two stents were approved under the provision for humanitarian device exemption by the FDA based on two clinical trials.[60,61] Both trials selected centers and operators with considerable experience although no formal criteria were defined. The Stenting of Symptomatic Atherosclerotic Lesions in the Vertebral or Intracranial Arteries (SSYLVIA) trial[60] was conducted in ten centers in the USA and Europe. Before treating the first patient under the protocol, each interventionalist took part in a didactic and practical training program. The second study[61] conducted in 12 centers in Europe and Asia assessed the safety and performance of Wingspan stent system (Boston Scientific Corp.). The Brain Attack Coalition[13] considered intracranial angioplasty or stent placement for cerebrovascular disease an optional component for a comprehensive stroke center, although there are selected cases in which such techniques may be of value. If a center offers this procedure, it was recommended that cases be entered into a registry to track outcomes.

Summary and recommendations

There are no available data to support specific training requirements for intracranial angioplasty or stent placement. Given the complexity of treating intracranial stenosis, the minimum requirements specified for cervical carotid intervention are not adequate. A minimum of 50 procedures requiring microcatheter and microwire placement in intracranial vessels beyond intracranial internal carotid artery or vertebral artery are required to gain expertise in navigating the intracranial vasculature. At least half of them should be performed as a primary operator under supervision. It is also recommended that physicians perform at least 25 endovascular procedures for intracranial stenosis under supervision prior to requesting privileges for performing these procedures. This specific requirement is in addition to meeting the training period and overall case volume requirements set by ACGME for endovascular surgical neuroradiology residency education. The committee recognizes that most practicing and graduating interventionalists will not train in an ACGME accredited program in surgical endovascular neuroradiology due to the recent institution of the accreditation process and current lack of accredited programs. Therefore, compliance with the ACGME requirements for overall case volume and training period in the absence of a formal accreditation (by relevant ACGME residency review committee) are considered adequate. Prior to using specific stents, the recommended training required by manufacturers must be completed.

Embolization of brain arteriovenous malformations

Technical advances in interventional neurology have afforded new alternatives in the treatment of brain arteriovenous malformations. Flow-directed and flow-assisted microcatheters have allowed more accurate delivery of embolic materials. Current embolic materials are divided into solid or liquid agents. Solid agents consist of polyvinyl alcohol particles, fibers, microcoils, and microballoons. Liquid agents consist of cyanoacrylic monomers such as IBCA (I-butyl cyanoacrylate) and NBCA (N-butyl cyanoacrylate) and polymer solutions such as ethylene vinyl alcohol (EVAL copolymer).[2,62]

Training in treatment of arteriovenous malformations is confounded by the small number of procedures performed and heterogeneity of presentations and treatment paradigms. To provide a scope of therapeutic embolization practice, the numbers of potential embolization procedures were estimated using a nationally representative sample of hospitals (Nationwide Inpatient Sample 2001) in the USA 15. The total number of patients with arteriovenous malformation (ICD-9 diagnosis code 387.3) who underwent embolization (ICD-9 procedure codes 39.72 or 39.53) in year 2001 was only 240. Based on these considerations, both animal and inanimate model systems have been used in the training of neuro-interventional procedures. The advantages of inanimate model systems include reduced expense and lowered demand for animal models.[63,64] The standardization inherent in a model (e.g., same resistance, same inflow and draining vessel dimensions, and so on) is useful. The arteriovenous malformation training models allow users to develop skills at their own rates, and permits safe "failure-mode" learning. Similarly, if different materials are being evaluated with a standard technique, a standardized model will highlight intrinsic differences in the materials.

The best recommendations beyond the broad guidelines of the ACGME curriculum are those given by the FDA at the time of approval of liquid embolic agents. In May 2000, premarket approval application for the Trufill® (Cordis Neurovascular, Miami Lakes, FL) n-butyl cyanoacrylate for the presurgical treatment of arteriovenous malformations was reviewed by the neurological devices panel.[65] The panel reviewed the training program provided by the manufacturer that covered the use of device and included a didactic session, case studies, and a hands-on workshop. The panel thought the sponsor-provided training was adequate but suggested the sponsor might wish to consider entry criteria and a periodic review course. The panel recommended that completion of the current physician training program should be required prior to allowing an individual to use the device.

At another advisory meeting held on August 5, 2003,[65] the Neurological Devices Panel recommended that Micro Therapeutics premarket approval for the Onyx Liquid Embolic System be approved subject to submission to, and approval by, the Center for Device and Radiological Health (CDRH) of a training program with hands-on training using in vitro and in vivo models under fluoroscopic visualization. Additionally, newly trained physicians would be required to have one proctored case and if the physician's first case were deemed a failure, the physician must conduct another proctored case. The physician training program, which consisted of a didactic session, a hands-on in vitro workshop, case review, and case observation by an experienced user, was presented to the panel. Some panel members believed that the training information was insufficient to address the reported poor penetration and visualization of the device. However, the panel concurred that training is critically important, and it should include a mandatory hands-on component, proctoring, monitoring of the program's effectiveness, and mandatory supervision by someone who could remove the catheter should it become stuck.

Summary and recommendations

Given the complexity of treating intracranial arteriovenous malformations, the minimum requirements specified for carotid intervention are not adequate. A minimum of 50 procedures requiring microcatheter and microwire placement in intracranial vessels beyond intracranial internal carotid artery or vertebral artery are considered necessary to gain expertise in navigating endovascular devices in intracranial vasculature. At least half of them should be performed as primary operator under supervision. It is also recommended that physicians perform at least 15 endovascular procedures for brain arteriovenous malformation under supervision prior to requesting privileges for performing these procedures. This specific requirement is in addition to meeting the training period and overall case volume requirements set by ACGME for endovascular surgical neuroradiology residency education. The committee recognizes that most practicing and graduating interventionalists will not train in an ACGME accredited program in surgical endovascular neuroradiology due to the recent institution of the accreditation process and current lack of accredited programs. Therefore, compliance with the ACGME requirements for overall case volume and training period in the absence of a formal accreditation (by relevant ACGME residency review committee) are considered adequate. Prior to using specific liquid agents, the recommended training provided by the manufacturers must be completed.

Other neuro-interventional procedures

Certain neurointerventional procedures are not included under specific credentialing requirements. In general, specific requirements beyond meeting the training period and overall case volume requirements set by ACGME for endovascular surgical neuroradiology residency education are not necessary for the procedures mentioned below.

Extracranial endovascular procedures

Endovascular treatment of patients with symptomatic extracranial vertebral stenosis involves similar techniques but is technically less challenging than intracranial angioplasty and stent placement and carries a lower risk of peri-procedural complications. Therefore, the committee feels that expertise in intracranial angioplasty and stent placement is adequate qualification for performing endovascular treatment of extracranial vertebrobasilar, ostial carotid, subclavian, and brachiocephalic disease presenting with cerebrovascular symptoms. Endovascular treatment involving extracranial vessels includes embolization for scalp and neck vascular malformations, head, neck, and spine vascular tumors, epistaxis, and trauma. These procedures involve similar techniques, but are technically less challenging than intracranial embolization and carry a lower risk of peri-procedural complications. Therefore, the committee feels that expertise in intracranial embolization is adequate qualification for performing endovascular treatment involving extracranial vessels.

Spinal endovascular procedures

Angiography and embolization of spinal arteriovenous malformations are considered an important part of the training in neurointerventional procedures and the committee feels the expertise obtained through training for diagnostic angiography and embolization of intracranial arteriovenous malformations is adequate for spinal interventional procedures.

Provocative and occlusion tests

Intracranial or extracranial balloon test occlusion, or intraarterial injection of intracarotid sodium amobarbital or other pharmacological agents for provocative testing (e.g., WADA testing) are procedures that are performed during neurointerventional training and are less challenging and carry less periprocedural risk than intracranial procedures. The committee feels that interventional neurologists with proper fellowship training are qualified to perform these procedures.

Conclusions

The guidelines are intended to help hospitals, medical staff, interventional neurologists, and other responsible individuals and organizations foster quality patient care by assuring the qualifications of interventional neurologists involved in performing neurointerventional procedures. They are subject to the limitations noted and are provided for informational purposes. These guidelines are not intended to replace the local institutional policies for determining individual physician's qualifications using peer review processes. Currently, the ACGME requirements for overall case volume and training period in the absence of a formal accreditation (by relevant ACGME residency review committee) are considered adequate but training in ACGME accredited programs maybe desirable over a 5-year period subject to the availability of accredited programs. Some of these recommendations will be modified as new data will be generated through future studies. Further efforts are required to define competence based on patient outcomes after adjustment for disease severity in addition to the operator experience.

References

1. Qureshi AI, Abou-Chebl A, Jovin TG. Qualification requirements for performing neurointerventional procedures: a Report of the Practice Guidelines Committee of the American Society of Neuroimaging and the Society of Vascular and Interventional Neurology. *J Neuroimaging* 2008;**18**: 433–47.

2. Qureshi AI. Endovascular treatment of cerebrovascular diseases and intracranial neoplasms. *Lancet* 2004;**363**:804–13.

3. ACGME. Program requirements for residency education in endovascular surgical neuroradiology.

4. Connors JJ, 3rd, Sacks D, Furlan AJ, *et al.* Training, competency, and credentialing standards for diagnostic cervicocerebral angiography, carotid stenting, and cerebrovascular intervention: a joint statement from the American Academy of Neurology, American Association of Neurological Surgeons, American Society of Interventional and Therapeutic Radiology, American Society of Neuroradiology, Congress of Neurological Surgeons, AANS/CNS Cerebrovascular Section, and Society of Interventional Radiology. *Radiology* 2005;**234**:26–34.

5. AI Q. Interventional section 2006–2007: American Academy of Neurology. In: *58th Annual Meeting of the American Academy of Neurology*; 2006; San Diego, CA, April 1–8, 2006; 2006.

6. Johnston SC. Who belongs inside the carotid arteries? *Neurology* 2005;**64**: 188–9.

7. (Accessed Last accessed on June 20th, 2006., at http://www.asitn.org/docs/pdf/2006_Fellowship_Programs.pdf.)

8. Rosenfield K, Babb JD, Cates CU, *et al.* Clinical competence statement on carotid stenting: training and credentialing for carotid stenting–multispecialty consensus recommendations: a report of the SCAI/SVMB/SVS Writing Committee to develop a clinical competence statement on carotid interventions. *J Am Coll Cardiol* 2005;**45**:165–74.

9. Connors JJ, 3rd, Sacks D, Furlan AJ, *et al.* Training, competency, and credentialing standards for diagnostic cervicocerebral angiography, carotid stenting, and cerebrovascular intervention: a joint statement from the American Academy of Neurology, the American Association of Neurological Surgeons, the American Society of Interventional and Therapeutic Neuroradiology, the American Society of Neuroradiology, the Congress of Neurological Surgeons, the AANS/CNS Cerebrovascular Section, and the Society of Interventional Radiology. *Neurology* 2005;**64**:190–8.

10. JCAHO. *The Comprehensive Accreditation Manual for Hospitals 1997*, 1997.

11. Levin DC, Becker GJ, Dorros G, *et al.* Training standards for physicians performing peripheral angioplasty and other percutaneous peripheral vascular interventions. A statement for health professionals from the Special Writing Group of the Councils on Cardiovascular Radiology, Cardio-Thoracic and Vascular Surgery, and Clinical Cardiology, the American Heart Association. *Circulation* 1992;**86**:1348–50.

12. ACGME. Program requirements for residency education in vascular neurology. In.

13. Alberts MJ, Latchaw RE, Selman WR, *et al.* Recommendations for comprehensive stroke centers: a consensus statement from the Brain Attack Coalition. *Stroke; J Cereb Circ* 2005;**36**:1597–616.

14. Cerebral arteriography. A report for health professionals by the Executive Committee of the Stroke Council, American Heart Association. *Circulation* 1989;**79**:474.

15. Qureshi AI. Ten years of advances in neuroendovascular procedures. *J Endovasc Ther* 2004;**11** Suppl 2:II1–4.

16. Quality improvement guidelines for adult diagnostic neuroangiography. Cooperative study between the ASNR, ASITN, and the SCVIR. American Society of Neuroradiology. American Society of Interventional and Therapeutic Neuroradiology. Society of Cardiovascular and Interventional Radiology. *Am J Neuroradiol* 2000;**21**:146–50.

17. Gomez C, Kinkel P, Masdeu J, *et al.* American Academy of Neurology guidelines for credentialing in neuroimaging. Report from the task force on updating guidelines for credentialing in neuroimaging. *Neurology* 1997;**49**:1734–7.

18. White RA, Hodgson KJ, Ahn SS, Hobson RW, 2nd, Veith FJ. Endovascular interventions training and credentialing for vascular surgeons. *J Vasc Surg* 1999;**29**:177–86.

19. White RA. Endovascular credentialing. Endovascular Surgery Credentialing and Training Subcommittee. *J Vasc Interv Radiol* 1995;**6**:287–9.

20. Higashida RT, Hopkins LN, Berenstein A, Halbach VV, Kerber C. Program requirements for residency/fellowship education in neuroendovascular surgery/interventional neuroradiology: a special report on graduate medical education. *Am J Neuroradiol* 2000;**21**:1153–9.

21. ACGME. Program Requirements for Residency Education in Neuroradiology.

22. Johnston DC, Chapman KM, Goldstein LB. Low rate of complications of cerebral angiography in routine clinical practice. *Neurology* 2001;**57**:2012–14.

23. Dion JE, Gates PC, Fox AJ, Barnett HJ, Blom RJ. Clinical events following neuroangiography: a prospective study. *Stroke* 1987;**18**:997–1004.

24. Sacks D, Connors JJ, 3rd. Carotid stenting, stroke prevention, and training. *J Vasc Interv Radiol* 2004;**15**:1381–4.

25. Berteloot D, Leclerc X, Leys D, Krivosic R, Pruvo JP. [Cerebral angiography: a study of complications in 450 consecutive procedures]. *Journal de radiologie* 1999;**80**:843–8.

26. Willinsky RA, Taylor SM, TerBrugge K, Farb RI, Tomlinson G, Montanera W. Neurologic complications of cerebral angiography: prospective analysis of 2,899 procedures and review of the literature. *Radiology* 2003;**227**:522–8.

27. Mani RL, Eisenberg RL, McDonald EJ, Jr., Pollock JA, Mani JR. Complications of catheter cerebral arteriography: analysis of 5,000 procedures. I. Criteria and incidence. *Am J Roentgenol* 1978;**131**:861–5.

28. McIvor J, Steiner TJ, Perkin GD, Greenhalgh RM, Rose FC. Neurological morbidity of arch and carotid arteriography in cerebrovascular disease. The influence of contrast medium and radiologist. *Br J Radiol* 1987;**60**:117–22.

29. Grzyska U, Freitag J, Zeumer H. Selective cerebral intraarterial DSA.

Complication rate and control of risk factors. *Neuroradiology* 1990;**32**:296–9.

30. Qureshi AI, Suri MFK, Nasar A, *et al.* Thrombolysis for ischemic stroke in the United States: data from National Hospital Discharge Survey 1999–2001. *Neurosurgery* 2005;**57**:647–54; discussion 654.

31. Adams HP, Jr., Adams RJ, Brott T, *et al.* Guidelines for the early management of patients with ischemic stroke: A scientific statement from the Stroke Council of the American Stroke Association. *Stroke* 2003;**34**:1056–83.

32. Adams HP, Jr., del Zoppo G, Alberts MJ, *et al.* Guidelines for the early management of adults with ischemic stroke: a guideline from the American Heart Association/American Stroke Association Stroke Council, Clinical Cardiology Council, Cardiovascular Radiology and Intervention Council, and the Atherosclerotic Peripheral Vascular Disease and Quality of Care Outcomes in Research Interdisciplinary Working Groups: the American Academy of Neurology affirms the value of this guideline as an educational tool for neurologists. *Stroke* 2007;**38**:1655–711.

33. Hacke W, Kaste M, Fieschi C, *et al.* Intravenous thrombolysis with recombinant tissue plasminogen activator for acute hemispheric stroke. The European Cooperative Acute Stroke Study (ECASS)[see comment]. *J Am Med Assoc* 1995;**274**:1017–25.

34. Katzan IL, Furlan AJ, Lloyd LE, *et al.* Use of tissue-type plasminogen activator for acute ischemic stroke: the Cleveland area experience.[see comment]. *J Am Med Assoc* 2000;**283**:1151–8.

35. Katzan IL, Hammer MD, Furlan AJ, Hixson ED, Nadzam DM, Cleveland Clinic Health System Stroke Quality Improvement T. Quality improvement and tissue-type plasminogen activator for acute ischemic stroke: a Cleveland update. *Stroke* 2003;**34**:799–800.

36. Qureshi AI, Harris-Lane P, Kirmani JF, *et al.* Intra-arterial reteplase and intravenous abciximab in patients with acute ischemic stroke: an open-label, dose-ranging, phase I study. *Neurosurgery* 2006;**59**:789–96; discussion 96–7.

37. Qureshi AI, Janjua N, Kirmani JF, *et al.* Mechanical disruption of thrombus following intravenous tissue plasminogen activator for ischemic stroke. *Journal of Neuroimaging* 2007;**17**:124–30.

38. Abou-Chebl A, Bajzer CT, Krieger DW, Furlan AJ, Yadav JS. Multimodal therapy for the treatment of severe ischemic stroke combining GPIIb/IIIa antagonists and angioplasty after failure of thrombolysis. *Stroke* 2005;**36**: 2286–8.

39. Combined intravenous and intra-arterial recanalization for acute ischemic stroke: the Interventional Management of Stroke Study. *Stroke; a journal of cerebral circulation* 2004;**35**:904–11.

40. Barr JD, Connors JJ, 3rd, Sacks D, *et al.* Quality improvement guidelines for the performance of cervical carotid angioplasty and stent placement. *J Vasc Interv Radiol* 2003;**14**:S321–35.

41. Bates ER, Babb JD, Casey DE, Jr., *et al.* ACCF/SCAI/SVMB/SIR/ASITN 2007 clinical expert consensus document on carotid stenting: a report of the American College of Cardiology Foundation Task Force on Clinical Expert Consensus Documents (ACCF/SCAI/SVMB/SIR/ASITN Clinical Expert Consensus Document Committee on Carotid Stenting). *J Am Coll Cardiol* 2007;**49**:126–70.

42. Beller GA, Bonow RO, Foster V. ACC revised recommendations for training in adult cardiovascular medicine. Core Cardiology Training II (COCATS 2). (Revision of the 1995 COCATS training statement). *J Am Coll Cardiol* 2002;**39**:1242–6.

43. Creager MA, Goldstone J, Hirshfeld JW, Jr., *et al.* ACC/ACP/SCAI/SVMB/SVS clinical competence statement on vascular medicine and catheter-based peripheral vascular interventions: a report of the American College of Cardiology/American Heart Association/American College of Physician Task Force on Clinical Competence (ACC/ACP/SCAI/SVMB/SVS Writing Committee to develop a clinical competence statement on peripheral vascular disease). *J Am Coll Cardiol* 2004;**44**:941–57.

44. Hobson RW, 2nd, Howard VJ, Roubin GS, *et al.* Credentialing of surgeons as interventionalists for carotid artery stenting: experience from the lead-in phase of CREST. *J Vasc Surg* 2004;**40**:952–7.

45. Qureshi AI. Carotid angioplasty and stent placement after EVA-3S trial. *Stroke* 2007;**38**:1993–6.

46. Yadav JS. Carotid stenting in high-risk patients: design and rationale of the SAPPHIRE trial. *Cleveland Clinic J Med* 2004;**71** Suppl 1:S45–6.

47. Mas JL, Chatellier G, Beyssen B, *et al.* Endarterectomy versus stenting in patients with symptomatic severe carotid stenosis. *N Engl J Med* 2006;**355**:1660–71.

48. Ringleb PA, Allenberg J, Bruckmann H, *et al.* 30 day results from the SPACE trial of stent-protected angioplasty versus carotid endarterectomy in symptomatic patients: a randomised non-inferiority trial. *Lancet* 2006;**368**:1239–47.

49. Gray WA, Yadav JS, Verta P, *et al.* The CAPTURE registry: results of carotid stenting with embolic protection in the post approval setting. *Catheter Cardiovasc Interv* 2007;**69**:341–8.

50. FDA. www.fda.gov/ohrms/dockets/ac/03/minutes/3975m1_Sum%20Min.pdf.

51. Schreiber TLCS, Massop D, Kumar V, Davis T, Ramee S.. Report of the CASES-PMS study: patient demographics and 30-day major adverse events for the Cordis PRECISE nitinol stent and AngioguardTM Emboli capture guidewire condition of approval surveillance study. In: American College of Cardiology 55th Annual Scientific Session; March 11th–14th, 2006 Atlanta, Georgia; March 11th – 14th, 2006.

52. Qureshi AI, Janardhan V, Hanel RA, Lanzino G. Comparison of endovascular and surgical treatments for intracranial aneurysms: an evidence-based review.

53. Qureshi AI, Suri MFK, Nasar A, *et al.* Trends in hospitalization and mortality for subarachnoid hemorrhage and unruptured aneurysms in the United States. *Neurosurgery* 2005;**57**:1–8; discussion 1–8.

54. Qureshi AI, Suri MFK, Nasar A, *et al.* Changes in cost and outcome among US patients with stroke hospitalized in 1990 to 1991 and those hospitalized in 2000 to 2001. *Stroke* 2007;**38**:2180–4.

55. Molyneux A, Kerr R, Stratton I, *et al.* International Subarachnoid Aneurysm Trial (ISAT) of neurosurgical clipping versus endovascular coiling in 2143 patients with ruptured intracranial

aneurysms: a randomised trial. *Lancet* 2002;**360**:1267–74.

56. Molyneux AJ, Kerr RS, Yu LM, *et al.* International subarachnoid aneurysm trial (ISAT) of neurosurgical clipping versus endovascular coiling in 2143 patients with ruptured intracranial aneurysms: a randomised comparison of effects on survival, dependency, seizures, rebleeding, subgroups, and aneurysm occlusion. *Lancet* 2005;**366**:809–17.

57. Singh V, Gress DR, Higashida RT, Dowd CF, Halbach VV, Johnston SC. The learning curve for coil embolization of unruptured intracranial aneurysms. *Am J Neuroradiol* 2002;**23**:768–71.

58. Hoh BL, Rabinov JD, Pryor JC, Carter BS, Barker FG, 2nd. In-hospital morbidity and mortality after endovascular treatment of unruptured intracranial aneurysms in the United States, 1996–2000: effect of hospital and physician volume. *AJNR Am J Neuroradiol* 2003;**24**:1409–20.

59. Qureshi AI, Ziai WC, Yahia AM, *et al.* Stroke-free survival and its determinants in patients with symptomatic vertebrobasilar stenosis: a multicenter study. *Neurosurgery* 2003;**52**:1033–9; discussion 9–40.

60. Investigators SS. Stenting of Symptomatic Atherosclerotic Lesions in the Vertebral or Intracranial Arteries (SSYLVIA): study results.[see comment]. *Stroke* 2004;**35**:1388–92.

61. Bose A, Hartmann M, Henkes H, *et al.* A novel, self-expanding, nitinol stent in medically refractory intracranial atherosclerotic stenoses: the Wingspan study. *Stroke* 2007;**38**:1531–7.

62. Ogilvy CS, Stieg PE, Awad I, *et al.* AHA Scientific Statement: Recommendations for the management of intracranial arteriovenous malformations: a statement for healthcare professionals from a special writing group of the Stroke Council, American Stroke Association. *Stroke* 2001;**32**:1458–71.

63. Kerber CW, Hecht ST, Knox K. Arteriovenous malformation model for training and research. *Am J Neuroradiol* 1997;**18**:1229–32.

64. Massoud TF, Ji C, Vinuela F, *et al.* Laboratory simulations and training in endovascular embolotherapy with a swine arteriovenous malformation model. *AJNR Am J Neuroradiol* 1996;**17**:271–9.

65. FDA. http://www.fda.gov/ohrms/dockets/ac/cdrh00.htm.

481

Index